GABBARD'S TEXTBOOK OF

PSYCHOTHERAPEUTIC TREATMENTS

SECOND EDITION

GABBARD'S TEXTBOOK OF
PSYCHOTHERAPEUTIC TREATMENTS

SECOND EDITION

EDITED BY

Holly Crisp, M.D.
Glen O. Gabbard, M.D.

AMERICAN PSYCHIATRIC ASSOCIATION PUBLISHING

Note: The authors have worked to ensure that all information in this book is accurate at the time of publication and consistent with general psychiatric and medical standards and that information concerning drug dosages, schedules, and routes of administration is accurate at the time of publication and consistent with standards set by the U.S. Food and Drug Administration and the general medical community. As medical research and practice continue to advance, however, therapeutic standards may change. Moreover, specific situations may require a specific therapeutic response not included in this book. For these reasons and because human and mechanical errors sometimes occur, we recommend that readers follow the advice of physicians directly involved in their care or the care of a member of their family.

Books published by American Psychiatric Association Publishing represent the findings, conclusions, and views of the individual authors and do not necessarily represent the policies and opinions of American Psychiatric Association Publishing or the American Psychiatric Association.

If you wish to buy 50 or more copies of the same title, please go to www.appi.org/specialdiscounts for more information.

Second Edition

Manufactured in the United States of America
26 25 24 23 22 5 4 3 2 1
ISBN 978-1-61537-326-0 (hardcover), 978-1-61537-406-9 (ebook)

American Psychiatric Association Publishing
800 Maine Avenue SW, Suite 900
Washington, DC 20024-2812
www.appi.org

Library of Congress Cataloging-in-Publication Data
A CIP record is available from the Library of Congress.

British Library Cataloguing in Publication Data
A CIP record is available from the British Library.

Contents

PART V
Supportive Psychotherapy

PART VI
Family, Couple, and Group Psychotherapy

PART VII
Racial and Ethnic Diversities in Psychotherapy

PART VIII
Gender and Sexualities in Psychotherapy

PART IX
Special Issues in Psychotherapy

Contributors

Mohsin Ahmed, M.D., Ph.D.
Assistant Professor of Psychiatry, Department of Psychiatry, Vagelos College of Physicians and Surgeons, Columbia University, New York, New York

Anthony Bateman, M.A., FRCPsych
Visiting Professor, Research Department of Clinical, Educational and Health Psychology, University College London, London, UK; The Anna Freud Centre, London, UK; Honorary Professorship in Psychotherapy, University of Copenhagen, Copenhagen, Denmark

Seamus Bhatt-Mackin, M.D.
Director, Program for Clinical Group Work, U.S. Veterans Affairs Mid-Atlantic Mental Illness, Research Education Clinical Core (MIRECC); Consulting Associate, Duke University Department of Psychiatry and Behavioral Sciences, Durham, North Carolina

Tali Boritz, Ph.D., C.Psych.
Assistant Professor, Department of Psychology, York University; Collaborator Scientist, Borderline Personality Disorder Clinic, Centre for Addiction and Mental Health, Toronto, Ontario, Canada

Nicola Brown, Ph.D., C.Psych.
Private practice, Winnipeg, Manitoba, Canada

Eve Caligor, M.D.
Clinical Professor of Psychiatry, Vagelos College of Physicians and Surgeons of Columbia University; Adjunct Professor of Psychiatry, Weill Medical College of Cornell University, New York, New York

Chloe Campbell, Ph.D.
Deputy Director, Psychoanalysis Unit, University College London, London, UK

David A. Casey, M.D.
Professor and John J. and Ruby B. Schwab Endowed Chair in Social, Community, and Family Psychiatry, Department of Psychiatry and Behavioral Sciences, University of Louisville School of Medicine, Louisville, Kentucky

Alexander L. Chapman, Ph.D., R.Psych.
Professor, Department of Psychology, Simon Fraser University, Burnaby, British Columbia, Canada

Calvin R. Chin, Ph.D.
Director, Counseling and Psychological Services, Princeton University, Princeton, New Jersey

Lois W. Choi-Kain, M.D., M.Ed.
Director, Gunderson Personality Disorders Institute; Assistant Professor of Psychiatry, Harvard Medical School, Cambridge, Massachusetts

David A. Clark, Ph.D.
Professor Emeritus, Department of Psychology, University of New Brunswick, Fredericton, New Brunswick, Canada

John F. Clarkin, Ph.D.
Clinical Professor of Psychology in Psychiatry and Codirector, Personality Disorders Institute, Weill Medical College of Cornell University, New York, New York

Jean Cottraux, M.D., Ph.D.
Honorary Psychiatrist and Former Head, Anxiety Disorders Unit, Hôpital Neurologique, Lyon, France

Holly Crisp, M.D.
Clinical Associate Professor of Psychiatry, Baylor College of Medicine, Houston, Texas

Mantosh Dewan, M.D.
President and SUNY Distinguished Service Professor, State University of New York Upstate Medical University, Syracuse, New York

Keith S. Dobson, Ph.D.
Professor of Clinical Psychology, Department of Psychology, University of Calgary, Calgary, Alberta, Canada

David J.A. Dozois, Ph.D.
Professor, Department of Psychology, University of Western Ontario, London, Ontario, Canada

Jack Drescher, M.D.
Clinical Professor of Psychiatry, Department of Psychiatry, Columbia University, New York, New York

Matthew Fadus, M.D.
Instructor, Department of Psychiatry, Harvard Medical School, Massachusetts General Hospital, Boston, Massachusetts

Peter Fonagy, Ph.D.
Professor of Contemporary Psychoanalysis and Developmental Science, University College London, London, UK

Glen O. Gabbard, M.D.
Clinical Professor of Psychiatry, Baylor College of Medicine, Houston, Texas

Rosa Garcia, M.S.
Graduate student, The Family Institute at Northwestern, Evanston, Illinois

Daniel Gaztambide, Psy.D.
Assistant Professor, Department of Psychology, The New School for Social Research, New York, New York

Michael Goldstein, M.D.
Physician-in-Charge, Neuroscience Education, Department of Psychiatry and Behavioral Sciences, Beth Israel Medical Center, New York, New York; Assistant Clinical Professor, Department of Psychiatry and Behavioral Sciences, Albert Einstein College of Medicine, Bronx, New York

Anton Hart, Ph.D.
Faculty, Training and Supervising Psychoanalyst, William Alanson White Institute, New York, New York

Mary Hepworth, Ph.D.
Professor of Psychoanalysis, University College London, London, UK

Alison Heru, M.D.
Professor of Psychiatry, Department of Psychiatry, University of Colorado Denver, Denver, Colorado

Daniel Jackson, M.D.
Forensic Fellow, Department of Psychiatry, State University of New York, Upstate Medical University, Syracuse, New York

Gurmeet Kanwal, M.D.
Clinical Associate Professor, Department of Psychiatry, Weill Medical College of Cornell University; Teaching Faculty and Supervising Psychoanalyst, William Alanson White Institute, New York, New York

Erin A. Kaufman, Ph.D.
Assistant Professor, Department of Psychology, University of Western Ontario, London, Ontario, Canada

Robert L. Leahy, Ph.D.
Director, American Institute for Cognitive Therapy, New York, New York

Jay L. Lebow, Ph.D., ABPP
Clinical Professor of Psychology, The Family Institute at Northwestern and Northwestern University, Evanston, Illinois

Falk Leichsenring, D.Sc.
Professor, Department of Psychotherapy and Psychosomatics, Justus Liebig University of Giessen, Giessen, Germany; Professor, Department of Psychosomatics and Psychotherapy, University of Rostock, Rostock, Germany

Molyn Leszcz, M.D.
Professor of Psychiatry, University of Toronto, Toronto, Ontario, Canada

Csilla Nani Lippert, M.D., Ph.D.
Staff Physician, Psychiatry, VA Palo Alto Health Care System, Palo Alto, California

Joshua D. Lipsitz, Ph.D.
Professor, Department of Psychology, Ben-Gurion University of the Negev, Marcus Family Campus, Beer-Sheva, Israel; Professor, Department of Psychiatry, College of Physicians and Surgeons, Columbia University, New York, New York, United States

Ilana Lipsitz-Odess, Ph.D.
Department of Psychology, University of Haifa, Haifa, Israel

Barbara F. Marcus, Ph.D.
Assistant Clinical Professor of Psychology in Psychiatry, Yale University School of Medicine, and Training and Supervising Analyst, Western New England Institute for Psychoanalysis, New Haven, Connecticut

John C. Markowitz, M.D.
Research Psychiatrist, New York State Psychiatric Institute; Professor of Clinical Psychiatry, Columbia University Vagelos College of Physicians and Surgeons, New York, New York

Benjamin McCommon, M.D.
Assistant Clinical Professor of Psychiatry, Columbia University, New York, New York

Amanda M. McEpplan, Ph.D.
Clinical Psychologist, Alberta Health Services, Calgary, Alberta, Canada

Christopher McIntosh, M.D., FRCPC
Associate Professor of Psychiatry, University of Toronto, Toronto, Ontario, Canada

Shelley McMain, Ph.D., C.Psych.
Associate Professor and Director of Psychotherapy, Humanities and Psychosocial Interventions (PHPI) Division, Department of Psychiatry, University of Toronto; Clinician Scientist and Head, Borderline Personality Disorder Clinic, Centre for Addiction and Mental Health, Toronto, Ontario, Canada

David Mintz, M.D.
Director of Psychiatric Education, The Austen Riggs Center, Stockbridge, Massachusetts

Diana E. Moga, M.D., Ph.D.
Assistant Clinical Professor of Psychiatry, Columbia University Center for Psychoanalytic Training and Research, New York, New York

J. Christopher Muran, Ph.D.
Associate Dean and Professor, Gordon F. Derner School of Psychology, Adelphi University, Garden City, New York; Director, Mount Sinai Beth Israel Brief Psychotherapy Program, New York, New York

Dionne R. Powell, M.D.
Clinical Assistant Professor of Psychiatry and Assistant Attending Psychiatrist, The New York-Presbyterian Hospital, Weill Cornell Medical College; Training and Supervising Psychoanalyst, Psychoanalytic Association of New York and Columbia University Center for Psychoanalytic Training and Research, New York, New York

Diana Punko, M.D., M.S.
Attending Physician, Department of Psychiatry, Massachusetts General Hospital; Instructor in Psychiatry, Harvard Medical School, Boston, Massachusetts

Romy A. Reading, Ph.D.
Private practice; Candidate, New York University Postdoctoral Program in Psychotherapy and Psychoanalysis, New York, New York

Jessica Reis, M.D.
Assistant Professor and Associate Director, Residency Training Program, Department of Psychiatry and Behavioral Sciences, University of Louisville School of Medicine, Louisville, Kentucky

Laura Weiss Roberts, M.D., M.A.
Katharine Dexter McCormick and Stanley McCormick Memorial Professor, Stanford University; Chair, Department of Psychiatry and Behavioral Sciences, Stanford University School of Medicine, Stanford, California

John S. Rolland, M.D., M.P.H.
Professor of Psychiatry and Behavioral Sciences, Feinberg School of Medicine, Northwestern University; Cofounder and Codirector, Chicago Center for Family Health, Chicago, Illinois

Richard N. Rosenthal, M.D.
Director, Division of Addiction Psychiatry, Department of Psychiatry and Behavioral Health, SUNY Stony Brook University Medical Center; Professor of Psychiatry, Department of Psychiatry and Behavioral Health, Renaissance School of Medicine at Stony Brook University, Stony Brook, New York

Jay Shore, M.D., M.P.H.
Director, Office of Telehealth and Technology Implementation for Behavioral Health Practice and Science, Department of Psychiatry, Aurora, Colorado

Anne Sonley, M.D., FRCPC
Lecturer, Department of Psychiatry, University of Toronto; Psychiatrist and Clinician Scientist, Borderline Personality Disorder Clinic, Centre for Addiction and Mental Health, Toronto, Ontario, Canada

Julia F. Sowislo, Ph.D.
Instructor of Psychology in Psychiatry, Weill Medical College of Cornell University, New York, New York

Christiane Steinert, Ph.D.
Professor, International Psychoanalytic University Berlin, Berlin, Germany; Professor, Department of Psychotherapy and Psychosomatics, Justus Liebig University of Giessen, Giessen, Germany

Lynn Stormon, Ph.D.
Clinical Psychologist and Psychoanalyst in private practice, Cazenovia, New York; Clinical Assistant Professor, Department of Psychiatry, SUNY Upstate Medical University, Syracuse, New York

Beverly J. Stoute, M.D.
Co-chair, Holmes Commission on Racial Equality in the American Psychoanalytic Association, New York, New York; Training and Supervising Analyst, Emory University Psychoanalytic Institute, Atlanta, Georgia; Child and Adolescent Supervising Analyst, New York Psychoanalytic Institute, New York, New York; Adjunct Associate

Professor of Psychiatry and Behavioral Sciences, Emory University School of Medicine, Atlanta, Georgia; Adjunct Clinical Associate Professor of Psychiatry and Behavioral Sciences, Morehouse School of Medicine, Atlanta, Georgia

Donna M. Sudak, M.D.
Professor of Psychiatry, Drexel University, Philadelphia, Pennsylvania

Holly A. Swartz, M.D.
Professor, Department of Psychiatry, University of Pittsburgh School of Medicine, Pittsburgh, Pennsylvania

Charles Swenson, M.D.
Department of Psychiatry, University of Massachusetts Medical School, Worcester, Massachusetts

Pratyusha Tummala-Narra, Ph.D.
Director of Community-Based Education, Albert & Jesse Danielsen Institute; Research Professor, Department of Psychological and Brain Sciences, Boston University, Boston, Massachusetts

Jasmine Ueng-McHale, Ph.D.
Princeton, New Jersey

Brandon Unruh, M.D.
Medical Director, Gunderson Residence; Director, Mentalization-Based Treatment Clinic, McLean Hospital; Instructor in Psychiatry, Harvard Medical School, Cambridge, Massachusetts

Adelya A. Urmanche, M.A., Ph.D.
Postdoctoral Fellow, Department of Psychiatry and Behavioral Sciences, Mount Sinai Beth Israel, New York, New York

Susan Vaughan, M.D.
Director, Columbia University Center for Psychoanalytic Training and Research; Associate Professor of Psychiatry at CUIMC, Department of Psychiatry, Vagelos College of Physicians and Surgeons, Columbia University, New York, New York

Froma Walsh, Ph.D.
Mose and Sylvia Firestone Professor Emerita, Crown Family School and Department of Psychiatry, Pritzker School of Medicine, University of Chicago; Cofounder and Codirector, Chicago Center for Family Health, Chicago, Illinois

Priyanthy Weerasekera, M.D., M.Ed.
Professor Emeritus, Psychiatry and Behavioural Neurosciences, McMaster University, Hamilton, Ontario, Canada

Arnold Winston, M.D.
Professor Emeritus of Psychiatry, Icahn School of Medicine, Mount Sinai Hospital System; Chairman Emeritus, Department of Psychiatry, Mount Sinai-Beth Israel Medical Center, New York, New York; Professor of Psychiatry and Associate Chairman of Psychiatry, St. George's Medical School, Grenada, West Indies

Jesse H. Wright, M.D., Ph.D.
Professor and Gotfried and Gisela Kolb Endowed Chair in Outpatient Psychiatry, Department of Psychiatry and Behavioral Sciences; Director, UofL Depression Center, University of Louisville School of Medicine, Louisville, Kentucky

Peter Yellowlees, M.D., M.B.B.S.
Chief Wellness Officer and Professor of Psychiatry, UC Davis Department of Psychiatry, University of California Davis, Sacramento, California

Disclosures

The following contributors to this book have indicated a financial interest in or other affiliation with a commercial supporter, a manufacturer of a commercial product, a provider of a commercial service, a nongovernmental organization, and/or a government agency, as listed below:

John C. Markowitz, M.D., receives salary support from the New York State Psychiatric Institute and some grant support from private foundations (the Bob Woodruff Foundation). He also receives minor book royalties from American Psychiatric Publishing, Basic Books, and Oxford University Press for books related to interpersonal psychotherapy, which is the focus of the section in which his introduction and chapter appear.

Holly A. Swartz, M.D., receives royalties from Wolters Kluwer, research support from Myriad Genetics, honorarium from Novus Medical Education, and an editorial stipend from American Psychiatric Association Publishing.

Jesse H. Wright, M.D., Ph.D., is an author of the *Good Days Ahead* program used in investigations cited in Chapter 8, "Techniques of Cognitive-Behavioral Therapy," and has an equity interest in Empower Interactive and MindStreet, developers and distributors of *Good Days Ahead*. His conflict of interest is managed with an agreement with the University of Louisville. He receives book royalties from American Psychiatric Association Publishing, Guilford Press, and Simon and Schuster.

The following contributors have indicated that they have no financial interests or other affiliations that represent or could appear to represent a competing interest with their contributions to this book:

Nicola Brown, Ph.D., C.Psych.; Eve Caligor, M.D.; Calvin R. Chin, Ph.D.; Holly Crisp, M.D.; David J.A. Dozois, Ph.D.; Jack Drescher, M.D.; Matthew Fadus, M.D.; Glen O. Gabbard, M.D.; Anton Hart, Ph.D.; Gurmeet Kanwal, M.D.; Jay L. Lebow, Ph.D., ABPP; Falk Leichsenring, D.Sc.; Csilla Nani Lippert, M.D., Ph.D.; Ilana Lipsitz-Odess, Ph.D.; Benjamin McCommon, M.D.; Diana Punko, M.D., M.S.; Romy A. Reading, Ph.D.; Pratyusha Tummala-Narra, Ph.D.; Adelya A. Urmanche, M.A.

Preface

It has been 12 years since the first edition of the *Textbook of Psychotherapeutic Treatments* was published. A sea change has occurred in the field during that time frame. We have a much more sophisticated understanding of the interface of brain and mind, and we now know from an abundance of empirical data collected that rigorous support for the efficacy of all the major forms of psychotherapy exists. As a result, this second edition features updated work on each of the empirically validated psychotherapies, including psychodynamic therapies, mentalization-based treatment, transference-focused therapy, cognitive-behavioral therapy, supportive psychotherapy, and interpersonal psychotherapy. The section on group, couple, and family psychotherapy has also been updated from the first edition.

In addition, we have added a new section on racial and ethnic diversity in psychotherapy. The relationship of race and culture to psychotherapy has historically been underplayed and neglected. The killing of George Floyd during the preparation of this textbook stirred the country to recognize that racism itself is a central part of the plague that we have all endured during the coronavirus SARS-CoV-2 disease (COVID-19) pandemic and highlighted the long-standing impact of systemic and institutionalized racism. Limited access to vaccines and discrimination regarding housing and hiring were deeply disturbing manifestations of the twin plagues of racism and COVID-19. Dr. Dionne Powell, the section editor of this new addition to the textbook, points out that in the twenty-first century, a competent clinician must advocate for cultural humility, informed inquiry, and an ongoing reflection on one's own internalized views about both what is familiar and what appears to be part of the "other." How clinicians think about these issues is critically important in regard to the formation of a therapeutic alliance, the understanding of countertransference, and the experience of affective states.

Another new section on diversity, this one involving gender and sexuality, reflects a commitment to move away from the shameful historical era when gay, lesbian, bisexual, and transgender patients were seen as requiring intensive psychotherapy to change their orientation. In recent years, a growing body of research has contributed to a thoroughgoing acceptance of lesbian, gay, transgender, and gender-diverse people. Dr. Jack Drescher, the section editor of this portion of the book, points out that although an LGBTQ+ identity may not necessarily be the primary focus of therapy in many cases, its impact on the course of treatment should not be underestimated or overlooked. Some therapists may believe that treating LGBTQ+ patients requires no specialized knowledge and may claim that they treat their LGBTQ+ patients like everyone else. However, this view may overlook the fact that growing up lesbian, gay, bisexual, or transgender is a different cultural experience from growing up heterosexual and cisgender.

One of the most sweeping changes in the history of psychotherapy was brought on by the rapid spread of COVID-19 throughout the world. In a veritable twinkling of the eye, psychotherapists shifted to virtual modalities to conduct their psychotherapeutic treatments. Indeed, the virus disrupted the way that we all live and practice. In many centers, mental health professionals shifted to treat most patients with videoconferencing and phone therapy. All of us struggled to adjust to screens and/or to hearing a voice on the phone unaccompanied by a visual component. On the other hand, some therapists note that there is nothing more intimate than a voice in one's ear and that phone therapy may free up some patients to be more revealing than they ever could be if they had to endure a therapist staring at them in an office each session. The ongoing experiences of trauma in the aftermath of the pandemic will continue to increase the need for psychotherapy and mental health treatment.

The COVID-19 era has brought about wide-ranging changes in all aspects of our lives. At the beginning of the pandemic, the streets of major cities were deserted. Both therapists and patients were wearing masks, a signal of potential danger that many worried would not be contained. In-person therapy has now become more controversial as a result. Debates about returning to the office versus continuing with phone therapy or virtual videoconferencing are raging in all parts of the country and abroad. Some colleagues have adjusted to the new modalities and find them just as effective as the in-person approaches. Some patients are fond of the changes because they no longer have to fight traffic to see their therapist. On the other hand, a significant number of therapists feel more comfortable returning to the way they were trained and argue that more information about the patient, however subtle, is available in the office. We cannot know at this time what the ultimate outcome will be. As we write this preface, many places in the world are managing the virus, whereas others are battling with serious outbreaks and variants that may require innovative strategies to defeat them. We fully recognize that our authors are writing in medias res.

Only time will tell, of course, but we decided to provide a comprehensive chapter on this subject in the final section of the book to summarize what has happened. The material in Chapter 34, "Psychotherapy and Cyberspace," can be applied to whatever psychotherapy challenges await the therapist. Other chapters in the final section include a new one on supervision and consultation that did not appear in the first edition. Also in this final section is a chapter on the interface of neuroscience and psychotherapy, one on ethics and boundaries in therapy, and one on the clinical strategies to integrate psychotherapy and medication in clinical practice.

Glen O. Gabbard, M.D.

Holly Crisp, M.D.

PART I

Individual Psychodynamic Psychotherapy

Section Editors: Glen O. Gabbard, M.D., and Holly Crisp, M.D.

Since the first edition of this textbook was published, the evidence base for psychodynamic psychotherapy has continued to expand. There was a time not so long ago when critics of psychodynamic psychotherapy would disparage the rigor of this approach by arguing that there was no empirical evidence of its efficacy. As the reader can see in Chapter 6, "Applications of Psychodynamic Psychotherapy to Specific Disorders," there is now an impressive evidence base for psychodynamic psychotherapy and a growing understanding regarding which interventions may be most effective in specific situations.

In the first chapter, "Theoretical Models of Psychodynamic Psychotherapy," Peter Fonagy, Mary Hepworth, and Chloe Campbell present the various models and schools of thought that comprise the overarching picture of psychodynamic therapy today. They argue that the fundamental activity that works in psychodynamic therapy relates to the enactment of a critical human behavior, "the alignment of minds based on shared mental states and focused on a shared objectivity, co-mentalizing, or joint intentionality" (p. 3).

In Chapter 2, "Techniques of Psychodynamic Psychotherapy," we provide an outline of the basic principles of psychodynamic therapy and clinical tools that are practical and useful for the clinician. Since the first edition of this textbook in 2009, psychodynamic psychotherapists and psychoanalysts have continued to become more flexible in their approaches to tailoring the treatment to the patient and to the specific dyad of the patient and the therapist. We outline key psychodynamic principles in the approach to assessment, formulation, and goal setting, while also considering the roles of transference, countertransference, and resistance in psychodynamic psychotherapy.

Mantosh Dewan, Priyanthy Weerasekera, Lynn Stormon, and Daniel Jackson have authored Chapter 3, "Techniques of Brief Psychodynamic Psychotherapy." Using vivid clinical examples, they outline fundamental skills and strategies from a variety of theoretical approaches used in brief dynamic therapy. The growing efficacy of brief modalities has been impressive since the first edition of this text.

In the years between the first edition and this volume, mentalization-based treatment (MBT) has been recognized as an effective modality for many conditions and has expanded our therapeutic armamentarium. Hence, we feel that it deserves a chapter of its own in this second edition. As a result, Chapter 4, "Theory and Practice of Mentalization-Based Treatment," has been added to this section, which allows Anthony Bateman, Lois W. Choi-Kain, and Brandon Unruh to present their vision of MBT and its application across a range of clinical conditions and settings. In addition, they review the core principles of mentalizing approaches and consider the similarities and differences between MBT and other therapies.

In Chapter 5, "Transference-Focused Psychotherapy For Levels of Personality Pathology Severity," John F. Clarkin, Eve Caligor, and Julia F. Sowislo delineate the goals and premises of transference-focused psychotherapy (TFP). They also discuss the nuances of TFP practice and its approach to psychotherapeutic treatment for a range of personality disorder diagnoses and severities, as well as depression and other symptoms that may emerge in association with personality pathology.

In the last chapter in this section, Chapter 6, "Applications of Psychodynamic Psychotherapy to Specific Disorders," Falk Leichsenring and Christiane Steinert provide an in-depth look at the empirical evidence for psychodynamic psychotherapy. After clarifying the criteria for evidence-based medicine and empirically supported treatments, they provide an impressive review of efficacious randomized controlled trials and meta-analyses of psychodynamic psychotherapies in specific mental disorders.

CHAPTER 1

Theoretical Models of Psychodynamic Psychotherapy

Peter Fonagy, Ph.D.
Mary Hepworth, Ph.D.
Chloe Campbell, Ph.D.

In the past decade or so since the first edition of this book was published, psychotherapeutic models of treatment have been bolstered by a growing research base showing their effectiveness, particularly in the treatment of depression (Cuijpers et al. 2020; Driessen et al. 2010) but also for a range of other diagnoses, such as borderline personality disorder (BPD; Cristea et al. 2017) and eating disorders (Grenon et al. 2019). Interpersonal psychotherapy (IPT) has come to the fore as a successful approach for a range of disorders (Cuijpers et al. 2011, 2016) and has become an increasingly popular model for practitioners (Weissman et al. 2017). Research, evidence building, and theorizing about psychotherapy have proliferated—a healthy development for the field, although one that is informed by a context of increasing concern about the prevalence of psychological distress, with rising rates among young people, particularly women (Patalay and Gage 2019), serving as a reminder of the imperative to think about models in terms of practical treatment value.

The major theoretical models for psychotherapy remain the same since the first edition of this book was published in 2009, but in this revised chapter, ahead of an account of these major models, we attempt to draw together what it is about these approaches that works. We argue that although many theories and many models exist, the core activity remains the same, and the reason is that effective psychotherapy, no matter how innovative the model, works because it enacts a paradigmatic human behavior—the alignment of minds based on shared mental states and focused on a shared objectivity, co-mentalizing, or joint intentionality. These thoughts draw on the work of Michael Tomasello (2018, 2019), who described how humans possess an evolutionarily unparalleled capacity to transfer information between agents.

We suggest that in order to understand the significance of social communication and the alignment of minds, and how they might both generate the risk of psychopathology and suggest ways of treating it, it is useful to unpack what is going on at such moments of thinking together. Tomasello described this joining of minds, or shared intentionality, in which two (or more) minds focus together on the same object, as a dual structure-activity intentionality (Tomasello 2020): it involves both a shared focus and individual, separate perspectives on the same thing (Tomasello 2016). The idea of the different perspectives is crucial—shared intentionality is so powerful because it does not involve separate minds melding and sharing the same thoughts in the task of thinking together; rather, it is bolstered by an awareness of separate perspectives, allowing for the mobilization of other people's ideas, thoughts, and viewpoints. The experience of shared intentionality has been described as generating a particular category of cognition, described as the *we-mode* (Gallotti and Frith 2013, p. 160). Winnicott (1956), in his account of the mother in the mirror role, described the same phenomenon and recognized its importance in developing the infant's sense of self, and Bion (1962) emphasized, through the container-contained concept, meaning being inherently mediated by social communication.

This seam of thinking increasingly locates human sociality at the heart of understanding the evolution of higher-order cognition (Gallotti and Frith 2013). Domains such as episodic memory (Mahr and Csibra 2017), reason and logic (Mercier and Sperber 2017), and human consciousness (Fonagy and Allison 2016) have all been reconsidered as intrinsically social: their evolutionary and individual acquisitions are in the service of complex social functioning. We have increasingly sought to reconsider psychopathology, and the role of psychotherapeutic treatment, within this framework of ideas, suggesting that in the context of emerging research evidence indicative of a general psychopathology factor (the *p* factor; Caspi and Moffitt 2018), disruptions in social communication may constitute an underpinning general vulnerability (Fonagy et al. 2017a, 2017b). In particular, features of BPD may constitute an archetypical expression of such a general vulnerability—as supported by research on BPD and the *p* factor (Gluschkoff et al. 2021; Sharp et al. 2015).

Psychotherapy might best be understood as an umbrella term for a range of approaches that seek to generate shared intentionality and we-mode cognition. The subject of focus in psychotherapy, which the patient and therapist join together in considering, is mental states themselves. The way in which mental states may be discussed may vary according to different models and therapeutic strategies, but at their core they involve the dual structure described by Tomasello. The work of generating the we-mode, of aligning minds in this way, will constitute an important part of the therapeutic process—for some patients, entering into we-mode and acknowledging joint intentionality while holding on to awareness of the separateness of the other's mind may in itself be an aversive, alien, or frightening experience. Such experience of shared intention is by its very nature dependent on some base level of trust: accepting collaboration and openness to another's mind while accepting that one cannot control or even with complete certainty know its contents fully, and still subjugating individual agency to this shared experience, is a developmental achievement in its own right. However, this is not the final end of psychotherapy; it is, in fact, just a step, albeit an essential one, of the therapeutic process, intimately tied to what is perhaps poorly named the therapeutic alliance (Safran and Muran 2006). The alliance is often presented as an end in itself—a predictor of outcome because it contains some secret ingredient of the change process. But its significance also arises from the benefits of the dramatic shift of mental processing that joint intentionality can bring. We suggest that the possible benefit of the therapeutic alliance arises from the significance of the alliance in co-mentalizing (or the we-mode), where two minds—the therapist's and the patient's—are jointly seeing to the outcome (Tuomela 2005, 2007). The state of shared intentionality, the experience of the we-mode, is a mutual creation. It naturally comes and goes, lost in noncooperative interactions and restored continually in the cultivation of epistemic trust—the opening of the mind to influence and learning. The we-mode is an experience that forms the basis for cooperation and commitment to shared goals and catalyzes the development of epistemic trust and trustworthiness (Allen 2021).

We began this discussion by describing how the capacity for thinking together is the mechanism that makes human sociality possible and brings with it all the benefits of social cooperation. It forms the basis for epistemic trust—openness to taking in socially communicated knowledge—which brings with it the potential for abandoning rigidly held archaic views and, in signaling alignment with another, a readiness to internalize a new perspective on reality that could generate improved social functioning that is associated with meaningful change. One study in the United Kingdom showing the benefits of psychoanalytic psychotherapy for the treatment of depression reported the intriguing finding that notable differences between treated and untreated groups emerged in the 18 months following the end of treatment (Fonagy et al. 2015), implying that the benefit was experienced not in the consulting room but in the social environment the patients encountered in their postclinical everyday life. The benefit accrued through the salutogenic effects available to individuals who are more open to social communication and accessing the consolations and regulatory support that epistemic trust can provide. In the next section, we aim to identify the common features of psychodynamic approaches that serve to ensure the potential for change we have described.

Core Components of Psychodynamic Therapy

All psychodynamic therapies aim to strengthen patients' capacity to understand the motivations and meanings of their own and others' subjective experiences, behavior, and relationships. The therapist aims to expand patients' conscious awareness of these mechanisms and influences so that they are better able to use their increased emotional awareness to manage continuing pressures.

The following eight assumptions may be considered core to modern psychodynamic therapy. Although some are not unique to the psychodynamic approach, other orientations would be unlikely to embrace all eight wholeheartedly.

1. *Notion of psychological causation.* At the heart of the psychodynamic approach is the assumption that the problems that people bring to psychotherapy can be usefully discussed in terms of thoughts and feelings. It is assumed that mental disorders

can be conceptualized as specific organizations of conscious or unconscious beliefs, thoughts, and feelings. This is an orientation toward a mentalizing, or, more accurately, co-mentalizing, stance in therapy.

2. *Limitations of consciousness and the influence of nonconscious mental states.* Psychodynamic clinicians generally assume that to understand conscious experiences, we need to refer to other mental states of which the individual is unaware. Further, in key instances, such a lack of awareness is not coincidental but rather is motivated by a wish to maximize the experience of safety by making parts of our personal narrative subdominant to the personal narrative driven by consciousness. Identifying these preconscious narratives driven out of consciousness because of their disruptive (anxiety-provoking) potential may be helpful in its own right, but their joint discovery with another mind whose shared focus with the patient's mind is the creation of an integrated self-narrative for the patient is in itself potentially therapeutic, enhancing a willingness to trust and collaborate. This should not be taken to imply a diminution of the emphasis placed by the theory on consciousness. Helping patients to become aware of the unconscious expectations underlying their behavior can help them to gain control of previously unmanageable emotions and behavior. However, it should be remembered that in the context of therapy, this is not a solitary experience but an intensely social (not to say intimate) experience.
3. *Assumption of internal representations of interpersonal relationships.* Psychodynamic clinicians consider interpersonal relationships, particularly attachment relationships, to be central to the organization of personality. Mental representations of these intense relationship experiences are assumed to be aggregated across time to form schematic mental structures. These structures are seen as shaping interpersonal expectations and self-representations. Particular individual histories, the accumulation of adverse experiences for the most part, leave such structures maladapted to collaboration and create tensions as individuals attempt to join a social world through emotional experiences of excessive suspicion, inappropriate feelings of guilt, and distressing experiences of shame. When epistemic trust is absent, these structures are not open to change even when communication from others implies that expectations of self or of others that may historically have been an appropriate adaptation are no longer so in a changed environment.
4. *Ubiquity of psychological conflict.* Psychodynamic approaches assume that wishes, affects, and ideas will sometimes be in conflict. These conflicts are seen as key causes of distress. Not only are conflicts thought to cause distress; they are also considered potentially to undermine the normal development of key psychological capacities that in turn reduce the person's ability to resolve incompatible ideas. The conflicts reflect the complexity of our models of mind—our own and those of others. We may have incompatible self-narratives, or our self-narrative may be at variance with how we construe the contents of the mind of an important figure in our life. The metacognition underpinning a self-narrative may also conflict with the personal second-order narrative of how we see others seeing us. The complexity of the thoughts and feelings we can ascribe to ourselves and others will inevitably mean that deep fissures are created and our mind becomes compartmentalized and particular lines of thought become separate from others, putting the resolution of the conflicting ideas beyond our reach. Living with the incompatibilities

may be a sound solution until reality forces us to confront what are simultaneously held incompatible views.

5. *Assumption of psychic defenses.* Historically, the psychodynamic approach has been particularly concerned with defenses: mental operations that distort conscious mental states to reduce their potential to generate anxiety. It is generally accepted that self-serving distortions of mental states relative to an external or internal reality are a ubiquitous feature of human information processing. The implicit assumption behind the supposition of psychic defenses is the driving force of an internal value system that sets standards for action, thought, and feeling that must be met to avoid negative emotional experiences. Shame and guilt are powerful feelings and can drive wholesale defensive distortions of denial or repression, whereas more subtle modifications of representations (e.g., ascribing agency for one's feelings to another agent, that is, projection) may serve to increase a sense of safety and well-being and to achieve a reduction in anxiety created by metacognitive awareness of mental states incompatible with one's self-narrative.
6. *Assumption of complex meanings.* Psychodynamic approaches assume that behavior can be understood in terms of mental states that are not explicit in action or within the awareness of the person concerned. In general, the theories specify particular constructions of experience assumed to account for psychological problems (e.g., grandiosity and vulnerable self-esteem associated with narcissistic personality disorder). It is striking that different psychodynamic orientations find different types of meanings concealed behind the same symptomatic behaviors. Within a contemporary context, it is the effort of seeking further personal meaning, rather than giving the patient insight in terms of any particular meaning structure, that would be considered most significant therapeutically. Within our preferred way of looking at this process, the shared discovery of these constructions with another person creates the most important opportunity for the we-mode experience, which in turn generates trust, which, if generalized extraclinically, can be invaluable in changing social relationships and bringing about the kind of permanent changes in internal representations of interpersonal relationships that can be life-changing for individuals with histories of trauma and adversity.
7. *Emphasis on the therapeutic relationship.* There is consensus that it is helpful for patients to establish an attachment relationship with a clinician. Different therapeutic schools explain this differently, but converging theorization and research data suggest that engagement with an understanding adult will trigger a basic set of human capacities for relatedness that appears to be therapeutic, apparently almost regardless of content (PDM Task Force 2006). However, controlled trials have repeatedly demonstrated that therapeutic alliance without theoretical content is insufficient (Dew and Bickman 2005); therapeutic impact seems to depend on an elaborated rationale in the therapist's mind that the patient expects to add meaning to their experience. The relationship in and of itself will bring little even if the patient develops powerful feelings for the therapist that are similar in form and content to those experienced in relation to primary caregivers. We need to take a further step regarding what functions attachment serves in the context of human development to see how and why the intense feelings that can evolve in relation to the therapist serve the purpose of healing. It is in this context that our social learning model may be of value. In human development, attachment may be one

of a number of routes by which a sense of belonging is created that signals that epistemic vigilance may be lowered and that opportunity has arisen for updating outdated knowledge structures. The trustworthiness of the therapist (Allen 2021) is critical, and so is the quality of the relationship. How the therapist is able to establish themselves in this light remains an issue of therapeutic technique, which is perhaps best seen in the context of an art—or, to follow Holmes's (2010) description, a craft—rather than a science.

8. *Developmental perspective.* Psychodynamic psychotherapists are invariably oriented to the developmental aspects of their patients' problems (when and how a problem started, how it relates to an idealized "normal" developmental sequence) and work at least in part to optimize developmental processes. They work along a developmental pathway where the joining of minds occurs with increasing complexity and early models are incorporated into more developmentally complex processes. The schematic development of co-mentalizing may serve as an example. Sharing emotions is present from early infancy and reflects the tendency of the human mind to resonate the affect of those in physical proximity. Joint intentionality is present from about 9 months but depends on recognition of the other as an intentional agent. Collective intentionality emerges developmentally from the fourth year, when sharing becomes generalized and goes beyond the dyadic, and the capacity to align with a group, principally of peers, arises as the person becomes embedded in culture. The relationship between therapist and patient in psychoanalytic psychotherapy involves all these developmental stages. Given this common framework, we take the developmental perspective in our review of psychodynamic theories.

In the above assumptions we aimed to apply a simple schematic model to the extraordinary richness and complexity of ideas that psychodynamic theories and practice of therapy represent. Although most of the above assumptions are certainly central to all psychodynamic theories, the theories differ in terms of the particular nonconscious meanings, developmental periods, patterns of interpersonal relations, qualities of the therapeutic relationship, and even models of mental function that they consider to be central when working clinically with troubled individuals. Historically, the theories were developed to fill gaps in understanding particular conditions or to justify shifts in therapeutic approaches. The degree to which they gained acceptance was due largely to their usefulness to (or fit with) the practical approach to therapy adopted by individual psychodynamic clinicians. Although all aim at providing comprehensive psychological models, none can be considered a definitive statement, simply because the nature of fresh, alternative accounts is to highlight the gaps in prior conceptualizations. Were we to consider theories that try to provide comprehensive accounts, we would have to conclude that none can be true. In reality, psychodynamic theory requires multiple theories in much the same way that we need multiple definitions of most complex constructs. Each captures unique aspects of a psychotherapeutic approach to human problems, and by considering each seriously, we acquire a more rounded view of both the person and the clinical process. In this chapter we briefly describe the most popular theoretical models of psychodynamic psychotherapy and establish their unique contributions. These descriptions provide not only a theoretical framework for the various methods of psychodynamic psychotherapy but also the historical contexts and discourses from which they arose and how the theories differ and borrow from each other.

Freudian Psychoanalysis and Developmental Theory

Sigmund Freud was the first to give meaning to mental disorder by linking it to childhood experiences (Breuer and Freud 1895) and to the vicissitudes of the developmental process (Freud 1900/1953). Freud's discoveries radically altered our perception of the child from one of idealized innocence to that of a person struggling to achieve control over their biological needs and make them acceptable to society through the microcosm of their family. Freud tried to explain all behavior in terms of the failure of the child's mental apparatus to deal adequately with the pressures inherent in a maturationally predetermined sequence of drive states. Adult psychopathology, dreaming, jokes, and slips of the tongue were all seen as the revisiting of unresolved childhood conflicts over sexuality (Freud 1900/1953, 1901/1960, 1905/1960). Freud later gave equal place to aggression as an ultimately unassimilable residue of normal development and, consequently, an explanation of psychological disturbance (Freud 1920/1955). Furthermore, Freud's innovative and enduring structural model of the psyche gave a prominent place to the influence of the social environment in analytic theory (Freud 1923/1961). This developmental framework is based around the tripartite structural schema of id, ego, and superego (Freud 1923/1961). The hypothesis that conflicts within the human mind are chiefly organized around three themes—wish versus moral injunction, wish versus reality, and internal reality versus external reality—has had extraordinary explanatory power. Notably, the ego's capacity to create defenses became the cornerstone of psychoanalytic theorization and clinical work by Heinz Hartmann in the United States (Hartmann et al. 1946) and by Anna Freud in the United Kingdom (Freud 1936/1966).

There are many limitations to Freud's model; the sheer variety of later psychoanalytic theories bears witness to cultural differences in psychological theory, suggesting that to some extent Freud's theories were applicable to only a certain time and place. Although Freud made significant contributions to the field, many others moved away from psychoanalysis—often at the expense of the wider recognition that seemed to be afforded to Freud alone. For example, Jung's rejection of libido theory led to a neglect of his undoubted advances in the understanding of narcissism and his development of a theory of the self throughout the life cycle (Jung 1923).

In spite of the diversity of psychoanalytic schools, subsequent psychoanalytic theories have continued the developmental motif. Anna Freud (1965) provided a comprehensive model of psychopathology based on the dimensions of normal and abnormal personality development. Melanie Klein (1935/1975, 1930/1948) offered a radically different perspective both on severe mental disorders and on early child development. Hartmann et al. (1946) focused on the evolution of mental structures necessary for adaptation and elaborated on the common developmental conflicts between mental structures in early childhood. Mahler et al. (1975) provided a dynamic map of the first 3 years of life and framed a model for the developmental origins of personality disorders. Kernberg (1975) drew on previous work by Klein, Hartmann, and others to furnish a developmental model of borderline and narcissistic disturbances; Kohut (1971) constructed a model of narcissistic disturbances based on presumed deficits of early parenting. Although their advocates were initially almost hostile to the developmental model, relational intersubjectivity theories have increasingly emphasized that the earliest experiences create a template for social communication (Mitchell 2000). Psychoanalytic schema theories represent a renaissance of interest in development, particularly infant development (Stern 1985), and mentalization-based approaches, which originate from an attachment theory perspective and complete the current survey (Fonagy et al. 2002).

As we can see, psychodynamic theoretical accounts have centered on children and childhood experiences ever since Freud: pathology is believed to be rooted in and made up of recapitulated ontogeny (our origins and development), and disorders of the mind are often understood as maladaptive residues of childhood experience or as developmentally "primitive" modes of mental functioning. The developmental perspective is acknowledged by all genuinely psychoanalytic theories to some degree. Longitudinal, epidemiological birth cohort studies have provided dramatic confirmation that psychoanalysts were on the right track when they emphasized the developmental perspective in their understanding of the clinical problems they faced with their adult patients (e.g., Hofstra et al. 2002; Kim-Cohen et al. 2003). These studies have shown that in the vast majority of cases adult psychopathology is antedated by diagnosable childhood disturbance. Across adult disorders, 75% of patients with a mental health disorder had a diagnosable childhood problem (Kim-Cohen et al. 2003).

However, although development is central to psychodynamic theories, potential problems arise with taking them too literally. There is arguably unjustified confidence in tracing particular forms of psychopathology to specific phases (e.g., the link between BPD and Mahler's rapprochement subphase of separation-individuation), as well as a likely overemphasis in psychoanalysis on early experience, which is frequently found to be at odds with developmental data (O'Connor 2006). Other objections include problems with *adultomorphizing infancy*, which is the tendency to use hypotheses about later states of psychopathology to describe early stages of development. Furthermore, because we cannot know what the infant experiences, some argue that it is hard to see how empirical evidence in support of psychoanalytic claims can ever be compiled (Green 2000).

In spite of these cogent arguments against the wholesale integration of studies of infant behavior into psychoanalytic theory, we can make excellent use of developmental data to deepen our psychoanalytic understanding of psychological disturbance. Empirical evidence provides good support for a developmental model that bears an uncanny resemblance to Freud's. Westen and Gabbard (2002) demonstrated substantial empirical support for Freud's core construct: that human consciousness cannot account for its maladaptive actions. A similar position was adopted by the neuroscientist and Freud scholar Mark Solms (Panksepp et al. 2017; Solms 2018a; Solms and Turnbull 2002). Good evidence exists, for example, for Freud's basic proposition that much of complex mental life is not conscious, that people can think, feel, and experience motivational forces without being aware of them and can therefore also experience psychological problems that they find puzzling (Mikulincer and Shaver 2007; Solms 2018b). Freud's claim that unconsciously, we are in some ways capable of more complex mental operations is supported by literally thousands of research findings, even if the unconscious that such studies point to is composed of processing structures that have little in common with Freud's original postulate of nonconscious mentation.

Structural Approach

Following Freud's argument that the self has a tripartite structure, comprising id, ego, and superego, the structural approach to psychoanalysis and to psychodynamic psychotherapy has concentrated on addressing problems in the ego; for clinicians using structural theory, disorder originates in faulty ego development (Rangell 1955). The structural approach has come to be referred to as ego psychology. Ego psychology proved to be popular among analysts in North America, where it became a complex, conceptually rigorous, and varied school before, regrettably, waning in influence in recent years.

In general, the structural model argues that neurosis and psychosis originate at the point when an individual adult's urge to gratify drives reverts to a previously outgrown infantile mode of satisfaction. The symptoms that arise are compromises reflecting the many attempts of the ego to restore equilibrium between the opposing agencies of external reality, superego, and the unacceptable drive representations. As a result of psychological or organic problems, the ego itself may regress, with resultant pathology. In psychosis a threat of total dissolution of the ego exists. If the ego resumes functioning characteristic of early childhood, it will come to be dominated by irrational, magical thoughts and poorly controlled impulses. Mental illness can thus be viewed as a failure of the ego to maintain harmonious interaction between psychic agencies at age-appropriate levels.

Key figures in the history of structural theory include Heinz Hartmann, Erik Erikson, René Spitz, Edith Jacobson, Jacob Arlow, Charles Brenner, and Hans Loewald. Hartmann proposed the key developmental assumption of *change of function*, whereby behavior originating at one point in development may serve an entirely different function later on (Hartmann 1939/1958). Thus, persistence of behavior should not be treated as simple repetition. A particular behavior with infantile origin can be independent of the drive originally motivating it when observed in an adult, thereby attaining a *secondary autonomy*. Furthermore, Hartmann disagreed with Freud by saying that the ego evolved out of an undifferentiated matrix from which the id and superego also emerged (as opposed to emerging gradually from the id; see Hartmann et al. 1946); the ego remains linked to the id to some degree because it uses energy from the drives. Hartmann's theory can be seen as psychosocial in that he conceived of development as relying on an *average expectable environment* that affirms the importance of the actual parent.

Erikson (1950), meanwhile, was concerned primarily with the interaction of social norms and biological drives in generating self and identity. He also conceived of development as covering the entire life cycle, as seen in his description of eight developmental stages, with later stages assuming the mastery of earlier ones. In his developmental sequence of identity formation, Erikson also described the syndrome of identity diffusion, that is, a lack of temporal continuity of self experience in social contexts. With this in mind, Erikson proposed that the organizing construct of self was based not on excitement but on interpersonal dealings and transactions, which he described as a question of developing basic trust over basic mistrust. Westen (1998) considered investigations of Eriksonian concepts of identity (Marcia 1994), intimacy (Orlofsky 1993), and generativity (Bradley 1997) to have been some of the most methodologically sound studies inspired by psychoanalytic theories of development.

René Spitz (1959) proposed that major shifts in psychological organization, marked by the emergence of new behaviors and new forms of affective expression (organizers), occur when functions are brought into new relation with one another and are linked into a coherent unit. He was also one of the first to ascribe primary importance to the mother-infant interaction as a force in quickening the development of the child's innate abilities. Jacobson (1964) creatively assumed that because early drive states shift continuously between the object and the self, a state of primitive fusion exists between early object and self representations. Finally, Loewald (1973/1980) proposed that *integrative experience* is at the center of development. His fundamental assumption was that all mental activity is relational (both interactional and intersubjective). Internalization (learning) is the basic psychological process that propels development (Loewald 1973/1980). As Friedman (1986) noted, Loewald also shifted emphasis from structures to processes and generated a subtle revision of the classical structural model so that it had internalization, understanding, and interpretation at its center.

Modern developmental observations raise questions about the structural approach. For example, although structural theorists see psychotic symptoms as regressions to normal but very early functioning, such arguments are inconsistent with empirical studies that fail to find a "normal" confusional state between self and object (Gergely 2000). It has been shown that from birth, infants are able to identify their mothers accurately and even to imitate facial gestures (Meltzoff and Moore 1997). Even if putative pathogenic mechanisms such as identity diffusion in some way represented early modes of thought, this in no way implies that their reemergence in adult mental functioning is indicative of a developmental timetable. In a review of psychoanalytic theorization about schizophrenia, Willick (2001) provided a number of examples from the literature that illustrate that this criticism applies not only to past psychoanalytic theory but also to some more recent work.

Changes in the notion of the id foreshadowed the demise of structural theory. The original model was criticized in the 1970s and 1980s for its quasi-physiological character, for its homophobic outlook, and for the primacy it gave to sexuality in explanations of psychopathology. As a result, structural theorists had to reinterpret Freud's concept of the id from being a container of all biologically based intense physical desires to being an organization related to reality and human figures (see, e.g., Loewald 1978).

By no means all psychoanalysts accepted the shift of the basic psychoanalytic model from the classical Freudian structural model to object relations theory. In North America, a number of psychoanalysts remain fully committed to modifications of the structural approach as proposed, for example, by Brenner (2002). Other influential writers such as Harold Blum (1983) and Len Shengold (1981) have managed to retain a perspective broadly focused on ego psychology while selectively adopting certain object relations ideas. None of these writers have, however, wished to advance a psychoanalytic model that may serve as an alternative to object relations theory. Only relational theorists, self psychologists, and writers in the interpersonalist tradition have aspired to do this.

More recent reviews have tempered the tendency to dismiss the structural approach as reductionist, biologically naive, and overinfluenced by the naive physiology of nineteenth-century central Europe. For example, experimental work (Birbaumer et al. 2005; Sterzer et al. 2005) confirmed Reich's (1933/1972) and Fenichel's (1941) suggestions that the presence of anxiety (autonomic reactivity, amygdala activity) in antisocial youth reduces the risk of adult criminal behavior. Furthermore, Howard Shevrin (1997) has linked the *wanting system*, identified as abnormally sensitized or oversensitive in drug-dependent individuals, to the ego psychological notion of psychic energy and drives—an argument that gained support from Panksepp (1998). Finally, the neuropsychological work of Solms (2000) also suggested that the neural systems that activate dreaming and craving are identical. Each and every dream, therefore, starts in the neural structure that most closely fits Freud's concept of instinctual drive states, the ventral tegmental area.

An enduring legacy of the structural approach is found in the work of three psychoanalytic theorists who drew on the structural approach in elaborating their developmental theories, each of whom, to a greater or lesser extent, brought psychoanalysis closer to object relations. They are Anna Freud, Margaret Mahler, and Joseph Sandler.

Work of Anna Freud, Margaret Mahler, and Joseph Sandler

Sigmund Freud's daughter Anna Freud should, perhaps, be described as a modern structural theorist. Her model is fundamentally developmental, with an emphasis placed on observational methods; she saw developmental progress as a child coming to terms with developmentally expectable conflicts, in which the child has to find a compromise among diverse wishes, needs, perceptions, physical and social realities, and object relations. Although she maintained the classic Freudian position that the individual's drives are the main factor in the construction of the ego and superego, she did carry her father's theories forward by identifying ways that child-rearing contributes to this process (Freud 1965).

Anna Freud's theory focused on the metaphor of developmental *lines*, which stressed the continuity and cumulative character of child development. The main lines that she developed were from dependency to emotional self-reliance and adult relationships, from egocentrism to social partnerships, from sucking to rational eating, and from irresponsibility to responsibility in body management, as well as, latterly, lines from animate to inanimate objects and from irresponsibility to guilt (Freud 1974/1981). For Anna Freud, pathology is assessed in terms of large discrepancies among the lines and notable lags with respect to normal progress along each line. Arrest in or regression along a particular developmental line can lead to the formulation of a problem.

Anna Freud also identified disturbances of narcissism, object relatedness, and the absence of control over aggressive or self-destructive tendencies alongside a range of deficiencies of development before suggesting that there is a developmental aspect to the emergence of anxiety problems in childhood. She also distinguished between objective anxiety (e.g., fear of any aspect of the external world, including the parents' real reactions) and fear of the internal world (impulses, wishes, feelings), building on her earlier work with infants at the Hampstead War Nurseries, where she found that children were less likely to be traumatized by being bombed if they were with their mothers during this experience and the mothers remained calm (Freud and Burlingham 1944/1973). A carefully conducted study of children's reactions to Scud missile attacks in Israel provided more recent support for this finding (Laor et al. 1996).

Traditions of study of the development of competence and psychopathology are present in the history of both psychiatry and psychoanalysis but are not commonly integrated, the former being the concern of developmental psychology and the latter being the concern of child and adult psychiatry. Anna Freud's work is notable for bridging the gap between the two.

Margaret Mahler was the first thoroughgoing developmentalist of the North American tradition. She elaborated a psychoanalytic model of development based on observations of children ages 6 months to 3 years. Her developmental model sees object relations and the self as elaborations of instinctual vicissitudes. Her focus is on the move from the unity of *I* and *not I* to eventual separation and individuation (Mahler et al. 1975). Separation, in Mahler's model, refers to the child's emergence from a symbiotic fusion with the mother, whereas "individuation consists of those achievements marking the child's assumption of his own individual characteristics" (Mahler et al. 1975, p. 4).

Mahler's developmental model involves "normal autism" during the first weeks of life, followed by a symbiotic phase, after which separation-individuation begins with the subphase of differentiation. The second subphase of individuation (practicing) takes place from 9 months to about 15–18 months, followed by a rapprochement subphase (the second half of the second year), during which the infant needs to be with the mother. Finally, the fourth subphase of separation-individuation is the consolidation of individuality that begins with the third year of life.

Mahler's work has been used extensively by clinicians working with adults with personality disorder (see Kramer and Akhtar 1988; Pine 1985). Narcissistic personality disorders are linked to inadequate soothing ministrations of the mother during the symbiotic phase and inadequate refueling during separation-individuation. Therefore, the omnipotence of the practicing subphase is never completely renounced. Cross-cultural research on parent-child relationships, however, suggests that prolonging the symbiotic union between mother and infant does not undermine the individual's capacity to achieve autonomy (Rothbaum et al. 2000). Individuals with BPD are often thought to experience residues of rapprochement subphase conflicts, with persistent longings for and dread of fusion with the other associated with either aggression or withdrawal on the part of the mother. Masterson (1985) suggested that the object, who is desperate to feel needed, rewards the toddler for demanding and clinging behavior. Limited evidence is available to support the suggestion that BPD is a transgenerational disorder. A study found that mothers with BPD were more intrusively insensitive toward their 2-month-old infants than were mothers without psychiatric disorders (Crandell et al. 2003).

Mahler described her work as enabling clinicians treating adults to make more accurate reconstructions of the preverbal period, thereby making patients more accessible to psychotherapeutic interventions. However, although Mahler's model has been highly influential, systematic experimental research with infants casts serious doubt on the dual notions of normal autism and self-object merger (Gergely 2000). That said, Mahler's developmental framework could well be appropriate for the truly psychological world of the human infant: the infant is aware of themself and the object as separate in the physical (bodily) domain but assumes that psychological states extend beyond physical boundaries (Fonagy et al. 2002). Similarly, Mahler's theories concerning childhood schizophrenia seem unlikely to be explained by the notion of a developmental fixation in the symbiotic phase, but her original contributions to the understanding of BPD have been most lasting. Her view of patients with BPD as fixated in a rapprochement, wishing to cling but fearing the loss of their fragile sense of self and wishing to be separate but also fearing to move away from the parental figure, has been crucial to both clinical intervention and theoretical understanding.

Joseph Sandler was a student of Anna Freud and played an instrumental role in the modernization of psychoanalysis, preparing its integration with the developmental sciences and finding common ground between American ego psychology and British object relations theory. Many of his ideas have been seamlessly integrated into modern core theory. Sandler introduced the frame of reference of the representational world, an approach very similar to the schema theory that has come to dominate social and cognitive-behavioral psychology (Sandler and Rosenblatt 1962). Sandler placed feeling states rather than psychic energy at the center of the psychoanalytic theory of motivation and introduced the revolutionary concept of the background of safety, within which the aim of the ego is to maximize safety or security rather than to avoid anxiety (Sandler 1960). He did not get rid of drives but explained their influence on behavior through the impact they had on feelings.

Sandler described how patients tend to create relationships to actualize unconscious fantasies by casting themselves and their therapists in specific relationship patterns and, by extension, offered an entirely new theory of internal object representations. Sandler differentiated the deeply unconscious hypothetical structures assumed by classical psychoanalysis to develop early in life that have no chance of directly emerging into consciousness (the past unconscious) from the present unconscious, which he believed worked as Freud described (irrationally, only partly observing the reality principle but principally concerned with current rather than past experience) (Sandler and Sandler 1984). The second system, the present unconscious, consists of here-and-now adaptations to conflicts and anxieties triggered in the first system, which is a genuine continuation of the past into the present. Sandler linked pleasure in experiencing particular styles of perceptual and cognitive functions with specific forms of pathology. For example, obsessionality, painful though it may be, is linked to pleasure in childhood. The developmental model of depression that Sandler proposed also made use of the representational world construct.

In further clinical formulations, Sandler explained the concept of projective identification without making the extravagant assumptions that many Kleinian authors have made (see the next section). The other can come to enact the patient's fantasy because the patient attempts to modify or control the behavior of the other so that it conforms to their distorted representation of the other. The patient's representation of the other comes to be distorted through the mechanism of projection, in which the other is experienced as owning unwanted aspects of the self-representation. This model is helpful in explaining therapeutic phenomena such as countertransference and phenomena identified by emotional developmental research, such as the transgenerational transmission of patterns of mother-infant interaction (Fraiberg et al. 1975).

Although Sandler's theories were, and are, extensively used, those who use his ideas are often unaware that they are doing so. Thus, no psychoanalytic school bears his name. He advanced thinking by clarifying a range of psychoanalytic concepts but was unable to excite his colleagues with the novelty of his contributions.

Object Relations Theory and the Klein-Bion Model

Object relations theory has had several incarnations, several of which grew to be immensely popular in the 1980s. Broadly speaking, object relations theory moves toward an understanding of psychopathology in terms of mental representations of self-and-object relationships, which are rooted in past relationships and are at first dyadic, later triadic, and still later multiple relationship representations. The increased interest in relationships is part of an underlying refocusing of psychoanalysis away from the study of intrapsychic conflict toward an experientially based perspective emphasizing the individual's experience of being with others and with the therapist during analytic work.

According to object relations theory, the ego is defined in relation to other objects, both internal and external, and as a result it is assumed that the child's mind is initially shaped by early experiences with the caregiver and becomes increasingly complex with development. These early object relations are thought to set patterns that are repeated and therefore become fixed in later life. In some versions of object relations theory (e.g., attachment theory) the individual is seen as possessing an *autonomous relationship drive*, whereas other versions derive relationships from drive theory (Winnicott) or derive drives from object relations (Kernberg). Friedman (1988) differentiated object relations theories along these lines into *hard* and *soft* categories, the former being characterized by the work of Melanie Klein, Ronald Fairbairn, and Otto Kernberg and the latter the work of Michael Balint, D.W. Winnicott, and Heinz Kohut.

Central to object relations theories are the ideas of Melanie Klein and Wilfred Bion, who offered highly speculative, often controversial, but remarkably influential accounts of pathology, particularly self-destructive and relatively immutable behaviors. Klein and Bion both highlighted the negative aspects of emotional development. Klein combined the structural model with an object relations model of development, which in turn puts strong emphasis on constitutional vulnerability rather than caregiver behavior as the prime determinant of developmental pathways. Klein's (1935/1975, 1940/1984) papers on the depressive position, her paper on the paranoid-schizoid position (Klein 1946), and her book *Envy and Gratitude* (Klein 1957/1975) all play a significant part in the Klein-Bion model, which builds on Freud's idea of a self-destructive death drive and postulates two modes of mental functioning: the paranoid-schizoid position and the depressive position.

The paranoid-schizoid position is dominated by tendencies to separate the good and the bad, the idealized and the persecutory; the depressive position entails a more mature, balanced recognition of the bad in the good and one's own role in unrealistically and self-servingly distorting the world into idealized and denigrated components. Klein's metaphor for these two states of mind is the perception of the mother as separately idealized and persecuting in the paranoid-schizoid state and as a whole person who accounts for both good and bad experiences in the depressive position. Recognition in the depressive position that the loved good object and the hated and feared bad object are one and the same gives rise to feelings of guilt and *depressive anxiety*, whereas the paranoid-schizoid position is characterized by *persecutory anxieties*.

An important contribution of the Klein-Bion model is the concept of projective identification; that is, the individual externalizes segments of the ego and attempts to gain control over these unwanted possessions, often through highly manipulative behavior toward the object (i.e., making the other identify with the projections). Projective identification is best characterized not as a defensive mechanism but rather as an interpersonal process whereby the self gets rid of feelings by evoking the same feelings in another self (Bion 1962). The roots of this process are found in infancy (Bion 1959).

Klein suggested that children innately possess ruthless and sadistic fantasies, which are not a reaction to frustration but pay lip service to the parent's capacity to mitigate the influence of the child's constitutional tendencies. Given its thesis that violent tendencies are innate rather than caused by environmental influences, the Klein-Bion model has been influential in psychological models of the mediation of genetic vulnerability. Evidence suggests that physical aggression and destructiveness are, indeed, particularly marked in the early years and naturally decline in most children over the course of the first decade, with violent children manifesting an absence of this expectable so-called taming rather than an emergence of aggression de novo in response to environmental impingement (Shaw et al. 2003; Tremblay 2000; Tremblay et al. 1999).

By and large, the Kleinian model of psychopathology understands mental disorder in terms of the depressive and paranoid-scizhoid positions described above. A predominance of the paranoid-schizoid position leads to mental disorder, whereas the relative stability of the depressive framework reflects mental health (although Bion [1957] argued that the depressive position is never permanently achieved). In psychotic states, annihilatory/persecutory anxieties are intense, and the object with whom the patient attempts to projectively identify is *reintrojected*, that is, experienced as entering the ego, creating a delusion of the mind or the body being under external control. Neurotic problems are seen as consequences of unresolved depressive anxiety. For example, depression arises because the experience of loss reminds the person of the damage they felt they caused to the good object. Chronic depression arises when the person cannot escape the fear of injuring the loved object and therefore has to repress all aggressiveness, generating a relentless self-persecution. Narcissistic character structure, meanwhile, is considered a defense against envy and dependence. The narcissist's relationship with others is highly destructive; narcissists make ruthless use of others and deny their need of them (Rosenfeld 1987).

Klein's ideas have provoked considerable controversy and ill feeling. Concerns have included her attribution of adult psychological capacities to infants and dating of pathology to such early stages (Bibring 1947). Because the mental states of infancy are extremely hard to observe, the postulation of crucial pathogenic processes in infancy is extremely unlikely to be disproved. Psychoanalytic infant observation (Bick 1964) permits widely differing interpretations. However, evidence that most of the important mental disorders of adulthood are, indeed, foreshadowed in the biological processes of infancy is accumulating (e.g., Hemmi et al. 2011; Marenco and Weinberger

2000), and early brain development is increasingly being seen as pivotal (Kao et al. 2010; Schore 2003).

British Independent School: Fairbairn and Winnicott

The so-called British Independent School comprises several theorists working individually, all of whom explicitly refrained from establishing schools of followers. Fairbairn and Guntrip were the theory builders, with major contributions from Winnicott, Balint, Klauber, Khan, and Bollas.

The core ideas of this somewhat heterogeneous group of theories might be summarized as follows: There is a primary drive for creating object relationships (Fairbairn 1952), and insufficient intimacy with the primary object can give rise to a *splitting* in the self; it is the persistence of incompatible ideas and lack of integration that is at the root of psychological disorder. Holding, or the capacity to comprehend the infant's mental states, is key to intimacy and integration (Winnicott 1960/1965); holding is communicated by mirroring that is never perfect but is good enough and permits repair (Winnicott 1967). The infant "conjures the mother" through the use of a physical object (e.g., a blanket), which is known as a *transitional object* (Winnicott 1953); the self emerges through nonintrusive interactions with the mother, which facilitate the infant's illusion that the object/mother is a product of the infant's creative gestures and therefore is controlled and controllable. If the mother cannot comprehend the infant, a *false (compliant) self* will develop to protect the true self (Winnicott 1960/1965); it is the lack of (recognition of) love between mother and child, rather than a primary destructiveness, that will lead the child to believe that their hate has destroyed the object/mother (Fairbairn 1952).

Fairbairn proposed that early trauma is stored in memories that are "frozen" or dissociated from a person's central ego or functional self, an idea of particular relevance to understanding narcissistic personality disorder and BPD. Fairbairn saw the roots of all pathology as being in a schizoid reaction to the trauma of not being known or loved. Winnicott and Fairbairn both associated schizophrenia with total privation—that is, the complete absence of a "good enough" mother, which makes the infant view their love as bad and destructive and leads them to withdraw from emotional contact with the outer world, ultimately creating a highly disturbed sense of external reality. Severe personality disorder could be seen as the result of having had a good enough mother who has subsequently disappeared. Schizoid personality (Fairbairn 1952) arises out of the infant's feeling that love for the mother is destroying her and therefore has to be inhibited along with all intimacy. Patients with BPD were considered by Winnicott to share defenses with psychotic patients: that is, they have no sense of others and respond with intense anger if their sense of omnipotence is threatened (Winnicott 1960/1965). Empirical studies have shown that patients with BPD do, indeed, have a specific deficit in mental state awareness in the context of attachment relationships (Petersen et al. 2016).

The British Independents' general approach to development, the description of the infant as biologically prepared to attend to environmental events that respond to them, has been very well supported by infant research (Meltzoff and Moore 1998; Watson 2001). Winnicott's views on the importance of sensitive maternal care are broadly supported by developmental research; for example, research on affective interactions between infant and mother supports the notion of a dual unit of infant and mother, in which the mother and infant mutually create the infant's moods (Jaffe et al. 2001; Tronick 2007; Tronick and Beeghly 2011). However, general dissatisfaction exists around the fuzziness of the concept of maternal sensitivity (De Wolff and van Ijzendoorn 1997), and the British Independent School has only partially stood the test of time.

Winnicott was correct to examine environmental influences on normal and pathological development. Research on long-term outcomes for a population of severely emotionally deprived Romanian infants adopted in late childhood supports Fairbairn's and Winnicott's assumptions, as do studies on the long-term impact of neglect more generally (Kumsta et al. 2015). Such levels of deprivation do appear to be associated with possible neurophysiological and neuroanatomical deficits (Jacoby et al. 2016; Mackes et al. 2020; Nelson et al. 2011; Pollak et al. 2010), but Winnicott seemed to overstate the case. For example, research does not support Winnicott's exclusive concern with the infant-mother relationship because many other factors, particularly genetic influences, shape a child's personality (Bolton et al. 2006). Winnicott's assumption that the relationship between infant and mother provides the basis for all serious mental disorders also flies in the face of accumulating evidence suggesting that genetic factors account for some of the observed association of environmental deprivation and pathological outcome (Plomin and McGuffin 2003; Rutter et al. 1999).

The major weakness in Winnicott's argument, however, remains his naive reconstruction of infancy in the adult mind. To an extent, this is characteristic of the entire British object relations tradition. Human development is far too complex for infantile experiences to have direct links to adult pathology. In fact, longitudinal studies of infancy suggest that personality organization is subject to reorganization throughout development on the basis of both positive and negative influences (Bleidorn et al. 2018; Borghuis et al. 2020; Pinquart et al. 2013).

Heinz Kohut and Self Psychology

Self psychology emerged from the thinking of Heinz Kohut (1977). Initially concentrating on problems of narcissism, self psychology was soon applied to other mental disorders and involved a specific therapeutic approach foregrounding empathy. Although Kohut's theories changed over time, his key assumptions included the following. Narcissistic development proceeds along a path of its own, and parents serve as selfobjects (people in the environment who perform particular functions for the self). Empathic responses from the mirroring selfobject allow the unfolding of exhibitionism and grandiosity; frustration permits a gradual modulation of infantile omnipotence through a *transmuting internalization* of this mirroring selfobject, which in turn leads gradually to a consolidation of the nuclear self. The idealization of selfobjects, also through internalization, leads to the development of ideals. Kohut (1977, 1984) latterly believed that a cohesive self was a goal to be attained, as opposed to there being a self that changes over time. Finally, the *enfeebled self* (to whom the selfobject has typically failed emotionally to attune) turns defensively toward pleasure aims (drives), and anxiety is primarily the self's experience of a defect or lack of continuity.

From the above description, self psychology emerges as a theory based on deficiency. A deficiency of facilitating experiences is assumed to lead to a primary psychic deficit, an inadequately developed self. Fear of losing the sense of who one is underlies all pathology. Diagnostic distinctions are made in terms of characteristics of the self: psychosis precludes a cohesive sense of self, patients with personality disorder have an enfeebled self vulnerable to temporary fragmentation, and neurotic pathology is thought to be associated with the robustness of self structure. Narcissistic personality, meanwhile, is a developmental arrest at the stage of the grandiose exhibitionistic self, which fails to be neutralized by the parent's age-specific mirroring responses, and BPD results from an inability psychologically to hold on to selfobjects that might otherwise be soothing to the self. Furthermore, drug addiction is thought to fill a missing gap in the psyche (Kohut 1977).

Like Winnicott, Kohut has proven influential, and although some evidence he used to support his theories is far-fetched, at other times his work seems prescient. For example, a large body of evidence supports the central role of self-esteem in the generation of psychological disturbance (Brown et al. 1995). Self psychologists have also felt supported by the identification of so-called *mirror neurons* in the primate brain (Gallese et al. 2004; Rizzolatti and Craighero 2004). These cells appear to be activated when a rhesus monkey identifies a movement analogous to its own in the world (it should be borne in mind that monkeys do not recognize themselves in the mirror; the suggestion here is for a predisposition to identifying environmental events pertaining to the self). Although prima facie this is consistent with a developmental emphasis on mirroring, it is somewhat far-fetched to consider it a direct confirmation of self psychological ideas.

Kohut's model has often, and appropriately, been criticized as "parent blaming"—and again like Winnicott, Kohut is open to criticism for overemphasizing environmental influences, especially in the face of increasing evidence of genetically rooted personality traits. Correlations between characteristics of early parenting and later child behavior can be reinterpreted given that any association may be attributable to the 50% genetic overlap between a parent and a biological child. This has been termed *passive genotype-environment correlation*. In a landmark investigation of genetic and environmental influences on adolescent development, Reiss and colleagues (2000) found that of 52 statistically significant associations between family relationship (e.g., parental warmth, sibling relationships) and measures of adjustment (e.g., depression, antisocial behavior), 44 showed genetic influences that accounted for more than half of the common variance. In almost half of the 52, little association between family relations and adolescent functioning remained once genetic influence was taken into consideration. Contemporary behavioral genetics is not compatible with a naively environmentalist position (Plomin et al. 2016). However, genetically informed studies do repeatedly find that qualities of the family environment moderate genetic influence, which is, for example, greater for antisocial behavior the more negative the parenting is (Feinberg et al. 2007; Pinquart 2017). Kohut seems also to have been criticized not only for his radical revision of psychoanalytic ideas but also for failing to recognize the work of others working in similar areas, including Winnicott and Loewald.

Otto Kernberg and Structural Object Relations

Primarily put forward by Otto Kernberg, structural object relations involves a synthesis of the Klein-Bion model and the work of the modernizers of structural theory (Sandler, Mahler, Loewald). Through his work, which offers a comprehensive reconsideration of psychological disorders, Kernberg has become the most cited living analyst and one of the most influential in the history of the field.

Following Sandler, Kernberg (1982) considered affects to be the primary motivational system. That is to say, representations of the interactions between self and object, colored by particular affects, constitute the basic building blocks of psychic structure; drives come about from the accumulations of types of self-object-affect triads—not the other way around—although eventually, drives do become motivators of behavior and are not replaced by object relations structures. The psychic structures (id, ego, superego) come about through various processes of *internalization*: through introjection, whereby entire interactions between self and other are internalized in their affective context; through identifications that recognize the variety of role dimensions that exist in interactions with others; and through ego identity, which denotes the overall organization of introjections and identifications (Kernberg 1976). As a child develops, the ego separates good images from bad ones to protect one from the other, before these images become integrated into complete object and self representations in the third year. Failure to integrate these separated images can lead to pathology, in which splitting as opposed to repression remains the principal coping mechanism. After a child reaches age 3, Kernberg's theory follows the structural model of development. For Kernberg, all disorders originate in the early stages of self-object dyadic configurations—that is, before self and object have emerged as integrated units.

The originality of Kernberg's approach to neurotic problems consists of focusing on the current state of the patient's thinking rather than attempting to identify the origin of currently dominant pathogenic conflicts and structural organizations. He uses psychiatric diagnostic categories as predictors of treatment response, arguing that twice-weekly expressive psychotherapy is a better treatment for severe character problems than psychoanalysis. Kernberg's contribution to understanding personality disorders is his most distinctive and valuable work. At mild levels of character pathology, not only is the ego poorly organized and unstable, but the superego is harsh and sadistic. The patient who feels that they are the victim of criticism (from the therapist) can suddenly turn into the vicious unreasonable critic. At severe levels of character pathology, primitive dissociation or splitting of internalized object relations is marked, with a consequent lack of integration of self and object representations. The individual insists on consistently constructing either idealized or persecutory self and object relations, making relationships with such individuals confused or chaotic (Kernberg 1984). The root cause of personality disorder is the intensity of destructive and aggressive impulses and the relative weakness of ego structures available to handle them. Wisely, Kernberg leaves open the question of whether such excessive aggressiveness is inborn or associated with particularly malevolent early environments.

Kernberg's treatment approach to BPD (transference-focused psychotherapy) is one of the few psychodynamic approaches that has a strong theoretical framework, is fully operationalized, and has been carefully evaluated (Kernberg et al. 2008; Perez et al. 2016; Taylor et al. 2018; Yeomans et al. 2015). The most recent findings suggest that transference-focused psychotherapy is at least as effective as dialectical behavior therapy and probably more efficacious than supportive psychotherapy (Clarkin et al. 2007; Levy et al. 2006; Perez et al. 2016; Taylor et al. 2018; Yeomans et al. 2015).

Kernberg's genius lies in marrying the structural (or *metapsychological*) to the phenomenological. For example, if a patient with BPD shows signs of idealization, devaluation, or denial (phenomena), these signs also indicate the organization (structure) of intrapsychic relationship representations, as well as the individual's failure to generate more advanced mental mechanisms. Kernberg also goes beyond traditional ego psychology in that the explanation in terms of *ego weakness* is no longer circular; for Kernberg, ego weakness is coterminous with an active defensive process that leads to the split-ego organizations that cannot withstand close contact with bad object representations.

Because Kernberg's theory leaves a place for innate factors in development, it can accommodate emerging evidence concerning the powerful genetic influences that appear to be present in BPD (Amad et al. 2014; Distel et al. 2008, 2011). In addition, his hypotheses concerning the ego weakness of patients with BPD have received empirical support from work within and outside the Personality Disorders Institute (Goldstein et al. 2007; Levy 2005; Rothbart et al. 2000). De Panfilis et al. (2016) showed how patients with BPD are high in negative affect and low in effortful control and how they benefit from psychotherapy in relation to their improved capacity to represent mental states in an attachment context.

It may be that Kernberg's etiological hypotheses share some of the general weaknesses of psychoanalytic formulations, but his contribution remains a landmark, not just because of his advancement of the psychoanalytic developmental framework for personality disorder but also because it brought about a major shift in the epistemic stance taken by psychoanalysts influenced by him—from a clinical hermeneutic perspective toward an empirical one.

Interpersonal Relational Approach

Stephen A. Mitchell (1988) introduced the framework for a range of theoretical developments that collectively may be termed *relational psychoanalytic theories*. This framework formed a relational matrix consisting of three dimensions—a self pole, an object pole, and an interactional pole—that could, in turn, be configured and reconfigured to create multiple new theories. Taking cues from Sullivan (1953) and linked to British object relations, this approach emphasizes the active role played by both or all parties in relationships, and important contributors to the approach include Benjamin (1998), Bromberg (1998), Hoffman (1994), McLaughlin (1991), Ogden (1994), and Renik (1993). Notions of objective truth are supplemented or replaced with subjectivity, the intrapsychic is supplemented or replaced with the intersubjective, and fantasy (poetics) is supplemented by or replaced with pragmatics (descriptions of experience); concepts of truth and distortion are supplemented with perspectivism, and a reliance on strong theories is replaced by attempts to avoid theoretical bias. Each of the major relational theorists offered a slightly different integration of the relational matrix (e.g., Mitchell's relational conflict theory, Ogden's intersubjectivity, Hoffman's social constructivism, Greenberg's (1991) dual-drive theory), meaning that there is no single, unifying relational psychoanalytic theory. Relational theories are metatheories, in which human relations are considered to play a superordinate role in the creation of human character.

Sullivan (1953) felt that psychoanalysis ignored the relationship-seeking aspect of human character and proposed that conflict was produced not in the individual but by conflicting and contradictory signals and values in the environment. For Sullivan, the causes of needs are interpersonal, as are those of anxiety, the development of which leads to psychopathology. Despite the different terminology, Sullivan's concepts have close ties to the psychodynamic domain: *security operations* seem to be the same as defenses, and *parataxic distortions* appear to be analogous to internal object relations. But here the therapist does not seek to impart understanding so much as explore the nature of and the reasons for patterns of behavior in an active and participatory manner. Whereas for self psychology the nuclear self is conceived as intrapsychic, here an individual's mind is a contradiction in terms because subjectivity is invariably rooted in intersubjectivity.

The relational model starts from the assumption that subjectivity is interpersonal—that is, the intersubjective replaces the intrapsychic (Mitchell 1988). This renders the human mind a contradiction in terms because subjectivity is invariably rooted in an intersubjective matrix of relational bonds in which personal meanings are embedded (Mitchell 2000), as opposed to being rooted in biological drives. Thus, the internal and the external are not discrete but are anticipated by the primacy of the interpersonal field, which includes the idea that the organism exists in relation to its environment. However, unlike most other psychoanalytic theories, the relational psychoanalytic model lacks a specific explanation for how relationality and intersubjectivity may develop.

In this way, sexuality, for example, not only is a powerful biological and physiological force but also emerges from an interpersonal context, which is mutually regulatory, intersubjective, or relational. Its power is derived not from organ pleasure but from its meaning in a relational matrix (Mitchell 1988). A result of this approach is that it privileges observable behavior and actuality over fantasy, meaning that reality is not behind the appearance; it is in the appearance.

According to Mitchell (2000), psychiatric disorders can come about in any of four groups of manners. The first way psychiatric disorders can arise is through nonreflective, presymbolic behavior that leads to the organization of relational fields around reciprocal influence and mutual regulation. The second way is through affective permeability, or the shared experience of intense affect across permeable boundaries where direct resonances emerge in interpersonal dyads. The third way is through the organization of experience into self-other configurations, as extensively discussed by Kernberg and other object relations theorists. The fourth way is through intersubjectivity, or the mutual recognition of self-reflective agents identified by relationally oriented psychoanalytic feminists such as Chodorow (1989) and Benjamin (1995). The theory embraces the notion that the absence of a sensitive object causes a child precociously to fulfill a missing parental function, but it is critical of the developmental arrest model. According to Mitchell, we privilege the earliest periods at the risk of overlooking current relationship needs. Relational theory also finds a middle ground between Kohut and Kernberg in recognizing both the child's need for the narcissistic illusion of grandiosity (Kohut) and the idea that the narcissistic illusion is defensive (Kernberg). Because the approach focuses on the present relationship between patient and therapist, controversy has arisen concerning the readiness with which therapists disclose their own feelings (Ehrenberg 1993).

Relational analysts have adapted infant research to apply the principle of ongoing dyadic regulation to the therapeutic situation (Beebe and Lachmann 1994; Stern et al. 1998). The therapist and the patient supposedly create a dyadic state of consciousness through mutual affect regulation; each patient-therapist dyad is different but will influence future exchanges for both parties—both with each other and with other people. Therapy happens when already extant states of consciousness are reintegrated and reconfigured for the patient. Current relational thinking often uses psychopathological accounts of trauma to highlight the relational aspects of actual experience (e.g., Davies 1996). "What really happened" is combined with attention to the subjective experience of the patient, not to separate veridical events from distortions associated with unconscious fantasy but rather to elaborate the overwhelming nature of the experience itself—especially because the context of trauma is assumed to preclude awareness of its meanings. The inherent paradox of attachment trauma (that is, an apparently unintended trauma perpetrated by a figure on whom one depends) is that a stance of "not knowing what one knows" (Bowlby 1988, p. 99) might be adopted to keep the crucial relationship intact. Relational psychoanalytic and attachment-inspired clinical descriptions provide similar formulations of dissociation linked with traumatic experience.

Substantial developmental and clinical evidence exists that psychopathology is accompanied by relational problems and that good interpersonal relations have a protective influence (e.g., Laub 1998; Lipsitz and Markowitz 2013; Santini et al. 2015a, 2015b). Peer awareness of unpopularity forecasts the emergence of conduct disorder in children, for example (Chen et al. 2015); similarly, poor peer relationships are strongly implicated in ADHD (Mikami and Normand 2015). More generally, peer relations predict the course of psychological disturbance (Parker et al. 2015). Risk of depression has long been shown to be related to exposure to difficult life events (Brown et al. 1998; Goodyer 1995). Of further significance is the strong evidence showing that supportive relationships offer protection against psychological problems associated with various forms of risk across the life course (Cohen et al. 2015; Wang et al. 2018).

Since the publication of the first edition of this book, the influence of the relational approach has grown considerably, with IPT emerging as one of the most widely practiced models of psychotherapy (Weissman et al. 2017). IPT is now included in various treatment guidelines internationally and is, for example, central to the United Kingdom's national Improving Access to Psychological Therapies program for the treatment of depression (National Collaborating Centre for Mental Health 2018). After cognitive-behavioral therapy, IPT probably stands as the psychotherapy with the next most comprehensive evidence base for treatment of depression (Cuijpers et al. 2011; Fonagy et al. 2020). Although neither the developers of IPT nor psychoanalysts pursuing the interpersonal/relational approach would accept a close affinity between these approaches to theory or practice, the shared emphasis on the representations of actual social relationships as a focus for interventions cannot be denied.

The quality of research evidence supporting psychodynamic therapies is undoubtedly strongest for interpersonal therapies (e.g., Cuijpers et al. 2011; Markowitz et al.

2006). IPT (Weissman et al. 2017) has a particularly strong evidence base in the literature on depression in adults and adolescents (Cuijpers et al. 2011; Fonagy et al. 2020; Mychailyszyn and Elson 2018), and, as a result, IPT is recommended by the U.K. National Institute for Health and Care Excellence's guidelines for the treatment of depression in adults (National Institute for Health and Care Excellence 2009), children (using family IPT), and young people (using IPT for adolescents) (National Institute for Health and Care Excellence 2019).

Psychoanalytic Schema Theories

Some theorists have attempted to combine psychoanalysis with systems theory (e.g., Boesky 1988; Peterfreund 1971; Rosenblatt and Thickstun 1977), whereas others have combined British object relations theory and cognitive science research with systems theory to create person schema theory (Horowitz et al. 1995). Anthony Ryle, for example, has advanced a model of psychotherapy based on the realization that unconscious relationship procedures can be described and the resulting descriptions can be of considerable value in psychotherapy (Ryle and Kerr 2002). Cognitive analytic therapy identifies and represents a relatively small number of underlying relationship patterns, including issues of care, dependency, control, submission, love, and anger, as *reciprocal role procedures*. Reciprocal role procedures are addressed explicitly by the therapy, including through formal correspondence between therapist and patient. The most widely cited psychoanalytic schema theorist is Daniel Stern.

Although Stern's account of self-development (Stern 1985) does not come with an immediate set of clinical applications, it has been widely used in accounts of the development of personality disorder and neurosis. For Stern, there are four phases of development, each linked to a different sense of self, although prior selves condition later stages of self development: 1) the emerging self from birth to 2 months; 2) the core self at 2–6 months, which is characterized by the emergence of a sense of agency and continuity across time; 3) a sense of subjective self, emerging between 9 and 18 months, when intentions may be shared and awareness of emotion in the other arises; and 4) the narrative self, marked by the emergence of language. Damasio (1999) also developed a similar model of development.

Stern described the subjective integration of all aspects of lived experience as *emergent moments* that derive from a range of schematic representations (event representations, semantic representations, perceptual schemas, sensorimotor representations) in conjunction with a representation of *feeling shapes* (patterns of arousal across time) and *proto-narrative envelopes* that give a proto-plot to an event with an agent, an action, instrumentality, and context. These are conceptualized in combination as the *schema of a-way-of-being-with-another*. Distortions in this basic schema lead to vulnerability to psychopathology. These schemas come closest to providing a neuropsychologically valid way of depicting a psychoanalytic model of the development of interpersonal experience.

Stern's model fits well with developmental data on infancy, but extensions of the model to childhood and adult psychopathology are less solid. The adult is not an infant, and continuities from infancy at the level of mental representation are quite unlikely, although they are possible at the procedural implicit level highlighted by Stern and his colleagues. It is in the realm of mental processes that continuity can seemingly be established from early childhood and through into adulthood.

Mentalizing Theory

Mentalizing refers to a person's ability (or lack thereof) to conceive of their own and others' mental states as explanations of behavior. In the psychodynamic model developed by Fonagy, Bateman, Target, and their colleagues (Bateman and Fonagy 2016; Fonagy et al. 2002), this capacity is seen as an index of the development of an agentive self. Rooted in attachment theory, the mentalizing-focused approach claims a further evolutionary rationale for the human attachment system in the opportunity that proximity to concerned adults affords for the development of social intelligence and meaning-making. Mentalization-based treatment (MBT) is interpersonally focused and makes use of cognitive strategies to explore preconscious thoughts and feelings (i.e., they are accessible, but the individual is unaware of them).

This approach explicitly rejects the classical Cartesian assumption that emotional and other internal mental states are from the start directly experienced introspectively. It is suggested that in the first instance, mental states are discovered through contingent mirroring interactions with the caregiver (Target and Fonagy 1996). Repeated experience of affect-reflective caregiver reactions is seen as essential for the infant to become sensitized to and to construct differentiated representations of their internal self-states, a process Gergely and Watson (1996) termed social biofeedback. Such experiences vitally contribute to the emergence of early mentalizing capacities, allowing the infant to discover or find their psychological self in the social world.

Two conditions need to be met to enable the infant to discover their psychological self: 1) reasonable congruency of mirroring, whereby the caregiver accurately matches the infant's mental state, and 2) *markedness* of the mirroring, whereby the caregiver is able to express an affect while indicating that the caregiver is not expressing their own feelings. Consequently, two impingements can occur: 1) in the case of incongruent mirroring, the infant's representation of the internal state will not correspond to a constitutional self state (nothing real), and a predisposition to a narcissistic (false-self) structure might be established; 2) in cases of unmarked mirroring, the caregiver's expression may be seen as externalization of the infant's experience, and a predisposition to experiencing emotion through other people (a borderline personality structure) might be established (Fonagy et al. 2002).

Mentalizing theory has always maintained that when our immediate social context, conceptualized dyadically, fails to mentalize us and we are not recognized as agentive, we are vulnerable to the development of psychopathology (Fonagy and Luyten 2009; Luyten et al. 2020). More recently, this emphasis on the interpersonal nature of mentalizing has led to a wider focus on the relationship between the individual and their social and cultural environment. This is partly informed by the work of developmentalists such as Tomasello on the social origins and orientation of high-order cognition, in particular the idea that the human capacity to learn and communicate culture is made possible by mentalizing (Tomasello 2018, 2019). We have argued that disruptions in social communication and an individual's inability to experience joint thinking and the we-mode (described in the introduction) may be heavily implicated in the prevalence of psychopathology. Exclusion from joint thinking may be a product of an interaction among individual developmental experiences, a nonmentalizing social system, and temperamental inclination; the consequences of such exclusion involve the loss of agentiveness, difficulties in self-regulation, and compromised access to social support through working with other minds. As such, it is proposed that a mentalizing approach may work by reintroducing the patient to joint thinking, stimulating their capacity for epistemic trust and social learning, thus enabling them to develop the salutogenic experience of improved social functioning in their wider social environment (Fonagy et al. 2021).

MBT was originally developed as a program for the treatment of BPD in a partial hospital setting. In the first randomized controlled trial of MBT (Bateman and Fonagy 1999), the MBT treatment group showed a statistically significant decrease on all measures, whereas the control group (routine psychiatric care) showed limited change or deterioration. Follow-up at 8 years (Bateman and Fonagy 2008) showed that patients in the MBT group continued to do better, although they remained somewhat compromised in the area of general social functioning. Significantly more patients who had been treated with MBT were in employment or full-time education than patients in the comparison group, and only 14% still met diagnostic criteria for BPD, compared with 87% of those in the comparison group who were available for interview. The original study was partially replicated and found good results in mental health services independent of the treatment developers (Bales et al. 2012, 2015, 2017).

An outpatient version of MBT was developed and was studied in a randomized controlled trial (Bateman and Fonagy 2009) that measured an 18-month program of MBT against a structured clinical management approach to BPD (Bales and Bateman 2012). Both groups showed good improvements across all outcomes, but those randomly assigned to MBT showed better outcomes, with a significantly greater reduction in both self-reported and clinically measured problems, such as suicide attempts and hospitalization. Both groups were found to have maintained these improvements at follow-up at 8 years, with the MBT sample retaining better outcomes than the control group (Bateman et al. 2021). A 2020 Cochrane review identified MBT as one of two therapies—the other being dialectical behavior therapy—with a reasonable evidence base for BPD (Storebø et al. 2020).

Conclusions and the Future

In the course of this review we have shown that each psychoanalytic model has produced a perspective on development. In many cases one cannot help concluding that psychoanalytic theoreticians were developmental reductionists, oversimplifying complex developmental processes and omitting a comprehensive exploration of how an early deficit could be expected to affect subsequent development. Even where infantile modes of thought and the adult mind in distress seem to share characteristics, it is unwise to assume that later development would not have altered both the mechanism and function of early structures to a point where similarities are superficial. For this reason, as psychodynamic psychotherapy has evolved, classical psychoanalytic theories have been supplemented by schema theory, systemic approaches, interpersonal approaches, and attachment theory, which have all contributed to the elaboration of more sophisticated developmental models.

Psychoanalysis studies human subjectivity at its most complex. It therefore provides an essential counterweight to advances in neuroscience and molecular genetics. In order to reach an adequate understanding of the interaction between genes and the environment we must retain our grasp of the full complexity of how the human mind grapples with the challenges of adaptation. Whether or not specific environmental factors trigger the expression of a gene may depend not only on the nature of those factors but also on the way the infant or child experiences them, which will be an intrapsychic function, determined by conscious or unconscious attribution of meaning to these experiences. The quality of this experiential filter may, in turn, be a function of either genetic or environmental influences or their interaction (Kandel 1998). In this context, it is essential that we do not neglect the nonconscious domain of human experience.

Psychoanalysis, with its focus on the representation of subjectivity and how this emerges from attachment relationships in early development, has much to contribute to the understanding of how individual differences in the quality of functioning of basic mental mechanisms arise. Cognitive psychology and cognitive-behavioral therapy have increasingly converged with psychoanalytic interest in the study of the influence of relationship representation patterns on human conduct. Schema theory, systemic approaches, interpersonal approaches, and attachment theory have converged on this problem from the mid-1980s. A full understanding of the interaction between individual mentalized representations of life experience and the expression of genetic dispositions is the task of psychoanalytic psychotherapy of the next decades. Kandel (1999, p. 508) cited François Jacob (1998): "The century that is ending has been preoccupied with nucleic acids and proteins. The next one will concentrate on memory and desire. Will it be able to answer the questions they pose?"

As it stands, evidence in favor of psychodynamic psychotherapies (Fonagy et al. 2005; Leichsenring et al. 2004, 2015), as well as most theory-based structured interventions (Roth and Fonagy 2005), continues to accumulate. Developmental psychopathology will play an increasingly important role in treatment because evidence suggests that adult psychiatric disorders have their roots in abnormalities that are already observable in childhood or adolescence.

That said, both psychoanalysis and psychodynamic psychotherapy as a whole have possible limitations. For example, the extent to which cultural context has a bearing not only on possible disorders but also on the treatment thereof is still to be proven. What is more, there is room for improvement in the measures of outcome used in many trials; because psychodynamic psychotherapy is not symptom oriented, limited evidence exists as to its efficacy (Gabbard et al. 2002). Perhaps the user/patient should play a larger part in devising therapies as well.

Once again, neuroscience will undoubtedly play a large role in addressing these issues, particularly if, as seems likely, scanning techniques are developed that allow the simultaneous imaging of two individuals interacting (King-Casas et al. 2005). Molecular biology similarly presents cause for optimism: for example, as molecular genetic findings unfold over the next few years, biological vulnerability likely will become increasingly detectable. Furthermore, large-scale biological investigations will not only help prevention but also enhance our understanding of biologically indicated psychosocial treatments. As we begin to understand the causal path that disease processes follow in the vulnerable brain, the need for specific psychosocial treatments to assist individuals with these vulnerabilities will become acute.

A further area of development for psychodynamic models of treatment is a more fully conceptualized and integrated framework for understanding the role of the social environment in the development and treatment of mental disorder. We know, for example, that socioeconomic deprivation is the strongest predictor of psychopathology (Lund et al. 2018), yet psychodynamic models have strikingly failed to consider—on a comprehensive theoretical level—the role of the social environment in developmental psychopathology. We suggest that the challenge for psychodynamic models in the future will be to create a way of understanding the risks and protections, the assaults and consolations, of the social context while avoiding the adoption of a naively materialist position. We hope that a psychoanalytically informed approach, with its capacity to consider the complexity, contradiction, and richly variant nature of human subjectivity in response to the minds around it, will have a uniquely valuable role in articulating how the social and cultural world interacts with individual psyches.

In other words, the future of psychodynamic psychotherapy lies not in rejecting but in embracing developments in biology and neuroscience, which, conversely, might also embrace psychodynamic psychotherapy with more open arms. For as it emerges that we cannot treat the brain in the same way that we treat the musculoskeletal system, it is quite possible that psychodynamic psychotherapy will similarly emerge (through an evidence-based and empirical psychology that incorporates imaging techniques, neuroanatomical methods, and human genetics) as the best means of understanding the human mind and helping it to help itself.

Key Points

- Clinicians can feel confident that the nonconscious is evidence based, that is, that referring to complex thoughts and feelings that appear to organize a patient's behavior outside the person's awareness cannot be rejected out of hand on scientific grounds.
- A range of excellent and internally coherent models specify the kinds of thoughts and feelings outside awareness that specific mental disorders might entail. From the perspective of clinical work, there seems to be little reason for favoring any one model over the others.
- The theoretical models come together in highlighting the significance for mental disorder of early development; current and past relationships with attachment figures; imagination and fantasy, particularly in relation to mental states; and enduring mental structures that derive from these experiences.
- Although the late 1980s and early 1990s saw a convergence of models around the so-called object relations school, early twenty-first-century dynamic theory is quite split again. Therapists who focus on facets of the relationships that the patient brings to therapy are more concerned with the

experiencing of these relationships than with the understanding that an insightful therapist could offer.

- The interface of psychiatry with neuroscience might create a new role for psychodynamic therapists as experts in the social brain, at least at the phenotypic level. These findings need to be reflected on rather than simply incorporated into the theory wholesale either as supporting evidence or as indications of the complexity of the phenomena under scrutiny.
- The interaction among the individual, the dyad, and the broader social environment might productively be considered more fully by new and existing models of psychodynamic psychotherapy.

Recommended Readings

Bateman AW, Allison E, Holmes J: Introduction to Psychoanalysis: Contemporary Theory and Practice, 2nd Edition. London, Routledge, 2022

Budd S, Rusbridger R (eds): Introducing Psychoanalysis: Essential Themes and Topics. London, Routledge, 2005

Cooper AM (ed): Contemporary Psychoanalysis in America. Washington, DC, American Psychiatric Publishing, 2006

Fonagy P, Target M: Psychoanalytic Theories: Perspectives From Developmental Psychopathology. London, Whurr, 2003

Gabbard GO: Psychodynamic Psychiatry in Clinical Practice, 4th Edition. Washington, DC, American Psychiatric Publishing, 2005

Gabbard GO, Gunderson JG, Fonagy P: The place of psychoanalytic treatments within psychiatry. Arch Gen Psychiatry 59(6):505–510, 2002

Holmes J, Bateman A: Integration in Psychotherapy: Models and Methods. Oxford, UK, Oxford University Press, 2002

Person ES, Cooper AM, Gabbard GO (eds): American Psychiatric Publishing Textbook of Psychoanalysis. Washington, DC, American Psychiatric Publishing, 2005

References

Allen JG: Trusting in Psychotherapy. Washington, DC, American Psychiatric Association Publishing, 2021

Amad A, Ramoz N, Thomas P, et al: Genetics of borderline personality disorder: systematic review and proposal of an integrative model. Neurosci Biobehav Rev 40:6–19, 2014 24456942

Bales D, Bateman A: Partial hospitalization settings, in Handbook of Mentalizing in Mental Health Practice. Edited by Bateman A, Fonagy P. Washington, DC, American Psychiatric Publishing, 2012, pp 197–226

Bales D, van Beek N, Smits M, et al: Treatment outcome of 18-month, day hospital mentalization-based treatment (MBT) in patients with severe borderline personality disorder in the Netherlands. J Pers Disord 26(4):568–582, 2012 22867507

Bales DL, Timman R, Andrea H, et al: Effectiveness of day hospital mentalization-based treatment for patients with severe borderline personality disorder: a matched control study. Clin Psychol Psychother 22(5):409–417, 2015 25060747

Bales DL, Timman R, Luyten P, et al: Implementation of evidence-based treatments for borderline personality disorder: the impact of organizational changes on treatment outcome of mentalization-based treatment. Pers Ment Health 11(4):266–277, 2017 28703383

Bateman A, Fonagy P: Effectiveness of partial hospitalization in the treatment of borderline personality disorder: a randomized controlled trial. Am J Psychiatry 156(10):1563–1569, 1999
Bateman A, Fonagy P: 8-year follow-up of patients treated for borderline personality disorder: mentalization-based treatment versus treatment as usual. Am J Psychiatry 165(5):631–638, 2008 18347003
Bateman A, Fonagy P: Randomized controlled trial of outpatient mentalization-based treatment versus structured clinical management for borderline personality disorder. Am J Psychiatry 166(12):1355–1364, 2009 19833787
Bateman A, Fonagy P: Mentalization-Based Treatment for Personality Disorders: A Practical Guide. Oxford, UK, Oxford University Press, 2016
Bateman A, Constantinou MP, Fonagy P, et al: Eight-year prospective follow-up of mentalization-based treatment versus structured clinical management for people with borderline personality disorder. Pers Disord 12(4):291–299, 2021 32584091
Beebe B, Lachmann FM: Representation and internalization in infancy: three principles of salience. Psychoanal Psychol 11(2):127–165, 1994
Benjamin J: Like Subjects, Love Objects. New Haven, CT, Yale University Press, 1995
Benjamin J: The Shadow of the Other: Intersubjectivity and Gender in Psychoanalysis. New York, Routledge, 1998
Bibring E: The so-called English school of psychoanalysis. Psychoanal Q 16(1):69–93, 1947
Bick E: Notes on infant observation in psychoanalytic training. Int J Psychoanal 45:558–566, 1964 14236194
Bion WR: Differentiation of the psychotic from the non-psychotic personalities. Int J Psychoanal 38(3–4):266–275, 1957 13438602
Bion WR: Attacks on linking. Int J Psychoanal 40:308–315, 1959
Bion WR: The psycho-analytic study of thinking: a theory of thinking. Int J Psychoanal 43:306–310, 1962 13968380
Birbaumer N, Veit R, Lotze M, et al: Deficient fear conditioning in psychopathy: a functional magnetic resonance imaging study. Arch Gen Psychiatry 62(7):799–805, 2005 15997022
Bleidorn W, Hopwood CJ, Lucas RE: Life events and personality trait change. J Pers 86(1):83–96, 2018 27716921
Blum HP: The position and value of extratransference interpretation. J Am Psychoanal Assoc 31(3):587–617, 1983 6681429
Boesky D: The concept of psychic structure. J Am Psychoanal Assoc 36:113–135, 1988
Bolton D, Eley TC, O'Connor TG, et al: Prevalence and genetic and environmental influences on anxiety disorders in 6-year-old twins. Psychol Med 36(3):335–344, 2006 16288680
Borghuis J, Bleidorn W, Sijtsma K, et al: Longitudinal associations between trait neuroticism and negative daily experiences in adolescence. J Pers Soc Psychol 118(2):348–363, 2020 30676043
Bowlby J: A Secure Base: Clinical Applications of Attachment Theory. London, Routledge, 1988
Bradley CL: Generativity-stagnation: development of a status model. Dev Rev 17(3):262–290, 1997
Brenner C: Conflict, compromise formation, and structural theory. Psychoanal Q 71(3):397–417, 2002 12116537
Breuer J, Freud S: Studies on Hysteria. London, Hogarth Press, 1895
Bromberg PM: Standing in the Spaces. Hillsdale, NJ, Analytic Press, 1998
Brown D, Scheflin AW, Hammond DC: Memory, Trauma Treatment, and the Law. New York, WW Norton, 1998
Brown GW, Harris TO, Hepworth C: Loss, humiliation and entrapment among women developing depression: a patient and non-patient comparison. Psychol Med 25(1):7–21, 1995 7792364
Caspi A, Moffitt TE: All for one and one for all: mental disorders in one dimension. Am J Psychiatry 175(9):831–844, 2018 29621902
Chen D, Drabick DA, Burgers DE: A developmental perspective on peer rejection, deviant peer affiliation, and conduct problems among youth. Child Psychiatry Hum Dev 46(6):823–838, 2015 25410430

Chodorow N: Feminism and Psychoanalytic Theory. New Haven, CT, Yale University Press, 1989
Clarkin JF, Levy KN, Lenzenweger MF, et al: Evaluating three treatments for borderline personality disorder: a multiwave study. Am J Psychiatry 164(6):922–928, 2007 17541052
Cohen JR, Spiro CN, Young JF, et al: Interpersonal risk profiles for youth depression: a person-centered, multi-wave, longitudinal study. J Abnorm Child Psychol 43(8):1415–1426, 2015 25907029
Crandell LE, Patrick MP, Hobson RP: "Still-face" interactions between mothers with borderline personality disorder and their 2-month-old infants. Br J Psychiatry 183:239–247, 2003 12948998
Cristea IA, Gentili C, Cotet CD, et al: Efficacy of psychotherapies for borderline personality disorder: a systematic review and meta-analysis. JAMA Psychiatry 74(4):319–328, 2017 28249086
Cuijpers P, Geraedts AS, van Oppen P, et al: Interpersonal psychotherapy for depression: a meta-analysis. Am J Psychiatry 168(6):581–592, 2011 21362740
Cuijpers P, Donker T, Weissman MM, et al: Interpersonal psychotherapy for mental health problems: a comprehensive meta-analysis. Am J Psychiatry 173(7):680–687, 2016 27032627
Cuijpers P, Karyotaki E, de Wit L, Ebert DD: The effects of fifteen evidence-supported therapies for adult depression: a meta-analytic review. Psychother Res 30(3):279–293, 2020 31394976
Damasio A: The Feeling of What Happens: Body and Emotion in the Making of Consciousness. New York, Harcourt Brace, 1999
Davies JM: Linking the "pre-analytic" with the postclassical—integration, dissociation, and the multiplicity of unconscious process. Contemp Psychoanal 32(4):553–576, 1996
De Panfilis C, Meehan KB, Cain NM, et al: Effortful control, rejection sensitivity, and borderline personality disorder features in adulthood. J Pers Disord 30(5):595–612, 2016 26623540
Dew SE, Bickman L: Client expectancies about therapy. Ment Health Serv Res 7(1):21–33, 2005 15832691
De Wolff MS, van Ijzendoorn MH: Sensitivity and attachment: a meta-analysis on parental antecedents of infant attachment. Child Dev 68(4):571–591, 1997 9306636
Distel MA, Trull TJ, Derom CA, et al: Heritability of borderline personality disorder features is similar across three countries. Psychol Med 38(9):1219–1229, 2008 17988414
Distel MA, Middeldorp CM, Trull TJ, et al: Life events and borderline personality features: the influence of gene-environment interaction and gene-environment correlation. Psychol Med 41(4):849–860, 2011 20594379
Driessen E, Cuijpers P, de Maat SCM, et al: The efficacy of short-term psychodynamic psychotherapy for depression: a meta-analysis. Clin Psychol Rev 30(1):25–36, 2010 19766369
Ehrenberg D: The Intimate Edge. New York, WW Norton, 1993
Erikson EH: Childhood and Society. New York, WW Norton, 1950
Fairbairn WRD: An Object-Relations Theory of the Personality. New York, Basic Books, 1952
Feinberg ME, Button TM, Neiderhiser JM, et al: Parenting and adolescent antisocial behavior and depression: evidence of genotype x parenting environment interaction. Arch Gen Psychiatry 64(4):457–465, 2007 17404122
Fenichel O: Problems of Psychoanalytic Technique. New York, Psychoanalytic Quarterly, 1941
Fonagy P, Allison E: Psychic reality and the nature of consciousness. Int J Psychoanal 97(1):5–24, 2016 26602060
Fonagy P, Luyten P: A developmental, mentalization-based approach to the understanding and treatment of borderline personality disorder. Dev Psychopathol 21(4):1355–1381, 2009 19825272
Fonagy P, Gergely G, Jurist E, Target M: Affect Regulation, Mentalization, and the Development of the Self. New York, Other Press, 2002
Fonagy P, Roth A, Higgitt A: The outcome of psychodynamic psychotherapy for psychological disorders. Clin Neurosci Res 4(5–6):367–377, 2005
Fonagy P, Rost F, Carlyle JA, et al: Pragmatic randomized controlled trial of long-term psychoanalytic psychotherapy for treatment-resistant depression: the Tavistock Adult Depression Study (TADS). World Psychiatry 14(3):312–321, 2015 26407787

Fonagy P, Luyten P, Allison E, et al: What we have changed our minds about: part 1: borderline personality disorder as a limitation of resilience. Borderline Personal Disord Emot Dysregul 4:11, 2017a 28413687

Fonagy P, Luyten P, Allison E, et al: What we have changed our minds about: part 2: borderline personality disorder, epistemic trust and the developmental significance of social communication. Borderline Personal Disord Emot Dysregul 4:9, 2017b 28405338

Fonagy P, Lemma A, Target M, et al: Dynamic interpersonal therapy for moderate to severe depression: a pilot randomized controlled and feasibility trial. Psychol Med 50(6):1010–1019, 2020 31084635

Fonagy P, Campbell C, Constantinou M, et al: Culture and psychopathology: an attempt at reconsidering the role of social learning. Dev Psychopathol Mar 26, 2021 33766162 Epub ahead of print

Fraiberg S, Adelson E, Shapiro V: Ghosts in the nursery: a psychoanalytic approach to the problems of impaired infant-mother relationships. J Am Acad Child Psychiatry 14(3):387–421, 1975 1141566

Freud A: The Ego and the Mechanisms of Defense. The Writings of Anna Freud, Vol 2 (1936). New York, International Universities Press, 1966

Freud A: Normality and Pathology in Childhood: Assessments of Development. Madison, CT, International Universities Press, 1965

Freud A: A psychoanalytic view of developmental psychopathology (1974), in The Writings of Anna Freud, Vol 8. New York, International Universities Press, 1981, pp 119–136

Freud A, Burlingham D: Infants Without Families: Reports on the Hampstead Nurseries. The Writings of Anna Freud, Vol 3 (1944). New York, International Universities Press, 1973

Freud S: The interpretation of dreams (1900), in Standard Edition of the Complete Psychological Works of Sigmund Freud, Vols 4 and 5. Translated and edited by Strachey J. London, Hogarth Press, 1953, pp 1–715

Freud S: The Psychopathology of Everyday Life. Standard Edition of the Complete Psychological Works of Sigmund Freud, Vol 6 (1901). Translated and edited by Strachey J. London, Hogarth Press, 1960

Freud S: Jokes and Their Relation to the Unconscious. Standard Edition of the Complete Psychological Works of Sigmund Freud, Vol 8 (1905). Translated and edited by Strachey J. London, Hogarth Press, 1960

Freud S: Beyond the pleasure principle (1920), in Standard Edition of the Complete Psychological Works of Sigmund Freud, Vol 18. Translated and edited by Strachey J. London, Hogarth Press, 1955, pp 1–64

Freud S: The ego and the id (1923), in Standard Edition of the Complete Psychological Works of Sigmund Freud, Vol 19. Translated and edited by Strachey J. London, Hogarth Press, 1961, pp 12–66

Friedman L: An appreciation of Hans Loewald's "On the therapeutic action of psychoanalysis." Paper presented at The Association for Psychoanalytic Medicine, December 2, 1986

Friedman L: The clinical popularity of object relations concepts. Psychoanal Q 57(4):667–691, 1988 3212108

Gabbard GO, Gunderson JG, Fonagy P: The place of psychoanalytic treatments within psychiatry. Arch Gen Psychiatry 59(6):505–510, 2002 12044192

Gallese V, Keysers C, Rizzolatti G: A unifying view of the basis of social cognition. Trends Cogn Sci 8(9):396–403, 2004 15350240

Gallotti M, Frith CD: Social cognition in the we-mode. Trends Cogn Sci 17(4):160–165, 2013 23499335

Gergely G: Reapproaching Mahler: new perspectives on normal autism, symbiosis, splitting and libidinal object constancy from cognitive developmental theory. J Am Psychoanal Assoc 48(4):1197–1228, 2000 11212188

Gergely G, Watson JS: The social biofeedback theory of parental affect-mirroring: the development of emotional self-awareness and self-control in infancy. Int J Psychoanal 77(Pt 6):1181–1212, 1996 9119582

Gluschkoff K, Jokela M, Rosenström T: General psychopathology factor and borderline personality disorder: evidence for substantial overlap from two nationally representative surveys of U.S. adults. Pers Disord 12(1):86–92, 2021 32584090
Goldstein M, Brendel G, Tuescher O, et al: Neural substrates of the interaction of emotional stimulus processing and motor inhibitory control: an emotional linguistic go/no-go fMRI study. Neuroimage 36(3):1026–1040, 2007 17509899
Goodyer IM: Life events and difficulties: their nature and effects, in The Depressed Child and Adolescent: Developmental and Clinical Perspectives. Edited by Goodyer IM. Cambridge, UK, Cambridge University Press, 1995, pp 171–193
Green A: Science and science fiction in infant research, in Clinical and Observational Psychoanalytic Research: Roots of a Controversy. Edited by Sandler J, Sandler A-M, Davies R. London, Karnac Books, 2000, pp 41–73
Greenberg J: Oedipus and Beyond: A Clinical Theory. Cambridge, MA, Harvard University Press, 1991
Grenon R, Carlucci S, Brugnera A, et al: Psychotherapy for eating disorders: a meta-analysis of direct comparisons. Psychother Res 29(7):833–845, 2019 29958509
Hartmann H: Ego Psychology and the Problem of Adaptation (1939). Translated by Rapaport D. New York, International Universities Press, 1958
Hartmann H, Kris E, Loewenstein RM: Comments on the formation of psychic structure. Psychoanal Study Child 2:11–38, 1946 20293622
Hemmi MH, Wolke D, Schneider S: Associations between problems with crying, sleeping and/or feeding in infancy and long-term behavioural outcomes in childhood: a meta-analysis. Arch Dis Child 96(7):622–629, 2011 21508059
Hoffman IZ: Dialectical thinking and therapeutic action in the psychoanalytic process. Psychoanal Q 63(2):187–218, 1994 8047630
Hofstra MB, van der Ende J, Verhulst FC: Child and adolescent problems predict DSM-IV disorders in adulthood: a 14-year follow-up of a Dutch epidemiological sample. J Am Acad Child Adolesc Psychiatry 41(2):182–189, 2002 11837408
Holmes J: Exploring in Security: Towards an Attachment-Informed Psychoanalytic Psychotherapy. New York, Routledge, 2010
Horowitz MJ, Eells T, Singer J, et al: Role-relationship models for case formulation. Arch Gen Psychiatry 52(8):625–632, 1995 7632110
Jacob F: Of Flies, Mice, and Men. Cambridge, MA, Harvard University Press, 1998
Jacobson E: The Self and the Object World. New York, International Universities Press, 1964
Jacoby N, Overfeld J, Binder E, et al: Stress neurobiology and developmental psychopathology, in Developmental Psychopathology, 3rd Edition, Vol 2: Developmental Neuroscience. Edited by Cicchetti D. New York, Wiley, 2016, pp 787–831
Jaffe J, Beebe B, Feldstein S, et al: Rhythms of dialogue in infancy: coordinated timing in development. Monogr Soc Res Child Dev 66(2):i–viii, 1–132, 2001 11428150
Jung CG: Psychological Types. London, Routledge/Kegan Paul, 1923
Kandel ER: A new intellectual framework for psychiatry. Am J Psychiatry 155(4):457–469, 1998 9545989
Kandel ER: Biology and the future of psychoanalysis: a new intellectual framework for psychiatry revisited. Am J Psychiatry 156(4):505–524, 1999 10200728
Kao WT, Wang Y, Kleinman JE, et al: Common genetic variation in neuregulin 3 (NRG3) influences risk for schizophrenia and impacts NRG3 expression in human brain. Proc Natl Acad Sci USA 107(35):15619–15624, 2010 20713722
Kernberg OF: Borderline Conditions and Pathological Narcissism. New York, Jason Aronson, 1975
Kernberg OF: Object Relations Theory and Clinical Psychoanalysis. New York, Jason Aronson, 1976
Kernberg OF: Self, ego, affects, and drives. J Am Psychoanal Assoc 30(4):893–917, 1982 6927244
Kernberg OF: Severe Personality Disorders: Psychotherapeutic Strategies. New Haven, CT, Yale University Press, 1984
Kernberg OF, Yeomans FE, Clarkin JF, et al: Transference focused psychotherapy: overview and update. Int J Psychoanal 89(3):601–620, 2008 18558958

Kim-Cohen J, Caspi A, Moffitt TE, et al: Prior juvenile diagnoses in adults with mental disorder: developmental follow-back of a prospective-longitudinal cohort. Arch Gen Psychiatry 60(7):709–717, 2003 12860775
King-Casas B, Tomlin D, Anen C, et al: Getting to know you: reputation and trust in a two-person economic exchange. Science 308(5718):78–83, 2005 15802598
Klein M: A contribution to the psychogenesis of manic-depressive states (1935), in The Writings of Melanie Klein, Vol 1: Love, Guilt, and Reparation. London, Hogarth Press, 1975, pp 236–289
Klein M: The psychotherapy of the psychoses (1930), in Contributions to Psychoanalysis, 1921–1945. London, Hogarth Press, 1948, pp 251–253
Klein M: Mourning and its relation to manic-depressive states (1940), in The Writings of Melanie Klein, Vol 1: Love, Guilt, and Reparation. New York, Macmillan, 1984, pp 344–369
Klein M: Notes on some schizoid mechanisms, in Developments in Psychoanalysis. Edited by Klein M, Heimann P, Isaacs S, et al. London, UK: Hogarth Press, 1946, pp 292–320
Klein M: Envy and gratitude (1957), in The Writings of Melanie Klein, Vol 3: Envy and Gratitude and Other Works. London, Hogarth Press, 1975, pp 176–235
Kohut H: The Analysis of the Self. New York, International Universities Press, 1971
Kohut H: The Restoration of the Self. New York, International Universities Press, 1977
Kohut H: How Does Analysis Cure? Chicago, IL, University of Chicago Press, 1984
Kramer S, Akhtar S: The developmental context of internalized preoedipal object relations: clinical applications of Mahler's theory of symbiosis and separation-individuation. Psychoanal Q 57(4):547–576, 1988 3212103
Kumsta R, Kreppner J, Kennedy M, et al: Psychological consequences of early global deprivation an overview of findings from the English and Romanian Adoptees Study. European Psychologist 20(2):138–151, 2015
Laor N, Wolmer L, Mayes LC, et al: Israeli preschoolers under Scud missile attacks: a developmental perspective on risk-modifying factors. Arch Gen Psychiatry 53(5):416–423, 1996 8624185
Laub JH: The interdependence of school violence with neighbourhood and family conditions, in Violence in American Schools: A New Perspective. Edited by Elliot DS, Hamburg B, Williams KR. New York, Cambridge University Press, 1998, pp 127–155
Leichsenring F, Rabung S, Leibing E: The efficacy of short-term psychodynamic psychotherapy in specific psychiatric disorders: a meta-analysis. Arch Gen Psychiatry 61(12):1208–1216, 2004 15583112
Leichsenring F, Leweke F, Klein S, et al: The empirical status of psychodynamic psychotherapy—an update: Bambi's alive and kicking. Psychother Psychosom 84(3):129–148, 2015 25833321
Levy KN: The implications of attachment theory and research for understanding borderline personality disorder. Dev Psychopathol 17(4):959–986, 2005 16613426
Levy KN, Meehan KB, Kelly KM, et al: Change in attachment patterns and reflective function in a randomized control trial of transference-focused psychotherapy for borderline personality disorder. J Consult Clin Psychol 74(6):1027–1040, 2006 17154733
Lipsitz JD, Markowitz JC: Mechanisms of change in interpersonal therapy (IPT). Clin Psychol Rev 33(8):1134–1147, 2013 24100081
Loewald HW: On internalization (1973), in Papers on Psychoanalysis. New Haven, CT, Yale University Press, 1980, pp 69–86
Loewald HW: Instinct theory, object relations, and psychic-structure formation. J Am Psychoanal Assoc 26(3):493–506, 1978 701735
Lund C, Brooke-Sumner C, Baingana F, et al: Social determinants of mental disorders and the sustainable development goals: a systematic review of reviews. Lancet Psychiatry 5(4):357–369, 2018 29580610
Luyten P, Campbell C, Allison E, et al: The mentalizing approach to psychopathology: state of the art and future directions. Annu Rev Clin Psychol 16:297–325, 2020 32023093
Mackes NK, Golm D, Sarkar S, et al: Early childhood deprivation is associated with alterations in adult brain structure despite subsequent environmental enrichment. Proc Natl Acad Sci USA 117(1):641–649, 2020 31907309

Mahler MS, Pine F, Bergman A: The Psychological Birth of the Human Infant: Symbiosis and Individuation. New York, Basic Books, 1975
Mahr J, Csibra G: Why do we remember? The communicative function of episodic memory. Behav Brain Sci 41:1–93, 2017 28100294
Marcia JE: The empirical study of ego identity, in Identity and Development: An Interdisciplinary Approach. Edited by Bosma HA, Graafsma TLG, Grotevant HD, et al. Thousand Oaks, CA, Sage, 1994, pp 67–80
Marenco S, Weinberger DR: The neurodevelopmental hypothesis of schizophrenia: following a trail of evidence from cradle to grave. Dev Psychopathol 12(3):501–527, 2000 11014750
Markowitz JC, Skodol AE, Bleiberg K: Interpersonal psychotherapy for borderline personality disorder: possible mechanisms of change. J Clin Psychol 62(4):431–444, 2006 16470711
Masterson JF: The Real Self: A Developmental, Self, and Object Relations Approach. New York, Brunner/Mazel, 1985
McLaughlin JT: Clinical and theoretical aspects of enactment. J Am Psychoanal Assoc 39(3):595–614, 1991 1939990
Meltzoff AN, Moore MK: Explaining facial imitation: a theoretical model. Early Dev Parent 6(3–4):179–192, 1997 24634574
Meltzoff AN, Moore MK: Infant intersubjectivity: broadening the dialogue to include imitation, identity and intention, in Intersubjective Communication and Emotion in Early Ontogeny. Edited by Braten S. Cambridge, UK, Cambridge University Press, 1998, pp 47–62
Mercier H, Sperber D: The Enigma of Reason: A New Theory of Human Understanding. London, Allen Lane, 2017
Mikami A, Normand S: The importance of social contextual factors in peer relationships of children with ADHD. Curr Dev Disord Rep 2:30–37, 2015
Mikulincer M, Shaver PR: Attachment in Adulthood: Structure, Dynamics and Change. New York, Guilford, 2007
Mitchell SA: Relational Concepts in Psychoanalysis: An Integration. Cambridge, MA, Harvard University Press, 1988
Mitchell SA: Relationality: From Attachment to Intersubjectivity. Hillsdale, NJ, Analytic Press, 2000
Mychailyszyn M, Elson D: Working through the blues: a meta-analysis on interpersonal psychotherapy for depressed adolescents (IPT-A). Child Youth Serv Rev 87:123–129, 2018
National Collaborating Centre for Mental Health: The Improving Access to Psychological Therapies Manual. June 4, 2018. Available at: www.england.nhs.uk/publication/the-improving-access-to-psychological-therapies-manual. Accessed February 11, 2022.
National Institute for Health and Care Excellence: Depression in adults: recognition and management. Clinical Guideline CG90, October 28, 2009. Available at: www.nice.org.uk/guidance/cg90. Accessed February 11, 2022.
National Institute for Health and Care Excellence: Depression in children and young people: identification and management. NICE Guideline NG134. June 25, 2019. Available at: www.nice.org.uk/guidance/ng134. Accessed February 11, 2022.
Nelson CAIII, Bos K, Gunnar MR, et al: The neurobiological toll of early human deprivation. Monogr Soc Res Child Dev 76(4):127–146, 2011 8005761
O'Connor T: The persisting effects of early experiences on social development, in Developmental Psychopathology, 2nd Edition, Vol 3: Risk, Disorder, and Adaptation. Edited by Cicchetti D, Cohen DJ. New York, Wiley, 2006, pp 202–234
Ogden TH: The analytic third: working with intersubjective clinical facts. Int J Psychoanal 75(Pt 1):3–19, 1994 8005761
Orlofsky J: Intimacy status: theory and research, in Ego Identity: A Handbook for Psychosocial Research. Edited by Marcia JE, Waterman AS, Matteson DR, et al. New York, Springer-Verlag, 1993, pp 111–133
Panksepp J: Affective Neuroscience: The Foundations of Human and Animal Emotions. Oxford, UK, Oxford University Press, 1998

Panksepp J, Lane RD, Solms M, et al: Reconciling cognitive and affective neuroscience perspectives on the brain basis of emotional experience. Neurosci Biobehav Rev 76(Pt B):187–215, 2017 27640756

Parker J, Rubin K, Erath S, et al: Peer relationships, child development, and adjustment: a developmental psychopathology perspective, in Developmental Psychopathology, Vol 1: Theory and Method. Edited by Cicchetti D, Cohen D. New York, Wiley, 2015, pp 419–493

Patalay P, Gage SH: Changes in millennial adolescent mental health and health-related behaviours over 10 years: a population cohort comparison study. Int J Epidemiol 48(5):1650–1664, 2019 30815691

PDM Task Force: Psychodynamic Diagnostic Manual. Silver Spring, MD, Alliance of Psychoanalytic Organizations, 2006

Perez DL, Vago DR, Pan H, et al: Frontolimbic neural circuit changes in emotional processing and inhibitory control associated with clinical improvement following transference-focused psychotherapy in borderline personality disorder. Psychiatry Clin Neurosci 70(1):51–61, 2016 26289141

Peterfreund E: Information, Systems, and Psychoanalysis: An Evolutionary Biological Approach to Psychoanalytic Theory. New York, International Universities Press, 1971

Petersen R, Brakoulias V, Langdon R: An experimental investigation of mentalization ability in borderline personality disorder. Compr Psychiatry 64:12–21, 2016 26608042

Pine F: Developmental Theory and Clinical Process. New Haven, CT, Yale University Press, 1985

Pinquart M: Associations of parenting dimensions and styles with externalizing problems of children and adolescents: an updated meta-analysis. Dev Psychol 53(5):873–932, 2017 28459276

Pinquart M, Feussner C, Ahnert L: Meta-analytic evidence for stability in attachments from infancy to early adulthood. Attach Hum Dev 15(2):189–218, 2013 23210665

Plomin R, McGuffin P: Psychopathology in the postgenomic era. Annu Rev Psychol 54:205–228, 2003 12172001

Plomin R, DeFries JC, Knopik VS, et al: Top 10 replicated findings from behavioral genetics. Perspect Psychol Sci 11(1):3–23, 2016 26817721

Pollak SD, Nelson CA, Schlaak MF, et al: Neurodevelopmental effects of early deprivation in postinstitutionalized children. Child Dev 81(1):224–236, 2010 20331664

Rangell L: The borderline case. J Am Psychoanal Assoc 3(2):285–298, 1955 14367185

Reich W: Character Analysis, 3rd Edition. Translated by Carfagno VR. New York, Farrar, Strauss and Giroux, 1933/1972

Reiss D, Neiderhiser J, Hetherington EM, et al: The Relationship Code: Deciphering Genetic and Social Patterns in Adolescent Development. Cambridge, MA, Harvard University Press, 2000

Renik O: Analytic interaction: conceptualizing technique in light of the analyst's irreducible subjectivity. Psychoanal Q 62(4):553–571, 1993 8284331

Rizzolatti G, Craighero L: The mirror-neuron system. Annu Rev Neurosci 27:169–192, 2004 15217330

Rosenblatt AD, Thickstun JT: Modern Psychoanalytic Concepts in a General Psychology. Part 1: General Concepts and Principles. Part 2: Motivation. New York, International Universities Press, 1977

Rosenfeld H: Impasse and Interpretation. London, Tavistock, 1987

Roth A, Fonagy P: What Works for Whom? A Critical Review of Psychotherapy Research, 2nd Edition. New York, Guilford, 2005

Rothbart MK, Ahadi SA, Evans DE: Temperament and personality: origins and outcomes. J Pers Soc Psychol 78(1):122–135, 2000 10653510

Rothbaum F, Pott M, Azuma H, et al: The development of close relationships in Japan and the United States: paths of symbiotic harmony and generative tension. Child Dev 71(5):1121–1142, 2000 11108082

Rutter M, Silberg J, O'Connor T, et al: Genetics and child psychiatry: I: advances in quantitative and molecular genetics. J Child Psychol Psychiatry 40(1):3–18, 1999 10102724

Ryle A, Kerr IB: Introducing Cognitive Analytic Therapy: Principles and Practice. Chichester, UK, Wiley, 2002
Safran JD, Muran JC: Has the concept of the therapeutic alliance outlived its usefulness? Psychotherapy (Chic) 43(3):286–291, 2006 22122099
Sandler J: The background of safety. Int J Psychoanal 41:352–356, 1960 13746183
Sandler J, Rosenblatt B: The concept of the representational world. Psychoanal Study Child 17(1):128–145, 1962
Sandler J, Sandler A-M: The past unconscious, the present unconscious, and interpretation of the transference. Psychoanal Inq 4:367–399, 1984
Santini ZI, Koyanagi A, Tyrovolas S, et al: The association between social relationships and depression: a systematic review. J Affect Disord 175:53–65, 2015a 25594512
Santini ZI, Koyanagi A, Tyrovolas S, et al: The association of relationship quality and social networks with depression, anxiety, and suicidal ideation among older married adults: Findings from a cross-sectional analysis of The Irish Longitudinal Study on Ageing (TILDA). J Affect Disord 179:134–141, 2015b 25863909
Schore A: Affect Regulation and the Repair of the Self. New York, WW Norton, 2003
Sharp C, Wright AG, Fowler JC, et al: The structure of personality pathology: both general ("g") and specific ("s") factors? J Abnorm Psychol 124(2):387–398, 2015 25730515
Shaw DS, Gilliom M, Ingoldsby EM, Nagin DS: Trajectories leading to school-age conduct problems. Dev Psychol 39(2):189–200, 2003 12661881
Shengold L: Insight as metaphor. Psychoanal Study Child 36:289–306, 1981 6171002
Shevrin H: Psychoanalysis as the patient: high in feeling, low in energy. J Am Psychoanal Assoc 45(3):841–864, 1997 9353708
Solms M: Dreaming and REM sleep are controlled by different brain mechanisms. Behav Brain Sci 23(6):843–850, discussion 904–1121, 2000 11515144
Solms ML: The neurobiological underpinnings of psychoanalytic theory and therapy. Front Behav Neurosci 12:294, 2018a 30564106
Solms M: The scientific standing of psychoanalysis. BJPsych Int 15(1):5–8, 2018b 29953128
Solms M, Turnbull O: The Brain and the Inner World: An Introduction to the Neuroscience of Subjective Experience. New York, Other Press, 2002
Spitz RA: A Genetic Field Theory of Ego Formation: Its Implications for Pathology. New York, International Universities Press, 1959
Stern DN: The Interpersonal World of the Infant: A View From Psychoanalysis and Developmental Psychology. New York, Basic Books, 1985
Stern DN, Sander LW, Nahum JP, et al: Non-interpretive mechanisms in psychoanalytic therapy: the "something more" than interpretation. Int J Psychoanal 79 (Pt 5):903–921, 1998 9871830
Sterzer P, Stadler C, Krebs A, et al: Abnormal neural responses to emotional visual stimuli in adolescents with conduct disorder. Biol Psychiatry 57(1):7–15, 2005 15607294
Storebø OJ, Stoffers-Winterling JM, Völlm BA, et al: Psychological therapies for people with borderline personality disorder. Cochrane Database Syst Rev 5(5):CD012955, 2020 32368793
Sullivan HS: The Interpersonal Theory of Psychiatry. New York, WW Norton, 1953
Target M, Fonagy P: Playing with reality: II: the development of psychic reality from a theoretical perspective. Int J Psychoanal 77(Pt 3):459–479, 1996 8818764
Taylor J, Gibson B, Taylor W, et al: Developing a paediatric advanced nurse practitioner led telephone clinic for children with acute lymphoblastic leukaemia. Pediatr Blood Cancer 65 (suppl 2):S634, 2018
Tomasello M: A Natural History of Human Morality. Cambridge, MA, Harvard University Press, 2016
Tomasello M: How children come to understand false beliefs: a shared intentionality account. Proc Natl Acad Sci USA 115(34):8491–8498, 2018 30104372
Tomasello M: Becoming Human: A Theory of Ontogeny. Cambridge, MA, Belknap Press of Harvard University Press, 2019
Tomasello M: The role of roles in uniquely human cognition and sociality. J Theory Soc Behav 50(1):2–19, 2020

Tremblay RE: The origins of violence (ISUMA). Canadian Journal of Policy Research 1(2):19–24, 2000
Tremblay RE, Japel C, Perusse D, et al: The search for the age of "onset" of physical aggression: Rousseau and Bandura revisited. Crim Behav Ment Health 9(1):8–23, 1999
Tronick E: The Neurobehavioral and Social-Emotional Development of Infants and Children. New York, WW Norton, 2007
Tronick E, Beeghly M: Infants' meaning-making and the development of mental health problems. Am Psychol 66(2):107–119, 2011 21142336
Tuomela R: We-intentions revisited. Philos Stud 125(3):327–369, 2005
Tuomela R: The Philosophy of Sociality: The Shared Point of View. Oxford, UK, Oxford University Press, 2007
Wang J, Mann F, Lloyd-Evans B, et al: Associations between loneliness and perceived social support and outcomes of mental health problems: a systematic review. BMC Psychiatry 18(1):156, 2018 29843662
Watson JS: Contingency perception and misperception in infancy: some potential implications for attachment. Bull Menninger Clin 65(3):296–320, 2001 11531128
Weissman MM, Markowitz JC, Klerman GL: The Guide to Interpersonal Psychotherapy: Updated and Expanded Edition. Oxford, UK, Oxford University Press, 2017
Westen D: The scientific legacy of Sigmund Freud: toward a psychodynamically informed psychological science. Psychol Bull 124(3):333–371, 1998
Westen D, Gabbard GO: Developments in cognitive neuroscience: I: conflict, compromise, and connectionism. J Am Psychoanal Assoc 50(1):53–98, 2002 12018875
Willick MS: Psychoanalysis and schizophrenia: a cautionary tale. J Am Psychoanal Assoc 49(1):27–56, 2001 11379725
Winnicott DW: Transitional objects and transitional phenomena; a study of the first not-me possession. Int J Psychoanal 34(2):89–97, 1953 13061115
Winnicott DW: Mirror role of mother and family in child development, in Playing and Reality. Edited by Winnicott DW. London, Tavistock, 1956, pp 111–118
Winnicott DW: Ego distortion in terms of true and false self (1960), in The Maturational Processes and the Facilitating Environment. Edited by Winnicott DW. New York, International Universities Press, 1965, pp 140–152
Winnicott DW: Mirror-role of the mother and family in child development, in The Predicament of the Family: A Psycho-Analytical Symposium. Edited by Lomas P. London, Hogarth Press, 1967, pp 26–33
Yeomans FE, Clarkin J, Kernberg OF: Transference-Focused Psychotherapy for Borderline Personality Disorder: A Clinical Guide. Washington, DC, American Psychiatric Publishing, 2015

CHAPTER 2

Techniques of Psychodynamic Psychotherapy

Glen O. Gabbard, M.D.
Holly Crisp, M.D.

Psychodynamic psychotherapy has been characterized by a variety of labels over the years: psychoanalytic psychotherapy, intensive psychotherapy, insight-oriented psychotherapy, expressive-supportive psychotherapy, and exploratory psychotherapy, to name a few. They are all essentially synonymous. This modality derives from the principles of psychoanalysis. Whereas psychoanalysis is generally conducted at a frequency of three to five times per week, with the patient supine on a couch, psychoanalytic psychotherapy is more typically provided once or twice per week, with the patient sitting up. In practice, most therapists today assume a continuum between psychoanalysis and psychodynamic psychotherapy, with the premise that therapist and patient together can determine both what frequency is best for the psychotherapy and also whether to have the patient face-to-face or on the couch. In psychodynamic psychotherapy, therapists emphasize the importance of flexibility rather than rigidity. Moreover, most therapists continue to modify their approach on the basis of the unique features of the therapeutic dyad.

Dynamic psychotherapy can be long-term and open-ended or short-term with a set number of sessions. Generally, we define *long-term psychodynamic psychotherapy* as lasting more than 24 sessions or longer than 6 months. *Short-term psychodynamic psychotherapy* entails all therapies of fewer than 24 sessions or lasting less than 6 months. A useful definition of psychodynamic psychotherapy is "a therapy that involves careful attention to the therapist-patient interaction, with carefully timed interpretation of transference and resistance embedded in a sophisticated appreciation of the therapist's contribution to the two-person field" (Gunderson and Gabbard 1999, p. 685).

In Chapter 1, "Theoretical Models of Psychodynamic Psychotherapy," Fonagy, Hepworth, and Campbell comprehensively lay out the various theoretical models subsumed under psychodynamic therapies. Each model emphasizes different aspects of techniques that follow logically from the theoretical assumptions. Although we note those emphases in passing as we present the fundamentals of technique in psychodynamic psychotherapy, our primary goal is to provide an introduction to common elements in psychodynamic technique, regardless of one's preferred theoretical model. These elements include the therapeutic alliance, specific types of interventions, transference, countertransference, resistance, working-through, and termination. Before discussing these technical principles, however, we first provide an overview of how to assess the patient's suitability for dynamic therapy, how to formulate the psychodynamic understanding of the patient, and how to collaborate with the patient on the establishment of treatment goals.

Assessment

In Chapter 6, "Applications of Psychodynamic Psychotherapy to Specific Disorders," Leichsenring and Steinert review the data from outcome studies of dynamic therapy and formulate indications for this modality. A core feature of psychodynamic thinking is that one must go beyond the DSM-5 diagnosis (American Psychiatric Association 2013) in assessing whether the patient is suitable for exploratory therapy. The patient's personality characteristics, defense mechanisms, motivation, and other capacities must be carefully evaluated before one reaches a conclusion about whether dynamic therapy is the optimal treatment. Several factors that go into this assessment are summarized in Table 2–1.

Above all, patients suited to psychodynamic therapy must be curious about themselves. They must be motivated to understand unconscious patterns in their lives that lead to suffering. They must be willing to work with the therapist collaboratively to figure out why they do things that are self-defeating or why they hurt others they do not wish to hurt. These qualities are often referred to as *psychological mindedness*—in other words, these patients can see the internal origins of their difficulties rather than seeing themselves as simply a leaf buffeted in the wind without a sense of agency.

Defense Mechanisms

In the classic model of ego psychology, defense mechanisms prevent a person from becoming aware of sexual or aggressive wishes or the anxiety that is connected with them. In addition, defenses preserve self-esteem in the face of shame and narcissistic vulnerability and externalize internal threats onto others. Defenses are also embedded in relatedness in that they make relationships more manageable by providing an illusion of control over what happens in an interaction with significant people in the patient's life.

Defense mechanisms are generally divided into those that are primitive or immature and those that are higher level or neurotic. Table 2–2 provides some of the common defenses in these two categories. The lists in Table 2–2 are by no means exhaustive. Moreover, everyone uses primitive defenses, such as denial and splitting, when under

TABLE 2–1. Elements of assessment for psychodynamic psychotherapy

DSM-5 diagnoses (American Psychiatric Association 2013)
Capacity and motivation to actively collaborate with the therapist in pursuit of understanding
Typical defense mechanisms
Mentalizing capacity
Quality of object relations
Ego strengths and weaknesses
Presence of intrapsychic conflicts
Developmental deficits

stress. There are also mature defenses that are not generally regarded as pathological. These include sublimation, anticipation, humor, suppression, and altruism.

Assessment of the defense mechanisms in Table 2–2 guides the psychodynamic clinician regarding how much support the patient needs versus how much insight the patient can tolerate. Thus, dynamic psychotherapy is practiced with an expressive-supportive continuum in mind (Gabbard 2014, 2017) (see Figure 2–1 later in this chapter). The therapist recognizes that there must be a balance of interpretive and supportive comments with most patients, and part of the purpose of a careful assessment is to determine the extent to which the emphasis should be in one direction or the other.

Mentalizing Capacity

As Bateman, Choi-Kain, and Unruh stress in Chapter 4, "Theory and Practice of Mentalization-Based Treatment," the capacity for mentalizing grows out of attachment theory and refers to a person's ability to conceive of their own and others' mental states as explanations of behavior. Hence, it, too, is related to psychological mindedness. The psychodynamic clinician assesses the ability of a patient to see that their behavior grows out of a set of beliefs, feelings, and perspectives that are not necessarily the same as others'. Like empathy, mentalizing requires a capacity to sense what is going on in another's mind and respond accordingly. This capacity to be sensitive to what others are feeling and to know that one's internal states contribute to one's behavior augurs well for a more exploratory or interpretive approach in dynamic psychotherapy.

Object Relations

The cornerstone of dynamic therapy is observing how patterns of relationships in a patient's life recur in the relationship with the therapist. Patients who do not have meaningful outside relationships may be more difficult to treat with a psychodynamic approach. Patients who have more chaotic relationships may also present challenges to the therapist, who seeks to have the patient reflect on the details of difficulties in encounters with intimacy rather than simply react with action. Nevertheless, some data suggest that interpretations of the recurrence of these patterns in patients who have disturbed interpersonal relationships may result in significant improvement (Gabbard 2006; Høglend et al. 2006).

TABLE 2–2. **Primitive and higher-level defense mechanisms**

Mechanism	Description
Primitive defenses	
Splitting	Compartmentalizing internal representations of self and others so that conflict is avoided and integration is not possible
Projective identification	A defense involving subtle interpersonal pressure so that the target of a projection takes on characteristics of an aspect of the self or the internal object that is being projected
Projection	Externalizing unacceptable inner impulses and their derivatives by attributing them to someone else
Denial	Avoiding awareness of aspects of external realities that are difficult to face by dismissing perceptions that are obvious to everyone in the environment
Schizoid fantasy	Retreating into one's private, internal world to avoid anxiety about interpersonal situations
Higher-level defenses	
Displacement	Shifting feelings associated with one idea or object to another that resembles the original in some way
Intellectualization	Using excessive and abstract ideation to avoid difficult feelings
Isolation of affect	Separating an idea from its associated affect states to avoid emotional turmoil
Sexualization	Endowing an object or behavior with sexual significance to turn a negative experience into an exciting and stimulating one
Reaction formation	Transforming an unacceptable wish or impulse into its opposite
Repression	Expelling unacceptable ideas or impulses, thus blocking them from entering consciousness (repression is more closely linked with inner states, whereas denial involves external sensory data)

Ego Strengths and Weaknesses

The ego is the executive organ of the psyche and is involved in a host of regulatory functions. Someone with high ego strengths tends to have good control of impulses and the capacity to tolerate intense affects such as anxiety, anger, or grief. Other ego strengths involve the capacity to anticipate consequences of one's actions (judgment) and to sustain activity such as work or school despite setbacks and adversities. Patients with these ego capacities are likely to be able to tolerate the frustration and anxiety brought about by exploration of the darkest corners of the psyche that have long been avoided or defended against. By contrast, those with ego weaknesses, such as impulsivity, impaired judgment, difficulties testing reality, and poor tolerance of affect states, will be less likely to endure the stresses of psychotherapy and may even drop out soon after beginning.

Intrapsychic Conflict and Developmental Deficits

In classic psychoanalytic ego psychology, intrapsychic conflict involves a wish or an impulse opposed by a defense. The id may seek pleasure, whereas the superego prohibits the impulse to enjoy oneself. In object relations theory, conflict may involve the disparate wishes or urges of different representations of the self and other. Whatever theoretical model one uses, internal conflict is a source of a great deal of suffering and often causes one to seek psychodynamic therapy. The conflict is often unconscious and appears as a symptom such as inhibition of love or work relationships.

Developmental deficits may occur through early experiences of abuse, neglect, or parental failure to respond empathically to the child's needs. Self psychology is a deficit model theory that postulates, for example, the absence of mirroring responses from the child's parents or caregiver (see Chapter 1). In the terms of British object relations theory, the self is intruded on by the mother, resulting in the creation of a false self to protect the true self (Winnicott 1965). Patients who have greater degrees of deficit may require more support to be able to tolerate insight, whereas those whose problems have a greater emphasis on intrapsychic conflict may respond more readily to interpretation and insight. The majority of patients have varying degrees of conflict and deficit that are joined in unique and idiosyncratic ways based on the patient's background, genetic vulnerabilities, and resilience.

In our current understanding of psychodynamic practice, we do not see patients merely through the lens of conflict or solely through the perspective of deficit. Psychodynamic therapists expect to see aspects of both conflict and deficit in the experiences of their patients. In fact, we would conceptualize psychodynamic therapy as involving a thoroughgoing attunement to a *series* of dialectical tensions as therapists think about their patients—the dialectics between conflict and deficit, between focus on the past and focus on the present, between self and object, and between internal struggles and external struggles with people in the patient's life, to name only a few.

Biopsychosocial Formulation

Formulating an understanding of the patient who is beginning psychodynamic psychotherapy provides an initial road map that may be rewritten as the journey progresses. The formulation must involve an understanding of the relative contributions of biology, psychological factors, and sociocultural influences. Psychodynamic therapy cannot occur in a vacuum that emphasizes only the intrapsychic while ignoring such factors as genetic contributions, medical illnesses, and traumatic brain injury. In addition, the sociocultural context the patient brings to the consulting room must be considered and incorporated as part of the understanding of the individual. Recent thinking has expanded our notion of the biopsychosocial formulation to include emphasis on the roles of cultural factors, race, ethnicity, gender, and sexuality, as well as religious or spiritual beliefs. These elements are central to how patients experience themselves and their relationships to others. Most therapists conceptualize a brief formulation as they get to know a new patient, and this formulation may expand as they develop deeper understandings of a patient over time.

Biopsychosocial formulation generally involves three central components (Gabbard 2017; Kassaw and Gabbard 2002; Sperry et al. 1992): 1) a brief description of the nature of the clinical picture and the stressors that brought the patient to treatment; 2) an attempt to integrate the biological, intrapsychic, and sociocultural factors in terms of their relative contributions to the presenting problems; and 3) a succinct statement about how the contributing factors will inform the treatment and the prognosis. Hence, if you feel that an abusive father is a powerful internal representation, represented as a harsh superego, you might predict that the patient might see a male therapist in that light when the psychotherapy deepens. This perception, conscious or unconscious, may make it difficult for the patient to open up fully.

Goals

Patient and therapist need to work together at the outset to form mutually agreed-on goals that are realistic. A patient may come to a therapist with a goal of finding a partner and having a baby. The therapist cannot realistically promise that psychotherapy can achieve that goal. The therapist might need to reframe the goal as understanding internal and interpersonal conflicts that might interfere with the patient's achievement of meaningful mutual relationships and the exploration of inhibitions that might be involved in wanting to become a parent. Sometimes goals need to be discussed at some length before therapist and patient can agree on where the therapy is headed. Moreover, therapy often takes unexpected detours and circuitous routes that require the modification and rethinking of therapeutic goals.

Goals may be heavily influenced by the theoretical orientation of a dynamic psychotherapist. Table 2–3 lists a number of goals from the psychoanalytic and psychodynamic literature that reflect the varying theoretical models of psychopathology and therapeutic change.

Resolution of conflict derives from ego psychology and the structural model. By exploring impulses, wishes, and defenses against these impulses and wishes, patients may ultimately master conflicts (but not completely eliminate them). The search for authenticity and the truth about oneself may be central to dynamic therapy, reflecting the work of Winnicott (1962/1976), who spoke of the distinction between the true self and the false self that was adopted to please parental figures during childhood. Self psychology seeks to help the patient function with more appropriate selfobjects that validate their needs. Most therapies try to improve relationships. Object relations theory would explicitly argue that those aspects of the self or object representations that are projected onto others must be "re-owned" so that the patient feels a more integrated sense of self and a more satisfying sense of relatedness with others. Meaning is also a goal of many therapies, but some models, such as relational theory (Mitchell 1997), suggest that the therapeutic dialogue is specifically designed to discover unconscious meanings and create new meanings through the conversation of patient and therapist. Finally, enhancement of mentalizing capacity is a central goal for therapies influenced by attachment theory. One is able to achieve a greater sense of intersubjectivity rather than assuming that one's one way of thinking is endorsed by everyone (Fonagy and Target 2000).

An ever-present peril in all psychotherapies is the imposition of the therapist's goals on the patient. A central tenet of psychodynamic therapy is that therapists must respect the patient's autonomy rather than trying to control how the patient behaves, thinks, and feels. When differences occur, a patient's goals generally supersede the therapist's goals, provided the former are reasonable. Too much emphasis on goals

TABLE 2–3. Goals of psychodynamic psychotherapy

Resolution of intrapsychic conflict
A search for truth about oneself
An improved capacity to seek out appropriate selfobjects
Improved relationships as a result of gains in understanding about one's internal object relationships
Generation of meaning in one's life as a result of therapeutic dialogue
Improved mentalizing capacity

Source. Gabbard 2017.

may also lead a patient to become oppositional. Many patients need a period without goals to explore themselves in the course of psychotherapy. One overarching goal for psychodynamic psychotherapy is for patients to feel more comfortable in their own skin—in other words, being more self-aware, having more agency and comfort with their own decisions, and finding meaning and purpose in their lives.

The cataloging of goals in Table 2–3 reflects another feature of psychodynamic psychotherapy technique: it is less geared to removal of symptoms than are other modalities, such as exposure and response prevention, which derive from behavior theory. Although symptoms may be seen as an important target, the broader goal is to achieve fundamental characterological change and to change the vulnerabilities inherent in the patient's character or personality. For example, a psychodynamic therapist who treats someone with chronic or recurring depression may emphasize the types of stressors and the reactions to those stressors that constitute a recurrent theme in the patient's susceptibility to depression. Does depression generally follow a breakup in a relationship in which the patient feels diminished by the negative view of a romantic partner? Is there an ongoing perfectionistic expectation of the self that is repeatedly contributing to disappointment? In other words, does the patient always fall short of the expectation of achieving something that is forever out of reach?

This focus on vulnerability has become essential in contemporary discourse about recurrent depression (Ingram and Price 2002). Psychodynamic therapists often refer to *structural change* when they modify inherent vulnerability or conflicts between intrapsychic agencies so that the patient's functioning and subjective experience both globally improve.

Therapeutic Alliance

The *therapeutic alliance* is the envelope within which dynamic therapy takes place. Good therapists must attend to the therapeutic alliance from early in the treatment to ensure that the therapy is viable. Research has repeatedly demonstrated that the role of the therapeutic relationship is more important than any specific technique in producing positive therapeutic outcomes (Butler and Strupp 1986; Horvath 2005; Krupnick et al. 1996; Zuroff and Blatt 2006). The therapeutic alliance is variously defined, but components commonly linked to a good therapeutic alliance are the following: the patient feels attached to the therapist; the patient feels that the therapist is helpful; and the patient and therapist feel a sense of mutual collaboration in pursuing common therapeutic goals (Hilsenroth and Cromer 2007; Horwitz et al. 1996; Luborsky 1984; Luborsky and Luborsky 2006).

Few dynamic psychotherapy concepts have been more rigorously studied than the therapeutic alliance. An extensive body of research suggests that a strong therapeutic alliance is positively correlated with a good outcome, that the patient's assessments tend to be more predictive of outcome than are assessments by others, and that early alliance in therapy is a predictor of outcome that is as good as or better than assessments taken later (Horvath 2005; Martin et al. 2000). This research indicates that the therapeutic alliance is formed early in treatment, even as early as the first session, and predicts later outcome. Some research provides guidelines regarding what the clinician can do in the first few sessions to enhance the therapeutic alliance (Hilsenroth and Cromer 2007). First, therapists must listen sensitively and convey trust, warmth, and understanding. Exploring the in-session process and the patient's affect in a nonjudgmental manner also improves the alliance, as does speaking with both emotional and cognitive content. Finally, therapists who identify new clinical issues to foster deeper levels of understanding and insight may enhance the alliance.

The basic strategy of dynamic psychotherapy, once it has been launched, is to pay careful attention to ruptures that occur in the alliance. Ruptures are usually defined as some kind of breakdown or strain in the collaborative process between therapist and patient, a deterioration in communication between the two, or a general deterioration in the quality of the relationship (Safran and Muran 1996, 2006). Ruptures may involve the withdrawal of the patient from the therapeutic dialogue or an angry or accusatory statement about the therapy or the therapist. It is essential for therapists to identify these ruptures and fully explore them, lest the patient leave without elaborating on the reasons for the rupture. Therapists who can acknowledge their own contribution to the rupture, rather than blaming it on the patient, tend to be more successful in repairing the damage to the alliance. Ruptures in the alliance often provide a glimpse of underlying concerns about the therapy that have been concealed throughout most of the sessions. Hence, they are a valuable opportunity to address potentially disruptive factors in the therapy.

In addition to the therapeutic alliance, another highly relevant component of psychotherapy is insight, which has long been viewed as a key aspect of the therapeutic action in psychodynamic therapy as well as other forms of psychotherapy. Jennissen et al. (2018) defined insight as patients' understanding of associations between past and present experiences; typical relationships; and the relationship among interpersonal challenges, emotional experiences, and psychological symptoms. They established this link empirically through their study of 13,849 initially identified abstracts. The authors were able to extract 23 independent effect sizes. A meta-analysis revealed a significant moderate correlation between insight and treatment outcome.

Therapeutic Interventions

Cinematic stereotypes of psychoanalysis and psychodynamic therapy often portray the therapist as an aloof, silent, and cold figure whose facial expressions never change. However, the contemporary dynamic therapist is warm, empathic, and spontaneous; the "blank screen" therapist belongs to an earlier era. We now know from studies in nonverbal communication that it is impossible to entirely conceal one's feelings and probably not helpful even if one could do so. A psychodynamic therapist focuses on the patient, so self-disclosure is kept to a minimum unless saying something about here-and-now feelings or if an area of common interest is likely to enhance the therapy. In any case, the therapeutic atmosphere should be one of a spontaneous conversation in which the patient feels understood and helped. Terms such as *neutrality* in describing the therapist's attitude are often misunderstood as cold aloofness. A better understanding of the term would be conveyed by saying that the therapist assumes a nonjudgmental attitude of listening to the patient's concerns.

Although the therapeutic dialogue should have a spontaneous quality to it, it is useful to have in mind a continuum of interventions that are designed to promote therapeutic change. These categories will not encompass all of the therapist's comments, but they serve as useful guideposts to help the therapist tailor the technique to the patient. As noted in the "Defense Mechanisms" subsection, dynamic psychotherapy usually takes place along an expressive-supportive continuum. Interventions can be conceptualized as residing on that continuum, as shown in Figure 2–1. Therapists must remain flexible and tailor the approach to the patient. For example, with a highly insightful patient, the therapist may be able to focus interventions closer to the expressive end of the continuum. With a patient who needs more support and reassurance, the therapist may focus their interventions more toward the supportive end. It is important to remember that all therapists modify what they are doing on the basis of in-the-moment cues from the patient. For example, the therapist may need to assume a stance in the supportive range after a major life crisis or loss with a patient in intensive psychodynamic psychotherapy or psychoanalysis who usually is in an interpretive/expressive space in the therapy. Similarly, the therapist who generally takes a more supportive approach with a patient may wait for moments of openness on the part of the patient when a more expressive or interpretive technique is indicated. The therapist moves back and forth along the continuum from moment to moment, session to session, and patient to patient.

Interpretation

The term *expressive* is used synonymously with *exploratory* or *interpretive*. Hence, at the left end of the continuum is *interpretation*, the most expressive or insight-producing comment in the therapeutic armamentarium. The intent is to make patients aware of things that are currently outside their awareness. Interpretations may bring to consciousness something that was previously unconscious, or they may explain a linkage that was outside the patient's awareness in a way that produces insight. An example of an interpretation is the following:

> **Therapist:** You seem to hold yourself back from succeeding because you worry that your mother will be envious and retaliate against you.

As this example illustrates, interpretation usually involves explaining something to the patient. An interpretation is more likely to be received with an open mind if it is presented to the patient in a tentative way, as a possibility rather than as a definitive statement from an oracular source of knowledge.

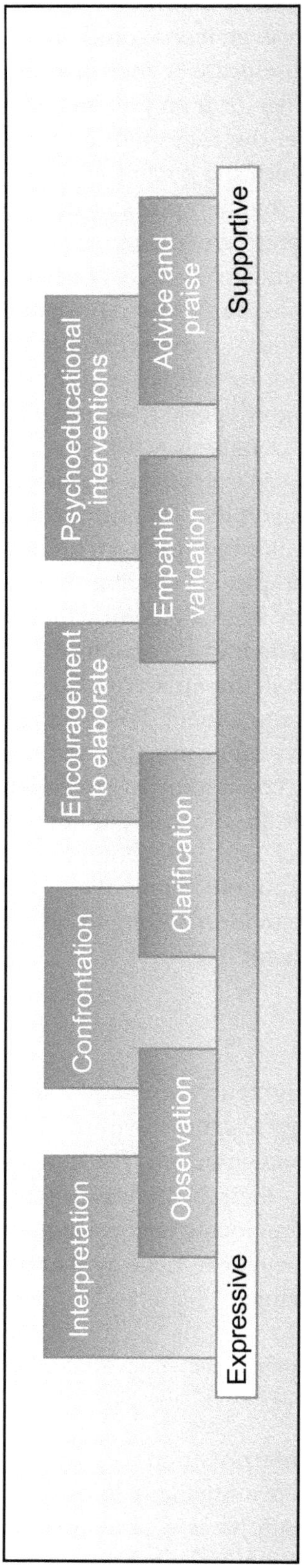

FIGURE 2–1. Expressive-supportive continuum of interventions.

Source. Reprinted from Gabbard GO: *Long-Term Psychodynamic Psychotherapy: A Basic Text,* Third Edition. Arlington, VA, American Psychiatric Association Publishing, 2017. Copyright © 2017 American Psychiatric Association Publishing. Used with permission.

Observation

Interpretation, by definition, explains a link between one thing and another. Observation stops short of making a linkage or explaining an underlying motivation. Hence, it calls the patient's attention to something that is outside their awareness. An example might be a simple comment such as "Have you noticed that you almost always yawn as you enter the office and greet me?" Observations frequently focus on nonverbal communications or unconscious enactments that are visible to the therapist but to which the patient has blind spots.

Confrontation

Whereas observations target behavior that is outside the patient's conscious awareness, confrontation generally points out something that is being avoided but that is within the conscious awareness of the patient. For example, a narcissistic patient came to a psychotherapy session on September 11, 2001, and made no reference to the terrorist attacks on the World Trade Center and the Pentagon that had occurred several hours earlier. As the patient went on and on about how his girlfriend had mistreated him, the therapist said, "I notice that you have not mentioned the terrorist attacks today." The avoidance of that topic led to a productive exploration of how the patient wished to deny the impact of the event on him because it terrified him. Confrontation may also involve the placing of limits for patients who are pushing the limits of the treatment setting. Confrontation may also involve the placing of limits for patients who are pushing the limits of the treatment setting. For example, one patient asked the therapist, "Could we take a walk instead of just doing therapy today? It is such a beautiful day, and it would be great to be outdoors with you instead of in the confines of this stuffy office talking about all my usual problems." The therapist was able to confront the patient on their wish to avoid their problems and the unconscious wish to perhaps soften the boundaries of the therapeutic relationship by getting out of the usual treatment setting. Instead, they stayed in the office and were able to dig into what was being avoided.

Clarification

Much of the therapist's activity involves clarifying what the patient is getting at. Patients may be vague or uncertain about what they are feeling or thinking, and therapists often try to summarize or repackage what the patient is saying in a way that clarifies it for both patient and therapist: "It sounds like what you're really saying is that you can't decide whether you really want to stay in this relationship or leave it." Often the therapist's voice has a questioning tone: "Do I understand correctly that you really didn't see your father from the age of 6 to 8?"

Encouragement to Elaborate

In the middle of the continuum is the intervention known as *encouragement to elaborate*. Perhaps the most common form of communication from the therapist, this intervention is designed to elicit further commentary from the patient. The principle of free association stemming from psychoanalysis is applied to dynamic therapy as well. Therapists do whatever they can to stimulate the patient's uncensored, open reporting of whatever comes to mind. Hence, a frequent intervention is "I'd like to hear more about that." Sometimes the patient is stopped at a moment when the therapist feels more needs to be said: "I'm sure you must have other feelings about it than those you have told me so far. Could you say a little more?" Generally, this kind of intervention is open-ended, but it may also be directed at something specific: "I'd like to hear more about your mother's father. I don't know much about him."

Empathic Validation

Although self psychology regards empathy as central to technique, therapists of all persuasions must be alert to patients' need for empathic validation. Often, patients have had their internal experiences invalidated or denied by parents as they grew up, leading to a need to present a facade or a false self to the family. Therapists can be particularly helpful when they validate that the patient has a right to certain feelings and that the patient's response is legitimate in light of what has happened to the patient. An empathically validating comment could be "It is completely understandable to me that you would be angry at your father after he said that to you." Such interventions can also be applied to the here-and-now situation: "You have every reason to be mistrustful of me, given what you've experienced from authority figures in the past."

Psychoeducational Interventions

Near the supportive end of the continuum, psychotherapy becomes more akin to teaching. Dynamic psychotherapy always has an educational aspect because patients learn about themselves in the process of trying to express the nature of their problems. Sometimes patients require specific forms of education about the nature of their illness, the goals of psychotherapy, or the limits of psychotherapy. One patient needed to be told that "I really can't accept your donation to my research because it would be unethical for me to take advantage of our therapeutic relationship by soliciting donations from you." Another dynamic therapist said to a patient with anxiety, "Most of the research on anxiety indicates that there are probably both a genetic component and contributions based on adverse environmental experiences."

Advice and Praise

The most supportive interventions in dynamic psychotherapy are those that directly praise the patient for specific behaviors or comments or offer advice to the patient on a particular course of action. There has long been a myth in psychodynamic therapy that the therapist does not give advice or praise. On the contrary, these supportive interventions may be useful and alliance building if done with reflectiveness and consideration. Patients who are in a state of crisis may need specific advice related to the immediate problem. However, therapists must avoid a stance of knowing what is best for the patient. Wise therapists use caution before stepping in to offer advice on life-changing decisions. For example, it would be prudent for the therapist to encourage the patient to explore potential benefits and losses, rather than give specific advice, if a patient asks, "Do you think I should quit my job?" We must be aware that we do not actually walk in the patient's shoes, and they, not we, must live with the decisions that they make. Clinicians must attune themselves to countertransference dynamics in patients who are actively seeking praise or unconsciously engaging the therapist for advice. Praise can facilitate the therapeutic alliance and can help the patient feel that they are participating in therapy effectively. A typical comment involving praise is "I think you've come up with a very important insight there that I hadn't thought about before." Praise often involves a therapist's statement of positive regard for the patient: "I'm proud of you for having the courage to speak directly to your mother about this problem instead of concealing it."

Transference

As the definition at the beginning of this chapter reveals, the focus on transference is a hallmark of psychodynamic psychotherapy. A simple definition of *transference* is the displacement of feelings and thoughts associated with a figure in the patient's past onto the therapist. Transference is often unconscious, at least initially, and the patient is bewildered by behavior toward the therapist because it does not make sense on the basis of who the therapist really is. Hence, the enactment of missing a session or of coming late to a session may reveal unconscious transference. A patient may say, "I have no idea why I forgot to come today. I'm not aware of any negative feelings about you." Whereas the original definition assumed that a kind of template in the unconscious was taken from the patient's mind and superimposed on the therapist without much alteration, today, the prevailing view is that the therapist's actual behavior is always influencing the patient's experience of the therapist (Hoffman 1998). Hence, the transference to the therapist is based partly on real characteristics and partly on figures from the patient's past—a combination of old and new relationships.

Beginning therapists can err on the side of calling too much attention to the transference too soon. As a general principle, the therapist should postpone the interpretation of transference until it becomes a resistance and until it is close to the patient's awareness (Gabbard 2017). In other words, if things are going reasonably well, it makes no sense to interpret transference. If the patient develops, for example, erotized or highly negative feelings, which impede the process of the therapy, interpretation may be essential. Many therapists regard treatment that focuses on transference as more exploratory than therapy geared to extratransference relationships. In supportive therapy, interpretation of the transference may be minimized, although the therapist may silently interpret the transference as a way of increasing their understanding of the patient.

The following dialogue illustrates the evolution of transference in one therapy session and its management by the therapist:

Patient: I need to tell you what happened in my conversation with Mom last night. She tries to control everything I do. She wants me to be a clone of herself.

Therapist: What exactly happened last night?

Patient: She said she wanted to take me to dinner, so I went. Then, when I tried to order, I just about lost it. She insisted that I get the special, which was what she was ordering. She told me that she specifically took me to the restaurant so I would try a particular dish. I've told her a hundred times that I'm trying to get red meat out of my diet, and the special was some kind of beef bourguignon that I simply did not want to eat. So we had an argument right there in front of the people at the next table, who were listening in.

Therapist: I know that you are exasperated right now, but as I've told you before, part of you unconsciously sets up that situation because you get something out of the conflict with your mother. I think you could have written last night's scenario before you went to the restaurant.

Patient: Why would I want to interact with my mother in such an annoying and argumentative way?

Therapist: I don't think we fully understand that yet.

Patient: We don't understand it because it's not true. There's nothing whatsoever appealing about that type of interaction.

Therapist: I think we go through the same type of "dance" here. It's very hard for you to accept what I say because you imagine I'm like your mother, believing that I insist that you think just like I do.

In this dialogue, the patient begins to recreate the relationship with her mother in the therapeutic setting. Dynamic therapists assume that patients will reestablish their family situation in therapy, just as they do in intimate relationships outside therapy. One way that the therapist helps is by *interpreting transference,* a process designed to illustrate to the patient that what happens in the therapeutic relationship is similar to what happens *outside* therapy. Many patients feel shamed or caught when the therapist interprets this type of repetition, so the therapist must be judicious in using transference interpretations.

Transference has many manifestations. Dreams may reveal feelings toward the therapist that otherwise do not enter into the process. Patients may talk about another doctor or professional in highly emotional terms as a way of displacing transference feelings elsewhere. Patients who have concealed erotic feelings toward their therapist may engage in an intense erotic relationship with someone who resembles the therapist.

Transferences also may vary in the course of psychotherapy. In contemporary psychoanalytic and psychodynamic discourse, it is generally recognized that there are multiple transferences—stemming from parents, siblings, and other figures—and not simply one specific transference. Moreover, some patients do not work well within the transference and do not feel intense feelings toward the therapist—a situation known as *resistance to the awareness of transference*—so the therapist will need to work interpretively on outside relationships until the patient feels comfortable enough to bring material into the therapeutic relationship. Other patients go through an entire psychotherapy and benefit greatly without a focus on the transference. Hence, therapists must adapt the types of interventions and the degree of transference work to the specific patient.

Countertransference

The original use of *countertransference,* as described by Freud (1910/1957), was the analyst's transference to the patient. In other words, the patient might remind the therapist of someone from the therapist's past, so the therapist starts to treat the patient as though they were that figure. Over time, this view of countertransference was broadened to include the total emotional reaction of the therapist to the patient. Today, it is recognized that countertransference is jointly created—it partly involves the therapist's past relationships, but it also involves feelings induced in the therapist by the patient's behavior. The part of the countertransference induced by the patient is generally referred to as *projective identification*. This process involves two steps: 1) a self or object representation within the patient is projectively disavowed by its unconsciously being placed onto someone else, and 2) the projector exerts internal pressure that nudges the other person to experience or unconsciously identify with whatever has been projected. One could say that step 1 is a type of transference, whereas step 2 is a countertransference reaction. In a psychotherapeutic context, a third step occurs: 3) the recipient of the projection, the therapist, contains and tolerates the affective state and the projection of the self or object representation associated with the affect until the patient can take them back and "own" what has been projected. In this manner, projective identification can be regarded as both an interpersonal communication and an intrapsychic defensive operation.

Projective identification often feels obligatory. Therapists may feel that an alien force is taking them over and may feel that they cannot avoid enacting the role that the patient has thrust on them. This state of affairs can be therapeutically useful, however, because the therapist is experiencing something that others in the patient's life experience.

Some therapists may use the countertransference as a step on the road to interpreting something useful to the patient. For example, the therapist might say, "I notice myself feeling a bit frustrated because I keep asking you questions to try to find out what you are thinking or feeling, but you tell me very little. This sounds like what goes on with your husband at home quite frequently." Pointing out the interpersonal process, the therapist can help the patient reflect on how they take an active role in creating a situation that may be unpleasant or difficult in relationships outside of therapy.

The therapist uses self-disclosure of countertransference to promote therapeutic gains in the patient. This type of self-disclosure must be used judiciously because disclosure of some countertransference feelings may be harmful to the process. For example, it is rarely useful to say to the patient, "I hate you" or "I feel bored by what you are telling me." The patient has no obligation to entertain the therapist, and the revelation of such feelings to the patient may inflict a severe wound that leaves the patient unable to trust the therapist. Revealing sexual feelings toward the patient is rarely useful. The patient may feel that the therapeutic setting is no longer a safe place if the therapist begins to express sexual desire toward them. In our current cultural milieu, in the wake of the MeToo movement, there is an important, necessary, and broader awareness of the perils of inequalities in power structure, particularly involving sexualized feelings, actions, or words. However, in the therapeutic relationship, the power differential and the professional boundaries required to protect the patient have been longstanding.

Positive countertransference feelings can be present without the therapist knowing it. Positive regard toward the patient may be seen as simply a caring posture that facilitates the therapy. However, countertransference blind spots can grow out of positive feelings. Therapists may be reluctant to confront the patient about aggression or other problems if they do not want to "rock the boat" and cause the patient to have negative feelings toward them. Similarly, a need to rescue the patient may keep the patient from developing their own resources for problem solving.

Resistance

The identification and management of *resistance* are also fundamental to the technique of psychodynamic psychotherapy. Dynamic therapists recognize that patients are ambivalent about changing. They unconsciously oppose the therapist's efforts to offer insight and therapeutic change. Defense mechanisms that defend against uncomfortable feelings are activated by the therapy as resistances.

Resistance is not necessarily spoken. It may take the form of a conscious admission of not wishing to go where the therapist wants the patient to go, but it may also appear as a failure to show up on time, a tendency to forget sessions, lapses into silence for no apparent reason, or a preference for discussing matters that appear to be quite irrelevant to the therapeutic goals. However, dynamic therapists know that the way the patient resists is a revelation of something important about the patient—often a highly significant internal object relationship from the patient's past, transported into the present moment with the therapist (Friedman 1991).

In this regard, many resistances are *transference resistances*. The patient may be opposing the therapist's efforts because of unconscious feelings or thoughts about the therapist based on figures from the patient's past. Patients may feel that the therapist may shame them if they open up or may criticize them for their shortcomings. A good psychodynamic therapist, however, does not directly confront the resistance and try to get the patient to "knock it off." Rather, the therapist attempts to understand why the patient is resisting and encourages the patient to develop a reflectiveness about what is being resisted and why.

When patients say that they cannot think of anything else to talk about or that they cannot reveal certain things about themselves, psychodynamic therapists generally do not directly pursue what is being withheld. Instead, they seek to examine the resistance before the content. Instead of saying, "Tell me what you're withholding," they might say, "Do you have any idea what you're worried about if you were to reveal this to me?" They might also ask, "How do you imagine I'd react if you were to reveal what you're concealing?"

Another form of resistance is acting out rather than talking. Patients often repeat in action what they cannot remember (Freud 1914/1958), and therapists study their nonverbal enactments carefully to understand their meaning.

In self psychology, resistances are regarded in a more positive way, as a way of safeguarding the self. Therapists of this persuasion suggest that it is best to empathize and respect the patient's need for defenses rather than to challenge the patient about their defensiveness. Most therapists generally agree with this position, given that confronting resistances head-on rarely causes them to fade away.

Most defenses are embedded in character, so characterological resistances are present in many patients. For example, a patient with obsessive-compulsive personality disorder who uses isolation of affect, reaction formation, and intellectualization as characteristic defenses will resist the therapy by intellectualizing and conveying the opposite of what they feel. Working on these resistances embedded in the personality is the bread and butter of psychodynamic work. Systematically analyzing these resistances may open a window into the characteristic patterns of relatedness and the underlying anxieties that activate the defenses.

Working-Through and Therapeutic Strategies

Working-through in many ways is the heart of psychodynamic psychotherapy. Characteristic patterns of defenses and internal object relations emerge again and again in different contexts and are repetitively clarified, confronted, observed, and interpreted. By pointing out repetitive patterns that occur in the transference and in outside relationships, as well as their derivation in childhood relationships, therapists ultimately help patients begin to see their own responsibility for creating situations in their life. Hence, one of the outcomes of working-through is an enhanced sense of agency whereby patients start to feel like authors of their own life experiences. Much of working-through involves systematic analysis of the patient's conscious and unconscious fantasies as they emerge in the treatment, as well as recurrent themes in their dreams.

A number of strategies are useful in promoting a productive working-through process. Exploring the core conflictual relationship theme (CCRT), developed by Luborsky (1984; Luborsky and Luborsky 2006), can be a fruitful course to pursue to help a patient increase self-observation and self-understanding. The CCRT involves a recurrent fantasy of relationships: a statement of the patient's wish, an expected imagined or actual response from the significant other, and a corresponding response from the self. The response from the self involves both behaviors and actions, as well as self-states and feelings that may not be expressed. The CCRT emerges as the therapist listens to themes in the patient's narratives about life outside the therapy. Exploring the specifics of disappointments and expectations often reveals the CCRT. The following example illustrates how these patterns emerge.

> A 28-year-old graduate student had completed all of his coursework but became stuck when it came to completing his dissertation. He told his therapist that he really wanted to get the Ph.D. and couldn't understand why he couldn't make himself sit down and complete the dissertation. He said he had finished about half of it but had lost his motivation and couldn't force himself to concentrate. The therapist asked him what he was afraid of. The patient hesitated and responded, "I'm not exactly sure, but I feel so much pressure from my dissertation adviser and my dad that it's driving me nuts." The therapist asked him to elaborate on the pressure he felt. In both the narrative involving his father and the narrative involving his dissertation adviser, the patient spoke as though they would expect more and more of him if he actually got his Ph.D. He felt his father was never satisfied. He recalled one time when he brought home a report card with all As except one B. His father's total focus was on why he got a B in the one course. The patient described his dissertation adviser as similarly hard-driving and demanding. With the help of his therapist, the patient was able to develop the following CCRT: He had a strong wish to succeed to please his father, but he feared that, ultimately, nothing would please his father (or his dissertation adviser) and that they would only expect more. To avoid placing himself under even greater pressure, he retreated from the task and shut down all his creative efforts. When the therapist pointed this out to the patient, the patient said he instantly felt understood, although he had never put the three aspects of the CCRT together on his own.

Another useful strategy is to follow the patient's affect states and make interventions that facilitate emotional expression. A survey of the psychodynamic therapy research literature (Diener and Hilsenroth 2008) showed considerable empirical support for the notion that emotion-focused techniques are positively linked to favorable outcomes. Among these techniques are the following: 1) increasing the patient's awareness of their emotions; 2) facilitating the patient's emotional experience by focusing specifically on affective indicators in the patient, such as crying, or shifts in the patient's mood; and 3) making specific references to these indicators. One has to be careful not to intervene too quickly when a patient cries, lest one inadvertently communicate that strong affect is too disturbing to handle. Diener and Hilsenroth recommend sitting with the sadness for a bit before attempting to interpret its meaning for the patient.

Another technique associated with positive outcome is to frame an interpretation as clarification in a manner that increases the patient's affect. An example would be to point out that feelings are not being expressed or to empathically validate the reason for the feelings.

Yet another strategy is to promote mentalization by helping patients to see situations from an alternative perspective. Goldberg (1999) emphasized the need to shift from a first-person perspective to a third-person perspective in the course of working through. Therapists need to validate the patient's "I" experience while also bringing to bear their own outside experience from a third-person perspective. Therapists can tactfully bring in their own views on what the patient brings up so that the patient gradually begins to appreciate alternative perspectives.

Therapists can enhance mentalization by calling attention to the patient's mental state, even when the patient may not be aware of the nature of that state. If, for example, a patient has a clenched fist, the therapist might observe that the patient appears angry. Then the therapist can illustrate how anger might influence the patient's perception. Moreover, if an impulsive behavior occurs, the therapist may ask the patient what was going on at the time that precipitated the behavior. By calling attention to internal states and specific kinds of actions in order to promote mentalization, the therapist helps the patient track and monitor their current state of mind. The therapist assumes a curious stance with the patient and actively inquires about mental states and alternative perspectives. Helping the patient focus on the therapist's mind is also a useful approach to improve the capacity for mentalization. As Bateman, Choi-Kain, and Unruh note in Chapter 4, "Theory and Practice of Mentalization-Based Treatment," therapists should focus on mentalizing the patient and creating an awareness of representations of self and other in the patient, along with moving toward a *we-ness* in the therapy, a "representational capacity of the relationship as something more than self and other" (p. 99).

After summarizing the various techniques and strategies of psychodynamic therapy, it is important to stress that there is almost always an improvisational aspect to effective therapy. Clinicians recognize that there is not one specific way to do psychodynamic psychotherapy "correctly" (Gabbard 2020). Those of us who practice dynamic therapy must always doubt our thinking and our interventions, and we must constantly adjust what we think and say to three factors: the person of the patient, the person of the therapist, and, today, the zeitgeist of the era. For example, those therapists treating patients during the 2020 coronavirus SARS-CoV-2 disease (COVID-19) pandemic found themselves adjusting to the reality of the danger as well as the shifting from in-person to virtual approaches. Flexibility is crucial. Therapists must know when to back off from their therapeutic zeal and must recognize that by pursuing symptom eradication, therapists can come off as coercive and moralizing. In the end, patients must do the therapy the way they have to do it. Therapists who insist on a technique they learned may promote deadness and discourage the patient (Ogden and Gabbard 2010).

Termination

Termination is often mythologized in discussions of ideal cases of psychotherapy or psychoanalysis. The reality is that therapy ends in all different kinds of ways, often with practical considerations such as changes in financial circumstances, relocation of the patient or therapist, or an impasse in the treatment. There is no such thing as a perfect or idealized termination; at best, we aim for a *good enough* termination (Gabbard 2009). One of the values of setting goals is that patient and therapist can together gauge the progress of the treatment by assessing how many of the goals have been accomplished and to what extent.

Therapists must avoid the countertransference position of idealizing termination and expecting a perfect outcome. Indeed, a major goal of therapy is to help patients internalize the process of inquiry that therapy represents so that patients can continue much of the work on their own. Studies of psychodynamic psychotherapy (Bateman and Fonagy 2001; Svartberg et al. 2004) suggest that there is a *timed-release* aspect to dynamic therapy. Patients' improvement continues after termination because the patient-therapist relationship has been internalized so that the work continues.

When patients are dead set on terminating for whatever reasons, it is rarely useful for the therapist to insist that they continue. Psychodynamic psychotherapy is noncoercive. Patients should be there because they want to be there, not because they have to be. It is far better to allow the patient to leave with the idea that the door is always open. Then the patient can return when they feel the need.

Many patients return periodically for a few sessions or for more extended therapy, depending on new challenges in their lives. Still other patients end up as "therapeutic lifers" who see the therapist once every 6 months or so to maintain their gains. Wallerstein (1986) found that in the follow-up of the Menninger Psychotherapy Research Project, some of the patients did well as long as they were never expected to terminate therapy. The ongoing tie to the therapist appeared to have a beneficial effect, rather than simply encouraging dependency. The varieties of termination are multiple and often unexpected (Table 2–4).

It is important for therapists to remember that we cannot know in advance how a patient will do after termination, and sometimes patients who choose unilateral termination may ultimately benefit as much as those who have mutual termination. Some patients may need to have an ending date established by the therapist because they feel they can never terminate. Above all, termination must be individualized in collaboration with the patient. Many themes recur in the course of the termination phase of therapy, and psychotherapists themselves often feel a sense of genuine loss, not just in the sense of losing a patient but also in the sense of losing a significant human relationship. For this reason, countertransference must be carefully monitored so that the therapist does not attempt to transform a therapeutic relationship into a personal one (Gabbard 2017).

TABLE 2–4. **Varieties of termination**

Mutual agreement of therapist and patient based on achievement of goals
Preplanned termination based on number of sessions
Forced termination because one of the following occurs:
• Therapist graduates or changes clinical assignment
• Patient relocates
• Patient's third-party payer discontinues reimbursement
Unilateral termination in which one of the following occurs:
• Patient feels there is no value in continuing
• Therapist feels there is no value in continuing (and refers patient elsewhere)
Failed attempt at termination, leading to "therapeutic lifer "status
End setting as a therapeutic strategy

Source. Adapted from Gabbard 2017.

Conclusion

Psychodynamic psychotherapy cannot be adequately characterized by its specific techniques. It fundamentally involves a human relationship in which one person tries to understand the other in an empathic, nonjudgmental manner that facilitates increasing levels of disclosure and trust. Although most of the therapist's comments can be categorized along the expressive-supportive continuum noted in this chapter, therapists should think about the time with the patient as a form of conversation that has spontaneity and responsiveness. Therapists who simply adhere to the technique as though it were a requirement of the therapy might lose the patient by appearing excessively rigid and scripted. Flexibility is a key feature of a good dynamic therapist, and therapists must adapt the treatment to the patient rather than the patient to the treatment.

Key Points

- The patient's personality characteristics, defense mechanisms, motivations, and other capacities must be carefully evaluated before a conclusion can be reached about whether dynamic therapy is the optimal treatment.
- A biopsychosocial formulation involving contributions from biology, psychology, and sociocultural influences guides the therapist in the initial stages of the treatment and serves to predict possible developments during therapy.
- Reasonable goals for the therapy must be collaboratively derived from negotiation between patient and therapist.
- Much attention should be paid to the development of the therapeutic alliance because it is one of the most powerful predictors of outcome in dynamic therapy.
- Insight regarding past and present relationship themes, interpersonal challenges, and recurrent psychological symptoms is a key aspect of therapeutic action.

- Interventions used in dynamic psychotherapy reside on an expressive-supportive continuum, and the therapist must shift flexibly along that continuum according to the patient's needs.
- Transference generally is not interpreted until it becomes a resistance.
- Countertransference is a joint creation caused by preexisting issues in the therapist's past and what is induced in the therapist by the patient's behavior.
- Resistance is the manifestation of the patient's defense mechanisms as they are activated in therapy. These manifestations are a major focus of dynamic psychotherapy.
- The working-through process is the heart of dynamic therapy and involves strategies that are tailored to the individual patient.
- Termination occurs in a variety of ways, and the therapist must be flexible in adapting the termination to the patient's situation.

Recommended Readings

Gabbard GO: Psychodynamic Psychiatry in Clinical Practice, 5th Edition. Washington, DC, American Psychiatric Publishing, 2014

Gabbard GO: Long-Term Psychodynamic Psychotherapy: A Basic Text, 3rd Edition. Arlington, VA, American Psychiatric Association Publishing, 2017

McWilliams N: Psychoanalytic Psychotherapy. New York, Guilford, 2004

References

American Psychiatric Association: Diagnostic and Statistical Manual of Mental Disorders, 5th Edition. Arlington, VA, American Psychiatric Association, 2013

Bateman A, Fonagy P: Treatment of borderline personality disorder with psychoanalytically oriented partial hospitalization: an 18-month follow-up. Am J Psychiatry 158(1):36–42, 2001 11136631

Butler FF, Strupp HH: Specific and nonspecific factors in psychotherapy: a problematic paradigm for psychotherapy research. Journal of Self Psychotherapy 23:30–39, 1986

Diener MJ, Hilsenroth MJ: Affect-focused techniques in psychodynamic psychotherapy, in Evidence-Based Psychodynamic Psychotherapy. Edited by Levy R, Ablon S. Totowa, NJ, Humana Press, 2008

Fonagy P, Target M: Playing with reality: III. The persistence of dual psychic reality in borderline patients. Int J Psychoanal 81 (Pt 5):853–873, 2000 11109573

Freud S: The future prospects of psycho-analytic therapy (1910), in The Standard Edition of the Complete Psychological Works of Sigmund Freud, Vol 11. Translated and edited by Strachey J. London, Hogarth Press, 1957, pp 139–152

Freud S: Remembering, repeating and working-through (further recommendations on the technique of psycho-analysis II) (1914), in The Standard Edition of the Complete Psychological Works of Sigmund Freud, Vol 12. Translated and edited by Strachey J. London, Hogarth Press, 1958, pp 145–156

Friedman L: A reading of Freud's papers on technique. Psychoanal Q 60(4):564–595, 1991 1758912

Gabbard GO: When is transference work useful in dynamic psychotherapy? Am J Psychiatry 163(10):1667–1669, 2006 17012669

Gabbard GO: What is a "good enough" termination? J Am Psychoanal Assoc 57(3):575–594, 2009 19620466
Gabbard GO: Psychodynamic Psychiatry in Clinical Practice, 5th Edition. Washington, DC, American Psychiatric Publishing, 2014
Gabbard GO: Long-Term Psychodynamic Psychotherapy: A Basic Text, 3rd Edition. Arlington, VA, American Psychiatric Association Publishing, 2017
Gabbard GO: The analyst and the virus. J Am Psychoanal Assoc 68(6):1089–1099, 2020 33439683
Goldberg A: Between empathy and judgment. J Am Psychoanal Assoc 47(2):350–365, discussion 365–400, 1999 10422046
Gunderson JG, Gabbard GO: Making the case for psychoanalytic therapies in the current psychiatric environment. J Am Psychoanal Assoc 47(3):679–704, discussion 704–740, 1999 10586398
Hilsenroth MJ, Cromer TD: Clinician interventions related to alliance during the initial interview and psychological assessment. Psychotherapy (Chic) 44(2):205–218, 2007 22122211
Hoffman IZ: Ritual and Spontaneity in the Psychoanalytic Process: A Dialectical-Constructivist View. Hillsdale, NJ, Analytic Press, 1998
Høglend P, Amlo S, Marble A, et al: Analysis of the patient-therapist relationship in dynamic psychotherapy: an experimental study of transference interpretations. Am J Psychiatry 163(10):1739–1746, 2006 17012684
Horvath AO: The therapeutic relationship: research and theory: an introduction to the special issue. Psychother Res 15:3–7, 2005
Horwitz L, Gabbard GO, Allen JG, et al: Borderline Personality Disorder: Tailoring the Psychotherapy to the Patient. Washington, DC, American Psychiatric Press, 1996
Ingram RE, Price JM (eds): Vulnerability to Psychopathology: Risk Across the Lifespan. New York, Lippincott Williams & Wilkins, 2002
Jennissen S, Huber J, Ehrenthal JC, et al: Association between insight and outcome of psychotherapy: systematic review and meta-analysis. Am J Psychiatry 175(10):961–969, 2018 30068262
Kassaw K, Gabbard GO: Creating a psychodynamic formulation from a clinical evaluation. Am J Psychiatry 159(5):721–726, 2002 11986123
Krupnick JL, Sotsky SM, Simmens S, et al: The role of the therapeutic alliance in psychotherapy and pharmacotherapy outcome: findings in the National Institute of Mental Health Treatment of Depression Collaborative Research Program. J Consult Clin Psychol 64(3):532–539, 1996 8698947
Luborsky L: Principles of Psychoanalytic Psychotherapy: A Manual for Supportive-Expressive Treatment. New York, Basic Books, 1984
Luborsky L, Luborsky E: Research and Psychotherapy: The Vital Link. New York, Jason Aronson, 2006
Martin DJ, Garske JP, Davis MK: Relation of the therapeutic alliance with outcome and other variables: a meta-analytic review. J Consult Clin Psychol 68(3):438–450, 2000 10883561
Mitchell S: Influence and Autonomy in Psychoanalysis. Hillsdale, NJ, Analytic Press, 1997
Ogden TH, Gabbard GO: The lure of the symptom in psychoanalytic treatment. J Am Psychoanal Assoc 58(3):533–544, 2010 20852143
Safran JD, Muran JC: The resolution of ruptures in the therapeutic alliance. J Consult Clin Psychol 64(3):447–458, 1996 8698936
Safran JD, Muran JC: Has the concept of the therapeutic alliance outlived its usefulness? Psychotherapy (Chic) 43(3):286–291, 2006 22122099
Sperry L, Gudeman JE, Blackwell B, et al: Psychiatric Case Formulations. Washington, DC, American Psychiatric Press, 1992
Svartberg M, Stiles TC, Seltzer MH: Randomized, controlled trial of the effectiveness of short-term dynamic psychotherapy and cognitive therapy for cluster C personality disorders. Am J Psychiatry 161(5):810–817, 2004 15121645
Wallerstein RS: Forty-Two Lives in Treatment: A Study of Psychoanalysis and Psychotherapy. New York, Guilford, 1986

Winnicott DW: The aims of psychoanalytic treatment (1962), in The Maturational Processes and the Facilitating Environment: Studies in the Theory of Emotional Development. London, Hogarth Press, 1976, pp 166–170

Winnicott DW: Ego distortion in terms of true and false self, in The Maturational Processes and the Facilitating Environment: Studies in the Theory of Emotional Development. New York, International Universities Press, 1965, pp 140–152

Zuroff DC, Blatt SJ: The therapeutic relationship in the brief treatment of depression: contributions to clinical improvement and enhanced adaptive capacities. J Consult Clin Psychol 74(1):130–140, 2006 16551150

CHAPTER 3

Techniques of Brief Psychodynamic Psychotherapy

Mantosh Dewan, M.D.
Priyanthy Weerasekera, M.D., M.Ed.
Lynn Stormon, Ph.D.
Daniel Jackson, M.D.

All brief therapies, not just brief psychodynamic psychotherapy (BPP), evolved from psychoanalytic roots. Sigmund Freud reported on psychoanalytic therapies that lasted 1 week (Katherine), 7 weeks (Emmy von N), and 9 weeks (Lucie R) and the cure of Gustav Mahler's impotence in a single 4-hour session (Breuer and Freud 1893–1895/1955; Jones 1957). Freud's followers defined and formally introduced the key ingredients of brief therapy: increased therapist activity; limited time and/or number of sessions; defined, narrow treatment focus; and restricted patient criteria. Sándor Ferenczi's (1920/1926) advocacy of *active therapy* and Alexander and French's (1946) active creation of corrective emotional experiences stand as notable contributions to increased therapist activity as a constituent of BPP. Limiting treatment duration and/or the number of sessions is another hallmark of BPP. Otto Rank limited time to 9 months but did not restrict the number of sessions (O'Dowd 1986); Malan (1979) set a firm end date at the first session with a flexible number of sessions, which averaged 18, and Mann (1973) set a firm end date and limited sessions to 12. A more defined, narrow treatment focus was envisioned as the focal conflict (French 1970), focal psychotherapy (Balint et al. 1972; Malan 1976), the core neurotic problem (Sifneos 1972), and the core conflictual relationship theme (Luborsky 1984). The restricted patient criteria ranged from accepting patients who were simply willing, as practiced by Rank (O'Dowd 1986), to accepting those who not only were motivated but could easily form an alliance (Malan 1976; Sifneos 1972). A divergent approach, with broadening of criteria, was taken by Davanloo (1980), who focused on patients with more severe pathology, including that of personality. Gregory et al. (2008) applied his approach to patients with borderline personality disorder and substance abuse.

Research has validated these theoretical underpinnings of BPP, and practitioners are extending the reach of this approach by introducing innovative techniques, by working in new settings, and by treating new populations. For instance, Davanloo's intensive short-term dynamic psychotherapy aims for a major unlocking of the unconscious by an insistent, intense attack on defenses, which can be done as block therapy, with each session lasting up to 7 hours (Caldiroli et al. 2020; Davanloo 2004). Milrod et al.'s (2007) panic-focused psychodynamic psychotherapy effectively treats patients with panic disorder, including those with comorbid personality disorders (Keefe et al. 2018). Gregory et al. (2008) demonstrated the efficacy of dynamic deconstructive psychotherapy in patients with borderline personality disorder with comorbid alcohol use disorder. Furthermore, de Roten et al.'s (2017) inpatient BPP combines approaches from Busch et al. (2004) and Despland et al. (2010), just one example of how BPP is being used in new settings via the syncretism of techniques.

Finally, BPP has been proven to be effective—and as effective as long-term therapy—for a wide variety of disorders, including depression (Busch et al. 2016), panic and anxiety disorders (Busch et al. 2012; Milrod et al. 2007), somatic symptom and related disorders, perinatal depression, functional dyspepsia, eating disorders, substance-related disorders, borderline personality disorder, and Cluster C personality disorders (Ben-Itzhak et al. 2012; Driessen et al. 2013; Faramarzi et al. 2013; Knekt et al. 2010; Laaksonen et al. 2013; Lindfors et al. 2012; Maljanen et al. 2012; McCarthy et al. 2018; Nanzer et al. 2012; Sattel et al. 2012; Sørensen et al. 2011; Zlotnick et al. 2020). The effectiveness of BPP is detailed in Chapter 6, "Applications of Psychodynamic Psychotherapy to Specific Disorders."

In this chapter, we address factors that are common to all types of BPP. To be consistent with other chapters in this text, we define BPPs as therapies that continue for less than 6 months or involve fewer than 24 sessions. We then describe the three main schools of brief psychodynamic therapies and illustrate how practitioners of each approach would conceptualize and treat the same patient.

Features Common to All Brief Psychodynamic Therapies

The goals of BPP are relief from distressing symptoms; resolution of key conflicts; and, in some cases, changes in character pathology. Research has demonstrated that BPP is efficacious in treating a variety of psychiatric disorders (Leichsenring 2005; see also Chapter 6) and that specific therapist and patient factors, as well as in-session interventions, predict the outcome of BPP (Crits-Christoph and Connolly 1999; Leichsenring 2005).

There are three major schools of brief dynamic psychotherapy: the *drive/structural model,* the *relational model,* and the *integrative/eclectic model* (Messer and Warren 1995). Several features that are common to all BPPs and that differentiate this modality from long-term psychodynamic psychotherapy are listed in Table 3–1. After outlining a ge-

TABLE 3–1. **Differences between brief and long-term psychodynamic psychotherapy**

Brief dynamic therapy	Long-term dynamic therapy
Rapid alliance formation	Gradual alliance formation
Narrow problem focus	Broad range of problems
Higher level of therapist activity	Moderate therapist activity
Ability to tolerate separation	Variable ability to tolerate separation
Good object relationships	Poor to good object relationships
Less severe pathology	More severe pathology
Here-and-now focus	Past-and-present focus

neric approach to BPP, we consider variations according to each specific school (Book 1998; Budman 1981; Dewan et al. 2019; Messer and Warren 1995).

Structural Elements

All types of BPP have the following structural elements in common:

- *Engagement*—rapid formation of a therapeutic alliance and translation of presenting problems into focal goals
- *Discrepancy*—provision of novel skills, insights, and experiences that challenge patient patterns and facilitate new understandings and actions
- *Consolidation*—rehearsal of new patterns in varied contexts, accompanied by feedback, to ensure internalization and prevent relapse (Dewan et al. 2019)

Patient Characteristics: Initial Interview and Patient Selection

A full psychiatric and psychodynamic assessment is completed in order to select only those patients who are most likely to benefit from this treatment (Table 3–2). Several patient characteristics have been identified that are considered essential for BPP. These include motivation for treatment, ability to identify a circumscribed problem, good object relationships (presence of past and current relationships), ability to rapidly form a therapeutic alliance, and capacity to tolerate separation. Patients lacking these characteristics would likely benefit from other approaches or long-term psychodynamic therapy (Book 1998).

Narrowed Problem Focus

After conducting a full assessment, the therapist converts the patient's presenting problem into a psychodynamic formulation, in which major themes center on conflicts that are based on drives, impulses, defenses, relational patterns, wishes, and other universal conflictual situations. Sifneos (1981, p. 49) illustrated an oedipal problem focus from the structural school:

> A graduate student complaining of difficulties with both men and women stated that he had a tendency to cover up his feelings, to wear "a mask," as he put it, so that others would not know what he truly was like. He attributed this tendency to his relationship

TABLE 3–2. Brief dynamic psychotherapy inclusion and exclusion criteria

	Inclusion	Exclusion
Diagnoses	Depression: mild to moderate[a]	Severe depression, bipolar disorder, psychosis, suicidality
	Anxiety: PTSD, social anxiety disorder (social phobia), panic disorder[a]	OCD
	Somatoform disorders[a]	Severe somatizing disorders
	Eating disorders[a]	Severe eating disorders
	Opioid dependence[a]	
Patient characteristics	Good object relationships (has had at least one relationship)	Poor object relationships
	Highly motivated, willing patient	Poor motivation
	Narrow symptom or problem focus	Chronic, severe character pathology; diffuse, ill-defined symptomatology
	Interpersonal difficulties[a]	

[a]Criteria supported by randomized controlled trials (Leichsenring 2005).
Note. OCD=obsessive-compulsive disorder.

> with his parents. As a result of his strong attachment to his mother, whose favorite he was, and competition with his father, he felt he had to hide his true feelings for both of them. This attitude interfered with his daily life.

Levenson (2018, p. 270) provided an example of a four-part *cyclical maladaptive pattern* (CMP) from the relational school:

1. *Acts of self*: "When I meet strangers, I think they wouldn't want to have anything to do with me."
2. *Expectations of others' reactions*: "If I go to the dance, no one will ask me to dance."
3. *Acts of others toward self*: "When I went to the dance, guys asked me to dance but only because they felt sorry for me."
4. *Acts of self toward the self (introjection)*: "When no one asked me to dance, I told myself that it is because I'm fat, ugly, and unlovable."

Mann (1981, p. 34) gave an example of a problem focus representing the integrated school of BPP:

> **Therapist:** You are a man who has been enormously successful despite many serious difficulties. What hurts you now and has always been a source of hurt to you is the difference you feel between your public image and the private feelings that you have about yourself.

The problem focus is presented to the patient, and a therapeutic contract is developed to work through the problem. This is one of the most important variables in the development of the therapeutic alliance (Horvath and Symonds 1991). If the patient does not agree with the problem focus, it is important that the problem be reexamined, reformulated, and presented to the patient for reconsideration (Book 1998). Because therapy is time-limited, the focus is limited to one or two attainable goals. Specific goals could be symptom relief or working-through of conflictual relationships (but with limited character change).

Increased Therapist Activity and Techniques

One key therapist variable that differentiates long-term psychodynamic psychotherapy from BPP is *therapist activity level.* Given that BPP typically lasts 4–6 months or less, it is essential that the therapist be active and promote the emergence of material in session. Because the problem focus is presented to the patient in the initial session, subsequent sessions single-mindedly focus on the problem as it is worked through. The specific techniques used depend on the model of therapy followed. The techniques that follow are common to all psychodynamic schools.

Interpretation

Psychodynamic psychotherapy focuses on the unconscious dimensions of the patient's experience. An *interpretation* is a statement made by the therapist that connects the patient's present-day thoughts, feelings, and behavior to their unconscious origins in past relationships (Levy 2002).

Therapist: I wonder whether your anger toward your boss has something to do with the experience of being criticized by your father. You're trying hard to please him and get his approval, like you did with your father.

Patient: He's an arrogant jerk! I can't stand his superior attitude. It's not my fault that I'm late sometimes!

Therapist: I think it might be easier to feel angry at him than hurt by his feedback or scared of being rejected, feelings you had when your father got angry and criticized you when you disappointed him.

Use of Transference

Transference is the term Freud (1905/1953) gave to his discovery that the patient *transfers* to the therapist unconscious patterns of relationship that have been internalized through interactions with important people, primarily within the family (Goldberg 2012). In the transference, the patient relives past experiences with the therapist, who interprets the patient's fantasies, conflicts, and defenses. This process increases the patient's awareness of the impact of the past on the present and transforms unconscious dynamics into conscious insight, which can alleviate symptoms and help the patient develop new patterns of experience.

Patient: (*The patient is 20 minutes late to the session and slammed the door on the way out of the last session.*) I was busy with a report. It's late, and my boss is pressuring me to finish it. I didn't notice it was time to leave (*falls silent, looks away, seems upset*).

Therapist: I get the feeling that you're angry at me. As we've discussed, sometimes you're late after a difficult session. Did my remarks about how you handled the feedback from your boss about your lateness make you feel criticized, like you felt criticized by your father?

Patient (*looking close to tears*): I feel like I can't get it right. I never measured up, I always let him down. I feel that way here, too. I try so hard, but I'm always screwing up.

Use of Countertransference

Countertransference is a term coined by Freud (1910/1953) to describe the therapist's unconscious reactions to the patient. This concept has since been greatly expanded in elaborating how the therapist may use their conscious and unconscious responses to understand the patient's inner world, including how the patient might pressure the therapist into enacting rather than understanding the transference (Brown 2012). In this regard, the therapist's own treatment is invaluable.

Therapist: (*Feeling frustrated and irritated by the patient's repeated absences and lateness, he pauses to reflect on the work he's done in therapy on his relationship with his own father. He feels pulled into an enactment in which he tells the patient he needs to get his act together but interprets instead.*) I get the feeling that by being late you're provoking me to tell you to get here on time. You're frequently late to work and in meeting deadlines as well, which provokes your boss into giving you a hard time. At least that way, you know we care about you and want you to do well. Your father never gave you the feeling he believed in you. He was frequently late to your games and school events because of business or didn't come at all. You felt that you weren't important to him.

Clarification

A *clarification* is a statement made by the therapist to the patient that restates what the patient has said to reflect back to the patient what the therapist has heard. The aim of clarification is to make sure the therapist has understood the meaning of the patient's communication.

Therapist: If I understand what you're saying, you're doing the best you can, but you're struggling. You're angry and disappointed in yourself for not being able to do better. Is that right?

Suggestion and Advice

The therapist can suggest alternative ways to understand a situation or advise the patient on a different course of action. These techniques should be used with care, given the power differential in the therapeutic relationship, especially if the patient idealizes the therapist or is excessively dependent or compliant. An example of appropriate advice is as follows:

Therapist: You've been unhappy in your job for quite some time. It's not entirely clear what the problem is. You might think about talking to Human Resources about your issues with your boss. Working with a career counselor to talk about your long-term career goals might also be helpful.

An example of *inappropriate* advice is as follows:

Patient: My boss is constantly on my back. I can't take it anymore.
Therapist: I think you should just quit your job.

These techniques are used in all forms of psychodynamic psychotherapy, although the frequency of use depends on the specific school because differences exist with respect to what is emphasized in the theory and in the therapeutic encounter with the patient (Table 3–3).

TABLE 3–3. **Brief dynamic models of psychotherapy**

Drive/structural model	Relational model	Integrative model
Focuses on drives and conflicts, including oedipal conflicts	Focuses on relationships	Focuses on both conflicts and relationships and also on loss
Challenges defenses	Focuses on interactional patterns	Focuses on conflicts, relationships, and self-esteem needs
Confrontational	Nonconfrontational	Nonconfrontational
Anxiety provoking	Non–anxiety provoking	Non–anxiety provoking
Patient experiences seen as conflicts related to impulses connected to the past	Patient experiences accepted at face value	Patient experiences accepted at face value
Addresses intrapsychic conflicts	Addresses deficits and conflicts	Addresses deficits and conflicts
Therapist as objective observer	Therapist as participant	Therapist as participant

Termination

Although the end of brief therapy is often defined by time, such as 6 months, or the number of sessions, such as 24, therapy ends appropriately only when the identified problem focus has been resolved and when newly acquired psychological skills have been internalized so that they can be readily applied to a variety of other situations.

Specific Approaches to Brief Psychodynamic Psychotherapy

Although all brief psychodynamic psychotherapeutic approaches have features in common, they differ in their understanding of the nature of psychological problems and in the emphasis they place on the focus of treatment. Three models can be described on the basis of their primary model: the drive/structural model, the relational model, and the integrative model.

Drive/Structural Model

Sigmund Freud's structural model divides the mind into the id, ego, and superego. A detailed discussion of this model can be found in Chapter 1, "Theoretical Models of Psychodynamic Psychotherapy." In brief, the id, housed primarily in the unconscious, contains all the psychic energy and focuses on gratifying instinctual drives. The id's pursuit of pleasure creates tension, and alternative ways to discharge this tension are carried out by the ego (Freud 1923/1961). The ego, however, is pragmatic, with no moral sense, thereby requiring the superego to provide a moral code for behavior. Conflict arises as the id's need to gratify all of the senses' desires becomes prohibited by the superego's morality. As described by Anna Freud (1936/1966), the ego uses a variety of defense mechanisms to transform the id's psychic energy into a less threatening form. Sigmund Freud also described oedipal conflicts that involve the child's attraction to the parent of the opposite sex, which, if not properly resolved, lead to specific interpersonal problems in young adulthood. These unresolved issues become the focus of therapy in later adulthood.

Formal BPP was developed in the 1960s, with Habib Davanloo, David Malan, and Peter Sifneos promoting their own brands of BPP according to Freud's drive/structural model (Malan 1979). Patients with adjustment disorders and less severe forms of depression, anxiety, or personality disorders are all considered appropriate candidates for therapy. Malan and Sifneos excluded those patients with more severe pathology, whereas Davanloo included a broader range of patients. Malan added additional exclusion criteria, including 1) difficulties in forming an alliance due to severe dependency issues or poor transferences, 2) highly rigid defenses, 3) poor motivation, and 4) complicated ingrained characterological issues. According to Malan, the purpose of therapy is to resolve just one conflict or a few conflicts. The specific conflict typically relates to unacceptable feelings or impulses toward a person in the patient's life; these feelings produce anxiety, which is defended against by a variety of mechanisms.

Malan's approach uses the two traditional psychoanalytic *triangles of insight*—a triangle of conflict and a triangle of persons—which help conceptualize the problem and guide treatment (Figure 3–1). The main goal is to make a connection between the patterns in the triangle of conflict (comprising anxiety, defenses, and impulses or feelings) and a person in the triangle of persons (comprising the therapist, a person in a current relationship with the patient, and a person in a past relationship), until all three persons are linked. Clarifying each pattern in the significant relationships, the therapist moves through both triangles. Malan's approach attends carefully and interprets along the line of the conflict, challenging defenses until the conflict is worked through (Malan 1979).

Sifneos (1972, 2004), in his *short-term anxiety-provoking psychotherapy*, emphasized the importance of presenting the key psychodynamic focus to the patient, which usually involves either oedipal conflicts or separation and grief issues. Using an anxiety-provoking confrontational style, the therapist addresses the patient's impulses, feelings, defenses, and resistances and clearly deals with transference. Despite the confrontational style of therapy, the therapist pays attention to the therapeutic alliance and works to provide a corrective emotional experience for the patient. When the patient is able to demonstrate a clear understanding of their difficulties and also a change in behavior, termination is considered (Budman 1981).

Davanloo (1980, 2004), on the other hand, employed an initial 1-hour- to several-hours-long *trial therapy*, during which the therapist works on *unlocking the unconscious* and establishes whether therapy is appropriate for the patient. The therapist rapidly develops a positive therapeutic alliance by carefully aligning with the patient against their pathology, which is made ego-dystonic. The therapist consistently focuses on the main problem by using a direct, confrontational style, which insistently challenges the patient's defenses and quickly clarifies resistance. Davanloo also recommended that therapists use the psychoanalytic triangles of insight and actively address transference, but, unlike other theorists, he did not suggest rigidly conforming to working out one triangle before moving on to the other. Rather, the therapist moves from the transference to past and present relationships as they work through

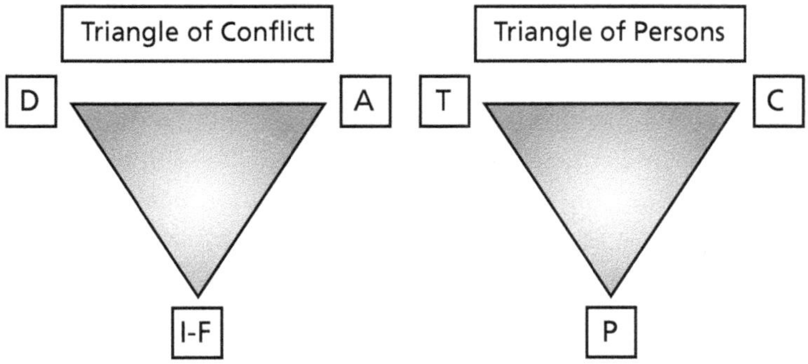

FIGURE 3–1. Traditional psychoanalytic triangles of insight.
A=anxiety; C=person in current relationship; D=defenses; I-F=impulse or feeling; P=person in past relationship; T=therapist.

the triangle of persons. Despite his confrontational style, Davanloo emphasized providing support and empathy and stated that this process facilitates openness, which permits unacknowledged feelings and conflicts to be brought into awareness and worked through. A strong therapeutic alliance is essential if one is to undertake such a confrontational style, and not all patients are able to tolerate this particular approach. Davanloo's inclusion criteria allow inclusion of patients with more serious character pathology and more severe illness than most other brief psychodynamic therapies allow. To increase the mobilization of the unconscious, Davanloo practiced *block therapy*, which consists of 5- to 7-hour-long sessions each day in blocks of 3 consecutive days (Davanloo 2004). These blocks are repeated 1–3 months apart.

The drive/structural model of BPP focuses on those key conflicts as originally described by Freud, with Davanloo, Malan, and Sifneos all developing their own brands of brief treatment. Each approach differs with respect to therapeutic style, patient inclusion criteria, and focus of treatment.

We illustrate how the techniques of the traditional drive/structural model would be applied to a patient, Ms. B (see "Case Vignette: Ms. B" and the discussion in the subsection "Therapy Approach 1: The Drive/Structural Model"). We also illustrate the treatment of the same patient according to the two other main schools, relational (see the subsection "Therapy Approach 2: Relational Time-Limited Dynamic Psychotherapy") and integrative (see the subsection "Therapy Approach 3: Mann's Integrative Time-Limited Psychotherapy").

Relational Model

Freud first used the term *object* to represent the aim of an individual's libidinal and aggressive drives. This view was further elaborated by the British Independent School of object relations theory, which gave primacy to the development and pathology of the self within the *relational* matrix between the self and the object. The primary motivating force of human behavior is seen not as pleasure seeking but as object seeking or relationship seeking. From birth, the infant seeks a relationship with the mother, first with parts of her (e.g., voice, touch) and then with the whole, integrated object (Greenberg and Mitchell 1983).

This significant shift in emphasis to the *relationship* between infant and mother was pioneered by Melanie Klein (1959/1975) and later developed by Fairbairn (1949/1959/1999), Winnicott (1965), Mahler et al. (1975), and Bowlby (1988). Departing radically from Freud's drive-conflict theory, Fairbairn posited that the motivational force driving human behavior is the fundamental need to relate with the object, a relationship considered necessary for survival. He viewed the primary developmental task of the infant as separating from the object and viewing self and object (or mother) as two distinct whole objects. He developed a sophisticated theory outlining this process and explained how individuals become involved in repeated destructive relationships. He provided a prescription for healthy functioning that permits an individual to participate in a mature relationship where true intimacy—with giving and receiving—is possible (Fairbairn 1949/1959/1999).

Following Fairbairn, Winnicott described the fundamental relational conditions necessary for a child to develop independence, creativity, and a true sense of self that permits creativity and healthy relationships (Winnicott 1965). The emphasis on separation, individuation, and differentiation was further elaborated by Mahler and, later, by Bowlby (1988). Bowlby systematically researched the mother-child relationship and, digressing from the language of the object relations school, focused on the *attachment* between the mother and child. He showed that early attachment patterns (secure, anxious-ambivalent, anxious-avoidant) produce a template or imprint for future relationships (Daniel 2006).

Object relations theory thereby shifted the focus from intrapsychic conflicts and a drive/structural model to include a deficit model in which specific environmental precursors predict future personality development, psychopathology, and future relationships, including the therapeutic relationship. Although conflict still remains important in this model, it is conflict between representations of the self and representations of the object within the self. The importance given to the object and the object relationship offers a *relational* and interpersonal dimension, illustrating our inherent human longing to connect with and relate to another. Personality is understood in terms of the individual's internal representation of self and other; greater attention is given to current as well as past experiences, and the therapist is viewed as a participant in an interactional process rather than as a passive, objective observer.

The approaches to brief psychodynamic therapy that follow the relational model were developed by Strupp and the Vanderbilt group (Strupp and Hadley 1979; Strupp et al. 1977) and later by Strupp and Binder (1984), Weiss et al. (1986), Luborsky and Crits-Christoph (1990), Horowitz (1991), and Levenson (2017). Strupp and colleagues (1977) proposed an interpersonal model that focused on CMPs, which are seen as the patient's repetitive maladaptive behaviors that induce negative behaviors from others. This pattern is reenacted in transference and is the focus of treatment, which emphasizes the here and now and the interpersonal dynamics of the session (Messer and Warren 1995).

Strupp and Binder's (1984) time-limited dynamic psychotherapy (TLDP) was further developed by Levenson (2017). As in other brief relational approaches, less emphasis is placed on interpretation to promote insight, and more is placed on experiential learning in the session. The therapeutic relationship is considered key in resolving dysfunctional interactional patterns, and transference is viewed as the patient's perception of the therapist based on actual previous experiences. Similarly, countertransference is seen as the therapist's natural response to the interpersonal process set up by the patient. According to TLDP, certain past experiences promote maladaptive relationship patterns, which are then reinforced in the present as a result of the patient engaging in similar maladaptive interactions. These patterns become alive in the therapeutic relationship because the therapist cannot help but become part of the maladaptive interactional dynamics. The therapeutic focus, then, is to help the patient work through these dynamics with the therapist so that what is learned can be transferred to outside relationships. The hope is for the therapist to offer a new relational experience for the patient. When several maladaptive relational patterns exist, it is important to focus on the one that creates the most difficulty (Levenson 2017).

Borrowing concepts from cognitive psychology, Horowitz (1991) described patients' *schemas, self-schemas,* and *role relationships.* Psychopathology is conceptualized as developing from the overuse of a maladaptive schema, with the main focus on stress response, loss, and mourning. Supportive as well as explorative techniques are used, with particular attention given to catharsis and the promotion of emotional expression.

The most researched approach is that based on Luborsky's core conflictual relationship theme (CCRT). Luborsky operationalized transference in his CCRT model and demonstrated that interpersonal struggles can be understood in terms of three components: a wish, a response from others, and a response from self (Luborsky and Crits-Christoph 1990). These components represent the core of the interpersonal struggle in the patient's real world and in the transference relationship and form the focus of treatment. Luborsky and Mark (1991) have identified key techniques specific to the CCRT method, which are divided into supportive and expressive techniques. Supportive techniques promote the development of a positive therapeutic alliance and include therapist-delivered acceptance, hope and encouragement, respect, and warmth. Expressive techniques focus on listening for the relationship patterns, on subsequent formulation and delivery of the CCRT to the patient as the central focus of treatment, and on the therapist's explanation of the CCRT's connection to the patient's presenting problem.

Book (1998) identified several patient variables important for treatment, including the following:

- Motivation for treatment
- Capacity to trust
- Ability to explore feelings
- Current experience of emotional suffering
- Ability to examine interpersonal conflicts
- Ability to maintain clear boundaries

In-session techniques emphasize giving greater attention to the present; to current relationships, including the therapeutic relationship; and to the interpersonal process occurring between patient and therapist as a way of understanding the patient's past and current relationship issues. Although interpretation of transference is important, the therapist is seen as providing a *corrective emotional experience* for the patient, which allows the patient to feel safe and explore painful issues. Compared with the drive/structural model, the relational model places less emphasis on insight and on the interpretation and confrontation of drives and defenses (Messer and Warren 1995).

The shift in the therapeutic stance of the therapist participating in the process is very obvious. Patients' accounts of their early developmental years and interpersonal relations are accepted at face value rather than interpreted according to oedipal fantasies (Cashdan 1988). Hanna Levenson (personal communication, December 2007) presented a case (see "Case Vignette: Ms. B") and illustrated the techniques used in a relationally oriented brief dynamic psychotherapy, TLDP (see the subsection "Therapy Approach 2: Relational Time-Limited Dynamic Psychotherapy").

Integrative Model

Bellak (1992), Garfield (1989), Gustafson (1986), andMann (1991) all developed eclectic approaches that integrate techniques from a variety of traditions. Mann developed an integrative model of brief dynamic psychotherapy that incorporates concepts from both the structural and the relational models. Using a developmental perspective, he identified separation-individuation as the main theme of brief therapy. His model identifies four universal conflicts that center on the management of loss: 1) independence versus dependence, 2) activity versus passivity, 3) development versus loss of self-esteem, and 4) unresolved versus delayed grief (Mann 1991). After developing a central focus, the therapist pays particular attention to the patient's self-esteem needs and to the therapeutic alliance. The therapist helps soothe the patient's anxiety rather than increasing it by confronting the patient about defenses and resistances, akin to the relational rather than the drive/structural model. Individuals with the following are all suitable for this approach:

- Adjustment disorders
- Anxiety reactions
- Maladaptive hysterical, depressive, or obsessional character structures
- Unsatisfactory relationship patterns
- Problems in interpersonal relationships
- Work problems
- Transitions in life

Patients should also have good ego strength, be able to engage in a therapeutic relationship, and be able to tolerate loss (Messer and Warren 1995). The therapist using Mann's integrative approach is very active, particularly in the early sessions, because therapy lasts only 12 sessions. Fundamental listening and validating skills are used in the early sessions to create a supportive therapeutic environment that facilitates self-disclosure. As therapy progresses, the therapist deals with the patient's disappointment that therapy is limited and is unable to provide an answer to all the problems they are experiencing. The therapist gently confronts and clarifies and offers interpretations around the core issues. As termination approaches, increased attention is paid to separation issues, and transference interpretations related to the past and present are offered. Therefore, Mann saw the therapist as providing self-object functions that reinforce self-esteem and a sense of mastery over the conflictual issue (Mann 1991). In the subsection "Therapy Approach 3: Mann's Integrative Time-Limited Psychotherapy," we illustrate how the technique based on Mann's integrative model would be applied to the patient described in the following case vignette.

Application of Approaches to a Specific Case

Case Vignette: Ms. B[1]

Ms. B, a 59-year-old married, white administrative assistant and mother of two grown sons, was sent to therapy by her physician because he suspected that her weight loss, multiple vague symptomatic complaints, and fatigue were symptoms of depression. Although Ms. B compliantly came for her first appointment, she made it very clear that she was "quite happy"; however, she did admit to having "some stress" in her life. Although she was well-groomed, her slumped shoulders and monotone voice made her appear lifeless.

Ms. B grew up in a strict, religious household. Her parents focused most of their attention on her "wild" sister because Ms. B "was such an easy child." She married at an early age and supported her husband, Tom, while he finished dentistry school. Their marriage was described as "normal." However, Ms. B and her husband did not spend much time together outside of going to church. Of late, her husband was spending more and more time on the computer.

Ms. B said she was a devoted mother. Although her sons were grown and out of the house, neither of them was yet financially independent, and this caused Ms. B great concern. However, she minimized her worry by saying they "just haven't found themselves yet." Ms. B hesitatingly said she suspected her younger son of having a gambling problem. Further inquiry revealed that over the past 2 years, her parents' health had deteriorated, and Ms. B had become their main source of social, financial, and health care support. Ms. B has worked almost her entire adult life. Recently, she had been experiencing much stress at work, where her duties had markedly increased after the office staff was downsized. Given all of this, she steadfastly maintained that "my life is good and I am blessed."

Therapy Approach 1: The Drive/Structural Model

The (male) therapist obtains a complete history, paying particular attention to Ms. B's interpersonal relationships. He uses open-ended questions in the first session to find out about her goals for treatment and her expectations of the therapist. It quickly becomes clear that she does not feel comfortable taking the initiative but rather expects the therapist to tell her what to do. This early manifestation of transference informs the therapist about patterns of compliance and pleasing behavior in relation to male authority figures.

In the second session, Ms. B reveals that her husband complains about feeling neglected and unappreciated. He spends a lot of time on the internet, on eBay, and usually does not come to bed until after she is asleep. Ms. B rationalizes this by saying that he has a stressful job and deserves to relax after work. The therapist decides to use Sifneos's short-term anxiety-provoking psychotherapy approach to confront Ms. B's avoidance of the problems in her marriage. He combines open-ended with forced-choice questions, which arouses Ms. B's anxiety but also reveals Ms. B as "Daddy's little girl" who consults her father on all decisions, which leaves her husband feeling

[1] This case vignette was kindly provided by Hanna Levenson, Ph.D.

sidelined and unimportant. Ms. B's mother is submissive and passive-aggressive, reacting against her husband's dominance with back pain that leaves her periodically bedridden. Ms. B's father habitually turns to Ms. B for companionship, complaining bitterly about her mother's inadequacies as a wife. When Ms. B talked to her father about her husband's excessive internet use, her father replied that he never thought that her husband was good enough for her—after all, dentists aren't real doctors—but that she shouldn't complain because she has a good life. Ms. B's father had worked long hours in a blue-collar job and always felt envious of her husband's success.

From very early on, Ms. B deployed defenses such as repression, reaction formation, isolation of affect, and rationalization to avoid her negative feelings in order to maintain her parents' positive regard, especially her father's. The therapist's persistent exploration of Ms. B's feelings about her husband's nighttime internet activity is actively defended against as she continues to maintain that her husband is a good provider and that she is content even as their sex life dwindles to nothing.

Therapist: How do you feel about competing with eBay for your husband's attention?

Ms. B: Well (*laughs nervously, somewhat taken aback*), I wouldn't say I am competing! He collects antique toy soldiers, something he enjoys a lot, and he works hard—he should have some fun, too.

Therapist: I agree, but it seems that this fun is coming at your expense—you're working extra hard at your job, taking care of your parents and your sons out of your own paycheck, and he's staying up late buying expensive toys while you go to bed alone.

Ms. B: It's not that bad.... I have a good life, nothing to complain about really...not like some people who have real problems.

Therapist: I'd say having no sex life is a "real" problem, wouldn't you?

Ms. B: Well...maybe that's normal...after all, we're not young anymore. He's a good, hard-working man...at least he's home and not out like some husbands.

Therapist: Sex is a normal part of a healthy marriage throughout the life cycle. Are you really satisfied that while he's home he ignores you?

Ms. B (*looking tearful*): We used to be closer that way, I guess, but...I spend most evenings taking care of my mother when she's not feeling well—I feel so horrible when I feel angry and resentful of her. Or I'm out to dinner with my father, who's miserable with her. Then there are the boys, who always need something. I feel wrung out at the end of the day and exhausted. (*She breaks down and cries.*) I feel so lonely.... I don't blame him for not wanting to be with me.... I look like a wreck and I feel that way, too.

The therapist recognizes the oedipal dynamic and summarizes it for Ms. B:

Therapist: All your life, you have had to distance yourself from your mother in order to protect your special status with your father. Now you distance yourself from your husband—whom your father does not like, just as he does not like your mother—perhaps as a way to maintain closeness with your father.

Ms. B is startled when she realizes that she is repeating the relationship that she has with her parents with her sons, in whom she confides and to whom she complains about her husband. Ms. B and the therapist agree that the problems in her marriage stem from her overly close relationship with her father. They agree that the task is to help Ms. B distance herself from her father and limit her involvement with her sons so that she has more time and energy to work on her marriage.

Initially, Ms. B appears compliant with the treatment goal, although she postpones talking to her husband. The therapist sees the positive paternal transference as a resistance because Ms. B pressures the therapist to reassure her that everything will turn out well while rationalizing waiting to talk to her husband until he is less stressed at work.

Therapist: I think you want me to be like your father, telling you what to do and how to feel, instead of paying attention to your own thoughts and feelings.
Ms. B (*flustered*): I just want to know that things are going to be OK.
Therapist: I think how things turn out depends on your being able to take a risk in asking for the affection and attention you need from your husband.
Ms. B (*crying helplessly*): But what if he says he's too tired from work to spend time with me at night?

The therapist persistently confronts her resistance while monitoring his countertransference for sadistic impulses or sexual arousal in response to her crying.

Soon, Ms. B begins to interact more with her husband, initiating dinner dates and other activities outside of church attendance, and feels more optimistic about the marriage; the therapist understands this as a reaction formation and a *flight into health* given that she has not initiated a discussion about the internet activity and their sex life is still nonexistent. The therapist actively confronts Ms. B's avoidance of conflict with her husband and with her father, who continues to make inordinate demands on her time.

Therapist: Have you talked to your husband yet?
Ms. B: Not yet, he's so stressed out....
Therapist: And you're not?
Ms. B: Well, yes, but it's better now that we've been going out to dinner....
Therapist: I think what you've been saying is that you need more—more love and affection, not just dinners out.
Ms. B (*after a long moment of reflection*): That's true...maybe I can come home earlier from work today, just call my parents instead of stopping by, turn off the phone, and make a nice dinner at home...candles and nice music might put us both in a more relaxed mood to talk.

Ms. B's husband reacts warmly. He acknowledges that he has been frustrated by her indifference to him, which makes him feel old and lonely. He tells her that he has enjoyed the extra time they now spend together and is pleasantly surprised that they are talking openly for the first time in their marriage.

As treatment intensifies, Ms. B gets in touch with her anger, first at the therapist and then at her husband, not only for his internet activity but also for not helping her more with their children and her parents. She then also feels anger at her father for demeaning her husband, for inappropriate demands on her time, and for criticizing her mother. Successfully working through these feelings helps Ms. B create more mature relationships with her parents and husband.

After 5 months of treatment, Ms. B is ready for termination as her attention shifts to her renewed, and increasingly healthy, relationship with her husband. A flexible date for termination is set. The therapist addresses Ms. B's feelings of separation and loss. Ms. B seesaws between feeling ready to go and needing reassurance from her therapist when she experiences conflict with her husband. The therapist encourages her to take on the role he has been playing in questioning her behavior and gives her time to feel ready to terminate treatment. Ms. B resolves her ambivalence and decides that she can handle things on her own. She ends therapy with sadness and gratitude.

Therapy Approach 2: Relational Time-Limited Dynamic Psychotherapy[2]

In keeping with a relational time-limited approach, the first aim is to develop a good working alliance. The therapist tries to acknowledge Ms. B's self-presentation and explore how important it is for her to perform at such a high level with all of her responsibilities. The therapist then begins to discern and to explore the interpersonal context related to Ms. B's story. In order to facilitate deriving a dynamic formulation concerning the relational themes (in content and in process) in her life, a method of organizing clinical information around the CMP (Levenson 1995) is used. With this method, the therapist is particularly interested in what the patient has to say about her own thoughts, wishes, feelings, and behaviors toward others (e.g., "I wish I could do a better job at work"); her expectations of others' behaviors (e.g., "My husband would not like it if I interrupted him while he is on the computer"); the behavior of others (e.g., "My sister leaves me to take care of our parents"); and how she treats and views herself (e.g., "I feel ashamed that sometimes I feel resentful"). These are placed into a narrative that describes the interlocking, interpersonal framework of how one's expectations about how one will be treated by others lead to certain behaviors that then invite others' complementary behaviors, which in turn reinforce a sense of self that leads to further unrewarding actions and expectations, thus becoming a self-fulfilling prophecy—the cyclical pattern of maladaptive behavior. In addition, as part of the TLDP approach, the therapist needs to be very aware of their own internal and external reactions to Ms. B—what the therapist is pulled or pushed to do as they interact with the patient (i.e., interactive countertransference).

Several themes in Ms. B's description of her life and in her style of interacting both in and out of the therapy room emerge, even during the first few sessions, with a recurring interpersonal scenario. Ms. B had always been the good daughter, wife, mother, and worker. Growing up, her place in her family was that of the easy child, for which she got much praise. As she matured, she found that her taking care of everyone else's needs and meeting others' expectations reinforced this role to the extent that she lost touch with what she needed and who she was. Others viewed her as a "can do" type of person and relied on her resourcefulness and consideration. She has seen herself as someone who is ready to make personal sacrifices, and this was congruent with her own self-image. But on the cusp of her sixtieth birthday, Ms. B is feeling resentful of how little time she has for herself and how little attention she has received in her life. Whenever her frustrations "leak out" in an abrupt tone of voice or an angry word, she feels guilty and ashamed. As a consequence, she is quite conflicted about exploring other facets of herself and allowing herself to have a broader range of feelings. Thus, she becomes depressed but can acknowledge it to herself only in the form of somatic complaints, for which she has sought medical treatment.

---

[2] Discussion of this therapy approach was kindly provided by Hanna Levenson, Ph.D.

In the initial session, the therapist experiences Ms. B as very willing to be the "good patient." She readily consents to the therapist's request to videotape her and is reluctant to ask for a different appointment time even though the one given to her was not convenient. In terms of interactive countertransference, the therapist is already aware of wanting something more from her (i.e., more congruent affect, more of a sense of entitlement), just as do others in her life. Her smiling affably while talking of how many demands people place on her and how she tries to meet them all makes the therapist want to shake her and shout, "Don't be such a doormat!" However, her sad eyes and slumped shoulders also pull for compassion.

The primary experiential goal for the therapy, derived from the CMP, is to make use of experiences within the therapy, where Ms. B can put her needs first and not be punished or shamed by the therapist. The therapist also tries to encourage Ms. B's risking this new behavior outside the therapy session and then processing how it goes in the sessions. Consistent with this approach, another goal is to help Ms. B experience and express a wider range of feelings (e.g., anger, joy, pride). In keeping with the relational, recursive model of TLDP, as Ms. B takes a more assertive stance in life, others do not take her as much for granted and come to respect and notice her more. For example, she makes it clear to her husband that she wants to spend more time with him, and he is able to do this, with the result that the marriage is more rewarding for both of them. At work, she is able to set limits on some of her duties and is in the process of asking for a raise when the therapy ends. In session, such changes are also evident. For example, Ms. B becomes irritated with something her therapist says and is able to tell the therapist directly. Ms. B's more active, straightforward behaviors and the resultant changes in how others react to her dramatically affect her sense of self. She comes to see herself as more powerful. She begins to draw again (something she has not done since high school) and is thinking of taking some art classes. Her depression is markedly reduced. Although she is somewhat anxious about "breaking all these old molds," she also leaves therapy after 18 sessions, feeling as if she has a "new lease on life."

The elements of TLDP illustrated in this vignette are the following:

- Need to develop a good alliance quickly
- Delineation of the core cyclical dynamic pattern, which becomes the focus of the work
- Development of experiential goals
- Use of interactive countertransference to inform the formulation as well as to direct the nature of the change
- Opportunity to practice new relational behaviors and attitudes inside and outside the therapy room (i.e., corrective interactive emotional experiences)

Therapy Approach 3: Mann's Integrative Time-Limited Psychotherapy

The therapist using an integrative time-limited approach first conducts several initial interviews to clarify what Ms. B is seeking from therapy and to collect details about her history with which to formulate the central issue, which includes time, affects, and her negative self-image and is stated as follows: "You are a competent, capable, hard-working woman whom others have always been able to depend on. However, you now feel and have always felt unimportant and unworthy." Next, the therapist gauges Ms. B's reaction to the statement, which, in keeping with her compliant attitude, is to agree with the statement, although she says she is surprised and does not know why she feels this way because her life is good and she has been blessed. The therapist then asks Ms. B to agree to a 12-session treatment schedule, informs her of the date and duration of each session, including the date of the final session, and asks for her response. Ms. B says that she's worried she will not know what to talk about because she does not think she has any real problems compared with other people's suffering.

In the first two sessions, a positive transference develops as the therapist encourages Ms. B to talk about the increased demands on her time at work, in caring for her parents, and in helping her sons and as the therapist empathizes with her feelings of chronic fatigue and ill health. Ms. B reports that she looks forward to sessions, and by the third or fourth session she starts to feel better and do more for herself. The therapist maintains a steady focus on the central issue—Ms. B's tendency to sacrifice her own needs for the needs of others, which maintains their dependency and prevents her from experiencing separation and loss through typical developmental phases. During this phase of treatment, the therapist learns a great deal more about the roots of Ms. B's problem in not being allowed to separate and individuate in her original family while growing up. She also begins to talk about her secret fantasy of quitting her job and becoming a travel agent. As the therapist continues to return Ms. B's attention to the central issue by interrupting her fantasies and suggesting they work on the problem at hand, her initial enthusiasm changes to irritation. Now in the middle of the treatment, she experiences the therapist in terms of earlier ambivalence toward her parents, who did not attend to her needs but rather demanded that she be "good" while they focused on her sister, who got the lion's share of their attention while Ms. B was pushed to the sidelines, where she enviously watched her sister's adventures and exploits.

A negatively toned transference develops, and Ms. B begins to resist the treatment. Characteristic defenses such as reaction formation, somatization, and isolation of affect reappear, along with denial of the seriousness of her situation, couched in a religious idiom. In the last set of sessions, Ms. B cancels one because of a vague somatic complaint. When the therapist queries her awareness of the impending end of treatment, she denies remembering that a date for termination was scheduled at the outset and becomes uncharacteristically irritable, complaining that there is not enough time left to solve her problems. She begins to talk about being angry with her boss, who has shifted a number of onerous responsibilities to her job description without taking time to teach her new skills or give her direction. The therapist interprets her anger at her boss and at her parents for expecting too much and not helping her more. He observes that this pattern is being repeated at work, where "being good" has resulted in more work for the same pay without adequate support and guidance.

By now it is obvious that Ms. B's problems stem from her inability to say no to the unreasonable demands of others, especially her parents, who have an extensive social network and sufficient financial resources not to have to rely on her exclusively, and her sons, who are well educated and able-bodied. This situation has alienated her husband, who has retreated into online computer games and perusing eBay. The therapist makes interpretations directed to Ms. B's negative self-image, which has developed over years of subordinating her needs to the needs of others while never being recognized or rewarded for her self-sacrifice and hard work.

The termination phase in time-limited psychotherapy typically involves strong affects. In the next-to-last session, Ms. B questions her faith and rails at God as she unconsciously experiences the therapist as abandoning her. In the last session, Ms. B is more sad than angry and has positive feelings about what she has learned in therapy as she separates from the therapist.

During a 6-month follow-up interview, the interviewer discovers that after an initial period of disorganization and emotional upset, Ms. B did make significant changes in her life in terms of being able to set boundaries with her parents and sons, which freed up time to take a long-postponed vacation with her husband. With his support and encouragement, she asked for a raise and got it, which enhanced her self-esteem. Although she still attends church on Sundays, she continues to question her faith and its demands for unquestioning obedience to authority. As she begins to assert herself, Ms. B's somatic complaints, depression, and fatigue subside, and she has more energy and enthusiasm for life.

Conclusion

The development of brief dynamic psychotherapy has followed a path similar to that of long-term psychodynamic therapy, with drive/structural models adhering to classic psychoanalysis, relational models adhering to the British object relations theory, and integrative models being connected to contemporary psychodynamic theories. Although these approaches have distinctly different flavors, all of them 1) pay attention to the therapeutic relationship, 2) have an active therapeutic stance, 3) emphasize the development of a clear but narrow focus for treatment, 4) have restrictive patient inclusion criteria, and 5) limit the length of therapy and/or number of sessions. Advances in technique have enabled BPP to become an effective treatment for a widening range of patients and disorders (Beutel et al. 2014; Chavooshi et al. 2016; Faramarzi et al. 2013; Mooney et al. 2019; Nanzer et al. 2012; Sattel et al. 2012). Reviews of randomized controlled studies revealed that BPP outcomes are equal to those of long-term therapy and cognitive-behavioral therapy (CBT; Abbass et al. 2014, 2020; Caldiroli et al. 2020; Lilliengren et al. 2016). This is a positive trend given that not all patients require long-term therapy and that some do not respond to other brief therapies such as CBT, interpersonal psychotherapy, and experiential therapies. Studies suggested that BPP can be integrated synergistically with other psychotherapies, medications, and even electroconvulsive therapy to obtain more robust results (Abbass et al. 2013, 2019; de Jonghe et al. 2001; Orvati Aziz et al. 2020; Zhang et al. 2020). Furthermore, the emergence of evidence-based short-term, manualized psychodynamic treatments has interesting implications for reimagining the importance and practicality of psychodynamic training in psychiatry residency education (Sandberg et al. 2012).

Finally, coronavirus SARS-CoV-2 disease (COVID-19) has forced adoption of remote therapy, in which patient and therapist meet virtually. However, a more dramatic advance is in internet-based therapies, in which the therapy is automated and the therapist provides minimal support (Andersson and Carlbring 2018). Good evidence exists that internet-based BPP is effective for depression and anxiety disorders. It is also as effective as internet-based CBT and in one study was chosen more often than CBT (Johansson et al. 2013; Lindegaard et al. 2020; Lindqvist et al. 2020). Clearly, BPP has emerged from the shadow of the better-studied cognitive-behavioral and interpersonal therapies. The decision as to which approach to select for a specific patient should be based on the empirical literature and patient preference rather than the therapist's personal preference. This literature is emerging at a rapid pace and will no doubt support exciting opportunities for both trainees and patients.

Key Points

- There are various models of brief psychodynamic psychotherapy.
- Drive/structural models adhere to Freud's classic psychoanalytic theory.
- Relational models focus on object relations principles.
- Integrative models attend to both classic and object relations principles.
- These models differ according to many variables, such as the therapist's involvement as participant versus observer.
- Most therapies consist of fewer than 24 sessions and last less than 6 months.
- Techniques used in long-term dynamic therapy are also used in brief dynamic therapy.
- Attention is given to rapid formation of a therapeutic alliance.
- Brief therapies can be useful for many patients with a variety of psychiatric problems.
- Randomized controlled trials have demonstrated the efficacy of BPP.

References

Abbass AA, Town JM, Bernier DC: Intensive short-term dynamic psychotherapy associated with decreases in electroconvulsive therapy on adult acute care inpatient ward. Psychother Psychosom 82(6):406–407, 2013 24080831

Abbass AA, Kisely SR, Town JM, et al: Short-term psychodynamic psychotherapies for common mental disorders. Cochrane Database Syst Rev Jul 1 (7):CD004687, 2014 24984083

Abbass A, Town J, Johansson R, et al: Sustained reduction in health care service usage after adjunctive treatment of intensive short-term dynamic psychotherapy in patients with bipolar disorder. Psychodyn Psychiatry 47(1):99–112, 2019 30840559

Abbass A, Town J, Holmes H, et al: Short-term psychodynamic psychotherapy for functional somatic disorders: a meta-analysis of randomized controlled trials. Psychother Psychosom 89(6):363–370, 2020 32428905

Alexander F, French TM: Psychoanalytic Therapy: Principles and Application. New York, Ronald Press, 1946

Andersson G, Carlbring P: Internet-based brief therapies, in The Art and Science of Brief Psychotherapies, 3rd Edition. Edited by Dewan M, Steenbarger B, Greenberg R. Washington, DC, American Psychiatric Association Publishing, 2018, pp 315–326

Balint M, Ornstein PH, Blaint E: Focal Psychotherapy: An Example of Applied Psychoanalysis. London, Tavistock, 1972
Bellak L: Handbook of Intensive Brief and Emergency Psychotherapy, 2nd Edition. Larchmont, NY, CPS, 1992
Ben-Itzhak S, Bluvstein I, Schreiber S, et al: The effectiveness of brief versus intermediate duration psychodynamic psychotherapy in the treatment of adjustment disorder. J Contemp Psychother 42(4):249–256, 2012
Beutel ME, Weißflog G, Leuteritz K, et al: Efficacy of short-term psychodynamic psychotherapy (STPP) with depressed breast cancer patients: results of a randomized controlled multicenter trial. Ann Oncol 25(2):378–384, 2014 24347520
Book H: Guidelines for the practice of brief psychodynamic psychotherapy, in Standards and Guidelines for the Psychotherapies. Edited by Cameron P, Ennis J, Deadman J. Toronto, ON, Canada, University of Toronto Press, 1998, pp 150–180
Bowlby J: A Secure Base: Parent-Child Attachment and Healthy Human Development. New York, Basic Books, 1988
Breuer J, Freud S: Studies on Hysteria. The Standard Edition of the Complete Psychological Works of Sigmund Freud, Vol 2 (1893–1895). Translated and edited by Strachey J. London, Hogarth Press, 1955
Brown LJ: Countertransference: an instrument of the analyst, in Textbook of Psychoanalysis, 2nd Edition. Edited by Gabbard G, Litowitz B, Williams P. Arlington, VA, American Psychiatric Publishing, 2012, pp 79–92
Budman S (ed): Forms of Brief Psychotherapy. New York, Guilford, 1981
Busch FN, Rudden M, Shapiro T: Psychodynamic Treatment of Depression. Washington, DC, American Psychiatric Publishing, 2004
Busch FN, Milrod BL, Singer M, et al: Manual of Panic Focused Psychodynamic Psychotherapy—Extended Range. New York, Routledge, 2012
Busch FN, Rudden M, Shapiro T: Psychodynamic Treatment of Depression, 2nd Edition. Arlington, VA, American Psychiatric Association Publishing, 2016
Caldiroli A, Capuzzi E, Riva I, et al: Efficacy of intensive short-term dynamic psychotherapy in mood disorders: a critical review. J Affect Disord 273:375–379, 2020 32560931
Cashdan S: Object Relations Therapy: Using the Relationship. New York, WW Norton, 1988
Chavooshi B, Mohammadkhani P, Dolatshahi B: A randomized double-blind controlled trial comparing Davanloo intensive short-term dynamic psychotherapy as internet-delivered vs treatment as usual for medically unexplained pain: a 6-month pilot study. Psychosomatics 57(3):292–300, 2016 27017450
Crits-Christoph P, Connolly MB: Alliance and technique in short-term dynamic therapy. Clin Psychol Rev 19(6):687–704, 1999 10421952
Daniel SI: Adult attachment patterns and individual psychotherapy: a review. Clin Psychol Rev 26(8):968–984, 2006 16545897
Davanloo H (ed): Short-Term Dynamic Psychotherapy. New York, Jason Aronson, 1980
Davanloo H: Intensive short-term dynamic psychotherapy, in Comprehensive Textbook of Psychiatry, 8th Edition. Edited by Sadock B, Sadock V. Baltimore, MD, Lippincott Williams & Wilkins, 2004, pp 2628–2652
de Jonghe F, Kool S, van Aalst G, et al: Combining psychotherapy and antidepressants in the treatment of depression. J Affect Disord 64(2–3):217–229, 2001 11313088
de Roten Y, Ambresin G, Herrera F, et al: Efficacy of an adjunctive brief psychodynamic psychotherapy to usual inpatient treatment of depression: results of a randomized controlled trial. J Affect Disord 209:105–113, 2017 27894036
Despland J, Michel L, de Roten Y: Brief Psychodynamic Intervention [in French]. Paris, Elsevier-Masson, 2010
Dewan MJ, Steenbarger BN, Greenberg RP: Brief psychotherapies, in The American Psychiatric Publishing Textbook of Psychiatry, 7th Edition. Edited by Roberts LW. Washington, DC, American Psychiatric Association Publishing, 2019, pp 899–924
Driessen E, Van HL, Don FJ, et al: The efficacy of cognitive-behavioral therapy and psychodynamic therapy in the outpatient treatment of major depression: a randomized clinical trial. Am J Psychiatry 170(9):1041–1050, 2013 24030613

Fairbairn WRD: Steps in the development of an object relations theory of the personality (1949), in Psychoanalytic Studies of the Personality (1959). London, Routledge, 1999, pp 152–161
Faramarzi M, Azadfallah P, Book HE, et al: A randomized controlled trial of brief psychoanalytic psychotherapy in patients with functional dyspepsia. Asian J Psychiatr 6(3):228–234, 2013 23642981
Ferenczi S: The further development of an active therapy in psycho-analysis (1920), in Further Contributions to the Theory and Technique of Psycho-Analysis. Compiled by Rickman J. Translated by Suttie JI. London, Hogarth Press/Institute of Psycho-Analysis, 1926, pp 198–216
French TM: Psychoanalytic Interpretations: The Selected Papers of Thomas M. French. Chicago, IL, Quadrangle Books, 1970
Freud A: The Ego and the Mechanisms of Defense. The Writings of Anna Freud, Vol 2 (1936). New York, International Universities Press, 1966
Freud S: Fragments of an analysis of a case of hysteria (1905), in The Standard Edition of the Complete Psychological Works of Sigmund Freud, Vol 7. Translated and edited by Strachey J. London, Hogarth Press, 1953, pp 7–122
Freud S: The future prospects of psycho-analytic therapy (1910), in The Standard Edition of the Complete Psychological Works of Sigmund Freud, Vol 11. Translated and edited by Strachey J. London, Hogarth Press, 1953, pp 7–12
Freud S: The ego and the id (1923), in The Standard Edition of the Complete Psychological Works of Sigmund Freud, Vol 19. Translated and edited by Strachey J. London, Hogarth Press, 1961, pp 12–66
Garfield SL: The Practice of Brief Psychotherapy. New York, Pergamon, 1989
Goldberg SH: Transference, in Textbook of Psychoanalysis, 2nd Edition. Edited by Gabbard G, Litowitz B, Williams P. Arlington, VA, American Psychiatric Publishing, 2012, pp 65–77
Greenberg JR, Mitchell SA: Object Relations in Psychoanalytic Theory. Cambridge, MA, Harvard University Press, 1983
Gregory RJ, Chlebowski S, Kang D, et al: A controlled trial of psychodynamic psychotherapy for co-occurring borderline personality disorder and alcohol use disorder. Psychotherapy (Chic) 45(1):28–41, 2008 22122363
Gustafson JP: The Complex Secret of Brief Psychotherapy. New York, WW Norton, 1986
Horowitz M: Short term dynamic therapy of stress response syndromes, in Handbook of Short-Term Dynamic Psychotherapy. Edited by Crits-Christoph P, Barber JP. New York, Basic Books, 1991, pp 166–198
Horvath AO, Symonds BD: Relation between working alliance and outcome in psychotherapy: a meta-analysis. J Couns Psychol 38:139–149, 1991
Johansson R, Nyblom A, Carlbring P, et al: Choosing between internet-based psychodynamic versus cognitive behavioral therapy for depression: a pilot preference study. BMC Psychiatry 13:268, 2013 24139066
Jones E: The Life and Work of Sigmund Freud. New York, Basic Books, 1957
Keefe JR, Milrod BL, Gallop R, et al: What is the effect on comorbid personality disorder of brief panic-focused psychotherapy in patients with panic disorder? Depress Anxiety 35(3):239–247, 2018 29212135
Klein M: Our adult world and its roots in infancy (1959), in The Writings of Melanie Klein, Vol 3. London, Hogarth Press, 1975, pp 247–263
Knekt P, Laaksonen MA, Raitasalo R, et al: Changes in lifestyle for psychiatric patients three years after the start of short- and long-term psychodynamic psychotherapy and solution-focused therapy. Eur Psychiatry, 25(1):1–7, 2010 19553088
Laaksonen MA, Knekt P, Sares-Jäske L, et al: Psychological predictors on the outcome of short-term psychodynamic psychotherapy and solution-focused therapy in the treatment of mood and anxiety disorder. Eur Psychiatry 28(2): 117–124, 2013 22705035
Leichsenring F: Are psychodynamic and psychoanalytic therapies effective? A review of empirical data. Int J Psychoanal 86 (Pt 3):841–868, 2005 16096078
Levenson H: Time-Limited Dynamic Psychotherapy: A Guide to Clinical Practice. New York, Basic Books, 1995

Levenson H: Brief Dynamic Therapy, 2nd Edition. Washington, DC, American Psychological Association, 2017

Levenson H: Time-limited dynamic psychotherapy: an integrative perspective, in The Art and Science of Brief Psychotherapies, 3rd Edition. Edited by Dewan MJ, Steenbarger BN, Greenberg RP. Washington, DC, American Psychiatric Association Publishing, 2018, pp 259–300

Levy ST: Principles of Interpretation: Mastering Clear and Concise Interventions in Psychotherapy. Northvale, NJ, Jason Aronson, 2002

Lilliengren P, Johansson R, Lindqvist K, et al: Efficacy of experiential dynamic therapy for psychiatric conditions: a meta-analysis of randomized controlled trials. Psychotherapy (Chic) 53(1):90–104, 2016 26390013

Lindegaard T, Hesslow T, Nilsson M, et al: Internet-based psychodynamic therapy vs cognitive behavioural therapy for social anxiety disorder: a preference study. Internet Interv 20:100316, 2020 32257826

Lindfors O, Knekt P, Virtala E, Laaksonen MA: The effectiveness of solution-focused therapy and short- and long-term psychodynamic psychotherapy on self-concept during a 3-year follow-up. J Nerv Ment Dis 200(11):946–953, 2012 23124178

Lindqvist K, Mechler J, Carlbring P, et al: Affect-focused psychodynamic internet-based therapy for adolescent depression: randomized controlled trial. J Med Internet Res 22(3):e18047, 2020 32224489

Luborsky L: Principles of Psychoanalytic Psychotherapy: A Manual for Supportive-Expressive Treatment. New York, Basic Books, 1984

Luborsky L, Crits-Christoph P: Understanding Transference: The Core Conflictual Relationship Theme Method. New York, Basic Books, 1990

Luborsky L, Mark D: Short-term supportive-expressive psychoanalytic psychotherapy, in Handbook of Short-Term Dynamic Psychotherapy. Edited by Barber JP, Crits-Christoph P. New York, Basic Books, 1991, pp 110–136

Mahler M, Pine F, Bergman A: The Psychological Birth of the Human Infant: Symbiosis and Individuation. New York, Basic Books, 1975

Malan DH: The Frontier of Brief Psychotherapy: An Example of the Convergence of Research and Clinical Practice. New York, Plenum, 1976

Malan DH: Individual Psychotherapy and the Science of Psychodynamics. Toronto, ON, Canada, Butterworths, 1979

Maljanen T, Paltta P, Harkanen T, et al: The cost-effectiveness of short-term psychodynamic psychotherapy and solution-focused therapy in the treatment of depressive and anxiety disorders during a one-year follow-up. J Ment Health Policy Econo 15(1):13–23, 2012 22611089

Mann J: Time-Limited Psychotherapy. Cambridge, MA, Harvard University Press, 1973

Mann J: The core of time-limited psychotherapy: time and the central issue, in Forms of Brief Therapy. Edited by Budman SH. New York, Guilford, 1981, pp 25–43

Mann J: Time-limited psychotherapy, in Handbook of Short-Term Dynamic Psychotherapy. Edited by Crits-Christoph P, Barber JP. New York, Basic Books, 1991, pp 17–44

McCarthy KS, Chambless DL, Solomonov N, et al: Twelve-month outcomes following successful panic-focused psychodynamic psychotherapy, cognitive-behavioral therapy, or applied relaxation training for panic disorder. J Clin Psychiatry 79(5):17m11807, 2018 30256548

Messer SB, Warren CS: Models of Brief Psychodynamic Therapy: A Comparative Approach. New York, Guilford, 1995

Milrod B, Leon AC, Busch F, et al: A randomized controlled clinical trial of psychoanalytic psychotherapy for panic disorder. Am J Psychiatry 164(2):265–272, 2007 17267789

Mooney A, Roberts A, Bayston A, et al: The piloting of a brief relational psychodynamic protocol (psychodynamic addiction model) for problem gambling and other compulsive addictions: a retrospective analysis. Couns Psychother Res 19(4):484–496, 2019

Nanzer N, Sancho Rossignol A, Righetti-Veltema M, et al: Effects of a brief psychoanalytic intervention for perinatal depression. Arch Women Ment Health 15(4):259–268, 2012 22610758

O'Dowd WT: Otto Rank and time-limited psychotherapy. Psychotherapy (Chic) 23(1):140–149, 1986

Orvati Aziz M, Mehrinejad SA, Hashemian K, et al: Integrative therapy (short-term psychodynamic psychotherapy and cognitive-behavioral therapy) and cognitive-behavioral therapy in the treatment of generalized anxiety disorder: a randomized controlled trial. Complement Ther Clin Pract 39:101122, 2020 32379661

Sandberg L, Busch F, Schneier F, et al: Panic-focused psychodynamic psychotherapy in a woman with panic disorder and generalized anxiety disorder. Harv Rev Psychiatry 20(5):268–276, 2012 23030215

Sattel H, Lahmann C, Gündel H, et al: Brief psychodynamic interpersonal psychotherapy for patients with multisomatoform disorder: randomised controlled trial. Br J Psychiatry 200(1):60–67, 2012 22075651

Sifneos P: Short-Term Psychotherapy and Emotional Crisis. Cambridge, MA, Harvard University Press, 1972

Sifneos P: Short-term anxiety-provoking psychotherapy, in Forms of Brief Therapy. Edited by Budman S. New York, Guilford, 1981, pp 45–81

Sifneos P: Short-Term Dynamic Psychotherapy: Evaluation and Technique, 2nd Edition. New York, Springer, 2004

Sørensen P, Birket-Smith M, Wattar U, et al. A randomized clinical trial of cognitive behavioural therapy versus short-term psychodynamic psychotherapy versus no intervention for patients with hypochondriasis. Psychol Med 41(2):431–441, 2011 20380779

Strupp HH, Binder JL: Psychotherapy in a New Key. New York, Basic Books, 1984

Strupp HH, Hadley SW: Specific vs nonspecific factors in psychotherapy: a controlled study of outcome. Arch Gen Psychiatry 36(10):1125–1136, 1979 475546

Strupp HH, Hadley SW, Gomes-Schwartz B: Psychotherapy for Better or Worse. New York, Jason Aronson, 1977

Weiss J, Sampson J, Mount Zion Psychotherapy Research Group: The Psychoanalytic Process: Theory, Clinical Observations, and Empirical Research. New York, Guilford, 1986

Winnicott DW: The Maturational Processes and the Facilitating Environment: Studies in the Theory of Emotional Development. New York, International Universities Press, 1965

Zhang Z, Gao X, Zhou Y, et al: Study on the combination of brief psychodynamic psychotherapy with Viagra in the treatment of non-organic ED. Gen Psychiatr 33(5):e100184, 2020 32875271

Zlotnick E, Strauss AY, Ellis P, et al: Re-evaluating ruptures and repairs in alliance: between- and within-session processes in cognitive–behavioral therapy and short-term psychodynamic psychotherapy. J Consult Clin Psychol 88(9):859–869, 2020 32672994

CHAPTER 4

Theory and Practice of Mentalization-Based Treatment

Anthony Bateman, M.A., FRCPsych
Lois W. Choi-Kain, M.D., M.Ed.
Brandon Unruh, M.D.

Mentalization-based treatment (MBT) was initially developed for the treatment of borderline personality disorder (BPD) (Bateman and Fonagy 2004, 2006a, 2016) and is now recognized in guidelines as an empirically supported treatment (Storebø et al. 2020). Adaptations of the core model of MBT for BPD have been investigated in randomized controlled trials for the treatment of other complex mental health disorders such as antisocial personality disorder (Bateman et al. 2016), eating disorders (Robinson et al. 2016), drug addiction (Philips et al. 2018), and depression (Jakobsen et al. 2014); have been applied to different age groups with specific problems such as self-harming adolescents (Rossouw and Fonagy 2012); and have been implemented in different settings such as day hospitals (Bales et al. 2012; Bateman and Fonagy 1999), inpatient units, prisons (Bateman and Fonagy 2019), and schools (Fonagy et al. 2009). In this chapter we explore why MBT has generated widespread interest and is applied in such a range of conditions and contexts, summarize core principles underpinning mentalizing interventions, and discuss similarities and differences between MBT and other specialist treatments for personality disorder.

MBT as a Generic Mental Health Treatment

The breadth of contexts and the range of conditions in which MBT is delivered are perhaps partly a result of the nature of mentalizing as a higher-order mental process that intersects extensively with all other psychological processes. Even at the biological level, mentalizing relates to brain structure at the top of a hierarchy of layers of abstraction and is a top-down influence on lower orders of this neural pyramid. It has the capacity and function to rearrange processes within the brain and ensure "business as usual" even under adverse conditions. Mentalizing facilitates effective responses to life challenges by generating a psychological understanding of our own actions and those of others in terms of underlying thoughts and feelings. It involves a blend of both cognitive and emotional responses to a challenge, awareness of one's own current experience alongside the experiences of others, and attention to both externally observable and internally subjective aspects of interpersonal interaction (Fonagy and Allison 2014). Mentalizing involves both the process of arriving at this psychological knowledge and the process of responding to such knowledge by designating it as "just thoughts or feelings" not requiring further consideration or, by contrast, a target worthy of serious reflection and a wellspring of purposeful action. Thus, mentalizing operates as an interpersonally contextualized metareflective process including, but not limited to, cognitive appraisal and emotional identification, experiencing, and regulation.

The aim of a mentalizing therapy is to enhance mentalizing processes regardless of the setting in which it is organized, to whom it is delivered, and what condition is being treated. The mentalizing therapist is not primarily or directly aiming to facilitate cognitive restructuring, growth of insight, or behavioral alteration. The focus is more broadly on engaging higher-order processes of the mind. Cognitive and behavioral changes do happen in MBT, and patients may recognize the underlying meaning of their problems and identify causes for why they are the way they are. Such changes, however, are an epiphenomenal consequence of more basic changes in mentalizing, rather like a positive side effect. Here again, mentalizing is a metaconcept, an umbrella term for a whole group of basic psychological operations relevant to treatment process and outcome. Good mentalizing generally enhances the quality of therapeutic interaction because a patient who feels their subjective experience is well understood is more likely to be receptive to therapeutic actions of any kind (Fonagy et al. 2019). Positive changes in mentalizing occurring throughout treatment catalyze further change in cognitions, emotions, and behavior—good mentalizing begets better mentalizing and healthier psychological functioning in general.

This catalyst model of mentalizing is not the whole story about the expansive applicability and efficacy of mentalizing and MBT. Evidence has accrued that individuals who have specific deficits in mentalizing in the context of attachment relationships are those who are currently defined as having a personality disorder (Fonagy and Bateman 2008). This finding is reflected in the Alternative DSM-5 Model for Personality Disorders (American Psychiatric Association 2013), which defines personality functioning as consisting of 1) an intact sense of self that allows coherent identity and effective self-directedness and 2) interpersonal functioning that enables good capacity for empathy and rewards intimacy with others. Mentalizing is the process through which we create a stable and operational sense of self while being able to accurately represent and understand the behavior of others in social contexts through cognitive and affective recognition of their mental states. Therefore, mentalizing is at the heart of both identity and interpersonal aspects of resilient personality function, without which mental health is easily compromised.

A disordered sense of self and dysfunctional interpersonal relationships, driven by problems in mentalizing, may be powerful criteria for personality disorder itself. However, this toxic mix created by mentalizing vulnerabilities encompasses a broader set of challenges beyond the restricted domain of BPD. Because mentalizing is a developmental capacity subject to adaptive changes occurring throughout childhood and adolescence, distortions in the growth of mentalizing are likely to cause problems well beyond personality disorder. This developmental view suggests that individuals with other mental health problems might benefit from their mentalizing problems being directly addressed. In addition, it implies that mentalizing as a fundamental psychological process of development will interface with any major mental disorder that originates in vulnerabilities during childhood and adolescence.

It is therefore not surprising that mentalizing treatments may improve well-being across a range of disorders, earning a place alongside the use of reinforcement or any other general psychological principle with generic applicability. Whatever the source of pathology, whether mentalizing is central or not, disordered mental processes will affect or be affected by the capacity to think and to represent affective experiences. In light of the evidence that a robust sense of self, effective interpersonal relationships, and the capacity to process attachment trauma are dependent on stable mentalizing, it is unsurprising that BPD itself, a disorder of interpersonal relationships, emotional control, and impulsivity, can be conceptualized within a mentalizing framework.

Mentalizing Model of Borderline Personality Disorder

BPD is viewed from a mentalizing standpoint as a disorder of the self that is in line with the contemporary definitions in DSM-5 (American Psychiatric Association 2013) and ICD-11 (World Health Organization 2018). The mentalizing model of BPD asserts that the characteristic interpersonal, emotional, and behavioral problems that make up BPD are the fallout from a central vulnerability in maintaining mentalizing of self and others when challenged with stressors, particularly those that trigger attachment anxiety, such as actual or perceived rejection by a romantic partner or lack of a reassuring response from a friend who seems distant.

The self develops in the affect regulatory context of early relationships and is rooted in attachment processes. Bowlby's (1988) attachment theory and its further elaboration by developmental psychologists highlight the importance of a reciprocity of emotional signaling between the infant and caregiver. Infants instinctively seek to regulate a distressing experience by signaling this distress to an attachment figure through attachment bids such as crying or seeking proximity. The establishment of a coherent and trustworthy sense of self requires these emotional signals to be accurately, or contingently, mirrored by an attachment figure. Mirroring is a misnomer because optimal responding by caregivers displays not a perfect mirror image of the infant's distress but a slightly distorted and even exaggerated expression of what the infant is expressing. Ideal caregiver responses are thus not only contingent but also marked to ensure the infant understands that the caregiver's display is a representation of the infant's emotional experience rather than an expression originating purely within the caretaker (Gergely 2007). In this way the infant will gradually build coherent representations of their own states of mind and those of others to form a robust and discrete sense of self. The absence or unreliable availability of marked contingent mirroring is associated with later development of disorganized attachment in which infants may show behaviors such as freezing (dissociation) and self-harm (e.g., head banging) and may even go on to develop oppositional highly controlling behavioral tendencies in middle childhood. By adulthood the results of the wayward trajectory across development become increasingly variable, with hyperactivation of disorganized and insecure attachment strategies becoming a key pathway to an unstable sense of self in individuals with BPD.

Attachment and mentalizing are loosely coupled developmental systems. Stimulation of attachment inhibits mentalizing, and excessive mentalizing deactivates attachment. Typical experiences of fragmentation within the self-structure related to attachment activation are reduced by the concurrent activation of mentalization. The key to personality function is maintaining effective mentalizing while attachment is triggered and yet being able to let mentalizing go when intimacy is achieved. This balance is disrupted in people with BPD who are unable to harness mentalizing adequately to inhibit fragmentation of self and to manage their attachment anxiety, resulting in an existential crisis with overwhelming emotion that can be managed only through externalization and immediate action, for example, self-harm or violence, to reinstate a stable sense of self and to control emotion.

The most important cause of disruption in the development of effective mentalization in the context of attachment relationships is psychological and/or physical trauma in the context of neglect, early or late in childhood, that undermines the capacity to think about mental states or generate meaningful yet tolerable narrative accounts of one's past relationships (Luyten et al. 2020). Psychological trauma may impair a child's capacity for mentalizing in a number of related ways. In BPD a continual search for attachment security within relationships is paradoxically coupled with a sensitivity to and distrust of others. This combination fosters frantic searching for attachment security or self-protective avoidance. Where the attachment relationship has itself been traumatizing, emotional arousal and epistemic vigilance are exacerbated because seeking proximity to the traumatizing attachment figure may invite further trauma or retraumatization. As a consequence, the attachment system becomes hypersensitive, perpetuating mentalizing impairments within emotionally intense relationship contexts (Bateman and Fonagy 2004). The mentalizing model of BPD therefore requires that therapeutic interventions focus on the patient's capacity to mentalize in the context of attachment relationships if both behavioral and affective aspects of BPD are to change.

Modes for Organizing Subjectivity

Individuals with BPD are "normal" mentalizers, albeit sometimes with a lower base level than others, except in the context of attachment relationships provoking heightened emotion and misreading of mental states within self and others. This is when the phenomenology of BPD appears as a consequence of inhibited mentalizing, which in turn allows the emergence of one or more of three prementalistic *modes* of organizing subjectivity that have the power to disorganize and destroy the narrative coherence of self experience and relationships that is sustained by normal mentalization. These have been termed psychic equivalence, the teleological mode, and the pretend mode (Bateman and Fonagy 2010).

In the mode of *psychic equivalence*, mental experience is rigid and inflexible, such that alternative or additional perspectives cannot be considered, there is no experience of "as if," and everything appears to be "for real." Thoughts and feelings are treated as facts. Mental reality is conflated with outer reality. This adds power and drama to the experience because even an image or fragmented memory (e.g., of an earlier traumatic experience) has the power of current reality and leads to a reaction that appears to others to be an exaggerated response to apparently small events but for the patient is justified by the seriousness with which they suddenly experience their own and others' thoughts and feelings. Psychic equivalence is accompanied by a subjective sense of certainty and finality about one's own views—there is no further room for reflection or reconsideration because the verdict is in about what is happening, what it means, and how one should respond.

Psychic equivalence is often paired with *teleological mode* functioning, in which experience is felt to be valid only when its consequences are externally visible or physically apparent. Mental states are understood primarily from what happens in the real world: the outside determines the inside. For example, affection is felt to be genuine only if it is accompanied by physical expression, or its magnitude is judged by the speed of responsiveness to a text message. One's own experiences are real only if communicated to others through behavior ("I cut myself so that you would see and understand"), and one grasps what others feel or mean only on the basis of their external action or its consequences ("you hurt me, so you must have meant to"). This perspective generates an exquisite sensitivity and skewed responsiveness not just to generally observable behavior but also to subtler cues of facial expression, tone of voice, and gaze. For example, a quick glance of the therapist toward the clock seems to communicate a total lack of investment and care.

Finally, in the *pretend mode*, thoughts and feelings become disconnected to the point of near meaninglessness. In this state patients discuss psychological experiences without contextualizing them in any kind of physical or material reality. The patient is in a world of their own and may attribute extensive and complex motives to their own actions and those of others with little grounding in any reality. Often, there is overrecruitment of cognitive processing systems without any integration with subjective affective experience, resulting in excessive intellectualization, rationalization, jargon, or detailed or aimless narration. Attempting psychotherapy with patients who are in this mode can lead the therapist to lengthy but inconsequential discussions of internal experience that have no impact on or link to genuine experience.

So far we have discussed mentalizing as if it is a unitary or unidimensional phenomenon. But in fact, these modes of ineffective mentalizing are the product of a rigid imbalance of the *dimensions,* or subcomponents, of mentalizing. Mentalizing is a multidimensional construct (Fonagy and Luyten 2009), and when the poles of each dimension become over- or underused or are inappropriately applied, the ineffective mentalizing modes become dominant and lead to disordered interpersonal interaction and disorganization of the self. Adaptive mentalizing, then, is the capacity to flexibly recruit and move between the poles of each dimension as called for by the situation one is in at any given time.

Multidimensional Nature of Mentalizing

Neuroscientists have identified four different mentalizing components, or dimensions, with balanced poles at either end (Lieberman 2007) that reflect different social-cognitive processes. In MBT it is helpful to distinguish the dimensions during clinical assessment of mentalizing along with the dominant default modes because they have significant clinical applications. The dimensions are as follows:

1. Automatic versus controlled mentalizing
2. Mentalizing the self versus mentalizing others
3. Cognitive versus affective mentalizing
4. Internal versus external focus for mentalizing

Mentalizing effectively requires the individual not only to be able to maintain a balance across these dimensions of social cognition but also to apply them appropriately and flexibly according to context (Fonagy and Luyten 2009). From this perspective, different types of psychopathology can be distinguished on the basis of different combinations of impairments along the four dimensions. In an adult with BPD, for example, consistently imbalanced mentalizing in at least one of these four dimensions would be evident. The clinician's dimensional assessment of the mentalizing process during initial sessions begins an individualized approach to the patient. A personalized case formulation is further developed as the clinician and patient collaboratively map out how the interaction between attachment and mentalizing plays out in the patient's life. This formulation is explicitly shared with the patient and written down as the *personal mentalizing profile* (Bateman and Fonagy 2019). It contains, at minimum, an outline of how for a given patient the mentalizing dimensions become imbalanced, how the nonmentalizing modes emerge and operate, and how the patient's attachment strategies are activated by common interpersonal and emotional challenges. This personal mentalizing profile provides the basis of treatment in both individual and group MBT and is repeatedly invoked and revamped as treatment progresses to facilitate steady focus on the patient's presenting or emerging problems.

The most fundamental dimension to mentalizing is the spectrum between *automatic* (or *implicit*) and *controlled* (or *explicit*) mentalizing. Automatic mentalizing involves fast processing; tends to be reflexive; and requires little or no attention, intention, awareness, or effort. Controlled mentalizing reflects a serial and relatively slower process, which is typically verbal and demands reflection, attention, awareness, intention, and effort. Most experts agree that automatic and controlled mentalizing systems arise from different neurocognitive mechanisms, both of which are specialized for thinking about and interpreting mental states (Apperly 2011). The automatic system develops early and tracks mental states in a fast and efficient way, whereas the explicit system develops later, operates more slowly, and makes greater demands on executive functions such as working memory and inhibitory control. In day-to-day life, ordinary social interaction, and therapy, mentalizing tends to be mostly automatic because most straightforward exchanges do not require more attention. In fact, the use of the controlled mentalizing style might hinder such interactions, slowing them down and making them ponderous and uncomfortably overdetailed (hypermentalized) (Sharp and Vanwoerden 2015).

Mentalizing difficulties arise when an individual relies exclusively on automatic assumptions about the mental states of the self or others that are overly simplistic or when applying automatic assumptions creates disharmony and confusion. The switching or rebalancing of this dimension of mentalizing is particularly effective in a secure attachment environment. In contrast, in insecure and disorganized attachment interaction, either an individual relies too much on automatic mentalizing, with no switching to controlled mentalizing when needed, or automatic mentalizing is deactivated through excessive use of controlled mentalizing or hypermentalizing. The task in MBT is to grasp and monitor automatic assumptions, challenging those that appear distorted; the patient should make these assumptions conscious and deliberately reflect on them in partnership with the clinician. This intervention is known as a *contrary move*—a basic MBT intervention that stimulates the opposite pole of a dimension to rebalance mentalizing along that dimension and thereby stimulate synchronous and adaptive activation of all poles of all dimensions (Bateman and Fonagy 2016). Contrary moves are therefore applied when a patient appears to be overusing or underusing any pole of any mentalizing dimension.

Balanced mentalizing further requires the capacity to consider and reflect on experiential states within both *self* and *others*, in various equivalent or mixed proportions, in a way that is adaptive within a particular setting. The two capacities of mentalizing one's own experiences and mentalizing those of others are closely interrelated, such that an imbalance at one pole signals vulnerability at the other. Nevertheless, individuals with mentalizing difficulties are likely to preferentially focus at a given time on one end of the self-other spectrum even though they are impaired at both. Individuals with grandiose or thick-skinned narcissistic traits often display an overly developed self-focus, prioritizing their own experiences while displaying limited concern for or interest in the experiences of others, except when their own self-states are fueled by regarding others' minds in particular ways. In contrast, those with BPD may defer to others' emotional requirements and relegate their own needs to a level of unimportance that creates vulnerability to exploitation. An MBT therapist identifies these mentalizing imbalances early on in the personal mentalizing profile and deploys contrary moves to explore how overuse and underuse of the poles lead to significant problems.

Cognitive mentalizing involves the ability to name, recognize, and reason about mental states (in oneself or others), whereas *affective* mentalizing involves the ability to access and experience the feeling of such states (again, in oneself or others). The latter is necessary for any genuine experience of empathy toward others or any full sense of self. Some individuals give undue weight to either cognitive or affective mentalizing. Patients with BPD may have a deficit of cognitive empathy (Harari et al. 2010; Ritter et al. 2011) coupled with heightened sensitivity toward any kind of emotional cue (Lynch et al. 2006). This suggests that these patients may have an emotional processing advantage, perhaps linked to a combination of amygdala overactivation and orbitofrontal cortex and prefrontal cortex regulatory deficits (Domes et al. 2009). In contrast, patients with narcissistic personality disorder may demonstrate intact cognitive empathy alongside impaired or disengaged emotional empathy (Drozek and Unruh 2020) in that they may accurately identify what others are feeling but do not grasp a corresponding feeling within themselves (Ritter et al. 2011).

Finally, the internal versus external dimension of mentalizing can dominate the clinical process and the daily challenges of people with personality disorder. Good mentalizing along this dimension involves balancing inferences from the *external* indicators of a person's mental states (e.g., facial expressions, tone of voice, body posture) with figuring out someone's *internal* subjective experience from what one knows about them and the situation they are in. It also includes a flexible, balanced analysis of one's own internal and external states. However, an individual with BPD who has poor access to and great uncertainty about their own subjective experience may come to a conclusion about what is felt from observing their own behavior as well as the concrete reactions of others. For instance, a man on a first date decides he is feeling anxious while sensing restlessness in his legs, but soon after that realization, a nervous glance from his partner during their conversation convinces him that instead he must be feeling angry. Another common mentalizing vulnerability in BPD is the conflation of external aspects of others' behavior with the totality of their internal experience, often leading to unbalanced interpersonal responsiveness. For example, a schoolteacher becomes convinced that his students' talking among themselves during the lesson indicates that they hate him, and he explodes at them in a fit of rage and then goes to quit on the spot.

From the perspective of clinical assessment, the internal-external distinction is particularly significant. There has been considerable research on BPD patients' hypersensitivity to facial cues; their performance in the Reading the Mind in the Eyes Test can outperform the norm, creating an impression in clinicians that their patients are better than average mind readers (sometimes called the borderline empathy paradox; Dinsdale and Crespi 2013). This conclusion from the research misses the point that a focus on external features in the absence of reflective mentalizing makes an individual with BPD highly vulnerable in social contexts because it generates the kind of interpersonal hypersensitivity well described by Gunderson and Lyons-Ruth (2008). In MBT, mentalizing interventions often need to start with a clinician examining the patient's interpretations of a person based on external cues and then helping the patient consider an expanded range of plausible associated states of mind while encouraging them to take into account the subtleties and complexities of people's internal worlds (Flasbeck et al. 2017).

MBT Treatment

Principles of MBT

As treatment begins using this model of BPD, MBT clinicians attend carefully to the interface of mentalizing and its relationship with contingency and marking systems in interpersonal interaction, attachment process, representation of self and others, emotional management, and personal affective narratives. The structure of MBT as a manualized clinical intervention with detailed descriptions of the intervention process is fully described elsewhere (Bateman and Fonagy 2006b, 2016), so only some principles will be outlined here.

Coherence of treatment is maintained by a commonality of purpose: all intervention has a primary purpose of facilitating and building robust mentalizing as the driver of epistemic vigilance and learning in the social world. To this end the MBT clinician gives considerable weight to treatment process rather than the content of sessions. Moment-to-moment interventions focus on the way session content is managed mentally, how thoughts are processed, the coherence of self-integration and differentiation from others, the level of congruity of emotion and cognition, and the tolerance of uncertainty and ambiguity. These interventions stabilize the patient's internal processing as well as the reciprocity of interaction between clinician and patient. Only then are trauma history, narrative content, and relational processes brought to the foreground and explored in detail.

MBT is delivered as an individual or group treatment or a combination of both, with research studies suggesting it is most effective for patients who show severe BPD and other personality disorders with co-occurring conditions such as substance use disorders, eating disorders, and PTSD and who have extensive social problems with chronic unemployment (Bateman and Fonagy 2013). Assessment follows a structured pathway, with a psychiatric evaluation followed by an assessment of the patient's personal mentalizing profile as discussed in the section "Multidimensional Nature of Mentalizing," which forms the core of the initial MBT formulation along with an agreement centered on the patient's value system.

Clarifying values is particularly important in MBT for antisocial personality disorder because interactions between patients and the criminal justice system create a clash of values and cultures in which patients experience the "system" as being coercive and forcing them to behave and think in ways that do not fit them. This is contrary to the mentalizing approach, which does not aim at controlling behavior or enforcing social conformity. Because mentalizing is developmentally acquired within a specific social context, the particular contours of any individual's mentalizing process will evince the priorities of its environmental origins. Hence, a joint mentalizing process in which both patient and clinician harness appreciation for each other's subjectivity is, perhaps, the only valid approach to appreciating cultural differences, recognizing alternative perspectives, and accepting different value systems. Thus, MBT's central focus on subjectivity steers therapist and patient together toward the core of human nature as biologically embedded in the intimately related constructs of community, trust, culture, and cooperation. Mentalizing is not bound in any one culture or limited by a rigid set of values but rather serves to bind groups together to form culture, understand cultural differences, and share values. The start of this process in treatment is for the patient and clinician to explicitly formulate their values and to use those values to determine the aims of treatment.

Once a formulation is collaboratively established, treatment begins with an introductory group socializing the patient to the model through psychoeducation about effective and ineffective mentalizing, attachment, emotions, and the treatment process itself. The topics discussed in the group are somewhat tailored to patient characteristics. For example, highly suicidal and self-harming patients work on safety and managing their actions, antisocial patients work on the relationship between mentalizing problems and violence and coercive control of others, and patients with eating disorders reframe eating problems in terms of difficulties with mentalizing bodily experiences and a tendency to retreat from a socially interactive world. At the end of the engagement period the clinician and patient share a value system, a treatment approach, and recognition of the centrality of mentalizing in addressing the problems they have defined together in the formulation.

MBT as a Principle-Driven Intervention

The practitioner's powerful commitment to the patient's subjectivity has intrinsic value in any treatment. At the core of the clinical practice of MBT lie a consistent focus on the subjective reality of the patient and a consistent effort to convey that the therapist is working to grasp the world from the patient's perspective. To maintain this focus, clinicians implementing MBT follow a structured intervention process during sessions on the basis of a series of principles. These principles are listed in Table 4–1.

Mentalizing and anxiety interact in ways that show a particularly strong interrelationship between attachment anxiety and quality of mentalizing. Mentalizing improves initially with increasing anxiety until a tipping point is reached, beyond which mentalizing decreases rapidly, leaving anxiety untethered and likely to overwhelm and trigger fight or flight. Patients with BPD, albeit primarily those with attachment or interpersonal challenges, reach this intrinsic tipping point more quickly and in a wider range of circumstances than others. Once a fight-or-flight state is in progress, patients cannot easily recover mental stability. Hence, these patients frequently experience emotional dysregulation and desperately attempt to restabilize and regulate through actions such as self-harm. Given that highly destabilizing interpersonal interactions result from insecure ambivalent attachment patterns being triggered in those with BPD, escalating anxiety and emotional expression are treated with great care to support mentalizing rather than undermine it.

But the converse situation of insufficient anxiety is also a danger for the clinician because the patient's attachment/mentalizing system will not be productively stimulated, leading to the patient not learning how to manage feelings, maintain mentalizing in relationships, and change. Some patients, such as those with more antisocial characteristics, downregulate or deactivate attachment anxiety with varying degrees of success. In the absence of attachment anxiety, mentalizing works to some extent, but it becomes restricted, for example, by excessive use of cognitive mentalizing with limited activation of affective mentalizing.

An imbalance in this direction of the cognitive/affective dimension leads to calm but an inability to use mentalizing flexibly. Cognitive rigidity ensues and generates the cold, calculated calm of the person with antisocial personality disorder and psychopathic traits who may have excessive cognitive mentalizing with no access to self-affective states and subjective experience of others with which they emotionally empathize (Bateman et al. 2013). For mentalizing to flourish in social and personal interaction, attachment and anxiety are necessary yet need to be kept within a range—not too much and not too little. Therefore, the first principle that MBT clinicians follow in treatment is to maintain anxiety within a range that encourages rather than inhibits mentalizing. A variety of techniques may be used to titrate the level of anxiety up or down as needed on the basis of shifting here-and-now assessments of how close a patient may be to their mentalizing tipping points or to losing sufficient arousal needed to foster mentalizing.

The second principle is to use contrary moves to rebalance mentalizing across the four dimensions of automatic/controlled, self/other, cognitive/affective, and internal/external when necessary in the context of attachment anxiety. For example, when patients with BPD are anxious, they show difficulties with separating self and other as a result of low levels of mentalizing, so the task is to help them reinstate a separateness and distinction between what they feel versus what others feel. The problem and solu-

TABLE 4–1. Principles to follow in mentalization-based treatment

Do
Manage anxiety and titrate attachment anxiety (relational/practical/functional mentalization)
Maintain flexibility of mentalizing dimensions with contrary moves such as the following:
Affect–cognitive dimension balance for deactivation and hyperactivation functioning
Self-other focus to generate *we-ness*
Intervene with contingent and marked responses to patient mental state as initial intervention
Follow the affect if mentalizing is stable; otherwise, use a contrary move to activate cognitive processing
Roll with the reaction of patient to emotional narratives
Do not
Join with nonmentalizing
Take over patient mentalizing
Mentalize nonmentalizing
Meet patient's low mentalizing with clinician's high mentalizing
Respond to patient as if they were mentalizing

tion are different in patients with narcissistic personality disorder, who may overinflate their self-experience and derogate others' experience, so the task is to use contrary moves to either rekindle the vestigial pole of regard for others or puncture gently (with careful concurrent empathic validation) the inflated pole of self-valuation (Drozek and Unruh 2020).

The third principle is to elevate mentalizing of self and other toward representing and effectively responding to what is happening within the current therapeutic relationship. This begins with ensuring that the representational levels of both self-experience and experience of the other are activated, separated, differentiated within affective experience, and, when possible, elevated to a *we-ness* experience that is a representational capacity of the relationship as something more than self and other. This is a perspective that transcends what occurs within the separate selves of *you* and *me* to represent what is occurring for the relational unit of *us* (Gallotti and Frith 2013; O'Madagain and Tomasello 2021; Tomasello 2016).

Higher levels of mentalizing go beyond individuality. Effective social interaction is partly dependent on groups of individuals seeing their actions as collaboratively directed in pursuit of a shared goal (as a *we*). This sense of we-ness is a striking feature of the psychology of collective behavior because individuals share their minds in a collective mode, and in doing so create another mind that is neither me nor you nor any of us. It is this collective mode of cognition that is called the we-mode in MBT. We-ness in the clinical interaction is distinct from either patient or clinician individual self/other perspectives. As an inherently relational representation, it is a state actively developed and promoted in MBT, starting with the joint formulation and personal mentalizing profile, followed by working explicitly not only with the mind states of the patient but also with those of the clinician. MBT clinicians openly present their mind states and their counterrelational responses to the patient, clarifying that neither person in the therapeutic interaction has a monopoly on valid views of reality and both must accept that each side experiences interpersonal interactions only impressionistically. The patient is asked to mentalize the clinician just as the clinician has to mentalize the patient. A sense of we-ness emerges as both are beholden to the shared task of mentalizing both self and other. In MBT groups, a sense of we-ness is additionally generated as participants define "our" group values at the outset and then revisit and reformulate the group project around those values at regular intervals (Bateman et al. 2021).

A fourth principle is for clinicians to make sure they do not join in at a process level when patients are in a low mentalizing state. It is all too easy for a clinician to start persuading a patient that their self-criticism is incorrect or lacking in evidence or to argue with their subjective experience that someone rejected them by pointing out their social sensitivity only to find that this makes matters worse, making the patient angry and leaving them feeling misunderstood.

In order not to join with the low mentalizing process, the clinician follows the fifth principle of intervening, initially using contingent and marked responses (Gergely 2007; Watson 1995) of *empathic validation* to facilitate a we-ness organized first around seeing things jointly from the patient's perspective. Humans are sensitive to the existence of contingencies between their behavior and environmental events and are equally sensitive to their own mental state intention and the mental response from others. It is our contention that contingency detection as an aspect of interpersonal interaction is crucially involved in progressively developing awareness of internal affective states. More specifically, the caregiver's contingent reflections of the patient's expressive displays while the patient struggles to mentalize play a central causal role in the development of emotional self-awareness and control, which is a central aspect of mentalizing but requires scaffolding and support in people with personality disorder. Thus, the clinician operates within a framework of empathic validation of the patient's experience as the foundation for all other interventions.

The final group of principles can be joined together. It is necessary to ensure that the therapeutic process remains a joint creation between patient and therapist while ensuring that the clinician not only recognizes low-level mentalizing but also does not take over mentalizing for the patient or mentalize nonmentalizing. None of these principles is as easy to follow as it sounds. All too often, clinicians are tricked into believing that the pretend mode is psychological insight when it takes the form of subtle hypermentalizing in which the motives of others and one's own contribution to problems are asserted in seemingly reflective complexity but with no grounding in reality. Clinicians have robust mentalizing capacities and may take over the patient's struggle to explore problems by giving constructive solutions to their concerns. It is natural to support and to offer help and provide alternative perspectives and solutions for the patient's challenges, but the patient's mentalizing muscle is never going to be exercised and strengthened unless it is used. Clinicians need to desist from doing the mentalizing for the patient and instead work consistently to trigger the patient's mentalizing and then help them maintain it.

MBT and Other Specialist Treatment for Borderline Personality Disorder

The fact that the diverse evidence-based treatments for BPD yield comparable improvements in this difficult-to-treat diagnostic population may suggest that their common features are generically responsible for their major effects more so than their unique components. Shared features of these specialist approaches include a well-specified formulation of BPD; a highly structured treatment with a selective focus, clear aims, and consistent procedures; and the activation of a strong and durable treatment relationship (Bateman 2012; Gabbard 2007). Dialectical behavior therapy (DBT; Linehan 1993) and schema-focused therapy (SFT; Young et al. 2003) both evolved from the observation that patients with BPD do not typically respond as usual to cognitive-behavioral therapy and require specially tailored adjustment to avoid the negative therapeutic reactions that expectably interfere with treatment effectiveness. Transference-focused psychotherapy (TFP; Clarkin et al. 2006) developed from the empirical findings of the Menninger Foundation's Psychotherapy Research Project that patients with BPD had greater responsiveness to an approach combining a focus on transference interpretations with a well-delineated treatment framework compared with both standard psychoanalytic psychotherapy and supportive psychotherapy (Kernberg et al. 2008). The central concepts and tools defining MBT overlap significantly with those found in DBT, SFT, and TFP. Arguably, all of these treatments work by enabling more steady reflection about mental states in oneself and others and likely generate epistemic trust and social learning via their endeavor to recognize and make clear sense of key problems that patients with BPD face. Therefore, all of these approaches are considered to be effective in promoting mentalization by stabilizing emotional expression, enhancing relational functioning, and evaluating needed change. Here we review the overlaps among these alternative specialist treatments to illustrate their intrinsically mentalizing effects as well as crucial differences that operate to preserve their coherence.

DBT consists of an abundance of ready-made protocols and skills that enable individuals with BPD to better comprehend and then more effectively problem solve emotional challenges. DBT formulates borderline personality as a disorder of emotional dysregulation, which results from chronic exposure of emotionally sensitive individuals with insufficient coping skills to invalidating responses from others that reinforce avoidance of emotions and self-damaging behavior. Therefore, validation is a technical starting point for DBT therapists because it reduces the putative symptom-generating effects of critical rejecting responses. Empathic validation in MBT also reduces BPD symptoms that threaten the goals of treatment but does so by providing marked and contingent mirroring of the patient's inner experience, which ultimately makes attention to and appreciation of mental states tolerable, so that the self-monitoring metacognition needed for reappraisal of one's own views as well as the realistic appreciation of what occurs in others' minds can be activated. In both approaches, validation becomes a primer for different but equally essential tasks of psychotherapy. Dialectical thinking in DBT and contrary moves in MBT also similarly operate to join fragmented and contradictory aspects of the patient's experience together in a more coherent depiction of reality and relationships. These functionally balancing maneuvers counteract black-and-white thinking and establish more consistent access to a continuous understanding of oneself. In the same vein, exercising attentional regulation of and detachment from mental states is a central aim of both mindfulness practice and mentalization, which inherently facilitate self-awareness, integration of emotionality and rationality, and self-control. Both mindfulness and mentalization therefore build agency and self-esteem. Mindfulness does so by reinforcing effective and self-affirming decision-making, whereas mentalization does so via the formation of a coherent self-narrative and steady navigation of one's social world.

Although mentalization is a more explicitly interpersonal construct than mindfulness and, overall, MBT is a more relationally focused treatment in comparison with DBT (Swenson and Choi-Kain 2015), their distinctive techniques overlap in their effect, possibly working via resultant improvements in mentalizing. Theoretically, the incorporation of MBT elements into DBT treatments could potentiate DBT's mentalizing effects (Swenson and Choi-Kain 2015). In fact, the addition of MBT group therapy to DBT was shown to reduce fearful attachment and increase mentalization of affect more than DBT alone (Edel et al. 2017). However, the degree of focus on specific skills content and predetermined protocols for self-examination inherent in DBT may be incompatible with MBT's insistence on generating a mentalizing process over any predetermined content.

The other remaining therapies, SFT and TFP, share a focus on early disruptive attachment experiences and impaired representational capacities as the basis of BPD pathology. However, SFT and TFP both diverge from MBT more completely in their process and techniques. SFT identifies four modes, or codified expressions of affect, thought, and relating, that drive the symptomatic expressions of persons with BPD: the abandoned and abused child, the angry impulsive child, the detached protector, and the punitive parent. These modes problematically remain unintegrated and fluctuating in individuals with BPD in the context of a deficiently developed, uninternalized healthy adult mode that provides thoughtful consideration and effective problem solving (i.e., executive functions), alongside clear boundaries containing healthy relationships (Kellogg and Young 2006). The therapeutic procedure linked to SFT's formulation of BPD involves the identification of these modes, joined with efforts by the therapist to supply the healthy adult presence and support that was lacking earlier. The ultimate goal of SFT's limited reparenting intervention is to allow the patient to internalize a more consistent healthy adult mode, which confers identity, confidence, and sense of agency that was previously fragmented and undeveloped.

TFP emphasizes identity diffusion and disturbed object relations as the key drivers of personality pathology. The primitive defense of splitting, caused by the patient's avoidance of the inherent anxieties and ambivalence of a more integrated way of viewing oneself in relation to others, promotes fragmentation and interferes with the patient's capacity to realistically represent themselves and others in relationships (i.e., mentalize). As a result, what is observed is an unstable oscillation between aggressive and idealized objects relations, which disrupts the patient's capacity for stable intimacy, professional development, and social functioning. TFP's explicit treatment frame introduces a necessary delineation of what is expectable and prohibited in the scope of the therapeutic interaction, which, when combined with restraint regarding supportive interventions, provokes frustrations that inevitably activate the patient's split internalized object relations. The TFP therapist then aims to confront and interpret the fragmented contradictory nature of these oscillating self-object representations to counteract defensive avoidance of their more realistic, but sobering, integration.

Both SFT and TFP prescribe interventions, namely, the identification of specified schemas or modes and interpretation of transference, that position the therapist, rather than the patient, as the predominant mentalizing force, who issues independently formed reflections on how patients function and why they act as they do. These techniques convey a degree of unrealistic certainty and privilege to the therapist's perspective as reflecting insight that patients should adopt. These maneuvers are potentially iatrogenic in terms of inducing the pretend mode in patients with BPD, who, according to the mentalizing model, may not comprehend, relate to, or gain meaningful self-understanding from sharing insight or being given skills directives. Furthermore, these techniques presume that patients have a level of intact mentalizing symbolically at play in SFT and at a level to understand interpretations of transference enactments in TFP that are potentially unrealistic for individuals with BPD.

Despite these technical differences, SFT and TFP still result in the promotion of the patient's capacity to make more coherent sense of themselves and others in terms of more nuanced appreciation of mental states and, through their distinctive techniques, promote a process of reappraisal, refinement, and integration that is inherently mentalizing. Evidence that TFP promotes reflective functioning has suggested that mentalizing might be a key mechanism of the symptomatic change it generates in individuals with BPD (Levy et al. 2006). Furthermore, psychotherapy process research has also indicated that mentalizing processes are significantly correlated with DBT and TFP specifically and cognitive-behavioral therapy and psychodynamic approaches more broadly (Goodman 2013). Although mentalizing is compatible with these various specialist treatments for BPD, we remain cautious about eclectic integration of their components, considering the likelihood that their coherent discrete formulations, well-structured focus, and related techniques act as a package to provide the major foundation of their established efficacy.

Key Points

- Mentalizing vulnerabilities are central to personality dysfunction.
- Loss of mentalizing results in psychiatric symptoms, impulsivity, and problems of interpersonal and social function.
- Mentalization-based treatment is a principle-driven treatment with a primary aim of stabilizing and enhancing mentalizing.
- All effective treatments for personality disorder enable steady reflection on mental states of self and others and generate epistemic trust and social learning.

References

American Psychiatric Association: Diagnostic and Statistical Manual of Mental Disorders, 5th Edition. Arlington, VA, American Psychiatric Association, 2013

Apperly IA: Mindreaders: The Cognitive Basis of "Theory of Mind." Hove, UK, Psychology Press, 2011

Bales D, van Beek N, Smits M, et al: Treatment outcome of 18-month, day hospital mentalization-based treatment (MBT) in patients with severe borderline personality disorder in the Netherlands. J Pers Disord 26(4):568–582, 2012 22867507

Bateman AW: Treating borderline personality disorder in clinical practice. Am J Psychiatry 169(6):560–563, 2012 22684591

Bateman A, Fonagy P: Effectiveness of partial hospitalization in the treatment of borderline personality disorder: a randomized controlled trial. Am J Psychiatry 156(10):1563–1569, 1999 10518167

Bateman A, Fonagy P: Psychotherapy for Borderline Personality Disorder: Mentalization-Based Treatment. Oxford, UK, Oxford University Press, 2004

Bateman A, Fonagy P: Mentalizing and borderline personality disorder, in Handbook of Mentalization-Based Treatment. Edited by Allen JG, Fonagy P. Chichester, UK, Wiley, 2006a, pp 185–200

Bateman AW, Fonagy P: Mentalization-Based Treatment for Borderline Personality Disorder: A Practical Guide. Oxford, UK, Oxford University Press, 2006b

Bateman A, Fonagy P: Mentalization based treatment for borderline personality disorder. World Psychiatry 9(1):11–15, 2010 20148147

Bateman A, Fonagy P: Impact of clinical severity on outcomes of mentalisation-based treatment for borderline personality disorder. Br J Psychiatry 203(3):221–227, 2013 23887998

Bateman A, Fonagy P: Mentalization-Based Treatment for Personality Disorders: A Practical Guide. Oxford, UK, Oxford University Press, 2016

Bateman A, Fonagy P (eds): Handbook of Mentalizing in Mental Health Practice, 2nd Edition. Washington, DC, American Psychiatric Association Publishing, 2019

Bateman A, Bolton R, Fonagy P: Antisocial personality disorder: a mentalizing framework. Focus Am Psychiatr Publ 11(2):178–186, 2013

Bateman A, O'Connell J, Lorenzini N, et al: A randomised controlled trial of mentalization-based treatment versus structured clinical management for patients with comorbid borderline personality disorder and antisocial personality disorder. BMC Psychiatry 16:304, 2016 27577562

Bateman A, Campbell C, Fonagy P: Rupture and repair in mentalization-based group psychotherapy. Int J Group Psychother 71(2):371–392, 2021

Bowlby J: A Secure Base: Parent-Child Attachment and Healthy Human Development. New York, Basic Books, 1988

Clarkin JF, Yeomans FE, Kernberg OF: Psychotherapy for Borderline Personality: Focusing on Object Relations. Washington, DC, American Psychiatric Publishing, 2006

Dinsdale N, Crespi BJ: The borderline empathy paradox: evidence and conceptual models for empathic enhancements in borderline personality disorder. J Pers Disord 27(2):172–195, 2013 23514182

Domes G, Schulze L, Herpertz SC: Emotion recognition in borderline personality disorder—a review of the literature. J Pers Disord 23(1):6–19, 2009 19267658

Drozek RP, Unruh BT: Mentalization-based treatment for pathological narcissism. J Pers Disord 34(suppl):177–203, 2020 32186985

Edel MA, Raaff V, Dimaggio G, et al: Exploring the effectiveness of combined mentalization-based group therapy and dialectical behavior therapy for inpatients with borderline personality disorder—a pilot study. Br J Clin Psychol 56(1):1–15, 2017 27897326

Flasbeck V, Enzi B, Brüne M: Altered empathy for psychological and physical pain in borderline personality disorder. J Pers Disord 31(5):689–708, 2017 28072040

Fonagy P, Allison E: The role of mentalizing and epistemic trust in the therapeutic relationship. Psychotherapy (Chic) 51(3):372–380, 2014 24773092

Fonagy P, Bateman A: Attachment, mentalization, and borderline personality disorder. European Psychotherapy 8(1):35–47, 2008

Fonagy P, Luyten P: A developmental, mentalization-based approach to the understanding and treatment of borderline personality disorder. Dev Psychopathol 21(4):1355–1381, 2009 19825272

Fonagy P, Twemlow SW, Vernberg EM, et al: A cluster randomized controlled trial of child-focused psychiatric consultation and a school systems-focused intervention to reduce aggression. J Child Psychol Psychiatry 50(5):607–616, 2009 19207633

Fonagy P, Allison E, Campbell C: Mentalizing, resilience, and epistemic trust, in Handbook of Mentalizing in Mental Health Practice, 2nd Edition. Edited by Bateman A, Fonagy P. Washington, DC, American Psychiatric Association Publishing, 2019, pp 63–77

Gabbard GO: Do all roads lead to Rome? New findings on borderline personality disorder. Am J Psychiatry 164(6):853–855, 2007 17541040

Gallotti M, Frith CD: Social cognition in the we-mode. Trends Cogn Sci 17(4):160–165, 2013 23499335

Gergely G: The social construction of the subjective self: the role of affect-mirroring, markedness, and ostensive communication in self development, in Developmental Science and Psychoanalysis: Integration and Innovation. Edited by Mayes L, Fonagy P, Target M. London, Karnac Books, 2007, pp 45–82

Goodman G: Is mentalization a common process factor in transference-focused psychotherapy and dialectical behavior therapy sessions? J Psychother Integration 23(2):179–192, 2013

Gunderson JG, Lyons-Ruth K: BPD's interpersonal hypersensitivity phenotype: a gene-environment-developmental model. J Pers Disord 22(1):22–41, 2008 18312121

Harari H, Shamay-Tsoory SG, Ravid M, et al: Double dissociation between cognitive and affective empathy in borderline personality disorder. Psychiatry Res 175(3):277–279, 2010 20045198

Jakobsen JC, Gluud C, Kongerslev M, et al: Third-wave cognitive therapy versus mentalisation-based treatment for major depressive disorder: a randomised clinical trial. BMJ Open 4(8):e004903, 2014 25138802

Kellogg SH, Young JE: Schema therapy for borderline personality disorder. J Clin Psychol 62(4):445–458, 2006 16470629

Kernberg OF, Diamond D, Yeomans FE, et al: Mentalization and attachment in borderline patients in transference focused psychotherapy, in Mind to Mind: Infant Research, Neuroscience, and Psychoanalysis. Edited by Jurist EL, Slade A, Bergner S. New York, Other Press, 2008, pp 167–201

Levy KN, Meehan KB, Kelly KM, et al: Change in attachment patterns and reflective function in a randomized control trial of transference-focused psychotherapy for borderline personality disorder. J Consult Clin Psychol 74(6):1027–1040, 2006 17154733

Lieberman MD: Social cognitive neuroscience: a review of core processes. Annu Rev Psychol 58:259–289, 2007 17002553

Linehan MM: Cognitive-Behavioral Treatment of Borderline Personality Disorder. New York, Guilford, 1993

Luyten P, Campbell C, Fonagy P: Borderline personality disorder, complex trauma, and problems with self and identity: a social-communicative approach. J Pers 88(1):88–105, 2020 31066053

Lynch TR, Rosenthal MZ, Kosson DS, et al: Heightened sensitivity to facial expressions of emotion in borderline personality disorder. Emotion 6(4):647–655, 2006 17144755

O'Madagain C, Tomasello M: Joint attention to mental content and the social origin of reasoning. Synthese 198:4057–4078 2021

Philips B, Wennberg P, Konradsson P, et al: Mentalization-based treatment for concurrent borderline personality disorder and substance use disorder: a randomized controlled feasibility study. Eur Addict Res 24(1):1–8, 2018 29402870

Ritter K, Dziobek I, Preissler S, et al: Lack of empathy in patients with narcissistic personality disorder. Psychiatry Res 187(1–2):241–247, 2011 21055831

Robinson P, Hellier J, Barrett B, et al: The NOURISHED randomised controlled trial comparing mentalisation-based treatment for eating disorders (MBT-ED) with specialist supportive clinical management (SSCM-ED) for patients with eating disorders and symptoms of borderline personality disorder. Trials 17(1):549, 2016 27855714

Rossouw TI, Fonagy P: Mentalization-based treatment for self-harm in adolescents: a randomized controlled trial. J Am Acad Child Adolesc Psychiatry 51(12):1304–1313.e3, 2012 23200287

Sharp C, Vanwoerden S: Hypermentalizing in borderline personality disorder: a model and data. J Infant Child Adolesc Psychother 14(1):33–45, 2015

Storebø OJ, Stoffers-Winterling JM, Völlm BA, et al: Psychological therapies for people with borderline personality disorder. Cochrane Database Syst Rev 5(5):CD012955, 2020 32368793

Swenson CR, Choi-Kain LW: Mentalization and dialectical behavior therapy. Am J Psychother 69(2):199–217, 2015 26160623

Tomasello M: A Natural History of Human Morality. Cambridge, MA, Harvard University Press, 2016

Watson JS: Self-orientation in early infancy: the general role of contingency and the specific case of reaching to the mouth, in The Self in Infancy: Theory and Research. Edited by Rochat P. Amsterdam, Elsevier, 1995, pp 375–393

World Health Organization: ICD-11 for Mortality and Morbidity Statistics. Geneva, World Health Organization, 2018

Young JE, Klosko JS, Weishaar ME: Schema Therapy: A Practitioner's Guide. New York, Guilford, 2003

CHAPTER 5

Transference-Focused Psychotherapy for Levels of Personality Pathology Severity

John F. Clarkin, Ph.D.
Eve Caligor, M.D.
Julia F. Sowislo, Ph.D.

Transference-focused psychotherapy (TFP) is a principle-driven, transdiagnostic psychodynamic psychotherapy for treatment of personality pathology. Although TFP was originally articulated (Clarkin et al. 1999), developed (Yeomans et al. 2015), and empirically validated (Clarkin et al. 2001, 2007; Doering et al. 2010) as an intensive individual psychotherapy for the treatment of patients with the categorical diagnosis of borderline personality disorder (BPD), the treatment has since been adapted to meet the clinical needs of a wide range of personality disorder presentations and levels of severity, ranging from subsyndromal personality pathology through severe personality disorder (Caligor et al. 2018). This evolution from a diagnosis-specific to a transdiagnostic treatment model reflects developments in the understanding of personality pathology, within which the categorical diagnosis of BPD is now seen as part of a large general factor of disordered personality functioning (Sharp et al. 2015). This general factor is characterized by deficits in self-functioning and interpersonal functioning, which may range from minor to severe, and is conceptually similar to Kernberg's (1984) borderline personality organization. In concert with these developments, TFP and its procedures have been articulated for the treatment and improvement of self- and interpersonal functioning of individuals who present with a range of personality disorders at different levels of functional severity (Caligor et al. 2018), as well as various symptom conditions such as depression that frequently emerge in the setting of personality pathology (Simon et al. 2015).

As a general principle, TFP is focused on treating the self-functioning and interpersonal functioning specific to a distressed individual rather than on a particular, categorical DSM diagnosis. This general principle is consistent with the growing focus on precision medicine (Cohen and DeRubeis 2018). In TFP, techniques are not applied in a lockstep approach with the same sequence and content for every patient but rather are flexibly applied, taking into account the individual patient's level of personality dysfunction, unique transference patterns, personal environment, and therapeutic relationship. As stated succinctly by the authors of the evidence-based psychotherapy guidelines (Norcross and Lambert 2019), any influence of therapeutic technique depends on the nature of the relationship between patient and therapist. This is especially true of the treatment of individuals with personality disorder, who, by definition, have mild to severe difficulties in relating to others, including the therapist. With this in mind, the TFP therapist pays close attention to the evolving relationship between patient and therapist from moment to moment in each session and throughout the course of treatment. Techniques are flexibly introduced into the unique dialogue with the patient so that the patient's resistance is identified and reduced and reflection is enhanced.

Description of the Treatment Model and Clinical Approach

The techniques of TFP are grounded in an understanding of personality pathology based on object relations theory (Kernberg 1984; Kernberg and Caligor 2005) and in the general principles of psychodynamic therapy. Kernberg (2018) has described the basic technical interventions that characterize psychoanalytic treatment as interpretation, transference analysis, technical neutrality, and countertransference utilization. In TFP these basic techniques are used in the context of a carefully structured treatment frame and are systematically modified to meet the clinical needs of an individual patient with a particular level of severity of personality dysfunction (i.e., neurotic and high-, mid-, and low-level borderline organization) (Table 5–1).

Model of Personality Pathology: Central Mechanism and Nosology

The cornerstone of the object relations theory model of personality functioning and pathology is the construct of identity. Identity is seen as the central psychological structure organizing self- and interpersonal functioning, and pathology of identity formation is the defining feature of the personality disorders as a group (Kernberg 1984; Kernberg and Caligor 2005). Normal identity formation, or identity consolidation, corresponds to a core sense of self that is stable, coherent, realistic, and continuous across time; a commensurate stable and rich experience of significant others; and an affective experience that is complex and well modulated (Clarkin et al. 2020). In contrast, failure of identity consolidation corresponds to a sense of self and others that

TABLE 5–1. Severity of personality pathology: implications for assessment and treatment parameters

	Neurotic organization	High borderline personality organization	Mid borderline personality organization	Low borderline personality organization
Level of Personality Functioning Scale (LPFS)	Level 1	Level 2	Level 3	Level 4
Typical categorical diagnosis	Obsessive-compulsive PD, depressive PD, hysterical PD	Dependent PD, histrionic PD, avoidant PD, narcissistic PD	Narcissistic PD, borderline PD, paranoid PD, schizoid PD	Narcissistic, borderline, and paranoid PDs with antisocial features; antisocial PD
Nature of self-other functioning	Integrated, realistic, and continuous experience of self in relation to others Relationships characterized by mutuality, but OR related to area of conflict excluded from sense of self by means of repression-based defenses Rigid functioning in area of conflict	Somewhat superficial and/or polarized experience of self in relation to others Some capacity for dependency but with conflict	Superficial, extreme, polarized, and unstable sense of self in relation to others, with gross distortion Need-fulfilling relationships	Caricature-like, extreme, highly polarized, and chaotic sense of self in relation to others, with gross distortion Exploitative relationships
Clinical objectives of treatment	Flexible functioning in area of conflict	Greater depth and stability in experience of self and others	Resolution of destructive behavior Greater depth in experience of self and others	Behavior control Modulation of aggression
Prognosis	Excellent	Good	Fair	Very guarded
Structuring of the treatment	Less need for structured contract	Explicitly agreed-on treatment contract promotes productive clinical process	Carefully constructed treatment contract is essential	Contracting must be extensive Focus on secondary gain and safety of patient and therapist

TABLE 5–1. Severity of personality pathology: implications for assessment and treatment parameters *(continued)*

	Neurotic organization	High borderline personality organization	Mid borderline personality organization	Low borderline personality organization
Treatment process	Little to no risk of acting out	Risk of low-level acting out (e.g., poor attendance)	Risk of dangerous acting out (e.g., suicide gestures or attempts, substance misuse)	Potentially lethal acting out (e.g., threats of violence to therapist, lethal suicide attempts)
Alliance	Clarity about seeking help from expert Open to alliance	Ambivalence about seeking help and depending on expert interferes with initial alliance Early alliance unstable or superficial	Suspicion, with fear of critical attack or exploitation by therapist, interferes with alliance Alliance built during course of treatment	Relatively fixed view of therapist as corrupt, arrogant, and exploitative limits capacity to form an alliance

Note. OR=object relations; PD=personality disorder.
Source. Caligor et al. 2018.

is superficial, unstable, distorted, and poorly contextualized and coupled with affects that are poorly integrated and poorly regulated. Within this model, the central mechanism of personality pathology is the predominance of highly charged negative affect states that drive the activation of splitting-based, or dissociative, defenses. These processes interfere with normal identity integration. Representations of self and others associated with positive affective experience are dissociated from those associated with negative affective experience, and the resulting affectively charged, polarized internal representations fail to coalesce into an overarching sense of self and others. The resulting failure of identity consolidation accounts for the unstable and distorted sense of self and others that is the hallmark of the personality disorders.

The nosology of personality pathology that has been developed within the framework of object relations theory combines both dimensional and prototypical descriptions of personality functioning and dysfunction. *Level of personality organization* reflects the dimensional severity of personality pathology. Each level of personality organization is characterized by different dimensional values of identity, quality of object relations, defensive functioning, aggression, and moral values. Determination of the level of severity can be combined with a prototypical classification of personality pathology (see Table 5–1). This nosology has the advantage of emphasizing the severity of personality pathology while accommodating categories of personality disorder presentation for treatment planning and application. This nosology has received empirical support (Lenzenweger et al. 2008) and has been replicated (Yun et al. 2013), suggesting that the subtypes may be important to guide further efforts to understand underlying endophenotypes and genotypes. Furthermore, it has given rise to a method of reliable clinical assessment related to object relations theory (see subsection "Clinical Assessment and Case Formulation").

Model of Change

Given the centrality of negative affect in the TFP model of pathogenesis, the treatment model posits a central role for affect activation, followed by affect containment, in the clinical process (Caligor et al. 2009; Levy et al. 2006). The TFP treatment frame and the technically neutral stance assumed by the therapist support the emergence of affectively charged object relations in the treatment, in which the object relations can be safely contained within the structure of the treatment setting and the therapeutic relationship. These affectively charged perceptions of self and other, which may be expressed in the patient's interactions with the therapist and/or in their descriptions of current interpersonal relationships, are a focus of clinical attention in the therapy. For example, a therapist may call attention to a patient's conviction that the therapist dislikes them and wants to get rid of them; at another time, the therapist may put into words this same patient's experience of being very special to the therapist. As affectively charged perceptions of self in relation to others are identified and explored, affects are contained, and extreme, distorted, paranoid, and idealized perceptions of self and other are contextualized in relation to one another. The interpretive process, described and illustrated in the subsection "Process of Interpretation," organizes these developments and guides clinical interventions to promote affect containment, self-awareness, reflection on internal states, and mentalization, capacities that foster integrative processes. Over time, as affects are tempered and extreme perceptions of self and others are gradually modified, dissociated experiences of self and others coalesce, leading to identity consolidation.

Clinical Assessment and Case Formulation

Because the delivery of techniques of TFP is shaped by the level of severity of personality pathology, it is imperative that the assessor or therapist carefully evaluate the nature and severity of a patient's difficulties in self and interpersonal functioning. The clinical interview is the time-honored approach preferred by clinicians to make the first evaluation contact with a prospective patient. Kernberg (1984) revolutionized the initial evaluation by describing the structural interview as focusing on not only the chief complaint, presenting symptoms, and mental status but also personality functioning. The structural interview is a procedure that allows clinical assessment of current symptoms and interpersonal difficulties and capacities for identity, object relations, level of defensive functioning, modulation of aggression, and moral functioning. Judgments are made about the severity of impairment in each of these domains of functioning, leading to the diagnosis of level of personality organization (i.e., neurotic or high-, mid-, or low-level borderline personality organization). To assist clinicians and researchers who have not been trained in the structural interview, we have constructed the Structured Interview for Personality Organization—Revised (STIPO-R) to guide the assessment (J.F. Clarkin, E. Caligor, B.L. Stern, et al., "Structured Interview for Personality Organization—Revised [STIPO-R]," unpublished manuscript, Weill Cornell Medical College, January 2015).

The initial clinical assessment provides a diagnostic impression along with an indication of the level of severity of symptoms, personality organization, and current social functioning. This evaluation is necessary to gauge the range of techniques that need to be used in the individual treatment situation.

Principal Intervention Strategies and Techniques

Treatment Structure: Contracting

Following a thorough assessment, the TFP therapist shares the diagnostic impression with the patient, focusing on identity and personality functioning and linking them to the patient's presenting complaint. The therapist introduces a structured treatment frame that elaborates necessary conditions for treatment effectiveness. The degree of structure required in the treatment is directly related to the severity of personality pathology. Before the therapy formally begins, the TFP therapist articulates a verbal treatment agreement, or *treatment contract*, with the prospective patient in which the responsibilities of both therapist and patient are stated, and a discussion of each participant's responsibilities evolves from that contract. The patient is responsible for coming to the sessions on time and discussing as freely as possible what is on their mind. Procedures for managing any self-destructive or suicidal behavior are discussed. The patient is responsible for engagement in school or work, whether it is part-time volunteer work or full-time paid engagement, during the treatment period. This engagement is not relevant for patients with functioning neurotic personality organization and most patients with high-level borderline personality organization but is most important for poorly functioning patients with mid- and low-level borderline personality organization. The therapist is committed to listening intently to the feelings, thoughts, and concerns of the patient and commenting when the patient deems it helpful. By structuring the treatment with explicit roles and behaviors for therapist and patient, both effective interaction and deviations from it can be identified. It is only after the treatment frame has been articulated that one can identify and interpret deviations from the frame, which presupposes a patient motivated to overcome symptoms and difficulties with the assistance of a therapist who is not omniscient but helpful.

Case Vignette: Neutrality and First Level of Interaction

Mr. H, a 35-year-old male executive with a history of hypertension, came to treatment at the urging of his wife after being let go from yet another in a series of jobs. Although competent, he tended to be reactive and depreciative of people he worked with, both his bosses and colleagues, and was prone to hostile outbursts in the workplace. He had a pattern of provoking and alienating others without really understanding what he was doing or why he kept getting fired. Rather than being concerned or able to make changes, he simply felt angry and unfairly treated and also increasingly diminished and inadequate with each failure. His relationship with his wife was somewhat stormy but stable. He was often dismissive in their interactions and poorly tolerated "her bossy side" but described himself as very much in love with her. There were no antisocial features or significant pathology of moral values. In a joint meeting with Mr. H and his wife during the evaluation phase it emerged that he had a history of noncompliance with his antihypertensive medications, resulting in several visits to the emergency department in hypertensive crisis. His father had died of heart disease at age 42.

After the therapist shared her diagnostic impression (Table 5–2), organized in relation to problems with self- and interpersonal functioning (which were relatively mild) as a way to explain Mr. H's difficulties, they discussed Mr. H's goals for treatment. (See Caligor et al. 2018 for a discussion of sharing the diagnostic impression prior to starting TFP.) Mr. H's goals were to improve his interpersonal functioning in the workplace and to succeed in his current job. After reviewing treatment options, Mr. H and the therapist decided to begin a twice-weekly TFP treatment. Before beginning treatment, they discussed the treatment frame and necessary conditions for treatment, introduced in the form of a treatment agreement, or *treatment contract*. The therapist introduced the standard TFP agreement, focusing on the need for consistent attendance in sessions, the need to maintain at least 30 hours of structured activity out of sessions (in Mr. H's case, continued employment), the procedures for intersession contact and handling of cancellations and payment, and the request that the patient communicate honestly and openly. In contrast to procedures commonly introduced in the treatments of more severe pathology, there was no need to contract around suicidality, handling of emergencies, or substance abuse. However, in light of Mr. H's history of hypertensive crises in the setting of noncompliance with antihypertensive medication (deemed a form of self-injurious behavior), compliance with blood pressure medication as prescribed by his cardiologist was included as a necessary condition for treatment.

Therapist's Stance

The TFP therapist closely monitors the quality of the relationship with the patient. This relationship has been conceptualized in the classical psychoanalytic literature in terms of patient transference and therapist countertransference. Attention to the patient-therapist relationship is also emphasized in the evidence-based principles of

Table 5–2. Summary of Mr. H's case

- Diagnostic formulation: High borderline personality organization with prominent narcissistic, obsessional, and sadomasochistic features manifesting in specific difficulties in self- and interpersonal functioning that are most evident in the workplace
- Treatment goal: To improve interpersonal functioning in the workplace
- Specific elements in contract: Compliance concerning antihypertensive medication

therapeutic intervention that have received various degrees of empirical support in the psychotherapy outcome literature (Norcross and Wampold 2018).

Implicit in treatment contracting is the TFP therapist's stance, which is characterized by two seemingly contradictory approaches. On the one hand, the therapist pays intense attention to the patient's behavior and attitudes, supporting the patient's motivation for positive change. On the other hand, the therapist maintains a neutral stance in relation to the patient's conflicts. Therapeutic neutrality enables the therapist to explore both sides of a patient's conflicts thoroughly while keeping the responsibility for conflict resolution in the hands of the patient.

Process of Interpretation

In TFP, clinical intervention is organized in relation to the *interpretive process*, which focuses on exploring the patient's current relationships, with both the therapist and significant others, and on the patient's current functioning in their life. The process of interpretation is carried out repeatedly over time and throughout the course of treatment, titrated to the rise and fall of the patient's affective state and serving a variety of functions at different clinical moments and phases of treatment. Through the process of interpretation, the patient's self- and object representations are identified and labeled by the therapist and traced as they contribute to the patient's experience of interpersonal relationships and interactions with the therapist.

The overall objectives of the interpretive process are to expand the patient's level of self- awareness, to support their ability to observe themselves, to reflect on their internal experience and external behavior, and to put momentary perceptions of self and others associated with intense affective states into the larger context of a complex relationship. This self-reflective capacity enhances the patient's ability to pursue study and work and to maintain satisfying relations with others. The goal of the interpretive process is to increase mentalization, not in the broad sense (Bateman and Fonagy 2006) but in the more specific sense of the acquisition of realistic insight related to the patient's distorted self-representations and the corresponding faulty representations of significant others (Kernberg 2018, p. 66).

The interpretive process can be conceptualized in terms of four levels of intervention, with each sequential level preparing the patient to make use of subsequent levels (Caligor et al. 2009). In concert, the four levels of intervention constitute a complex process, involving much repetition and moving to and fro, and play out somewhat differently with each patient. The process of interpretation begins at the level of self- and other representations that organize the patient's interpersonal experience and self-states. The quality and nature of these representations reflect the individual's level of personality organization (Caligor et al. 2018; Kernberg and Caligor 2005) and characteristic personality style (Kernberg 2019).

First Level of Intervention

The first level of intervention entails defining the dominant object relations—the implicit perceptions that patients have of themselves in relationship to others, including the therapist, that organize their experience in the moment. The therapist begins by putting words to the patient's dominant affective experience, described in terms of an internal object relation or relationship pattern, in session. In the treatment of patients with BPD, the dominant object relation often takes the form of a victim in the hands of a persecutor. In the treatment of patients with narcissistic personality disorder (NPD), the dominant object relation is often composed of someone superior and devaluing in relation to someone inferior, dismissed, and inept. With patients with both BPD and NPD, the dominant affect is most commonly negative, colored by hostility. Regardless of the specific features of the dominant object relation, the TFP therapist begins by attempting to clarify the view of self and other organizing the patient's dominant conscious experience in the session. This process often leads to the crystallization of the dominant object relations in relation to the therapist, whose task is to help the patient put their experience into words. In this process, the therapist approaches the material through the patient's subjectivity, without calling into question the patient's experience. Done well, identifying and putting words to the dominant object relationship of patient to therapist or significant other can provide affective containment and promote self-observation on the part of the patient while communicating the therapist's empathy and wish to understand.

Case Vignette: Neutrality and First Level of Intervention

Mr. H had just come from his office, where his boss had given him negative feedback in his semiannual review in relation to his handling of a specific matter. Mr. H complained to the therapist that he was certain the boss, a "sadistic son of a bitch," had "enjoyed every moment." As Mr. H continued to complain about his boss's character, the therapist maintained a neutral stance. This entailed abstaining from joining in Mr. H's criticism of his boss or coaching Mr. H on how to better handle the boss and also called on the therapist to contain an internal pressure she was aware of to argue the boss's position. Instead, the therapist attempted to get a clearer understanding of what had happened in the review while maintaining a neutral, inquiring stance. In response, Mr. H only became increasingly agitated and impatient. The therapist called attention to Mr. H's attitude, stating that he seemed to be agitated by her questions and to find them irritating. He responded that the therapist couldn't possibly understand what it was like to be unfairly devalued and treated with contempt. "You're just an ivory tower bitch!" Mr. H's tone was both depreciative and hostile, and he seemed to be escalating. When the therapist attempted to empathize with Mr. H's distress and frustration with her, Mr. H quickly and repeatedly interrupted, dismissing her or contemptuously mocking her by parroting her words. In the countertransference the therapist noted feeling depreciated, attacked, and also angry; she noted, and contained, a developing impulse to depreciate Mr. H.

Making an effort to step out of her countertransference and taking a moment to observe her own internal experience and what was being enacted in the session, the therapist was able to identify in her own mind a familiar object relation, previously identified on multiple occasions in the treatment, organizing Mr. H's dominant experience in the moment. Making use of the first level of intervention, she put words to her understanding of Mr. H's dominant experience in the transference and his representation of her, along with the associated self-representation and affect state, while entering the material through Mr. H's subjective experience: "It seems you see me as looking down on you, feeling superior, and maybe even secretly enjoying your sense of humiliation.…I understand this leaves you angry and also makes it painful to be here." Mr. H visibly relaxed.

Second Level of Intervention

The next level of interpretation entails observing and identifying role reversals within the previously identified object relations dyads active in the session. In this process the therapist tactfully helps the patient to attend to aspects of their behavior and experience that have been dissociated, denied, and seen in the other. For example, at the same time that the patient may perceive themselves as a victim in the hands of a victimizing therapist, the patient may angrily attack the therapist; that is, the therapist becomes the victim of verbal attack at the hands of the patient. Or as commonly encountered in patients with NPD, at the same time the patient experiences the therapist as inattentive and uninterested, the patient uses the therapist as a sounding board, ignoring or interrupting whenever the therapist attempts to speak. Often, the patient is very aware of one configuration (as in the first example with the patient feeling like a victim at the hands of others or in the second example with the patient feeling dismissed by an uninterested and inattentive therapist) but is not consciously aware of the relationship with roles reversed (e.g., the patient victimizing the other or being dismissive and inattentive in relation to the therapist). By pointing out role reversals, the therapist is introducing a new and different perspective, inviting the patient to go beyond their immediate, in-the-moment, concrete experience to attend to aspects of their behavior and experience that have been dissociated and denied. This process promotes self-awareness along with the patient's capacity to step outside immediate, affectively charged experiences to entertain alternative perspectives. Individuals with NPD often have particular difficulty developing this capacity and may remain locked in a one-sided, rigid, and static view of the therapeutic interaction for extended periods of time (Diamond et al. 2011).

Case Vignette: Second Level of Intervention—Calling Attention to Reversal of Roles in the Dyad

In "Case Vignette: Neutrality and First Level of Intervention," as the therapist identified Mr. H's dominant experience in the session, in which she was superior and depreciative and secretly enjoying his humiliation, she was also aware that that same object relation with roles reversed was simultaneously being enacted between them. That is, in his dominant experience, Mr. H felt depreciated, but out of his awareness, he was himself depreciating the therapist and his boss, which he enacted but dissociated and denied. As the session continued, the therapist encouraged Mr. H to identify and explore his expectation that his humiliation was enjoyed by the therapist. With time, Mr. H came to seem more thoughtful and less paranoid. The therapist wondered if Mr. H might be in a sufficiently reflective state of mind to make use of the second level of intervention, which involved calling attention to the role reversal enacted in his behavior and attitude but denied by him earlier in the session: "At the same time you see me as looking down on you, it seems sometimes you behave in ways, perhaps out of your awareness, likely to leave me feeling put down or feeling that you hold me in contempt, for example, when you mocked me earlier in the session and described my comment as 'pathetic,' insisting that this treatment has been a total waste of time and I have no idea what I'm doing."

Third Level of Intervention

The third level of interpretation entails making connections between contradictory (typically idealized and persecutory) experiences of self in relation to others that have been defensively dissociated across time. Here the therapist invites the patient to observe and reflect on the polarized and contradictory nature of their experience, such as the contradiction that today the therapist is heartless and the patient is neglected and enraged, whereas only last session the therapist was infinitely caring and the patient was basking in the therapist's love (common in BPD) or that today the therapist is useless, totally ineffective, and an exploitative charlatan, whereas last session the therapist was a powerful genius, admired and feared (common in NPD). This third level of intervention begins by pointing to the instability of the patient's experience, a process that invites reflection and curiosity on the part of the patient about the relationship between their internal experience and external reality. Appreciation of the shifting and contradictory quality of their experience ultimately helps the patient appreciate that experience is subjective, internal, and constructed, in contrast to concrete; they have the opportunity to observe and reflect on how their mind works and how it influences their behavior and relationships, fostering a capacity for mentalization. Ultimately, the objective is to help the patient hold two contradictory states in mind, tolerating the anxiety generated by moments of transient integration.

Case Vignette: Third Level of Interaction—Making Connections Between Contradictory Dyads

Several weeks after the session described in "Case Vignette: Level 2," Mr. H began a session by commenting that he had had "a really good day." His boss had made a point of taking him aside and telling him that he had made excellent use of the feedback from his review to distinguish himself in his management of a tricky situation with a client. Recounting this to the therapist, Mr. H was beaming. He went on to say that he never could have done it without the therapist; he couldn't believe how lucky he had been with the referral to her, and the help was beyond anything he had thought possible. The therapist understood Mr. H's attitude to be genuine, but she was also mindful that this attitude was entirely discrepant and dissociated from a far more negative view of her and the treatment that Mr. H had articulated only a session earlier: "I can see that your attitude here today, expressing how lucky you feel to have me as your therapist, is clearly heartfelt, and I agree you are making very meaningful gains; at the same time, I can't help but remember our last session, when you were considering ending therapy, experiencing me as ineffective and totally unable to understand you."

Fourth Level of Intervention

The fourth level in the interpretive process moves to the level of symbolic meanings and unconscious motivations as the therapist offers hypotheses about how to understand the polarized and unstable quality of the patient's experience. For example, the therapist might suggest that a patient with BPD maintains maladaptive, contradictory, and polarized (idealized and persecutory) views of the therapist or significant others out of a wish to preserve the possibility of finding a perfect caretaker or that a patient with NPD clings to a devalued view of the therapist because the therapist being effective and able to help would constitute a humiliating confirmation of the patient's inferiority. This final step in the interpretive process that corresponds to conventional psychodynamic and psychoanalytic notions of *interpretation*, focusing on conveying understanding of unconscious meanings and motivations. This level of intervention is essentially explanatory and can be contrasted with earlier levels of interpretation that can be seen to focus on the designated (Tuckett 2019) or enacted (Joseph 2013) transferences active in the moment. TFP emphasizes that in the treatment of severe personality disorders, focusing on dissociative defenses enacted in the transference, first in the form of role reversals and then in the dissociation of idealized and paranoid sectors, is the cornerstone of the interpretive process. Exploration of unconscious meanings is the final step, and not necessarily the most critical one, in a complex process and is introduced only after earlier interventions have created a patient who is aware of, troubled by, able to reflect on, and curious about the dissociated nature of their experience. This final level of intervention can function to help the patient bind the anxiety motivating splitting-based defenses.

Case Vignette: Fourth Level of Interaction—Exploring Motivations for Defense

The therapist had begun the third level of intervention by calling Mr. H's attention to his highly discrepant and contradictory experiences of her—today, his experience was extremely positive (she was helpful, a lifesaver), in marked contrast to last session, when his experience was extremely negative (she was ineffective, unempathic). In her interventions, the therapist highlighted the black-and-white, extreme quality of both views and of Mr. H's corresponding views of himself—cared for and helped in contrast to mistreated and misunderstood—and she called attention to the discontinuous nature of his experience.

At a certain moment the therapist noted a subtle shift in Mr. H's attitude, that he seemed first genuinely struck by and then troubled by the unstable and polarized nature of his experience. His anxiety and effort to understand were palpable as he conveyed a deepening awareness that they were observing a problem within his mind that concerned him rather than a problem with the therapist and her behavior. He asked the therapist, seemingly thoughtfully, "Why does this happen to me? Does this happen to others? Why would my mind organize things this way?" Noting the developing ego-dystonicity of his defenses and his genuine curiosity and confusion, the therapist hazarded a formal interpretation: "Perhaps you feel a need to forget the negative view of our relationship you experienced last time, as if you fear those feelings could destroy the positive feelings you have today.…It is as if the negative feelings are too powerful and could too easily swamp these new and perhaps more fragile positive feelings."

Process of Treatment

The initial process of TFP is the same for all patients across the full range of personality pathology. As described in the preceding sections, treatment is preceded by careful diagnostic assessment of presenting symptoms and personal difficulties and the level of functioning in work/professional life and social relations, including friendships and intimate relations. Assessment of the level of personality organization determines the next steps in TFP.

After reviewing the assessment information and discussing treatment options, patient and therapist agree on a course of TFP if it is indicated. All that follows (treatment contracting, phases of TFP) depends on the level of personality organization of the individual patient. TFP begins at the level of adjustment of the individual patient.

The negotiation of a treatment contract follows. The lower the level of personality organization of the patient (i.e., the more severe the patient's personality pathology), the more careful and detailed the contract must be concerning treatment compliance and management of self-destructive behavior. As the early treatment phase begins, challenges to the treatment frame can be expected, especially in the more severe form with patients at mid and lower levels of borderline personality organization (e.g., potentially lethal behaviors, devaluation of the therapist and the therapy process). With the structure of the treatment frame, which the therapist reiterates, attenuation of out-of-session self-destructive behavior ensues, making it possible for the therapist to shift clinical attention to understanding the underlying conflicted object relations that drive these maladaptive behaviors. The patient's conflicted object relations now become focused in the treatment and, in particular, in the therapeutic relationship.

The rhythm and interaction of the patient talking about self and relations with others, therapist interventions as outlined above, and the patient's response to the therapist's intervention change and develop over time. Gradually, interventions focus more on advanced levels of the interpretive process because the patient is more alert to what the therapist says, is increasingly reflective, and is able to take in and expand on the therapist's interventions. Thus, both the transference to the therapist (from paranoid to more depressive) and patient activity (less resistance, more self-guided reflection) evolve.

The usual progression of change in TFP is first a reduction of symptoms and problem behaviors, followed by the patient's growing recognition of, and responsibility for, conflictual aspects of internal experience and external behavior. The specific nature of this progression is modified by the patient's level of personality organization and is related to the severity of problems in self- and interpersonal functioning at the beginning of treatment. Self-functioning and interpersonal functioning improve in neurotic-level patients as their perceptions of self and others are expanded to include aspects of experience previously defended against. In patients at borderline levels of organization, idealized and persecutory object relations become less extreme and affectively charged. Signs of the beginnings of transient coalescence emerge. These changes are reflected in the nature of the transference and improvement in work relations and friendships. The degree of change in work relations and intimate relations varies substantially on the basis of the initial severity.

Role of Peer Consultation

The field of psychotherapy research has emphasized the importance of treatment manuals to ensure homogeneity of the intervention and evidence supporting the adherent and competent delivery of the treatment in a therapy trial. There is no doubt that the description of treatment in a carefully constructed manual and ratings of adherence and competence are important procedures for clinical empirical advance. However, we have found some nuances in this process that have shaped our approach.

The idea that a therapist can be trained to a permanent level of adherence and competence is, we think, a false fantasy. We have clinical experience of finding senior adherent and competent therapists who become deskilled with interfering countertransference patterns with particular patients. This is quite consistent with the current emphasis on not only the categorical diagnosis but also the severity of the particular patient. Our current view is that initial training to adherence and competence is useful but must be followed by peer supervision, especially for the most severe cases.

Conclusion

In this chapter we have described the clinical and empirical development of TFP from a treatment for patients with BPD to a more comprehensive version applicable to a range of patients presenting with various personality disorders, all of whom have prominent difficulties in self-functioning and related interpersonal functioning. The three building blocks of TFP—object relations theory, assessment, and treatment structure—are intimately interrelated. Object relations theory places emphasis on the impact of internal representations of self and others that guide behavior. Clinical assessment of the severity of the key domains of personality organization is directly linked to central aspects of TFP treatment such as contract setting, relative focus on transference, and the process of interpretation.

TFP is a principle-driven approach for patients with difficulties in self- and interpersonal functioning tailored to the unique aspects of the individual, in line with current thinking concerning precision medicine. In a principle-driven treatment approach it is the task of the therapist to apply the strategies and techniques flexibly in relation to the individual patient.

Psychotherapy research will advance as the mechanisms of change are demonstrated both at the psychological level and at the level of neural functioning. Refinements in TFP are fostered by clinical experience with a range of personality pathology severity and increasing empirical information on the nature of functioning among these patients.

Key Points

- Transference-focused psychotherapy (TFP) is a transdiagnostic psychodynamic therapy treating problems of self-functioning and functioning with others, the core features of personality disorder.
- The focus of TFP is identification and exploration of the affectively charged relationship patterns, or object relations, that emerge in the treatment setting.
- Initial clinical assessment and case formulation are based on level of personality organization severity, which determines the structure and process of the treatment.
- The interpretive process in TFP is conceptualized in terms of four levels of intervention exploring the patient's self-states and related interpersonal experience while promoting reflective processes.

References

Bateman AW, Fonagy P: Mentalization-Based Treatment for Borderline Personality Disorder: A Practical Guide. Oxford, UK, Oxford University Press, 2006

Caligor E, Diamond D, Yeomans FE, et al: The interpretive process in the psychoanalytic psychotherapy of borderline personality pathology. J Am Psychoanal Assoc 57(2):271–301, 2009 19516053

Caligor E, Kernberg OF, Clarkin JF, et al: Psychodynamic Therapy for Personality Pathology: Treating Self and Interpersonal Functioning. Washington, DC, American Psychiatric Association Publishing, 2018

Clarkin JF, Yeomans FE, Kernberg OF: Psychotherapy for Borderline Personality. New York, Wiley, 1999

Clarkin JF, Foelsch PA, Levy KN, et al: The development of a psychodynamic treatment for patients with borderline personality disorder: a preliminary study of behavioral change. J Pers Disord 15(6):487–495, 2001 11778390

Clarkin JF, Levy KN, Lenzenweger MF, et al: Evaluating three treatments for borderline personality disorder: a multiwave study. Am J Psychiatry 164(6):922–928, 2007 17541052

Clarkin JF, Caligor E, Sowislo JF: An object relations model perspective on the alternative model for personality disorders (DSM-5). Psychopathology 53(3–4):141–148, 2020 32698184

Cohen ZD, DeRubeis RJ: Treatment selection in depression. Annu Rev Clin Psychol 14:209–236, 2018 29494258

Diamond D, Yeomans FE, Levy KN: Psychodynamic psychotherapy for narcissistic personality disorder, in The Handbook of Narcissism and Narcissistic Personality Disorder: Theoretical Approaches, Empirical Findings, and Treatment. Edited by Campbell K, Miller JD. New York, Wiley, 2011, pp 421–433

Doering S, Hörz S, Rentrop M, et al: Transference-focused psychotherapy v. treatment by community psychotherapists for borderline personality disorder: randomised controlled trial. Br J Psychiatry 196(5):389–395, 2010 20435966

Joseph B: Here and now: my perspective. Int J Psychoanal 94(1):1–5, 2013 23438980

Kernberg OF: Severe Personality Disorders: Psychotherapeutic Strategies. New Haven, CT, Yale University Press, 1984

Kernberg OF: Treatment of Severe Personality Disorders: Resolution of Aggression and Recovery of Eroticism. Washington, DC, American Psychiatric Association Publishing, 2018

Kernberg OF: Therapeutic implications of transference structures in various personality pathologies. J Am Psychoanal Assoc 67(6):951–986, 2019 32043388

Kernberg OF, Caligor E: A psychodynamic theory of personality disorders, in Major Theories of Personality Disorder. Edited by Lenzenweger MF, Clarkin JF. New York, Guilford, 2005, pp 114–156

Lenzenweger MF, Clarkin JF, Yeomans FE, et al: Refining the borderline personality disorder phenotype through finite mixture modeling: implications for classification. J Pers Disord 22(4):313–331, 2008 18684047

Levy KN, Meehan KB, Kelly KM, et al: Change in attachment patterns and reflective function in a randomized control trial of transference-focused psychotherapy for borderline personality disorder. J Consult Clin Psychol 74(6):1027–1040, 2006 17154733

Norcross JC, Lambert MJ: Psychotherapy Relationships That Work, Vol 1: Evidence-Based Therapist Contributions. Oxford, UK, Oxford University Press, 2019

Norcross JC, Wampold BE: A new therapy for each patient: evidence-based relationships and responsiveness. J Clin Psychol 74(11):1889–1906, 2018 30334258

Sharp C, Wright AG, Fowler JC, et al: The structure of personality pathology: both general ("g") and specific ("s") factors? J Abnorm Psychol 124(2):387–398, 2015 25730515

Simon S, Cain NM, Wallner Samstag L, et al: Assessing interpersonal subtypes in depression. J Pers Assess 97(4):364–373, 2015 25803309

Tuckett D: Transference and transference interpretation revisited: why a parsimonious model of practice may be useful. Int J Psychoanal 100(5):852–876, 2019 33952107

Yeomans FE, Clarkin JF, Kernberg OF: Transference-Focused Psychotherapy for Borderline Personality Disorder: A Clinician's Guide. Washington, DC, American Psychiatric Association Publishing, 2015

Yun RJ, Stern BL, Lenzenweger MF, et al: Refining personality disorder subtypes and classification using finite mixture modeling. Pers Disord 4(2):121–128, 2013 23046042

CHAPTER 6

Applications of Psychodynamic Psychotherapy to Specific Disorders

Falk Leichsenring, D.Sc.
Christiane Steinert, Ph.D.

Empirical outcome research in psychodynamic and psychoanalytic therapy is needed (Gabbard et al. 2002). In this chapter, we review the available evidence for psychodynamic therapy. In the first part, we discuss the procedures of evidence-based medicine and empirically supported treatments. In the second part, we present a review of the available randomized controlled trials (RCTs) and meta-analyses of psychodynamic therapy for specific mental disorders.

Evidence-Based Medicine and Empirically Supported Treatments

Several proposals have been made to grade the available evidence for both medical and psychotherapeutic treatments (Canadian Task Force on the Periodic Health Examination 1979; Chambless and Hollon 1998; Clarke and Oxman 2003; Cook et al. 1995; Guyatt et al. 1995; Nathan and Gorman 2015; Tolin et al. 2015). Apart from other differences, all available proposals regard RCTs (efficacy studies) as the gold standard for the demonstration that a treatment is effective. According to this view, only RCTs can provide level 1 evidence, which is the highest level of evidence (Oxford Centre, www.cebm.ox.ac.uk/resources/levels-of-evidence/oxford-centre-for-evidence-based-medicine-levels-of-evidence-march-2009). More recently, meta-analyses and systematic reviews of RCTs in the field of mental health outcomes have been emphasized (Fusar-Poli and Radua 2018; Tolin et al. 2015).

RCTs are conducted under controlled experimental conditions; thus, they allow researchers to control for variables systematically influencing the outcome, including the treatment condition. The defining feature of an RCT is the random assignment of subjects to the different conditions of treatment (Shadish et al. 2002). Randomization is regarded as indispensable in order to ensure that a priori differences between subjects are equally distributed. The goal of randomization is to attribute the observed effects exclusively to the applied therapy. Thus, randomization is used to ensure the internal validity of a study (Shadish et al. 2002). Gabbard et al. (2002) discussed different types of RCTs that provide different levels of evidence. The most stringent test of efficacy is achieved by comparison with rival treatments, thus controlling for specific and unspecific therapeutic factors (Chambless and Hollon 1998, p. 8). Furthermore, such comparisons provide explicit information regarding the relative benefits of competing treatments. Treatments that are found to be superior to rival treatments are more highly valued. However, more recently, it has consistently been shown that all bona fide treatments show similar outcomes—a finding that led to lively discussions about the so-called *Dodo bird verdict* (Wampold and Imel 2015), which assumes that all bona fide forms of psychotherapy are equally efficacious. Opponents of the Dodo bird verdict point to differences between treatments in efficacy. Differences are, however, usually small and clinically not significant.

The exclusive position of RCTs in psychotherapy research, however, has been questioned for several reasons (Beutler 1998; Fonagy 1999; Leichsenring 2004; Persons and Silberschatz 1998; Roth and Parry 1997; Rothwell 2005; Seligman 1995; Westen et al. 2004). RCTs have their strengths and limitations. Carried out under highly controlled conditions, RCTs usually have high internal validity. However, being carried out under controlled conditions may reduce their external validity; that is, the results may not be fully representative of clinical practice (Leichsenring 2004).

In contrast to RCTs, naturalistic studies (effectiveness studies) are conducted under the conditions of clinical practice. Thus, their results are more representative for clinical practice with regard to patients, therapists, and treatments, that is, external validity (Shadish et al. 2000). However, effectiveness studies cannot control for factors affecting the outcome to the same extent as RCTs (internal validity). However, the internal validity of effectiveness studies can be improved by quasi-experimental designs using methods other than randomization to rule out alternative explanations of the results (Leichsenring 2004; Shadish et al. 2002). According to several studies, there is evidence that effectiveness studies do not seem to overestimate effect sizes compared with RCTs (Benson and Hartz 2000; Concato et al. 2000; Shadish et al. 2000).

According to these considerations, efficacy and effectiveness studies address different research questions: RCTs examine the efficacy of a treatment under controlled experimental conditions, whereas effectiveness studies address the effectiveness under clinical practice conditions (Leichsenring 2004). As a consequence, the results of an efficacy study cannot be directly transferred to clinical practice and vice versa (Leichsenring 2004). From this perspective, a distinction is required between empirically supported therapies and RCT methodology (Leichsenring 2004; Westen et al.

2004), with the former including both efficacy and effectiveness studies. The relationship between RCTs and effectiveness studies should not be considered rivalrous; rather, it is complementary.

Meanwhile, the criteria for evidence-based psychotherapy proposed by Chambless and Hollon (1998) have been updated, taking into account several aspects critically put forward (Tolin et al. 2015). This update emphasizes a focus on systematic reviews rather than on individual studies, the quality of the studies, clinical significance in addition to statistical significance, long-term outcomes in addition to short-term efficacy, functional or other health-related outcomes in addition to symptoms, and generalization to nonresearch settings, deemphasizing diagnoses and emphasizing syndromes as well as mechanisms of psychopathology.

Evidence for Psychodynamic Psychotherapy in Specific Mental Disorders

The aim of this chapter is to identify for which mental disorders RCTs of both short-term and long-term psychodynamic psychotherapies are available. Here the criteria to define efficacious treatments proposed by the Task Force on Promotion and Dissemination of Psychological Procedures of the American Psychological Association (Task Force on Promotion and Dissemination of Psychological Procedures 1995) and modified by Chambless and Hollon (1998) are applied. Thus, one aim of this review is to examine the evidence for psychodynamic psychotherapy under the requirements of the criteria proposed by Chambless and Hollon (1998).

Definition of Psychodynamic Psychotherapy

Psychodynamic therapy focuses on the therapeutic relationship, expression of emotion, exploration of avoidance patterns, identification of recurring themes, discussion of past experiences, and interpersonal issues (Gabbard 2004). Many psychodynamic treatments, especially short-term variants, involve the development of a therapy focus according to a patient's presumed unconscious conflicts, internalized object relations, or structural impairments (e.g., Luborsky 1984).

Psychodynamic psychotherapy operates on an interpretive-supportive continuum. The use of more interpretive or supportive interventions depends on the patient's needs (Gabbard 2004; Wallerstein 1989). Whereas interpretive interventions enhance the patient's insight about repetitive conflicts sustaining his or her problems, supportive interventions aim to strengthen abilities (*ego functions*) that are not accessible because of acute stress or insufficient development (Luborsky 1984).

Gabbard (2004) suggested that therapies lasting more than 24 sessions or longer than 6 months should be regarded as long-term. In this review, the definitions of short-term and long-term psychodynamic psychotherapies given by Gabbard (2004) are applied. With regard to short-term psychodynamic psychotherapy (STPP), different models have been developed and were reviewed, for example, by Messer and Warren (1995). Gabbard's definition of long-term psychodynamic psychotherapy (LTPP) is the working model of this chapter (Gabbard 2004, p. 2): "a therapy that involves careful attention to the therapist-patient interaction, with thoughtfully timed interpretation of transference and resistance embedded in a sophisticated appreciation of the therapist's contribution to the two-person field."

Efficacy Studies of Psychodynamic Psychotherapy

Seventy RCTs providing evidence for psychodynamic psychotherapy are included in this review. These studies are presented in Table 6–1.

Evidence for the Efficacy of Psychodynamic Psychotherapy in Specific Mental Disorders

The studies of psychodynamic psychotherapy included here will be presented for the different mental disorders according to diagnostic manuals (e.g., DSM). However, from a psychodynamic perspective, the results of a therapy for a specific psychiatric disorder (e.g., depression, agoraphobia) are influenced by the underlying psychodynamic features (e.g., conflicts, defenses, personality organization), which may vary considerably within one category of psychiatric disorder (Kernberg 1996). These psychodynamic factors may affect treatment outcome and may be more important for outcome than the phenomenological DSM categories (Piper et al. 2001).

Specific Mental Disorders

Major Depression

The strictness of a test on efficacy depends on the comparator against which a treatment is tested. Waiting list conditions, for example, represent a relatively weak comparator, leading to larger effect sizes than for other comparators (Cuijpers et al. 2016; Huhn et al. 2014). In contrast, comparisons with placebo or treatment as usual (TAU) provide better estimates of the true efficacy of a treatment (Cuijpers et al. 2016), showing whether treatments have an additional gain compared with these conditions. From a health-economic perspective, they also provide information to see whether the efforts, costs, and side effects of specialized treatments pay off.

The strictest test is provided by a comparison with an already established treatment (Chambless and Hollon 1998). For these reasons the evidence for psychodynamic therapy will be presented by comparators.

In several RCTs, psychodynamic therapy was superior to waiting list control conditions or alternative treatments with regard to improving depression (Table 6–1) (Ajilchi et al. 2016; Knekt et al. 2008; Maina et al. 2005; Thompson et al. 1987). Psychodynamic therapy was superior to TAU for treatment-resistant depression (Town et al. 2017) and in specific groups of depressed patients, that is, patients with maternal depression (Cooper et al. 2003) and patients with breast cancer (Beutel et al. 2014). A small pilot study reported large effect sizes in favor of psychodynamic therapy compared with TAU, but the study was not sufficiently powered for a superiority trial, and the differences did not achieve statistical significance (Connolly Gibbons et al. 2012). Internet-guided psychodynamic self-help was reported to be superior to internet-delivered structured support (Johansson et al. 2012, 2013).

TABLE 6–1. Randomized controlled studies of manual-guided psychodynamic psychotherapy in specific mental disorders

Study	*N* (psychodynamic therapy)	Comparison group	Duration of psychodynamic therapy
Depressive disorders			
Major depressive disorder (MDD)			
Ajilchi et al. 2016	16	Waiting list: $N=16$	M=15 sessions
Barber et al. 2012	51	Pharmacotherapy: $N=55$ Placebo: $N=50$	20 sessions, 16 weeks
Barkham et al. 1996	18	CBT: $N=18$	8 vs. 16 sessions
Connolly Gibbons et al. 2012	21	TAU: $N=19$	12 sessions
Connolly Gibbons et al. 2016	118	CBT: $N=119$	16 sessions
Cooper et al. 2003	50	CBT: $N=43$ Counseling: $N=48$ TAU: $N=52$	10 sessions
de Jonghe et al. 2004	106	Psychodynamic therapy plus pharmacotherapy: $N=85$	16 sessions
Driessen et al. 2013	177	CBT: $N=164$	16 sessions
Johansson et al. 2012	46	Structured support: $N=46$	10 weeks
Salminen et al. 2008	26	Fluoxetine: $N=25$	16 sessions
Shapiro et al. 1994	58	CBT: $N=59$	8 vs. 16 sessions
Thompson et al. 1987; Gallagher-Thompson et al. 1990	24	BT: $N=25$ CBT: $N=27$ Waiting list: $N=19$	16–20 sessions
Town et al. 2017	30	TAU: $N=30$	20 sessions
Depressive disorders in patients with breast cancer			
Beutel et al. 2013	78	TAU: $N=79$	Up to 25 sessions

TABLE 6–1. Randomized controlled studies of manual-guided psychodynamic psychotherapy in specific mental disorders *(continued)*

Study	*N* (psychodynamic therapy)	Comparison group	Duration of psychodynamic therapy
Depressive disorders *(continued)*			
Dysthymic disorder			
Maina et al. 2005	10	Supportive therapy: *N*=10 Waiting list: *N*=10	15–30 sessions, M=19.6
Depressed caregivers			
Gallagher-Thompson and Steffen 1994	30	CBT: *N*=36	16–20 sessions
Psychodynamic therapy combined with pharmacotherapy for MD			
Burnand et al. 2002	35	Clomipramine: *N*=39	10 weeks
de Jonghe et al. 2001	72	Pharmacotherapy: *N*=57	16 sessions
Maina et al. 2007	18	Brief supportive therapy combined with pharmacotherapy: *N*=17	15–30 sessions
Mixed samples of patients with depressive and/or anxiety disorders			
Bressi et al. 2010	30	TAU: *N*=30	40 sessions, 1 year
Johansson et al. 2013[a]	50	Supportive interventions: *N*=50	10 weeks
Knekt et al. 2008[a]	STPP: 101 LTPP: 128	SFT: *N*=97	STPP: 18.5 sessions LTPP: 232 sessions SFT: 9.8 sessions
Complicated grief			
McCallum and Piper 1990	27	Waiting list: *N*=27	12 sessions
Piper et al. 2001	53	Supportive therapy: *N*=54	12 sessions
Anxiety disorders			
Social anxiety disorder			
Bögels et al. 2014	22	CBT: *N*=27 Waiting list: *N*=27	36 sessions
Knijnik et al. 2004	15	Credible placebo control group: *N*=15	12 sessions

TABLE 6–1. Randomized controlled studies of manual-guided psychodynamic psychotherapy in specific mental disorders *(continued)*

Study	*N* (psychodynamic therapy)	Comparison group	Duration of psychodynamic therapy
Leichsenring et al. 2013a, 2014	207	Cognitive therapy: *N*=209 Waiting list: *N*=79	30 sessions
Psychodynamic therapy combined with pharmacotherapy for social anxiety disorder			
Knijnik et al. 2008, 2009	29	Pharmacotherapy: *N*=29	12 sessions
Generalized anxiety disorder			
Andersson et al. 2012	27	ICBT: *N*=27 Waiting list: *N*=27	8 weeks
Leichsenring et al. 2009; Salzer et al. 2011	28	CBT: *N*=29	30 sessions
Panic disorder			
Beutel et al. 2013	36	CBT: *N*=18	24 sessions
Milrod et al. 2007	26	Applied relaxation: *N*=23	24 sessions
Milrod et al. 2016	80	CBT: *N*=81 Applied relaxation: *N*=39	19–24 sessions
Psychodynamic therapy combined with pharmacotherapy for panic disorder			
Wiborg and Dahl 1996	20	Pharmacotherapy alone: *N*=20	15 sessions
Obsessive-compulsive and related disorders			
Psychodynamic therapy combined with pharmacotherapy for obsessive-compulsive disorder			
Maina et al. 2010	27	Pharmacotherapy: *N*=30	10–16 sessions
Trauma- and stressor-related disorders			
PTSD			
Brom et al. 1989	29	Desensitization: *N*=31 Hypnotherapy: *N*=29 Waiting list: *N*=23	18.8 sessions
Steinert et al. 2016, 2017b	53	Waiting list: *N*=33	5 sessions

TABLE 6–1. Randomized controlled studies of manual-guided psychodynamic psychotherapy in specific mental disorders *(continued)*

Study	*N* (psychodynamic therapy)	Comparison group	Duration of psychodynamic therapy
Eating disorders			
Bulimia nervosa			
Bachar et al. 1999	17	Cognitive therapy: *N*=17 Nutritional counseling: *N*=10	46 sessions
Fairburn et al. 1986	11	CBT: *N*=11	19 sessions
Garner et al. 1993	25	CBT: *N*=25	19 sessions
Poulsen et al. 2014	34	CBT: *N*=36	PP: 73 sessions CBT: 20 sessions
Stefini et al. 2017	42	CBT: *N*=39	Up to 60 sessions
Binge-eating disorder			
Tasca et al. 2006	48	Group CBT: *N*=47 Waiting list: *N*=40	16 sessions
Anorexia nervosa			
Dare et al. 2001	21	Cognitive-analytic therapy: *N*=22 Family therapy: *N*=22 Routine treatment: *N*=19	M=24.9 sessions
Zipfel et al. 2014	80	Enhanced CBT: *N*=80 Optimized TAU: *N*=82	Psychodynamic therapy: 39.9 sessions Enhanced CBT: 44.8 sessions Optimized TAU: 50.8 sessions
Somatic symptom and related disorders			
Creed et al. 2003	59	Paroxetine: *N*=43 TAU: *N*=86	8 sessions
Faramarzi et al. 2013	24	Medical treatment: *N*=25	16 sessions
Guthrie et al. 1991	50	Supportive listening: *N*=46	8 sessions

TABLE 6–1. Randomized controlled studies of manual-guided psychodynamic psychotherapy in specific mental disorders *(continued)*

Study	*N* (psychodynamic therapy)	Comparison group	Duration of psychodynamic therapy
Guthrie et al. 1993	50	Supportive listening: *N*=46	8 sessions
Hamilton et al. 2000	37	Supportive therapy: *N*=36	7 sessions
Monsen and Monsen 2000	20	TAU/no therapy: *N*=20	33 sessions
Sattel et al. 2012	107	Enhanced medical care: *N*=104	12 sessions
Substance-related and addictive disorders			
Cocaine dependence			
Crits-Christoph et al. 1999, 2001	124	CBT+group DC: *N*=97 Individual DC: *N*=92 Individual DC+group DC: *N*=96	Up to 36 individual and 24 group sessions, 4 months
Opioid addiction			
Woody et al. 1983, 1990	31	DC: *N*=35 CBT+DC: *N*=34	12 sessions
Woody et al. 1995	57	DC: *N*=27	26 sessions
Personality disorders			
Borderline personality disorder			
Bateman and Fonagy 1999, 2001	19	TAU: *N*=19	18 months
Bateman and Fonagy 2009	71	Structured clinical management: *N*=63	18 months
Clarkin et al. 2007; Levy et al. 2006	30	Dialectical behavior therapy: *N*=30 Supportive psychodynamic therapy: *N*=30	12 months
Doering et al. 2010	43	Treatment by experienced community therapists: *N*=29	1 year
Giesen-Bloo et al. 2006	42	CBT: *N*=44	3 years with sessions twice a week
Gregory et al. 2008	15	TAU: *N*=15	M=24.9 sessions

TABLE 6–1. Randomized controlled studies of manual-guided psychodynamic psychotherapy in specific mental disorders *(continued)*

Study	*N* (psychodynamic therapy)	Comparison group	Duration of psychodynamic therapy
Personality disorders ***(continued)***			
Cluster C personality disorders			
Muran et al. 2005	22	Brief relational therapy: *N*=33 CBT: *N*=29	30 sessions
Svartberg et al. 2004	25	CBT: *N*=25	40 sessions
Avoidant personality disorder			
Emmelkamp et al. 2006	23	CBT: *N*=21 Waiting list: *N*=18	20 sessions
Heterogeneous personality disorders			
Abbass et al. 2008	14	Minimal contact: *N*=13	M=27.7 sessions
Hellerstein et al. 1998	25	Brief supportive psychotherapy: *N*=24	40 sessions
Vinnars et al. 2005	80	Community-delivered psychodynamic therapy: *N*=76	40 sessions
Winston et al. 1994	25	Brief adaptive psychotherapy: *N*=30 Waiting list: *N*=26	40 weeks, M=40.3 sessions
High users of psychiatric services			
Guthrie et al. 1999	55	TAU: *N*=55	8 sessions
Marital distress			
Snyder and Wills 1989; Snyder et al. 1991	30	Behavioral marital therapy: *N*=29 Waiting list: *N*=20	Up to 25 sessions

Note. BT=behavioral therapy; CBT=cognitive-behavioral therapy; DC=drug counseling; ICBT=internet cognitive-behavioral therapy; LTPP=long-term psychodynamic psychotherapy; M=mean; SFT=solution-focused therapy; PP=psychodynamic psychotherapy; STPP=short-term psychodynamic psychotherapy; TAU=treatment as usual.

[a]The outcome was evaluated separately for depressive and anxiety disorders; only results of STPP are included in this review because for LTTP no manuals were used.

With regard to comparisons with established treatments such as cognitive-behavioral therapy (CBT) or pharmacotherapy, three studies were sufficiently powered to test for equivalence or noninferiority (Connolly Gibbons et al. 2016; de Jonghe et al. 2004; Driessen et al. 2013). No statistically significant differences in outcome were found in these RCTs. However, the first study (de Jonghe et al. 2004) did not apply the two one-sided test procedure (Walker and Nowacki 2011) necessary to show equivalence, but rather used the traditional two-sided test (de Jonghe et al. 2004); the second RCT tested for noninferiority (Driessen et al. 2013). Driessen et al. (2013), however, could not show noninferiority of psychodynamic therapy compared with CBT for remission rates (21% vs. 24%), but for continuous measures of depression posttreatment. However, the difference in remission rates (21% vs. 24%) was minimal. In the third study, noninferiority was adequately tested, and psychodynamic therapy proved to be noninferior to CBT (Connolly Gibbons et al. 2016).

In addition, several RCTs reported no differences in outcome between psychodynamic therapy and treatments with established efficacy, but they were not sufficiently powered to demonstrate equivalence if a criterion of at least 70 patients per group, as previously suggested (Leichsenring et al. 2015b), is applied (Barber et al. 2012; Barkham et al. 1996; Gallagher-Thompson and Steffen 1994; Salminen et al. 2008; Shapiro et al. 1994). Meta-analyses achieve a higher statistical power than individual studies (Borenstein et al. 2011). For these reasons, it is of note that several meta-analyses found individual psychodynamic therapy to be efficacious for depressive disorders with no differences compared with other bona fide treatments (Abbass and Driessen 2010; Cuijpers et al. 2014; Driessen et al. 2010; Leichsenring et al. 2004, 2011).

Pathological Grief

In RCTs by McCallum and Piper (1990) and Piper et al. (2001), the treatment of prolonged or complicated grief by short-term psychodynamic group therapy was studied. In the first study, short-term psychodynamic group therapy was significantly superior to a wait list (McCallum and Piper 1990). In the second study, a significant interaction was found. With regard to grief symptoms, patients with a high quality of object relations improved more in interpretative therapy, and patients with a low quality of object relations improved more in supportive therapy. For general symptoms, clinical significance favored interpretive therapy over supportive therapy (Piper et al. 2001).

Anxiety Disorders

The efficacy of psychodynamic therapy in the treatment of anxiety disorders is supported by several RCTs (Table 6–1).

Social Anxiety Disorder

For social anxiety disorder, psychodynamic therapy was superior to a credible placebo and as efficacious as CBT (Bögels et al. 2014; Knijnik et al. 2004). One RCT found psychodynamic therapy to be superior to a waiting list and to be as efficacious as CBT in all outcomes, including social anxiety, general psychopathology, and defense mechanisms (Bögels et al. 2014). In this study, which the authors reported to be sufficiently powered to detect medium differences (Bögels et al. 2014, p. 370), success rates were above 50% and were found to be stable at the 3- and 12-month follow-ups. In a large multicenter RCT, both psychodynamic therapy and CBT were superior to a waiting list condition (Leichsenring et al. 2013a); no differences between psychodynamic therapy and CBT were found with regard to response rates and reduction of depression. CBT was superior with regard to remission rates, self-reported social anxiety, and interpersonal problems, yet these differences were small and below the threshold defined a priori as being clinically meaningful (Leichsenring et al. 2013a). Furthermore, no differences were found with regard to long-term effects on any outcome measure 6, 12, and 24 months after the end of therapy (Leichsenring et al. 2014). A review on social anxiety disorder was given by Leichsenring and Leweke (2017).

Panic Disorder

For panic disorder, psychodynamic therapy was superior to applied relaxation (Milrod et al. 2007). In an RCT by Milrod et al. (2016) comparing psychodynamic therapy, CBT, and applied relaxation for panic disorder, a significant site-by-treatment interaction was found, with CBT being superior in one site. When overall response rates were taken into account, no significant differences between CBT and psychodynamic therapy were found (63% vs. 59%; 46% for applied relaxation). In another RCT of psychodynamic therapy versus CBT for panic disorder, no significant differences in remission rates were found, but the study was not sufficiently powered to show equivalence (Beutel et al. 2013).

Generalized Anxiety Disorder

For generalized anxiety disorder, one RCT reported no significant differences between psychodynamic therapy and CBT in the primary outcome measure (Hamilton Anxiety Rating Scale), but the study was not sufficiently powered for an equivalence trial (Leichsenring et al. 2009). For secondary measures (e.g., worry, depression), CBT achieved significantly better outcomes (Leichsenring et al. 2009; Salzer et al. 2011). Treatment effects were stable 12 months after the end of therapy (Salzer et al. 2011). In another RCT, internet-guided psychodynamic self-help proved to be superior to a waiting list control condition for generalized anxiety disorder (Andersson et al. 2012). No differences from internet-guided CBT were reported, but this study was not sufficiently powered to demonstrate equivalence (Table 6–1).

Mixed Anxiety Disorders

The combination of psychodynamic therapy plus pharmacotherapy was shown to be superior to pharmacotherapy alone in the treatment of both social anxiety disorder (Knijnik et al. 2008, 2009) and panic disorder (Wiborg and Dahl 1996). For panic disorder, psychodynamic therapy combined with pharmacotherapy was superior to pharmacotherapy alone with regard to rates of remission and relapse prevention (Wiborg and Dahl 1996).

For a mixed sample including the various categories of anxiety disorders, STPP was superior to LTPP (and as efficacious as solution-focused therapy) with regard to recovery at 7-month follow-up (Knekt et al. 2008). In a mixed sample of patients with depressive and/or anxiety disorders, psychodynamic therapy was superior to TAU (pharmacotherapy) (Bressi et al. 2010).

A meta-analysis found psychodynamic therapy to be superior to inactive control conditions in anxiety disorders (Keefe et al. 2014). No differences were found between psychodynamic therapy and other bona fide treatments (Keefe et al. 2014). For this meta-analysis, the authors reported that large and medium effect sizes between psychodynamic therapy and alternative active treatments at termination could be detected with a power of about 1.00 regardless of the degree of heterogeneity (Keefe et al. 2014).

Obsessive-Compulsive Disorder

In an RCT by Maina et al. (2010) psychodynamic therapy combined with pharmacotherapy was not superior to pharmacotherapy alone for obsessive-compulsive disorder (Maina et al. 2010). An RCT comparing psychodynamic therapy with a waiting list for obsessive-compulsive disorder using a disorder-specific treatment manual is presently being carried out (Leichsenring and Steinert 2017b).

Posttraumatic Stress Disorder

In an early RCT by Brom et al. (1989), no statistically significant differences in outcome among psychodynamic therapy, hypnotherapy, and CBT were found for PTSD. However, this study was not sufficiently powered to show equivalence (Table 6–1). Psychodynamic therapy was superior to a waiting list in two of three measures and achieved the largest within-group effect sizes at follow-up. In an RCT carried out in Cambodia (Steinert et al. 2016, 2017b), resource-oriented psychodynamic therapy proved to be efficacious compared with a waiting list condition. A large-scale multicenter RCT comparing psychodynamic therapy and CBT for PTSD related to childhood maltreatment is presently being carried out (www.drks.de/drks_web/navigate.do?navigationId=trial.HTML&TRIAL_ID=DRKS00021142).

Somatoform Disorders

Several RCTs provide evidence for the efficacy of psychodynamic therapy in somatoform disorders, now referred to as somatic symptom and related disorders in DSM-5 (American Psychiatric Association 2013) (Table 6–1). Evidence from RCTs is available for irritable bowel syndrome (Creed et al. 2003; Guthrie et al. 1991, 1993), functional dyspepsia (Faramarzi et al. 2013; Hamilton et al. 2000), and somatoform pain disorder (Monsen and Monsen 2000; Sattel et al. 2012). In each of these RCTs, psychodynamic therapy was superior to TAU or supportive therapy. A meta-analysis found psychodynamic therapy to be efficacious in patients with somatic disorders (Abbass et al. 2009). A recent meta-analysis investigated STPP in functional somatic disorders (Abbass et al. 2020). Seventeen RCTs were included. STPP was significantly superior to control conditions (minimal attention, TAU, waitlist controls) with regard to measures of somatic symptoms posttreatment and at follow-up. As a limitation the authors stressed small samples and possible publication bias.

Eating Disorders

Bulimia Nervosa

Two RCTs (Fairburn et al. 1986; Garner et al. 1993) found no difference between psychodynamic therapy and CBT with regard to the primary outcome measure (bulimic episodes, vomiting), but, again, these studies were not sufficiently powered to demonstrate equivalence (Table 6–1). Differences in favor of CBT were found in secondary measures (Fairburn et al. 1986; Garner et al. 1993). Another RCT found psychodynamic therapy to be superior to cognitive therapy and nutritional counseling (Bachar et al. 1999). In a more recent RCT, CBT was superior to psychodynamic therapy (Poulsen et al. 2014). The study was controversially discussed because the psychodynamic therapy was not symptom focused, potentially disadvantaging the psychodynamic treatment (Poulsen and Lunn 2014; Tasca et al. 2014). In contrast, another RCT found psychodynamic therapy as efficacious as CBT in adolescents with bulimia nervosa (Stefini et al. 2017); unfortunately, the study was not sufficiently powered to demonstrate equivalence (Table 6–1).

Anorexia Nervosa

Two RCTs provide evidence for psychodynamic therapy for anorexia nervosa (Dare et al. 2001; Zipfel et al. 2014). The more recent RCT compared manual-guided psychodynamic therapy, enhanced CBT, and optimized TAU in the treatment of anorexia nervosa (Zipfel et al. 2014). At the end of treatment, significant improvements were found in all treatments, with no differences in the primary outcome measure (BMI). At 12-month follow-up, however, psychodynamic therapy was significantly superior to optimized TAU on rates of recovery, whereas enhanced CBT was not (Zipfel et al. 2014). Recovery rates were 35% for psychodynamic therapy, 19% for enhanced CBT, and 13% for optimized TAU. This study was sufficiently powered to show equivalence (Table 6–1).

Binge-Eating Disorder

For binge-eating disorder, psychodynamic therapy was found to be superior to a waiting list condition and to be as efficacious as CBT (Tasca et al. 2006). However, the study was not sufficiently powered to demonstrate equivalence to active treatments (Table 6–1).

Personality Disorders

Cluster C Personality Disorders

One RCT reported CBT as being more effective than waiting list control and psychodynamic therapy in the treatment of avoidant personality disorder (Emmelkamp et al. 2006). The study has attracted controversy because of possible biases (Emmelkamp 2007; Leichsenring and Leibing 2007), for example, whether a disorder-specific, manual-guided, bona fide version of psychodynamic therapy was used (Emmelkamp 2007; Leichsenring and Leibing 2007). Two RCTs found no differences in outcome relative to CBT (Muran et al. 2005; Svartberg et al. 2004). These studies were not sufficiently powered to demonstrate equivalence (Table 6–1).

Cluster B Personality Disorders

Five RCTs have demonstrated the efficacy of psychodynamic therapy for borderline personality disorder (Bateman and Fonagy 1999, 2001, 2009; Clarkin et al. 2007; Doering et al. 2010; Gregory et al. 2008; Levy et al. 2006). In their first RCT, Bateman and Fonagy (1999) found psychodynamic therapy (mentalization-based therapy [MBT]) to be superior to day TAU. In their second RCT, MBT was superior to a manual-guided structured clinical management (Bateman and Fonagy 2009). MBT was superior with regard to self-reported and clinically significant problems, including suicide attempts and hospitalization. Clarkin et al. (2007) compared two types of psychodynamic therapy (transference-focused therapy [TFP] and supportive psychodynamic therapy [SPT]) to dialectical behavior therapy (DBT). No differences were found among the three treatments across several outcome measures, but TFP was superior to DBT with regard to improvements in reflective functioning and attachment (Levy et al. 2006). Only TFP and SPT were associated with improvements in anger and impulsivity, and only TFP was associated with a change in irritability and verbal and direct assault (Clarkin et al. 2007). TFP demonstrated significant improvements in 10 of 12 outcome measures, DBT showed significant improvements in 5 of 12 measures, and SPT demonstrated significant improvements in 6 of 12 measures (Clarkin et al. 2007). The efficacy of TFP was corroborated by another RCT showing that TFP was superior to a treatment by experienced community therapists (Doering et al. 2010). Gregory et al. (2008) reported that psychodynamic therapy (deconstructive therapy) was superior to a TAU condition for borderline patients with co-occurring alcohol use disorder. Another RCT compared psychodynamic therapy (TFP) with schema-focused therapy (Giesen-Bloo et al. 2006). The authors reported statistically and clinically significant improvements for both treatments. However, schema-focused therapy was found to be superior to TFP in several outcome measures. Furthermore, significantly higher dropout was reported in TFP. Several concerns have been raised concerning this study, most prominently regarding the treatment integrity of TFP (Giesen-Bloo and Arntz 2007; Yeomans 2007). The two studies comparing psychodynamic therapy to another active treatment reported superiority of psychodynamic therapy or the comparison condition in at least some measures (Giesen-Bloo et al. 2006; Levy et al. 2006).

Heterogeneous Samples of Patients With Personality Disorders

Psychodynamic therapy was superior to waiting list or minimal-contact conditions in samples with heterogeneous personality disorders in two RCTs (Abbass et al. 2008; Winston et al. 1994). Another RCT found no differences in outcome between psychodynamic therapy and brief supportive therapy (Hellerstein et al. 1998). However, two of these studies (Hellerstein et al. 1998; Winston et al. 1994) were not sufficiently powered to detect possible differences between psychodynamic therapy and the comparator treatments. In a sufficiently powered study, manual-guided psychodynamic therapy was as effective as community-delivered psychodynamic therapy (Vinnars et al. 2005). Several meta-analyses found psychodynamic therapy to be efficacious in the treatment of personality disorders (Barber et al. 2013; Cristea et al. 2017; Keefe et al. 2020; Town et al. 2011). In the meta-analysis by Cristea et al. (2017) on borderline personality disorder, psychodynamic therapy and DBT were superior to control conditions, with effect sizes of $g=0.41$ and 0.34; for CBT this was not the case ($g=0.24$).

Substance-Related Disorders

Woody et al. (1983, 1995) studied the effects of STPP and CBT given in addition to drug counseling in the treatment of opioid dependence (Table 6–1). In their first RCT, STPP plus drug counseling yielded significant improvements in measures of drug-related symptoms and general psychiatric symptoms (Woody et al. 1983). At 7-month follow-up, STPP and CBT plus drug counseling were equally effective, and both treatments were superior to drug counseling alone. In the second RCT, psychodynamic psychotherapy of 26 sessions given in addition to drug counseling was also superior to drug counseling alone in the treatment of opioid dependence (Woody et al. 1995). By 6-month follow-up, most of the gains made by the patients who had received psychodynamic therapy remained.

In an RCT conducted by Crits-Christoph et al. (1999, 2001) psychodynamic psychotherapy of up to 36 individual sessions was combined with 24 sessions of group drug counseling in the treatment of cocaine dependence. The combined treatment yielded significant improvements and was as effective as CBT that was combined with group drug counseling as well. However, neither CBT nor psychodynamic psychotherapy plus group drug counseling was more effective than group drug counseling alone. Furthermore, individual drug counseling was significantly superior to both forms of therapy concerning measures of drug abuse. With regard to psychological and social outcome variables, all treatments were equally effective (Crits-Christoph et al. 1999, 2001).

In an RCT by Sandahl et al. (1998), STPP and CBT were compared with regard to their efficacy in the treatment of alcohol abuse. STPP yielded significant improvements in measures of alcohol abuse, which were stable at 15-month follow-up. STPP was significantly superior to CBT in the number of abstinent days and in the improvement of general psychiatric symptoms.

Long-Term Psychodynamic Psychotherapy for Complex Mental Disorders

According to several meta-analyses, LTPP, defined as involving at least 50 sessions or lasting for at least 1 year, was shown to be superior to shorter or less intensive forms of treatment for patients with complex mental disorders (defined as chronic mental disorders), personality disorders, or multiple comorbid disorders (Leichsenring and Rabung 2008, 2011b; Leichsenring et al. 2013b; Woll and Schönbrodt 2020). Improvements in target problems, general psychiatric symptoms, and social functioning were found to be superior. These results are consistent with data on dose-effect relations, which suggest that for many patients with chronic mental disorders or personality disorders, short-term psychotherapy is not sufficient (Howard et al. 1986). For these patients, long-term treatments seem to be more effective.

The results of the meta-analysis by Leichsenring and Rabung (2008) were controversially discussed, for example, with regard to statistical analysis and the included comparison conditions (Bhar et al. 2010). Several responses have addressed these concerns (Leichsenring and Rabung 2011a, 2011b; Leichsenring et al. 2013b). The results of the previous meta-analysis (Leichsenring and Rabung 2008) were corroborated if, for example, only active comparison conditions were included, studies previously not included were considered, or between-group effect sizes were analyzed (Leichsenring and Rabung 2011b; Leichsenring et al. 2013a). Results were independently replicated by Woll and Schönbrodt (2020). Thus, for complex mental disorders, LTPP again proved to be superior to shorter or less intensive treatments. Analogously, we expect other forms of long-term psychotherapy to be superior to shorter forms of these treatments for complex mental disorders. DBT and schema-focused therapy for borderline personality disorders, for example, are also long-term treatments (Clarkin et al. 2007; Giesen-Bloo et al. 2006).

Efficacy of Psychodynamic Therapy Compared With Other Treatments

Whether psychodynamic therapy is as efficacious as other treatments with established efficacy is a matter of controversy (Marcus et al. 2014; Tolin 2014, 2015; Zhou et al. 2015). One meta-analysis formally tested whether psychodynamic therapy is as efficacious as treatments established in efficacy for specific mental disorders (Steinert et al. 2017a). The authors controlled for researcher allegiance effects by including representatives of psychodynamic therapy and CBT, the main rival psychotherapeutic treatments (adversarial collaboration), and applied the formal criteria for testing equivalence, resulting in a particularly strict test that a priori defined a margin compatible with equivalence ($g=0.25$, a small effect), used the two one-sided test procedure, and ensured the efficacy of the comparator (in most cases CBT). The primary outcome was *target symptoms* (e.g., depressive symptoms in depressive disorders, anxiety symptoms in anxiety disorders). Twenty-three RCTs with more than 2,700 patients were included. The mean study quality of included trials was good, as demonstrated by reliable rating methods. Statistical analyses showed the equivalence of psychodynamic therapy to comparison conditions for target symptoms at posttreatment and at follow-up. Furthermore, for long-term outcome, no differences between psychodynamic therapy and alternative therapy were found (Kivlighan et al. 2015).

A Cochrane review comprising 33 RCTs found STPP to be superior to control groups in most primary outcomes (i.e., general, anxiety, and depressive symptom reduction) as well as in interpersonal problems and social adjustment. The only exception was somatic measures (Abbass et al. 2014). Generally, effect sizes increased in long-term follow-ups; however, some of these effects did not reach statistical significance. The authors emphasized that because of large heterogeneity findings should be interpreted with caution. Furthermore, for most of the common mental disorders psychodynamic therapy was shown to fulfill the criteria of empirically supported therapies (Leichsenring et al. 2015a).

Process-Outcome Relationship: Mechanisms of Change

Despite decades of process-outcome research, only a few replicable results have emerged (Crits-Christoph et al. 2013). Most evidence exists for the role of the alliance across a range of psychotherapies (Crits-Christoph et al. 2013). For psychodynamic therapy, improvements in self-understanding were found to be associated with improvements in symptoms (Crits-Christoph et al. 2013). Results have been replicated in several studies (Crits-Christoph et al. 2013).

Conclusion

According to the findings presented in this chapter, substantial evidence exists for the efficacy of psychodynamic therapy for depressive, anxiety, somatoform, eating, substance-related, and personality disorders. This is consistent with a Cochrane report that found psychodynamic therapy to be efficacious in common mental disorders (Abbass et al. 2014). In follow-up assessments the effects of psychodynamic therapy were found to be stable or even to have increased (Abbass et al. 2009, 2014; Leichsenring and Rabung 2008). In contrast to beliefs held by some psychodynamic researchers, however, psychodynamic therapy does not seem to be superior to alternative therapies in the long term (Kivlighan et al. 2015).

With regard to the comparison of psychodynamic therapy and CBT, no substantial differences in efficacy were found in those studies sufficiently powered for testing equivalence (Crits-Christoph et al. 1999; Driessen et al. 2013; Leichsenring et al. 2013a, 2014; Zipfel et al. 2014). The equivalence of psychodynamic therapy to treatments established in efficacy was explicitly tested and demonstrated (Steinert et al. 2017a). If future research confirms that no substantial differences in outcome exist among the different forms of bona fide psychotherapy for common mental disorders, the next question becomes which patients benefit more from which kind of therapy.

For specific mental disorders, further RCTs of psychodynamic therapy are required. This applies, for instance, to obsessive-compulsive disorder and PTSD. For PTSD, only two RCTs exist (Brom et al. 1989; Steinert et al. 2017b). More adequately powered equivalence trials are needed. In future studies of psychodynamic therapy, not only measures of symptoms or DSM criteria but also measures more specific to psychodynamic therapy should be applied. Future studies should also examine whether specific gains are achieved by only psychodynamic therapy, that is, the question of *added value*. Such an added value was demonstrated, for example, by Levy et al. (2006), who compared psychodynamic therapy with DBT with regard to improvements in reflective functioning and attachment. Future research should address the mechanisms of change of psychodynamic therapy to further improve the treatments.

In the RCTs included here, various methods of psychodynamic therapy were used. However, from an empirical perspective, it is not clear how different the various approaches really—that is, *empirically*—are. For the treatment of anxiety disorders and depressive disorders, the various approaches were shown to be consistent with each other and to overlap to a high degree (Leichsenring and Salzer 2014; Leichsenring and Schauenburg 2014; Leichsenring and Steinert 2018). Thus, developing unified or transdiagnostic protocols for the psychodynamic treatment of major mental disorders is possible and may be an important target for future research and practice.

At present, no method of psychotherapy can claim to be the gold standard (Leichsenring and Steinert 2017a). A plurality of evidence-based therapies is to be welcomed, both in treatment and in research. Only plurality allows for bridging the gap between the different approaches and for learning from each approach to further improve the treatment of patients with mental disorders (Roy-Byrne 2017).

Key Points

- There is evidence for psychodynamic therapy in most common mental disorders.
- For specific disorders (e.g,. for obsessive-compulsive disorder, posttraumatic stress disorder), further research is required. This is true for long-term psychodynamic therapy in complex mental disorders as well.
- Future research should identify the specific additional gain achieved by psychodynamic therapy (e.g., in such areas as reflective functioning or attachment).

References

American Psychiatric Association: Diagnostic and Statistical Manual of Mental Disorders, 5th Edition. Arlington, VA, American Psychiatric Association, 2013

Abbass A, Driessen E: The efficacy of short-term psychodynamic psychotherapy for depression: a summary of recent findings. Acta Psychiatr Scand 121(5):398–399, author reply 398–399, 2010 20064127

Abbass A, Sheldon A, Gyra J, et al: Intensive short-term dynamic psychotherapy for DSM-IV personality disorders: a randomized controlled trial. J Nerv Ment Dis 196(3):211–216, 2008 18340256

Abbass A, Kisely S, Kroenke K: Short-term psychodynamic psychotherapy for somatic disorders: systematic review and meta-analysis of clinical trials. Psychother Psychosom 78(5):265–274, 2009 19602915

Abbass AA, Kisely SR, Town JM, et al: Short-term psychodynamic psychotherapies for common mental disorders. Cochrane Database Syst Rev Jul 1 (7):CD004687, 2014 24984083

Abbass A, Town J, Holmes H, et al: Short-term psychodynamic psychotherapy for functional somatic disorders: a meta-analysis of randomized controlled trials. Psychother Psychosom 89(6):363–370, 2020 32428905

Ajilchi B, Nejati V, Town JM, et al: Effects of intensive short-term dynamic psychotherapy on depressive symptoms and executive functioning in major depression. J Nerv Ment Dis 204(7):500–505, 2016 27065106

Andersson G, Paxling B, Roch-Norlund P, et al: Internet-based psychodynamic versus cognitive behavioral guided self-help for generalized anxiety disorder: a randomized controlled trial. Psychother Psychosom 81(6):344–355, 2012 22964540

Bachar E, Latzer Y, Kreitler S, et al: Empirical comparison of two psychological therapies: self psychology and cognitive orientation in the treatment of anorexia and bulimia. J Psychother Pract Res 8(2):115–128, 1999 10079459

Barber JP, Barrett MS, Gallop R, et al: Short-term dynamic psychotherapy versus pharmacotherapy for major depressive disorder: a randomized, placebo-controlled trial. J Clin Psychiatry 73(1):66–73, 2012 22152401

Barber JP, Muran JC, McCarthy KS, et al: Research on psychodynamic therapies, in Bergin and Garfield's Handbook of Psychotherapy and Behavior Change, 6th Edition. Edited by Lambert MJ. New York, Wiley, 2013, pp 443–494

Barkham M, Rees A, Shapiro DA, et al: Outcomes of time-limited psychotherapy in applied settings: replicating the Second Sheffield Psychotherapy Project. J Consult Clin Psychol 64(5):1079–1085, 1996 8916639

Bateman A, Fonagy P: Effectiveness of partial hospitalization in the treatment of borderline personality disorder: a randomized controlled trial. Am J Psychiatry 156(10):1563–1569, 1999 10518167

Bateman A, Fonagy P: Treatment of borderline personality disorder with psychoanalytically oriented partial hospitalization: an 18-month follow-up. Am J Psychiatry 158(1):36–42, 2001 11136631

Bateman A, Fonagy P: Randomized controlled trial of outpatient mentalization-based treatment versus structured clinical management for borderline personality disorder. Am J Psychiatry 166(12):1355–1364, 2009 19833787

Benson K, Hartz AJ: A comparison of observational studies and randomized, controlled trials. N Engl J Med 342(25):1878–1886, 2000 10861324

Beutel ME, Scheurich V, Knebel A, et al: Implementing panic-focused psychodynamic psychotherapy into clinical practice. Can J Psychiatry 58(6):326–334, 2013 23768260

Beutel ME, Weißflog G, Leuteritz K, et al: Efficacy of short-term psychodynamic psychotherapy (STPP) with depressed breast cancer patients: results of a randomized controlled multicenter trial. Ann Oncol 25(2):378–384, 2014 24347520

Beutler LE: Identifying empirically supported treatments: what if we didn't? J Consult Clin Psychol 66(1):113–120, 1998 9489264

Bhar SS, Thombs BD, Pignotti M, et al: Is longer-term psychodynamic psychotherapy more effective than shorter-term therapies? Review and critique of the evidence. Psychother Psychosom 79(4):208–216, 2010 20424498

Bögels SM, Wijts P, Oort FJ, et al: Psychodynamic psychotherapy versus cognitive behavior therapy for social anxiety disorder: an efficacy and partial effectiveness trial. Depress Anxiety 31(5):363–373, 2014 24577880

Borenstein M, Hedges LV, Higgins JPT, et al: Introduction to Meta-Analysis. Chichester, UK, Wiley, 2011

Bressi C, Porcellana M, Marinaccio PM, et al: Short-term psychodynamic psychotherapy versus treatment as usual for depressive and anxiety disorders: a randomized clinical trial of efficacy. J Nerv Ment Dis 198(9):647–652, 2010 20823726

Brom D, Kleber RJ, Defares PB: Brief psychotherapy for posttraumatic stress disorders. J Consult Clin Psychol 57(5):607–612, 1989 2571625

Burnand Y, Andreoli A, Kolatte E, et al: Psychodynamic psychotherapy and clomipramine in the treatment of major depression. Psychiatr Serv 53(5)585–590, 2002 11986508

Canadian Task Force on the Periodic Health Examination: The periodic health examination. Can Med Assoc J 121(9):1193–1254, 1979 115569

Chambless DL, Hollon SD: Defining empirically supported therapies. J Consult Clin Psychol 66(1):7–18, 1998 9489259

Clarke M, Oxman AD (eds): Cochrane Reviewers' Handbook 4.1.6 (updated January 2003) (Cochrane Library, Issue 1). Oxford, UK, Update Software, 2003

Clarkin JF, Levy KN, Lenzenweger MF, et al: Evaluating three treatments for borderline personality disorder: a multiwave study. Am J Psychiatry 164(6):922–928, 2007 17541052

Concato J, Shah N, Horwitz RI: Randomized, controlled trials, observational studies, and the hierarchy of research designs. N Engl J Med 342(25):1887–1892, 2000 10861325

Connolly Gibbons MB, Thompson SM, Scott K, et al: Supportive-expressive dynamic psychotherapy in the community mental health system: a pilot effectiveness trial for the treatment of depression. Psychotherapy (Chic) 49(3):303–316, 2012 22962971

Connolly Gibbons MB, Gallop R, Thompson D, et al: Comparative effectiveness of cognitive therapy and dynamic psychotherapy for major depressive disorder in a community mental health setting: a randomized clinical noninferiority trial. JAMA Psychiatry 73(9):904–911, 2016 27487573

Cook DJ, Guyatt GH, Laupacis A, et al: Clinical recommendations using levels of evidence for antithrombotic agents. Chest 108(4 suppl):227S–230S, 1995 7555178

Cooper PJ, Murray L, Wilson A, et al: Controlled trial of the short- and long-term effect of psychological treatment of post-partum depression. I. Impact on maternal mood. Br J Psychiatry 182:412–419, 2003 12724244

Creed F, Fernandes L, Guthrie E, et al: The cost-effectiveness of psychotherapy and paroxetine for severe irritable bowel syndrome. Gastroenterology 124(2):303–317, 2003 12557136

Cristea IA, Gentili C, Cotet CD, et al: Efficacy of psychotherapies for borderline personality disorder: a systematic review and meta-analysis. JAMA Psychiatry 74(4):319–328, 2017 28249086
Crits-Christoph P, Siqueland L, Blaine J, et al: Psychosocial treatments for cocaine dependence: National Institute on Drug Abuse Collaborative Cocaine Treatment Study. Arch Gen Psychiatry 56(6):493–502, 1999 10359461
Crits-Christoph P, Siqueland L, McCalmont E, et al: Impact of psychosocial treatments on associated problems of cocaine-dependent patients. J Consult Clin Psychol 69(5):825–830, 2001 11680559
Crits-Christoph P, Connolly Gibbons MB, Mukherjee D: Psychotherapy process-outcome research, in Bergin and Garfield's Handbook of Psychotherapy and Behavior Change, 6th Edition. Edited by Lambert MJ. New York, Wiley, 2013, pp 298–340
Cuijpers P, Karyotaki E, Weitz E, et al: The effects of psychotherapies for major depression in adults on remission, recovery and improvement: a meta-analysis. J Affect Disord 159:118–126, 2014 24679399
Cuijpers P, Cristea IA, Karyotaki E, et al: How effective are cognitive behavior therapies for major depression and anxiety disorders? A meta-analytic update of the evidence. World Psychiatry 15(3):245–258, 2016 27717254
Dare C, Eisler I, Russell G, et al: Psychological therapies for adults with anorexia nervosa: randomised controlled trial of out-patient treatments. Br J Psychiatry 178:216–221, 2001 11230031
de Jonghe F, Kool S, van Aalst G, et al: Combining psychotherapy and antidepressants in the treatment of depression. J Affect Disord, 64(2–3)217–229, 2001 11313088
de Jonghe F, Hendricksen M, van Aalst G, et al: Psychotherapy alone and combined with pharmacotherapy in the treatment of depression. Br J Psychiatry 185:37–45, 2004 15231554
Doering S, Hörz S, Rentrop M, et al: Transference-focused psychotherapy v. treatment by community psychotherapists for borderline personality disorder: randomised controlled trial. Br J Psychiatry 196(5):389–395, 2010 20435966
Driessen E, Cuijpers P, de Maat SCM, et al: The efficacy of short-term psychodynamic psychotherapy for depression: a meta-analysis. Clin Psychol Rev 30(1):25–36, 2010 19766369
Driessen E, Van HL, Don FJ, et al: The efficacy of cognitive-behavioral therapy and psychodynamic therapy in the outpatient treatment of major depression: a randomized clinical trial. Am J Psychiatry 170(9):1041–1050, 2013 24030613
Emmelkamp P: Author's reply. Br J Psychiatry 190:80–81, 2007
Emmelkamp PM, Benner A, Kuipers A, et al: Comparison of brief dynamic and cognitive-behavioural therapies in avoidant personality disorder. Br J Psychiatry 189:60–64, 2006 16816307
Fairburn CG, Kirk J, O'Connor M, et al: A comparison of two psychological treatments for bulimia nervosa. Behav Res Ther 24(6):629–643, 1986 3800834
Faramarzi M, Azadfallah P, Book HE, et al: A randomized controlled trial of brief psychoanalytic psychotherapy in patients with functional dyspepsia. Asian J Psychiatr 6(3):228–234, 2013 23642981
Fonagy P: Process and outcome in mental health care delivery: a model approach to treatment evaluation. Bull Menninger Clin 63(3):288–304, 1999 10452192
Fusar-Poli P, Radua J: Ten simple rules for conducting umbrella reviews. Evid Based Ment Health 21(3):95–100, 2018 30006442
Gabbard GO: Long-Term Psychodynamic Psychotherapy. Washington, DC, American Psychiatric Publishing, 2004
Gabbard GO, Gunderson JG, Fonagy P: The place of psychoanalytic treatments within psychiatry. Arch Gen Psychiatry 59(6):505–510, 2002 12044192
Gallagher-Thompson D, Steffen AM: Comparative effects of cognitive-behavioral and brief psychodynamic psychotherapies for depressed family caregivers. J Consult Clin Psychol 62(3):543–549, 1994 8063980
Gallagher-Thompson D, Hanley-Peterson P, Thompson LW: Maintenance of gains versus relapse following brief psychotherapy for depression. J Consult Clin Psychol 58(3)371–374, 1990 2365900

Garner DM, Rockert W, Davis R, et al: Comparison of cognitive-behavioral and supportive-expressive therapy for bulimia nervosa. Am J Psychiatry 150(1):37–46, 1993 8417578

Giesen-Bloo J, Arntz A: Questions concerning the randomized trial of schema-focused therapy vs transference-focused psychotherapy—reply. Arch Gen Psychiatry 64:610–611, 2007

Giesen-Bloo J, van Dyck R, Spinhoven P, et al: Outpatient psychotherapy for borderline personality disorder: randomized trial of schema-focused therapy vs transference-focused psychotherapy. Arch Gen Psychiatry 63(6):649–658, 2006 16754838

Gregory RJ, Chlebowski S, Kang D, et al: A controlled trial of psychodynamic psychotherapy for co-occurring borderline personality disorder and alcohol use disorder. Psychotherapy (Chic) 45(1):28–41, 2008 22122363

Guthrie E, Creed F, Dawson D, et al: A controlled trial of psychological treatment for the irritable bowel syndrome. Gastroenterology 100(2):450–457, 1991 1985041

Guthrie E, Creed F, Dawson D, et al: A randomised controlled trial of psychotherapy in patients with refractory irritable bowel syndrome. Br J Psychiatry 163:315–321, 1993 8401959

Guthrie E, Moorey J, Margison F, et al: Cost-effectiveness of brief psychodynamic-interpersonal therapy in high utilizers of psychiatric services. Arch Gen Psychiatry 56(6):519–526, 1999 10359466

Guyatt GH, Sackett DL, Sinclair JC, et al: Users' guides to the medical literature IX: a method for grading health care recommendations. JAMA 274(22):1800–1804, 1995 7500513

Hamilton J, Guthrie E, Creed F, et al: A randomized controlled trial of psychotherapy in patients with chronic functional dyspepsia. Gastroenterology 119(3):661–669, 2000 10982759

Hellerstein DJ, Rosenthal RN, Pinsker H, et al: A randomized prospective study comparing supportive and dynamic therapies: outcome and alliance. J Psychother Pract Res 7(4):261–271, 1998 9752637

Howard KI, Kopta SM, Krause MS, et al: The dose-effect relationship in psychotherapy. Am Psychol 41(2):159–164, 1986 3516036

Huhn M, Tardy M, Spineli LM, et al: Efficacy of pharmacotherapy and psychotherapy for adult psychiatric disorders: a systematic overview of meta-analyses. JAMA Psychiatry 71(6):706–715, 2014 24789675

Johansson R, Ekbladh S, Hebert A, et al: Psychodynamic guided self-help for adult depression through the internet: a randomised controlled trial. PLoS One 7(5):e38021, 2012 22741027

Johansson R, Björklund M, Hornborg C, et al: Affect-focused psychodynamic psychotherapy for depression and anxiety through the internet: a randomized controlled trial. PeerJ 102:1–22, 2013 23862104

Keefe JR, McCarthy KS, Dinger U, et al: A meta-analytic review of psychodynamic therapies for anxiety disorders. Clin Psychol Rev 34(4):309–323, 2014 24786897

Keefe JR, McMain SF, McCarthy KS, et al: A meta-analysis of psychodynamic treatments for borderline and Cluster C personality disorders. Pers Disord 11(3):157–169, 2020 31804128

Kernberg OF: A psychoanalytic model for the classification of personality disorders, in Implications of Psychopharmacology to Psychiatry. Edited by Achenheil BBM, Engel R, Ermann M, et al. New York, Springer, 1996, pp 66–78

Kivlighan DM III, Goldberg SB, Abbas M, et al: The enduring effects of psychodynamic treatments vis-à-vis alternative treatments: a multilevel longitudinal meta-analysis. Clin Psychol Rev 40:1–14, 2015 26042927

Knekt P, Lindfors O, Härkänen T, et al: Randomized trial on the effectiveness of long-and short-term psychodynamic psychotherapy and solution-focused therapy on psychiatric symptoms during a 3-year follow-up. Psychol Med 38(5):689–703, 2008 18005493

Knijnik DZ, Kapczinski F, Chachamovich E, et al: Psychodynamic group treatment for generalized social phobia [in Portuguese]. Braz J Psychiatry 26(2):77–81, 2004 15517057

Knijnik DZ, Blanco C, Salum GA, et al: A pilot study of clonazepam versus psychodynamic group therapy plus clonazepam in the treatment of generalized social anxiety disorder. Eur Psychiatry 23(8):567–574, 2008 18774274

Knijnik DZ, Salum GAJ Jr, Blanco C, et al: Defense style changes with the addition of psychodynamic group therapy to clonazepam in social anxiety disorder. J Nerv Ment Dis 197(7):547–551, 2009 19597364

Leichsenring F: Randomized controlled vs. naturalistic studies: a new research agenda. Bull Menninger Clin 68:115–129, 2004

Leichsenring F, Leibing E: Cognitive-behavioural therapy for avoidant personality disorder. Br J Psychiatry 190:80, author reply 80–81, 2007 17197665

Leichsenring F, Leweke F: Social anxiety disorder. N Engl J Med 376(23):2255–2264, 2017 28591542

Leichsenring F, Rabung S: Effectiveness of long-term psychodynamic psychotherapy: a meta-analysis. JAMA 300(13):1551–1565, 2008 18827212

Leichsenring F, Rabung S: Double standards in psychotherapy research. Psychother Psychosom 80(1):48–51, author reply 53–54, 2011a 21088445

Leichsenring F, Rabung S: Long-term psychodynamic psychotherapy in complex mental disorders: update of a meta-analysis. Br J Psychiatry 199(1):15–22, 2011b 21719877

Leichsenring F, Salzer S: A unified protocol for the transdiagnostic psychodynamic treatment of anxiety disorders: an evidence-based approach. Psychotherapy (Chic) 51(2):224–245, 2014 24377407

Leichsenring F, Schauenburg H: Empirically supported methods of short-term psychodynamic therapy in depression—towards an evidence-based unified protocol. J Affect Disord 169:128–143, 2014 25194781

Leichsenring F, Steinert C: Is cognitive behavioral therapy the gold standard for psychotherapy? The need for plurality in treatment and research. JAMA 318(14):1323–1324, 2017a 28975264

Leichsenring F, Steinert C: Short-term psychodynamic therapy for obsessive-compulsive disorder: a manual-guided approach to treating the "inhibited rebel." Bull Menninger Clin 81(4):341–389, 2017b 28745949

Leichsenring F, Steinert C: Towards an evidence-based unified psychodynamic protocol for emotional disorders. J Affect Disord 232:400–416, 2018 29522960

Leichsenring F, Rabung S, Leibing E: The efficacy of short-term psychodynamic psychotherapy in specific psychiatric disorders: a meta-analysis. Arch Gen Psychiatry 61(12):1208–1216, 2004 15583112

Leichsenring F, Salzer S, Jaeger U, et al: Short-term psychodynamic psychotherapy and cognitive-behavioral therapy in generalized anxiety disorder: a randomized, controlled trial. Am J Psychiatry 166(8):875–881, 2009 19570931

Leichsenring F, Salzer S, Hilsenroth M, et al: Treatment integrity: an unresolved issue in psychotherapy research. Curr Psychiatry Rev 7:313–321, 2011

Leichsenring F, Salzer S, Beutel ME, et al: Psychodynamic therapy and cognitive-behavioral therapy in social anxiety disorder: a multicenter randomized controlled trial. Am J Psychiatry 170(7):759–767, 2013a 23680854

Leichsenring F, Abbass A, Luyten P, et al: The emerging evidence for long-term psychodynamic therapy. Psychodyn Psychiatry 41(3):361–384, 2013b 24001160

Leichsenring F, Salzer S, Beutel ME, et al: Long-term outcome of psychodynamic therapy and cognitive-behavioral therapy in social anxiety disorder. Am J Psychiatry 171(10):1074–1082, 2014 25016974

Leichsenring F, Leweke F, Klein S, et al: The empirical status of psychodynamic psychotherapy—an update: Bambi's alive and kicking. Psychother Psychosom 84(3):129–148, 2015a 25833321

Leichsenring F, Luyten P, Hilsenroth MJ, et al: Psychodynamic therapy meets evidence-based medicine: a systematic review using updated criteria. Lancet Psychiatry 2(7):648–660, 2015b 26303562

Levy KN, Meehan KB, Kelly KM, et al: Change in attachment patterns and reflective function in a randomized control trial of transference-focused psychotherapy for borderline personality disorder. J Consult Clin Psychol 74(6):1027–1040, 2006 17154733

Luborsky L: Principles of Psychoanalytic Psychotherapy: Manual for Supportive-Expressive Treatment. New York, Basic Books, 1984

Maina G, Forner F, Bogetto F: Randomized controlled trial comparing brief dynamic and supportive therapy with waiting list condition in minor depressive disorders. Psychother Psychosom 74(1):43–50, 2005 15627856

Maina G, Rosso G, Crespi C, Bogetto F: Combined brief dynamic therapy and pharmacotherapy in the treatment of major depressive disorder: a pilot study. Psychother Psychosom 76(5)298–305 2007 17700050
Maina G, Rosso G, Rigardetto S, et al: No effect of adding brief dynamic therapy to pharmacotherapy in the treatment of obsessive-compulsive disorder with concurrent major depression. Psychother Psychosom 79(5):295–302, 2010 20616624
Marcus DK, O'Connell D, Norris AL, et al: Is the Dodo bird endangered in the 21st century? A meta-analysis of treatment comparison studies. Clin Psychol Rev 34(7):519–530, 2014 25238455
McCallum M, Piper WE: A controlled study of effectiveness and patient suitability for short-term group psychotherapy. Int J Group Psychother 40(4):431–452, 1990 2228349
Messer SB, Warren CS: Models of Brief Psychodynamic Therapy: A Comparative Approach. New York, Guilford, 1995
Milrod B, Leon AC, Busch F, et al: A randomized controlled clinical trial of psychoanalytic psychotherapy for panic disorder. Am J Psychiatry 164(2):265–272, 2007 17267789
Milrod B, Chambless DL, Gallop R, et al: Psychotherapies for panic disorder: a tale of two sites. J Clin Psychiatry 77(7):927–935, 2016 27464313
Monsen K, Monsen TJ: Chronic pain and psychodynamic body therapy. Psychotherapy (Chic) 37:257–269, 2000
Muran JC, Safran JD, Samstag LW, Winston A: Evaluating an alliance-focused treatment for personality disorders. Psychotherapy (Chic) 42:532–545, 2005
Nathan PE, Gorman JM (eds): A Guide to Treatments That Work, 4th Edition. New York, Oxford University Press, 2015
Persons JB, Silberschatz G: Are results of randomized controlled trials useful to psychotherapists? J Consult Clin Psychol 66(1):126–135, 1998 9489266
Piper WE, McCallum M, Joyce AS, et al: Patient personality and time-limited group psychotherapy for complicated grief. Int J Group Psychother 51(4):525–552, 2001 11582899
Poulsen S, Lunn S: Response to Tasca et al. Am J Psychiatry 171(5):584, 2014 24788288
Poulsen S, Lunn S, Daniel SI, et al: A randomized controlled trial of psychoanalytic psychotherapy or cognitive-behavioral therapy for bulimia nervosa. Am J Psychiatry 171(1):109–116, 2014 24275909
Roth A, Parry G: The implications of psychotherapy research for clinical practice and service development: lessons and limitations. J Ment Health 6:367–380, 1997
Rothwell PM: External validity of randomised controlled trials: "to whom do the results of this trial apply?" Lancet 365(9453):82–93, 2005 15639683
Roy-Byrne P: Transdiagnostic cognitive-behavioral therapy and the return of the repressed. JAMA Psychiatry 74(9):867–868, 2017 28768336
Salminen JK, Karlsson H, Hietala J, et al: Short-term psychodynamic psychotherapy and fluoxetine in major depressive disorder: a randomized comparative study. Psychother Psychosom 77(6):351–357, 2008 18701831
Salzer S, Winkelbach C, Leweke F, et al: Long-term effects of short-term psychodynamic psychotherapy and cognitive-behavioural therapy in generalized anxiety disorder: 12-month follow-up. Can J Psychiatry 56(8):503–508, 2011 21878162
Sandahl C, Herlitz K, Ahlin G, et al: Time-limited group psychotherapy for moderately alcohol dependent patients: A randomized controlled clinical trial. Psychother Res 8:361–378, 1998
Sattel H, Lahmann C, Gündel H, et al: Brief psychodynamic interpersonal psychotherapy for patients with multisomatoform disorder: randomised controlled trial. Br J Psychiatry 200(1):60–67, 2012 22075651
Seligman ME: The effectiveness of psychotherapy: the Consumer Reports study. Am Psychol 50(12):965–974, 1995 8561380
Shadish WR, Matt GE, Navarro AM, et al: The effects of psychological therapies under clinically representative conditions: a meta-analysis. Psychol Bull 126(4):512–529, 2000 10900994
Shadish WR, Cook TD, Campbell DT: Experimental and Quasi-experimental Designs for Generalized Causal Inference. Boston, MA, Houghton Mifflin, 2002

Shapiro DA, Barkham M, Rees A, et al: Effects of treatment duration and severity of depression on the effectiveness of cognitive-behavioral and psychodynamic-interpersonal psychotherapy. J Consult Clin Psychol 62(3):522–534, 1994 8063978
Stefini A, Salzer S, Reich G, et al: Cognitive-behavioral and psychodynamic therapy in female adolescents with bulimia nervosa: a randomized controlled trial. J Am Acad Child Adolesc Psychiatry 56(4):329–335, 2017 28335877
Snyder DK, Wills RM: Behavioral versus insight-oriented marital therapy: effects on individual and interspousal functioning. J Consult Clin Psychol 57(1)39–46, 1989 2925973
Snyder DK, Wills RM, Grady-Fletcher A: Long-term effectiveness of behavioral versus insight-oriented marital therapy: a 4-year follow-up study. J Consult Clin Psychol 59(1):138–141, 1991 2002129
Steinert C, Bumke PJ, Hollekamp RL, et al: Treating post-traumatic stress disorder by resource activation in Cambodia. World Psychiatry 15(2):183–185, 2016 27265714
Steinert C, Munder T, Rabung S, et al: Psychodynamic therapy: as efficacious as other empirically supported treatments? A meta-analysis testing equivalence of outcomes. Am J Psychiatry 174(10):943–953, 2017a 28541091
Steinert C, Bumke PJ, Hollekamp RL, et al: Resource activation for treating post-traumatic stress disorder, co-morbid symptoms and impaired functioning: a randomized controlled trial in Cambodia. Psychol Med 47(3):553–564, 2017b 27804900
Svartberg M, Stiles TC, Seltzer MH: Randomized, controlled trial of the effectiveness of short-term dynamic psychotherapy and cognitive therapy for Cluster C personality disorders. Am J Psychiatry 161(5):810–817, 2004 15121645
Tasca GA, Ritchie K, Conrad G, et al: Attachment scales predict outcome in a randomized clinical trial of group psychotherapy for binge eating disorder: an aptitude by treatment interaction. Psychother Res 16:106–121, 2006
Tasca GA, Hilsenroth M, Thompson-Brenner H: Psychoanalytic psychotherapy or cognitive-behavioral therapy for bulimia nervosa. Am J Psychiatry 171(5):583–584, 2014 24788287
Task Force on Promotion and Dissemination of Psychological Procedures: Training and dissemination of empirically validated psychological treatments: report and recommendations. Clin Psychol 48:3–23, 1995
Thompson LW, Gallagher D, Breckenridge JS: Comparative effectiveness of psychotherapies for depressed elders. J Consult Clin Psychol 55(3):385–390, 1987 3597953
Tolin DF: Beating a dead Dodo bird: looking at signal vs. noise in cognitive-behavioral therapy for anxiety disorders. Clin Psychol Sci Pract 21(3):351–362, 2014
Tolin DF: Corrigendum to "Beating a dead Dodo bird: looking at signal vs. noise in cognitive-behavioral therapy for anxiety disorders." Clin Psychol Sci Pract 22(3):315–316, 2015
Tolin DF, McKay D, Forman EM, et al: Empirically supported treatment: recommendations for a new model. Clin Psychol Sci Pract 22:317–338, 2015
Town JM, Abbass A, Hardy G: Short-term psychodynamic psychotherapy for personality disorders: a critical review of randomized controlled trials. J Pers Disord 25(6):723–740, 2011 22217220
Town JM, Abbass A, Stride C, Bernier D: A randomised controlled trial of intensive short-term dynamic psychotherapy for treatment resistant depression: the Halifax Depression Study. J Affect Disord 214:15–25, 2017 28266318
Vinnars B, Barber JP, Norén K, et al: Manualized supportive-expressive psychotherapy versus nonmanualized community-delivered psychodynamic therapy for patients with personality disorders: bridging efficacy and effectiveness. Am J Psychiatry 162(10):1933–1940, 2005 16199841
Walker E, Nowacki AS: Understanding equivalence and noninferiority testing. J Gen Intern Med 26(2):192–196, 2011 20857339
Wallerstein RS: The psychotherapy research project of the Menninger Foundation: an overview. J Consult Clin Psychol 57(2):195–205, 1989 2708605
Wampold BE, Imel ZE: The Great Psychotherapy Debate: The Evidence for What Makes Psychotherapy Work, 2nd Edition. New York, Routledge, 2015

Westen D, Novotny CM, Thompson-Brenner H: The empirical status of empirically supported psychotherapies: assumptions, findings, and reporting in controlled clinical trials. Psychol Bull 130(4):631–663, 2004 15250817

Wiborg IM, Dahl AA: Does brief dynamic psychotherapy reduce the relapse rate of panic disorder? Arch Gen Psychiatry 53(8):689–694, 1996 8694682

Winston A, Laikin M, Pollack J, et al: Short-term psychotherapy of personality disorders. Am J Psychiatry 151(2):190–194, 1994 8296887

Woll CF, Schönbrodt FD: A series of meta-analytic tests of the efficacy of long-term psychoanalytic psychotherapy. Eur Psychol 25:51–72, 2020

Woody GE, Luborsky L, McLellan AT, et al: Psychotherapy for opiate addicts: does it help? Arch Gen Psychiatry 40(6):639–645, 1983 6847332

Woody GE, Luborsky L, McLellan AT, O'Brien CP: Corrections and revised analyses for psychotherapy in methadone maintenance patients. Arch Gen Psychiatry 47(8):788–789, 1990 2378551

Woody GE, McLellan AT, Luborsky L, et al: Psychotherapy in community methadone programs: a validation study. Am J Psychiatry 152(9):1302–1308, 1995 7653685

Yeomans F: Questions concerning the randomized trial of schema-focused therapy vs transference-focused psychotherapy. Arch Gen Psychiatry 64(5):609–610, author reply 610–611, 2007 17485613

Zhou X, Hetrick SE, Cuijpers P, et al: Comparative efficacy and acceptability of psychotherapies for depression in children and adolescents: a systematic review and network meta-analysis. World Psychiatry 14(2):207–222, 2015 26043339

Zipfel S, Wild B, Groß G, et al: Focal psychodynamic therapy, cognitive behaviour therapy, and optimised treatment as usual in outpatients with anorexia nervosa (ANTOP study): randomised controlled trial. Lancet 383(9912):127–137, 2014 24131861

PART II

Cognitive-Behavioral Therapy

Section Editors: Donna M. Sudak, M.D., and Seamus Bhatt-Mackin, M.D.

Cognitive-behavioral therapy (CBT) is a highly researched and effective treatment for numerous psychiatric conditions. Since its origin more than 40 years ago, the theory and practice of CBT have expanded research evidence for its underlying theoretical base and clinical efficacy. CBT has also evolved a number of specialized treatments and models. Alternative forms of the therapy have focused on acceptance and mindfulness, further emphasized the role of emotion, expanded skills training, and increased attention to powerful behavioral treatments. Such an expansion may help patients who do not respond to standard CBT and may increase dissemination to resource-poor environments. All of the therapies described in Part II share several fundamental characteristics: a commitment to rigorous empirical study; an understanding that the therapeutic relationship is of primary importance; and treatment models that consider the interrelationships among thoughts, emotions, and behaviors and the need to determine reinforcement for behavior in interpersonal and intrapersonal contexts.

In this part, three separate chapters give us a snapshot of the state of the art in CBT. In Chapter 7, "Cognitive-Behavioral Theories," Leahy et al. describe the evolution of Beck's approach to the cognitive model and the universe of current CBT approaches. In Chapter 8, "Techniques of Cognitive-Behavioral Therapy," Wright et al. provide us with a series of vivid illustrations of the major techniques of CBT treatment, including more contemporary approaches to complex conditions such as schizophrenia and suicidal behavior. Finally, in Chapter 9, "Indications, Applications, and Efficacy of Individual Cognitive-Behavioral Therapy to Specific Psychiatric Disorders," Bhatt-Mackin et al. provide a concise review of the substantial research evidence supporting

CBT for various conditions. For those of us who believe that psychotherapy should be chosen on the basis of current available evidence, this chapter will be of considerable help.

Many theorists have used the term *cognitive revolution* to describe the explosive growth of this paradigm for treatment. More accurately, these chapters help us to see that we have a *cognitive evolution* in our science and practice, with continued growth and development as a field whose goal is more effective relief of human suffering.

CHAPTER 7

Cognitive-Behavioral Theories

Robert L. Leahy, Ph.D.
David A. Clark, Ph.D.
David J.A. Dozois, Ph.D.

Cognitive-behavioral theory of emotional and behavioral disorders has evolved and expanded since it was first developed in the 1960s. In this chapter we focus on several leading contemporary models within the cognitive-behavioral tradition: Beck's cognitive theory, behavioral activation, exposure therapy, metacognitive theory, mindfulness-based cognitive therapy, and acceptance and commitment therapy. Space limitations prevent the review of other important approaches, including dialectical behavior therapy (Linehan 1993), cognitive processing therapy (Resick 2018), problem-solving therapy (D'Zurilla and Nezu 2001; Nezu 2004), rational emotive behavior therapy (Ellis and MacLaren 1998), the cognitive-behavioral analysis system of psychotherapy (McCullough et al. 2015), and motivational interviewing (Miller and Rollnick 2002).

Beck's Cognitive Theory

One of the earliest and most influential of the cognitive-behavioral theories is Aaron T. Beck's *cognitive theory*. Originally formulated as the conceptual basis for Beck's cognitive therapy of depression (Beck 1967), the model and its therapy have been refined and expanded to encompass major psychiatric conditions in adults and children, including anxiety disorders (Beck et al. 1985), substance abuse (Beck et al. 2001), personality disorders (Beck et al. 2015), and schizophrenia (Beck et al. 2011). Moreover, variants and adaptions of the core tenets of the model have been applied to other problems, including eating disorders, PTSD, obsessive-compulsive and related disorders, and relationship discord. Beck's cognitive theory (Beck 1963) is unparalleled in its influence on contemporary psychological explanations for and treatment of psychiatric conditions.

The enormity of Beck's theory cannot be covered adequately in just a few pages. Numerous publications are available that provide a fuller explanation and evaluation of Beck's cognitive theory (e.g., Beck 1991, 1996; Clark and Beck 2010a, 2010b; Clark et al. 1999; Dozois and Beck 2008; Leahy 2004). Here we review the earliest and best-known standard cognitive model, a newer iteration known as the generic model (Beck and Haigh 2014), and the most recent version, recovery-oriented cognitive therapy (CT-R) (Beck et al. 2020).

Standard Cognitive Model

Basic Assumptions and Definition

Beck's cognitive theory is based on seven tenets that are fundamental to its conceptual integrity:

1. Information processing and meaning representation are essential for survival and adaptation.
2. The structures, processes, and content of the information processing apparatus create an individualized construction of reality that varies in its adaptability.
3. Information processing guides emotion, behavior, and physical aspects of human experience.
4. Cognitive functioning reflects the interaction of stimulus-driven information and higher-order semantic processes.
5. Meaning-making structures (i.e., schemas) have differing thresholds of activation and capacity to dominate the information processing system.
6. Psychological disturbance is characterized by excessive and/or deficient activation of specific schemas.
7. Modification of meaning-making structures (beliefs, attitudes) is critical for human change.

On the basis of the basic assumptions and key concepts of the cognitive model, we offer the following definition:

> Beck's standard cognitive theory asserts that psychological disturbance can be understood in terms of enduring, idiosyncratic, and maladaptive meaning representations of the self, others, and world that are activated by matching life experiences, leading to biased processing of self-referent information, and consequent maladaptive thoughts, behavior, affect, and physical responses that manifest as specific psychopathological symptoms. Recovery from acute psychological disturbance requires remediation of the biased information processing of disorder-relevant experiences.

Schemas

From the cognitive model's earliest days, the notion of *schemas* has been its bedrock. Schemas are enduring semantic representations of stimuli, ideas, or experience that organize and integrate new information in a meaningful manner that determines how phenomena are perceived and conceptualized (Beck 1967; Clark et al. 1999; Williams et al. 1997). As hypothetical structures containing the stored representations of meaning, schemas guide the selection, encoding, organization, storage, and retrieval of information. Schematic content is evident in the beliefs, attitudes, and assumptions held by individuals. Because schemas assume this executive function, our beliefs and attitudes determine the type and intensity of emotional response through their symbolic representation of situations (Clark et al. 1999).

The two main types of schemas especially important in Beck's cognitive theory are *intermediate* and *core beliefs* (Beck 2011). Intermediate beliefs are rules and assumptions used to evaluate and guide our behavior as well as to influence our interpretation of other people and personal experience. They often occur in the form of conditional rules or if-then statements (e.g., "If I am to succeed, then I need to work harder than others"). Core beliefs are a smaller subset of schematic content that represent more basic ideas about the self, personal world, and others. They are often rigid, absolute, overgeneralized convictions that are rooted in early childhood development. It is thought that core beliefs must be addressed to achieve enduring change with cognitive therapy.

Biased Cognitive Processing

In psychopathological states, the activation of maladaptive schemas frequently biases processing information in overly negative ways, causing inaccurate appraisals of self, personal experience, and interpersonal relations. Cognitive theory characterizes this biased processing into several errors (Beck et al. 1979). They include *arbitrary inference* (drawing conclusions without evidence), *selective abstraction* (interpreting a specific detail out of context), *overgeneralization* (drawing a conclusion from an isolated incident), *dichotomous thinking* (classifying experience in extremes), *personalization* (assuming a self-focus to external events), and *magnification* and *minimization* (exaggerating or discounting the significance of an experience). Because cognitive errors contribute to the maintenance of emotional disturbance, their correction is an important therapeutic element.

Negative Automatic Thoughts

Maladaptive schemas and biased cognitive processing result in overly negative thinking that Beck (1967) called *negative automatic thoughts*. Such thoughts and images are specific to current concerns, transient, involuntary, and highly plausible to a person because they are congruent with that person's affective state or personality disposition. In depression, for example, automatic thinking is highly negative about the self, the world, and the future (Beck et al. 1979). Negative automatic thoughts are situation specific and laden with emotional intent. For example, an anxious student might have the automatic thought "I don't know anything; I'm going to fail," whereas a depressed executive might think "Everyone is bored by my presentations." Automatic thoughts and images may not be readily apparent, but individuals can learn to access them. Cognitive restructuring involves the identification, evaluation, and discovery of alternative interpretations to biased automatic thinking. This method to correct cognitive errors is a core therapeutic intervention in cognitive therapy.

Compensatory Responses

Behavioral responses that individuals use to cope with maladaptive core beliefs are called *compensatory responses* (Beck 2011). For example, in response to a negative core belief about the self (e.g., "I am unlovable"), a person might frequently please other people to gain their favor. Beck et al. (2015) also noted that certain beliefs might accompany these compensatory strategies. When possessing the belief "I am unlovable," the person might also believe "If I please other people, then they will tolerate me" while engaging in the compensatory behavior. In another case, a person who believes "I can't trust myself to make the right decision" might compensate by seeking the opinion and reassurance of others with the compensatory belief that "getting advice from others will ensure that I've made the right decision." Identification and correction of such compensatory strategies and associated beliefs are an important component of cognitive therapy, especially when treating personality disorders.

Cognitive Content Specificity

In the cognitive model, themes and content in automatic thoughts and images are disorder specific (e.g., Beck and Perkins 2001). Self-referential thoughts of loss, failure, and deprivation are most prevalent in depression, whereas thoughts of threat, danger, and helplessness are prominent in anxiety disorders. Content is also different among anxiety disorder subtypes; examples include misinterpretation of bodily sensations in panic disorder, preoccupation with negative evaluation by others in social anxiety, and worry about future catastrophic outcomes in generalized anxiety disorder. Content specificity of automatic thoughts and beliefs guides the cognitive therapist in assessment and formulation of a treatment plan tailored to the specific concerns of each individual.

Generic Cognitive Model

Beck and Haigh (2014) presented a transdiagnostic cognitive model of clinical and subclinical psychological disturbance that extended certain aspects of the standard model and addressed gaps and limitations in the original theory. This *generic cognitive model* (GCM) proposes that clinical disorders represent an exaggeration of typical adaptive functioning, that biased information processing involves an autonomous and reflective processing subsystem, that life goals and expectations play an integral role in psychopathology via activation of modes, and that highly energized or charged schemas dominate the information processing apparatus.

All beliefs, processing biases, and ways of thinking may be healthy if they help us adapt to a current life situation. However, when a negative bias exaggerates loss or threat or a positive bias exaggerates gain or pleasure in a way that is disproportionate to life experience, psychological disturbance is more likely. The GCM posits that exaggerated positivity bias can also be problematic, such as in bipolar manic episodes.

Beck and Haigh (2014) characterized the cognitive apparatus as an interaction between automatic and reflective processing systems, an elaboration of the same concepts introduced in the standard cognitive model of anxiety (Clark and Beck 2010a). As part of this automatic system, *protoschemas* (see also Beck 1996; Clark and Beck 2010a) provide an initial (preconscious) evaluation of stimuli as good or bad for survival. The reflective system, under higher-order executive function, is slower and more effortful, involving the activation of more complex schemas. In cognitive therapy, reflective processing enables the evaluation and correction of biased meanings assigned by the automatic system.

Beck (1996) introduced the concept of *modes* as a network of cognitive, affective, motivational, and behavioral schemas organized to deal with life demands important to survival and adaptation. Beck and Haigh (2014) emphasized that modes enable the pursuit of life goals and management of daily stresses and challenges. Two constructs emphasized in the GCM are the *self-expansive* and *self-protective* modes. The former is associated with the desire to increase one's personal value (achieve goals that bring status, affiliation, vital resources), whereas the latter is associated with early detection of and preparation for a possible threat or danger to survival and potential loss of vital resources. Clinical disorders are characterized by the expression of negative self-expansion (goal attainment thwarted) and inappropriate or exaggerated activation of the self-protective mode.

The GCM reaffirms the importance of schemas or beliefs, asserting that *primal beliefs* play a central role in clinical disorders. Such beliefs focus on basic issues of survival, health, identity, and relationships. Accessibility, conviction, conditionality, attribution, and bias are important features of primal schemas that determine their prominence in psychopathological conditions. Highly energized or *charged* schemas have greater influence over the information processing system, and they have lower activation thresholds. In addition, they are less amenable to change.

Beck and Haigh (2014) contended that the GCM is a more robust theoretical account of psychological disturbance than the standard cognitive model. They argued that it could improve diagnostic classification, be more amenable to empirical investigation, account for subclinical as well as clinical disorders, and provide the conceptual basis for a more transdiagnostic cognitive therapy. The GCM has sparked little research as yet, so its heuristic value remains untested.

Recovery-Oriented Cognitive Therapy

Beck and colleagues' most recent variant of the cognitive model comes from the treatment of individuals with severe mental illness (Beck et al. 2020). In CT-R, the therapist identifies attitudes and behaviors that block recovery goals and intervenes to encourage hope, skill, and mastery. CT-R works to strengthen the adaptive mode (see Beck and Haigh 2014) by focusing on positive emotions, beliefs, and action. The therapist collaborates in the development of positive experiences that relate to an individual's core life values and aspirations to strengthen adaptive beliefs about the self, others, and the future and empower the person to better manage psychological disturbances, life stressors, and challenges. CT-R may have a broader application to other psychological conditions, but this awaits findings from key treatment process studies. A complete description of CT-R, including clinical application, was recently published by Beck et al. (2020).

Behavioral Activation

Behavioral activation (BA), a critical component of cognitive-behavioral therapy (CBT) for depression (Beck et al. 1979), has strong efficacy data as a stand-alone treatment for this disorder (Martell et al. 2009). BA is based on a model that suggests that loss, reduction, or persistently low levels of positive reinforcement contribute to the onset and maintenance of depression (Manos et al. 2010). By countering avoidance, withdrawal, rumination, and inactivity, BA helps depressed individuals to reengage fully in their lives (Jacobson et al. 2001). Specific strategies are used to help patients increase functioning and engagement in behaviors that are sources of positive reinforcement (e.g., pleasure- and mastery-oriented experiences), reduce activities that maintain or exacerbate depression (e.g., avoidance, rumination), and learn how to effectively problem solve.

One important assumption of BA is that depression may be treated effectively when an individual learns to act from the outside in rather than the inside out (Martell et al. 2010). In other words, instead of permitting mood to dictate behavior, patients are encouraged to commit to act in antidepressant ways, despite how they are feeling, and in so doing, mood, energy, motivation, and life satisfaction improve. Acronyms such as getting out of the TRAP (Trigger, Response, Avoidance Pattern) and back on TRAC (Trigger, Response, Alternative Coping) (see Martell et al. 2010) facilitate such behavior.

BA neither advocates a "just do it" mentality nor encourages individuals to simply increase pleasure in their lives (which is insufficient for an antidepressant effect) (Dimidjian et al. 2011). Rather, activation is conducted ideographically and is based on a comprehensive functional analysis of the patient's day-to-day activities. BA therapists employ strategies to reduce cognitive and behavioral avoidance (Dimidjian et al. 2014; Martell et al. 2010), including assessment of the patient's goals and values, self-monitoring, activity scheduling, disrupting avoidance and escape behaviors, social skills training, graded task assignment, and problem solving (Dimidjian et al. 2014).

BA as a stand-alone treatment (e.g., Martell et al. 2001) and BA used in the context of CBT (Beck et al. 1979) apply common principles of behavior therapy. With BA as a stand-alone treatment, activation strategies change reinforcement contingencies, whereas with BA in CBT, the therapist also uses activation strategies to identify, test, and modify negative cognitions (Dimidjian et al. 2011; Hollon 2001). BA has also been applied to other psychological conditions (e.g., social anxiety, generalized anxiety disorder, PTSD, obsessive-compulsive disorder) in which avoidance and negative reinforcement are fundamental components (see Judah et al. 2020).

The conceptual foundations underlying BA stem from behavioral models of depression (for a review, see Dimidjian et al. 2014; Hopko et al. 2003; Quigley and Dobson 2017). Ferster (1973) observed that individuals with depression engage in avoidance behaviors that limit access to positive reinforcement, narrow attention inward, decrease attention to positive reinforcement, and constrain a repertoire of adaptive behaviors. Lewinsohn (1974) similarly contended that depression is caused by a low rate of, or decline in, response-contingent positive reinforcement or by inadequate social skills. Because individuals with depression experience fewer environmental reinforcers, avoidance increases and approach behaviors become extinguished, which further worsens depressed mood, increases passivity, and reduces opportunities for the reinforcement of activity. Research studies support this model in finding that reduced environmental rewards and fewer positive events correlate with increased depressive severity (e.g., Lewinsohn and Graf 1973), that individuals with depression engage in fewer pleasant activities and find them less rewarding compared with individuals who are not depressed (MacPhillamy and Lewinsohn 1974), and that the lives of individuals with depression are often devoid of gratification, a sense of accomplishment, rewarding social interactions, and social reinforcement (for a review, see Carvalho and Hopko 2011). On the basis of these findings, Lewinsohn et al. (1976) developed a comprehensive treatment manual that employed activity scheduling to mitigate deficits in reinforcement (e.g., enhancing the reward value of potentially pleasurable activities, reducing the aversiveness of unpleasurable events) and social skills training to improve behavioral deficits that contributed to a lack of positive reinforcement (Kanter et al. 2010; Quigley and Dobson 2017).

Beck et al.'s (1979) seminal treatment manual also emphasized BA strategies as an important component of cognitive therapy for depression. Beck's cognitive theory and therapy (see Beck and Dozois 2014) essentially eclipsed more focused behavioral conceptualizations and interventions (Carvalho and Hopko 2011; Hollon 2001) until publication of a groundbreaking dismantling study intended to test its active components. This study found that BA was as efficacious as fully implemented CBT (Jacobson et al. 1996). Moreover, BA treatment gains were maintained at 2-year follow-up (Gortner et al. 1998). These findings called into question the necessity of cognitive change interventions (or at least their efficiency) and led to the development of BA as a stand-alone treatment for depression (Lejuez et al. 2001, 2011; Martell et al. 2001, 2010; Nagy et al. 2020). As Martell et al. (2010, p. 200) argued, developments in BA "actually represent a return to the historical roots of the treatment" (also see Jacobson et al. 2001). BA may be an important factor in the success of CBT for depression (see Soucy Chartier and Provencher 2013). Data from randomized controlled trials and meta-analyses provide strong support for BA as an evidence-based treatment for depression (see Dimidjian et al. 2011; Martell et al. 2010).

Exposure Therapy

Exposure therapy is considered the most effective treatment for psychopathology associated with fear and anxiety (Abramowitz 2013; Craske et al. 2014; Frank and McKay 2019). Meta-analytic studies have yielded large effect sizes for exposure therapy for anxiety disorders (e.g., Cuijpers et al. 2016; Hofmann et al. 2012). Of note, more than one theoretical model exists; in this section, we first review overlapping core concepts, and then we review two models (emotion processing therapy and inhibitory learning theory) in more detail.

All models of exposure therapy involve systematically and repeatedly confronting feared stimuli (e.g., objects, situations, thoughts) that do not objectively pose a significant risk of physical danger. Individuals with social anxiety, for example, are encouraged to engage in avoided social interactions such as initiating a conversation or going to a party. The main treatment for obsessive-compulsive disorder involves exposure and ritual prevention (also called response prevention), meaning the person deliberately contacts the feared object or situation (e.g., germs) and then refrains from rituals (e.g., washing) that temporarily reduce anxiety (Franklin and Foa 2014). The treatment of panic disorder involves exposure to both external feared situations (in vivo exposure) and internal body sensations (interoceptive exposure) (Craske and Barlow 2014). For PTSD, the patient may be instructed to write about, describe, or recall the details of a traumatic event (imaginal exposure) to learn that the event—although horrific—is in memory rather than an ongoing occurrence (Resick 2018).

A number of anxiety and related disorders are believed to stem from conditioned fear—learning that occurs when an innocuous or neutral stimulus (the conditioned stimulus [CS]) precedes the onset of a frightening or aversive event (the unconditioned stimulus [UCS]). After repeated pairings of the CS and UCS, the previously neutral stimulus itself begins to elicit fear (conditioned response [CR]). Fear conditioning may, however, occur even after a single conditioning trial, and it can generalize rapidly to other situations, a process called stimulus generalization (see Maples-Keller and Rauch 2020). For example, someone who was assaulted (UCS) in a parking lot (CS) may quickly learn to fear all parking lots (CR).

Mowrer (1947) proposed that although fears may be acquired through classical conditioning (the pairing of conditioned and unconditioned stimuli), they are maintained via operant conditioning (the consequent reinforcement of reducing anxiety by avoidance or escape). In other words, the individual learns to reduce anxiety by avoiding the CS, a behavior that becomes negatively reinforced (see Antony 2019). Thus, avoidance is extremely effective in reducing anxiety in the short term, but it maintains or increases anxiety over the long term.

Exposure therapy is highly efficacious for reducing or eliminating conditioned fear responses by using the principles of extinction (repeatedly presenting the CS without the UCS occurring and blocking avoidance). Most researchers agree that exposure is the main therapeutic ingredient across all psychological interventions for anxiety and related disorders. Exposure therapy techniques are relatively easy to implement, but a comprehensive understanding of the conceptual models underlying the treatments is critical to optimizing outcomes (see Abramowitz 2013).

Emotion processing theory has been the prevailing model proposed for the mechanisms of exposure therapy (Foa and Kozak 1986; Foa et al. 2006). According to this model, fear is extinguished during exposure because the network of beliefs about the feared stimulus, response, and meaning that are stored in memory (the activated fear structure) is presented together with information that is discrepant or incompatible (corrective information). The decline in fear in the presence of the feared stimulus (habituation) is purported to result in a new (nonfear) structure that replaces or competes with the old fear structure (Abramowitz 2013; Blakey and Abramowitz 2016; Maples-Keller and Rauch 2020).

Habituation, however, does not fully account for the extinction of fears following exposure (e.g., fears can spontaneously return after a period of time or when the contextual circumstances change), and research data indicate that fearful associations are not necessarily unlearned (Abramowitz et al. 2018; Blakey and Abramowitz 2016). Newer models of inhibitory learning provide a more parsimonious account of the mechanisms of exposure therapy. According to *inhibitory learning theory* (Craske et al. 2014), exposure modifies memory structures such that feared stimuli now possess both the original fear-based interpretation and a new safety-based, inhibitory meaning (Blakey and Abramowitz 2016; Sewart and Craske 2020; Weisman and Rodebaugh 2018). Rather than unlearning feared associations, exposure therapy maximizes inhibitory learning by generating and retrieving new, nonthreat associations. In other words, patients learn that the CS no longer reliably predicts the UCS and to tolerate negative emotional and physiological experiences.

After inhibitory learning has occurred, therapists implement various strategies to enhance the retrieval and consolidation of these newly learned associations. In biological terms, over the course of treatment the prefrontal cortex begins to play more and more of an inhibitory role, attenuating limbic-related threat associations (Tolin 2019; also see Ouimet et al. 2009). Table 7–1 provides an overview of Craske et al.'s (2014) recommendations for enhancing inhibitory learning during exposure therapy. Rather than simply exposing patients to feared stimuli and having them remain in the situation until their fear dissipates, a key therapeutic principle in inhibitory learning is to design exposure assignments that maximize new learning about their fear-based predictions (Sewart and Craske 2020).

Metacognitive Therapy

The cognitive model advanced by Beck places emphasis on the content of thoughts. For example, the negative triad underlying depression reflects negative beliefs about self, experience, and the future. In contrast, the metacognitive model advanced by Adrian Wells proposes that it is the beliefs and strategies that an individual employs in response to unwanted thoughts that constitute the most significant problem and result in worry and rumination (Wells 2019; Wells and Fisher 2015; Wells and Papageorgiou 2004).

Wells advanced the self-regulatory executive function (S-REF) model that describes psychological problems arising through biases in executive function. A perseverative focus on negative information perpetuates attentional processes, which results in thinking that is continually focused on the content of one's own thoughts (labeled *metacognition*) (Wells 1995, 2008; Wells and Papageorgiou 2004). Thus, thinking turns on itself in a recurring, inflexible process. Wells described declarative beliefs and procedural beliefs; the former refer to beliefs about thinking ("worry is harmful"), and the latter refer to plans or procedures to engage thinking. Declarative beliefs are further divided into positive beliefs about thinking ("worry will prepare me") and negative beliefs ("my worry is uncontrollable") (Wells 2011). Wells described three aspects of thought underlying psychopathology (Wells 2000; Wells and Matthews 1996): repetitive thinking, worry and rumination, and threat monitoring. Wells also detailed unhelpful strategies to cope with thoughts such as worry, reassurance seeking, avoidance, substance abuse, and other behaviors. Moreover, Wells divided strategies and beliefs about worry into two categories, namely, type one (positive) and type two (negative).

According to Wells, worry and rumination are maintained and activated by a series of engagements and interpretations of thoughts that he labels the cognitive attentional syndrome. These include excessive attention to thoughts, attempts to suppress thoughts, and overengagement in the content of thoughts. Wells suggested that there are five factors that underlie worry. These include cognitive confidence (the belief that one cannot trust one's memory), cognitive self-consciousness (focus on and awareness of one's thoughts), control of thoughts (thoughts are viewed as being out of control), positive view of worry (worry helps one prepare for and solve problems), and negative beliefs about worry (worry can be harmful to the self) (Wells and Carter 2001; Wells and Cartwright-Hatton 2004).

TABLE 7–1. **Strategies for enhancing inhibitory learning during exposure therapy**

Strategy	Description
Expectancy violation	Test it out: Design exposures that violate the patient's expectations about the frequency or intensity of the feared outcome. For example, an individual who fears dogs because dogs will bite should use exposures to disconfirm this belief and learn that dogs will probably not bite.
Deepened extinction	Combine it: Whenever possible, expose the individual to multiple feared situations simultaneously after at least one has been successfully mastered. For example, if drinking coffee and entering a shopping mall are two separate situations that trigger feared bodily sensations (e.g., heart palpitations), exposure to both situations simultaneously may enhance learning.
Removal of safety behaviors	Throw it out: Decrease the use of safety behaviors while completing exposure exercises. Examples of safety behaviors include having medication to take if a panic attack occurs, rehearsing a conversation in advance to prevent saying the wrong thing and feeling socially anxious, and bringing a friend or therapist along for reassurance in a feared situation.
Variability	Vary it up: Vary stimuli and contexts in which exposures to the feared situation are experienced. This will increase the number of retrieval cues and enhance the ability to make and access newly learned responses to the feared situation.
Reinforced extinction	Face your fears: Occasionally present the feared outcome during exposures. For example, if a socially anxious individual avoids interacting with others for fear of rejection, deliberate experiencing of rejection can enhance exposure.
Attentional focus	Stay with it: Maintain attention on the target stimulus during exposure.
Affect labeling	Talk it out: Encourage patients to describe and label their emotional experience during exposures.
Mental reinstatement/ retrieval cues	Bring it back: Imagine previous successful exposures to help maintain the effectiveness of exposure therapy.

Source. Dozois DJA, Wilde J, Frewen PA: "Anxiety, obsessive-compulsive, and trauma-related disorders," in *Abnormal Psychology: Perspectives*, 6th Edition. Edited by Dozois DJA. Toronto, ON, Canada, Pearson, 2019, pp. 95–126 (adapted from Craske et al. 2014).

The metacognitive model of therapy begins with educating the patient that beliefs about unwanted thoughts may maintain worry or rumination. The therapist explores with the patient which strategies the patient has used to cope with unwanted thoughts, illustrating in this process how these attempts have not worked. The goal is to understand that unwanted thoughts may occur but do not require engagement; one can have unwanted thoughts and focus on other goals. If the patient believes an inability to successfully eliminate or suppress thoughts implies that they lack control, the therapist illustrates that attempting to suppress thoughts does not work and introduces a number of metacognitive techniques that encourage the patient to employ alternative strategies. These include postponing worry to a later time, imagining the intrusive thoughts as trains in a station that one observes but does not board, imagining thoughts as telemarketing calls that one does not take, or imagining thoughts as clouds in the sky that drift independently of the observer. Wells describes these techniques as mindful detachment, suggesting that the patient can observe without actively engaging. This is not equivalent to mindfulness training as in mindfulness-based cognitive therapy or other more traditional mindfulness practices. Rather, it is simply observing and "letting be," without engaging, challenging, or suppressing.

The variety of techniques employed address various components of the S-REF model. For example, the idea that one always has to be watching one's thoughts (cognitive self-consciousness) is contrasted with shifting attention to other stimuli. The belief that one has no control is contrasted with delaying worry to "worry time." The idea that worry has positive consequences such as preparation and avoiding surprise is challenged by illustrating that prior worry has not decreased worry, prepared the person, or avoided surprise. The idea that worry will drive someone insane or have other negative consequences is contrasted with the fact that the patient has not gone insane and is simply anxious. Finally, the lack of confidence in one's memory or thoughts is related to the fact that the individual is using up a lot of space to keep track of the worries. The therapist assists the patient in realizing that they do not have to get hijacked by their intrusive thoughts and can choose to treat them as background noise.

Mindfulness-Based Cognitive Therapy

Mindfulness-based cognitive therapy was first developed by Williams et al. (2000) and focused primarily on recurrent major depression. They observed that people prone to recurrent depression demonstrate overgeneralized autobiographical memory independent of depressed mood (Segal et al. 2002). For example, rather than recall that last summer "I went to the shore, and we went out on kayaks," individuals prone to recurrent depression might say, "I had a difficult summer." Recalling events in general, abstract, and vague terms makes it difficult to link emotions, behaviors, and interactions to specific stimuli and makes it difficult to change thoughts, behaviors, and interactions. Teasdale (1999) described cognitive processing as a hierarchy of three modes within the interacting cognitive systems: *mindless emoting*, *conceptualizing/doing*, and *mindful experiencing/being*. Referring to Rachman's (1980) emotional processing model, Teasdale argued that higher-order, abstract, conceptual processing does not facilitate the emotional processing needed to counter depression.

According to the mindfulness model, only the mindful experiencing mode facilitates emotional processing, whereas the other modes facilitate rumination and conceptual and emotionally avoidant processing. Thus, Williams et al. (2000) described a model to facilitate both awareness to specifics in the present situation and emotional processing (Teasdale et al. 2002). Williams and colleagues decided that attention training was needed to assist patients to attend to the details of current observations rather than form more abstract impressions. Drawing on the mindfulness training program developed by Kabat-Zinn et al. (1985), Williams et al. defined mindfulness as focused, present-oriented, purposeful, and nonjudgmental attention. Later, the definition of mindfulness was expanded to also incorporate elements of compassion, kindness, and acceptance.

Mindful awareness is employed to shift one's thoughts toward focused attention on specific stimuli in the current moment while continuing to observe what one had been observing, accepting it, and recognizing whether the mind drifts toward alternative thoughts, sounds, or sensations. Redirecting attention was the initial emphasis in the mindfulness model. Mindfulness approaches in CBT have since been expanded to generalized anxiety disorder, obsessive-compulsive disorder, depression, prevention of relapse in depression, substance abuse, and other disorders (for a review, see Wielgosz et al. 2019).

Acceptance and Commitment Therapy

Interest in acceptance and commitment therapy (ACT) as an alternative to strictly behavioral or strictly cognitive approaches has been increasing. Hayes (2016) characterized ACT as a third-wave CBT, after the initial first wave (behavioral) and second wave (cognitive). ACT focuses on values, flexibility, commitment to change, acceptance, and experiential avoidance, which have been proposed to underlie a wide range of psychopathology (Hayes et al. 2013). Hayes based ACT on his relational frame theory, which proposes that individuals learn the relation and context of language, concepts, and behavior, rather than a simple association, as suggested by earlier learning theory, such as Skinner's model (Hayes et al. 2001). According to relational frame theory and ACT, humans experience a wider range of psychopathology than do other animals because of their capacity to use language and symbolization to maintain a less direct relationship with experience and their inflexible following of rules and beliefs (Hayes et al. 2011). ACT is based on a contextual model of experience and knowledge such that the "truth" or even the function of an event depends on the specific context. Thus, one's behavior or thoughts are true depending on how they work in the specific context, and the self is viewed through the lens of different contexts. The self is viewed as I-here-now, rather than a persisting continuity of self that is independent of context, experience, or goals (Hayes et al. 2011).

The ACT therapist attempts to help patients experience life in a manner not tied to established intervening concepts—that is, having more direct experience, unmediated by language, which can facilitate change. ACT distinguishes between verbal knowledge (which is abstract) and experiential knowledge (which is more concrete, specific, and present oriented). The ACT model incorporates a wide range of concepts, conceptualizations, techniques, metaphors, and interventions. According to the model, problems are perpetuated by a process of self monitoring, evaluation, emotional response, and controlled efforts, in contrast to direct awareness, mindful nonjudgmental acceptance, and flexibility in accepting while still committing to valued action (Hayes et al. 2013). ACT encourages the patient to make room for unwanted or unpleasant internal experiences rather than to suppress, control, or eliminate those experiences. In ACT, one might say, "You have to go through it to get past it."

Fusion with thoughts and language is contrasted with diffusion, which is the ability to flexibly disentangle from the mediating function of thinking. Standing back, noticing, distancing, and decentering from thinking while observing and accepting the stream of thoughts and feelings in the moment are presumed to allow the individual to both accept and experience the present while not being controlled and limited by these internal processes (Hayes et al. 2006).

ACT uses a hexagon to describe psychological flexibility, which includes flexible attention to the present moment, chosen values, committed action, self as context, diffusion, and acceptance. Mindfulness is incorporated as a means whereby one can stop, become aware, and step back, nonjudgmentally, while accepting and letting go. This contrasts with more traditional cognitive models that identify and engage with thoughts in an attempt to make them less credible. ACT stresses identifying and living according to personal values and examining whether actions are moving one toward valued directions.

Conclusion

As is clear from our review, there is no single CBT. Active debate as to which approach should be preferred is ongoing. Each of the approaches we describe has empirical support, and there is no current clarity for one having a particular advantage for patients. Recently, an attempt was made to identify common processes (e.g., rumination, avoidance, emotional dysregulation), rather than focusing on DSM categories of diagnosis (Hofmann and Hayes 2019), such that the therapist might choose which approach might be better suited for which process for a specific patient. Cognitive-behavioral therapies have emerged as a dominant form of therapy, but there is no one CBT model that defines this school of therapy. As should be clear from this review, there are many approaches, some emphasizing the content of thoughts; others emphasizing behavioral activation and contingencies; others emphasizing how one thinks about one's thoughts; and still another that emphasizes clarifying values, examining the context of behavior, defusing thoughts from actions, and encouraging committed behavior. Despite the controversies and disagreements within the CBT tradition, each approach has been shown to be effective, and no one approach can claim uniform superiority.

Key Points

- Cognitive-behavioral therapies have emerged as a dominant form of therapy, but there is no one model that defines this school of therapy.
- Maladaptive schemas and biased cognitive processing result in negative automatic thoughts, which can be addressed through cognitive restructuring.
- Behavioral activation helps patients with depression increase functioning and engagement in positive behaviors through assessment of patient goals and values and self-monitoring and scheduling activities.
- Exposure therapy, in which patients systematically confront feared stimuli, is an effective treatment for anxiety disorders.
- Mindfulness allows patients to gain distance from and defusion of problematic thoughts.

- Acceptance and valued action provide greater flexibility and commitment to change.
- Metacognitive therapy addresses the beliefs and strategies patients use in response to unwanted thoughts.

References

Abramowitz JS: The practice of exposure therapy: relevance of cognitive-behavioral theory and extinction theory. Behav Ther 44(4):548–558, 2013 24094780

Abramowitz JS, Blakey SM, Reuman L, et al: New directions in the cognitive-behavioral treatment of OCD: theory, research, and practice. Behav Ther 49(3):311–322, 2018 29704962

Antony MM: Behavior therapy, in Current Psychotherapies. Edited by Wedding D, Corsini RJ. Boston, MA, Cengage Learning, 2019, pp 199–236

Beck AT: Thinking and depression I: idiosyncratic content and cognitive distortions. Arch Gen Psychiatry 9:324–333, 1963 14045261

Beck AT: Depression: Causes and Treatment. Philadelphia, University of Pennsylvania Press, 1967

Beck AT: Cognitive therapy: a 30-year retrospective. Am Psychol 46(4):368–375, 1991 2048795

Beck AT: Beyond belief: a theory of modes, personality, and psychopathology, in Frontiers of Cognitive Therapy. Edited by Salkovskis PM. New York, Guilford, 1996, pp 1–25

Beck AT, Dozois DJA: Cognitive theory and therapy: past, present and future, in Psychiatry: Past, Present, and Prospect. Edited by Bloch S, Green SA, Holmes J. Oxford, UK, Oxford University Press, 2014, pp 366–382

Beck AT, Haigh EAP: Advances in cognitive theory and therapy: the generic cognitive model. Annu Rev Clin Psychol 10:1–24, 2014 24387236

Beck AT, Rush AJ, Shaw BF, et al: Cognitive Therapy of Depression. New York, Guilford, 1979

Beck AT, Emery G, Greenberg RL: Anxiety Disorders and Phobias: A Cognitive Perspective. New York, Basic Books, 1985

Beck AT, Wright FD, Newman CF, et al: Cognitive Therapy of Substance Abuse. New York, Guilford, 2001

Beck AT, Rector NA, Grant P: Schizophrenia: Cognitive Theory, Research, and Therapy. New York, Guilford, 2011

Beck AT, Davis DD, Freeman A: Cognitive Therapy of Personality Disorders, 3rd Edition. New York, Guilford, 2015

Beck AT, Grant P, Inverso E, et al: Recovery-Oriented Cognitive Therapy for Serious Mental Health Conditions. New York, Guilford, 2020

Beck JS: Cognitive Behavior Therapy: Basics and Beyond, 2nd Edition. New York, Guilford, 2011

Beck R, Perkins TS: Cognitive content-specificity for anxiety and depression: a meta analysis. Cognit Ther Res 25:651–663, 2001

Blakey SM, Abramowitz JS: The effects of safety behaviors during exposure therapy for anxiety: critical analysis from an inhibitory learning perspective. Clin Psychol Rev 49:1–15, 2016 27475477

Carvalho JP, Hopko DR: Behavioral theory of depression: reinforcement as a mediating variable between avoidance and depression. J Behav Ther Exp Psychiatry 42(2):154–162, 2011 21315876

Clark DA, Beck AT: Cognitive Therapy of Anxiety Disorders: Science and Practice. New York, Guilford, 2010a

Clark DA, Beck AT: Cognitive theory and therapy of anxiety and depression: convergence with neurobiological findings. Trends Cogn Sci 14(9):418–424, 2010b 20655801

Clark DA, Beck AT, Alford B: Scientific Foundations of Cognitive Theory and Therapy of Depression, New York, Wiley, 1999

Craske MG, Barlow DH: Panic disorder and agoraphobia, in Clinical Handbook of Psychological Disorders. Edited by Barlow DH. New York, Guilford, 2014, pp 1–61

Craske MG, Treanor M, Conway CC, et al: Maximizing exposure therapy: an inhibitory learning approach. Behav Res Ther 58:10–23, 2014 24864005
Cuijpers P, Cristea IA, Karyotaki E, et al: How effective are cognitive behavior therapies for major depression and anxiety disorders? A meta-analytic update of the evidence. World Psychiatry 15(3):245–258, 2016 27717254
Dimidjian S, Barrera M Jr, Martell C, et al: The origins and current status of behavioral activation treatments for depression. Annu Rev Clin Psychol 7:1–38, 2011 21275642
Dimidjian S, Martell CR, Herman-Dunn R, et al: Behavioral activation for depression, in Clinical Handbook of Psychological Disorders. Edited by Barlow DH. New York, Guilford, 2014, pp 353–393
Dozois DJA, Beck AT: Cognitive schemas, beliefs, and assumptions, in Risk Factors in Depression. Edited by Dobson KS, Dozois DJA. Amsterdam, Elsevier, 2008, pp 121–143
Dozois DJA, Wilde J, Frewen PA: Anxiety, obsessive-compulsive, and trauma-related disorders, in Abnormal Psychology: Perspectives, 6th Edition. Edited by Dozois DJA. Toronto, ON, Canada, Pearson, 2019, pp 95–126
D'Zurilla TJ, Nezu AM: Problem-solving therapies, in Handbook of Cognitive-Behavioral Therapies. Edited by Dobson KS. New York, Guilford, 2001, pp 211–245
Ellis A, MacLaren C: Rational Emotive Behavior Therapy: A Therapist's Guide. San Luis Obispo, CA, Impact, 1998
Ferster CB: A functional anlysis of depression. Am Psychol 28(10):857–870, 1973 4753644
Foa EB, Kozak MJ: Emotional processing of fear: exposure to corrective information. Psychol Bull 99(1):20–35, 1986 2871574
Foa EB, Huppert JD, Cahill SP: Emotional processing theory: an update, in Pathological Anxiety: Emotional Processing in Etiology and Treatment. Edited by Rothbaum BO. New York, Guilford, 2006, pp 3–24
Frank B, McKay D: Introduction to the special series: clinical applications of the inhibitory learning model. Cognit Behav Pract 26:127–129, 2019
Franklin ME, Foa EB: Obsessive compulsive disorder, in Clinical Handbook of Psychological Disorders. Edited by Barlow DH. New York, Guilford, 2014, pp 155–205
Gortner ET, Gollan JK, Dobson KS, Jacobson NS: Cognitive-behavioral treatment for depression: relapse prevention. J Consult Clin Psychol 66(2):377–384, 1998 9583341
Hayes SC: Acceptance and commitment therapy, relational frame theory, and the third wave of behavioral and cognitive therapies. Behav Ther 47(6):869–885, 2016 27993338
Hayes SC, Roche B, Barnes-Holmes D: Relational Frame Theory: A Post-Skinnerian Account of Human Language and Cognition. New York, Plenum, 2001
Hayes SC, Luoma JB, Bond FW, et al: Acceptance and commitment therapy: model, processes and outcomes. Behav Res Ther 44(1):1–25, 2006 16300724
Hayes SC, Strosahl KD, Wilson KG: Acceptance and Commitment Therapy: The Process and Practice of Mindful Change. New York, Guilford, 2011
Hayes SC, Levin ME, Plumb-Vilardaga J, et al: Acceptance and commitment therapy and contextual behavioral science: examining the progress of a distinctive model of behavioral and cognitive therapy. Behav Ther 44(2):180–198, 2013 23611068
Hofmann SG, Hayes SC: The future of intervention science: process-based therapy. Clin Psychol Sci 7(1):37–50, 2019 30713811
Hofmann SG, Asnaani A, Vonk IJJ, et al: The efficacy of cognitive behavioral therapy: a review of meta-analyses. Cognit Ther Res 36(5):427–440, 2012 23459093
Hollon SD: Behavioral activation treatment for depression: a commentary. Clin Psychol 8:271–274, 2001
Hopko DR, Lejuez CW, Ruggiero KJ, et al: Contemporary behavioral activation treatments for depression: procedures, principles, and progress. Clin Psychol Rev 23(5):699–717, 2003 12971906
Jacobson NS, Dobson KS, Truax PA, et al: A component analysis of cognitive-behavioral treatment for depression. J Consult Clin Psychol 64(2):295–304, 1996 8871414
Jacobson NS, Martell CR, Dimidjian S: Behavioral activation treatment for depression: returning to contextual roots. Clin Psychol Sci Pract 8:255–270, 2001

Judah MR, Dahne J, Hershenberg R, et al: Behavioral activation, in Clinical Handbook of Fear and Anxiety: Maintenance Processes and Treatment Mechanisms. Edited by Abramowitz JS, Blakey SM. Washington, DC, American Psychological Association, 2020

Kabat-Zinn J, Lipworth L, Burney R: The clinical use of mindfulness meditation for the self-regulation of chronic pain. J Behav Med 8(2):163–190, 1985 3897551

Kanter JW, Manos RC, Bowe WM, et al: What is behavioral activation? A review of the empirical literature. Clin Psychol Rev 30(6):608–620, 2010 20677369

Leahy RL: Contemporary Cognitive Therapy: Theory, Research, and Practice. New York, Guilford, 2004

Lejuez CW, Hopko DR, Hopko SDA: A brief behavioral activation treatment for depression: treatment manual. Behav Modif 25(2):255–286, 2001 11317637

Lejuez CW, Hopko DR, Acierno R, et al: Ten year revision of the brief behavioral activation treatment for depression: revised treatment manual. Behav Modif 35(2):111–161, 2011 21324944

Lewinsohn PM: A behavioral approach to depression, in The Psychology of Depression: Contemporary Theory and Research. Edited by Friedman RM, Katz MM. New York, Wiley, 1974, pp 157–178

Lewinsohn PM, Graf M: Pleasant activities and depression. J Consult Clin Psychol 41(2):261–268, 1973 4147832

Lewinsohn PM, Biglan A, Zeiss AM: Behavioral treatment for depression, in Behavioral Management of Anxiety, Depression, and Pain. Edited by Davidson PO. New York, Brunner/Mazel, 1976, pp 91–146

Linehan MM: Cognitive-Behavioral Treatment of Borderline Personality Disorder. New York, Guilford, 1993

MacPhillamy DJ, Lewinsohn PM: Depression as a function of levels of desired and obtained pleasure. J Abnorm Psychol 83(6):651–657, 1974 4155711

Manos RC, Kanter JW, Busch AM: A critical review of assessment strategies to measure the behavioral activation model of depression. Clin Psychol Rev 30(5):547–561, 2010 20444531

Maples-Keller JL, Rauch SAM: Habituation, in Clinical Handbook of Fear and Anxiety: Maintenance Processes and Treatment Mechanisms. Edited by Abramowitz JS, Blakey SM. Washington, DC, American Psychological Association, 2020, pp 248–263

Martell CR, Addis ME, Jacobson NS: Depression in Context: Strategies for Guided Action. New York, WW Norton, 2001

Martell CR, Dimidjian S, Lewinsohn PM: Behavioral activation therapy, in Cognitive and Behavioral Theories in Clinical Practice. Edited by Kazantzis N, Reinecke AM, Freeman A. New York, Guilford, 2009, pp 193–217

Martell CR, Dimidjian S, Herman-Dunn R: Behavioral Activation for Depression: A Clinician's Guide. New York, Guilford, 2010

McCullough JP Jr, Schramm E, Penberthy JK: CBASP as a Distinctive Treatment of Persistent Depressive Disorder (CBT Distinctive Feature Series). London, Routledge, 2015

Miller WR, Rollnick S: Motivational Interviewing: Preparing People to Change, 2nd Edition. New York, Guilford, 2002

Mowrer OH: On the dual nature of learning—a reinterpretation of "conditioning" and "problem-solving." Harv Educ Rev 17:102–148, 1947

Nagy GA, Cernasov P, Pisoni A, et al: Reward network modulation as a mechanism of change in behavioral activation. Behav Modif 44(2):186–213, 2020 30317863

Nezu AM: Problem solving and behavior therapy revisited. Behav Ther 35:1–33, 2004

Ouimet AJ, Gawronski B, Dozois DJA: Cognitive vulnerability to anxiety: a review and an integrative model. Clin Psychol Rev 29(6):459–470, 2009 19552990

Quigley L, Dobson KS: Behavioral activation treatments for depression, in The Science of Cognitive Behavioral Therapy. Edited by Hofmann SG, Asmundson G. London, Academic Press, 2017, pp 291–318

Rachman S: Emotional processing. Behav Res Ther 18(1):51–60, 1980 7369988

Resick PA: Cognitive therapy for posttraumatic stress disorder, in Science and Practice in Cognitive Therapy: Foundations, Mechanisms, and Applications. Edited by Leahy RL. New York, Guilford, 2018, pp 358–377

Segal ZV, Williams JMG, Teasdale JD: Mindfulness-Based Cognitive Therapy for Depression: A New Approach to Preventing Relapse. New York, Guilford, 2002

Sewart AR, Craske MG: Inhibitory learning, in Clinical Handbook of Fear and Anxiety: Maintenance Processes and Treatment Mechanisms. Edited by Abramowitz JS, Blakey SM. Washington, DC, American Psychological Association, 2020, pp 265–285

Soucy Chartier I, Provencher MD: Behavioural activation for depression: efficacy, effectiveness and dissemination. J Affect Disord 145(3):292–299, 2013 22884236

Teasdale JD: Multi-level theories of cognition-emotion relations, in Handbook of Cognition and Emotion. Edited by Dalgleish T, Power MJ. Chichester, UK, Wiley, 1999, pp 665–681

Teasdale JD, Moore RG, Hayhurst H, et al: Metacognitive awareness and prevention of relapse in depression: empirical evidence. J Consult Clin Psychol 70(2):275–287, 2002 11952186

Tolin DF: Inhibitory learning for anxiety-related disorders. Cognit Behav Pract 26:225–236, 2019

Weisman JS, Rodebaugh TL: Exposure therapy augmentation: a review and extension of techniques informed by an inhibitory learning approach. Clin Psychol Rev 59:41–51, 2018 29128146

Wells A: Meta-cognition and worry: a cognitive model of generalized anxiety disorder. Behav Cogn Psychother 23:301–320, 1995

Wells A: Emotional Disorders and Metacognition: Innovative Cognitive Therapy. New York, Wiley, 2000

Wells A: Metacognitive Therapy for Anxiety and Depression. New York, Guilford, 2008

Wells A: Metacognitive therapy, in Acceptance and Mindfulness in Cognitive Behavior Therapy. Edited by Herbert JD, Forman EM. New York, Wiley, 2011, pp 83–108

Wells A: Breaking the cybernetic code: understanding and treating the human metacognitive control system to enhance mental health. Front Psychol 10:2621, 2019 31920769

Wells A, Carter K: Further tests of a cognitive model of generalized anxiety disorder: metacognitions and worry in GAD, panic disorder, social phobia, depression, and nonpatients. Behav Ther 32(1):85–102, 2001

Wells A, Cartwright-Hatton S: A short form of the metacognitions questionnaire: properties of the MCQ-30. Behav Res Ther 42(4):385–396, 2004 14998733

Wells A, Fisher PL: Metacognitive therapy: theoretical background and model of depression, in Depression Treatment: Metacognitive, Cognitive-Behavioural, Acceptance and Mindfulness Therapies. Edited by Wells A, Fisher PL. Chichester, UK, Wiley, 2015

Wells A, Matthews G: Modelling cognition in emotional disorder: the S-REF model. Behav Res Ther 34(11–12):881–888, 1996 8990539

Wells A, Papageorgiou C: Metacognitive therapy for depressive rumination, in Depressive Rumination: Nature, Theory, and Treatment. Edited by Wells A, Papageorgiou C. Chichester, UK, Wiley, 2004

Wielgosz J, Goldberg SB, Kral TRA, et al: Mindfulness meditation and psychopathology. Annu Rev Clin Psychol 15(1):285–316, 2019 30525995

Williams JMG, Watts FN, MacLeod C, et al: Cognitive Psychology and Emotional Disorders, 2nd Edition. Chichester, UK, Wiley, 1997

Williams JM, Teasdale JD, Segal ZV, et al: Mindfulness-based cognitive therapy reduces overgeneral autobiographical memory in formerly depressed patients. J Abnorm Psychol 109(1):150–155, 2000 10740947

CHAPTER 8

Techniques of Cognitive-Behavioral Therapy

Jesse H. Wright, M.D., Ph.D.
Jessica Reis, M.D.
David A. Casey, M.D.

Cognitive-behavioral therapy (CBT) methods are a direct outgrowth of the basic theories and experimental findings on cognitive and behavioral pathology in specific psychiatric disorders. Thus, cognitive-behavioral therapists implement procedures that are directly linked to core theoretical constructs. For example, the cognitive restructuring and exposure and response prevention interventions used for panic disorder with agoraphobia are designed to reverse pathologies of 1) overestimation of risk or danger, 2) underestimation of coping abilities, and 3) avoidance of feared situations.

CBT includes highly detailed treatment techniques that can be misapplied if the clinician puts too much emphasis on implementing specific methods without developing an effective case formulation or fully attending to the therapeutic relationship. We have observed this problem many times in trainees who rush to apply a technique such as a thought record or a behavioral intervention without developing a comprehensive treatment plan. Thus, we recommend that the techniques described in this chapter be used when consistent with the case formulation and when coordinated with the overall plan for therapy.

In this chapter, we describe general CBT methods such as the collaborative-empirical therapeutic relationship, structuring procedures, and psychoeducation. Commonly used cognitive and behavioral interventions are then defined and illustrated. After detailing basic methods for depression and anxiety, we then illustrate adaptations of CBT for other disorders or problems by briefly describing modifications for schizophrenia, eating disorders, and insomnia. Because of CBT's high relevance in reducing suicide attempts, we also outline CBT methods for suicide risk.

CBT interventions have been developed for a wide variety of other conditions and problems such as substance abuse (Beck et al. 1993; Ray et al. 2020), personality disorders (Beck et al. 2015), chronic pain (Bernard et al. 2018; Cheng and Cheng 2019; Ehde et al. 2014), irritable bowel syndrome (Hanlon et al. 2018; Kinsinger 2017; Li et al. 2014), and fibromyalgia (Bernardy et al. 2013, 2018; White and Nielson 1995). Also, CBT methods have been detailed for group (Bieling et al. 2009; White and Freeman 2000) and family (Dattilio 2013; Epstein 2002) applications and for treating children and adolescents (James et al. 2005; Muñoz-Solomando et al. 2008; Reinecke et al. 2003).

Readers who seek a more comprehensive description may wish to consult CBT textbooks that describe how to use standard cognitive therapy interventions in more detail (Beck 2020) and include video demonstrations of key CBT techniques (Wright et al. 2017) or may wish to consult texts on different disorders or applications. See "Recommended Readings" for a list of recommended resources for CBT.

General Methods Used in CBT

Therapeutic Relationship

The therapeutic relationship in CBT is characterized by a high degree of collaboration between patient and therapist and an empirical approach to the work of therapy. The therapist and patient work together as an investigative team. They jointly develop hypotheses about the validity of automatic thoughts and schemas or, alternatively, about the effectiveness of patterns of behavior. A series of exercises or experiments is then designed to test the validity of the hypotheses and, subsequently, to modify cognitions or behavior. Beck et al. (1979) termed this form of therapeutic relationship *collaborative empiricism.* Methods for developing a collaborative and empirical relationship are listed in Table 8–1.

Basic counseling skills that promote a sound therapeutic alliance are also important in CBT. Therapists strive to build genuineness, warmth, trust, and acceptance into the treatment relationship, in addition to showing sensitivity to sociocultural and gender influences (Davis and Wright 1994; Wright et al. 2017). Accurate empathy is another important component of the collaborative relationship in CBT (Wright et al. 2017). From a cognitive-behavioral perspective, accurate empathy involves the therapist's capacity to place themselves in the position of the patient so that they can sense what the patient is feeling and thinking while retaining objectivity for sorting out possible distortions, illogical reasoning, or maladaptive behavior that may be contributing to the patient's problems. Full expression of accurate empathy in CBT not only involves showing sensitive concern for patients but also includes a vigorous search for solutions and actions that reduce suffering and help the patient manage life problems.

Structuring Cognitive Therapy Sessions

One of the most important techniques for CBT is the use of a *therapy agenda* (Table 8–2). At the beginning of each session, the therapist and patient work collaboratively to derive a short list of topics, usually consisting of two to four items to be covered during the session. Generally, it is advisable to shape an agenda that 1) can be managed

TABLE 8–1. Methods of enhancing collaborative empiricism

Work together as an investigative team.
Promote essential nonspecific therapist variables (e.g., kindness, empathy, equanimity, positive general attitude).
Encourage self-monitoring and self-help.
Obtain accurate assessment of validity of cognitions and efficacy of behavior.
Develop coping strategies for real losses and actual deficits.
Provide and request feedback on a regular basis.
Be sensitive to sociocultural differences and issues.
Customize therapy interventions.
Use gentle humor.

Source. Adapted from Wright JH, Thase ME, Beck AT: "Cognitive-Behavioral Therapy," in *The American Psychiatric Association Publishing Textbook of Psychiatry*, 7th Edition. Edited by Roberts LW. Washington, DC, American Psychiatric Association Publishing, 2019, p. 964. Copyright © 2019 American Psychiatric Association Publishing. Used with permission.

TABLE 8–2. Structuring procedures for cognitive therapy

Set agenda for therapy sessions.
Give constructive feedback to direct the course of therapy.
Ask for feedback and summarization about the therapy from the patient.
Employ common cognitive therapy techniques on a regular basis.
Assign homework to link sessions together.

Source. Adapted from Wright JH, Thase ME, Beck AT: "Cognitive-Behavioral Therapy," in *The American Psychiatric Association Publishing Textbook of Psychiatry*, 7th Edition. Edited by Roberts LW. Washington, DC, American Psychiatric Association Publishing, 2019, p. 967. Copyright © 2019 American Psychiatric Association Publishing. Used with permission.

within the time frame of an individual session, 2) follows up on material from earlier sessions, 3) reviews any homework from the previous session and provides an opportunity for new homework assignments, and 4) contains specific items that are highly relevant to the patient but are not too global or abstract. This is particularly important in early sessions. Agenda setting facilitates problem-solving and keeps the therapy efficient and focused on salient issues. Also, agenda setting may counteract hopelessness by breaking overwhelming problems into more manageable segments.

Cognitive-behavioral therapists provide and ask for *feedback* during each therapy session in order to build structure into the therapy session, enhance learning, and provide a forum for examining and correcting distortions about the content and process of the therapy. Areas of inquiry used to solicit feedback include the following: What are the patient's reactions to the therapist? What things are going well in the therapy? What would the patient like to change? In addition to initiating explicit, direct conversations about feedback, cognitive-behavioral therapists also are sensitive to nonverbal forms of feedback. Is the patient engaged in the therapeutic process? Has there been a change in mood? Cognitive-behavioral therapists monitor and then inquire about the patient's thoughts when these clues are noted.

Cognitive-behavioral therapists regularly *summarize* to enhance the patient's understanding of the main points of the therapy session. For example, patients are asked to identify key elements of the session or to explain what they understand about a specific intervention. Such points are often written down to enhance learning. A good question to ask near the end of the session is "What are the main takeaways from today's session?" Therapists may need to assist patients in this process if important information is not recalled or if patients have difficulty in providing summaries.

The use of *specific cognitive and behavioral techniques* in and between sessions contributes additional structure to the therapy. Examples include activity scheduling, graded task assignments, and use of thought change records. These interventions, and others of similar nature, provide a clear and understandable method for reducing symptoms and changing behaviors. The repeated use of procedures such as recording, labeling, and modifying automatic thoughts helps to link sessions together, especially if they are introduced in therapy and then used as part of action plans for work outside sessions.

Psychoeducation

One of the core principles of CBT is a focus on psychoeducation to teach patients basic concepts and skills (Wright et al. 2017). The educational process in sessions may be especially effective if it is woven into therapeutic work on recent, emotionally resonant situations and if it provides a real-life demonstration connected to CBT principles. For example, a 55-year-old businessperson with depression and anger problems reported in his second session that he felt very guilty about "exploding" at his assistant earlier in the day. The therapist capitalized on this opportunity to educate the patient by having him detail the triggering event ("He showed me a lot of new reports that he thought were important, but I was busy doing something else"), identify specific automatic thoughts ("I can't deal with another single thing.... He will drive me crazy....I'm on total overload"), and define emotions and physiological symptoms that were experienced in the situation (anger, anxiety, physical tension). In this first attempt to teach the patient about the basic CBT model, the therapist diagrammed the relationship between events, cognitions, and emotions. Then the therapist used this diagram to explain the nature of automatic thoughts. Because the situation was very important to the patient and it stimulated intense emotion, the lessons taught in the therapeutic interchange were more likely to be remembered and used.

Therapists can employ several very useful education methods to give patients work between sessions. Readings in self-help books, pamphlets, or handouts are used frequently and extensively in CBT (Table 8–3). We recommend that therapists read several of the commonly used books or pamphlets and be prepared to make customized recommendations that will best suit the needs and the cognitive capacities of the individual patient. Suggesting that a patient read a specific chapter or portion of a publication may be more helpful than assigning an entire book. When patients are deeply depressed or have high levels of anxiety, assigning too much reading may be overwhelming and lead to discouragement. Thus, we typically suggest reading in a stepped fashion, increasing the volume or complexity on the basis of the patient's grasp of previous material and the degree of cognitive and symptomatic improvement.

Computer programs for CBT are particularly valuable resources for providing psychoeducation. In addition, they improve the efficiency of treatment by acting as a "ther-

TABLE 8–3. Psychoeducational materials and programs for cognitive-behavioral therapy

Title	Authors	Description
Coping With Depression	Beck AT, Greenberg RL, Beck J	Booklet, The Beck Institute, 1995
Feeling Good: The New Mood Therapy	Burns DD	Book with self-help program, 1999
Getting Your Life Back: The Complete Guide to Recovery From Depression	Wright JH, Basco MR	Book with self-help program, 2002; integrates cognitive therapy and biological approaches
Good Days Ahead: The Multimedia Program for Cognitive Therapy	Wright JH, Wright AS, Beck AT	Computer-assisted therapy and self-help program, Empower Interactive, 2012
Mastery of Your Anxiety and Panic, 4th Edition	Barlow DH, Craske MG	Self-help workbook for anxiety, 2007
Mind Over Mood: Change How Your Feel by Changing the Way You Think, 2nd Edition	Greenberger D, Padesky CA	Self-help workbook, 2016
Never Good Enough: How to Use Perfectionism to Your Advantage Without Letting It Ruin Your Life	Basco MR	Book on perfectionism, 2000
The Worry Cure: Seven Steps to Stop Worry From Stopping You	Foa EB, Wilson R	Self-help book for obsessive-compulsive disorder, 2001
The Bipolar Workbook: Tools for Controlling Your Mood Swings, 2nd Edition	Basco MR	Self-help workbook

Source. Adapted from Wright JH, Thase ME, Beck AT: "Cognitive-Behavioral Therapy," in *The American Psychiatric Association Publishing Textbook of Psychiatry*, 7th Edition. Edited by Roberts LW. Washington, DC, American Psychiatric Association Publishing, 2019, p. 969. Copyright © 2019 American Psychiatric Association Publishing. Used with permission.

apist's assistant." Computer-assisted CBT (CCBT) can reinforce learning, deepen the patient's understanding of CBT principles, and promote the use of self-help methods. A large number of studies of CCBT have shown that this newer method of treatment delivery, if supported by a modest amount of clinician effort, is as effective as standard CBT for depression (Andersson et al. 2014; Andrews et al. 2018; Richards and Richardson 2012; Wright et al. 2019b, 2019c). Examples of such programs are *Good Days Ahead* (Thase et al. 2018; Wright et al. 1995, 2004), *Beating the Blues* (Proudfoot et al. 2004), and *Deprexis* (Meyer et al. 2015). The *Good Days Ahead* program (coauthored by one of the authors of this chapter, J.H.W.) features large amounts of video and audio, along with interactive self-help exercises. Research on this program has demonstrated excellent acceptance by patients and substantial effects in reducing symptoms of depression (Thase et al. 2018; Wright et al. 2002, 2005, 2022). In a large multicenter randomized controlled trial, CCBT with *Good Days Ahead* was found to be as effective as a full course of up to 20 sessions of standard face-to-face CBT, even though clinician contact was reduced by two-thirds in CCBT (Thase et al. 2018).

CCBT usually involves a series of lessons or modules that cover the core methods and skills of CBT. Thus, a course of CCBT is designed to be a full immersion in CBT. In contrast, many mobile apps are targeted at specific self-help techniques such as breathing training, meditation, or developing an adaptive mantra. Studies of mobile apps in behavioral health have underscored the need for caution in evaluating the integrity, content, and security of such apps (Huguet et al. 2016; Monteith and Glenn 2016; Wright and Mishkind 2020). For example, an analysis of a large number of apps that claimed to be based on CBT found that only 10% were consistent with CBT methods. Wright and Mishkind (2020) discussed evaluations of mobile apps for psychiatric treatment and recommended several for use with patients (Table 8–4).

Case Formulation

The case formulation is used as a road map for therapy. The patient's unique history is understood through the lens of cognitive-behavioral theory in order to select specific methods that match individual problems, symptoms, assets, and potentials (Wright et al. 2017).

The Academy of Cognitive and Behavioral Therapies (www.academyofct.org) recommends that the case formulation include 1) an outline of the most salient aspects of the history and mental status examination; 2) details of at least three examples from the patient's life of the relationship between events, automatic thoughts, emotions, and behaviors (illustrations of the cognitive model as it pertains to this patient); 3) identification of important schemas; 4) a listing of strengths; 5) a working hypothesis that weaves together all of the information in items 1–4 with the cognitive and behavioral theories that most closely fit the patient's diagnosis and symptoms (e.g., models for anxiety disorders, depression, eating disorders, psychoses, other conditions); and 6) a treatment plan that is based on the working hypothesis. Detailed methods, worksheets, and examples of the use of this formulation method are described elsewhere (Wright et al. 2017), and they can be downloaded from the American Psychiatric Association Publishing website (www.appi.org/wright).

TABLE 8–4. Mobile apps for depression

Mobile app	Features	Source
Day to Day	Daily tips on cognitive-behavioral therapy skills such as challenging negative thoughts and behavioral activation	Intellicare, Northwestern University
Headspace	Mindfulness	Headspace.com
My Mantra	Mantra creation	Intellicare, Northwestern University
Positive Activity Jackpot	Behavioral activation	U.S. Department of Defense
Thought Challenger	Modifying negative thoughts	Intellicare, Northwestern University
Virtual Hope Box	Coping skills for unpleasant emotions and thoughts	U.S. Department of Defense

Note. All apps are available through the App Store or Google Play except for Headspace, which is available at www.headspace.com, and My Mantra, which is available at https://intellicare.cbits.northwestern.edu/app/mantra.

Source. Adapted from Wright JH, Mishkind M: "Computer-Assisted CBT and Mobile Apps for Depression: Assessment and Integration Into Clinical Care." *Focus* 18(2):162–168, 2020. Copyright © 2020 American Psychiatric Association Publishing. Used with permission.

Cognitive Techniques

The cognitive interventions used in CBT are designed to first identify and then modify dysfunctional thinking at two main levels of cognitive processing: automatic thoughts (Table 8–5) and core beliefs (also called schemas). We describe here some of the most commonly used procedures for recognizing and changing maladaptive cognitions.

Guided Discovery

Guided discovery is the most frequently used technique to help patients articulate automatic thoughts in sessions. This process involves gentle eliciting, exploring, and questioning of the patient's thinking. Instead of trying to debate, convince, or sell patients on an idea, therapists ask Socratic-type questions that encourage the patient to expand their perspective and become actively involved in the learning process.

Patient: My anxiety is off the chart this week; I just can't settle down.
Therapist: Did something happen this week that seemed to trigger it?
Patient: I just feel tense all of the time.
Therapist: In the last 24 hours, when was your anxiety the worst, and what were you doing at the time? [*being specific*]
Patient (*pauses*): I guess I was at my house alone watching television, and I started having that tingling and a weird sensation up here again (*pointing all around his chest*).
Therapist: And what were you thinking at that point?
Patient: My chest feels strange.

TABLE 8–5. **Working with automatic thoughts**

Techniques to identify automatic thoughts	Techniques to modify automatic thoughts
Guided discovery	Examining the evidence
Recognizing mood shifts	Reattribution techniques
Imagery and role-play exercises	Identifying cognitive errors
Checklists for automatic thoughts	Thought change records
Thought recording	

Source. Wright et al. 2019a.

Therapist: What did you think was going to happen next as a result of your discomfort? [*probing for automatic thoughts*]

Patient: I felt like, "Is this the big one? Is this my heart attack?" I know that I'm 35 and have been worked up a bunch of times at the emergency room, but I just can't help thinking this.

Therapist: Was the sensation bearable? [*probing for more automatic thoughts*]

Patient: No, it was terrible, I couldn't stand it. I felt that my chest was going to just open up and explode. [*automatic image*]

Therapist: So it sounds as if you were thinking when this sensation occurred that you were going to die, you were having a heart attack, the sensation was terrible and unbearable, and that you had an image of your chest actually opening up from the excruciating pain. Did I hear that right?

Patient: Yes, I hate it when these attacks come. I am never sure if it is the big one or not.

As shown, guided discovery allows for active participation on the part of the patient and facilitation from the therapist.

Recognizing Mood Shifts

One of the most powerful ways to teach patients to detect automatic thoughts is to find a real-life example of how automatic thoughts influence their emotional responses. A shift in mood during a therapy session is often an opportune time for the therapist to facilitate the identification of automatic thoughts. When the therapist observes that a strong emotion such as sadness, anxiety, or anger has appeared, prompts to describe the thoughts that "went through your head" just prior to the mood shift are frequently successful because during periods of affective arousal, automatic thoughts and schemas may be especially potent and accessible. Hence, cognitive therapists capitalize on spontaneously occurring mood shifts during sessions and may also pursue lines of questioning that are likely to elicit intense emotional responses.

Imagery and Role-Play

Imagery and role-play are two methods for uncovering cognitions when direct questions are unsuccessful (or only partially successful) in generating suspected automatic thinking (Beck et al. 1979). With some patients, imagery can be implemented by simply asking them to imagine themselves back in the particularly troubling or emotion-provoking situation and then to describe the thoughts that occurred. Other patients may need facilitating questions that "set the scene." The therapist may ask the patient to describe the details of the setting: When and where did the incident take place? What happened immediately before the incident? How did the characters in the scene appear? What were the main physical features of the setting? These questions bring the memory to life in the patient's mind and facilitate recall of cognitive responses to the situation.

The objectives of role-play are similar. With this procedure, the therapist first asks a series of questions to try to understand an upsetting situation that involves an interpersonal relationship or other social interchange. With the permission of the patient, the therapist then briefly steps into the role of the individual in the scene and facilitates playing out a typical response set. Roles can be reversed if needed to further enhance recall of significant automatic thoughts.

Checklists for Automatic Thoughts

Checklists for automatic thoughts provide an additional method to help patients identify their dysfunctional cognitions. The Automatic Thought Questionnaire (Hollon and Kendall 1980) is a comprehensive list of dysfunctional thoughts that has been used primarily in research studies. Similar lists may be used in clinical settings when patients are having difficulty detecting their automatic thoughts (for an example, see Wright et al. 2017). CBT computer programs can also be used to teach patients to develop their own customized list of negative automatic thoughts and other cognitions (Wright et al. 2004).

Thought Recording

Thought recording is a standard CBT procedure for identifying automatic thoughts (Beck 2020; Wright et al. 2017). Although patients can log their thoughts in a number of ways, most begin by using the two-column technique shown in Figure 8–1. In this example, the patient was asked to write down automatic thoughts that occurred in situations that she associated with her depressed mood. Alternatively, a three-column exercise could include a description of the situation, a list of automatic thoughts, and a list of associated emotions. Thought recording helps the patient recognize the effects of underlying automatic thoughts and understand how the basic CBT model (i.e., relationship among situations, thoughts, feelings, and behaviors) applies to personal experiences.

Modifying Automatic Thoughts

Generally, there is no sharp distinction between the processes of eliciting and modifying automatic thoughts. As patients begin to recognize the nature of their dysfunctional thinking, they typically develop some increased degree of objectivity regarding the validity of their automatic thoughts and begin to question and revise their cognitive distortions. However, additional techniques are usually needed to promote durable changes in automatic thoughts. Methods discussed in this chapter for revising automatic thoughts include 1) examining the evidence, 2) reattribution techniques, 3) identifying cognitive errors, and 4) thought change records (Beck 2020; Beck et al. 1979; Wright et al. 2017).

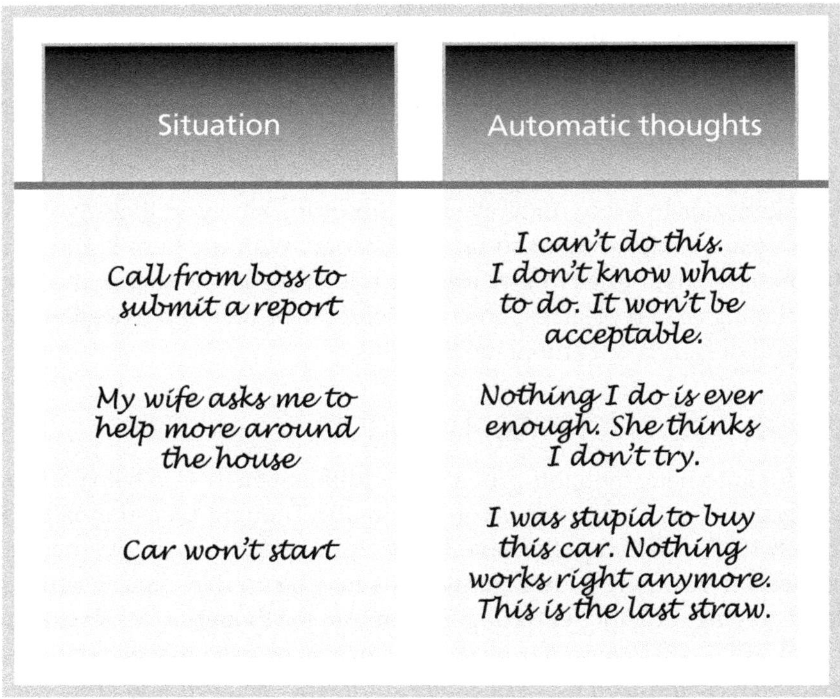

FIGURE 8–1. Two-column thought recording.

Source. Adapted from Wright JH, Thase ME, Beck AT: "Cognitive-Behavioral Therapy," in *The American Psychiatric Association Publishing Textbook of Psychiatry*, 7th Edition. Edited by Roberts LW. Washington, DC, American Psychiatric Association Publishing, 2019, p. 972. Copyright © 2019 American Psychiatric Association Publishing. Used with permission.

Examining the Evidence

Examining the evidence is a technique in which the therapist and patient collaboratively explore the evidence for and the evidence against a specific thought or belief (Wright et al. 2017). When working through the exercise, the therapist typically writes the thought or belief at the top of a piece of paper and then labels two columns with "evidence for" and "evidence against." Then the patient is guided to methodically explore and write down each piece of evidence. At the end of this procedure, the evidence for the cognition is quantified and estimated (e.g., 30%), as well as the evidence against (e.g., 70%). Often, cognitive errors can be identified in the evidence for maladaptive automatic thoughts or schemas. Typically, examining the evidence stimulates a rethinking of dysfunctional cognitions and the development of a more rational thinking style. A case example is provided in the section "Schizophrenia."

Reattribution Techniques

The reattribution method is based on research that shows that depressed individuals often have negatively biased attributions (meanings attached to events) in three dimensions (Abramson et al. 1978): internal versus external (excessive blame toward self for negative events), global versus specific (circumscribed negative events that are overgeneralized and allowed to define one's entire self-concept), and fixed versus variable (hopeless view of likelihood of positive change in the future). CBT therapists employ several different types of reattribution procedures, including psychoeducation about the attributional process, Socratic questioning to stimulate reattribution, the use of scales or graphs to recognize and reinforce alternative attributions, and homework assignments to test out the accuracy of attributions. The basic thrust of this work is to help patients make reasonable attributions about life events so that they do not blame themselves excessively or unnecessarily, give too much weight to negative events, or develop a sense of immutability about their lives. Actual flaws or negative events are recognized, but a more accurate assessment of their meaning is encouraged.

Identifying Cognitive Errors

The thought processes of persons with emotional disorders are frequently characterized by a high frequency of errors in logic (Lefebvre 1981; Watkins and Rush 1983). Aaron T. Beck and others described six main categories of cognitive errors: selective abstraction, arbitrary inference, absolutistic (dichotomous or all-or-nothing) thinking, magnification and minimization, personalization, and catastrophic thinking (Beck et al. 1979; Clark et al. 1999). Definitions and examples of each of these cognitive errors are provided in Table 8–6.

Patients can be taught to spot characteristic cognitive errors to help modify their automatic thoughts. We find most patients need a brief period in session reviewing a basic handout on the definitions of cognitive errors as well as reading about cognitive errors in CBT books written for the general public (see Table 8–3 for a list of resources). Once patients have been exposed to these materials and have practiced spotting their errors in session, they often are able to recognize typical cognitive errors in their thinking. However, repeated practice may be needed before they can use this skill on a routine basis.

Thought Change Records

Self-monitoring with thought change records (TCRs) is a standard element of CBT for most emotional disorders (Beck et al. 1979; Wright et al. 2017). The TCR helps patients 1) observe and recognize their automatic thoughts, 2) apply methods to modify their distorted thoughts, and 3) recognize positive outcomes in their emotions and behavior that result from changes in their thinking.

The TCR (Figure 8–2) is a five-column table with the following headings: Situation, Automatic thoughts, Emotion(s), Rational response, and Outcome. Patients use the first two columns to write down an event, their associated automatic thoughts, and the degree (0%–100%) of their belief in the automatic thoughts. The third column is used to identify the specific emotion linked with each automatic thought and the degree or level of each emotion (0%–100%). The fourth column is used to record rational alternatives to distorted thoughts. This step is a critical element in the use of the TCR because it stimulates patients to learn to assess the validity of their own thoughts. A number of methods to modify automatic thoughts can be used to generate a list of alternative rational thoughts. For example, the technique of identifying cognitive errors

TABLE 8–6. **Cognitive errors**

Error	Description
Selective abstraction (sometimes termed *mental filter*)	Drawing a conclusion based on only a small portion of the available data
Arbitrary inference	Coming to a conclusion without adequate supporting evidence or despite contradictory evidence
Absolutistic thinking ("all-or-nothing" thinking)	Categorizing oneself or personal experiences into rigid dichotomies (e.g., all good or all bad, perfect or completely flawed, success or total failure)
Magnification and minimization	Overvaluing or undervaluing the significance of a personal attribute, a life event, or a future possibility
Personalization	Linking external occurrences to oneself (e.g., taking blame, assuming responsibility, criticizing oneself) when little or no basis exists for making these associations
Catastrophic thinking	Predicting the worst possible outcome while ignoring more likely eventualities

Source. Adapted from Wright JH, Thase ME, Beck AT: "Cognitive-Behavioral Therapy," in *The American Psychiatric Association Publishing Textbook of Psychiatry*, 7th Edition. Edited by Roberts LW. Washington, DC, American Psychiatric Association Publishing, 2019, p. 959.

can be one of the methods used to generate alternative thoughts. Examining the evidence, reattribution, and a variety of other methods can be suggested as ways of generating rational thoughts for the TCR.

The fifth column, Outcome, is used to record any changes that have occurred as a result of revising and modifying automatic thoughts. In the case illustration of a TCR in Figure 8–2, a significant decrease in dysphoric mood occurred. Although the use of the TCR will usually lead to the development of a more adaptive set of cognitions and a reduction in painful affect, on some occasions the initial automatic thoughts will prove to be accurate. In such situations, the therapist helps the patient take a problem-solving approach, including the development of an action plan, to manage the stressful or upsetting event.

Identifying Schemas

The process of identifying and modifying schemas is usually more difficult than changing negative automatic thoughts because these core beliefs are more deeply embedded, may be largely out of the patient's awareness, and usually have been reinforced through years of life experience. A variety of cognitive techniques are used to work at the schema level (Beck et al. 1979; Wright et al. 2017), many of which overlap with the methods used by therapists to identify automatic thoughts (Table 8–7). Two specific methods are discussed in this section: the downward arrow technique and identifying repetitive patterns of automatic thoughts. A more detailed review of methods to identify and modify core beliefs is available (Wright et al. 2017).

Downward Arrow Technique

The downward arrow technique is a powerful cognitive method to assist patients in uncovering negative core beliefs. The therapist asks a series of questions directed at

Situation	Automatic thoughts	Emotion(s)	Rational response	Outcome
Describe 1. Actual event leading to unpleasant emotion; or 2. Stream of thoughts, daydream, or recollection leading to unpleasant emotion; or 3. Unpleasant physiological sensations	1. Write automatic thought(s) that preceded emotion(s). 2. Rate belief in automatic thought(s), 0%–100%.	1. Specify sad, anxious, angry, etc. 2. Rate degree of emotion, 0%–100%.	1. Identify cognitive errors. 2. Write rational response to automatic thought(s). 3. Rate belief in rational response, 0%–100%.	1. Once again, rate belief in automatic thought(s), 0%–100%. 2. Specify and rate subsequent emotion(s), 0%–100%.
Tuesday				
I am reviewing policies and procedures at work, and I am immediately concerned about the amount of work.	*1. I should have completed this weeks ago.*	*Sad: 80%* *Anxious: 50%*	*1. <u>Personalization</u>. Although it is true that the project is overdue, I am not the only one assigned to this project. Two other people have been assigned to work on it and are just as responsible as I am. (80%)*	*Sad: 30%* *Anxious: 20%*
	2. I always wait until the last minute to start things.		*2. <u>All-or-nothing thinking</u>. Although I wanted to start on this project earlier in the month, I was busy with other important duties that the company was asking me to complete. (90%)*	
	3. I'll never complete it.		*3. <u>Catastrophic thinking</u>. Last year this was a big project, and I assisted in completing it. I have also completed other big projects for the company. The project is about 50% complete. (70%)*	

FIGURE 8–2. Thought change record: an example.

Source. Adapted from Wright JH, Thase ME, Beck AT: "Cognitive-Behavioral Therapy," in *The American Psychiatric Association Publishing Textbook of Psychiatry,* 7th Edition. Edited by Roberts LW. Washington, DC, American Psychiatric Association Publishing, 2019, p. 974. Copyright © 2019 American Psychiatric Association Publishing. Used with permission.

TABLE 8–7. Methods for identifying and modifying schemas

Questioning methods (including the downward arrow technique)
Imagery and role-play
Identifying repetitive patterns of automatic thoughts
Using a schema checklist
Psychoeducation
Examining the evidence
Listing advantages and disadvantages
Generating alternatives
Cognitive rehearsal

Source. Adapted from Wright JH, Thase ME, Beck AT: "Cognitive-Behavioral Therapy," in *The American Psychiatric Association Publishing Textbook of Psychiatry*, 7th Edition. Edited by Roberts LW. Washington, DC, American Psychiatric Association Publishing, 2019, p. 976.

revealing increasingly deeper levels of thinking. Questions are first aimed at automatic thoughts that are uncovered around an activating event. The therapist infers that an underlying schema is present and constructs a chain of linked questions that builds on the supposition that the distorted cognitions are, in fact, true. Most questions take on the following format: "If this thought were true, what would it mean about you (or about others or the future)?" This type of questioning needs to be done in a highly collaborative and supportive manner. In the following example, the therapist uses this technique to uncover a key schema in a patient with body dysmorphic disorder.

Therapist: You mentioned that you had a plastic surgeon evaluate your nose for another surgery in the last week and that you are noticing a lot of the different imperfections. Did I get that right?

Patient: Yes. I know we have talked about my concern about my body, but it just doesn't look right. There is a big and rounded point here (*pointing to a place on his nose*).

Therapist: Let's see if there is a larger meaning to these thoughts. If it were true that your nose was truly disfigured, what would that mean?

Patient: I would be ugly and unattractive.

Therapist: What if that were true?

Patient: I don't think Julie or any other woman would be interested in dating me.

Therapist: And if others were not interested in going out with you, what would that mean about you or your future?

Patient: I would be alone, and I am not sure I could ever be happy without being in a relationship (*tearing up*).

Therapist: So one thing that might be behind your multiple plastic surgeries is a belief that you are unattractive and that you are going to end up alone and not in an intimate relationship. If this were true what would this mean about you?

Patient: I'm unlovable.

Therapist: Am I hearing that you think you are ultimately unlovable?

Patient: I guess I have never thought of it in that way, but that is the way it feels now.

This example demonstrates how the downward arrow uncovers core beliefs that were out of the patient's awareness.

Identifying Repetitive Patterns of Automatic Thoughts

As the patient gains experience in recognizing automatic thoughts, repetitive patterns may begin to emerge that may suggest the presence of underlying schemas. Looking for patterns in automatic thoughts can be used as a specific therapy activity or homework assignment. Good sources for material for these reviews can be previous work with TCRs, examining the evidence, or other CBT written exercises. Once a pattern is identified, patients are asked if there is a particular theme to the thoughts that suggests an underlying core belief.

Schema Checklists

In a manner similar to the use of automatic thought checklists, patients can be asked to review lists of commonly endorsed core beliefs. An example of an inventory of maladaptive and adaptive schemas is provided in *Learning Cognitive-Behavior Therapy: An Illustrated Guide* (Wright et al. 2017). Using a checklist can help patients recognize schemas that otherwise may have gone undetected. This type of exercise can be particularly useful for identifying positive or healthy core beliefs that have been obscured by depression, anxiety, or other symptoms of mental disorders. Recognition of adaptive schemas can provide good building blocks for enhancing self-esteem and self-efficacy.

Modifying Schemas

Interventions used to modify schemas include examining the evidence, generating alternatives, using cognitive rehearsal, and listing advantages and disadvantages. After a schema is identified, the therapist may ask the patient to use the two-column procedure described in the subsection "Thought Recording" for examining the evidence for an automatic thought. This intervention is used to stimulate doubt in the validity of the schema and to start the patient thinking of alternative explanations.

An intervention based on examining the evidence is often combined with another step of schema modification, generating alternatives. The list of alternative schemas will usually include several different options, ranging from rather minor adjustments to extensive revisions in the schema. The therapist uses Socratic questioning and other CBT techniques such as imagery and role-play to help the patient recognize potential alternative schemas. A brainstorming attitude is encouraged. Instead of trying to be sure that a revised schema is entirely accurate at first glance, the therapist usually suggests that the patient try to generate a variety of modified schemas without initially considering their validity or practicality. This stimulates creativity and gives the patient further encouragement to step aside from rigid, long-standing schemas.

After alternatives are generated and discussed, the therapy turns toward examining the potential consequences of changing basic attitudes. Cognitive rehearsal can be used in the therapy session to test a schema modification. This may be followed by homework assignments to try out the revised schema in vivo. Usually, specific behavioral changes, consistent with the revised schema, need to be practiced repeatedly before modified core beliefs are fully accepted and put into action.

In addition to these techniques, patients can be taught to list the advantages and disadvantages of a schema. This procedure is designed to bring into awareness the hidden motivations that keep patients from fully accepting a more adaptive schema. Once these risks and benefits are clear, the patient can choose either to maintain the schema or to replace it with a more adaptive one.

Some schemas (e.g., "I'm stupid"; "I'll always lose in the end") appear to have few, if any, advantages, but many schemas (e.g., "If I decide to do something, I must succeed"; "I always have to work harder than others, or I'll fail") have both positive and negative features. The latter group of schemas may be maintained even in the face of their dysfunctional aspects because they encourage hard work, perseverance, or other behaviors that are adaptive. However, the absolute and demanding nature of the schemas ultimately leads to excessive stress, failed expectations, low self-esteem, or other deleterious results. Listing advantages and disadvantages can help the patient to examine the full range of effects of a schema and often encourages modifications that can make the schema both more adaptive and less damaging. The illustration in Figure 8–3 demonstrates how Mr. A, a 43-year-old businessperson, examined the advantages and disadvantages of a perfectionistic schema.

Behavioral Methods for Symptoms of Depression and Anxiety

Behavioral methods may be used to address many of the problems encountered in depression, anxiety, and other psychiatric conditions. Low energy, difficulty completing tasks, avoidance, lack of enjoyment in activities, and poor problem solving are among the issues that may be effectively addressed using the behavioral components of CBT. Several of the more commonly used behavioral activation methods are described here. Video illustrations and detailed instructions for using these methods are provided elsewhere (Wright et al. 2017).

Behavioral Action Plans

For patients who are in the early stage of therapy and/or are highly symptomatic, behavioral activation may involve assigning a specific action. This is usually a circumscribed realistic task that the patient is avoiding but that may stimulate increased activity and energy. Examples include making a commitment to walk for 20 minutes twice a week, agreeing to cook one meal in the next week, or accepting an invitation from a friend to go to the movies. More demanding activities can be used for behavioral activation later in therapy or for patients who are less symptomatic.

The choice of a problem to tackle with a behavioral action plan entails identifying a problem of sufficient magnitude to make the effort meaningful for which the chances of success are also high. Collaboration is critical to success in choosing an activity. Whenever possible, patients should take the lead in selecting the intervention target and giving an honest appraisal of their capabilities in completing the assignment. Therapists can often increase the chances of a good outcome by helping patients identify barriers to completing the task. A good question to ask is "What might get in the way of you following this plan?" If barriers or obstacles can be identified, then the therapist can assist the patient in developing solutions. Another good question to ask is "What is your estimate of the percentage likelihood that you will follow

Advantages	Disadvantages
I got my MBA.	I feel overburdened, depressed, and anxious. I can never relax.
My company knows they can count on me.	Everyone says, "He walks on water." With these expectations, I don't feel I can share my real self with others, and I feel lonely.
I am the "go-to guy."	I never feel as if I can get away from work. They even call me when I am on vacation.
Life is predictable and controlled.	Everything is planned, and nothing ever is a surprise or spontaneous.
I can count on myself to get things done.	It prevents me from counting on others to get things done.

FIGURE 8–3. Mr. A's list of advantages and disadvantages for the belief "I must be perfect."

this plan?" If the patient responds with a low percentage, then the therapist can spend more time trying to overcome obstacles or can assist with choosing another activity that is more likely to be completed.

Activity Scheduling

Activity scheduling is frequently used in CBT when patients have low energy and anhedonia. It is a mainstay in the treatment of depression but can also be useful in treating any clinical condition that causes patients to have difficulty organizing their time. Activity scheduling includes an assessment of the patient's current activity, with the explicit goal being to increase mastery and pleasure. In this context, mastery ratings may be used to measure the patient's sense of accomplishment in completing activities. Pleasure ratings are used to indicate the level of enjoyment experienced while participating in activities. Ratings may be made on a 0- to 10-point scale, in which 10 represents maximum mastery or pleasure and 0 represents no mastery or pleasure.

Typically, patients are introduced to an activity log during a therapy session and instructed how to complete it (see Wright et al. 2017 for a template for an activity schedule log). Examples of specific activities from the recent past can be used to highlight the relationship between participation in activities and the patient's experience of mastery and pleasure. To illustrate, a severely depressed man had earlier reported that he could not "enjoy anything." However, when asked to rate his experiences while watching his son's soccer game, he noted a pleasure rating of 6 and a mastery rating of 7.

For some patients, a full week of activity scheduling can be a fruitful assignment. But the exercise can be scaled down to only a day or part of a day for patients who are severely depressed or are having problems with concentration or very low energy.

After collecting baseline activity schedules with mastery and pleasure ratings, therapists can help patients organize a daily schedule to enhance a sense of mastery and pleasure. They can try to increase activities that receive higher ratings of mastery and pleasure and also brainstorm for stimulating or productive activities to add to the schedule. Problems or deficits in mastery or pleasure are discussed, and strategies are formulated to address these problems. The patient's management of time may also become a fruitful topic of discussion.

Reviewing an activity schedule may reveal a host of negative thoughts, cognitive distortions, or schemas that contribute to the behavioral manifestations of depression or anxiety. This interplay between the cognitive and behavioral aspects of treatment is an important element of CBT. For example, a 50-year-old salesperson had a depressive episode after being fired from his job. He became withdrawn and lost interest in activities. The therapist introduced the concept of activity scheduling by asking him to keep a simple log of his activities during the week between sessions. During the following session, the therapist reviewed the log with the patient and introduced the concept of rating activities. Maladaptive cognitions about behavioral activity became readily apparent as the patient reported such thoughts as "What's the use of doing anything?," "I'm too ashamed to go out in public," and "I'll never succeed." The therapist needed to help the patient reverse hopeless cognitions in order to effectively implement activity scheduling.

Graded Task Assignments

Graded task assignments involve taking seemingly overwhelming tasks and breaking them down into manageable pieces. Developing a graded task assignment may require a cognitive analysis of the task to identify distortions prior to initiating a behavioral plan. Often, several iterations of the process are required as the patient and therapist collaborate to make each component of the task appear workable. The plan should begin with smaller tasks and gradually move toward larger, more difficult ones. Patients may need coaching on ways to complete steps in the assignment.

Use of a graded task assignment is illustrated in the treatment of a depressed woman who reported that her home was completely full of clutter, dirty dishes, and laundry. She felt overwhelmed and totally unable to tackle the task of cleaning up the mess. Her assessment of her incapacity contributed to a downward spiral of depression in which negative cognitions were reinforcing maladaptive behavioral patterns, which in turn were worsening her low self-esteem. The patient and therapist agreed on a plan that divided the cleaning into manageable segments with gradually building levels of effort. Successful progression through the steps appeared to be a catalyst in the patient's overall recovery from depression.

Relaxation Training

Relaxation techniques are commonly used to treat anxiety symptoms, especially if the patient exhibits muscle tension. A frequently used method is known as progressive relaxation. In this approach, the patient is instructed to systematically relax muscle groups throughout the body, one by one. This technique may be combined with imagery, meditation, or breathing techniques. During relaxation training, the patient may report the emergence of cognitions that require further exploration. Relaxation techniques can be taught and practiced during sessions and then used by the patient between sessions.

Exposure and Response Prevention

Because avoidance is a central feature of anxiety disorders, exposure techniques are a major component of CBT for these conditions. Typically, exposure methods are graded so that the patient starts by facing stimuli that trigger lower levels of anxiety and then progressively experiences stimuli that may produce higher amounts of anxiety. A multiple-step hierarchy involving exposure to the stimulus is constructed in collaboration with the patient. Often, a simple rating scale of 0–100 is used to rate the expected amount of anxiety associated with each progressive step. The exposure may be performed using imagery or in vivo. Virtual reality programs are available for simulating anxiety-producing situations (e.g., fear of flying, PTSD, social phobia) in the therapist's office.

In using these methods, therapists and patients work collaboratively to increase the patient's exposure to anxiety-provoking experiences they are avoiding. This provides a context in which therapists can help patients test out their maladaptive beliefs about anxiety, their vulnerability, or their resources. The response prevention component of exposure therapy involves a detailed analysis of all avoidance behaviors, including misguided attempts to cope with anxiety-provoking stimuli that actually reinforce avoidance (called *safety behaviors*), and collaborative agreements to stop using such maladaptive behaviors.

CBT Methods for Specific Disorders

Schizophrenia

The first reported case of CBT for schizophrenia occurred in 1952 when Aaron T. Beck described successful treatment of delusions in a patient with schizophrenia (Beck 1952). However, systematic exploration of the possible role of CBT in treatment of schizophrenia and other psychoses did not begin until the early 1990s (Kingdon and Turkington 1991; Tarrier et al. 1993). Over the past three decades, several books have been published that detail methods for performing CBT with patients with psychosis (Chadwick et al. 1996; Kingdon and Turkington 2005; Wright et al. 2009), numerous outcome studies have been completed (McKenna et al. 2019; Morrison et al. 2018), and CBT applications for schizophrenia have gained increased acceptance. In the United Kingdom, where much of the research on CBT for psychoses has been conducted, the National Institute for Health and Care Excellence (2014) guidelines for treatment of schizophrenia recommended a course of CBT for all patients with this condition.

CBT methods for schizophrenia use the same basic strategies employed in treatment of nonpsychotic disorders. However, there are modifications in the therapeutic relationship, the pace of therapy, targets for interventions, and implementation of techniques. Because patients with schizophrenia often have difficulty engaging in therapy and can be stigmatized by this illness, considerable effort is expended early in CBT on building a collaborative therapeutic relationship. A gentle, nonthreatening questioning style is used in which the therapist tries to set the patient at ease.

Psychoeducation that includes the normalizing rationale is a key element of the beginning stages of CBT for schizophrenia (Kingdon and Turkington 1991, 2005; Wright et al. 2009). One part of this process is for therapists to ask patients to give their explanations of symptoms. Often, the responses reflect dysfunctional beliefs (e.g., "The devil is talking to me," "I have done something terribly wrong and deserve to be punished," "Nobody else hears voices," "All doctors want to do is push pills—I won't take them") and thus offer useful opportunities for educating and/or destigmatizing.

The *normalizing rationale* can be a centerpiece of efforts to help patients understand their illnesses in more rational and affirming ways (Kingdon and Turkington 1991, 2005; Wright et al. 2009). The cognitive-behavioral therapist explains that experiences such as having paranoia or hearing voices are very common and can be induced by lack of sleep, sensory deprivation, medical illnesses, and other stresses. The discussion can then lead to presentation of a stress-vulnerability model for symptoms. The goal of this process is to help patients develop a conceptualization that has the following core elements: 1) Psychotic symptoms can occur in a wide range of people and thus can be a part of "normal" experience. 2) Stress can interact with a biological vulnerability to produce or worsen symptoms. 3) Problems can be reduced or solved by learning ways to manage symptoms and cope with stress. If this conceptualization is understood and accepted, therapeutic work on reducing delusions and hallucinations and reversing negative symptoms is more likely to succeed.

CBT for delusions relies primarily on the use of Socratic questioning and guided discovery to gradually help patients see different perspectives. *Examining the evidence* can be a quite useful specific technique. For example, a patient might be asked to list the evidence for and against a belief that his food is being poisoned, people are following him, or there are hidden microphones in the heating ducts. After examining the evidence in a therapy session, the therapist and patient can develop homework assignments to test out the belief or to obtain further information. It is important for therapists to maintain an empirical stance when doing this type of work. Instead of the therapist trying to persuade the patient to give up a delusion, the therapist and patient function as an investigative team. Together, they explore evidence and attempt to draw the most rational conclusion.

Figure 8–4 provides an example of using the technique of examining the evidence with a woman with paranoid schizophrenia. As often happens in performing this type of exercise, the *evidence for* the delusional belief contains numerous cognitive er-

Examining the evidence for a delusional belief:
people in red cars are trying to get me

Evidence For	Evidence Against
I see red cars going past my house every day.	*There are so many red cars on the road; how could they all be after me?*
It seems like people in red cars are staring at me.	*No one in a red car has actually ever threatened me or hurt me.*
A teacher who hated me drove a red car.	*My chemical imbalance can make me afraid of things that won't harm me.*
Someone in a red car slows down when she drives past my house.	*I trust my sister, and she says that I don't need to be afraid of red cars.*

My plan

I'll slowly check out this fear with these steps:

1. *Take a walk in my neighborhood with my sister and walk past some red cars.*
2. *Take a drive with my sister and drive by some red cars on purpose.*
3. *If I am comfortable with the first two steps, I'll try to go to the mall. I'll walk through the parking lot and get used to seeing lots of red cars.*

FIGURE 8–4. Examining the evidence for a delusional belief.

rors that can be discussed in the therapy session. The intervention plan developed with this patient employed graded exposure in a manner similar to the stepped approach used for anxiety disorders. The patient had been isolating herself in a darkened house with all of the shades drawn. Thus, a combined cognitive and behavioral intervention was used to decrease the intensity of her delusional belief and help her resume normal activities.

The CBT approach to hallucinations uses the educating and normalizing process outlined earlier to help patients understand these symptoms in the most adaptive way possible. The patient's attributions (explanation of causality) about these perceptions are elicited and discussed with the goal of developing an explanatory model that assists with coping. For example, a patient who first explained his auditory hallucinations as "coming from the devil" was eventually able to articulate and accept a much more adaptive construct: "I have an illness that affects my thinking and makes me hear voices.... I don't need to pay attention to the voices or do what they say.... The voices get softer and less bothersome when I pay less attention to them."

Therapeutic work with hallucinations may also involve developing lists of behaviors that either aggravate or reduce the intensity of the symptom. For example, a patient might note that lack of sleep, arguments with parents, and spending time alone with nothing to do can make her voices worse. Conversely, listening to soothing music, socializing with a friend, working on crafts projects, and going out to eat may reduce the hallucinations. Behavioral plans can be made to cope with aggravating influences and to use identified coping methods more frequently. If patients have difficulty finding ways to reduce hallucinations, it can be helpful to provide them with a list of commonly used strategies (see the Appendix to Wright et al. 2009 for a list of 60 coping methods, which can be downloaded at www.appi.org/wright).

Cognitive and behavioral interventions for negative symptoms are less direct than techniques for positive symptoms. Kingdon and Turkington (2005) recommended a "go slow" approach for negative symptoms. Instead of trying to aggressively push patients to break patterns of social isolation or apathy, therapists gradually build the therapeutic relationship and assist patients in meeting their goals for change, even if these goals are rather modest. When patients are ready to begin changing negative symptoms, therapists may suggest techniques such as graded task assignments to help them take sequential steps toward improvement.

Grant and colleagues have developed a recovery-oriented form of CBT for psychosis that emphasizes methods to reduce defeatist and asocial beliefs while increasing positive beliefs and meaning in life. These methods also target negative symptoms and withdrawal from community and social activities for change. Research on this form of CBT for psychosis has shown promising early results (Chang et al. 2014; Grant et al. 2012).

Eating Disorders

CBT is recommended as the first-line treatment for adults with bulimia nervosa and binge-eating disorder, and CBT is recognized as one of several effective psychological interventions for anorexia nervosa (American Psychiatric Association 2006; National Institute for Health and Care Excellence 2017). Empirical evidence supports enhanced cognitive-behavioral therapy (CBT-E) as an efficacious and effective treatment for adults and older adolescents with a range of eating disorder diagnoses (Atwood and Friedman 2020; de Jong et al. 2018; Linardon et al. 2017).

CBT-E is based on the transdiagnostic theory that posits that a common psychopathology is central to the maintenance of all eating disorders. The psychological process involves overevaluation of the body, perfectionistic standards, and the idea of control. The treatment has four stages that are typically delivered over 20 sessions (Fairburn 2008; Murphy et al. 2010).

The first phase of treatment aims to engage and educate the patient while introducing behavioral modifications, including regular eating, weekly weighing, and self-monitoring with food records. During this early phase of treatment, a strong emphasis should be placed on the therapeutic relationship and psychoeducation about normal eating.

In the second stage, the patient and therapist jointly review progress, identify problems and emerging barriers, and revise the formulation and treatment plan if indicated. The third stage encompasses the main body of treatment and aims 1) to address concerns about body image, 2) to modify dietary restraint, and 3) to enhance the patient's ability to tolerate day-to-day events and moods. A central focus in CBT-E is understanding the overevaluation of body shape and its impact on eating disorder behaviors. Patients are educated about the impact of body checking and how to use mirrors appropriately. The patient and therapist collaborate to enhance the importance of other domains for self-evaluation. These include helping the patient engage in aspects of life that have been marginalized because of the eating disorder. Once normal eating has been reestablished, food experiments can be useful for testing beliefs about feared foods. For example, if a patient believes she will gain 5 pounds if she eats a doughnut, she may be asked to eat the doughnut and then weigh herself. The patient is taught to recognize cues or triggers and develop lists of healthy coping strategies for managing the negative emotions that lead to eating disorder behaviors. The therapist may also help the patient address interpersonal problems and modify deeply rooted schemas with themes of perfectionism and low self-worth that commonly drive eating disorder behaviors.

The final phase focuses on maintaining the progress that has been made and developing a comprehensive relapse prevention plan. Identifying high-risk situations, recognizing early warning signs of a relapse, and developing a list of recovery behaviors are essential in relapse prevention.

Insomnia

Cognitive behavioral therapy for insomnia (CBT-I) is recognized by the American College of Physicians (Qaseem et al. 2016), the National Institutes of Health (2005), and the American Academy of Sleep Medicine (Morgenthaler et al. 2006) as the first-line treatment for adults with chronic insomnia. A growing body of evidence supports the efficacy of CBT-I in the treatment of primary insomnia as well as insomnia associated with comorbid medical and psychiatric conditions (Koffel et al. 2015; Wu et al. 2015).

CBT-I is a multicomponent treatment approach that combines behavioral and cognitive methods to address maladaptive behaviors and dysfunctional attitudes that interfere with sleep (Sharma and Andrade 2012). A sleep diary is used in the early part of CBT-I to collect baseline sleep data in order to tailor behavioral and cognitive interventions to the patient's needs.

Stimulus Control

Stimulus control counseling is based on the premise that insomnia is a conditioned response. Repeatedly lying in bed awake pairs the bed or bedroom with wakefulness, anxiety, and frustration about sleep. Stimulus control attempts to break this pairing and recondition patient to pair the bed and bedroom with rapid sleep onset (Bootzin and Perlis 2011). Instructions for stimulus control include using the bed exclusively for sleep and sexual activity, getting out of bed if not asleep within 20 minutes, engaging in nonstimulating activities and returning to bed when sleepy, and avoiding falling asleep outside the bedroom.

Sleep Restriction

The goal of sleep restriction is to improve sleep efficiency (total sleep time/total time in bed). Curtailing the amount of time spent in bed to equal the recently reported sleep time results in partial sleep deprivation and increased sleepiness the following day (Morgenthaler et al. 2006). Time in bed is then slowly titrated on the basis of calculations of sleep efficiency. Sleep restriction is contraindicated for individuals with bipolar disorder, untreated sleep apnea, parasomnias, or seizure disorder (Perlis et al. 2011).

Relaxation Training and Biofeedback

Most individuals with insomnia experience somatic or cognitive arousal. Relaxation training aims to reduce somatic tension and intrusive thoughts at bedtime that interfere with sleep. Relaxation strategies include meditation, guided imagery, breathing exercises, passive body focusing, and mindfulness (Perlis et al. 2011). Sufficient evidence exists to support biofeedback as an effective intervention for chronic insomnia. Biofeedback provides visual or auditory information to patients to help them control some physiological parameters (e.g., muscle tension) in order to seek reduction in somatic arousal (Morgenthaler et al. 2006).

Paradoxical Intention

Paradoxical intention (trying to stay awake instead of trying to fall asleep) and lying in bed passively awake are two strategies recommended for sleep initiation insomnia (Perlis et al. 2011). These two strategies seek to eliminate performance anxiety that can develop and contribute to hyperarousal (Morgenthaler et al. 2006).

Cognitive Restructuring

CBT seeks to alter beliefs, attitudes, and attributions about sleep that are presumed to contribute to chronic insomnia. Cognitive restructuring aims to refute the irrational belief that poor sleep causes catastrophic outcomes. One technique involves exploring the validity of these beliefs by examining the actual occurrence rate of the perceived negative consequence. For example, an individual may believe that if they do not get a good night of sleep, they will have a horrible day at work. Reflecting on the number of nights with poor sleep and the number of horrible days at work highlights the discrepancy between beliefs and actual outcomes (Perlis et al. 2011).

A standard course of CBT-I is delivered over six to eight weekly sessions by a trained therapist. Finding a therapist who is trained in CBT-I may be a barrier to treatment. Alternative delivery models have emerged and include internet-based programs, applications, and self-help manuals. A small, but growing, body of evidence demonstrates that internet-delivered programs can effectively decrease insomnia severity and contribute to overall sleep improvement (Ritterband et al. 2009).

CBT for Suicide Risk Reduction

CBT has emerged as a primary, evidence-based method of reducing suicide risk (Brown et al. 2005; Stanley et al. 2009, 2018; Wright et al. 2017). In a study done at the University of Pennsylvania, a CBT intervention for persons who had attempted suicide led to an almost 50% reduction in subsequent suicide attempts compared with a control condition (Brown et al. 2005). Research on safety planning, a core feature of CBT for suicide risk, found that brief safety planning in emergency departments substantially lowered the rate of later suicide attempts (Stanley et al. 2018).

The CBT methods described by Brown and colleagues (Brown et al. 2005; Wright et al. 2017) begin with a thorough assessment of suicide risk and development of a commitment to treatment. The therapist provides information about CBT and explains that suicide risk can rise or fall. A goal of treatment is for the patient to gain skills that can be used to cope with and survive suicidal crises. Thus, the patient is asked to agree to work collaboratively to develop these skills.

Hopelessness is often targeted as an early focus of CBT for suicide risk because of the association between this common symptom of depression and suicide. If patients see little or no hope that their suffering will end, therapists can use standard CBT methods such as Socratic questioning and examining the evidence to elicit reasons to have hope. Therapists may discuss the positive results of CBT and other methods for relieving depression. A particularly useful line of questioning is to ask patients about their reasons to live. If a patient cannot verbalize any genuine reasons to live and indicates the belief that trying is pointless, concern about suicide risk should be high. If CBT is ineffective in helping the patient view the future differently, precautions such as hospitalization may be needed. Conversely, if the patient identifies significant reasons to live and the therapist can bolster their strength with CBT methods, these positive, future-oriented cognitions may reduce the risk of suicide.

Safety planning involves a series of specific steps described in a written action plan that patients take with them for use between sessions. Clinicians can record the safety plan in the health care record to be used in follow-up visits and to document implementation of this valuable method of reducing the risk of suicide attempts. The steps in building a safety plan are shown in Table 8–8.

Another component of the CBT approach for suicide risk reduction is the development of a hope kit. The patient is asked to think of photos, images, music, and/or objects that could stimulate a sense of hope or remind them of reasons to live and to store them in a box or kit. The box can be a tangible object or can be virtually created on a mobile app. Socratic questions and other CBT methods can be used to help patients consider possible additions to the hope kit. For example, the therapist might ask, "What might you have put in the kit before you became so depressed?" or "What would a loved one or a close friend suggest you put in your kit?"

The therapist and patient work on standard CBT skill building such as learning how to spot and modify automatic thoughts and how to use behavioral activation techniques. Progress with these interventions can help reduce hopelessness and other symptoms of depression while giving the patient tools to manage stressors and triggers for relapse. Brown and coworkers (2005) also recommended that therapists use cognitive-behavioral rehearsal to prepare for possible future crises. When the patient

TABLE 8–8. Safety planning steps

Step 1. ***Identify warning signs.*** Work with the patient to elicit warning signs for increased suicide risk. If the warning signs are vague, explain that it is important to be specific in order to increase the likelihood of recognizing the beginning of the crisis.

Step 2. ***Develop coping strategies.*** Explain how distraction from suicidal thoughts can help to lower risk. Ask "What can you do if you become suicidal again to help yourself not to act on your thoughts or urges?" Identify at least three specific strategies. Determine whether these strategies are safe and will not increase distress and whether they are feasible. Assess barriers to using these strategies, if any, and use a collaborative, problem-solving approach to address potential roadblocks.

Step 3. ***Identify social contacts and social settings.*** Ask the patient to identify individuals who would help to distract them from their problems and who could help them feel better. Also, identify social settings that may help distract the patient from their problems. Determine the likelihood that they would be able to talk with someone or go somewhere during a time of crisis. Assess the barriers to using these strategies and identify ways to resolve roadblocks or identify alternatives.

Step 4. ***Contact family members or friends.*** Ask the patient to determine family members or friends who could be contacted for help during a crisis. Assess the likelihood that they will be able to reach out to each identified person. If doubt is expressed about contacting others, assess the barriers and address potential roadblocks or identify others to contact.

Step 5. ***Contact professionals or agencies.*** Identify any mental health professionals who can be contacted during a crisis. Explain how to contact the National Suicide Prevention Lifeline (1-800-273-8255) or go to the hospital or urgent care setting during a crisis. Assess the likelihood the patient will contact each professional, agency, or crisis line; identify potential obstacles and problem solve.

Step 6. ***Make the environment safe.*** Explain that making the environment safer will help to lower the risk of acting on suicidal feelings. Ask the patient whether they have access to a firearm. If an individual has identified other potentially lethal methods, then determine whether they have access to them. For each lethal method, collaboratively develop a plan to make the environment safer so that the patient will be less likely to use this method. For firearms, consider asking a family member or friend who is authorized to possess a firearm to remove it or consider locking up the firearm and ammunition separately.

Step 7. ***Identify and build up reasons to live.*** Spend enough time with the patient to recognize and amplify these especially valuable protective factors against suicide.

Source. Adapted from Wright JH, Brown GK, Thase ME, et al: *Learning Cognitive-Behavior Therapy: An Illustrated Guide*, 2nd Edition. Arlington, VA, American Psychiatric Association Publishing, 2017, pp. 221–222. Copyright © 2017 American Psychiatric Association Publishing. Used with permission.

describes a worst-case scenario such as relational infidelity, unemployment, or the death of a loved one, the therapist is empathic but then assists the patient in rehearsing cognitive and behavioral methods that could help the patient get through the crisis. By preparing in advance, the patient will be armed with useful methods to reduce the risk of suicide.

Conclusion

CBT methods are based directly on core theories of altered information processing and associated maladaptive behavior in psychiatric disorders. Therapists select techniques on the basis of the patient's diagnosis, an individualized CBT formulation, and the objectives that are collaboratively determined during each session. Nonspecific features of all effective psychotherapies are also important in CBT. Thus, therapists work to promote understanding, trust, genuineness, and accurate empathy. The CBT relationship is highly collaborative and active. Specific emphasis is placed on psychoeducation, structuring sessions, and enhancing learning and skill acquisition. A variety of cognitive techniques such as thought recording, examining the evidence, and rehearsal are used to modify dysfunctional automatic thoughts and schemas. In addition, behavioral methods such as activity scheduling, graded task assignments, and exposure and response prevention are used routinely in CBT sessions.

CBT has been studied extensively in randomized controlled trials. Detailed treatment principles and techniques have been described for most psychiatric conditions. Future challenges for CBT include study of methods to further enhance treatment results, detailed examination of predictors for outcome, incorporation of new developments in computer-assisted learning or other technologies, and research on best practices for dissemination of CBT methods to trainees across health care disciplines and in various health care settings.

Key Points

- CBT methods are constructed from the basic theories and experimental findings on cognitive and behavioral pathology in specific psychiatric disorders.
- Prior to the selection and implementation of CBT techniques, the unique history of each patient is understood through the lens of cognitive and behavioral theory. Specific methods are then selected that match the patient's problems, symptoms, assets, and potential.
- General CBT methods such as a collaborative-empirical therapeutic relationship and structuring procedures are used across sessions and incorporated into the treatment of all disorders.
- CBT treatment plans aim to modify and change maladaptive automatic thoughts and schemas. A variety of cognitive methods enable patients to engage in this process.
- Methods that target problematic behaviors associated with depression and anxiety include activity monitoring, behavioral activation, and exposure and response prevention. These are also incorporated into the treatments of other disorders.
- CBT methods for schizophrenia include many of the typical procedures for depression and anxiety conditions. However, the *normalizing rationale* is central in assisting patients to understand their illness in a more rational and affirming way.
- CBT methods for eating disorders focus on maladaptive beliefs about food, weight, body image, self-worth, and dysfunctional behaviors.
- CBT is a first-line treatment for insomnia that employs stimulus control, sleep restriction, relaxation, cognitive restructuring, and other CBT methods to improve sleep onset and maintenance.

- The CBT approach to suicide risk reduction focuses on improving a sense of hope; developing a specific and practical safety plan, including reasons to live; building core CBT skills; and preparing in advance for possible future crises.

Recommended Readings

Barlow DH, Cerney JA: Psychological Treatment of Panic (Treatment Manuals for Practitioners). New York, Guilford, 1988

Basco MR, Rush AJ: Cognitive-Behavioral Therapy for Bipolar Disorder, 2nd Edition. New York, Guilford, 2007

Beck AT, Rush AJ, Shaw BF, et al: Cognitive Therapy of Depression. New York, Guilford, 1979

Beck AT, Wright FD, Newman CF, Liese BS: Cognitive Therapy of Substance Abuse. New York, Guilford, 1993

Beck AT, Davis DD, Freeman A: Cognitive Therapy of Personality Disorders, 3rd Edition. New York, Guilford, 2015

Beck JS: Cognitive Therapy: Basics and Beyond, 3rd Edition. New York, Guilford, 2020

Brownell K, Walsh BT (eds): Eating Disorders and Obesity: A Comprehensive Handbook, 3rd Edition. New York, Guilford, 2017

Clark DA, Beck AT: The Anxiety and Worry Workbook: The Cognitive Behavioral Solution, Illustrated Edition. New York, Guilford, 2012

Clark DA, Beck AT, Alford BA: Scientific Foundations of Cognitive Theory and Therapy of Depression. New York, Wiley, 1999

Kingdon DG, Turkington D: Cognitive Therapy for Schizophrenia (Guides to Individualized Evidence-Based Treatment). New York, Guilford, 2008

Linehan MM: Cognitive-Behavioral Treatment of Borderline Personality Disorder. New York, Guilford, 1993

Meichenbaum DB: Cognitive-Behavior Modification: An Integrative Approach. New York, Plenum, 1977

Reinecke MA, Dattilio FM, Freeman A (eds): Cognitive Therapy With Children and Adolescents: A Casebook for Clinical Practice, 2nd Edition. New York, Guilford, 2003

Wilkes TCR, Belsher G, Rush AJ, et al: Cognitive Therapy for Depressed Adolescents. New York, Guilford, 1994

Wright JH, Turkington D, Kingdon D, et al: Cognitive-Behavior Therapy for Severe Mental Illness: An Illustrated Guide. Washington, DC, American Psychiatric Publishing, 2009

Wright JH, Sudak D, Turkington D, et al: High-Yield Cognitive-Behavior Therapy for Brief Sessions: An Illustrated Guide. Washington, DC, American Psychiatric Publishing, 2010

Wright JH, Brown GK, Thase ME, et al: Learning Cognitive-Behavior Therapy: An Illustrated Guide, 2nd Edition. Arlington, VA, American Psychiatric Association Publishing, 2017

References

Abramson LY, Seligman MEP, Teasdale JD: Learned helplessness in humans: critique and reformulation. J Abnorm Psychol 87(1):49–74, 1978 649856

American Psychiatric Association: Practice Guideline for the Treatment of Patients With Eating Disorders, 3rd Edition. Washington, DC, American Psychiatric Publishing, 2006

Andersson G, Cuijpers P, Carlbring P, et al: Guided internet-based vs. face-to-face cognitive behavior therapy for psychiatric and somatic disorders: a systematic review and meta-analysis. World Psychiatry 13(3):288–295, 2014 25273302

Andrews G, Basu A, Cuijpers P, et al: Computer therapy for the anxiety and depression disorders is effective, acceptable and practical health care: an updated meta-analysis. J Anxiety Disord 55:70–78, 2018 29422409

Atwood ME, Friedman A: A systematic review of enhanced cognitive behavioral therapy (CBT-E) for eating disorders. Int J Eat Disord 53(3):311–330, 2020 31840285

Basco MR: The Bipolar Workbook: Tools for Controlling Your Mood Swings. New York, Guilford, 2006

Beck AT: Successful outpatient psychotherapy of a chronic schizophrenic with a delusion based on borrowed guilt. Psychiatry 15(3):305–312, 1952 12983446

Beck AT, Rush AJ, Shaw BF, et al: Cognitive Therapy of Depression. New York, Guilford, 1979

Beck AT, Wright FW, Newman CF, Liese BS: Cognitive Therapy of Substance Abuse. New York, Guilford, 1993

Beck AT, Davis DD, Freeman A: Cognitive Therapy of Personality Disorders, 3rd Edition. New York, Guilford, 2015

Beck JS: Cognitive Therapy: Basics and Beyond, 3rd Edition. New York, Guilford, 2020

Bernard P, Romain AJ, Caudroit J, et al: Cognitive behavior therapy combined with exercise for adults with chronic diseases: systematic review and meta-analysis. Health Psychol 37(5):433–450, 2018 29698018

Bernardy K, Klose P, Busch AJ, et al: Cognitive behavioural therapies for fibromyalgia. Cochrane Database Syst Rev Sep 10 (9):CD009796, 2013 24018611

Bernardy K, Klose P, Welsch P, et al: Efficacy, acceptability and safety of cognitive behavioural therapies in fibromyalgia syndrome: a systematic review and meta-analysis of randomized controlled trials. Eur J Pain 22(2):242–260, 2018 28984402

Bieling PJ, McCabe RD, Antony MM: Cognitive-Behavioral Therapy in Groups. New York, Guilford, 2009

Bootzin R, Perlis M: Stimulus control therapy, in Behavioral Treatments for Sleep Disorders. Edited by Perlis M, Aloia M, Kuhn B, et al. New York, Academic Press, 2011, pp 21–30

Brown GK, Ten Have T, Henriques GR, et al: Cognitive therapy for the prevention of suicide attempts: a randomized controlled trial. JAMA 294(5):563–570, 2005 16077050

Burns DD: Feeling Good: The New Mood Therapy. New York, Signet, 1980

Chadwick P, Birchwood M, Trower P: Cognitive Therapy of Voices, Delusions, and Paranoia. Chichester, UK, Wiley, 1996

Chang NA, Grant PM, Luther L, et al: Effects of a recovery-oriented cognitive therapy training program on inpatient staff attitudes and incidents of seclusion and restraint. Community Ment Health J 50(4):415–421, 2014 24337473

Cheng JOS, Cheng ST: Effectiveness of physical and cognitive-behavioural intervention programmes for chronic musculoskeletal pain in adults: a systematic review and meta-analysis of randomized controlled trials. PLoS One 14(10):e0223367, 2019 31600270

Clark DA, Beck AT, Alford BA: Scientific Foundations of Cognitive Theory and Therapy of Depression. New York, Wiley, 1999

Dattilio FM: Cognitive-Behavioral Therapy With Couples and Families. New York, Guilford, 2013

Davis D, Wright JH: The therapeutic relationship in cognitive-behavioral therapy: patient perceptions and therapist responses. Cognit Behav Pract 1:25–45, 1994

de Jong M, Schoorl M, Hoek HW: Enhanced cognitive behavioural therapy for patients with eating disorders: a systematic review. Curr Opin Psychiatry 31(6):436–444, 2018 30188385

Ehde DM, Dillworth TM, Turner JA: Cognitive-behavioral therapy for individuals with chronic pain: efficacy, innovations, and directions for research. Am Psychol 69(2):153–166, 2014 24547801

Epstein N: Couple and family therapy, in Comparative Treatments of Depression. Edited by Reinecke MA, Davison MR. New York, Springer, 2002, pp 358–396

Fairburn CG: Cognitive Behavioral Therapy and Eating Disorders. New York, Guilford, 2008

Grant PM, Huh GA, Perivoliotis D, et al: Randomized trial to evaluate the efficacy of cognitive therapy for low-functioning patients with schizophrenia. Arch Gen Psychiatry 69(2):121–127, 2012 21969420

Hanlon I, Hewitt C, Bell K, et al: Systematic review with meta-analysis: online psychological interventions for mental and physical health outcomes in gastrointestinal disorders including irritable bowel syndrome and inflammatory bowel disease. Aliment Pharmacol Ther 48(3):244–259, 2018 29901820

Hollon SD, Kendall PC: Cognitive self-statements in depression: development of an automatic thoughts questionnaire. Cognit Ther Res 4:383–395, 1980

Huguet A, Rao S, McGrath PJ, et al: A systematic review of cognitive behavioral therapy and behavioral activation apps for depression. PLoS One 11(5):e0154248, 2016 27135410

James A, Soler A, Weatherall R: Cognitive behavioural therapy for anxiety disorders in children and adolescents. Cochrane Database Syst Rev Oct 19 (4):CD004690, 2005 16235374

Kingdon DG, Turkington D: The use of cognitive behavior therapy with a normalizing rationale in schizophrenia. Preliminary report. J Nerv Ment Dis 179(4):207–211, 1991 2007891

Kingdon D, Turkington D: Cognitive Therapy for Schizophrenia. New York, Guilford, 2005

Kinsinger SW: Cognitive-behavioral therapy for patients with irritable bowel syndrome: current insights. Psychol Res Behav Manag 10:231–237, 2017 28790872

Koffel EA, Koffel JB, Gehrman PR: A meta-analysis of group cognitive behavioral therapy for insomnia. Sleep Med Rev 19(2):6–16, 2015 24931811

Lefebvre MF: Cognitive distortion and cognitive errors in depressed psychiatric and low back pain patients. J Consult Clin Psychol 49(4):517–525, 1981 6455451

Li L, Xiong L, Zhang S, et al: Cognitive-behavioral therapy for irritable bowel syndrome: a meta-analysis. J Psychosom Res 77(1):1–12, 2014 24913335

Linardon J, Wade TD, de la Piedad Garcia X, et al: The efficacy of cognitive-behavioral therapy for eating disorders: a systematic review and meta-analysis. J Consult Clin Psychol 85(11):1080–1094, 2017 29083223

McKenna P, Leucht S, Jauhar S, et al: The controversy about cognitive behavioural therapy for schizophrenia. World Psychiatry 18(2):235–236, 2019 31059624

Meyer B, Bierbrodt J, Schröder J, et al: Effects of an internet intervention (Deprexis) on severe depression symptoms: randomized controlled trial. Internet Interv 2(1):48–59, 2015

Monteith S, Glenn T: Automated decision-making and big data: concerns for people with mental illness. Curr Psychiatry Rep 18(12):112–123, 2016 27783339

Morgenthaler T, Kramer M, Alessi C, et al: Practice parameters for the psychological and behavioral treatment of insomnia: an update: an American Academy of Sleep Medicine report. Sleep 29(11):1415–1419, 2006 17162987

Morrison AP, Pyle M, Gumley A, et al: Cognitive behavioural therapy in clozapine-resistant schizophrenia (FOCUS): an assessor-blinded, randomized controlled trial. Lancet Psychiatry 5(8):633–643, 2018 30001930

Muñoz-Solomando A, Kendall T, Whittington CJ: Cognitive behavioural therapy for children and adolescents. Curr Opin Psychiatry 21(4):332–337, 2008 18520736

Murphy R, Straebler S, Cooper Z, et al: Cognitive behavioral therapy for eating disorders. Psychiatr Clin North Am 33(3):611–627, 2010 20599136

National Institute for Health and Care Excellence: Psychosis and schizophrenia in adults: prevention and management. Clinical Guideline CG178. London, National Institute for Health and Care Excellence, February 12, 2014. Available at: www.nice.org.uk/guidance/cg178. Accessed September 2, 2021.

National Institute for Health and Care Excellence: Eating disorders: recognition and treatment. NICE Guideline NG69. London, National Institute for Health and Care Excellence, May 23, 2017. Available at: www.nice.org.uk/guidance/ng69. Accessed September 3, 2021.

National Institutes of Health: National Institutes of Health State of the Science Conference statement Manifestations and Management of Chronic Insomnia in Adults, June 13–15, 2005. Sleep 28(9):1049–1057, 2005 16268373

Perlis M, Aloia M, Kuhn B: Behavioral Treatments for Sleep Disorders: Practical Resources for the Mental Health Professional. New York, Academic Press, 2011

Proudfoot J, Ryden C, Everitt B, et al: Clinical efficacy of computerised cognitive-behavioural therapy for anxiety and depression in primary care: randomised controlled trial. Br J Psychiatry 185:46–54, 2004 15231555

Qaseem A, Kansagara D, Forciea MA, et al: Management of chronic insomnia disorder in adults: a clinical practice guideline from the American College of Physicians. Ann Intern Med 165(2):125–133, 2016 27136449

Ray LA, Meredith LR, Kiluk BD, et al: Combined pharmacotherapy and cognitive behavioral therapy for adults with alcohol or substance use disorders: a systematic review and meta-analysis. JAMA Netw Open 3(6):e208279, 2020 32558914

Reinecke MA, Dattilio FM, Freeman A (eds): Cognitive Therapy With Children and Adolescents: A Casebook for Clinical Practice, 2nd Edition. New York, Guilford, 2003

Richards D, Richardson T: Computer-based psychological treatments for depression: a systematic review and meta-analysis. Clin Psychol Rev 32(4):329–342, 2012 22466510

Ritterband LM, Thorndike FP, Gonder-Frederick LA, et al: Efficacy of an internet-based behavioral intervention for adults with insomnia. Arch Gen Psychiatry 66(7):692–698, 2009 19581560

Sharma MP, Andrade C: Behavioral interventions for insomnia: theory and practice. Indian J Psychiatry 54(4):359–366, 2012 23372241

Stanley B, Brown G, Brent DA, et al: Cognitive-behavioral therapy for suicide prevention (CBT-SP): treatment model, feasibility, and acceptability. J Am Acad Child Adolesc Psychiatry 48(10):1005–1013, 2009 19730273

Stanley B, Brown GK, Brenner LA, et al: Comparison of the safety planning intervention with follow-up vs usual care of suicidal patients treated in the emergency department. JAMA Psychiatry 75(9):894–900, 2018 29998307

Tarrier N, Beckett R, Harwood S, et al: A trial of two cognitive-behavioural methods of treating drug-resistant residual psychotic symptoms in schizophrenic patients: I. Outcome. Br J Psychiatry 162:524–532, 1993 8481745

Thase ME, Wright JH, Eells TD, et al: Improving the efficiency of psychotherapy for depression: computer-assisted versus standard CBT. Am J Psychiatry 175(3):242–250, 2018 28969439

Watkins JT, Rush AJ: Cognitive response test. Cognit Ther Res 7(5):125–126, 1983

White J, Freeman A: Cognitive-Behavioral Group Therapy for Specific Problems and Populations. Washington, DC, American Psychological Association, 2000

White KP, Nielson WR: Cognitive behavioral treatment of fibromyalgia syndrome: a followup assessment. J Rheumatol 22(4):717–721, 1995 7791170

Wright JH, McCray LW: Breaking Free From Depression: Pathways to Wellness. New York, Guilford, 2012

Wright JH, Mishkind M: Computer-assisted CBT and mobile apps for depression: assessment and integration into clinical care. Focus (Am Psychiatr Publ) 18(2):162–168, 2020 33162853

Wright JH, Salmon P, Wright AS, et al: Cognitive Therapy: A Multimedia Learning Program. Louisville, KY, MindStreet, 1995

Wright JH, Wright AS, Salmon P, et al: Development and initial testing of a multimedia program for computer-assisted cognitive therapy. Am J Psychother 56(1):76–86, 2002 11977785

Wright JH, Wright AS, Beck AT: Good Days Ahead: The Multimedia Program for Cognitive Therapy. Louisville, KY, MindStreet, 2004

Wright JH, Wright AS, Albano AM, et al: Computer-assisted cognitive therapy for depression: maintaining efficacy while reducing therapist time. Am J Psychiatry 162(6):1158–1164, 2005 15930065

Wright JH, Turkington D, Kingdon D, et al: Cognitive-Behavior Therapy for Severe Mental Illness: An Illustrated Guide. Washington, DC, American Psychiatric Publishing, 2009

Wright JH, Brown GK, Thase ME, et al: Learning Cognitive-Behavior Therapy: An Illustrated Guide, 2nd Edition. Arlington, VA, American Psychiatric Association Publishing, 2017

Wright JH, Beck AT, Thase ME: Cognitive-behavior therapy, in The American Psychiatric Association Publishing Textbook of Psychiatry, 7th Edition. Edited by Roberts LW. Washington DC, American Psychiatric Association Publishing, 2019a, pp 955–998

Wright JH, Mishkind M, Eells TD, et al: Computer-assisted cognitive-behavior therapy and mobile apps for depression and anxiety. Curr Psychiatry Rep 21(7):62, 2019b 31250242

Wright JH, Owen JJ, Richards D, et al: Computer-assisted cognitive-behavior therapy for depression: a systematic review and meta-analysis. J Clin Pschyiatry 80(2):18r12188, 2019c 30900849

Wright JH, Owen J, Eells TO, et al: Effect of computer-assisted cognitive behavior therapy vs usual care on depression among adults in primary care: a randomized clinical trial. JAMA Netw Open 5(2):e2146716, 2022 35142833

Wu JQ, Appleman ER, Salazar RD, et al: Cognitive behavioral therapy for insomnia comorbid with psychiatric and medical conditions: a meta-analysis. JAMA Intern Med 175(9):1461–1472, 2015 26147487

CHAPTER 9

Indications, Applications, and Efficacy of Individual Cognitive-Behavioral Therapy to Specific Psychiatric Disorders

Seamus Bhatt-Mackin, M.D.
Amanda M. McEpplan, Ph.D.
Keith S. Dobson, Ph.D.
Jean Cottraux, M.D., Ph.D.

Cognitive-behavioral therapy (CBT) is a psychotherapeutic approach grounded in science-based clinical research and practice (Hofmann et al. 2013). It is one of the most commonly used psychotherapeutic treatments of psychiatric disorders in adults (Leichsenring et al. 2006), is "the most actively researched system of psychotherapy over the past decade" (Prochaska and Norcross 2018, p. 257), and is widely used to develop psychotherapists in professional training programs (Dozois et al. 2019). CBT has been identified as an empirically supported therapy for most psychiatric disorders and many medical conditions with psychological components. In this chapter we review outcome research as applied to the major psychiatric disorders by focusing on meta-analyses of randomized controlled trials (RCTs). Limitations and knowledge gaps within the current empirical literature are discussed, along with suggestions for future research and applications.

Indications for Cognitive-Behavioral Therapy

The term *CBT* often refers to a variety of approaches that employ both cognitive and behavioral strategies. It refers to both standard cognitive therapy (CT) (cf. Beck et al. 1979) and an atheoretical combination of cognitive and behavioral therapies. Thus, in this chapter we consider all forms of CBT and CT in reviewing the indications, efficacy, and applications of CBT. CBT is a general model that can be applied to a wide variety of specific problems (see Chapter 8, "Techniques of Cognitive-Behavioral Therapy," for a description of CBT techniques). The efficacy of CBT has been studied in a broad range of psychiatric disorders and problems (Hofmann et al. 2012), including depression and dysthymia, bipolar disorder, anxiety disorders, personality disorders, substance use disorders, schizophrenia and other psychotic disorders, somatoform disorders, eating disorders, insomnia, anger and aggression, criminal behaviors, general distress, distress due to general medical conditions, chronic pain, and fatigue. CBT has also been studied as an adjunctive treatment in a wide variety of medical conditions and in direct comparison with psychotropic medications for a number of disorders. In addition, medications have been proposed to potentiate or inhibit the efficacy and effectiveness of CBT. Although CBT has also been adapted for and used with child, adolescent, and geriatric populations, in this chapter we focus on only those psychiatric disorders that have received the greatest attention in the literature in adult populations. Given the large number and wide range of disorders and problems to which CBT has been applied, the scope of this chapter does not allow for a comprehensive review.

Review Methodology

Because of the large volume of the literature on CBT, we focus our review on meta-analyses of RCTs in an attempt to aggregate the available data (cf. Kazdin 2002). RCTs are the most rigorous science-based evaluation of treatment outcome because they allow clinical researchers to control for confounding variables. This method increases confidence that treatment outcome is related to the study intervention. Without a control condition, covariant factors beyond the intervention under study can contribute to treatment outcome. An advantage of meta-analysis is that it takes into account the sample size and the magnitude of the effect size for the interventions compared in each study (Rosenthal 1998), although it does minimize the variable methodological details across studies.

We include three types of meta-analyses in this review. *Efficacy studies* examine the outcome of a treatment within an experimental setting (Kazdin 2002), and we include two types of efficacy studies. *Absolute efficacy* studies compare an active CBT treatment with a no-treatment alternative or standard care (also called *treatment as usual*). These trials establish that CBT has a clinical effect. *Relative efficacy* studies compare CBT with other interventions, which can be different psychotherapies or pharmacotherapy. Research on the role of common factors in psychotherapy outcomes (Wampold 2015) and how medications and psychotherapy can complement (Dunlop 2016) or inhibit (Guina et al. 2015) one another is ongoing, and these studies contribute to that work.

Last, *effectiveness studies* examine treatment outcomes in the real world (Kazdin 2002), with fewer control conditions to allow for greater external validity.

Applications of Cognitive-Behavioral Therapy

Mood Disorders

Unipolar Depression

Absolute efficacy. CBT for adult unipolar depression has been studied extensively. The first meta-analysis on CT for adult depression examined 28 studies and revealed strong evidence for the superiority of CT relative to a no-treatment or wait list control condition (Dobson 1989). In more recent meta-analytic work looking at CBT for adult depression (Cuijpers et al. 2013), 115 RCTs met inclusion criteria and strongly supported and sustained the finding that CBT is an efficacious treatment for adult depression, with an effect size in the high moderate range (Hedges' $g=0.71$, 95% CI 0.62–0.79).

Relative efficacy. Cuijpers et al. (2013) also looked at other comparisons. In 46 studies, CBT could be directly compared with other psychotherapies, and effect sizes ranged from −0.02 to 0.25; 20 studies were identified in which CBT was compared with pharmacotherapy, with effect sizes that ranged from −0.13 to 0.18, showing no significant overall difference between the different forms of treatment (CBT, other psychotherapy, pharmacotherapy) for adult unipolar depression.

Effectiveness. Atop this solid foundation of established efficacy, Hans and Hiller (2013) aggregated 34 CBT effectiveness studies on the treatment of adult unipolar depression. Their work showed large effect sizes on depressive severity in both completer (Cohen's $d=1.13$) and intention-to-treat ($d=1.06$) samples.

Bipolar Disorder

Bipolar disorder is a complex psychiatric condition characterized by persistent mood episodes minimally influenced by environmental cues (Miklowitz and Gitlen 2014) such that nagging depressive cognitions persist in the face of good news and expansive, optimistic cognitions persist in the face of trials and tribulations (Dodd et al. 2011). Treatment is complicated by the fact that it must address multiple acute pathological mood states (manic, hypomanic, depressive, mixed). Chiang et al. (2017) included 19 RCTs with a total of 716 patients and 668 control subjects in their meta-analysis of the efficacy of CBT for bipolar disorder (including bipolar I and bipolar II). Their study assessed four outcome measures (depression, mania, relapse rate, and psychosocial functioning), but conclusions were hampered by large heterogeneity in the analysis. Chatterton et al. (2017) completed a network meta-analysis of all psychosocial treatments used in concert with medication for bipolar disorder and found that psychoeducation plus CBT significantly reduced manic symptoms and increased global assessment of function. No intervention was associated with a significant reduction in depressive symptoms, and only interventions that involved family members affected relapse rates.

Summary: Mood Disorders

There is ample and strong evidence that CBT is an efficacious treatment for unipolar depression and that it is as efficacious as both other psychological treatments and pharmacotherapy. In addition, there is substantial evidence that CBT for depression has demonstrated effectiveness in real-world settings. Clinical research support has increased for the use of CBT as an adjunctive treatment for bipolar disorder in conjunction with pharmacotherapy and in conjunction with psychosocial interventions that involve the family system.

Anxiety Disorders

CBT has been evaluated as a treatment for a broad range of anxiety disorders and typically includes psychoeducation; cognitive restructuring; and exposure to the anxiety-provoking stimulus, situation, memory, or physiological experience (Barlow 2004). The study of these treatments has a 50-year history (Öst 2008) with a sustained track record demonstrating efficacy. Some meta-analytic studies have included all DSM-5 (American Psychiatric Association 2013) anxiety disorders in a single category (not following DSM-5 in recategorizing obsessive-compulsive disorder and PTSD outside the anxiety disorders section). For example, Carpenter et al. (2018) included 41 studies in which CBT was used to treat acute stress disorder, generalized anxiety disorder (GAD), obsessive-compulsive disorder (OCD), panic disorder, PTSD, or social anxiety disorder and found a moderate effect on target disorder symptoms ($g=0.56$) as compared with placebo control. They found variability across disorders, with small to moderate effect sizes for PTSD, social anxiety disorder, and panic disorder and large effect sizes for OCD, GAD, and acute stress disorder. Given this heterogeneity, we review each of these disorders in turn. We also treat OCD and PTSD separately because they have been removed from the anxiety disorders category.

Panic Disorder With or Without Agoraphobia

Absolute efficacy. Several meta-analytic reviews of the treatment outcome literature for panic disorder with or without agoraphobia were conducted in the past decade, although some meta-analyses have exclusively examined behavioral treatments. Oei et al. (1999) conducted both a qualitative and a quantitative review of the literature. They found that CBT was effective at reducing self-reported agoraphobic symptoms, and its clinical efficacy was substantially demonstrated with community norms. Long-term treatment effects were roughly equal to acute treatment effects, although follow-up duration was not reported. Pompoli et al. (2016) conducted a network meta-analysis with 54 studies across different theoretical orientations that showed well-replicated evidence in support of CBT for panic disorder.

Relative efficacy. Gould et al. (1995) conducted a standard meta-analysis comparing pharmacotherapy, CBT, their combination, and a control (no treatment, wait list, drug, or psychological placebo) for panic disorder with or without agoraphobia. All three types of active treatment were superior, at acute treatment, to the control condition. Mitte (2005) conducted a comprehensive meta-analysis of 124 studies involving pharmacotherapy and/or CBT psychotherapy for panic disorder and found that CBT was at least as effective as pharmacotherapy and, depending on the type of analysis, sometimes was even significantly more effective. The relationship between medications and CBT for panic disorder is different from that for some other disorders. Some medications (e.g., benzodiazepines) have been suggested to interfere with CBT psychotherapy (Otto et al. 2016). Other medications (e.g., D-cycloserine) initially described in a small study as improving the effectiveness of CBT psychotherapy (Ressler et al. 2004) likely have a more complex and differential effect (Hofmann 2014) than initially proposed.

Maximizing efficacy. Dismantling studies examine different parts of the treatment package to assess which components are involved with effective treatment. Pompoli and colleagues (2018) included 72 studies with 4,064 participants. Interoceptive exposure and a face-to-face setting were associated with better treatment efficacy and acceptability. Muscle relaxation and virtual reality exposure were associated with significantly lower efficacy. Finally, Heuzenroeder et al. (2004) showed CBT psychotherapy to be more cost-effective than pharmacotherapy.

Generalized Anxiety Disorder

Absolute efficacy. Gould et al. (1997b) compared CBT with no treatment and wait list, drug, or psychological placebo control groups. Short-term (less than or equal to 16 weeks) treatment outcome findings indicated that CBT is highly efficacious at reducing symptoms of anxiety and depression. No significant differences were found between group and individual therapy formats, and a longer duration of treatment was not associated with better outcomes. Gould et al. (1997b) also found some limited evidence for the long-term (minimum of 6 months) maintenance of treatment gains in terms of reduced anxiety symptoms.

The meta-analytic literature also supports the efficacy of CBT for GAD. Because of the obscure nature of external triggers for the anxiety associated with GAD, it has not been amenable to the same exposure methods that have been effective for the other anxiety disorders (Deacon and Abramowitz 2004). Research methods have become more nuanced over time, as exemplified by a meta-analysis of CBT for pathological worry among patients with GAD in which Covin et al. (2008) included 10 studies that used a specific, validated outcome measure (the Penn State Worry Questionnaire). They found a large effect size ($g=1.15$) when CBT was compared with a control group.

Relative efficacy. Gould et al. (1997b) found that CBT had superior outcomes to relaxation training with biofeedback. They also compared CBT with pharmacotherapy and found no differences between the two on measures of change in anxiety severity, but CBT was favored over pharmacotherapy on change in depressive symptoms. Cuijpers et al. (2014) reviewed all psychological treatments for GAD and found a moderate effect size in which 31 of the 41 papers reviewed included a CBT treatment arm. There were not sufficient other forms of treatment to make meaningful conclusions about relative efficacy in psychological treatment.

Social Anxiety Disorder (Social Phobia)

Absolute efficacy. Treatments for social anxiety disorder frequently include exposure, social skills training, cognitive restructuring, or a combination of these strategies (Abramowitz et al. 2005). Mayo-Wilson et al. (2014) published a systematic review and network meta-analysis of 101 trials with 13,164 participants across 41 interventions or control conditions with 17 different classes. Individual CBT was associated with a large effect size (standardized mean difference [SMD]=1.19) compared with wait list and a moderate effect size (SMD=0.56) compared with psychological placebo.

Relative efficacy. In the same study, Mayo-Wilson et al. (2014) demonstrated that CBT had a greater effect than psychodynamic psychotherapy, interpersonal psychotherapy, mindfulness, and supportive therapy. They concluded that CBT is the best intervention for the initial treatment of social anxiety disorder and that selective serotonin reuptake inhibitors (SSRIs) and serotonin-norepinephrine reuptake inhibitors should be offered to individuals who decline psychological interventions.

Specific Phobia

No meta-analysis is available in the literature for the treatment of specific phobia with CBT. However, a comprehensive systematic review by Choy et al. (2007) showed that in vivo exposure therapy is the most robust treatment for most of the specific phobia subtypes. However, there is evidence that specific phobias are not equally responsive across their subtypes and that CT is the most helpful in claustrophobia.

Summary: Anxiety Disorders

Strong empirical support exists for the use of CBT for panic disorder, GAD, and social anxiety disorder, and moderate support exists for its use in specific phobia. A recent meta-analysis of 69 randomized clinical trials (van Dis et al. 2020) demonstrated sustained improvement at 6 months and 12 months for patients treated with CBT for GAD, panic disorder, social anxiety disorder, specific phobia, PTSD, and OCD. High-quality treatment studies of longer duration are needed.

Obsessive-Compulsive Disorder

Absolute Efficacy

The efficacy of CBT for OCD has been studied extensively. Exposure and response prevention (ERP) is the most widely studied treatment technique for OCD (Abramowitz 1997). Although ERP is typically categorized as a behavioral procedure, it involves cognitive elements and overlapping procedures (Allen 2006). It is possible that CT and ERP use similar mechanisms of change (Abramowitz 1997).

In an early meta-analysis, Van Balkom et al. (1994) found that both CT and CBT were more effective than placebo therapy for self- and assessor-rated obsessive-compulsive symptoms and that treatment effects persisted at 6 and 12 months. In more recent work, Olatunji et al. (2013) included 16 studies in a meta-analysis with a very large effect size (g=1.39) in comparison with control conditions.

Relative Efficacy

Abramowitz (1997) found small and nonsignificant differences in treatment outcomes between CT and ERP. Whittal et al. (2005) also failed to find significant differences between ERP and CBT posttreatment and at 3 months in their randomized trial. They found that CBT resulted in a higher (but nonsignificant) percentage of recovered participants than ERP posttreatment and at 3 months. Cottraux et al. (2001) conducted an RCT comparing CT with intensive ERP. They found that although both groups improved significantly and the rate of response was similar in the two groups, CT demonstrated a greater effect at reducing depressive symptoms at posttest. Improvements were retained at 1-year follow-up without any between-group differences. The intent-to-treat analysis (Last Observation Carried Forward) found no between-group differences in obsessions, rituals, or depression. Kobak et al. (1998) performed a meta-analysis comparing CBT, pharmacotherapy (SSRIs), and their combination in the treatment of OCD. Although CBT was reported to be superior to SSRIs, this difference disappeared when the outcomes were controlled by the year of publication of the studies and the CBT methods that were used (see also Abramowitz 1997). These results suggest common mechanisms of action between the treatments. More recently, Foa et al. (2005) categorized ERP as a form of CBT in their RCT comparing CBT, pharmacotherapy, and their combination. They found that intensive CBT alone and CBT and clomipramine combined had comparable short-term effects and that both were more efficacious than clomipramine alone. In a meta-analysis of 37 RCT psychotherapeutic and pharmacological studies from 1993 to 2014, Öst et al. (2015) found that CBT was significantly better than medication ($g=0.55$) and that the combination of CBT and medication was not significantly better than CBT plus placebo.

PTSD

Absolute Efficacy

In the most recent *Guidelines for the Prevention and Treatment of Posttraumatic Stress Disorder* from the International Society for Traumatic Stress Studies (Bisson et al. 2020), CBT has been given the highest recommendation ("strong recommendation") when delivered in the form of cognitive processing therapy, CT, individual CBT with a trauma focus, or prolonged exposure. This position was developed after review and inclusion of 361 RCTs (see Bisson et al. 2019). In support of this position, Watts et al. (2013) found large effect sizes for CT ($g=1.63$) and exposure therapy ($g=1.08$) in their meta-analysis.

Relative Efficacy

Gerger et al. (2014) reviewed 66 RCTs to compare psychological interventions for adults with PTSD. No single intervention was consistently superior to other specific psychological interventions; however, a wide range in the robustness of evidence across the psychological interventions was found, with the most robust evidence for CBT and exposure therapy. Merz et al. (2019) compared the efficacy and acceptability of pharmacological, psychotherapeutic, and combination treatments in adults with PTSD in a network meta-analysis involving 12 RCTs. They found that the long-term benefits of psychotherapeutic and combined treatments were superior to pharmacological treatments across six randomized clinical trials that reported follow-up data. However, critiques of their methodology (Sonis and Cook 2020; Stein and Norman 2019; Zheng et al. 2020) pointed to the inclusion of studies of lower quality. More high-quality research is required.

Effectiveness

In addition to its effectiveness for single-event trauma in adult life (e.g., motor vehicle accidents), trauma-focused CBT has been shown to be effective for complex trauma such as that following armed conflict, forcible displacement, childhood sexual abuse, and domestic violence (Coventry et al. 2020).

Schizophrenia

CBT has been studied as an adjunctive treatment to pharmacotherapy and case management (routine care) for schizophrenia. Gould et al. (2001) conducted a meta-analysis of the effects of CT on decreasing psychotic symptoms (hallucinations and delusions) and modifying core dysfunctional beliefs in schizophrenia, schizoaffective disorder, or delusional disorder. They found large acute treatment effects for CT across seven controlled studies, and these effects were maintained, and even increased in some cases, over time. More recently, the impact of CBT was reviewed in meta-analyses that examined positive symptoms in medication-resistant psychosis (Burns et al. 2014), negative symptoms (Marder and Galderisi 2017), functioning, distress, and quality of life (Laws et al. 2018).

The *positive symptoms* of schizophrenia are treated primarily with antipsychotic medications. However, the effectiveness of these medications has been shown to be less than robust, even with second-generation antipsychotics (Lieberman et al. 2005). In those cases, adjunctive treatment with CBT was associated with a moderate effect size (g=0.47, 95% CI 0.35–0.70) in 12 RCTs. The effect was maintained at follow-up. In addition, Eichner and Berna (2016) reviewed 15 studies of *metacognitive training*, which is a form of treatment based on the principles of CBT that focuses in particular on problematic thinking styles that are associated with the development and maintenance of positive symptoms (Moritz et al. 2010). The meta-analysis showed a small to moderate effect (g=0.34, 95% CI 0.15–0.53) on positive symptoms, a small to moderate effect (g=0.41, 95% CI 0.07–0.74) on delusions, and a large effect (g=0.84, 95% CI 0.15–0.53) on the acceptance of the intervention.

CBT interventions have been developed to treat the *negative symptoms* of schizophrenia because of their key role in functional impairment (Marder and Galderisi 2017). However, in one meta-analysis (Velthorst et al. 2015), the pooled effect size across 30 trials from 1993 to 2013 showed a small effect size (g=0.093, 95% CI –0.028 to 0.214) that was not statistically significant (P=0.13). In a review of 36 RCTs (27 assessing functioning, 8 on distress, and 10 on quality of life), Laws et al. (2018) found that CBT for schizophrenia had a small therapeutic effect on functioning at the end of trial (g=0.25, 95% CI 0.14–0.33) that was not sustained at follow-up, a small effect on reducing distress (g=0.37, 95% CI 0.05–0.69), and no effect on quality of life.

Personality Disorders

The efficacy of CBT for personality disorders has not been widely studied, but borderline personality disorder (BPD) has been the most thoroughly investigated. Clinical research into cognitive-behavioral treatment of parasuicidal behaviors in patients with BPD led to the development of dialectical behavior therapy (Linehan 1993, 2015; see also Chapter 12, "Dialectical Behavior Therapy: Efficacy, Applications, and Adaptations").

Davidson et al. (2006) compared CBT plus treatment as usual (CBT+TAU) with TAU alone for BPD. They did not find significant differences between the two groups at 12–24 months in the outcome of scores on depression, trait anxiety, other psychiatric symptoms, interpersonal functioning, or quality of life. In addition, although all patients demonstrated gradual and sustained improvement, levels of distress and dysfunction remained relatively high over the course of the study (2 years). However, at 1 year the CBT+TAU group had greater improvement than the TAU group in symptom distress and at 2 years showed greater improvement in dysfunctional core beliefs and state anxiety. The mean number of suicidal acts over the course of the study was also significantly reduced for the CBT+TAU group. Although Davidson et al.'s (2006) findings were mixed, a smaller uncontrolled trial (Brown et al. 2004) found that CT for BPD was associated with significant and clinically important improvements on measures of suicide ideation, hopelessness, depression, number of borderline symptoms, and dysfunctional beliefs at the end of treatment and at 6-month follow-up.

Giesen-Bloo et al. (2006) compared the effectiveness of Young's schema-focused CT (SFCT; Young et al. 2003) with the psychodynamically based transference-focused psychotherapy in patients with BPD. They conducted a randomized two-group design in four general community mental health centers in the Netherlands over a 3-year period. Results revealed that significantly more SFCT patients recovered or showed reliable clinical improvements on the Borderline Personality Disorder Severity Index, in levels of general psychopathological dysfunction, and on quality-of-life measures. In addition, the dropout rate was higher for transference-focused psychotherapy than for SFCT. Schema therapy has been reviewed and described as an effective treatment for avoidant, dependent, and obsessive-compulsive personality disorders; however, no meta-analysis is available to include in this review. In a multicenter RCT of the clinical effectiveness of schema therapy for personality disorders, Bamelis et al. (2014) found that a significantly greater proportion of patients recovered in schema therapy compared with TAU and clarification-oriented psychotherapy.

CBT has been applied to antisocial personality disorder with some limited effects (Gibbon et al. 2020). Svartberg et al. (2004) randomly assigned patients with a diagnosis of one or more Cluster C personality disorders to either short-term dynamic psychotherapy or CT. Both psychotherapies demonstrated significant patient improvements on all measures during treatment, and these improvements were maintained after treatment. There were no significant differences between groups on any of the measures during any of the time periods. However, patients who received dynamic psychotherapy showed significant changes in symptom distress posttreatment, but those who received CT did not.

Limitations, Knowledge Gaps, and Future Directions

In this chapter we relied on meta-analyses of RCTs to report on what is known about the efficacy and effectiveness of CBT as applied across psychiatric disorders. Well-conducted RCT studies employ an elegant research design that allows the researcher to make reasonable conclusions about the treatment(s) under investigation. Nonetheless, this form of research does have limitations. For example, the generalizability of RCT results to routine clinical practice is sometimes limited because of the level of control exerted over the experimental situation (Leichsenring et al. 2006). Another concern about efficacy research is researcher allegiance, or the tendency of the authors of a comparative treatment study to prefer one treatment over another, introducing bias in favor of the preferred treatment (Butler et al. 2006).

In addition, meta-analysis has itself been critiqued as a method because the outcome measures employed across different studies often differ. The choice of outcome measure (e.g., self-report vs. clinician rated) can bias the relative strength of a treatment effect. Thus, the total effect size for a particular treatment calculated by meta-analysis will be biased by the inclusion of various dependent measures (Gould et al. 1997a).

With the expansion of research work, research trial and meta-analytic methods continue to evolve and improve. Clinical researchers continue to make efforts in the following additional identified areas: publication bias, control conditions, input and output, diverse populations, treatment labeling, short- and long-term outcomes, combined treatments, and live and digital delivery.

Publication Bias

Publication bias is present in a scientific field when the publication of studies depends on the direction and statistical significance of the results (van Aert et al. 2019). Publication bias can be addressed through trial registration to decrease selective outcome reporting. This practice is not yet routine in clinical research (Bradley et al. 2017).

Control Conditions

The choice of control condition in a given psychotherapy research trial will affect the results and so is an important consideration in trial design, in subsequent interpretation, and in the use of studies to construct clinical practice guidelines (Gold et al. 2017). The authors of meta-analyses must also decide whether to include all relevant studies across all control conditions or to restrict inclusion to selected control conditions (no treatment or wait list, treatment as usual, supportive or nondirective treatment, or active comparison treatment). This issue is also complex when comparing psychotherapy and pharmacotherapy.

Input and Output

The quality of a meta-analysis is dependent on both the quality of the included RCTs and the methodology of that meta-analytic review. As noted in the response to Merz et al.'s (2019) study comparing psychotherapy and pharmacotherapy for PTSD, disagreement can arise about what constitutes sufficient quality to include in a study, including whether to take a comprehensive or selective approach, the methodology of the meta-analysis, and, ultimately, whether conclusions are warranted (Sonis and Cook 2020; Stein and Norman 2019; Zheng et al. 2020).

Diverse Populations

As described by Henrich et al. (2010), behavioral scientists regularly make general claims about human psychology, behavior, and treatment based on work conducted entirely on WEIRD (Western, educated, industrialized, rich, and democratic) populations. A weakness of the current review chapter is that the meta-analytic reviews obscure differences among subsets of the population and can be composed of nonrepresentative samples.

Treatment Labeling

The issue of treatment labeling stands out as a significant concern in the literature. Behavioral therapies are sometimes classified as *behavioral* and sometimes as *cognitive-behavioral*, even when they employ highly similar treatment elements, confounding comparisons among studies. Moreover, the distinctions among variants of CBT or other kinds of psychotherapy may be blurred in some trials.

Short- and Long-Term Outcomes

The long-term evidence base for the majority of psychiatric disorders represents another knowledge gap in the literature on the efficacy of CBT. Many studies do not assess long-term outcomes at all, some provide only relatively short-term outcomes, and others do not explicitly report the time points at which follow-ups were conducted. Difficulties in conducting long-term outcome assessments include ethical restrictions on maintaining participants in control conditions for extended periods of time. Most studies that incorporate waitlist control subjects provide treatment to control participants after a period of time, thereby obviating comparative assessment of long-term outcomes between treatment groups and control subjects. Further research comparing the long-term efficacy of different active treatments is indicated.

Combined Treatments

The combination and sequencing of medications and psychotherapy remain an understudied and challenging area. This includes established psychiatric medications (SSRIs, antipsychotics, benzodiazepines) and psychedelic psychotropics (3,4-methylenedioxymethamphetamine [MDMA], psilocybin) that have seen a resurgence in study. Examples of RCTs of psychotropics include MDMA-assisted cognitive-behavioral conjoint psychotherapy for PTSD (Wagner et al. 2019) and psilocybin-assisted CBT for smoking cessation (Johnson et al. 2017). The amount and quality of this research do not yet warrant a meta-analytic review; however, it is a potential future direction for the field.

Live and Digital Delivery

In the setting of the worldwide coronavirus SARS-CoV-2 disease (COVID-19) pandemic, providing psychotherapy online through videoconferencing has become more common, in some cases despite the interest and attitudes of clinicians and therapists (Békés and Aafjes-van Doorn 2020), out of necessity. New strategies and techniques in the areas of boundary maintenance (Drum and Littleton 2014), working alliance (Norwood et al. 2018), telepresence (Hilty et al. 2019), and other areas have been developed. As in other areas of psychotherapy practice, internet-delivered CBT is among the best-studied digital mental health interventions (Titov et al. 2018). This method of delivery will likely increase in the future, and continued research should guide best practices.

Summary and Conclusions

The empirical literature on CBT has continued to expand, and new developments have led to the use of CBT in an even wider variety of contexts. Broadly speaking,

CBT is an efficacious treatment across a range of psychiatric disorders. Findings differ within and among disorders for the efficacy of CBT compared with other psychotherapies and pharmacotherapy. The evidence base for the efficacy of CBT is greatest in the treatment of unipolar depression. The literature indicates that CBT is highly superior to control conditions in the treatment of anxiety disorders, and it is roughly comparable with behavior therapy. However, a particular source of confusion in the literature is that interventions involving the same procedures are sometimes referred to as *behavioral* and sometimes as *cognitive-behavioral* (Abramowitz et al. 2005). It is difficult to make conclusive statements about the relative efficacy of CBT compared with pharmacotherapy in the treatment of anxiety disorders and long-term outcomes in general. Further research in these domains is needed.

In addition to being highly efficacious in the treatment of a wide assortment of psychiatric disorders, CBT has numerous other strengths. For example, CBT has lower dropout rates than pharmacotherapy in the treatment of panic disorder (Gould et al. 1995) and bulimia nervosa (Whittal et al. 1999) and lower dropout rates than exposure and response prevention in the treatment of OCD (Abramowitz et al. 2005). Compared with exposure-based interventions, CBT is also perceived as being less aversive or intrusive to individuals being treated for specific phobias. Thus, research indicates that CBT is both a highly efficacious and an acceptable treatment choice. Although the research base for CBT is quite extensive, limitations and knowledge gaps need to be addressed. In summary, a considerable and growing body of evidence generally supports the continued use of CBT as a treatment for a wide variety of disorders.

Key Points

- CBT is one of the most common psychotherapies practiced and the most common psychotherapy in training and can be applied to a wide variety of psychiatric disorders and problems.
- CBT for adult unipolar depression clearly is highly efficacious and effective, and as an adjunctive treatment to pharmacotherapy in bipolar disorder, CBT can reduce relapse rates in the short term and can improve symptoms acutely and longer term.
- CBT is highly superior to control conditions and roughly comparable with behavior therapy for the treatment of anxiety disorders, has a large effect size in the treatment of OCD, and is significantly more efficacious than medications for OCD. CBT has a large effect size in treating PTSD, and some data suggest its effect is comparable to or larger than the effect of medications.
- CBT for schizophrenia as an adjunct to medication has demonstrated small to moderate effects on positive symptoms; small transient effects on negative symptoms; and no sustained effect on functioning, distress, and quality of life.
- CBT is the most researched treatment for personality disorders and has moderate to strong support. Schema therapy also has empirical support.

Recommended Readings

Beck AT: The current state of cognitive therapy: a 40-year retrospective. Arch Gen Psychiatry 62(9):953–959, 2005 16143727

Chambless DL, Ollendick TH: Empirically supported psychological interventions: controversies and evidence. Annu Rev Psychol 52:685–716, 2001 11148322

Dobson KS, Dozois DJA (eds): Handbook of Cognitive-Behavioral Therapies, 4th Edition. New York, Guilford, 2019

Hofmann SG, Asnaani A, Vonk IJ, et al: The efficacy of cognitive behavioral therapy: a review of meta-analyses. Cognit Ther Res 36(5):427–440, 2012 23459093

Roth A, Fonagy P (eds): What Works for Whom? A Critical Review of Psychotherapy Research, 2nd Edition. New York, Guilford, 2005

References

Abramowitz JS: Effectiveness of psychological and pharmacological treatments for obsessive-compulsive disorder: a quantitative review. J Consult Clin Psychol 65(1):44–52, 1997 9103733

Abramowitz JS, Taylor S, McKay D: Potentials and limitations of cognitive treatments for obsessive-compulsive disorder. Cogn Behav Ther 34(3):140–147, 2005 16195053

Allen A: Cognitive-behavior therapy and other psychosocial interventions in the treatment of obsessive-compulsive disorder. Psychiatr Ann 36(7):474–479, 2006

American Psychiatric Association: Diagnostic and Statistical Manual of Mental Disorders, 5th Edition. Arlington, VA, American Psychiatric Association, 2013

Bamelis LL, Evers SM, Spinhoven P, et al: Results of a multicenter randomized controlled trial of the clinical effectiveness of schema therapy for personality disorders. Am J Psychiatry 171(3):305–322, 2014 24322378

Barlow DH: Psychological treatments. Am Psychol 59(9):869–878, 2004 15584821

Beck AT, Rush AJ, Shaw BF, et al: Cognitive Therapy of Depression. New York, Guilford, 1979

Békés V, Aafjes-van Doorn K: Psychotherapists' attitudes toward online therapy during the COVID-19 pandemic. J Psychother Integration 30(2):238–247, 2020

Bisson JI, Berliner L, Cloitre M, et al: The International Society for Traumatic Stress Studies new guidelines for the prevention and treatment of posttraumatic stress disorder: methodology and development process. J Trauma Stress 32(4):475–483, 2019 31283056

Bisson JI, Lewis C, Roberts N: ISTSS PTSD Prevention and Treatment Guidelines: recommendations, in Effective Treatments for PTSD: Practice Guidelines From the International Society for Traumatic Stress Studies. Edited by Forbes D, Bisson JI, Monson CM, Berliner L. New York, Guilford, 2020, pp 109–114

Bradley HA, Rucklidge JJ, Mulder RT: A systematic review of trial registration and selective outcome reporting in psychotherapy randomized controlled trials. Acta Psychiatr Scand 135(1):65–77, 2017 27690210

Brown GK, Newman CF, Charlesworth SE, et al: An open clinical trial of cognitive therapy for borderline personality disorder. J Pers Disord 18(3):257–271, 2004 15237046

Burns AM, Erickson DH, Brenner CA: Cognitive-behavioral therapy for medication-resistant psychosis: a meta-analytic review. Psychiatr Serv 65(7):874–880, 2014 24686725

Butler AC, Chapman JE, Forman EM, et al: The empirical status of cognitive-behavioral therapy: a review of meta-analyses. Clin Psychol Rev 26(1):17–31, 2006 16199119

Carpenter JK, Andrews LA, Witcraft SM, et al: Cognitive behavioral therapy for anxiety and related disorders: a meta-analysis of randomized placebo-controlled trials. Depress Anxiety 35(6):502–514, 2018 29451967

Chatterton ML, Stockings E, Berk M, et al: Psychosocial therapies for the adjunctive treatment of bipolar disorder in adults: network meta-analysis. Br J Psychiatry 210(5):333–341, 2017 28209591

Chiang KJ, Tsai JC, Liu D, et al: Efficacy of cognitive-behavioral therapy in patients with bipolar disorder: a meta-analysis of randomized controlled trials. PLoS One 12(5):e0176849, 2017 28472082

Choy Y, Fyer AJ, Lipsitz JD: Treatment of specific phobia in adults. Clin Psychol Rev 27(3):266–286, 2007 17112646

Cottraux J, Note I, Yao SN, et al: A randomized controlled trial of cognitive therapy versus intensive behavior therapy in obsessive compulsive disorder. Psychother Psychosom 70(6):288–297, 2001 11598428

Coventry PA, Meader N, Melton H, et al: Psychological and pharmacological interventions for posttraumatic stress disorder and comorbid mental health problems following complex traumatic events: systematic review and component network meta-analysis. PLoS Med 17(8):e1003262, 2020 32813696

Covin R, Ouimet AJ, Seeds PM, Dozois DJ: A meta-analysis of CBT for pathological worry among clients with GAD. J Anxiety Disord 22(1):108–116, 2008 17321717

Cuijpers P, Berking M, Andersson G, et al: A meta-analysis of cognitive-behavioural therapy for adult depression, alone and in comparison with other treatments. Can J Psychiatry 58(7):376–385, 2013 23870719

Cuijpers P, Sijbrandij M, Koole S, et al: Psychological treatment of generalized anxiety disorder: a meta-analysis. Clin Psychol Rev 34(2):130–140, 2014 24487344

Davidson K, Norrie J, Tyrer P, et al: The effectiveness of cognitive behavior therapy for borderline personality disorder: results from the Borderline Personality Disorder Study of Cognitive therapy (BOSCOT) trial. J Pers Disord 20(5):450–465, 2006 17032158

Deacon BJ, Abramowitz JS: Cognitive and behavioral treatments for anxiety disorders: a review of meta-analytic findings. J Clin Psychol 60(4):429–441, 2004 15022272

Dobson KS: A meta-analysis of the efficacy of cognitive therapy for depression. J Consult Clin Psychol 57(3):414–419, 1989 2738214

Dodd AL, Mansell W, Morrison AP, et al: Extreme appraisals of internal states and bipolar symptoms: the Hypomanic Attitudes and Positive Predictions Inventory. Psychol Assess 23(3):635–645, 2011 21500923

Dozois DJA, Dobson KS, Rnic K: Historical and philosophical bases of the cognitive-behavioral therapies, in Handbook of Cognitive-Behavioral Therapies, 4th Edition. Edited by Dobson KS, Dozois DJA. New York, Guilford, 2019, pp 3–31

Drum KB, Littleton HL: Therapeutic boundaries in telepsychology: unique issues and best practice recommendations. Prof Psychol Res Pr 45(5):309–315, 2014 25414540

Dunlop BW: Evidence-based applications of combination psychotherapy and pharmacotherapy for depression. Focus Am Psychiatr Publ 14(2):156–173, 2016 31975799

Eichner C, Berna F: Acceptance and efficacy of metacognitive training (MCT) on positive symptoms and delusions in patients with schizophrenia: a meta-analysis taking into account important moderators. Schizophr Bull 42(4):952–962, 2016 26748396

Foa EB, Liebowitz MR, Kozak MJ, et al: Randomized, placebo-controlled trial of exposure and ritual prevention, clomipramine, and their combination in the treatment of obsessive-compulsive disorder. Am J Psychiatry 162(1):151–161, 2005 15625214

Gerger H, Munder T, Gemperli A, et al: Integrating fragmented evidence by network meta-analysis: relative effectiveness of psychological interventions for adults with post-traumatic stress disorder. Psychol Med 44(15):3151–3164, 2014 25066766

Gibbon S, Khalifa NR, Cheung NH, et al: Psychological interventions for antisocial personality disorder. Cochrane Database Syst Rev 9(9):CD007668, 2020 32880104

Giesen-Bloo J, van Dyck R, Spinhoven P, et al: Outpatient psychotherapy for borderline personality disorder: randomized trial of schema-focused therapy vs transference-focused psychotherapy. Arch Gen Psychiatry 63(6):649–658, 2006 16754838

Gold SM, Enck P, Hasselmann H, et al: Control conditions for randomised trials of behavioural interventions in psychiatry: a decision framework. Lancet Psychiatry 4(9):725–732, 2017 28396067

Gould RA, Otto MW, Pollack MH: A meta-analysis of treatment outcome for panic disorder. Clin Psychol Rev 15(8):819–844, 1995

Gould RA, Buckminster S, Pollack MH, et al: Cognitive-behavioral and pharmacological treatment for social phobia: a meta-analysis. Clin Psychol Sci Pract 4:291–306, 1997a

Gould RA, Otto MW, Pollack MH, et al: Cognitive behavioral and pharmacological treatment of generalized anxiety disorder: a preliminary meta-analysis. Behav Ther 28:285–305, 1997b

Gould RA, Mueser KT, Bolton E, et al: Cognitive therapy for psychosis in schizophrenia: an effect size analysis. Schizophr Res 48(2–3):335–342, 2001 11295385

Guina J, Rossetter SR, DeRhodes BJ, et al: Benzodiazepines for PTSD: a systematic review and meta-analysis. J Psychiatr Pract 21(4):281–303, 2015 26164054

Hans E, Hiller W: Effectiveness of and dropout from outpatient cognitive behavioral therapy for adult unipolar depression: a meta-analysis of nonrandomized effectiveness studies. J Consult Clin Psychol 81(1):75–88, 2013 23379264

Henrich J, Heine SJ, Norenzayan A: The weirdest people in the world? Behav Brain Sci 33(2–3):61–83, discussion 83–135, 2010 20550733

Heuzenroeder L, Donnelly M, Haby MM, et al: Cost-effectiveness of psychological and pharmacological interventions for generalized anxiety disorder and panic disorder. Aust N Z J Psychiatry 38(8):602–612, 2004 15298582

Hilty D, Randhawa K, Maheu M, et al: Therapeutic relationship of telepsychiatry and telebehavioral health: ideas from research on telepresence, virtual reality and augmented reality. Psychol Cogn Sci 5:14–29, 2019

Hofmann SG: D-cycloserine for treating anxiety disorders: making good exposures better and bad exposures worse. Depress Anxiety 31(3):175–177, 2014 24677604

Hofmann SG, Asnaani A, Vonk IJ, et al: The efficacy of cognitive behavioral therapy: a review of meta-analyses. Cognit Ther Res 36(5):427–440, 2012 23459093

Hofmann SG, Asmundson GJ, Beck AT: The science of cognitive therapy. Behav Ther 44(2):199–212, 2013 23611069

Johnson MW, Garcia-Romeu A, Griffiths RR: Long-term follow-up of psilocybin-facilitated smoking cessation. Am J Drug Alcohol Abuse 43(1):55–60, 2017 27441452

Kazdin AE: Research Design in Clinical Psychology, 4th Edition. New York, Allyn & Bacon, 2002

Kobak KA, Greist JH, Jefferson JW, et al: Behavioral versus pharmacological treatments of obsessive compulsive disorder: a meta-analysis. Psychopharmacology (Berl) 136(3):205–216, 1998 9566805

Laws KR, Darlington N, Kondel TK, et al: Cognitive behavioural therapy for schizophrenia—outcomes for functioning, distress and quality of life: a meta-analysis. BMC Psychol 6(1):32, 2018

Leichsenring F, Hiller W, Weissberg M, et al: Cognitive-behavioral therapy and psychodynamic psychotherapy: techniques, efficacy, and indications. Am J Psychother 60(3):233–259, 2006 17066756

Lieberman JA, Stroup TS, McEvoy JP, et al: Effectiveness of antipsychotic drugs in patients with chronic schizophrenia. N Engl J Med 353(12):1209–1223, 2005 16172203

Linehan MM: Cognitive-Behavioral Treatment of Borderline Personality Disorder. New York, Guilford, 1993

Linehan MM: DBT Skills Training Manual, 2nd Edition, New York, Guilford, 2015

Marder SR, Galderisi S: The current conceptualization of negative symptoms in schizophrenia. World Psychiatry 16(1):14–24, 2017 28127915

Mayo-Wilson E, Dias S, Mavranezouli I, et al: Psychological and pharmacological interventions for social anxiety disorder in adults: a systematic review and network meta-analysis. Lancet Psychiatry 1(5):368–376, 2014 26361000

Merz J, Schwarzer G, Gerger H: Comparative efficacy and acceptability of pharmacological, psychotherapeutic, and combination treatments in adults with posttraumatic stress disorder: a network meta-analysis. JAMA Psychiatry 76(9):904–913, 2019 31188399

Miklowitz DJ, Gitlen MJ: Clinician's Guide to Bipolar Disorder: Integrating Pharmacology and Psychotherapy. New York, Guilford, 2014

Mitte K: A meta-analysis of the efficacy of psycho- and pharmacotherapy in panic disorder with and without agoraphobia. J Affect Disord 88(1):27–45, 2005 16005982

Moritz S, Vitzthum F, Randjbar S, et al: Detecting and defusing cognitive traps: metacognitive intervention in schizophrenia. Curr Opin Psychiatry 23(6):561–569, 2010 20683332

Norwood C, Moghaddam NG, Malins S, et al: Working alliance and outcome effectiveness in videoconferencing psychotherapy: a systematic review and noninferiority meta-analysis. Clin Psychol Psychother 25(6):797–808, 2018 30014606

Oei TPS, Llamas M, Devilly GJ: The efficacy and cognitive processes of cognitive behaviour therapy in the treatment of panic disorder with agoraphobia. Behav Cogn Psychother 27:63–88, 1999

Olatunji BO, Davis ML, Powers MB, et al: Cognitive-behavioral therapy for obsessive-compulsive disorder: a meta-analysis of treatment outcome and moderators. J Psychiatr Res 47(1):33–41, 2013 22999486

Öst LG: Cognitive behavior therapy for anxiety disorders: 40 years of progress. Nord J Psychiatry 62 (suppl 47):5–10, 2008 18752112

Öst LG, Havnen A, Hansen B, et al: Cognitive behavioral treatments of obsessive-compulsive disorder: a systematic review and meta-analysis of studies published 1993–2014. Clin Psychol Rev 40:156–169, 2015 26117062

Otto MW, Pollack MH, Dowd SM, et al: Randomized trial of D-cylcoserine enhancement of cognitive-behavioral therapy for panic disorder. Depress Anxiety 33(8):737–745, 2016 27315514

Pompoli A, Furukawa TA, Imai H, et al: Psychological therapies for panic disorder with or without agoraphobia in adults: a network meta-analysis. Cochrane Database Syst Rev 4(4):CD011004, 2016 27071857

Pompoli A, Furukawa TA, Efthimiou O, et al: Dismantling cognitive-behaviour therapy for panic disorder: a systematic review and component network meta-analysis. Psychol Med 48(12):1945–1953, 2018 29368665

Prochaska JO, Norcross JC: Systems of Psychotherapy: A Transtheoretical Analysis, 9th Edition. Belmont, CA, Brooks/Cole, 2018

Ressler KJ, Rothbaum BO, Tannenbaum L, et al: Cognitive enhancers as adjuncts to psychotherapy: use of D-cycloserine in phobic individuals to facilitate extinction of fear. Arch Gen Psychiatry 61(11):1136–1144, 2004 15520361

Rosenthal R: Meta-analysis: concepts, corollaries and controversies, in Advances in Psychological Science, Vol 1: Social, Personal and Cultural Aspects. Edited by Adair J, Belanger D, Dion KL. Hove, UK, Psychology Press, 1998, pp 371–384

Sonis J, Cook JM: Concerns regarding a meta-analysis comparing psychotherapy with medications for posttraumatic stress disorder. JAMA Psychiatry 77(2):214–215, 2020 31577331

Stein MB, Norman SB: When does meta-analysis of a network not work? Fishing for answers. JAMA Psychiatry 76(9):885–886, 2019 31188403

Svartberg M, Stiles TC, Seltzer MH: Randomized, controlled trial of the effectiveness of short-term dynamic psychotherapy and cognitive therapy for Cluster C personality disorders. Am J Psychiatry 161(5):810–817, 2004 15121645

Titov N, Dear B, Nielssen O, et al: ICBT in routine care: a descriptive analysis of successful clinics in five countries. Internet Interv 13:108–115, 2018 30206525

van Aert RCM, Wicherts JM, van Assen MALM: Publication bias examined in meta-analyses from psychology and medicine: a meta-meta-analysis. PLoS One 14(4):e0215052, 2019 30978228

Van Balkom AJLM, van Oppen P, Vermeulen AWA, et al: A meta-analysis on the treatment of obsessive-compulsive disorder: a comparison of antidepressants, behavior, and cognitive therapy. Clin Psychol Rev 14:359–381, 1994

van Dis EAM, van Veen SC, Hagenaars MA, et al: Long-term outcomes of cognitive behavioral therapy for anxiety-related disorders: a systematic review and meta-analysis. JAMA Psychiatry 77(3):265–273, 2020 31758858

Velthorst E, Koeter M, van der Gaag M, et al: Adapted cognitive-behavioural therapy required for targeting negative symptoms in schizophrenia: meta-analysis and meta-regression. Psychol Med 45(3):453–465, 2015 24993642

Wagner AC, Mithoefer MC, Mithoefer AT, et al: Combining cognitive-behavioral conjoint therapy for PTSD with 3,4-methylenedioxymethamphetamine (MDMA): a case example. J Psychoactive Drugs 51(2):166–173, 2019 30890035

Wampold BE: How important are the common factors in psychotherapy? An update. World Psychiatry 14(3):270–277, 2015 26407772

Watts BV, Schnurr PP, Mayo L, et al: Meta-analysis of the efficacy of treatments for posttraumatic stress disorder. J Clin Psychiatry 74(6):e541–e550, 2013 23842024

Whittal ML, Agras WS, Gould RA: Bulimia nervosa: a meta-analysis of psychosocial and pharmacological treatments. Behavior Therapy 30(1):117–135, 1999

Whittal ML, Thordarson DS, McLean PD: Treatment of obsessive-compulsive disorder: cognitive behavior therapy vs. exposure and response prevention. Behav Res Ther 43(12):1559–1576, 2005 15913543

Young J, Klosko J, Weishaar M: Schema Therapy: A Practitioner's Guide. New York, Guilford, 2003

Zheng W, Qi H, Xiang YT: Concerns regarding a meta-analysis comparing psychotherapy with medications for posttraumatic stress disorder. JAMA Psychiatry 77(2):215–216, 2020 31577338

PART III

Dialectical Behavior Therapy

Section Editor: Shelley McMain, Ph.D., C.Psych.

Dialectical behavior therapy (DBT) is a broad-based approach that integrates cognitive-behavioral therapy with acceptance-based approaches. Dialectical philosophy informs the practice of treatment and its contradictory synthesis of acceptance and change strategies. Marsha Linehan, the founder of DBT, originally designed the approach as an outpatient treatment to address the unique needs of chronically suicidal people diagnosed with borderline personality disorder. Over the past three decades DBT has been disseminated widely across a diverse range of health care contexts and adapted to a range of clinical populations characterized by severe and complex problems and problems of emotional dysregulation. Knowledge of DBT is important and timely given its appeal and effectiveness with complex and severe clinical populations.

DBT has a robust empirical base. Trained as a behaviorist, Linehan is a fierce advocate of empiricism and has done an enormous service in helping to establish a treatment informed by the science of behavior and behavior change. Through the establishment of an annual international DBT research meeting, she inspired and supported a cadre of dedicated researchers who helped contribute to the accumulation of numerous studies supporting the efficacy of DBT across a range of psychiatric disorders. The empirical base of DBT continues to evolve rapidly, with a growing number of well-controlled randomized trials and replication studies across diverse clinical populations and settings. Growing evidence supporting the effectiveness of DBT with a range of complex clinical presentations (e.g., borderline personality disorder, complex PTSD, self-harming adolescents) has contributed to increased optimism about the prognoses of many disorders that were previously considered treatment refractory.

This section on DBT includes three chapters that provide a concise and comprehensive summary of a substantial body of research findings, the theoretical foundation of the therapy, and a description and illustration of DBT in clinical practice. In Chapter 10, "Theory in Dialectical Behavior Therapy," Alexander Chapman and Erin Kaufman trace the theoretical foundations of DBT and explain key concepts emphasizing DBT's biosocial theory and the centrality of emotional dsysregulation. In Chapter 11, "Techniques of Dialectical Behavior Therapy," Charles Swenson describes and illustrates the practice of DBT, emphasizing its structure and flexibility, use of cognitive-behavioral strategies, validation, and dialectical strategies. He illustrates how specific principles guide interventions. Finally, in Chapter 12, "Dialectical Behavior Therapy: Efficacy, Applications, and Adaptations," Anne Sonley, Tali Boritz, and Shelley McMain review and critique the empirical support for effectiveness of DBT for borderline personality disorder, substance use disorders, eating disorders, PTSD, mood disorders, and ADHD as well as emerging evidence with special populations.

CHAPTER 10

Theory in Dialectical Behavior Therapy

Alexander L. Chapman, Ph.D., R.Psych.
Erin A. Kaufman, Ph.D.

Case Vignette

Miranda arrives 15 minutes late for her therapy session, smelling of alcohol and appearing disheveled. She begins sobbing, describes a terrible fight with her partner, exclaims she has no place to live and has been couch surfing for the past week or so, and collapses on the sofa. She hands the therapist her crumpled diary card (a weekly self-monitoring form used in dialectical behavior therapy [DBT]). It indicates she attempted suicide via overdose 5 days ago, and her current urges to quit therapy are 4 out of 5 (on a scale where 0=no urges and 5=highest possible urges). With her head in her hands, Miranda says that treatment isn't working and she wants to quit. When the therapist asks her questions about what has been happening, Miranda shakes her head and says, "I don't know."

Treating persons with severe emotional dysregulation can be a turbulent ride. Individual clients and individual sessions vary greatly. The therapist often must juggle so many urgent priorities that it is hard to know where to begin or how to proceed. Moreover, clients and therapists alike often get in the way of effective therapy. In the case vignette, Miranda's arriving intoxicated and having strong urges to quit therapy reflect what we call *therapy-interfering behaviors*. Somehow, the therapist must deftly juggle various treatment targets and goals, move therapy along consistently, and help clients learn how to build lives they experience as worth living.

When navigating the often rocky terrain of therapy with clients who have complex mental health concerns (e.g., co-occurring psychopathology and severe emotional dsyregulation), a coherent theoretical framework is an invaluable guide. The therapist must flexibly respond to challenges as they arise, and the theoretical model acts as a North Star, keeping the work on course.

The framework underlying DBT can be conceptualized on a hierarchy, with different levels of theory going from more general to more specific (Figure 10–1). At the broadest level, DBT includes assumptions about the nature of reality, informed by Zen practice and dialectical theory. Miranda's therapist can use the wisdom of Zen practice to accept and validate her behaviors, thoughts, and feelings as they are in the moment and help her accept them as well. At the same time, dialectical theory proposes that reality is constantly changing and encourages the therapist to balance acceptance and validation with essential change-based strategies, coping skills, and problem-solving. Both acceptance and change are needed to help Miranda reduce her emotional dysregulation, engage in therapy effectively, and improve her life.

The next level of theoretical influence on DBT consists of foundational behavioral principles that help us understand, identify, and change factors that cause and maintain behavior. From this perspective, all behavior is understandable, often serves important purposes or functions, and must be understood in view of contextual influences, the person's traits and learning history, and the transaction of the individual with the environment. In the case vignette, the therapist might try to determine the antecedents and reinforcing consequences of Miranda's recent suicide attempt and understand the context and function of her statement that she wants to quit therapy. The DBT therapist would use behavioral assessment strategies to help develop a useful conceptualization of the problems Miranda is trying to solve by attempting suicide or quitting therapy. The therapist and Miranda can then identify interventions stemming from this conceptualization and help Miranda change her behavior and work toward important goals.

Finally, the most specific level of theory informing DBT practice draws on our understanding of factors contributing to the development and maintenance of severe emotional dysregulation and associated concerns (e.g., borderline personality disorder [BPD], self-inflicted injury [SII], suicidality). The biosocial developmental theory (Crowell et al. 2009, 2014b; Linehan 1993a) suggests that emotional dysregulation plays a critical role in Miranda's difficulties. Resulting interventions will aim to help her understand and effectively regulate emotions that are difficult to tolerate or that interfere with her goals. Miranda and her therapist will apply these strategies both in session (e.g., when she is sobbing and nonresponsive) and in Miranda's daily life (e.g., through phone coaching when she is dealing with interpersonal conflict).

In this chapter, we describe and discuss key theoretical underpinnings of DBT. We begin with a brief history of DBT's development. This serves to provide context for how treatment aims were created and how dialectics, Zen practice, behaviorism, and the biosocial theory became theoretical pillars of DBT. Subsequently, we describe each of these areas of DBT theory and how they translate into application.

Brief History of DBT

Marsha Linehan's lived experiences with severe mental illness informed the creation of DBT (Linehan 2020). In her late adolescence and young adulthood, while suffering from severe mental health problems, Linehan was admitted to a psychiatric hospital, where she became well-acquainted with the potentially harmful effects of the 1960s version of inpatient treatment. Indeed, she has described the experience of "hell" as be-

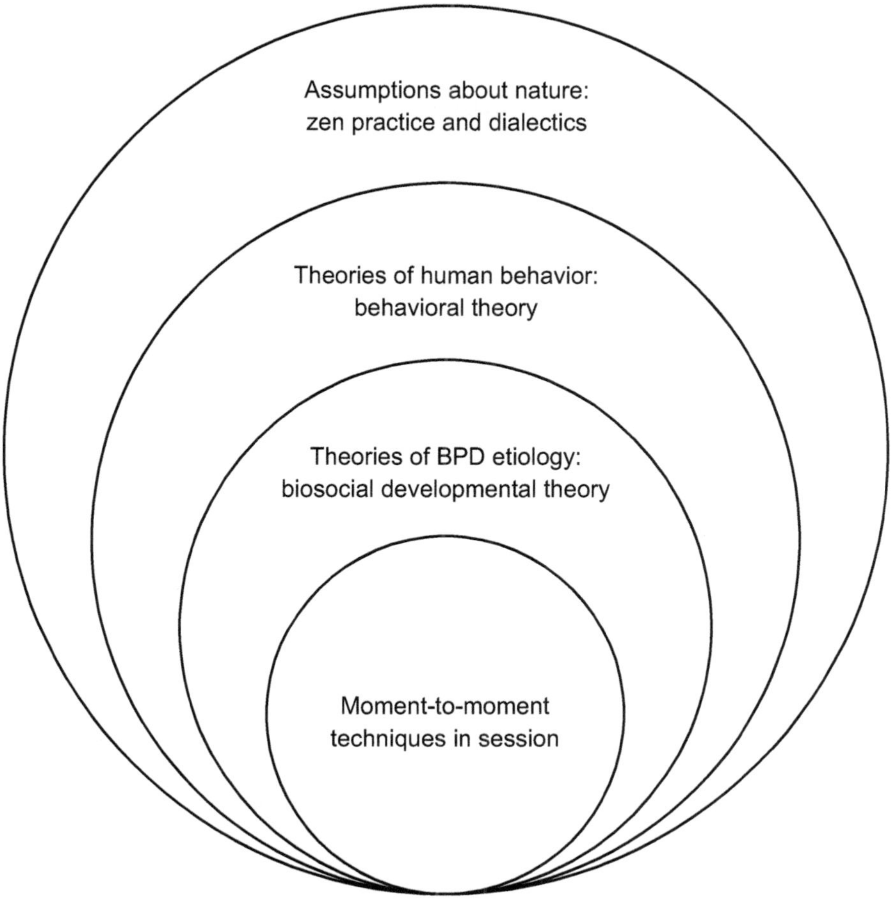

FIGURE 10–1. **Hierarchy of dialectical behavior therapy theory.**

ing trapped in a sterile white room much like those she resided in during her hospitalizations (Linehan 2020). Through a combination of treatment and spiritual practice, Linehan began to overcome these difficulties. She made a commitment to helping others learn to escape from hell and learn to develop lives that are worth living. She reasoned that chronically suicidal individuals were likely the most intensely suffering people in the mental health community and resolved to learn how to help them.

To accomplish this aim, Linehan pursued a degree in psychology, and during her postdoctoral studies with Gerald Davison, she began to apply cutting-edge behavioral intervention strategies to highly suicidal individuals. Her recently published memoir (Linehan 2020) includes an excerpt from a colleague describing his visit to the home of a suicidal man who was holed up in his bathroom with a gun. He describes Linehan calmly entering the bathroom, convincing the man to give up the gun, giving it to her colleague to disarm (this was apparently not within his skill set), and conducting on-the-spot suicide risk assessment and intervention. By combining her courageous nature, clinical talent, and personal understanding of intense emotional pain, Linehan used her formative postdoctoral training to assemble the building blocks of an effective treatment. While she was systematically testing this emerging approach with suicidal clients, the theory and practice of DBT began to take shape in unexpected ways.

As an assistant professor at the University of Washington in the 1970s, Linehan established a treatment development center, the Behavioral Research and Therapy Clinics (BRTC). She and her trainees at the BRTC began to treat chronically suicidal clients using both behavioral interventions and cognitive strategies (Beck et al. 1979). Through a trial-by-fire process with life-or-death stakes, Linehan's team learned that the unrelenting focus on change of cognitive-behavioral therapy (CBT) failed miserably among clients with intense, complex, and persistent mental health problems. Chronically suicidal clients found that traditional CBT strategies invalidated the extent and complexity of their suffering. Many of them withdrew, became frustrated with the therapist, or terminated treatment.

Linehan's clients often included individuals with severe emotional dysregulation, interpersonal challenges, and histories of severe invalidation or trauma. Intense emotional arousal makes it challenging to process information, view thoughts objectively, and consider alternative interpretations of upsetting events (McRae and Zarolia 2020; Tyng et al. 2017). Thus, cognitive strategies encouraging the logical gathering or examining of evidence often went unheeded. Moreover, many CBT mainstays (e.g., building coping skills, engaging in more pleasurable activities, facing fears through exposure) often came across as oversimplified and ineffective solutions to complex client problems. Scheduling time to engage in pleasant activities, for example, may seem ridiculous to a chronically suicidal client with persistent depression for 15 years and a history of severe childhood abuse. Recognizing that to solve complex problems, both clients and therapists must first understand and accept the problems, Linehan and her research team began to systematically incorporate acceptance-based strategies into DBT (Linehan 1993a). They also developed a separate skills-focused group component to help clients learn essential skills to address the many problems that accompany severe emotional dysregulation (Linehan 1993b). Many clients came to find the resulting combination of acceptance, change, and practical skills to build a life worth living to be realistic, acceptable, and effective.

Zen, Mindfulness, and Acceptance in DBT

Zen, Mindfulness, and Acting "As If"

Many of DBT's acceptance-oriented skills, interventions, and therapeutic styles derived from Zen mindfulness practices. While developing DBT, Linehan went on sabbatical to a Zen monastery. On her return, she collaborated with Zen masters in the United States and Germany to translate Zen practice into concrete, practical behavioral skills for clients. She reasoned that skills stemming from Zen were unlikely to chafe against clients' spiritual beliefs and developed several core mindfulness skills that all derive directly from Zen practices (Linehan 1993b, 2015).

The core Zen practice is called *zazen* and most commonly involves sitting and paying attention to experiences of the present moment (e.g., breathing, observing sounds and sights in the room, feeling one's cushion or chair; Suzuki 1970). During zazen, the student experiences sensations of the present moment (e.g., thoughts; emotions;

bodily sensations; physical and emotional discomfort; the boredom of observing the rise and fall of one's breath; urges to move, scratch an itch, or run screaming from the room), while avoiding attachment to any particular state or experience.

Zen often involves a student working with a teacher or master. The student describes their practice and experiences during mindfulness; the teacher provides guidance and verifies or corroborates the student's experiences. This process is mirrored to some extent in DBT, whereby the therapist asks the client to describe their experience while practicing mindfulness or another skill and guides them toward more effective practice.

From a Zen perspective, suffering arises from attachment. All things are viewed as impermanent, including the self. Clinging to a particular state of existence, even to the experience of oneself as a separate and permanent being, is futile. Therefore, Zen practice involves continually experiencing and accepting things exactly as they are. This idea of accepting without attachment eventually evolved into the DBT distress tolerance skill of *radical acceptance*, or completely accepting the experience of the present moment (Linehan 1993b, 2015).

Although Zen practice is sometimes misunderstood as a way to *attain* enlightenment, the goal of zazen is simply to practice zazen—not to strive to achieve a particular goal or attain anything. In Zen, the practitioner does not attain enlightenment at all. There is nothing to attain. Rather, engaging in the practice is considered an expression of our true nature (Suzuki 1970). We are all impermanent, both separate and unified with each other and the universe. Zen students, therefore, practice "as if" they are already enlightened, wise, compassionate, and so forth, and in the process, they might notice that they are (Aitken 1982).

Practicing "as if" is woven into the fabric of DBT and can help address the severe emotional dysregulation that is at the heart of many forms of psychopathology. The DBT skill of opposite action involves behaving in a manner that is opposite to what the client feels like doing when emotionally dysregulated. A client who becomes enraged during a work meeting, for example, might practice opposite action by behaving as if they have compassion for their coworkers or by gently avoiding heated discussions (Chapman and Gratz 2016; Linehan 2015). A client who is ashamed of their physical features or sexual orientation may act as if these characteristics are not shameful (e.g., by encountering people without hiding their body; openly disclosing their sexual orientation). Likewise, therapists must treat clients as if they can change and are able to develop lives that are worth living.

Validation

Linehan also incorporated acceptance-oriented therapeutic styles and strategies, including validation, into DBT. To effectively address severe problems with emotional dysregulation, therapists need to understand and accept their clients and convey such acceptance and understanding. Indeed, in DBT, one of the key functions of validation is to help clients regulate their emotions. Accurately validating a client's emotional experiences helps reduce emotional arousal. Over time, the therapist becomes a model for how clients can use validation with themselves under conditions of high emotional arousal or dysregulation. One of us, for example, saw a client, Linda, who regularly invalidated her emotional reactions, even when they were perfectly understandable (e.g., feeling sad and angry with her mother for repeatedly criticizing her weight). Her emotions intensified when she invalidated herself, and maladaptive secondary emotions emerged, such as shame, which then increased her acute risk of SII. Over time, Linda noticed that her emotional responses resolved much more quickly once she began to practice the DBT skill of mindfulness of current emotion (Linehan 2015) by stepping back and observing and describing her emotions and then asking herself, "How do these feelings make sense?"

Although validation has always been a pillar of psychotherapy, Linehan identified and organized specific therapeutic behaviors into seven different categories, or *levels of validation* (Linehan 1993a; Linehan et al. 2007). Clearly operationalizing such behaviors facilitates learning and practicing validation for therapist and client alike (e.g., in the context of therapy, daily life, and with important others)—much like other behavioral skills in DBT. DBT therapists seek to balance validation and acceptance with behavior change strategies. Dialectical theory serves as a framework for this acceptance-change interplay.

Dialectical Theory

Assuming a dialectical worldview is an essential and fairly unique characteristic of the DBT model. *Dialectic* refers to seemingly incompatible concepts, feelings, behaviors, or perspectives that are simultaneously true. Any extreme position contains its own antithesis or opposite position (e.g., right and wrong, positive and negative charge). For example, a key dialectical assumption in DBT is that clients are doing the best they can, and they need to work harder, try harder, and be more motivated to change (Linehan 1993a). Although these ideas are seemingly in competition, it is helpful to believe that both of them are valid. Doing so diminishes the pull for therapists to blame clients when they struggle to change while also highlighting clients' responsibility to actively engage in therapy. The therapist embraces a worldview in which they can hold the position of completely accepting the client as they are while simultaneously moving urgently for change.

Dialectical poles are often extreme and maladaptive when considered in isolation or adhered to rigidly. When considered together, each position offers some truth that the other is missing (Koerner 2012). Dialectical theory holds that the process of change involves balancing and synthesizing opposite positions. For every thesis, there is an equally valid antithesis. Put another way, from a dialectical perspective, the opposite of a good idea is another good idea. Growth occurs through acknowledging and retaining the truths in opposing perspectives and bringing these truths together to form a more complete picture of reality.

In practice, generating and discussing dialectics function to reduce emotional dysregulation through promoting synthesis and emotional balance and shifting the client's attention when their emotional arousal is high. Adopting a dialectical stance also counters the tendency for the therapist and client to become mired in arguments, polarizing positions, and black-and-white thinking. When confused or stuck, client and therapist work together to assess what is being left out and search for validity in each position. By adopting a dialectical stance, the therapist strives to consider many relevant influences on behavior, bring mindful awareness to tension(s) between contrasting views, and find a balanced approach forward. Balancing dialectics functions to increase psychological flexibility and creativity and ideally leads to more effective solutions.

In DBT, there are many ways to construe a situation, feeling, behavior, or emotion. For example, the client who dwells on suicidal thoughts and becomes angry when their therapist suggests otherwise has a valid point: Suicidal thoughts are comforting—providing a sense that the client's suffering will end and that suicidal behavior sometimes has desirable consequences (e.g., needed treatment, increased concern or support from loved ones). Why would a client wish to continue living a life that is not worth living? At the same time, the therapist has a valid point: It is very difficult to engage in therapy and build a life worth living when suicide remains on the table. If the client's efforts are spent considering, rationalizing, and preparing for suicide, they may have little time and energy to engage in alternative behavior. The challenge for the DBT therapist is to synthesize these perspectives by helping the client change a life that is not worth living *and* remove suicide as a viable option. Building a life worth living meets both needs.

Dialectics permeates DBT treatment philosophy, general practice, and specific in-session strategies. The concept of dialectics, however, can be challenging to apply for several reasons. Humans naturally categorize their experiences, stimuli, and other people. Many societies apply dichotomizing and evaluative language that reinforces extreme positions (e.g., the common saying "you either love it or you hate it"). In DBT, language is consciously and deliberately selected. Words that synthesize (e.g., *both, and*) are typically preferred over those that dichotomize (e.g., *either, or*) and those that imply a "correct" perspective. For example, the word *should* suggests an objective and universally preferable process or outcome (when this is rarely the case) and places undue pressure on the individual. Client and therapist each strive to articulate truths that may be getting left out or going unsaid. For example, a client who has difficulty identifying or acknowledging negative feelings can love their partner and feel angry at them. One does not cancel out the other. Finding a path forward that honors both perspectives will be most effective.

Foundations of DBT: Behavioral Theory and Emotion Science

Behavioral Theory

The next level of theoretical influence on DBT pertains to how we conceptualize the factors causing and maintaining behavior. In this regard, behavioral theory is woven throughout the treatment. Although there are various schools of behavioral theory, each focuses on the following: understanding contextual influences on human behavior, the role of operant and respondent (classically conditioned) learning processes, and generating *testable* formulations of clinically relevant behaviors. DBT shares these features of other behavioral approaches and places particular emphasis on emotions and behavioral skills.

Linehan was influenced by the work of Arthur Staats and his theory of social behaviorism (Staats 1975), later elaborated in his book *Psychological Behaviorism* (Staats 1995). In that text, Staats emphasized integrating behavioral theory with other areas of psychology, such as cognitive, developmental, and personality theories (Chapman and Linehan 2005; Staats 1995). Within this framework, person × environment transactions shape the development of *basic behavioral repertoires*, consisting of a person's characteristic patterns of actions, emotions, thoughts, and urges in particular situations. Consistent with this approach, DBT therapists tend to emphasize a skills deficit model, whereby clients' basic behavioral repertoires are conceptualized as missing some key strategies that would improve their lives. In the case vignette, Miranda's tendency to experience shame, shut down, and avoid talking when asked questions about her suicidal behavior suggests that she could learn alternative skills to better address her needs (e.g., identifying and regulating shame, actively addressing and solving problems).

A precise understanding of the contingencies surrounding clinical target behaviors is absolutely essential for identifying deficits and learning to apply skills effectively. A common method of assessment in DBT is the chain analysis (Linehan 1993a, 1993b; Rizvi 2019), which is essentially the same as a functional analysis used more broadly in other behavioral approaches (Farmer and Chapman 2016). Repeated chain analyses can form the building blocks of an effective behavioral case formulation and highlight effective directions for treatment.

A common rubric for formulating clinically relevant behaviors is the S-O-R-C model, first described by Goldfried and Davison (1976): stimuli, organismic variables, responses, and consequences. A variation on this model names these phenomena antecedents (conditions cueing particular behavior[s]), person variables (including learning history, biological characteristics, and other individual differences), behaviors (relevant actions, emotions, thoughts, and urges [including the behavior that is the target of the formulation]), and consequences that might increase (reinforcement) or decrease (extinction, punishment) the target behavior (Farmer and Chapman 2016). In the case vignette, when Miranda put her head down during the chain analysis of her most recent suicide attempt and said, "I don't know," a behavioral formulation might include the following:

- **Antecedents**—Being asked specific questions about events leading up to the suicide attempt, shame, and feeling tense and overwhelmed
- **Person variables**—A learning history of being invalidated for expressing certain emotions and chastised for "out of control" behavior; a propensity for intense anxiety, influenced by biologically mediated trait negative affectivity; deficits in skills to manage anxiety and identify and name emotions
- **Behaviors**—Looking down, resting her head in her hands, and saying "I don't know."
- **Consequences**—The therapist asks more questions for a period, validates how difficult it is to talk about Miranda's suicidal behavior, withdraws, and changes the topic when she persists in stating, "I don't know." Should these consequences occur, Miranda's behavior is reinforced because she is able to escape an uncomfortable discussion of her suicide attempt. Unless the therapist is vigilant, she may learn that it is aversive to ask about Miranda's suicide attempt and eventually be punished out of asking for further details.

With this formulation in mind, the therapist generates hypotheses about Miranda's behavior. In doing so, it would be important to know that it is more typical for Miranda to actively answer questions and engage in therapy discussions when such discussions are not focused on her suicidal or self-injurious behavior. One hypothesis is that withdrawing and saying, "I don't know" occurs specifically in contexts where she is asked to discuss her problem behavior. In her youth, Miranda had difficulty stopping herself from getting into trouble in various ways, and on the basis of her history of invalidation and others' punitive reactions to her impulsive behavior, she may feel heightened shame. Looking down and disengaging could be consistent with the shame-related tendency to hide or conceal oneself or one's behavior. When Miranda enacts this behavior, the therapist appears to validate and soothe her and discontinue the distressing questioning. As such, the therapist may be inadvertently positively (validating, soothing) and negatively (reducing demands to engage in a difficult discussion) reinforcing Miranda's behaviors.

The next step in a behavioral formulation for Miranda is to collaboratively design interventions that address the specific factors contributing to her behaviors, per the hypotheses generated by the assessment. Success or failure of these interventions would either support or refute the therapist's hypotheses. The clinician might, for example, have Miranda practice the DBT skill of opposite action while talking about her suicide attempt by sitting upright, making direct eye contact, and providing details about what happened. These behaviors are inconsistent with shame. Should Miranda practice these new behaviors repeatedly over time, her shame would likely decrease because she would have the opportunity to learn that the therapist does not chastise or reject her because of her problem behavior. Within a DBT framework, shame occurs in contexts involving threats of rejection (Linehan 1993b, 2015). Given that the therapist's actions might reinforce Miranda's withdrawal from discussions, she and Miranda could agree that when Miranda looks down and says, "I don't know," the therapist will not back off and instead will coach her to practice opposite action. To reinforce the alternative behavior (engaging in the discussion), the therapist might allow Miranda extra time to discuss desired topics such as problems with her partner or some other preferred topic. Testing the effects of these strategies will help to support or refute the therapist's hypotheses. If the therapist avoids backing off when Miranda shuts down, and Miranda continues to shut down, the therapist's backing off might not be an important negative reinforcer for Miranda's behavior. From a behavioral perspective, therefore, assessment, formulation, and treatment are intimately intertwined, and the DBT therapist revises and improves their case formulation iteratively throughout treatment.

A behavioral framework also influences the focus and style of DBT. As with other behavioral approaches, DBT is a learning-oriented therapy. The therapist looks for opportunities to help the client learn new, effective behaviors and skills. Whenever possible, therapists seize the opportunity for clients to practice new behavior in the moment as problem behaviors arise during therapy sessions (as indicated in the example of Miranda practicing opposite action). This illustrates how DBT is an active, action-oriented approach. We have often told our supervisees that if they are simply spending most of their sessions talking with the client, they are not doing DBT. In keeping with a skills deficit model, DBT therapists seek to prompt new behavior, coach clients on how to perform skills more effectively, and have them practice skills repeatedly within and outside therapy sessions. This helps clients generalize the skills they are learning to everyday life. Even in very difficult moments, when a client is emotionally dysregulated, threatening, or yelling at the therapist, it would be consistent with DBT to help the client learn how to communicate differently, on the spot. One skill with multiple components to cultivate is the DEAR MAN (describe the situation, express feelings and opinions, assert oneself, reinforce positive effects, mindfully focus, appear confident, negotiate). Let's say Miranda became fed up with chain analysis:

> **Miranda:** Stop trying to talk to me about this! I already feel badly enough. Don't you know anything? I'm going to leave if you don't quit it!
>
> **Therapist:** I know this is incredibly hard, and I want to find a way to both understand what led to the suicide attempt and respect your wishes. I also want to help you avoid avoiding stuff that's hard to talk about. How about this? If you want a short break from the chain, try asking me without yelling at me or threatening to leave. Remember your DEAR MAN skills, and try them out right now here with me.

In the case vignette, the therapist validates Miranda's experiences and then prompts her to use an alternative skill to get what she wants. If Miranda were to do so effectively (or even close to effectively, following behavioral shaping principles), the therapist would likely allow a short break from the chain and return to it later to ensure she is not reinforcing avoidance. For further discussion and examples of behavioral theory's influence on DBT, please see Chapman (2018).

Emotion Science

As is hopefully apparent from the discussion in the previous subsection, DBT incorporates information and theory about emotions into case formulation as well as intervention. DBT is an emotion-focused therapy, based on the notion that people with complex mental health problems often have difficulty recognizing, understanding, accepting, tolerating, and regulating emotions. To truly understand a client in a manner that guides effective interventions, it is crucial to assess the role of emotions and emotion regulation in their behavior.

Consistent with prevailing emotion theory and empirical evidence, DBT therapists conceptualize emotions as systemic responses that involve a variety of physiological, cognitive, and behavioral components (Gross 2014; Lazarus 1991; Linehan 1993a, 2015; Mauss et al. 2005; Scherer et al. 2001). Emotional responses serve important social and behavioral functions, produce changes across various bodily systems (i.e., central and peripheral nervous systems, hormonal systems), and are accompanied by physiological sensations and action tendencies. At the same time, emotions influence, and are influenced by, the person's perceptions, appraisals, and other cognitive processes (McRae and Zarolia 2020).

Emotions also can motivate us to meet our goals or needs. Walking down a forested path and hearing a heavy rustling in the bushes is a motivationally relevant situation that is likely to precipitate fear for the first author (A.L.C.), who lives near the mountains, with a sizable population of black bears. Miranda's goal is to be accepted by others and feel interpersonally connected. This makes publicly discussing behaviors that she perceives to be shameful a motivationally relevant and emotionally evocative situation. From a DBT perspective, emotional dysregulation emerges when clients' emotion-related experiences and behaviors interfere with achieving their goals (Chapman and Hope 2020). Miranda's experience of shame following interpersonal conflict may be overwhelming, and self-injury or suicidal behavior may emerge as a means of escape. Within therapy sessions, her emotional responses to chain analyses make it difficult to discuss ways to reduce suicidal behavior and improve her life.

From a DBT perspective, emotion regulation involves changes to various elements of the emotion system. This is similar to James Gross's definition of emotion regulation as the ways in which we alter our experience or expression of emotion (Gross 1998). Emotions have many different components, such as physiological signatures (increased heart rate for fear or excitement), associated urges (avoidance when afraid), and associated thoughts, that are functionally interconnected. Changes to any singular input or component can affect the entire system. Emotion regulation, therefore, can involve changing the situations that give rise to emotional responses (e.g., situation selection); modifying perceptions, valuations, or appraisals of emotionally evocative events (e.g., cognitive reappraisal); directing attention toward or away from emotional material (e.g., attention deployment); regulating emotional expressions (e.g., suppressing or enhancing emotional expressions); or directly altering the emotional response (e.g., through coping strategies that alter physiological responses, use of medications). There are many roads to Rome.

All of these emotion regulation options require some kind of change in behavior. Although cognitive reappraisal and DBT skills involving cognitive change can be very effective, with emotionally dysregulated clients, we often front-load skills that help clients change their actions. Because emotions affect cognition and attention, efforts to "talk Miranda out of" feeling ashamed and angry during a chain analysis or help her reappraise the situation might go unheeded in the heat of the moment. Once Miranda's emotions are less intense, she and her therapist might create a plan for her to use cognitive strategies in the future *before* she becomes dysregulated. In sum, the emotion science literature heavily influences DBT theory and practice. DBT's focus on emotions and emotion regulation also derives directly from what we know about the development of complex mental health conditions such as SII and BPD.

Biosocial Developmental Theory of BPD, Self-Inflicted Injury, and Emotional Dysregulation

Linehan proposed a biosocial model of the etiology of BPD that has become highly influential (Linehan 1993a). This model can be applied to problems characterized by emotional dysregulation more broadly (Linehan et al. 2007). Consistent with other leading psychopathology models, the biosocial theory proposed that biologically based vulnerabilities interact with specific environmental processes over time to result in severe and chronic emotional dysregulation, SII, and BPD (Linehan 1993a). The key biological vulnerability factor in this model included a predisposition toward emotion *vulnerability*, consisting of heightened sensitivity to emotional cues, intense emotional responses, and a slow return to emotional baseline following an emotional response. People who are emotionally vulnerable may be more easily and intensely distressed and take a longer amount of time to recover from their distress relative to those without this predisposition. Increased vulnerability to intense emotional responses (negative affectivity more specifically) is a common precursor to many types of clinical problems; most forms of psychopathology are characterized by maladaptive emotional experiences and expressions. Linehan hypothesized that emotion vulnerability transacts with an invalidating caregiving environment to raise the risk that an individual will develop SII and/or BPD specifically.

Invalidating environments are characterized by caregiver(s) repeatedly ignoring, rejecting, or minimizing their child's emotion-related expressions. This includes overtly problematic behaviors such as threatening, bullying, and shaming. Invalidation, however, is not always intentional and can be quite subtle. For example, a parent who scoffs and says, "It's nothing to get upset over" when their son cries loudly may unintentionally invalidate their sensitive child. The message the child may receive is that his feelings are wrong or unacceptable to others. Thus, he may attempt to inhibit expressing his emotions in the future. Because a vulnerable child's emotional expressions are often intense and overwhelming, their emotional needs may often exceed the family's capacity to provide support and validation.

Invalidating environments also intermittently reinforce extreme emotional expressions. Although not always effective, negative outbursts may function to elicit emotional support or allow the child to delay or avoid parental demands. Coercive processes also often arise in families where parent and child reciprocally escalate aversive behaviors and negative affect during their interactions. For example, a child crying for candy in a supermarket may initially stop in response to a parent raising their voice yet may cry longer and louder the next time, until the parent gives in and buys them a chocolate bar. Over time, these patterns become more intense and frequent, resulting in poor emotional and behavioral control, difficulties with resolving conflict, and maladaptive interpersonal strategies (e.g., silent treatments, making demands, yelling, threatening, destroying possessions, physical confrontations). Youth and caregiver shape one another into using aversive behaviors to meet their own needs. Because intense escalated actions are often reinforced and such actions include intense emotional expression (e.g., emotional outbursts, yelling, screaming), invalidating environments shape emotional lability.

In her original publication of the biosocial model, Linehan focused on emotional dysregulation as *the* core mechanism underlying the risk for BPD, with SII and suicidality typically emerging as strategies to reduce emotional distress. An updated version of her model, developed with Sheila Crowell and Ted Beauchaine, incorporates trait impulsivity as another, even earlier-emerging and highly heritable vulnerability for emotional dysregulation, BPD, and SII (Crowell et al. 2009). In this revision, the authors focused on creating a set of testable hypotheses for the biosocial theory across development and spanning multiple levels of analysis (e.g., genetic, physiological functioning, family functioning).

The revised biosocial developmental model suggests that impulsivity confers vulnerability to behavioral disorders (e.g., oppositional defiant disorder, ADHD), along with a particular susceptibility to the negative effects of invalidating or adverse childhood environments. Over time, through coercive processes, the environment shapes and reinforces emotional dysregulation. In early adolescence, harmful coping (substance use, SII, suicidal behavior) emerges to cope with emotional lability. SII and suicidal behavior in particular often portend the emergence of the trademark cognitive, behavioral, and emotional features of BPD in later adolescence (Crowell et al. 2009, 2014b).

Since the publication of Linehan's theory, empirical support has accumulated for the role of the invalidating environment in the development of BPD, SII, and related problems. For example, studies find that familial rejection confers a substantial increase in suicide risk (Ryan et al. 2009); elevated parental criticism and emotional overinvolvement are each linked to adolescent SII (Wedig and Nock 2007); and markers of youth risk appear across genetic, central, autonomic, and behavioral levels of analysis (e.g., Belsky et al. 2012; Crowell et al. 2005, 2013, 2014a; Kaufman et al. 2020). Patterns of negative reinforcement of emotional lability and conflict escalation are also each well documented in families of adolescents with SII and BPD (Crowell et al. 2013, 2017; Fruzzetti et al. 2005).

The biosocial model influences DBT practice in several ways. First, in DBT, there is a strong emphasis on helping clients understand and manage emotional dysregulation. Emotion regulation skills explicitly address these concerns by helping clients learn to identify and manage emotions. Distress tolerance skills help clients avoid acting in maladaptive ways in the context of emotional dysregulation. Individual therapists also address emotional dysregulation as it arises in therapy sessions by helping clients to observe, describe, and regulate emotions in the moment. Second, DBT therapists weave didactics on the biosocial model, emotions, and behavioral science into their work as needed to help clients better understand factors related to emotional dysregulation. Third, as mentioned earlier, the systematic use of validation in DBT can help emotionally dysregulated clients with histories of pervasive invalidation learn to experience their reactions as understandable, trust their appraisals without judgment, and validate others. Fourth, interpersonal effectiveness skills can help the client learn alternatives to the coercive interpersonal processes that often characterized their earlier rearing environments. In sum, an understanding of how severe emotion regulation deficits develop is essential for identifying fruitful intervention targets.

Conclusion and Future Directions

In this chapter, we introduced several theoretical underpinnings that inform DBT practice. A combination of Marsha Linehan's lived experience and the lessons learned from applying standard CBT approaches to complex, suicidal clients shaped the evolution of DBT theory. Zen practice informed the development of acceptance-oriented approaches, and dialectics emerged as a way to effectively balance and synthesize perspectives and treatment strategies. Behavioral theory and emotion science form the foundation of behavior change strategies in DBT, and the evolving biosocial developmental theory helps to tailor the treatment to the specific needs of complex clients with severe emotional dysregulation.

Clinicians with a solid grounding in these conceptual frameworks will be prepared to apply DBT strategies and principles effectively—particularly in unexpected or very challenging circumstances. Keeping the tenets of Zen, dialectics, behaviorism, emotion science, and biosocial theory in mind through the assessment, treatment planning, and intervention stages of DBT will guide a coherent application of DBT principles to the many new and interesting challenges presented by emotionally dysregulated clients. As the treatment, science, and theory evolve, it will be crucial for clinicians to remain theoretically grounded while flexibly incorporating new information and strategies into the treatment. Indeed, Marsha Linehan has often stated that if a better treatment comes along, she will do that treatment. It is crucial, therefore, to remain focused on the ultimate goal of DBT: to help clients learn to build lives worth living.

Key Points

- Dialectical behavior therapy (DBT) was originally developed to help chronically suicidal clients and has evolved into a helpful treatment for complex clients with emotion regulation problems more broadly.
- Dialectical theory and Zen practice inform the worldview underlying DBT, the balance of treatment styles and strategies, and the use of acceptance and mindfulness-based practices.
- Behavioral theory and emotion science inform the DBT view of factors causing and maintaining behavior and guide the use of evidence-based interventions.
- The biosocial developmental theory places complex problems with emotion regulation within a developmental context and highlights the need to help clients learn to understand and effectively regulate emotions.

References

Aitken R: Taking the Path of Zen. New York, North Point, 1982

Beck AT, Rush AJ, Shaw BF, et al: Cognitive Therapy of Depression. New York, Guilford, 1979

Belsky DW, Caspi A, Arseneault L, et al: Etiological features of borderline personality related characteristics in a birth cohort of 12-year-old children. Dev Psychopathol 24(1):251–265, 2012 22293008

Chapman AL: Phone Coaching in Dialectical Behavior Therapy. New York, Guilford, 2018

Chapman AL, Gratz KL: The DBT Skills Workbook for Anger. Oakland, CA, New Harbinger, 2016

Chapman AL, Hope N: Dialectical behavior therapy and treatment of emotion dysregulation, in Oxford Handbook of Emotion Dysregulation. Edited by Beauchaine T, Crowell S. Oxford, UK, Oxford University Press, 2020, pp 463–476

Chapman AL, Linehan MM: Dialectical behavior therapy for borderline personality disorder, in Borderline Personality Disorder. Edited by Zanarini M. Boca Raton, FL, Taylor & Francis, 2005, pp 211–242

Crowell SE, Beauchaine TP, McCauley E, et al: Psychological, physiological, and serotonergic correlates of parasuicidal behavior among adolescent girls. Dev Psychopathol 17(4):1105–1127, 2005 16613433

Crowell SE, Beauchaine TP, Linehan MM: A biosocial developmental model of borderline personality: elaborating and extending Linehan's theory. Psychol Bull 135(3):495–510, 2009 19379027

Crowell SE, Baucom BR, McCauley E, et al: Mechanisms of contextual risk for adolescent self-injury: invalidation and conflict escalation in mother-child interactions. J Clin Child Adolesc Psychol 42(4):467–480, 2013 23581508

Crowell SE, Baucom BR, Yaptangco M, et al: Emotion dysregulation and dyadic conflict in depressed and typical adolescents: evaluating concordance across psychophysiological and observational measures. Biol Psychol 98:50–58, 2014a 24607894

Crowell SE, Kaufman EA, Beauchaine TP: A biosocial model of BPD: theory and empirical evidence, in Handbook of Borderline Personality Disorder in Children and Adolescents. Edited by Sharp C, Tackett JL. New York, Springer, 2014b, pp 143–157

Crowell SE, Butner JE, Wiltshire TJ, et al: Evaluating emotional and biological sensitivity to maternal behavior among self-injuring and depressed adolescent girls using nonlinear dynamics. Clin Psychol Sci 5(2):272–285, 2017 28924493

Farmer RF, Chapman AL: Behavioral Interventions in Cognitive Behavior Therapy: Practical Guidance for Putting Theory Into Action, 2nd Edition. Washington, DC, American Psychological Association, 2016
Fruzzetti AE, Shenk C, Hoffman PD: Family interaction and the development of borderline personality disorder: a transactional model. Dev Psychopathol 17(4):1007–1030, 2005 16613433
Goldfried MR, Davison GR: Clinical Behavior Therapy. New York, Holt, Rinehart, and Winston, 1976
Gross JJ: The emerging field of emotion regulation: an integrative review. Rev Gen Psychol 2(3):271–299, 1998
Gross JJ: Emotion regulation: conceptual and empirical foundations, in Handbook of Emotion Regulation, 2nd Edition. Edited by Gross JJ. New York, Guilford, 2014, pp 3–20
Kaufman EA, Puzia ME, Godfrey DA, et al: Physiological and behavioral effects of interpersonal validation: a multilevel approach to examining a core intervention strategy among self-injuring adolescents and their mothers. J Clin Psychol 76(3):559–580, 2020 31742683
Koerner K: Doing Dialectical Behavior Therapy: A Practical Guide. New York, Guilford, 2012
Lazarus RS: Emotion and Adaptation. Oxford, UK, Oxford University Press, 1991
Linehan M: Cognitive-Behavioral Treatment of Borderline Personality Disorder. New York, Guilford, 1993a
Linehan M: Skills Training Manual for Treating Borderline Personality Disorder. New York, Guilford, 1993b
Linehan M: DBT Skills Training Manual, 2nd Edition. New York, Guilford, 2015
Linehan M: Building a Life Worth Living: A Memoir. New York, Random House, 2020
Linehan MM, Bohus M, Lynch TR: Dialectical behavior therapy for pervasive emotion dysregulation, in Handbook of Emotion Regulation, 2nd Edition. Edited by Gross JJ. New York, Guilford, 2007, pp 581–605
Mauss IB, Levenson RW, McCarter L, et al: The tie that binds? Coherence among emotion experience, behavior, and physiology. Emotion 5(2):175–190, 2005 15982083
McRae K, Zarolia P: Cognition and emotion in emotion dysregulation, in The Oxford Handbook of Emotion Dysregulation. Edited by Beauchaine TP, Crowell SE. New York, Oxford University Press, 2020, pp 39–52
Rizvi SL: Chain Analysis in Dialectical Behavior Therapy. New York, Guilford, 2019
Ryan C, Huebner D, Diaz RM, et al: Family rejection as a predictor of negative health outcomes in white and Latino lesbian, gay, and bisexual young adults. Pediatrics 123(1):346–352, 2009 19117902
Scherer KR, Schorr A, Johstone T: Appraisal Processes in Emotion: Theory, Methods, Research. New York, Oxford University Press, 2001
Staats AW: Social Behaviorism. Oxford, UK, Dorsey, 1975
Staats AW: Paradigmatic behaviorism and paradigmatic behavior therapy, in Theories of Behavior Therapy: Exploring Behavior Change. Edited by O'Donohue WT, Krasner L. Washington, DC, American Psychological Association, 1995, pp 659–693
Suzuki S: Zen Mind, Beginner's Mind. New York, Weatherhill, 1970
Tyng CM, Amin HU, Saad MNM, Malik AS: The influences of emotion on learning and memory. Front Psychol 8:1454, 2017 28883804
Wedig MM, Nock MK: Parental expressed emotion and adolescent self-injury. J Am Acad Child Adolesc Psychiatry 46(9):1171–1178, 2007 17712240

CHAPTER 11

Treatment Techniques in Dialectical Behavior Therapy

Charles Swenson, M.D.

This chapter begins with a focus on problem-solving techniques of dialectical behavior therapy (DBT), which is based on cognitive-behavioral therapy (CBT). Next, I discuss acceptance-oriented strategies, including validation, and then, finally, dialectical strategies. Although the main focus is on the use of DBT techniques in the context of individual therapy, it is important to recognize that the same repertoire of strategies is used in all DBT treatment modes, such as group skills training sessions; telephone calls to the therapist for skills coaching; and among therapists in the DBT consultation team. For instance, group skills training classes begin with a review of patients' homework practice from the prior week. The skills group leader uses validation strategies in the service of strengthening the connection between therapist and patient, then uses a range of change-oriented techniques to improve the patient's skillful capacities. The skills training group leader, for instance, briefly uses behavioral chain analysis to assess problems in homework compliance or ineffective skills use, then intervenes with brief, targeted problem-solving practices to strengthen compliance, effective use of skills, and generalization of the learning to the natural environment. Later in the same group meeting, while teaching the new skill of the week, the leader draws from the whole package of problem-solving, validation, and dialectical strategies to heighten skills acquisition and strengthening. The chapter concludes with brief comments on how to bring the three paradigms and the multitude of strategies together in therapy sessions.

Strategic Core of Dialectical Behavior Therapy

It was Marsha Linehan's intention to create a cognitive-behavioral treatment for individuals with repetitive suicide attempts and self-injurious behaviors, eventually including individuals with borderline personality disorder (Linehan 1993a). She expected that her work would result in a 12- to 16-week protocol based on standard CBT techniques: behavioral analysis, skills training, contingency procedures, cognitive restructuring, and exposure and response prevention. If her expectations had been met successfully, DBT would never have been developed.

Certain features in the clinical presentation of patients with borderline personality disorder made it impossible to use standard CBT effectively. First, the patients presented not only with high-risk behaviors but also with chronic and severe disturbances in emotion regulation. They were exquisitely sensitive, highly reactive emotionally, and impulsive. They presented not only with borderline personality disorder but also commonly with substance use disorders, eating disorders, anxiety disorders, PTSD, dissociative disorders, and at least a smattering of antisocial traits. These biologically based emotional vulnerabilities mitigated against the level of discipline, cooperation, and commitment optimal for successful CBT treatments. Linehan adapted to this challenge in three ways. She built a comprehensive skills training curriculum to remedy the patients' emotion regulation deficits. She created a targeting template and staged system that could accommodate all treatment targets within one treatment, prioritizing them from most severe to less severe. Finally, she found a user-friendly way to package and engage with a huge array of CBT techniques that could be used to address almost any clinical twists and turns in the treatment. Emphasizing the principles behind the techniques as much as the techniques themselves enables therapists to apply them with a high degree of flexibility and fluidity.

For example, when I was assessing the chain of events that led to a self-cutting incident by a young adult patient, Abby, she reported that she had been standing in a parking lot in the rain, overcome by self-loathing thoughts and deep shame. I hypothesized that this episode had been instrumental to the eventual cutting incident, so in aiming to address Abby's self-loathing, I asked about antecedent events. She reported that she had no idea what happened or why she was in a parking lot. The last thing she remembered was in the early evening the night before when she was talking with a male friend. As she put it, she "woke up" cutting herself in the rain in the parking lot. I started the session targeting the self-harm, then shifted to targeting the self-loathing. Next, I assessed the factors leading Abby into a dissociative state. As she tried to engage with me about the dissociation, she began to dissociate in the session, becoming more withdrawn, distant, and confused about what was going on. Suddenly, I was assessing a dissociative episode in real time, orienting Abby to reality, walking her through some mindfulness-based grounding skills, and maintaining our connection as best as I could. Soon she had reestablished presence and stability and we could return to the focus on the primary target, self-cutting. The framework of prioritized treatment targets allowed me to shift as different targets came into view, and the wide range of treatment techniques allowed me to have approaches to each of the situations.

In addition to the impact of biologically based emotional vulnerabilities on treatment, another factor is the significant degree to which many of these patients have been subjected to pervasive invalidating environments, the degree to which they invalidate themselves, and the degree to which they are sensitive to even slight manifestations of invalidation. Change-oriented techniques easily and often lead them to feel invalidated, which sets off reactions against the treatment, against the therapist, and against themselves, all of which interfere with CBT techniques. This was such a significant impediment to treatment that Linehan created and applied a robust set of acceptance-oriented techniques to use before, during, and following the change techniques. At first Linehan emphasized that validation was the "sugar coating" that would help the change-oriented medicine go down. With years of experience and research on validation, she came to understand validation as a potent change-oriented intervention in its own right, perhaps the most potent strategy for reducing emotional dysregulation. Validation is an active ingredient alongside problem-solving, and the therapist moves back and forth between validation and problem-solving throughout the session.

The third feature of these patients that stood in the way of standard CBT was the fact that they often presented with extreme behavioral responses, black-and-white thinking, passive as well as rigid styles of problem-solving, and the tendency to engage in polarized and polarizing relationships. Stalemates and logjams were frequent, bringing therapy to a halt from which both parties were at risk of spiraling into burnout. Just as Linehan had created the validation strategies package to deal with invalidation and suffering, she created a package of dialectical strategies designed to resolve stalemates and turmoil that were associated with extreme behavioral responses, rigid thinking patterns, and polarized relationship transactions.

By the late 1980s, when the full tripartite package was in place, the therapist targeted the patient's problematic behavioral patterns from three angles, using 1) problem-solving techniques to change behaviors; 2) validation and other acceptance strategies to reduce suffering, to remedy misunderstandings, and to strengthen the therapy relationship; and 3) dialectical principles and strategies to address stalemates and polarization. Each aspect of treatment provides an active ingredient in the search for behavioral changes that will lead each patient to a self-defined life worth living. Each ingredient can be used for multiple purposes: problem-solving will sometimes help with acceptance, validation will sometimes help with problem-solving, and dialectics is, in its essence, an amalgam of change and acceptance techniques.

Linehan's initial goal was to develop a treatment for adult women with self-injurious and suicidal behaviors, but she soon broadened the target population to include all individuals with borderline personality disorder. In the past 20 years, the treatment has been applied successfully to other populations: males; adolescents; people with substance use disorders, eating disorders, dissociative disorders, and complex PTSD; forensic patients; and, most recently, children and families.

Supplementary Strategy Groups

Surrounding and extending the tripartite strategic core of DBT are several groups of strategies, each with a particular purpose. *Structural treatment strategies* define how the therapist establishes the frame of the therapy, including agreements, assumptions, functions, treatment modes, and a few rules. They guide the therapist in structuring not only the overall treatment but also each therapy session in establishing and sticking to a target-driven agenda.

Stylistic communication strategies define styles of interacting with patients that provide the atmosphere that will support the work of the moment. Two styles are defined: one that accompanies and strengthens a problem-solving approach and one that accompanies and reinforces an acceptance-oriented approach. The former is called the *irreverent communication style* and includes such strategies as confrontation, calling the patient's bluff, and "jumping in where angels fear to tread." The latter is the *reciprocal communication style,* and prescribes warmth, genuineness, responsiveness, and strategically used self-disclosure within limits.

Case management strategies provide guidance for the therapist regarding how to interact with the patient's social, familial, and professional networks, again defining two approaches: one that is more change oriented and one that is more acceptance oriented. The change-oriented approach is to consult with patients as individuals so that their ability to manage their own lives is enhanced; the acceptance-oriented approach, *environmental intervention,* defines certain circumstances in which the therapist supports and advocates for the patient in the environment when the outcome is important but the patient has neither the power nor the skills to effect the outcome.

Finally, there is an array of *special treatment strategies* in which the DBT techniques are applied to particular situations. These protocols and strategies are used for assessing and managing heightened suicide risk, for managing in-session dysfunctional behaviors and therapy-interfering behaviors, and for managing the therapeutic relationship.

Changing Behavior: Cognitive-Behavioral Techniques in Dialectical Behavior Therapy

Problem-Solving Protocol

Essentially, DBT uses a wide range of cognitive and behavioral strategies based largely on four foundational theories of behavioral change in CBT: classical conditioning, operant conditioning, cognitive mediation, and skills deficit theory. Linehan has organized the comprehensive array of behavioral and cognitive techniques into a step-by-step problem-solving protocol so that even when faced with chaotic situations, the therapist can stay on track and have the change techniques at their fingertips. Once a given behavior is identified and targeted, whether at the beginning of the session or when recognized midsession, the therapist proceeds to implement the steps in the protocol. The problem-solving protocol can double as a study guide for therapists learning the basic approaches in CBT that are used in DBT. When I was learning to practice DBT, having been trained primarily in psychoanalysis and psychodynamic psychotherapy, this protocol became the syllabus of contents for my study of cognitive-behavioral techniques.

Therapy sessions in DBT begin with a process of determining which treatment targets have been active since the prior session and which will be the focus of the current session. To make that determination, the therapist reviews the patient's diary card, a daily tracking form to capture the presence of target behaviors. The problem-solving might then begin with a statement such as "It looks like the highest-priority target behavior from the week was the suicide attempt you made yesterday. Let's figure out what happened and see what you can do in the future to find better solutions. OK?" At other times, the problem behavior is identified midsession when it comes to light or if it occurs as an in-session behavior. For example, "I noticed that a few minutes ago you stopped talking and you became really withdrawn. It's happened in here before. Let's see if we can figure out what caused it and how best to deal with it so it doesn't get in the way of your treatment."

When the problem-solving protocol is used, two caveats are relevant. First, it will not always be the case that every step of the protocol is to be followed; the protocol establishes a rough algorithm to guide the therapist, not to promote rigid adherence to every step. Second, none of these techniques will be effective unless there is a good therapeutic relationship, the development and maintenance of which is a crucial part of DBT. Table 11–1 lists the steps in the protocol; the following subsections discuss each step and associated behavioral change techniques.

Behavioral Chain Analysis

As a psychotherapist who discovered DBT after many years of practicing psychoanalytic psychotherapy with patients with borderline personality disorder, I was accustomed to thinking "vertically." The essence of the problem, I thought, lay beneath the surface; the role of psychoanalysis was to clarify the intrapsychic structure, to make the unconscious conscious, to foster insight, and to resolve defenses and conflicts. In contrast, a DBT therapist looks for the driving forces of functional or pathological behaviors represented horizontally as links on a chain moving from left to right. Rather than psychoanalysis, the DBT therapist uses behavioral chain analysis. Rather than searching for unconscious entities that control behaviors, the DBT therapist searches for controlling variables among *links*—emotions, cognitions, actions, and environmental events—that are discoverable on the behavioral chain. The chain leading up to and following a self-injurious behavior, for instance, will be constructed collaboratively by therapist and patient. Out of an episode shrouded in uncertainty, confusion, negative emotions, and perhaps chaos, the behavioral chain brings clarity, order, and understanding. Alternatively, the therapist can work with the patient on the construction of a chain leading up to a functional behavior in order to locate the controlling variables of adaptive functioning rather than just focusing on pathology.

The chain as a template has five segments (Figure 11–1). From left to right, the segments are 1) *vulnerability factors* rendering the patient vulnerable to the upcoming prompting event; 2) the *prompting event*, usually an encounter with the environment but sometimes an internal, private event; 3) the various *links in the chain* occurring from the prompting event until the problem behavior; 4) the *problem behavior* itself; and 5) the *consequences* of the problem behavior, in particular those that were contingent on the problem behavior.

The DBT therapist gets the detailed information to assemble the chain within this template by joining with the patient to do so. Even in an exhaustive analysis, it is assumed that there are undiscovered links that are outside the patient's awareness.

TABLE 11–1. **Problem-solving protocol**

Step	Purpose
1. Behavioral chain analysis	Assess the problem behavior
2. Insight strategies	Recognize recurring patterns in the chain and arrive at hypotheses to explain them
3. Solution analysis strategies	Select appropriate solutions from among four overarching behavioral change procedures, guided by the hypotheses
4. Change procedures	
Skills training	Used if skills deficits contribute to the problem
Contingency procedures	Used if problematic contingencies contribute to the problem
Exposure procedures	Used if classically conditioned intense emotions contribute to the problem
Cognitive modification procedures	Used if problematic cognitions contribute to the problem
5. Didactic strategies	Teach the patient about the behaviors or their treatment
6. Orienting strategies	Orient the patient to roles and expectations of treatment procedures
7. Commitment strategies	Strengthen the patient's commitment to the treatment or a particular treatment procedure

Sometimes the missing links are key to solving the problems, and the therapist and patient search to find them. For instance, whereas a psychoanalyst may posit that the patient's surface presentation suggests the presence of unconscious hostility along with unconscious defenses against it, a DBT therapist might search the chain for evidence of emotional dysregulation, thoughts, and actions that are the way they are because of a combination of emotion regulation skills deficits, dysfunctional beliefs, emotionally salient conditioned cues eliciting powerful emotional responses, and reinforcers of the problematic behavioral response. Building a chain representing a chaotic series of events has the effect of creating a coherent story, which is beneficial in many ways.

After identifying a problem behavior to be targeted, the therapist orients the patient to the conduct of chain analysis. This should be handled in a way that respects the patient and protects and strengthens the therapeutic relationship. With some patients, I will introduce the topic by saying, "OK, so let's do a chain analysis that will help us figure out what caused this to happen again, so we can come up with better alternatives or solutions." With other patients who might experience this proposal as overly clinical and intrusive, I am more likely to say, "So tell me what the story was, how this happened, so we can change the storyline in the future, OK?" In other words, chain analysis is a strategy that can be approached with different tactics that suit the situation.

On agreement to do the chain analysis, I usually inquire first into the details of the problem behavior and then try to locate the most salient prompting event, and from there "fill in" the rest of the chain, including the vulnerability factors, the links in the chain, and the consequences. There is no particular necessary order in eliciting the chain; although the clinician should aim for a rigorous and well-organized chain, this

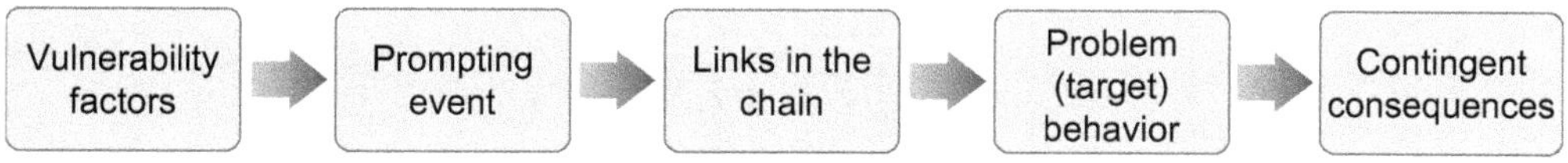
Vulnerability factors
Prompting event
Links in the chain
Problem (target) behavior
Contingent consequences

FIGURE 11–1. Template for behavioral chain.

need not be done in a rigid or highly organized manner. It is a way to help the therapist and patient think more about important links and controlling variables. Much more about the technical details of chain analysis can be found in several texts (Koerner 2011; Linehan 1993a; Rizvi 2019; Swenson 2016).

For the sake of illustration, consider the case of Julia, a 17-year-old girl with a target behavior of self-cutting. Several chain analyses of her self-cutting incidents have revealed a pattern, which is illustrated in Figure 11–2. Her treatment plan will aim to reinforce the functional behaviors in the chain (e.g., "tries skills to distract…") and to replace the dysfunctional links with more adaptive ones (e.g., using distress tolerance skills rather than "cuts herself on the arm…").

The chain analysis is primarily an assessment tool, but at the same time it is also a platform for problem-solving. For instance, when a problematic link in the chain is identified, the therapist might "get off the chain" to bring in possible solutions right then and there, returning to the chain after a problem-solving intervention. Or the therapist might get off the chain at a certain point in order to get a deeper account of the history or context of that link in the chain. As needed, the therapist might get off the chain to validate the patient for a particular action, emotion, or cognition, or to use a dialectical strategy to deal with polarization. In each case, the therapist then gets back on the chain, picking up where they left off. Within the chain there will also be functional, skillful behaviors that the therapist may immediately reinforce. The chain and the conduct of chain analysis are central to the assessment and treatment process in DBT; treatment can be thought of as a modification of the current dysfunctional chain with a more adaptive chain. The DBT therapist has chains on the mind in most sessions.

Insight Strategies

While conducting chain analysis, the therapist is alert to finding patterns of links within the chain that are characteristic of the patient and that are associated with the problem behavior. The discovery and highlighting of these patterns is the practice of insight strategies. *Insight* in this context simply refers to pattern recognition without an assumption of what causes those patterns or what functions they serve. As part of the insight strategies, the therapist engages the patient in generating hypotheses that might explain the origins or functions of the pattern and help in the search for solutions. For instance, regarding Julia, whose self-cutting is assessed in the chain described in the previous subsection, the brainstorming might go as follows.

Therapist: Now that we can see the pattern, I wonder what the function of the cutting was?
Julia: It's obvious. I was able to go to sleep.
Therapist: Yeah, right, I see that. I assume it helped you get rid of your tension and distress.
Julia: Right.

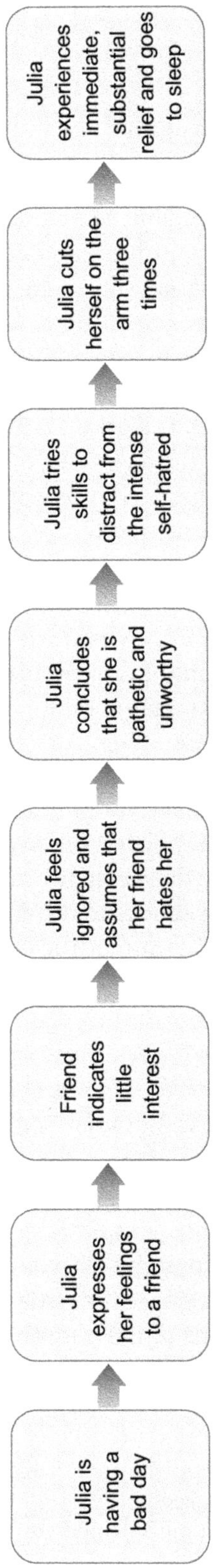

FIGURE 11–2. Sample chain analysis for a patient who engages in self-cutting.

Therapist: Do you think you would have had to cut yourself if you were having a good day?

Julia: Hmm. I don't know. Maybe not. I might have brushed it off if I felt better.

Therapist: Yeah, I wondered about that. Let me ask you something else. If you had been able to just allow yourself to feel rejected, and tell yourself that anyone would feel rejected in that situation, is it possible you would not have ended up feeling you were pathetic?

Julia: Maybe, but I don't think I can do that because I feel like I *am* pathetic.

Therapist: Yeah, I know, though I think that it is just a deep belief you have because of incidents like this, and the pattern goes around and around.

Julia: When I feel pathetic, I feel like I might just as well die.

Therapist: Yeah, it's incredibly painful. But here's one thing I take from this. If we could get it so that you stopped yourself in the middle of the chain, when you were thinking you were pathetic, and you could think about it in a different way, it might make all the difference. Are you willing to work on that, on how to feel not so pathetic even though you feel rejected?

Julia: I'm willing to try.

Solution Analysis

With chain analysis, once important patterns are recognized and spelled out and hypotheses are generated and put to the test, the therapist moves to the next step: finding solutions based on those hypotheses. This process is called *solution analysis* and involves several steps. In the dialogue above, for instance, the therapist hypothesized that Julia's belief that she was pathetic may have been a potent controlling variable leading to self-cutting. The next step would be to find solutions so that Julia either does not think of herself as pathetic or can temporarily tolerate that thought without needing to cut herself. In addition, or alternatively, solutions may be indicated for other controlling variables in that brief chain, such as the following:

1. How to get herself in a better mood on a bad day or to tolerate a bad mood
2. How to communicate her feelings to her friend in an effective way
3. How to be disappointed in what felt rejecting but without hating herself
4. How to experience disappointment and distress and notice the tendency to hate herself as pathetic but remind herself that these thoughts are not factual
5. How to use crisis survival skills to tolerate her distress and get relief without cutting

After brainstorming possible solutions with the patient, the next step in solution analysis is to select one or more solutions and put them into action. Whenever possible, the DBT therapist wants to elicit new behaviors from the patient during the session in order to practice the solutions.

Change Procedures

When seeking solutions for the patterns instrumental to the problem behavior, the therapist turns to a menu of four change procedures: skills training, contingency procedures, exposure procedures, and cognitive modification procedures, each of which is derived from an important foundational theory underlying CBT.

Skills Training

The presence of emotional and interpersonal skills deficits in the chain may prompt skills training solutions, such as the reinforcement of skills the patient has learned already or teaching new skills on the spot. In the case of Julia, relevant skills might include mindfulness skills for enhancing awareness, attention, and nonjudgmental thinking; distress tolerance skills for radically accepting her friend's response and her subsequent disappointment; crisis survival skills for tolerating distress without making things worse; emotion regulation skills for observing and describing her emotions and checking whether they were justified by facts or not; and interpersonal skills for asserting herself with her friend.

Contingency Procedures

Contingency procedures, derived from operant conditioning theory, proceed from the perspective that contingent consequences of a behavior can strengthen (reinforce) or weaken (extinguish, punish) that behavior. For Julia, the total relief and sleep that followed her self-cutting are a reinforcement of cutting. Although the therapist probably cannot take away this reinforcement, based as it is in Julia's physiology, it may be possible to link an additional contingent consequence to her cutting behavior, something more aversive. Some patients, for instance, find that knowing they will need to spend part of the next therapy session doing a chain analysis of their self-cutting is aversive enough to help them not cut themselves.

Throughout sessions, DBT therapists use opportunities to reinforce adaptive behaviors while extinguishing dysfunctional ones. I once had a patient who dreaded the ending of sessions. A pattern developed in which she brought up life-threatening scenarios in the final minutes of sessions, which I then reinforced by extending the sessions. Inadvertently, I was probably reinforcing the reporting of life-threatening behaviors at the end of sessions, possibly even prompting rehearsals in her mind of life-threatening behaviors. Once I recognized the pattern and oriented the patient, we came up with alternative ways for her to communicate and cope with her session-ending distress.

Exposure Procedures

Exposure procedures are based on classical conditioning theory. In particular, the mini storyline captured by this theory is a story of three terms: 1) a *cue* that is paired in the mind with a previous traumatic event, 2) the intense emotional response to the cue, and 3) the *escape behavior* that helps the patient to "escape" from the cue or the emotional response. Very often, the problem behavior serves as the escape behavior (e.g., self-cutting as an escape from emotional distress and tension). Some adaptive solutions serve to decrease the potency of the cue by having the patient deliberately avoid or modify it. Other solutions aim to decrease the intensity of the emotional response by deliberately and repeatedly exposing the patient to the cue or a situation that matches the cue, all while blocking the escape response and having a nonreinforcing (safe) outcome. With one of my patients for whom being alone was terrifying, we figured out a practice whereby I would leave her alone in the session while I stayed in the waiting room, first for just a few minutes but then graduating up to the point where she stayed alone for an entire session. From there, she was able to engage in practices of doing things alone in her daily life. Once a therapist understands the principles of formal exposure practices developed in the treatment of anxiety disorders, it is possible to import them into brief, informal exposure practices when conditioned behavioral patterns occur in sessions.

Cognitive Modification Procedures

According to cognitive mediational theory, changing intense emotions and actions requires changing the interpretations that a patient makes about reality. Effective protocols have been worked out in detail in cognitive therapies, using in-session interventions accompanied by homework practice that includes filling out worksheets and testing one's interpretations. Within the context of DBT, the same principles are applied but not usually using the worksheets and the formal homework assignments. It is already challenging enough to get these patients to do their practice assignments from their group skills training. Therefore, cognitive modification is more typically done in the moment in sessions, addressing problematic cognitions as they arise (which occurs frequently), emphasizing mindfulness of cognitions, and directly intervening with suggestions for alternative cognitions, rather than using the technique of Socratic questioning. The therapist might just intervene with a "brush stroke," such as "That's an interesting way to interpret that event." For a deep and recurring problematic cognition, such as the belief in one's own "badness," unlovability, or incompetence, the therapist is likely to orient the patient to the problem and work more deliberately within sessions to highlight the belief, challenge it, and arrive at alternative interpretations. Because of the patient's vulnerability to the experience of being invalidated, the DBT therapist might first need to validate the dysfunctional thought or belief before moving on to the standard steps of cognitive restructuring. For instance, the therapist might say, "No wonder you think all relationships will fall apart; you have had more than your share of tough endings."

Didactic and Orienting Strategies

DBT therapists are not shy about explaining things to patients in didactic terms. The therapist may share information from research or experience to enhance the patient's understanding of the nature of a problem behavior or the rationale for a treatment approach. For instance, the therapist of a patient with addictions might summarize some research about the implications of having intense cravings. Or in another case, the therapist might share research findings about the beneficial effects of mindfulness practices or exercise. Orienting strategies refer specifically to orienting the patient to what treatment will require, either DBT as a whole treatment package or the engagement in a particular change procedure or other technique. For instance, the therapist orients the patient to what is expected in skills training, exposure procedures, or cognitive modification procedures. Done effectively, orienting strengthens compliance with treatment and leads to the most effective behaviors.

Commitment Strategies

DBT therapists attend to the nature and degree of a patient's commitment to treatment goals and methods. *Commitment* does not refer to a simple on-off switch, switching from lack of commitment to a full commitment. Instead it is defined behaviorally, referring to those private and public behaviors that will help the patient succeed. Commitment can include privately stated intentions, publicly stated intentions, and actions taken in the service of the goal. The therapist assesses the variables that increase commitment in the patient and those variables that interfere with it and tries to strengthen commitment by addressing these variables. Linehan specified several specific commitment strategies to be used in this strengthening process:

1. Weighing pros and cons invites the patient to consider the advantages and disadvantages of making a commitment as well as the advantages and disadvantages of not making a commitment. This strategy helps the patient discover that making a commitment often brings long-term advantages while sacrificing short term advantages. This is similar to the interventions in motivational interviewing to increase patients' motivation to change (Miller and Rollnick 2013).
2. Highlighting the patient's freedom to choose in the absence of alternatives demonstrates that willingness to commit is a voluntary matter even if the alternative choices are not good.
3. The techniques of "door-in-the-face" and "foot-in-the-door" are used in conjunction with each other as a kind of bargaining with the patient to get the strongest possible commitment that is still realistic. In the door-in-the-face technique, the therapist asks the patient to make a commitment that may be beyond what the patient can do or will do and then to be willing to negotiate for less. In the foot-in-the-door technique, the therapist asks for a rather small commitment to which the patient can more easily consent and then ups the ante to a larger commitment.
4. In the technique of connecting present commitments to prior ones, the therapist elicits from or reminds the patient of previously made commitments that were successful for the patient as a way to draw from those successes and apply them to the current challenge.
5. Shaping, a standard contingency procedure, is used to reinforce any behaviors or features of the patient that are on the road to a stronger commitment. This could include highlighting the patient's courage, integrity, intelligence, sense of humor, or other positives, getting them to feel increasingly that they can do what is needed in treatment.
6. Devil's advocate technique is used if the therapist thinks the patient is giving lip service to commitment but does not grasp how difficult the process will be. The therapist turns the tables by saying something like, "Are you sure you want to commit to this? Do you realize how difficult it will be?" It is hoped that this will cause the patient to consider the commitment more seriously and to articulate why they need to make this commitment.

Acceptance-Oriented Techniques in DBT

Consider the following clinical example. I was assessing Kate, a 15-year-old girl with bipolar disorder and borderline personality disorder, on the first day of her admission to the psychiatric hospital after she was reported to the police by next-door neighbors. She had climbed up onto the roof of her family's house, hung onto the television antenna, and swung around while loudly singing all the songs from *West Side Story*.

Therapist: Can you tell me what you did that landed you in the hospital?

Kate: Yeah. My parents were fighting, as usual, and I couldn't stand it. So I left the house and climbed up the ladder onto the roof. And then I just started singing….

Therapist: And swinging.

Kate: Yeah. I just wanted to forget what was going on, and I love *West Side Story*.

Therapist: Were you thinking that it might be dangerous?

Kate: Not right then, but I know now that it could have been.

Therapist: Tell me more, if you can, about your decision to climb up on the roof.

Kate: My parents always fight with each other. It gets really loud until I can't stand it anymore. I just wanted to get away.

Therapist: Now that makes sense to me. It must be horrible to live with. But then what about climbing on the roof? What did you have in mind?

Kate: I just wanted to get away, and when I walked out of the house the ladder was there.

Therapist: OK, I can see how that happened. But then when you grabbed the antenna and started swinging around, and singing, what was that about?

Kate: I don't know. I just love *West Side Story* and I know all the songs, and it just kept me busy and helped me to forget that my parents were in the house fighting.

Therapist: I think I can understand it; in your mind it drowned out what your parents were doing.

Kate: Yeah, I could leave it all behind.

Therapist: Let me be clear: I think it was a terrible idea to do that. It put you in danger, and I don't want you to do it again. But at the same time, I can see your reasoning for each step. And you ended up in a hospital.

Kate: Yeah, but that might be a good thing.

Therapist: Oh yeah? How? How is it good to be in a hospital?

Kate: It might be the only way my parents will get some help, because they will have to come for meetings.

Therapist: Wow! You were thinking of all of that when you went up there?

Kate: No. But I'm thinking it now.

Therapist: You know what? You are an amazing person, really smart, and you care about your parents. Still, in spite of that, don't do it again. We can try to get your parents help.

Kate: I know. I won't.

Kate's behavior was chaotic, impulsive, and dangerous. Working with patients with these characteristics requires not only finding change-oriented solutions but also balancing that push for change with careful listening, understanding the hidden logic, and communicating acceptance for those elements in the chain that are, in a sense, valid. In Kate's case, I could validate her urge to get away from her parents' fight, to climb up the ladder that was right in front of her, to do something dramatic to help her drown out what was going on, and to see the hospitalization as a possible means for her parents to get help. To validate, which is the purest form of DBT's acceptance-oriented strategies, is to confirm and corroborate the wisdom and validity that one finds in the patient's emotions, thinking, and actions. As Linehan (1993b, p. 224) wrote, "validating a patient's response is like looking for a nugget of gold in every cup of sand."

Why validate behaviors when you find them adjacent to seriously problematic behaviors? There are several positive effects. Joining with the patient in looking for the nuggets of gold and sharing your understanding of why the patient did what they did will make them more likely to engage in treatment to change the problematic aspects. Validation communicates that you are taking the patient seriously as a meaningful and important person in their own right. Done routinely and skillfully, it strengthens the therapeutic bond—not a small accomplishment with a patient population whose treatment is known to lead to therapist burnout. Furthermore, validation is one of the most effective ways to regulate negative emotions even when looking at ways to change the chain of events. Perhaps most important of all, validation helps to confirm to the patients that they do, indeed, have the capacity for accurate perceptions, wisdom, and valid responses, in spite of a lifetime during which they have been repeatedly treated as if they do not have such capabilities. Validation provides the antidote to the invalidating environment, and the resulting self-invalidating internal environment, that these patients experience.

Validation can be communicated by explicit verbal statements, by nonverbal behaviors that communicate acceptance and compassion, and sometimes by actions that demonstrate an accurate understanding of the patient's current predicament. Common to all ways of communicating validation is the accurate recognition of what is going on and responding to the patient's predicament with the best response. We call it *functional validation.*

There are four types of targets of validation: emotions, cognitions, actions, and capabilities. To validate emotions means to take the patient's emotions very seriously, to hear the patient accurately, to seek out the causes of the emotions, and to encourage emotional expression by the patient. Many patients think that their emotions are inherently flawed and distorted; validating emotions helps to counter this cognition while also helping the patient take a closer look at the emotions. To validate cognitions emphasizes that even if cognitions are problematic, there is a reason for their existence, a history to their presence that makes them make sense. The therapist helps patients to recognize that cognitions have a life of their own and that they are interpretations of reality, not reality itself. This helps them to see that their cognitions, paradoxically, are both powerful in causing subsequent emotional and action responses and also quite insubstantial.

To validate actions means to help patients recognize the kernel of truth and wisdom in their actions even when the actions are part of a problematic sequence. This is apparent in the case of Kate. The therapist was able to find the kernels of wisdom within the chain, which probably increased Kate's willingness to acknowledge the dysfunction in other parts. A particular problem comes up if a therapist is validating some action of which the patient is ashamed. The patient is likely to reject the validating statement, to insist that they "should have done better." In these situations, the therapist may need to acknowledge and validate the patient's disappointment in their own actions and acknowledge and understand that they feel disappointed in themselves. Once this has happened, it may be possible to validate the actions as understandable given the circumstances. To validate capabilities, also known as *cheerleading* in DBT, is to find and highlight capabilities in the patient's behavior that they do not appreciate. I remember saying to a patient who was convinced that her problem behaviors were signs that she was doomed that her levels of courage and integrity and honesty were signs that she was going to succeed in her life.

Linehan articulated six levels through which therapists validate patients' behaviors. These can also be thought of as six strategies for validation. The first three levels are common to all forms of counseling and therapy, indeed probably to all good relationships. Level 1 validates through careful, "awake" listening, conveying that the patient is being taken very seriously, as a meaningful person with meaningful behaviors. Level 2 validates through reflecting back what is heard, often directly in the patient's words or with a close paraphrase. If the therapist's understanding of the patient is accurate, level 2 will indicate that to the patient. If the patient cannot confirm the accuracy of the therapist's reflection, validation is assumed not to have taken place, and the search for accurate validation continues. Validation takes place in the recipient, not in the person who delivers it. Level 3 is another type of reflection: The therapist reflects back something that the patient did not communicate verbally but may have communicated nonverbally. For instance, the therapist might reflect back to a patient that he looks sad even though he has not said so. This reflection also can be considered a type of mind-reading by the therapist.

Levels 4 and 5 are similar in that through each of them the therapist conveys that the patient's behavior—emotions, cognitions, actions—make sense to the therapist. With level 4 the therapist makes sense of the behavior by reference to the patient's particular history or biology. For instance, in the case of Kate, on the basis of the cumulative history of her parents' fights and the impact they had on her, it made sense that Kate fled the house. With level 5, the therapist finds the sense in the behavior by reference to realistic factors in the current situation that might have provoked a similar response in many people. In other words, level 5 highlights the normative aspects of the patient's behavior. Kate's therapist used a level 5 validation when suggesting to her that many people would have wanted to drown out the awareness of their parents' fighting. There is a high priority in DBT to find level 5 validations of patients as an antidote to their assumption that their behavior makes no sense.

Level 6 validation, known as *radical genuineness*, refers to the therapist's broader way of being within the relationship with the patient. If the therapist acts genuinely as who they actually are, in contrast to "acting like a therapist" with the patient, the patient is likely to feel more worthy, to feel that they are in the same class of being a human being as the therapist rather than being relegated to the "patient class." One hopes that radical genuineness is pervasive in the relationship, not just in response to certain emotions, cognitions, or actions.

Obviously, the therapist does not treat the patient's behaviors as if they are *all* valid. The problematic behaviors that are leading to bad outcomes can be seen as invalid behaviors insofar as they are obstacles to the patient's ultimate goals. Thus, the therapist uses validation for valid behaviors while invalidating invalid behaviors (pushing for change). This dance sometimes requires a good deal of agility and accuracy, validating one link in a chain and then invalidating the link adjacent to it. Perhaps most people think they already know what it is to validate, but it can be tricky. For instance, it is important to distinguish sharply between what it means to validate—

to communicate the wisdom or validity of a behavior—versus what it means to approve of a behavior or agree with it. One can validate a behavior (e.g., climbing up on a roof) without approving of it or agreeing with it.

Resolving Polarization and Conflict: Dialectical Strategies

Problem-solving strategies and validation strategies are considered the core strategy groups of DBT, one pushing insistently toward change and the other communicating understanding, acceptance, and compassion about things as they are or have been. The therapist pivots back and forth between these two paradigms—acceptance and change—again and again during a session and over time in treatment. Sticking with change strategies too much can invalidate, discourage, and aggravate a patient, who then pushes back against therapy and the therapist. Sticking with acceptance and compassion for too long, without offering ways to change the patient's situation or behavior, can generate discouragement and hopelessness. The alert therapist attuned to the evolving state of the patient will tack back and forth between change and acceptance; improvement never happens in a straight line.

Rapid movement between change and acceptance at the core of DBT, sometimes even to the point that change and acceptance are communicated simultaneously, is known as the first of the dialectical strategies, *balancing treatment* strategies. Dialectical philosophy holds the view that one force or proposition in reality will bring about its opposite. Then the opposites have come into being, each having a kernel of validity. When opposition, or polarization, is present, there is tension and conflict. The dialectical solution is to find a synthesis, a new construction that has within it the kernel of validity from both sides. Dialectical thinking is "both…and" thinking rather than "either…or" thinking. In the face of tension and conflict due to opposing forces, the dialectically based approach in DBT is to search for, or allow for the emergence of, the synthesis. Once the synthesis happens, it, too, will activate its opposite.

Given the patient population, DBT treatments are punctuated by collisions between opposing entities—often collisions between therapist and patient, as in the following examples:

Therapist: I think you need to go into a hospital.
Patient: I refuse.

or

Therapist: Can I see your diary card?
Elena: No way. I think diary cards are ridiculous.

Along with balancing treatment strategies, there are many other dialectical strategies to activate in sessions when facing polarized situations. Each of the dialectical strategies assumes that there is an unresolved conflict, that treatment is stuck as a result, and that each side of the conflict has validity. Each strategy is designed to create movement, to unbalance the standoff, and to move toward a synthesis. These strategies are not designed to accomplish the behavioral targets; they are designed to change the flow and upset the applecart temporarily so that a new equilibrium can be found. We bring each of several of the dialectical strategies to bear on the same situation, in which a patient named Elena is now unwilling to comply with the daily completion of the diary card. Let's see how the different strategies might work.

Making lemonade out of lemons helps to find the silver lining of an undesirable situation.

Therapist: Can I see your diary card?
Elena: I am not doing them anymore. They are stupid, just busywork.
Therapist: We went over why it is important in the treatment. Do you remember?
Elena: Of course! I'm no idiot. I just don't want to do them; they are tedious.
Therapist: I know they are. Actually, it's sort of perfect for you to refuse to do diary cards. After all, life is filled with "diary cards," the scut work of a job or a class at school or taking care of an apartment or a house, things that none of us like but we all have to do. Maybe if we can figure this out in relation to the diary card, you will be in good shape to handle the diary cards in your future.

Enter the paradox locates a contradiction that the patient, or the patient and therapist, find themselves in and names the contradiction without resolving it.

Therapist: So how about the diary card? Can I see it?
Elena: No. I don't do it anymore. There's no point. I told you before, I am refusing to do it.
Therapist: I don't want to try too hard to convince you to do it because you might end up doing it just to shut me up, and I don't want that. I think you should keep refusing until diary cards make sense to you. Since I believe in them, I should keep working with you to do the diary cards. It's an important conflict; let's not rush to solve it. Just keep refusing to do it until you see the wisdom in doing it, and we will talk about it each session.

Metaphor represents the opposing positions in the form of a metaphor. When the therapist and patient play with the metaphor together, movement that does not happen in ordinary discursive dialogue may be possible.

Elena: No, I still refuse to do the diary card. Don't you understand?
Therapist: Yeah, I've been thinking about it. It's like you and I are baking a cake, and the recipe lays out how we can make a fabulous cake, but you don't like following recipes because it just seems too tedious and boring.
Elena: Yeah, why don't we improvise? It's more fun that way anyway.
Therapist: Yeah, but this is the proven recipe for a great cake. I'd rather we do it right even if it's a little boring. Can't we just do the recipe right and find different ways to make it interesting? Maybe we can dance while we do the boring recipe?

Extending involves taking the patient's maladaptive behavior or intention further than they intended it to be taken, which then changes the dynamic.

Therapist: We are really stuck about this. You don't want to do the diary card. So since you don't want to do DBT, does that mean you don't want to work with me? Do we need to find you a different treatment?

Notice that these interventions do not themselves solve the problem. They focus much more on shifting the process, the balance between the opposing parties, in hopes of a new outcome, without knowing in what way it will shift. Dialectical strategies are done partly just to create movement in a tense standoff.

Elicit wise mind invites the patient to consider what their "wise mind" position would be in the current stalemate, in contrast to the current emotion mind position.

Therapist: Let me ask you something. Do you think that your refusal to do the diary card comes from emotion mind, reasonable mind, or wise mind?
Elena: I think you know it comes mostly from emotion mind. I just don't feel like doing it. But reasonable mind too, since I don't see why we have to do it.
Therapist: OK, I get that. But let me ask you something else. What do you think wise mind would do, if wise mind were in charge?
Elena: Probably just do the fucking diary card and tell you how stupid it is.

Allow natural change deals with the dilemma by just going with the forces in the conflict.

Therapist: You have been telling me for a while that you just don't see the sense in doing the diary card, which makes it a pain to do.
Elena: Right! Exactly!
Therapist: And I've been fighting you on it since from my perspective it is really valuable.
Elena: Believe me, I know what you think.
Therapist: So maybe we should just go with your point of view. Let's revise the whole diary card and the diary card system so that it makes sense to you. What do you think would work so that you can keep track of what's going on day by day and then report that to me each week?

The seven strategies covered above are most of the ones from the manual (Linehan 1993b), but after you grasp their function and the principles, you can come up with many more of your own.

Conclusion

DBT is a synthesis of techniques derived from three paradigms: change, acceptance, and dialectics. Change techniques are largely imported from cognitive-behavioral therapies, and their goal is to change behavioral patterns in a direction that matches the patient's ultimate goal to build a life worth living. Acceptance techniques are based largely on Zen mindfulness practices and empathic interventions such as those found in client-centered therapy. The function of acceptance techniques is to reduce suffering and to enhance the patient's willingness to engage in behavioral change techniques. As such, DBT is at its core a change-oriented therapy in a context of acceptance. Dialectical approaches and techniques, consistent with dialectical philosophy and inspired by family therapy models and martial arts practices, are used to create flexibility, movement, and synthesis in the face of rigid, extreme behavioral patterns and polarized relationship situations.

When doing therapy with such difficult-to-treat individuals, who are dealing with emotional intensity and high-risk situations, it is helpful to have a wide array of techniques coming from three different paradigms that supplement one another. But it is not helpful to try to think, "Which of the 85+ strategies should I use in this moment?" That is a paralyzing proposition. It is more helpful to think, in the moment, "Does this situation call for change, acceptance, or dialectics?" Once the therapist has chosen which of these three paths to take, they can then decide how to go in that direction and which techniques to use.

Key Points

- Core treatment techniques in dialectical behavior therapy (DBT) are practical applications of three underlying paradigms: behavioral change techniques, acceptance techniques, and dialectical techniques.
- The DBT therapist balances irreverence and reciprocal communication strategies, consulting to the client versus intervening in the client's environment, structural strategies defining how to conduct therapy sessions and treatment as a whole, and special treatment strategies such as dealing with suicide risk or in-session dysfunctional behaviors.
- Marsha Linehan found that problem-solving alone did not suffice in treating chronically emotionally dysregulated suicidal clients. She made a number of modifications over time, including the inclusion of acceptance and dialectics, which ultimately resulted in DBT.
- DBT's change techniques derive from four foundational frameworks out of which cognitive-behavioral therapies arose: classical conditioning, operant conditioning, cognitive mediation, and skills deficit models.
- DBT's change techniques are usually applied in a step-by-step manner using behavioral chain analysis, insight, solution analysis, didactics, orientation, and commitment.
- DBT's purest form of reality acceptance is embodied in validation strategies. Successful validation paves the way to reduced dysregulation, enhanced willingness to problem-solve, a stronger therapeutic alliance, and compassion toward self and others.
- Dialectical strategies were brought into DBT from family therapy models, martial arts practices, paradoxical thinking, and metaphor. These strategies give the therapist an arsenal of techniques that promote balance, flexibility, and the search for synthesis of opposing forces and propositions. As a result, a therapy caught in a "logjam" can be shifted and moved forward again.

References

Koerner K: Doing Dialectical Behavior Therapy: A Practical Guide. New York, Guilford, 2011

Linehan MM: Cognitive Behavioral Therapy for Borderline Personality Disorder. New York, Guilford, 1993a

Linehan MM: Cognitive Behavioral Treatment of Borderline Personality Disorder. New York, Guilford 1993b

Miller WR, Rollnick SR: Motivational Interviewing: Helping People Change. 3rd Edition. New York, Guilford, 2013

Rizvi SL: Chain Analysis in Dialectical Behavior Therapy. New York, Guilford, 2019

Swenson CR: DBT Principles in Action: Acceptance, Change, and Dialectics. New York, Guilford, 2016

CHAPTER 12

Dialectical Behavior Therapy

Efficacy, Applications, and Adaptations

Anne Sonley, M.D., FRCPC
Tali Boritz, Ph.D., C.Psych.
Shelley McMain, Ph.D., C.Psych.

Dialectical behavior therapy (DBT) was originally designed as a treatment for people at risk of suicide (Linehan 1993) and has been most extensively studied in adults with borderline personality disorder (BPD) engaging in self-harm and suicidal behaviors (Cristea et al. 2017; Stoffers et al. 2012; Storebø et al. 2020). However, a growing literature is establishing its efficacy for a wide range of other psychiatric disorders and with specific populations, such as children, adolescents, and forensic populations. In this chapter we outline promising new applications of DBT and review the evidence for its efficacy in treating various disorders and specific populations, focusing primarily on evidence from randomized controlled trials (RCTs) published in English. The studies described here were located through searches of studies in the Medline, Embase, and PsycInfo databases conducted in June 2020.

Applications of Dialectical Behavior Therapy

DBT and Borderline Personality Disorder

The efficacy of DBT for BPD has been well established. A Cochrane review in 2012 followed by an updated review in 2020 found DBT to be significantly more effective than treatment as usual (TAU) in treating BPD severity and self-harm and improving psychosocial functioning (Stoffers et al. 2012; Storebø et al. 2020). To date there have been a total of 20 RCTs comparing DBT with TAU or active comparisons. Of these RCTs, eight involved standard DBT, three involved shortened 6-month DBT, four involved skills-only DBT groups, two involved individual DBT, and three involved inpatient DBT.

Standard DBT, originally developed as an outpatient treatment for chronically suicidal women, consists of 1 year of treatment involving four modes of intervention: weekly individual therapy, weekly DBT skills group, a weekly therapist consultation team, and coaching calls between sessions as needed. There have been eight RCTs of standard 1-year DBT in adult populations with BPD; RCTs of BPD and substance use disorders are discussed in the next subsection. Three of the eight RCTs compared DBT with TAU (Feigenbaum et al. 2012 [*N*=42]; Linehan et al. 1991 [*N*=44]; Priebe et al. 2012 [*N*=40]), four compared it with an active control treatment (Clarkin et al. 2007 [*N*=90]; Linehan et al. 2006 [*N*=101]; McMain et al. 2009 [*N*=180]; Walton et al. 2020 [*N*=162]), and one was a component analysis that compared standard DBT with DBT skills training plus case management or with DBT individual therapy plus activities group (Linehan et al. 2015 [*N*=99]). In seven of these studies, participants showed significant reduction in self-harm, suicidality, BPD symptoms, or health care use with standard DBT, with the only exception being the study by Feigenbaum and colleagues, which showed no significant reduction in self-harm or health care use with standard DBT. The component analysis by Linehan and colleagues showed that standard DBT, DBT skills training plus case management, and DBT individual therapy plus activities group all resulted in significant improvements in suicide and self-harm behaviors, depression, and anxiety at 1-year follow-up; however, the DBT individual therapy plus activities group had significantly more dropouts and less improvement in acute health care use, and improvements occurred more slowly than in standard DBT (Linehan et al. 2015).

Other trials have evaluated modified forms of DBT. Two RCTs compared shortened 6-month DBT with TAU and showed significantly greater improvement in the DBT group (Carter et al. 2010 [*N*=73]; Koons et al. 2001 [*N*=20]). A third compared 5 months of DBT with acceptance and commitment therapy (ACT) or a combination of DBT, ACT, and functional analytic psychotherapy and found significant improvements in all three groups (Reyes-Ortega et al. 2020). Two RCTs compared a 20-week DBT program consisting of only a skills group (i.e., no individual therapy) with wait list or TAU (Kramer et al. 2016 [*N*=41]; McMain et al. 2017 [*N*=84]), and two RCTs compared 8- to 13-week skills groups with an active control (Lin et al. 2019 [*N*=82]; Soler et al. 2009 [*N*=59]). These four studies found decreases in BPD-related symptoms such as general psychopathology and depression. Only two of the studies measured self-harm behavior or acute health care use. Soler and colleagues found no significant group differences in self-harm or acute health care use, whereas McMain and colleagues found significant differences in self-harm but not acute health care use (McMain et al. 2017; Soler et al. 2009). Two RCTs have studied DBT in an individual therapy format (i.e., no skills group component). Turner (2000) compared 1 year of client-centered therapy versus individual DBT in 23 adults with BPD and found that patients in the DBT condition showed significant decreases in self-harm and suicide behavior and acute health care use compared with client-centered therapy. Andión and colleagues (2012) studied 37 patients randomly assigned to individual DBT and 14 patients randomly assigned to standard DBT and found no significant differences between the groups on any of the posttreatment evaluations.

Three RCTs have looked at DBT modified for inpatient settings. The two studies that compared 3 months of inpatient DBT with a waitlist control (Bohus et al. 2004 [*N*=50]; Roepke et al. 2011 [*N*=40]) found significant improvements in psychopathology in the inpatient DBT condition compared with the wait list. In a larger study comparing inpatient DBT with an active control (Sinnaeve et al. 2018 [*N*=84]), patients were randomly assigned to either 12 months of standard outpatient DBT or a step-down model involving 3 months of inpatient DBT followed by 9 months of outpatient DBT. Both groups showed significant improvements in self-harm and borderline symptoms; however, the authors concluded that the step-down condition was neither more effective nor more cost-effective than standard DBT.

DBT and Substance Use Disorders

The high rate of overlap between BPD and substance use disorders led to the development of DBT for substance use disorders (DBT-S), which is tailored to address the unique characteristics associated with substance abuse, including high rates of treatment attrition and intense physiological and psychological triggers. Adaptations from standard DBT include additional strategies to address problems related to treatment engagement, dialectical methods to enhance motivation to eliminate substance misuse, and a modified target hierarchy that prioritizes a focus on substance use. Patients are trained in skills to address common addictive behaviors such as denial, craving, and urges to manage cues to substance use and to enhance community reinforcers. DBT-S has also been examined for the treatment of individuals with substance use disorders and comorbid conditions other than BPD.

To date, two RCTs have evaluated the efficacy of DBT-S in patients with comorbid substance use disorders and BPD, one has evaluated standard DBT in this population, and one has evaluated online DBT-S in patients with substance use disorders and comorbid conditions other than BPD. These four trials are reviewed below. Most were delivered in an outpatient format, provided therapy for 1 year, and excluded individuals with severe comorbid mental illness such as a psychotic disorder, bipolar I disorder, significant cognitive impairment, or traumatic brain injury.

The two RCTs that examined DBT-S in patients with BPD were conducted by Marsha Linehan, the developer of both DBT and DBT-S. In the first RCT (Linehan et al. 1999), participants were randomly assigned to receive 1 year of either DBT-S (*n*=12) or community TAU (*n*=16). Treatment retention was significantly higher in the DBT-S group: 64% compared with 27% of the TAU group. Over the 12 months of treatment and at a 16-month follow-up, patients in the DBT-S group showed lower levels of drug use compared with the TAU group, and at follow-up, they scored better on measures of social functioning and global adjustment. In a similar small-scale RCT conducted a few years later (Linehan et al. 2002), patients with BPD and opioid dependence were randomly assigned to 1 year of either DBT-S (*n*=11) or comprehensive validation therapy augmented by a 12-step facilitation intervention (CVT+12-step; *n*=12). The latter treatment, which was drawn from Project MATCH (Matching Alcoholism to Treatment to Client Heterogeneity; Nowinski et al. 1999), included weekly individual therapy and a weekly therapist consultation meeting. Additionally, patients were encouraged to attend 12-step meetings. This study involved a dismantling of DBT's two core strategies, validation and behavioral change, and was designed to test the effects of validation. Treatment retention was lower in the DBT-S group, with four patients (36.4%) withdrawing versus none in the CVT+12-step group. Both groups showed significant reductions in opioid use over the first 8 months of treatment, but over the past 4 months, the CVT+12-step group showed significant increases in opioid use, whereas the DBT-S group maintained their reduced use. At the end of treatment, the DBT-S group showed lower symptom distress and better social and global functioning.

In the only RCT of DBT conducted in this population that was independent of the treatment developer, Verheul et al. (2003) examined the effectiveness of standard DBT (i.e., not DBT-S) in an outpatient sample in the Netherlands in women with BPD, some but not all of whom had comorbid substance dependence. Patients were randomly assigned to receive DBT (n=27) or TAU (n=31). The DBT group was superior with respect to treatment retention (63% vs. 23%) and reduction of self-mutilating behaviors, self-damaging impulsive behaviors, and alcohol problems; however, there were no group differences with respect to reduction of drug use.

Wilks et al. (2018) conducted the only trial of DBT delivered virtually. Individuals with suicidal ideation and problematic alcohol use were randomly assigned to an internet-based DBT (i-DBT) skills training group (n=30) or a waitlist control (n=29). The 8-week i-DBT intervention consisted of 30- to 50-minute sessions that included a didactic presentation and an interactive and guided practice focusing on teaching mindfulness, emotion regulation, and distress tolerance skills. Compared with the waitlist group, the i-DBT group showed greater reductions in alcohol consumption and a lower rate of heavy episodic drinking.

DBT and Eating Disorders

DBT has been widely implemented in clinical settings for the treatment of eating disorders, including binge-eating disorder (BED) and bulimia nervosa (BN). This has been driven partly by the theoretical conceptualization that emotional dysregulation problems underlie eating disorder behaviors (Lavender et al. 2015) and partly by the high rate of overlap (21%) between BN and BPD (Cassin and von Ranson 2005).

Adaptations of DBT for BED have amassed the most evidence. Three RCTs randomly assigned patients to either wait list or a 20-session DBT skills group that was modified to address BED symptoms (Dastan et al. 2019 [N=40]; Rahmani et al. 2018 [N=60]; Telch et al. 2001 [N=44]). All three studies reported significant improvements in the DBT arm. A fourth RCT (Safer et al. 2010) compared a 20-week DBT for BED skills group with a supportive therapy group (N=101). The DBT group showed a faster response to treatment and had a lower dropout rate (4% vs. 33%); however, there were no significant group differences in binge-eating behaviors at 12-month follow-up. A subsequent secondary analysis found that people with an earlier age at onset of eating disorder symptoms and those with comorbid avoidant personality disorder achieved better outcomes in the DBT arm (Robinson and Safer 2012). Self-help DBT has also been shown to be helpful for treating BED. In a study by Masson and colleagues (2013), 60 patients were randomly assigned to either wait list or to guided self-help using a DBT-BED skills manual; significant improvements were reported in the DBT arm. In a study by Carter and colleagues (2020), 73 patients were randomly assigned to 12 weeks of guided self-help with a DBT-BED skills manual, unguided self-help with the same manual, or unguided self-help with a self-esteem manual. All three groups showed significant improvements in BED symptoms, with large effect sizes.

Two RCTs looked at DBT adaptations for the treatment of BN. Both included people with subthreshold BN (one episode a week of binging and purging rather than two), with about 80% of participants meeting the full criteria for BN. The first of these (Safer et al. 2001) randomly assigned patients ($N=31$) to either a wait list or 20 sessions of individual psychotherapy aimed at teaching emotion regulation skills to reduce binge eating and purging. The other (Hill et al. 2011) randomly assigned patients ($N=32$) to either a wait list or 12 individual sessions aimed at teaching appetite awareness techniques and DBT skills. In both studies, the DBT adaptations resulted in significantly greater improvement in binge-eating and purging behaviors.

Two RCTs examined DBT adaptations in mixed BN and BED samples. Klein et al. (2013) compared two different types of a modified 16-week DBT program—one that included a skills group with coaching calls and one that included a diary card condition—in people with either BED ($n=25$) or BN ($n=11$). Subjects in both treatment groups showed decreases in binge eating, but the decreases were significantly greater in the DBT skills group condition. Chen et al. (2017) randomly assigned individuals with either BED ($n=78$) or BN ($n=31$) who had not previously responded to 4 weeks of guided self-help cognitive-behavioral therapy (CBT) to either in-person CBT or DBT. There were no significant group differences in terms of overall treatment response, but there was a medium effect on vomiting frequency in the DBT group versus no effect in the CBT group.

DBT and PTSD

Two adapted forms of DBT have been developed for the treatment of comorbid BPD and PTSD: Dialectical Behavior Therapy Prolonged Exposure (DBT PE) and dialectical behavior therapy for posttraumatic stress disorder (DBT-PTSD). DBT PE is an evidence-based PTSD treatment that includes in vivo exposure to feared situations, imaginal exposures to trauma memories, and trauma processing (i.e., in-depth discussion of the past trauma) (Foa et al. 2007); in DBT PE, developed by Melanie Harned, PE is added to DBT. In a pilot RCT that compared DBT PE with standard DBT in 26 female patients with BPD, PTSD, and recent self-injury (Harned et al. 2014), both treatments showed significant reduction in suicide attempts and nonsuicidal self-injury (NSSI) behaviors, but patients who completed the DBT PE protocol were twice as likely as those in standard DBT to achieve diagnostic remission from PTSD at posttreatment (80% vs. 40%). At 3-month follow-up, remission rates had decreased to 60% and 0%, respectively. Among treatment completers, moderate to large effect sizes favored DBT PE for improvements in dissociation, trauma-related guilt cognitions, shame, anxiety, depression, and global functioning.

DBT-PTSD is a modular treatment developed by Martin Bohus and colleagues that integrates DBT with trauma-focused cognitive and exposure-based interventions, as well as with specific techniques from compassion-focused therapy (Gilbert 2010) and ACT (Hayes 2016). In one RCT, 74 female inpatients with PTSD related to childhood sexual abuse were randomly assigned to either a 12-week residential DBT-PTSD program or a TAU wait list (TAU-WL; Bohus et al. 2013). The DBT-PTSD patients showed significantly larger reductions in PTSD symptoms, problems with global social functioning, and depression compared with participants in the TAU-WL condition, but there were no significant group differences in general symptom severity, dissociative experiences, or borderline symptoms. A second RCT evaluated an adaptation of DBT-PTSD in an outpatient setting compared with cognitive processing therapy (CPT; Bohus et al. 2020), an evidence-based treatment for PTSD. Participants were 193 women with PTSD related to childhood trauma who also met at least three DSM-5 criteria for BPD (American Psychiatric Association 2013). In both groups, participants showed improvement in PTSD symptoms (pre-post effect sizes $d=1.35$ for DBT-PTSD and $d=0.98$ for CPT), with a small but significant effect favoring the DBT-PTSD group. Both groups showed decreases in the duration of dissociation, but participants in the DBT-PTSD group also showed a significant decline in the intensity of dissociative symptoms and demonstrated greater reductions in BPD symptoms.

DBT and Mood Disorders

DBT has been studied as an adjunctive treatment for both major depressive disorder (MDD) and bipolar disorder. To date, there have been three RCTs of skills-only DBT for treating MDD. Harley et al. (2008) randomly assigned patients with treatment-resistant depression ($N=24$) to either a 16-week DBT skills group or to a wait list and found that the skills group participants had significantly greater improvements in depressive symptoms, with large effect sizes. In the other two studies, depressed older adults were randomly assigned to approximately 6 months of either medication management alone or medication management with a DBT skills group. One of these two studies (Lynch et al. 2003 [$N=34$]) found that significantly more patients in the DBT group achieved remission, but the other (Lynch et al. 2007 [$N=37$]) found no significant difference between the groups. Of note, participants in the second study had at least one personality disorder and had not responded to antidepressant medication in an initial 8-week open trial. Radically Open DBT (RO-DBT), an adaptation of DBT for disorders characterized by excessive self-control, has also been studied in people with treatment-resistant MDD (Lynch et al. 2020 [$N=250$]). In this large study, there was a significant difference between TAU and RO-DBT in terms of depressive symptoms posttreatment, but not at 6- and 12-month follow-up. An economic analysis of this treatment did not support it as cost-effective (Shearer et al. 2019).

There have been three RCTs of modified DBT as an adjunctive treatment for bipolar disorder. Goldstein et al. (2015) randomly assigned 20 adolescents with bipolar disorder (DSM-IV type I, II, or not otherwise specified; American Psychiatric Association 1994) to 1 year of either TAU or a modified DBT treatment comprising 18 individual sessions and 18 skills training sessions including family members. Patients in the DBT group demonstrated significant improvements in depressive symptoms and decreases in suicidal ideation as well as more weeks of euthymia; however, there were no between-group differences in manic symptoms. Van Dijk et al. (2013) randomly assigned 26 adults with type I or II bipolar disorder to either a 12-week DBT skills group or a waitlist control. In that study, participants in the DBT arm showed increased mindfulness and control over emotional states. Zargar and colleagues (2019) randomly assigned 50 adults with bipolar I disorder to medication management alone or medication management with a 12-week DBT skills group. Manic symptoms were significantly reduced in participants in the DBT condition compared with the control condition, but depressive symptoms were not significantly different. Finally, Afshari and colleagues (2020) randomly assigned 60 patients with type I or II bipolar disorder to wait list or a 12-session DBT skills group and found significant improvement in mania, depression, and emotional dysregulation in the DBT group posttreatment.

DBT and ADHD

DBT skills groups have also been studied as an adjunctive treatment for ADHD. In one RCT, 51 adults with ADHD who were stable in terms of medication management were randomly assigned to 14 weeks of either a DBT skills group or a discussion group (Hirvikoski et al. 2011). Only those in the DBT group showed a significant reduction in ADHD symptoms by the end of the study. In another RCT, 34 college students with ADHD, most of whom were being treated with medication, were randomly assigned either to attend an 8-week DBT skills group or to receive skills handouts (Fleming et al. 2015). Those in the DBT skills group condition showed significantly greater treatment response rates and clinical recovery rates in ADHD symptoms.

DBT and Special Populations

DBT in Forensic and Correctional Populations

Given the prevalence of personality disorders in individuals in forensic and correctional settings, the emphasis in DBT on skills to modulate strong emotions and behaviors, and the individualized approach of DBT to problem-solving tailored to criminogenic behaviors, there has been interest in examining the potential benefits of DBT for these populations.

Three RCTs have examined the efficacy of DBT in individuals in prison, on parole, or on probation. Rosenfeld et al. (2019) enrolled 109 adults who were in a criminal justice diversion program after being charged with stalking-related offenses and randomly assigned them to DBT modified for stalkers (n=57) or CBT for anger management (n=52). The 24-week DBT intervention consisted of once-weekly individual therapy sessions, a weekly 90-minute skills group, and phone consultation as needed. The CBT-based intervention consisted of 18 weekly 1-hour sessions that targeted anger management. Recidivism rates were assessed through renewed stalking, violent behaviors, and other offenses assessed at baseline and over a 1-year follow-up. Outcomes were measured via self-report questionnaires and criminal justice service records of renewed charges and arrests. The study results showed no significant differences between the groups. The overall treatment retention rate was good and did not differ between groups (71.93% for DBT; 78.85% for CBT). The rates of reoffense in both groups was small; the DBT group showed a slightly superior but nonsignificant benefit. There was no evidence to justify the implementation of DBT with this population, given the failure to find superiority of DBT and given its greater resource intensity and length.

Another RCT examined the clinical effectiveness of a DBT case management program for homeless women who had recently been released from incarceration (Nyamathi et al. 2017, 2018). This program was brief, consisting of six weekly group sessions and six individual treatment sessions, including coping skills to address substance use and employment. Participants were randomly assigned to DBT case management (n=65) or to a health promotion program (n=65). The DBT therapists included community health workers and nurses trained to deliver the intervention. Between-group comparisons at 6-month follow-up showed that recidivism was lower in the DBT group compared with the health promotion group (RR=0.59, 95% CI –0.26 to –1.35, P=0.208; Nyamathi et al. 2018), with the effect greater in those individuals who had a higher desire for help. DBT group participants also showed higher rates of abstinence from drug use (65.5% vs. 48.3%) and showed increased alcohol abstinence at 6 months.

A third RCT examined the effectiveness of DBT for women in a medium-security prison in the United States who had a history of sexual and physical abuse (Bradley and Follingstad 2003). Participants were randomly assigned to either 18 sessions of DBT skills training plus writing assignments (n=24) or a no-contact control (n=25). There were significant between-group differences favoring the DBT group on interpersonal functioning, depressive symptoms, and trauma symptoms (e.g., intrusive experiences, anxious arousal, dissociation, anger, impaired self-reference). The average pre-post effect sizes for the treatment group ranged from medium to large effects, whereas for the control group, they ranged from average to small effects.

DBT has also been widely implemented in forensic settings. One small randomized trial (N=21) examined the effectiveness of DBT in a forensic inpatient setting for men diagnosed with BPD (Bianchini et al. 2019). Participants were randomly assigned to 12 months of standard DBT as an adjunct to the therapeutic milieu or to the milieu setting only. Those receiving DBT showed greater improvement on impulsivity score and difficulties in emotion regulation; however, there were no differences between the groups in alexithymia.

Tomlinson and Hoaken (2017) conducted a randomized controlled (wait list) pre-follow-up crossover trial (N=15) of 6 months of DBT skills training with men in a medium-secure forensic psychiatric setting in Canada. They found no statistically significant changes between DBT and TAU groups on measures in the first 6 months. However, when DBT groups were combined, results showed a significant decrease in hostility in the first 6 months of DBT and in the 6 months following DBT.

DBT in Children and Adolescents

DBT has been modified specifically for adolescents (DBT-A). This form of DBT is typically briefer (approximately 16–19 weeks) and includes skills training delivered in a family format. To date, five RCTs have evaluated the effects of DBT-A, mostly in patients with high suicidality. All but one study were conducted in an outpatient setting, and all excluded participants with psychotic disorders, cognitive impairment, low intellectual functioning, and (with the exception of one study) bipolar disorder. Studies have been conducted in Norway, the United States, Spain, and Australia.

The first RCT of DBT-A for suicidal adolescents was a well-designed trial carried out in a public health care setting in Oslo, Norway (Mehlum et al. 2014). Multiproblem adolescents with chronic self-harm behaviors (*N*=77), ranging in age from 12–18 years, were randomly assigned to 19 weeks of either DBT-A (*n*=39) or an enhanced usual care condition (*n*=38). Treatment retention in both groups was good. At the end of treatment, DBT-A participants showed superior reductions in the frequency of self-harm behavior, suicidal ideation, and depression and continued to show superior reductions in self-harm behaviors at 1- and 3-year follow-ups. Postdischarge, there were no between-group differences on other outcomes because the enhanced usual care group caught up to the DBT-A group (Mehlum et al. 2016, 2019). Of note, the effects of DBT-A on self-harm reductions were mediated by decreases in hopelessness.

McCauley et al. (2018) enrolled 173 adolescents (95% female) ranging in age from 12 to 18 years who had one prior lifetime suicide attempt and elevated suicide ideation. Participants were randomly assigned to either DBT or a manualized treatment, involving individual and group supportive therapy, which is based on a client-centered approach and emphasizes connection and belongingness. Primary outcomes included reductions in suicide attempts, NSSI behaviors, and self-harm. The DBT group showed superior outcomes on all primary outcomes at end of treatment (6 months); however, the benefits of DBT had weakened and were no longer significant at final 12-month follow-up.

Santamarina-Perez et al. (2020) randomly assigned a sample of suicidal adolescents ages 12–18 years who were enrolled in a community outpatient program in Barcelona to 16 weeks of either DBT (*n*=18) or TAU plus group sessions (TAU+GS; *n*=17). Whereas DBT-A typically includes patients and their family members together in the skills training sessions, in this trial, the patients and family members attended these sessions separately. Primary outcomes, assessed at pretreatment and at 4, 8, 12, and 16 weeks of treatment, were suicidal self-injurious behavior and suicide attempts. Intent-to-treat analyses showed that the DBT-A group had superior outcomes to the TAU+GS group on the frequency of NSSI behavior (Cohen's *d*=0.73; medium effect), mean antipsychotic dosage, and global functioning (Cohen's *d*=1.26; large effect).

Growing interest in DBT for young people led to the modification of DBT for children with severe emotional dysregulation problems (Perepletchikova et al. 2017). DBT for children (DBT-C) incorporates the standard modes of DBT (individual therapy, skills training, phone coaching calls, therapist consultation team), and also includes parent training. The treatment consists of 32 weekly 90-minute sessions divided into child counseling, parent training, and skills training with both parties. One RCT has investigated DBT-C in preadolescent children with disruptive mood dysregulation disorder (Perepletchikova et al. 2017). Children ages 7–12 years were randomly assigned to receive either DBT-C (*n*=21) or a TAU psychosocial control condition with medication management (*n*=22). No participants in the DBT-C group dropped out of treatment prematurely, in contrast to 36.4% who dropped out of the TAU group. Compared with the TAU group, the DBT-C group showed a superior positive response on the Children's Global Assessment Scale (90.4% vs. 45.5%), had superior overall remission rates (52.4% versus 27.3%), and had a higher level of functioning that was seen at 32 weeks (after treatment) and maintained at 3-month follow-up. However, in this study, treatment was delivered free of charge to participants in the DBT-C but not the TAU group, which is a key confound.

DBT skills training has been evaluated as a mental health prevention intervention for school-age children and adolescents, and although the data are meager, they confirm some positive trends. In an Australian study (Burckhardt et al. 2018), 96 tenth-grade high school students ages 14–16 years were randomly assigned to either DBT skills intervention ($n=50$) consisting of 5 hours of workshops (6×50 minutes) that covered the four DBT skills modules (emotion regulation, mindfulness, distress tolerance, and interpersonal relationships) or a control condition that involved attending their usual classes ($n=46$). Assessments of emotion regulation, depression, anxiety, and anger were conducted at baseline, postintervention, and 6-month follow-up. There were no significant between-group differences on any postbaseline outcomes. However, an examination of qualitative data revealed that 74% of DBT participants reported positive benefits such as improved emotion regulation and getting less angry.

Katz et al. (2020) conducted a cluster-randomized (by school) trial to examine the efficacy of DBT skills training as a mental health prevention intervention in two Canadian cities. The sample consisted of 995 students across 40 third- to twelfth-grade classrooms. The intervention was delivered by trained classroom teachers and involved DBT skills (three lessons per each of the four skills modules) and mental health literacy. There were significant differences favoring the intervention schools compared with the control schools on self-concept, coping skills, and social support across the school year. The effect sizes were large for the intervention schools on all measures ($g=1.00$–1.39).

Emerging Evidence for DBT Adaptations in Other Specific Populations

In addition to the adaptations summarized previously, there have been promising preliminary RCTs investigating the use of DBT as an adjunctive treatment in several other populations, including patients with trichotillomania (Keuthen et al. 2012), multiple sclerosis (Blair et al. 2017), heart disease (Tavakoli et al. 2019), and obesity (Cancian et al. 2019). Additional RCTs in these areas are warranted.

Key Points

- Dialectical behavior therapy (DBT) was initially designed for treating suicidal behaviors and self-harm and has been most extensively studied in adults with borderline personality disorder (BPD). A Cochrane review recently updated in 2020 found DBT to be effective in treating BPD severity and self-harm and in improving psychosocial functioning.
- Modified forms of DBT have also been studied. Shortened 6-month DBT, skills group–only DBT, and individual-only DBT may be effective in reducing some BPD symptoms. There is some evidence that inpatient DBT may lead to symptom improvement; however, one larger trial has suggested that it is neither more effective nor more cost-effective than standard outpatient DBT.
- There is evidence that DBT-S for treating substance use is associated with improvements in drug and alcohol use, impulsivity, and self-harm behaviors and increases in treatment retention and social and general functioning.

- Modified DBT skills groups are more effective than waitlist for treating binge eating disorder and bulimia nervosa.
- Patients with comorbid BPD and PTSD can benefit significantly from DBT treatments that specifically target their PTSD symptoms.
- There is mixed evidence as to whether DBT skills groups may be an effective adjunctive treatment for depression. One large trial has suggested that Radically Open DBT is not effective or cost-effective for treatment-resistant depression. Modified DBT may be effective as an adjunctive treatment for certain symptoms of bipolar disorder.
- DBT skills training shows promise as an adjunctive treatment for ADHD symptoms.
- DBT shows promise for improving recidivism risk behaviors in individuals in forensic and correctional settings.
- DBT adapted for children shows promise based on preliminary evidence from one RCT. For adolescents, the results of several small RCTs provide support for the efficacy of DBT-A.
- Further RCT evidence is needed in support of the use of modified DBT for patients with trichotillomania, multiple sclerosis, heart disease, and obesity.

References

Afshari B, Omidi A, Ahmadvand A: Effects of dialectical behavior therapy on executive functions, emotion regulation, and mindfulness in bipolar disorder. J Contemp Psychother 50:123–131, 2020

American Psychiatric Association: Diagnostic and Statistical Manual of Mental Disorders, 4th Edition. Washington, DC, American Psychiatric Association, 1994

American Psychiatric Association: Diagnostic and Statistical Manual of Mental Disorders, 5th Edition, Arlington, VA, American Psychiatric Association, 2013

Andión Ó, Ferrer M, Matali J, et al: Effectiveness of combined individual and group dialectical behavior therapy compared to only individual dialectical behavior therapy: a preliminary study. Psychotherapy (Chic) 49(2):241–250, 2012 22642527

Bianchini V, Cofini V, Curto M, et al: Dialectical behaviour therapy (DBT) for forensic psychiatric patients: an Italian pilot study. Crim Behav Ment Health 29(2):122–130, 2019 30648303

Blair M, Ferreria G, Gill S, et al: Dialectical behavior group therapy is feasible and reduces emotional dysfunction in multiple sclerosis. Int J Group Psychother 67(4):500–518, 2017

Bohus M, Haaf B, Simms T, et al: Effectiveness of inpatient dialectical behavioral therapy for borderline personality disorder: a controlled trial. Behav Res Ther 42(5):487–499, 2004 15033496

Bohus M, Dyer AS, Priebe K, et al: Dialectical behaviour therapy for post-traumatic stress disorder after childhood sexual abuse in patients with and without borderline personality disorder: a randomised controlled trial. Psychother Psychosom 82(4):221–233, 2013 23712109

Bohus M, Kleindienst N, Hahn C, et al: Dialectical behavior therapy for posttraumatic stress disorder (DBT-PTSD) compared with cognitive processing therapy (CPT) in complex presentations of PTSD in women survivors of childhood abuse: a randomized clinical trial. JAMA Psychiatry 77(12):1235–1245, 2020 32697288

Bradley RG, Follingstad DR: Group therapy for incarcerated women who experienced interpersonal violence: a pilot study. J Trauma Stress 16(4):337–340, 2003 12895016

Burckhardt R, Manicavasagar V, Shaw F, et al: Preventing mental health symptoms in adolescents using dialectical behaviour therapy skills group: a feasibility study. Int J Adolesc Youth 23:70–85, 2018

Cancian ACM, de Souza LAS, Liboni RPA, et al: Effects of a dialectical behavior therapy-based skills group intervention for obese individuals: a Brazilian pilot study. Eat Weight Disord 24(6):1099–1111, 2019 29197947

Carter GL, Willcox CH, Lewin TJ, et al: Hunter DBT project: randomized controlled trial of dialectical behaviour therapy in women with borderline personality disorder. Aust N Z J Psychiatry 44(2):162–173, 2010 20113305

Carter JC, Kenny TE, Singleton C, et al: Dialectical behavior therapy self-help for binge-eating disorder: a randomized controlled study. Int J Eat Disord 53(3):451–460, 2020 31821592

Cassin SE, von Ranson KM: Personality and eating disorders: a decade in review. Clin Psychol Rev 25(7):895–916, 2005 16099563

Chen EY, Cacioppo J, Fettich K, et al: An adaptive randomized trial of dialectical behavior therapy and cognitive behavior therapy for binge-eating. Psychol Med 47(4):703–717, 2017 27852348

Clarkin JF, Levy KN, Lenzenweger MF, et al: Evaluating three treatments for borderline personality disorder: a multiwave study. Am J Psychiatry 164(6):922–928, 2007 17541052

Cristea IA, Gentili C, Cotet CD, et al: Efficacy of psychotherapies for borderline personality disorder: a systematic review and meta-analysis. JAMA Psychiatry 74(4):319–328, 2017 28249086

Dastan B, Zanjani S, Adl A, et al: The effectiveness of dialectical behaviour therapy for treating women with obesity suffering from BED: a feasibility and pilot study. Clinical Psychologist 24(2):133–142, 2019

Feigenbaum JD, Fonagy P, Pilling S, et al: A real-world study of the effectiveness of DBT in the UK National Health Service. Br J Clin Psychol 51(2):121–141, 2012 22574799

Fleming AP, McMahon RJ, Moran LR, et al: Pilot randomized controlled trial of dialectical behavior therapy group skills training for ADHD among college students. J Atten Disord 19(3):260–271, 2015 24874347

Foa EB, Hembree E, Rothbaum B: Prolonged Exposure Therapy for PTSD: Emotional Processing of Traumatic Experiences, Therapist Guide (Treatments That Work Series). New York, Oxford University Press, 2007

Gilbert P: An introduction to compassion focused therapy in cognitive behavior therapy. Int J Cogn Ther 3(2):97–112, 2010

Goldstein TR, Fersch-Podrat RK, Rivera M, et al: Dialectical behavior therapy for adolescents with bipolar disorder: results from a pilot randomized trial. J Child Adolesc Psychopharmacol 25(2):140–149, 2015 25010702

Harley R, Sprich S, Safren S, et al: Adaptation of dialectical behavior therapy skills training group for treatment-resistant depression. J Nerv Ment Dis 196(2):136–143, 2008 18277222

Harned MS, Korslund KE, Linehan MM: A pilot randomized controlled trial of dialectical behavior therapy with and without the dialectical behavior therapy prolonged exposure protocol for suicidal and self-injuring women with borderline personality disorder and PTSD. Behav Res Ther 55:7–17, 2014 24562087

Hayes SC: Acceptance and commitment therapy, relational frame theory, and the third wave of behavioral and cognitive therapies—republished article. Behav Ther 47(6):869–885, 2016 27993338

Hill DM, Craighead LW, Safer DL: Appetite-focused dialectical behavior therapy for the treatment of binge eating with purging: a preliminary trial. Int J Eat Disord 44(3):249–261, 2011 20196109

Hirvikoski T, Waaler E, Alfredsson J, et al: Reduced ADHD symptoms in adults with ADHD after structured skills training group: results from a randomized controlled trial. Behav Res Ther 49(3):175–185, 2011 21295767

Katz J, Mercer SH, Skinner S: Developing self-concept, coping skills, and social support in grades 3–12: a cluster-randomized trial of a combined mental health literacy and dialectical behavior therapy skills program. School Ment Health 12:323–335, 2020

Keuthen NJ, Rothbaum BO, Fama J, et al: DBT-enhanced cognitive-behavioral treatment for trichotillomania: a randomized controlled trial. J Behav Addict 1(3):106–114, 2012 26165460
Klein AS, Skinner JB, Hawley KM: Targeting binge eating through components of dialectical behavior therapy: preliminary outcomes for individually supported diary card self-monitoring versus group-based DBT. Psychotherapy (Chic) 50(4):543–552, 2013 24295464
Koons CR, Robins CJ, Lindsey Tweed J, et al: Efficacy of dialectical behavior therapy in women veterans with borderline personality disorder. Behav Ther 32:371–390, 2001
Kramer U, Pascual-Leone A, Berthoud L, et al: Assertive anger mediates effects of dialectical behaviour-informed skills training for borderline personality disorder: a randomized controlled trial. Clin Psychol Psychother 23(3):189–202, 2016 25864773
Lavender JM, Wonderlich SA, Engel SG, et al: Dimensions of emotion dysregulation in anorexia nervosa and bulimia nervosa: a conceptual review of the empirical literature. Clin Psychol Rev 40:111–122, 2015 26112760
Lin TJ, Ko HC, Wu JYW, et al: The effectiveness of dialectical behavior therapy skills training group vs. cognitive therapy group on reducing depression and suicide attempts for borderline personality disorder in Taiwan. Arch Suicide Res 23(1):82–99, 2019 29528807
Linehan MM: Cognitive-Behavioral Treatment of Borderline Personality Disorder: Diagnosis and Treatment of Mental Disorders. New York, Guilford, 1993
Linehan MM, Armstrong HE, Suarez A, et al: Cognitive-behavioral treatment of chronically parasuicidal borderline patients. Arch Gen Psychiatry 48(12):1060–1064, 1991 1845222
Linehan MM, Schmidt H III, Dimeff LA, et al: Dialectical behavior therapy for patients with borderline personality disorder and drug-dependence. Am J Addict 8(4):279–292, 1999 10598211
Linehan MM, Dimeff LA, Reynolds SK, et al: Dialectical behavior therapy versus comprehensive validation therapy plus 12-step for the treatment of opioid dependent women meeting criteria for borderline personality disorder. Drug Alcohol Depend 67(1):13–26, 2002 12062776
Linehan MM, Comtois KA, Murray AM, et al: Two-year randomized controlled trial and follow-up of dialectical behavior therapy vs therapy by experts for suicidal behaviors and borderline personality disorder. Arch Gen Psychiatry 63(7):757–766, 2006 16818865
Linehan MM, Korslund KE, Harned M, et al: Dialectical behavior therapy for high suicide risk in individuals with borderline personality disorder: a randomized clinical trial and component analysis. JAMA Psychiatry 72(5):475–482, 2015 25806661
Lynch TR, Morse JQ, Mendelson T, et al: Dialectical behavior therapy for depressed older adults: a randomized pilot study. Am J Geriatr Psychiatry 11(1):33–45, 2003 12527538
Lynch TR, Cheavens JS, Cukrowicz KC, et al: Treatment of older adults with co-morbid personality disorder and depression: a dialectical behavior therapy approach. Int J Geriatr Psychiatry 22(2):131–143, 2007 17096462
Lynch TR, Hempel RJ, Whalley B, et al: Refractory depression—mechanisms and efficacy of radically open dialectical behaviour therapy (RefraMED): findings of a randomised trial on benefits and harms. Br J Psychiatry 216(4):204–212, 2020 31317843
Masson PC, von Ranson KM, Wallace LM, et al: A randomized wait-list controlled pilot study of dialectical behaviour therapy guided self-help for binge eating disorder. Behav Res Ther 51(11):723–728, 2013 24029304
McCauley E, Berk MS, Asarnow JR, et al: Efficacy of dialectical behavior therapy for adolescents at high risk for suicide: a randomized clinical trial. JAMA Psychiatry 75(8):777–785, 2018 29926087
McMain SF, Links PS, Gnam WH, et al: A randomized trial of dialectical behavior therapy versus general psychiatric management for borderline personality disorder. Am J Psychiatry 166(12):1365–1374, 2009 19755574
McMain SF, Guimond T, Barnhart R, et al: A randomized trial of brief dialectical behaviour therapy skills training in suicidal patients suffering from borderline disorder. Acta Psychiatr Scand 135(2):138–148, 2017 27858962
Mehlum L, Tørmoen AJ, Ramberg M, et al: Dialectical behavior therapy for adolescents with repeated suicidal and self-harming behavior: a randomized trial. J Am Acad Child Adolesc Psychiatry 53(10):1082–1091, 2014 25245352

Mehlum L, Ramberg M, Tørmoen AJ, et al: Dialectical behavior therapy compared with enhanced usual care for adolescents with repeated suicidal and self-harming behavior: outcomes over a one-year follow-up. J Am Acad Child Adolesc Psychiatry 55(4):295–300, 2016 27015720

Mehlum L, Ramleth RK, Tørmoen AJ, et al: Long term effectiveness of dialectical behavior therapy versus enhanced usual care for adolescents with self-harming and suicidal behavior. J Child Psychol Psychiatry 60(10):1112–1122, 2019 31127612

Nowinski J, Baker S, Carroll K: Twelve Step Facilitation Therapy Manual: A Clinical Research Guide for Therapists Treating Individuals With Alcohol Abuse and Dependence. Project MATCH Monograph Series, Vol 1. Rockville MD, National Institute on Alcohol Abuse and Alcoholism, 1999. Available at: https://pubs.niaaa.nih.gov/publications/projectmatch/match01.pdf. Accessed September 7, 2021.

Nyamathi AM, Shin SS, Smeltzer J, et al: Achieving drug and alcohol abstinence among recently incarcerated homeless women: a randomized controlled trial comparing dialectical behavioral therapy-case management with a health promotion program. Nurs Res 66(6):432–441, 2017 29095374

Nyamathi A, Shin SS, Smeltzer J, et al: Effectiveness of dialectical behavioral therapy on reduction of recidivism among recently incarcerated homeless women: a pilot study. Int J Offender Ther Comp Criminol 62(15):4796–4813, 2018 30058395

Perepletchikova F, Nathanson D, Axelrod SR, et al: Randomized clinical trial of dialectical behavior therapy for preadolescent children with disruptive mood dysregulation disorder: feasibility and outcomes. J Am Acad Child Adolesc Psychiatry 56(10):832–840, 2017 28942805

Priebe S, Bhatti N, Barnicot K, et al: Effectiveness and cost-effectiveness of dialectical behaviour therapy for self-harming patients with personality disorder: a pragmatic randomised controlled trial. Psychother Psychosom 81(6):356–365, 2012 22964561

Rahmani M, Omidi A, Asemi Z, et al: The effect of dialectical behavior therapy on binge eating, difficulties in emotion regulation and BMI in overweight patients with binge-eating disorder: a randomized controlled trial. Ment Health Prev 9:13–18, 2018

Reyes-Ortega MA, Miranda EM, Fresán A, et al: Clinical efficacy of a combined acceptance and commitment therapy, dialectical behavioural therapy, and functional analytic psychotherapy intervention in patients with borderline personality disorder. Psychol Psychother 93(3):474–489, 2020 31246370

Robinson AH, Safer DL: Moderators of dialectical behavior therapy for binge eating disorder: results from a randomized controlled trial. Int J Eat Disord 45(4):597–602, 2012 21500238

Roepke S, Schröder-Abé M, Schütz A, et al: Dialectic behavioural therapy has an impact on self-concept clarity and facets of self-esteem in women with borderline personality disorder. Clin Psychol Psychother 18(2):148–158, 2011 20187169

Rosenfeld B, Galietta M, Foellmi M, et al: Dialectical behavior therapy (DBT) for the treatment of stalking offenders: a randomized controlled study. Law Hum Behav 43(4):319–328, 2019 31204832

Safer DL, Telch CF, Agras WS: Dialectical behavior therapy for bulimia nervosa. Am J Psychiatry 158(4):632–634, 2001 11282700

Safer DL, Robinson AH, Jo B: Outcome from a randomized controlled trial of group therapy for binge eating disorder: comparing dialectical behavior therapy adapted for binge eating to an active comparison group therapy. Behav Ther 41(1):106–120, 2010 20171332

Santamarina-Perez P, Mendez I, Singh MK, et al: Adapted dialectical behavior therapy for adolescents with a high risk of suicide in a community clinic: a pragmatic randomized controlled trial. Suicide Life Threat Behav 50(3):652–667, 2020 31944371

Shearer J, Lynch TR, Chamba R, et al: Refractory depression—cost-effectiveness of radically open dialectical behaviour therapy: findings of economic evaluation of RefraMED trial. BJPsych Open 5(5):e64, 2019 31352916

Sinnaeve R, van den Bosch LMC, Hakkaart-van Roijen L, et al: Effectiveness of step-down versus outpatient dialectical behaviour therapy for patients with severe levels of borderline personality disorder: a pragmatic randomized controlled trial. Borderline Personal Disord Emot Dysregul 5:12, 2018 30002832

Soler J, Pascual JC, Tiana T, et al: Dialectical behaviour therapy skills training compared to standard group therapy in borderline personality disorder: a 3-month randomised controlled clinical trial. Behav Res Ther 47(5):353–358, 2009 19246029

Stoffers JM, Völlm BA, Rücker G, et al: Psychological therapies for people with borderline personality disorder. Cochrane Database Syst Rev (8):CD005652, 2012 22895952

Storebø OJ, Stoffers-Winterling JM, Völlm BA, et al: Psychological therapies for people with borderline personality disorder. Cochrane Database Syst Rev 5(5):CD012955, 2020 32368793

Tavakoli F, Kazemi-Zahrani H, Sadeghi M: The effectiveness of dialectical behavior therapy on adherence to treatment and self-caring behavior in patients with coronary heart disease. ARYA Atheroscler 15(6):281–287, 2019 32206072

Telch CF, Agras WS, Linehan MM: Dialectical behavior therapy for binge eating disorder. J Consult Clin Psychol 69(6):1061–1065, 2001 11777110

Tomlinson MF, Hoaken PNS: The potential for a skills-based dialectical behavior therapy program to reduce aggression, anger and hostility in a Canadian psychiatric sample: a pilot study. Int J Forensic Ment Health 16:215–226, 2017

Turner RM: Naturalistic evaluation of dialectical behavior therapy-oriented treatment for borderline personality disorder. Cognit Behav Pract 7:413–419, 2000

Van Dijk S, Jeffrey J, Katz MR: A randomized, controlled, pilot study of dialectical behavior therapy skills in a psychoeducational group for individuals with bipolar disorder. J Affect Disord 145(3):386–393, 2013 22858264

Verheul R, Van Den Bosch LMC, Koeter MWJ, et al: Dialectical behaviour therapy for women with borderline personality disorder: 12-month, randomised clinical trial in The Netherlands. Br J Psychiatry 182:135–140, 2003 12562741

Walton CJ, Bendit N, Baker AL, et al: A randomised trial of dialectical behaviour therapy and the conversational model for the treatment of borderline personality disorder with recent suicidal and/or non-suicidal self-injury: an effectiveness study in an Australian public mental health service. Aust N Z J Psychiatry 54(10):1020–1034, 2020 32551819

Wilks CR, Lungu A, Ang SY, et al: A randomized controlled trial of an internet delivered dialectical behavior therapy skills training for suicidal and heavy episodic drinkers. J Affect Disord 232:219–228, 2018 29499504

Zargar F, Haghshenas N, Rajabi F, et al: Effectiveness of dialectical behavioral therapy on executive function, emotional control, and severity of symptoms in patients with bipolar I disorder. Adv Biomed Res 8:59, 2019 31673532

PART IV

Interpersonal Psychotherapy

Section Editor: John C. Markowitz, M.D.

Interpersonal psychotherapy (IPT) is a proven but underutilized psychotherapy. Developed more than 40 years ago, this manualized brief treatment has been tested in more than 100 clinical trials, with generally positive results that have led to its inclusion in treatment guidelines for mood disorders, eating disorders, and, most recently, PTSD. A fairly straightforward psychotherapy (as psychotherapies go), IPT focuses on the patient's life circumstances, emotional responses, and connections. It is an affect-focused rather than a cognitive-behavioral therapy. In helping patients to understand, accept, and use their affective responses to handle difficult interpersonal situations, IPT builds self-reflection, social skills, and crucial social support while relieving the target disorder.

Patients and therapists who become acquainted with IPT tend to like it, and most patients improve with IPT treatment. Nonetheless, IPT has been underused. For years it was a highly successful research treatment with little dissemination into community practice. Only in the past 10–15 years, building on that strong research base, has it finally begun to spread. The growing International Society of Interpersonal Psychotherapy (ISIPT; https://interpersonalpsychotherapy.org) holds biennial meetings, runs an active listserv, and certifies IPT trainers and supervisors.

In Part 4 of this textbook, the chapter authors do not provide the technical detail that an IPT treatment manual does, but the three chapters do cover important aspects of IPT and offer a general introduction to the approach. The authors address the theories behind the treatment (although IPT has always leaned more heavily on practical outcome than theory), its therapeutic techniques, and its clinical applications. These chapters should give the reader a good sense of the richness and efficiency of this potent, practical therapy.

CHAPTER 13

Theories of Interpersonal Therapy

Ilana Lipsitz-Odess, Ph.D.
Joshua D. Lipsitz, Ph.D.
John C. Markowitz, M.D.

Man is by nature a social animal.

—Aristotle, *Politics*

Interpersonal theory focuses on the patient as a social being interacting with others. This differs from many other psychological approaches that target intrapsychic phenomena. Several psychological theories can be classified as *interpersonal* because of their focus on interpersonal experience. The major theories among the many interpersonal approaches include attachment theory (Bowlby 1969), psychoanalytic object relations theories (Klein 1964; Winnicott 1965), and social learning theory

---

Joshua D. Lipsitz, Ph.D., was a clinical psychologist noted in his field, a prolific author of many and diverse journal publications. He maintained an affiliation with the Columbia University/New York State Psychiatric Institute Anxiety Disorders Clinic in New York City and subsequently was a tenured Professor at Ben Gurion University in Israel, where he was a beloved teacher and mentor. Josh had a special interest in interpersonal psychotherapy (IPT) and helped develop a paradigm to treat social anxiety with IPT. He introduced IPT in Israel and trained many therapists. Sadly, Josh was diagnosed with brain cancer and passed away (at age 55) in 2017, leaving behind a family and the vast work he contributed to the field of IPT. His daughter, Ilana Lipsitz-Odess, following in his footsteps, has completed her doctorate in clinical psychology. Together with Dr. John Markowitz, Josh's longtime colleague, they collaborated on this chapter, based on previous chapters on IPT theory Josh had authored.

(Bandura and Walters 1963). In this chapter we review the historical evolution of interpersonal theory and the major interpersonal approaches, with emphasis on the unique perspective of interpersonal psychotherapy (IPT; Klerman et al. 1984; Weissman et al. 2018).

Historical Evolution of Interpersonal Theory

Interpersonal theory can be seen as the joining of two streams of thought: the emerging disciplines of the social sciences and the clinical approach to patients and their problems. The fusion of these two streams produced an interpersonal outlook, a novel conceptualization of human behavior and psychopathology. In the early 1900s, developing theories of social psychology, sociology, and cultural anthropology began to focus on psychological health and illness, offering a radically different perspective from Kraepelin's (1919/1971) medical psychiatry or Freud's (1915–1916/1961) drive theory. For example, Emile Durkheim (1897/1951), a founder of sociology, examined the prevalence of suicide and concluded that anomie, or social disconnection, placed some social groups at higher risk of suicide than others. This laid a foundation for the implication that strong social ties help people survive periods of change and tumult in society.

At about the same time, the psychologist William James (1890/1950) proposed that human beings have a wide range of instincts, including play, curiosity, and sociability. George Herbert Mead (1913) posited that the individual was a product of the social environment. Charles Cooley's theory of social subjectivity went even further in seeing society and the individual as virtually inseparable (Cooley 1902/1983). The psychiatrist Adolf Meyer initiated the integration of these emerging disciplines into an interpersonal clinical theory, and Harry Stack Sullivan later expanded this into a comprehensive clinical theory.

The Psychobiology of Adolf Meyer

Meyer was a leading figure in American psychiatry in the first half of the twentieth century. He espoused an integrative approach to psychopathology, which he called *psychobiology*, also referred to as the genetic-dynamic approach (Meyer 1951). This concept combined the traditional medical psychiatry of Kraepelin with the broader perspectives of psychology and social science. Meyer insisted that he was interested in "the function of the total person" (Meyer 1951). His approach differed from Kraepelin's narrowly biological approach and Freud's rigid focus on drives and intrapsychic conflict. Meyer accepted that psychopathology occurred within the biological organism, but he dramatically widened the field of view by emphasizing how the organism adapted to its environment. In line with social Darwinism, Meyer believed that the social-interpersonal environment is the most important locus of the individual's adaptation.

From the early years of his clinical work, Meyer emphasized the significance of detailed empirical observation, another influence of the pragmatist school. His observations attended with equal precision to biological and psychosocial factors. One of

Meyer's most prominent contributions was the detailed life chart he introduced, highlighting chronological life events from the patient's history, incorporating both biological and psychosocial components. Another contribution was his recognition of the importance of the physician-patient relationship (Meyer 1951), setting the stage for the concept of the therapeutic alliance. Meyer's integrative model later became the basis for IPT's integrative model (Weissman et al. 2000).

Interpersonal Theory of Harry Stack Sullivan

Harry Stack Sullivan (1892–1949), the most influential figure in the development of the interpersonal theory of psychopathology, is often credited with bridging the gap between psychiatry and social science. Raised Irish Catholic in a largely Protestant area of upstate New York, he experienced prejudice and ostracization from his peers. Later in life he continued to experience feelings of loneliness and isolation. These experiences shaped Sullivan's views and helped him appreciate the prominent role of broader social forces in psychological distress (Perry 1982).

Sullivan was strongly influenced by Meyer's psychobiology but found his thinking limited in its focus on interpersonal factors from the individual's perspective. Whereas Meyer presented an interpersonally informed alternative to the psychoanalysis of Freud, Sullivan revolutionized psychoanalysis itself, creating an entirely new interpersonal approach to psychoanalytic work. Another strong influence on Sullivan's thinking was his close contact with members of the Chicago School of philosophy and social science, such individuals as George Herbert Mead, Charles Cooley, and Edward Sapir. Through these influences, Sullivan sought insights into the makeup and effects of the social system to which the individual adapts.

Sullivan (1953) concluded that human beings are intrinsically and unavoidably interpersonal. Sullivan did not believe the need for interpersonal relations is secondary to more basic biological needs; rather, he believed that it is the individual's most basic and important need. Mental health thus depends on healthy connections to other people. Psychopathology is, at its core, the study of human relationships. This approach, which remains an influential strain within psychoanalysis to this day, focuses on relationships rather than drives as the most fundamental aspect of human experience.

Karen Horney's Interpersonal Theory

Karen Horney was greatly influenced by Sullivan but had some revolutionary advances of her own. Horney (1967) presented the first feminist challenge to psychoanalysis, emphasizing the importance of societal and cultural roles rather than inherent psychological differences between men and women. Horney was the first psychiatrist to develop a comprehensive interpersonal personality typology (Horney 1950). In contrast to Sullivan and others who saw personality as dynamic and constantly influenced by different relationship experiences, Horney believed that personality is mainly stable and self-perpetuating after adolescence. This view influenced interpersonal theory toward fixed interpersonal personality patterns. Although Sullivanian and Horneyan therapies have faded as historical movements, the theories remain the basis for much of treatment today.

Kaiser Group

Hubert Coffee and colleagues from the Kaiser Foundation Psychology Research Project transformed existing interpersonal theories into a contemporary system of classification (Freedman et al. 1951; Leary 1957) for assessing and quantifying personality change during psychotherapy. One of the most important contributions was the interpersonal circle, measuring interpersonal experience across two axial dimensions: control-power (ranging from dominance to submission) and affiliation (ranging from hostility to affection) (Freedman et al. 1951; Leary 1957). These interpersonal classification systems formed the basis of some interpersonal personality models that remain prevalent.

Interpersonal Theory of Psychopathology

Sullivan's Theory

Harry Stack Sullivan (1949, 1953) developed the interpersonal theory of personality and psychopathology. Sullivan saw psychological symptoms and distress as intertwined with personality such that even in an optimally developed personality, problems could cause or signal signs of psychopathology. Thus, Sullivan developed an interpersonal developmental theory accentuating the significance of early interpersonal experience.

For Sullivan, the developing infant has two sets of needs. The first set involves the need for satisfaction, which initially relates to basic biological needs such as hunger. As the infant develops, however, satisfaction pertains with equal valence to emotional-relational needs. Sullivan organized the developmental phases around the specific emotional needs of each phase. From infancy to early childhood, the child seeks attachment-like needs from adults (e.g., the need for a parent to witness and approve of their activities). From ages 4 to 8 years, the child seeks competition and cooperation from playmates; from age 8 to adolescence, the youth seeks a "chum," a close friend and confidant; and from adolescence onward, the individual seeks romantic intimacy. Decades before Bowlby's elaborated attachment theory, Sullivan observed that the child's prolonged period of dependency magnified the importance of the social environment in satisfying basic needs, thus increasing the importance of the "mothering one" and her reactions for development.

Psychopathology

Psychopathology, according to Sullivan, is more closely tied to a second need, the need for security. The individual requires a sense of safety and competence in the interpersonal sphere, especially in response to the looming threat of interpersonal anxiety. For Sullivan, anxiety does not stem from frustration of biological needs but rather arises in the interpersonal relationship, namely, through the mother's (contagious) experience of anxiety. The mother's anxiety may be a response to the infant's behavior, but it may also be unrelated to the infant and its needs. The intense investment in this relationship passes the mother's anxiety on to the infant and assumes great importance. For Sullivan, this contagious anxiety lies at the core of psychopathological development. Its derivative negative emotions thus have their origin in the emotional atmosphere in the earliest interactions.

In response to the need for security, the individual implements *security operations*, loosely related to Freud's defense mechanisms. When behavior receives a positive response from the mother, associated feelings are experienced as a desirable part of the self (*good me*). An anxious maternal reaction may lead to the child's experiencing internal feelings as undesirable (*bad me*) or even untenable (*not me*). These feelings are dissociated, leading to personality dysfunction. Common security operations include selective inattention (the tendency to avoid noticing certain things to avoid feeling anxious), sublimation, and obsessionalism.

Importance of Social Roles

Influenced by the work of Mead and Cooley, Sullivan emphasized the importance of social roles and reactions of others in shaping the individual. Sullivan described the self as made up of *reflected appraisals*. Thus, not only interpersonal behavior per se, but also the person's place within the social environment, is important. In contrast to social psychology, which emphasized the impact of society in general and social institutions, Sullivan's approach focused on close individual relationships: the nuclear family, the extended family, the peer group, and the workplace.

Schizophrenia and the Therapeutic Community

Sullivan's clinical work focused on schizophrenia. For many years, he ran a schizophrenia ward in the Sheppard and Enoch Pratt Hospital in Maryland. Sullivan saw schizophrenia as essentially a disorder in ability to relate to other people. He believed schizophrenia could be reversed with proper psychotherapy aimed at integrating cut-off aspects of the patient's internal life. Sullivan argued that even the most bizarre psychotic content made sense when considered within the interpersonal context of the patient's life. If schizophrenia was an interpersonal disorder, it followed that the patient's condition would be influenced by social factors, including those of their current hospital surroundings. Therefore, Sullivan paid attention to many details in the overall social milieu for patients. This later came to be called the *therapeutic community*.

The goal of therapy, according to Sullivan, is to help the patient improve negative interpersonal patterns and integrate dissociated aspects of personality. Primary goals are to identify and elucidate interpersonal patterns in which distortions occur and to explore the origins of this interpersonal experience in interactions with significant people of the past. Identifying negative patterns involves analyzing patterns of communication and subtleties of language. For Sullivan, clinical observation is most keenly focused on interpersonal patterns as they emerge and are analyzed within the therapeutic relationship.

Therapist Stance

An essential component of Sullivan's theory concerns the therapist's role within the therapy or psychiatric interview. On the one hand, Sullivan felt it was important for the therapist to assume the role of expert. This would inspire the patient's respect in the clinician's competence and confidence and motivate the patient to continue the therapeutic process. However, this expert role does not imply aloofness on the part of the therapist. The therapist is a participant-observer in the relationship. Sullivan saw the therapeutic relationship as akin to any other relationship, in which all interactions are reciprocal and in which the therapist's own personal qualities and unconscious material would necessarily influence interactions. This contrasted with the then-prevailing psychoanalytic view that the therapist should try to remain objective ("a blank screen") by keeping his or her own personal psychological baggage out of the therapy. Sullivan also challenged the passive therapist stance commonly used to facilitate free association. Because Sullivan was interested in real events and real interactions (in addition to unconscious processes), he advocated the use of direct inquiry.

Object Relations

The British school of object relations, another influential strain within psychoanalysis, also identified human relationships as the most important arena of human experience and the primary focus of psychotherapy. As the term *object* suggests, this involves a more abstract view of internal representations of the other person and the patient within the relationship. Early theorists of this school, such as Melanie Klein (1964), tied their thinking closely to Freud's drive theory and focused predominantly on imagined-representative relationships within fantasy rather than on real relationships. However, some later adherents gave greater emphasis to real relationships. W.R.D. Fairbairn (1952), for example, suggested that personality problems arise when the infant's needs for attachment encounter absent, intrusive, or chaotic parents. Not unlike interpersonal psychoanalysis, an object relations therapy approach might examine both external relationships and the therapeutic relationship to uncover faulty internal templates and eventually ameliorate problematic interpersonal patterns. Given the understanding that detrimental effects derive from deficiencies in early nurturing, D.W. Winnicott (1965) proposed that psychotherapy may serve as a *corrective emotional experience* in which the therapist, through a caring, empathic relationship, helps compensate for lack of nurturance in earlier relationships.

Attachment and Loss

John Bowlby, whose background was in psychoanalytic object relations, is most responsible for making the concept of attachment prominent in typical and atypical development. Bowlby saw attachment as a complex, biologically determined system designed to keep the caregiver in close proximity. He observed that youngsters often seek out parents as a safe haven in times of distress and that attachment serves as a base from which to launch goal-oriented behaviors. A secure attachment early in life forms a foundation for later success in interpersonal relationships. Although the survival function of attachment is most acute in infancy, the system remains essential through the course of life in providing individuals with warmth, nurturance, and protection through relationships. In the object relational tradition, Bowlby emphasized *internal working models* that the child develops on the basis of early experiences. These models guide expectations and thus interpersonal behaviors in future relationships.

One insight into the importance of attachment came from observing what happens when the youngster is separated from the caretaker. Building on observations of Rene Spitz and Katherine Wolf (Spitz and Wolf 1946) and his own systematic observations of children separated from caretakers, Bowlby (1969) described a predictable and devastating sequence of emotional responses. First the separated infant would *protest*, a stage characterized by overt distress and increased motor activity; this was followed by *despair*, which involved crying and reduced motor activity; and finally, the infant showed *detachment*, withdrawing and seeming to lose interest in other people.

Bowlby saw emotional difficulties as originating from early disturbances in attachment: all anxiety is at its core anxiety about separation. Bowlby's work was later expanded by Ainsworth (1979) and colleagues, who conceptualized different *attachment styles* with which individuals approached and negotiated relationships. These internal templates were determined by the success or failure of early attachment experiences. They included secure, anxious-ambivalent, and avoidant attachment styles that would influence the quality of later adult relationships.

Real Relationships Versus Intrapsychic Factors

Both Sullivan's interpersonal psychoanalysis and the object relations approaches established interpersonal relationships as the primary subject matter for their respective psychotherapeutic work, differing from classic intrapsychic approaches. To varying degrees, these approaches focus attention on the patient's real relationships outside therapy. They all see internal factors—in the form of such elements as experiential residue, object representation, internal working models, and attachment styles—as determinants of real interpersonal problems. Thus, the patient's internal life and the role of early childhood experiences that determine it become the foci of the therapeutic work.

An individual may meet a new colleague and experience themself as helpless and flawed and the colleague as unrealistically powerful. This reflects the internal experience, which may have originated because of early contacts with a controlling parent. This internal template creates expectations and causes the individual to attend to some features of the interaction and not others. These internal factors also contribute to the real relationship unfolding in a certain way. For example, this individual might be overly deferential to the new colleague. The colleague, influenced by this behavior as well as their own internal experiences, may respond by acting more like a supervisor than a colleague. These psychoanalytic approaches would dismiss the superficial handling of an interpersonal predicament as being unlikely to have any lasting benefit for the patient.

From Interpersonal Theory to IPT

Interpersonal Theory of Depression

Of the various psychotherapies developed from interpersonal theory, IPT is by far the most studied (Cuijpers et al. 2016; Klerman et al. 1984). IPT is a time-limited, diagnosis-focused, present-centered treatment, initially developed to treat major depressive disorder. This unique approach was created in the context of important developments in the understanding of depression and the impact of interpersonal factors on this disorder. Interpersonal and object relational psychoanalytic approaches conceptualized depression as a fluid outgrowth of (dysfunctional) personality development. Sullivan himself related depression to repetitive patterns and internal vulnerabilities and rejected the depressed patient's attempts to tie their depression to a contemporaneous external event (Sullivan 1940). Cohen and colleagues (1954), of the interpersonal school, suggested that severe depression stems from a parent who resisted the child's striving for independence and excessively pressured the child to achieve. This led to dependency on the parent and alienation from peers, who are seen as competitors. Others (Fairbairn 1952; Klein 1964) theorized that depression results from early experiences of intense anger toward the frustrating but all-important internalized representation of the mother. This anger engenders feelings of ambivalence, guilt, helplessness, and, ultimately, depression.

Interpersonal Problem Areas in IPT

IPT organizes the therapeutic work around a central interpersonal problem area in the patient's life. In acute treatment for depression, the potential focal problem areas are grief, role disputes, role transition, and role deficits. In the following subsections, we briefly examine the conceptual basis for linking depression to these overall areas of interpersonal life, first by presenting an interpersonal link to depression and then by connecting it to an interpersonal problem area.

Bereavement and Depression

In "Mourning and Melancholia," Freud (1917 [1915]/1957) highlighted specific differences between grief reactions and clinical depression in the context of other obvious similarities. Lindemann's (1994) careful description of a large sample of bereaved individuals as having somatic distress, preoccupation with the deceased, guilt, and anger (all common depressive symptoms) further reinforced the association between bereavement and clinical depression. At the same time, Paykel et al.'s (1969) study showed that although bereavement was a common stressor prior to depression, most people who experience bereavement do not subsequently become depressed. Similarly, Clayton (1982) found that a preponderance of bereaved women do not go on to develop clinical depression. However, specific factors (e.g., younger age) make it more likely for clinical depression to occur among those who are bereaved. Depression may also be more likely to occur among bereaved individuals with poor social support (Maddison and Walker 1967).

IPT problem area: grief. On the basis of epidemiological data, IPT's developers found that bereavement is a potential precursor of clinical depression. Clinical depression that develops following the death of a significant other is evidence that the normal grief process has not taken its course. This means that these individuals are having an atypical, delayed or prolonged grief reaction. In these cases the work of IPT is to help the patient experience the normal grief process. IPT for grief differs from IPT for other problem areas in its substantially internal focus, at least in the initial stages. The goal is to resolve a problem in a real relationship. However, the relationship is with the deceased, and resolution means working through the grief reactions, letting go, and moving on.

Marriage and Depression

Weissman and Paykel (1974) identified interpersonal factors that characterize depressed women. They that found marital and family difficulties are the most prominent feature distinguishing these women. Furthermore, they found that these difficulties often persist after the depression improves, suggesting that the difficulty is not simply an effect of the patient's depressed mood. Marital difficulties were also associated with later depression in Brown and Harris's (1978) sample. Subsequent research supported the association between marital discord and depression (Downey and Coyne 1990; Hammen 2003; Hooley and Teasdale 1989). Although there is some evidence that depression may engender marital problems, evidence suggests that external factors (e.g., the depressed individual's spouse's personality issues) also contribute to marital difficulties.

IPT problem area: role dispute. A role dispute can occur in any important relationship. Disputes with life partners provide a compelling and clinically ubiquitous model of the potentially devastating and pervasive effects of a role dispute.

Stressful Life Events and Depression

When IPT was conceived, a growing body of evidence associated recent stressful life events with onset of depression. Thus, it was not necessary to trace internal distress and vulnerability to adverse experiences in infancy as in interpersonal psychoanalysis. Distress could arise from painful or challenging experiences in adulthood. Paykel et al. (1969), for example, noted that certain types of events are more frequently reported prior to onset of depression. These particularly include *exit events*, such as death of a loved one or separation from a spouse, and *negative events* such as physical illness, work problems, or sexual difficulties. Brown and Harris (1978) observed that stressful life events were associated with depression in working-class women.

Much research on stressful life events and depression has been conducted since IPT was first formulated (Hammen 2005). This more than 40-year interval has made evident the challenges and limitations of life events research. Some research indicated that a significant proportion of life events are themselves associated with genetic factors (Kendler and Karkowski-Shuman 1997) or other personal factors (Hammen 2006). Stressful life events seem more prominent in relation to the first episode of depression than to subsequent episodes (Kendler et al. 2000). However, the overall evidence from this now extensive body of research confirms that life events—particularly events of loss and separation—are associated with onset of depression (Paykel 2003). This complexity does not particularly affect IPT because the approach does not presume that stressful events "cause" depression, merely that illness episodes and life events are linked in individuals vulnerable to developing depression.

IPT problem area: role transition. Although specific stressful experiences are relevant to other IPT problem areas in the broadest sense (see next subsection), adjusting to stress and change in the social context requires a role transition. This might be the case in depression following such events as college graduation, birth of a child, retirement, medical illness, or divorce.

Social Support and Depression

One important contribution of Brown and Harris (1978) was their consideration of lasting features of the social context, including positive, potentially buffering features of this context, in determining whether depression would occur. In their study of working class women, lack of a close confidante was a strong risk factor for later depression. Around this time, Henderson and colleagues' (1978) pioneering work identified the association between weak social bonds or a poor social support network and neurosis (much of which was depression). Since then, numerous studies have identified a link between absence of perceived social support and depressive symptoms (Duer et al. 1988; Monroe et al. 1986). Here too, there are methodological challenges, and causal pathways are not entirely clear. Social support may buffer the effects of adversity, or it may constitute an independent positive factor important to psychological health (Overholser and Adam 1997). Conversely, loneliness itself may be a risk factor for depression (Dill and Anderson 1999; Green et al. 1992).

IPT problem area: interpersonal deficits. In this problem area, the patient's primary problem is identified as being a paucity of social connections. Relationships buffer against stressful life events and are important for psychological well-being. Attention to social support and a positive social network is a component of work in all the focal IPT problem areas. In role transition, the individual may need to renegotiate or start new relationships in order to obtain needed support within the new role. In role disputes, the individual may need to reach out positively to others—aside from the other person in the dispute—to help get through the dispute.

Impact of Depression on Interpersonal Relationships

Many clinicians have recognized that interacting with depressed patients often affects other people, including the therapist. Although depression initially may evoke sympathy, its excessive dependency and helplessness sometimes leave others frustrated or angry, which may cause them to withdraw from the depressed person. Some commentators have taken a decidedly unsympathetic view of the depressive mode of interacting, interpreting this as evidence of veiled hostility (Bonime 1976).

Coyne (1976) proposed an interactional theory of depression in which the depressed individual seeks reassurance from others close to them but is unable to accept this reassurance. This creates a vicious cycle of excessive reassurance seeking by the depressed person and increased frustration and irritation in friends and family, leading ultimately to these others distancing themselves from the depressed individual. This increases isolation and decreases social connections for the depressed person, which helps to maintain the depressive state. A more behavioral theory by Lewinsohn (1974) proposes that depressed persons lack the necessary social skills to meet their needs for social warmth and approval. Therapy would then involve helping these patient develop social skills sufficient to achieve their interpersonal needs.

Interpersonal Contexts Within a Diathesis-Stress Model

Interpersonal contexts have become increasingly prominent in understanding psychopathology. However, most individuals who experience stressful life events will not develop psychiatric disorders, meaning that circumstantial interpersonal contexts cannot fully explain causation of these disorders. Accumulating evidence has demonstrated that genetic and biological factors play a significant role in the etiology of various psychiatric disorders. The diathesis-stress (or vulnerability-stress) perspective fills this gap by viewing both external, environmental factors and internal, constitutional (including biological) factors as contributory. As the developers of IPT stated:

"Genetics, early life experience, environmental stress, and personality combine in complex ways to produce the etiology and pathogenesis of depression. These factors will operate in different degrees for individual patients" (Klerman et al. 1984, p. 38).

A vast amount of evidence has supported a diathesis-stress model as a general epidemiological approach to medical disease, among which is a range of disorders (Hankin and Abela 2005), including major depression. Research has begun to illustrate how environmental and biological factors interact and alter vulnerability and the course of psychiatric disorders (Caspi et al. 2003; Mitchell et al. 2014). Interpersonal factors such as stressful life events alone cannot explain the etiology of psychopathology such as major depression, but they can help to explain why, in the context of biological and other vulnerabilities, a depressive episode might develop at a specific time, persist longer, or recur sooner. Because diathesis factors are less resilient to psychological change, IPT focuses on the stress side of this framework: contextual interpersonal factors that precipitate and sustain psychiatric illness.

Interpersonal Problem as Framework and Change Process

IPT focuses on a core current interpersonal crisis in the patient's life, and the resolution of this crisis through the central interpersonal change process is the goal of therapy (Weissman et al. 2018). IPT targets helping the patient understand their feelings in interpersonal situations not as being negative or problematic but as informative to the interpersonal encounter. The therapy then uses these feelings to organize an appropriate interpersonal response, improving the handling of relationships. Most other individual therapy models identify the issue within the patient and seek to change some problematic aspect of the patient's personality, patterns, attachment styles, and so on. In contrast, IPT identifies the issue in the interpersonal context and does not attempt to fix a problem in the patient; rather, the goal is to assist the patient in fixing the problem in the interpersonal context and their relationship to this problem. This approach will help the patient solve the predicament and recover from the psychiatric disorder.

How does resolving the interpersonal problem alleviate psychiatric symptoms? Lipsitz and Markowitz (2013) proposed four mechanisms of change in IPT: enhancing social support, decreasing interpersonal stress, processing emotions, and improving interpersonal skills. Change can also occur via two additional mechanisms, mentalization and attachment.

Enhancing Social Support

Each IPT interpersonal problem area reflects a difficulty in the patient's environmental context and current social functioning that disrupts and undermines social support. Role disputes reflect conflict in a primary relationship, which may compromise the social support from this relationship. Role transitions (e.g., divorce, retirement, illness) are life changes that interfere with or interrupt established social ties. Grief denotes the loss of a primary social tie that previously may have provided support, belonging, and social value. Grief also may leave the individual emotionally distanced from others who do not share this grief, impeding development of alternative, compensatory ties. Interpersonal deficits reflect general isolation and lack of interpersonal connection and support. In all of these cases, resolving the interpersonal problem at hand entails meaningfully improving social support for the patient.

In its focus on resolving a specific interpersonal problem as a means of enhancing social support, IPT differs from supportive therapy (e.g., Pinsker 2002) and from systematic social support interventions, which seek to directly engender support more globally. IPT further differs from some relational psychoanalytic therapies (e.g., Winnicott 1965), which view supportive *holding* as a primary function of the therapist, believing that this will ultimately improve the patient's internal emotion regulation. IPT views the therapeutic relationship as an important transitional source of social support; however, it emphasizes this time-limited role and uses the therapeutic relationship as a springboard to develop, strengthen, renew, and deepen outside relationships. The therapist actively encourages the patient to develop supportive relationships outside therapy and helps the patient engage with and rely more on others through communication analysis and role-play.

Decreasing Interpersonal Stress

Each IPT interpersonal problem area constitutes an interpersonal stressor for the patient; hence, a primary goal is to reduce the patient's stress experienced in this context. Grief (death of a loved one) is among the most stressful life events (Holmes and Rahe 1967). IPT facilitates the grieving process so that the patient emotionally processes this loss and it gradually becomes less distressing. Role transitions strain the individual's existing modes of adaptation, as the earliest definition of stress suggests (Selye 1955). This may also occur with seemingly positive events, such as marriage, the birth of a baby, starting college, or a promotion. IPT seeks to help the patient reduce the stress of the transition by acknowledging and mourning losses, clarifying positive and negative aspects, identifying and processing strong feelings about the transition, and modifying interpersonal patterns. For role disputes, IPT attempts to lessen stress associated with ongoing friction, anger, shame, helplessness, and alienation that may occur in a discordant relationship. In interpersonal deficits, lessening the stress of loneliness and isolation (Cacioppo and Hawkley 2003) becomes the primary goal. IPT views the interpersonal problem itself as the primary culprit for current feelings of stress by changing stressful aspects of this reality or the patient's relationship to it.

Processing Emotions

Interpersonal losses, changes, and conflicts generate varied, powerful emotions that individuals with depression and other psychiatric disorders may have difficulty tolerating, understanding, and expressing (Markowitz and Milrod 2011). Like psychodynamic psychotherapy, IPT is an affect-focused treatment. The individual in a role dispute, feeling frustrated and angry, may need help accepting the legitimacy and appropriateness of these feelings; understanding their interpersonal meaning (e.g., anger often means someone is bothering you, failing to respond to you); and then expressing them, perhaps initially in sessions and role-plays with the therapist and later directly to the object of conflict. Someone experiencing a role transition, such as adjusting to a serious illness, may need to mourn the old role and adjust emotionally to the new role by increasing awareness;, acceptance; and ability to express uncomfortable feelings of sadness, anger, shame, and guilt. The therapist seeks to help the patient first acknowledge the presence and depth of these feelings, then verbalize them in an interpersonal encounter, all the while accepting their legitimacy, validity, and social utility. In complicated grief, emotional processing may be a central thrust of IPT as the patient needs help working through the loss before they can reinvest in existing connections or establish new ones. In interpersonal deficits, the novel experience of sharing and expressing uncomfortable emotions with the therapist may be an important first step in allowing openness and comfort in other relationships.

Improving Interpersonal Skills

IPT seeks to improve interpersonal skills primarily within the framework of the focal interpersonal problem area. In a role dispute, this may include learning to communicate feelings more directly, using constructive assertiveness, or learning to defuse tension. In role transitions, IPT focuses on skills needed to better adapt to the new interpersonal role. For a patient dealing with an illness, this may involve expressing their needs to others or setting limits with a caring but intrusive caretaker. For a retiree, this may include learning to initiate social contacts and activities. In grief, interpersonal skills may include independent functions previously managed by the deceased. Communication skills may play a more central role in interpersonal deficits, for which a range of skills might be needed to overcome social isolation.

Mentalization

Markowitz et al. (2019) proposed an additional underlying change mechanism in IPT. Mentalizing is the capacity to understand that mental processes such as thoughts, feelings, and wishes influence one's own and other people's behavior. Although not mentioned in the IPT manual, IPT may use mentalization as an underlying process for therapeutic change. IPT focuses on helping patients develop or renew social relationships by strengthening the patient's ability to understand the motives of significant others. IPT uses the emotions that arise in difficult situations and relationships to analyze communication patterns and then use role-playing to further facilitate patients' understanding of others and themselves. By inviting patients to reflect on their emotional understanding of interpersonal encounters, IPT implicitly employs mentalizing. Mentalizing can be considered a general capacity to understand emotional and relational aspects of human interactions. Improving this capacity may be a core ingredient of Lipsitz and Markowitz (2013)'s four mechanisms of change (mentioned previously) in IPT therapeutic processes.

Attachment

Similarly, IPT and perhaps all affect-based treatments are attachment based. Patients with depression, PTSD, and anxiety disorders present with at least state-dependent insecure attachment: they mistrust encounters with others and struggle to elicit or maintain beneficial social support. Intriguing data from a recent open trial of IPT for military veterans with PTSD found that these patients had high rates of comorbid separation anxiety disorder, which is a facet of attachment dysregulation (Milrod et al. 2020). Fourteen weeks of IPT treatment improved not only PTSD symptoms but also separation anxiety and symptom-specific reflective function, another attachment-related measure (Markowitz et al. 2009; Rudden et al. 2009). Separation anxiety improvement early in IPT predicted posttreatment improvement in depressive symptoms. These preliminary findings suggest that IPT might work through improving attachment dysregulation (Milrod et al. 2020).

Conclusion

The theory of interpersonal therapy provides a framework for clinical understanding and fills a gap for many clinicians and researchers who feel frustrated by the abstraction and therapist neutrality in psychoanalysis and by the focus exclusively on observable behaviors. IPT generated a novel outlook, bridging the self and the system, avoiding focusing exclusively on either. Interpersonal theory remains an important framework for explaining human motivation and behavior and for understanding the etiology and treatment of psychological problems; however, it needs to be bolstered by clinical evidence. Indeed, strong data exist indicating that psychological disorders and interpersonal problems have a reciprocal relationship (Alden and Taylor 2004; Coyne 1976). Interpersonal theory has generated a powerful and demonstrably effective treatment—IPT—for several disorders.

IPT is a first-tier evidence-based psychotherapy for unipolar depression, eating disorders, some anxiety disorders, and PTSD. IPT has accumulated an extensive evidence base for efficacy for depression; however, IPT requires more systematic study of problems and barriers that may be specific to disorders other than depression (Markowitz et al. 2014). In addition, IPT researchers are beginning to accumulate evidence to support underlying interpersonal mechanisms of change (Lipsitz and Markowitz 2013), but further research is needed to support these mechanisms. Analysis is needed both to better link IPT's efficacy to its focus on interpersonal stress and social support and to study more systematically the role of the interpersonal problem area. Finally, IPT requires more methodical efforts at dissemination so that more patients have access to this treatment.

References

Ainsworth MD: Infant-mother attachment. Am Psychol 34(10):932–937, 1979 517843

Alden LE, Taylor CT: Interpersonal processes in social phobia. Clin Psychol Rev 24(7):857–882, 2004 15501559

Bandura A, Walters RH: Social Learning and Personality Development. New York, Holt Rinehart & Winston, 1963

Bonime W: The psychodynamics of neurotic depression. J Am Acad Psychoanal 4(3):301–326, 1976 1025074

Bowlby J: Attachment and Loss, Vol 1: Attachment. New York, Basic Books, 1969.

Brown GW, Harris T: The Social Origins of Depression: A Study of Psychiatric Disorder in Women. New York, Free Press, 1978

Cacioppo JT, Hawkley LC: Social isolation and health, with an emphasis on underlying mechanisms. Perspect Biol Med 46(3 suppl):S39–S52, 2003 14563073

Caspi A, Sugden K, Moffitt TE, et al: Influence of life stress on depression: moderation by a polymorphism in the 5-HTT gene. Science 301(5631):386–389, 2003 12869766

Clayton PJ: Bereavement, in Handbook of Affective Disorders. Edited by Paykel ES. New York, Guilford, 1982, pp 403–415
Cohen MB, Baker G, Cohen RA, et al: An intensive study of twelve cases of manic-depressive psychosis. Psychiatry 17(2):103–137, 1954 13167224
Cooley CH: Human Nature and the Social Order (1902). Piscataway, NY, Transaction, 1983
Coyne JC: Toward an interactional description of depression. Psychiatry 39(1):28–40, 1976 1257353
Cuijpers P, Donker T, Weissman MM, et al: Interpersonal psychotherapy for mental health problems: a comprehensive meta-analysis. Am J Psychiatry 173(7):680–687, 2016 27032627
Dill JC, Anderson CA: Loneliness, shyness, and depression: the etiology and interrelationships of everyday problems in living, in The Interactional Nature of Depression. Edited by Joiner T, Coyne JC. Washington, DC, American Psychological Association, 1999, pp 93–125
Downey G, Coyne JC: Children of depressed parents: an integrative review. Psychol Bull 108(1):50–76, 1990 2200073
Duer S, Schwenk TL, Coyne JC: Medical and psychosocial correlates of self-reported depressive symptoms in family practice. J Fam Pract 27(6):609–614, 1988 3199089
Durkheim E: Suicide: A Study in Sociology (1897). London, Routledge & Kegan Paul, 1951
Fairbairn WRD: An Object Relations Theory of the Personality. New York, Basic Books, 1952
Freedman MB, Leary TF, Ossorio AG, et al: The interpersonal dimension of personality. J Pers 20(2):143–161, 1951 14918048
Freud S: The Standard Edition of the Complete Psychological Works of Sigmund Freud, Vol 15. Introductory Lectures on Psycho-analysis (Parts 1 and 2) (1915–1916). Translated and edited by Strachey J. London, Hogarth Press, 1961
Freud S: Mourning and melancholia (1917 [1915]), in The Standard Edition of the Complete Psychological Works of Sigmund Freud, Vol 14. Translated and edited by Strachey J. London, Hogarth Press, 1957, pp 237–260
Green BH, Copeland JRM, Dewey ME, et al: Risk factors for depression in elderly people: a prospective study. Acta Psychiatr Scand 86(3):213–217, 1992 1414415
Hammen C: Interpersonal stress and depression in women. J Affect Disord 74(1):49–57, 2003 12646298
Hammen C: Stress and depression. Annu Rev Clin Psychol 1:293–319, 2005 17716090
Hammen C: Stress generation in depression: reflections on origins, research, and future directions. J Clin Psychol 62(9):1065–1082, 2006 16810666
Hankin BL, Abela JRZ: Development of Psychopathology: A Vulnerability-Stress Perspective. Thousand Oaks, CA, Sage, 2005
Henderson S, Byrne DG, Duncan-Jones P, et al: Social bonds in the epidemiology of neurosis: a preliminary communication. Br J Psychiatry 132:463–466, 1978 656709
Holmes TH, Rahe RH: The social readjustment rating scale. J Psychosom Res 11(2):213–218, 1967 6059863
Hooley JM, Teasdale JD: Predictors of relapse in unipolar depressives: expressed emotion, marital distress, and perceived criticism. J Abnorm Psychol 98(3):229–235, 1989 2768657
Horney K: Neurosis and Human Growth: The Struggle Towards Self Realization. London, Routeledge & Kegan Paul, 1950
Horney K: Feminine Psychology. New York, Norton, 1967
James W: The Principles of Psychology (1890). New York, Dover, 1950
Kendler KS, Karkowski-Shuman L: Stressful life events and genetic liability to major depression: genetic control of exposure to the environment? Psychol Med 27(3):539–547, 1997 9153675
Kendler KS, Thornton LM, Gardner CO: Stressful life events and previous episodes in the etiology of major depression in women: an evaluation of the "kindling" hypothesis. Am J Psychiatry 157(8):1243–1251, 2000 10910786
Klein M: Love, Guilt and Reparation and Other Works 1921–1945. Edited by Love H, Klein RM, Riviere J. New York, Norton, 1964
Klerman GL, Weissman MM, Rounsaville BJ, et al: Interpersonal Psychotherapy of Depression. New York, Basic Books, 1984
Kraepelin E: Dementia Praecox (1919). New York, Churchill Livingston, 1971
Leary TF: Interpersonal Diagnosis of Personality. New York, Ronald Press, 1957

Lewinsohn PM: A behavioral approach to depression, in The Psychology of Depression: Contemporary Theory and Research. Edited by Friedman RM, Katz MM. New York, Wiley, 1974, pp 157–185

Lindemann E: Symptomatology and management of acute grief. 1944. Am J Psychiatry 151(6 suppl):155–160, 1994 8192191

Lipsitz JD, Markowitz JC: Mechanisms of change in interpersonal therapy (IPT). Clin Psychol Rev 33(8):1134–1147, 2013 24100081

Maddison D, Walker WL: Factors affecting the outcome of conjugal bereavement. Br J Psychiatry 113(503):1057–1067, 1967 6057373

Markowitz JC, Milrod BL: The importance of responding to negative affect in psychotherapies. Am J Psychiatry 168(2):124–128, 2011 21297048

Markowitz JC, Milrod B, Bleiberg K, et al: Interpersonal factors in understanding and treating posttraumatic stress disorder. J Psychiatr Pract 15(2):133–140, 2009 19339847

Markowitz JC, Lipsitz J, Milrod BL: Critical review of outcome research on interpersonal psychotherapy for anxiety disorders. Depress Anxiety 31(4):316–325, 2014 24493661

Markowitz JC, Milrod B, Luyten P, et al: Mentalizing in interpersonal psychotherapy. Am J Psychother 72(4):95–100, 2019 31752509

Mead GH: The social self. Journal of Philosophy, Psychology, and Scientific Methods 10:374–380, 1913

Meyer A: The Collected Papers of Adolf Meyer, Vol 2: Psychiatry. Edited by Winters EE. Baltimore, MD, Johns Hopkins University Press, 1951

Milrod B, Keefe JR, Choo TH, et al: Separation anxiety in PTSD: a pilot study of mechanisms in patients undergoing IPT. Depress Anxiety 37(4):386–395, 2020 32097526

Mitchell C, Hobcraft J, McLanahan SS, et al: Social disadvantage, genetic sensitivity, and children's telomere length. Proc Natl Acad Sci USA 111(16):5944–5949, 2014 24711381

Monroe SM, Bromet EJ, Connell MM, et al: Social support, life events, and depressive symptoms: a 1-year prospective study. J Consult Clin Psychol 54(4):424–431, 1986 3745594

Overholser JC, Adam DM: Stressful life events and social support in depressed psychiatric inpatients, in Clinical Disorders and Stressful Life Events. Edited by Miller TW. Madison, CT, International Universities Press, 1997, pp 121–141

Paykel ES: Life events and affective disorders. Acta Psychiatr Scand Suppl 108(418):61–66, 2003 12956817

Paykel ES, Myers JK, Dienelt MN, et al: Life events and depression: a controlled study. Arch Gen Psychiatry 21(6):753–760, 1969 5389659

Perry HS: Psychiatrist of America: The Life of Harry Stack Sullivan. Cambridge, MA, Belknap Press, 1982

Pinsker H: A Primer of Supportive Psychotherapy, 2nd Reprint Edition. London, Routledge, 2002.

Rudden MG, Milrod B, Meehan KB, et al: Symptom-specific reflective functioning: incorporating psychoanalytic measures into clinical trials. J Am Psychoanal Assoc 57(6):1473–1478, 2009 20068250

Selye H: Stress and disease. Laryngoscope 65(7):500–514, 1955 13243777

Spitz RA, Wolf KM: The smiling response: a contribution to the ontogenesis of social relations. Genet Psychol Monogr 34:57–125, 1946

Sullivan H: Conceptions of Modern Psychiatry. New York, Norton, 1940

Sullivan HS: Multidisciplined coordination of interpersonal data, in Culture and Personality. Edited by Sargent SS, Smith MW. New York, Viking, 1949, pp 175–194

Sullivan HS: The Interpersonal Theory of Psychiatry. New York, Norton, 1953

Weissman MM, Paykel ES: The Depressed Woman: A Study of Social Relationships. Chicago, IL, University of Chicago Press, 1974

Weissman MM, Markowitz JC, Klerman G: Comprehensive Guide to Interpersonal Psychotherapy. New York, Basic Books, 2000

Weissman MM, Markowitz JC, Klerman GL: The Guide to Interpersonal Psychotherapy. New York, Oxford University Press, 2018

Winnicott DW: The Maturational Processes and the Facilitating Environment: Studies in the Theory of Emotional Development. London, Hogarth Press, 1965

CHAPTER 14

Techniques of Individual Interpersonal Psychotherapy

Holly A. Swartz, M.D.

Interpersonal psychotherapy (IPT) is a practical, intuitively reasonable treatment for depression. Readers new to IPT will find that much of what is described in this chapter sounds familiar and overlaps with other psychotherapies. Thus, on one level, IPT demands few novel skills from therapists and is relatively easy to learn. The challenges of IPT lie not in any individual technique or strategy but in organizing these approaches to establish and maintain a coherent focus. Therapists who are used to less structured therapies may initially find it difficult to organize sessions around a specific IPT focus and to eschew the temptations of digressing into extraneous clinical material. Therapists accustomed to more prescriptive treatments may struggle to balance the exploratory aspects of IPT with the need to stay focused. Additional challenges arise from "unlearning" reflexive responses from prior training experiences such as transference-focused interventions (for psychodynamic therapists) or identifying automatic cognitions (for cognitive therapists).

In this chapter I focus on basic IPT strategies and techniques, highlighting aspects of treatment that may be challenging for clinicians learning IPT. I also clarify, from a practical standpoint, the relationship of IPT to other psychotherapies described in this textbook. The focus in this chapter is on IPT for major depression, the first and still best tested indication for IPT, although the same principles may apply to other disorders. For additional information about IPT, readers are referred to the IPT manual (Weissman et al. 2018).

Important Concepts

IPT is organized around six important concepts: 1) psychotherapy common factors, 2) an explicit link between mood and life events, 3) a focus on the here and now, 4) selection of an IPT problem area, 5) use of the medical model, and 6) blaming the depression (rather than the patient) for interpersonal difficulties. Each concept is explained below.

Common Factors

IPT therapists facilitate expression of affect; remain attentive to the emotional significance of the therapeutic experience; and maintain a supportive, encouraging stance. They pull for affect in sessions, focusing on patients' feelings in the context of recent life events. Therapists lean forward (unless the patient finds this intrusive), focus on particulars, and foster hope. IPT techniques facilitate a positive therapeutic alliance that is crucial to good outcome (Frank 1971).

Link Between Mood and Life Events

IPT spans two psychological domains: the patient's current mood state and recent interpersonal experiences. It helps patients understand connections between the two. Upsetting life events trigger depressive episodes in vulnerable individuals, and negative interpersonal encounters lower mood; conversely, depressed mood impairs social functioning. The putative mechanism of IPT is that as patients manage interpersonal experiences more effectively, mood improves (Lipsitz and Markowitz 2013). In an iterative fashion, improved mood then allows patients to more effectively manage interpersonal stressors. Thus, the sine que non of IPT is constant attention to the reciprocal links between mood and interpersonal life events.

Here and Now

IPT focuses on life events taking place in the here and now (in contrast to the "there and then"). Unlike psychodynamic psychotherapy, IPT does *not* focus on early childhood experiences and long-standing familial dynamics. Thus, current mood state is linked to recent experiences rather than those rooted in the distant past. IPT also does not focus on transferential events within the office, except in the relatively rare instances when problems arise in the therapeutic alliance. IPT highlights recent experiences *outside the office.*

IPT Problem Areas

Treatment focuses on one of four possible problem areas: *role transition* (a major life change, such as divorce, work promotion, or medical illness), *grief* (death of an important individual in the patient's life), *role dispute* (conflictual interpersonal relationship characterized by nonreciprocal expectations between two parties about their respective social roles), or *interpersonal deficits* (long-standing contentious or impoverished interpersonal relationships).

Medical Model

Unlike most psychotherapies, IPT's roots are in the medical tradition. Using a medical framework for understanding illness, therapists provide psychoeducation about depression, stressing its biological underpinnings. A diathesis-stress model provides a framework for understanding interactions between biological vulnerability and stressful life events, helping patients to understand that they are not responsible (or to blame) for their illness yet are in an excellent position to help themselves recover from depression.

Blame the Depression

Whereas patients with other medical diagnoses generally recognize that they are ill, depressed patients blame themselves. Although these biased views could be correctly characterized as negative cognitions, the IPT therapist does *not* systematically question and evaluate automatic negative thoughts. Unlike with cognitive therapy, IPT therapists neither employ thought records nor weigh the evidence to help patients reevaluate negative cognitions. Instead, they shift excessive guilt from the self to the illness. Without being disingenuous, the therapist seeks to "blame the depression" when patients falter and credit patients whenever they succeed, which often provides patients with immediate feelings of relief. Therapists then capitalize on this transient mood improvement by encouraging patients to take positive steps toward resolving interpersonal problems, which has more enduring effects on mood.

Phases of IPT

IPT is a time-limited psychotherapy. Like any acute antidepressant treatment, IPT strives for rapid relief of depression. Patients and therapists understand from the outset that therapy will last for a predetermined interval (typically 12–16 sessions) and that its goal is symptomatic relief, to be achieved by resolving an interpersonal crisis. The time limit pressures both patient and therapist to action. IPT is divided into three parts: initial phase, middle phase, and termination.

Initial Phase

The initial phase of treatment (sessions 1–3; see Table 14–1) identifies a specific treatment focus (IPT problem area), outlines IPT principles, and establishes the time limit. Many novice IPT therapists find the numerous tasks of the initial phase the most difficult part of IPT.

Diagnosis

The first step is to determine the patient's diagnosis. Using the medical model, the IPT therapist conducts a careful psychiatric assessment to yield a diagnosis consistent with DSM 5 criteria (American Psychiatric Association 2013). This process includes eliciting a medical history, probing for psychiatric symptoms, ruling out medical confounds, and establishing a diagnosis.

Systematic Review of Depressive Symptoms

A standardized rating scale such as the Hamilton Rating Scale for Depression (Hamilton 1960) or Beck Depression Inventory (Beck and Steer 1993) is used to evaluate severity of depressive symptoms. The therapist readministers the same rating scale at regular intervals, providing an assessment of baseline severity against which to measure improvement. Standardized ratings help to educate patients about the symp-

TABLE 14–1. **Techniques associated with the initial phase of interpersonal psychotherapy (IPT)**

Goal	Technique
Diagnosis	Psychiatric interview and assessment
Systematic review of depressive symptoms	Assessment with standardized depression rating scale
Induction to the sick role and the medical model of depression	Psychoeducation
Evaluation of interpersonal relationships	Interpersonal inventory
Selection of IPT problem area	Illness time line and interpersonal inventory
Treatment contract	IPT case formulation
Provision of hope	Psychoeducation and optimistic therapeutic stance

toms of depression and confer validity to the construct of depression as a real illness that can be reliably assessed and quantified.

Induction to the Sick Role

Parsons (1951) defined the sick role as a social role that absolves the patient from responsibilities that the illness precludes while presenting new responsibilities related to the illness. Following the medical model, the IPT therapist inducts the patient into the sick role by explaining that they are suffering from a medical illness—like influenza or diabetes—that may interfere with fulfilling social obligations such as entertaining friends, working every day (if the illness is very severe), or caring for an ailing relative. While offering a respite from some responsibilities, the therapist simultaneously confers on the patient requirements for self-care and illness management such as attending therapy appointments, taking medications (if prescribed), and addressing the identified IPT problem area. This dual message of relief and responsibility excuses patients from unmanageable obligations while prioritizing treatment.

Evaluation of Interpersonal Relationships

The cornerstone of IPT case formulation is the interpersonal inventory. Conducted over the course of one or two sessions, the inventory is a careful review of important people in the patient's life currently and the quality of those relationships. The goals are to determine available social supports and relationship difficulties that may be a cause or consequence of the depressive episode and to understand the patient's handling of intimacy, self-assertion, communication, and anger. Information collected in the interpersonal inventory allows therapists to select an appropriate IPT problem area. Beginning with open-ended questions, therapists ask progressively more directive questions as needed to obtain a complete picture of patients' social relationships:

Therapist: Tell me about the important people in your life. In whom do you confide? How well do you get along with your coworkers? Tell me about your romantic partner(s).

Although IPT does not focus on early childhood experiences and relationships, therapists ask about the family of origin and current relationships with family members as part of the interpersonal inventory.

An important IPT concept is *nonreciprocal role expectations*. This notion underscores that it is not expectations themselves that are problematic in relationships; rather, conflict arises when two individuals disagree about their expectations of one another. For instance, when a romantic couple inhabits traditionally gendered roles, conflict is unlikely if both agree on heteronormative social roles. Yet conflict is very likely if expectations are nonreciprocal, such as if one partner expects the other partner to handle most of the child-rearing and domestic responsibilities but the other partner expects these tasks to be jointly shared. Thus, beyond understanding who is central to the patient's life, it is important to explore the nature of expectations within relationships. Therapists elicit this information by asking questions such as the following:

Therapist: Are you satisfied in your relationship with your partner? What are sources of friction in your relationship? What happens when you disagree?

Selection of IPT Problem Area

To determine the treatment focus (IPT problem area), the therapist links the onset or maintenance of the depressive episode to an event in the patient's interpersonal life. Sometimes this is straightforward (e.g., "I became depressed after I was fired from my job"). In more complex cases, it may be helpful to construct a time line that charts the temporal sequence of mood changes and changing relationships or life events, allowing therapist and patient to identify the links between them. Information collected in the time line can be used to help clarify which life event is temporally linked to the onset of the current mood episode.

On the basis of information collected in the interpersonal inventory and from the time line, the therapist selects one of the four possible problem areas—role transition, grief, role dispute, or interpersonal deficits—as the treatment focus. Role transition is chosen when there are marked shifts in social roles (e.g., from health to sickness, from employed to unemployed). The grief problem area is reserved for an emotionally meaningful death; psychological losses (e.g., loss of a job or relationship) are defined as role transitions in IPT. Role dispute is chosen when the patient is involved in a problematic relationship characterized by nonreciprocal expectations between two parties about their respective social roles (e.g., around caretaking, financial responsibilities, sexual roles). Interpersonal deficits is the problem area of last resort, chosen when the other three options do not apply. When there is more than one reasonable option, the therapist suggests the problem area with maximal emotional valence for the patient.

Treatment Contract and Provision of Hope

Case formulation formally synthesizes the elements covered in the initial phase (Markowitz and Swartz 2007). The therapist reviews the patient's diagnosis, explicitly links the interpersonal problem area to the onset of the depressive episode, and obtains explicit agreement from the patient to focus on this problem area for the remainder of treatment, as in the following:

Therapist: You began to experience financial problems 2 years ago, but your mood did not deteriorate until these problems forced you and your children to move back home with your parents. Although you continue to view yourself as an independent adult who sets rules for your children, your mother believes that while you live in her house, she has ultimate authority over your children. Because you feel indebted to your parents, you are reluctant to argue with your mother about the rules she sets for your kids. Yet, you disagree with some of her decisions, like her allowing them unlimited screen time and using candy as incentive for them to do chores. You have been keeping these thoughts to yourself but feel angry inside. Although the financial issues were very stressful, you were managing OK until the problems with your mother started. We call this struggle between you a *role dispute.* You and your mother disagree about how to handle your children and who's in charge where they're concerned. This dispute is clearly connected to your depression: the more your mother undermines your parental authority, the worse your mood gets. I suggest that we spend the next nine sessions focusing on this dispute. My bet is that as your relationship with your mother improves, so will your mood. How does that sound to you?

The case formulation serves as a treatment contract, setting forth the planned focus of treatment and treatment duration. If not previously specified in an earlier session, the therapist can add information during the case formulation about expectations around treatment attendance, missed sessions, and payment.

Middle Phase

The middle phase is the working portion of IPT. During these sessions (typically, sessions 4–13), the therapist actively engages the patient in the process of resolving the focal interpersonal problem area and further exploring the links between the patient's mood and interpersonal focus. The following vignette describes general IPT techniques of the middle phase and specific techniques associated with each of the four problem areas (Table 14–2).

Case Vignette

Ms. G is a 31-year-old mother of two children whose husband, Jeff, works as director of sales for a small health care technology company. Ms. G's depression began when her husband's work responsibilities shifted, requiring him to travel frequently to solicit out-of-state customers. Ms. G described feeling sad and lonely during his absences but also angry that he was spending less time with her and the children. Mr. G, on the other hand, seemed to think that Ms. G should feel grateful because his increased responsibilities meant better compensation, which, in turn, helped the family financially. Ms. G begins IPT with Dr. E.

General Techniques

How have you been since we last met? This seemingly simple phrase opens all IPT sessions after the first session. By invoking the temporal frame "since we last met," the therapist focuses the patient's attention on recent (as opposed to past) events and mood states. With Ms. G, "How have you been?" elicits a response with either mood-related content ("I've been so-so") or life event–related content ("Jeff and I have been fighting nonstop"; "I tried to get the kids to listen to me, but it was hopeless").

TABLE 14–2. **Techniques of the middle phase of interpersonal psychotherapy (IPT)**

Goal	Technique
Focus on mood and recent life events	"How have you been since we last met?"
Systematic review of depressive symptoms	Assessment with standardized depression rating scale
Improved capacity for communication	Communication analysis and role-play
Exploration of options	Decision analysis
Focus on IPT problem area	Relate change in depressive symptoms to changes in interpersonal problem area
Enhanced understanding of depression as a medical illness	Psychoeducation
Protecting the therapeutic relationship	Use of reflective listening, empathic statements, and attention to affect within the session
Enhancing activation	Encourage increased socialization in a graded fashion; reinforce even small steps toward increased activity levels

During sessions, the therapist encourages the patient to expand on both mood and recent interpersonal experiences, helping them to see links between the two over the past week. If the patient responds with mood-related content, the therapist encourage the patient to elaborate on their symptoms:

> **Dr. E:** Tell me what you mean by "so-so." Can you rate your mood on a scale of 1 to 10? And how has your sleep been?

After obtaining a clear understanding of the patient's depressive symptoms over the past week, the therapist then links the mood state to the interpersonal problem area.

> **Dr. E:** It sounds like your depression has been worse this week. Tell me what's been going on in your role dispute with Jeff.

If the therapist chooses wisely in the initial phase, the patient's life events will connect to the problem area selected as the treatment focus.

> **Dr. E:** Tell me more about what has been happening between you and Jeff.

After exploring these interpersonal issues, the therapist helps the patient connect the events to their mood.

> **Dr. E:** Tell me how all this fighting [Jeff's absence] has affected your mood.

Alternatively, if the patient responds to the opening question by describing an event, the therapist asks the following:

> **Dr. E:** How did that make you feel?

Therapist and patient can then work on understanding what happened, the relationship of the event to the patient's mood, and potential solutions to the problematic situation. If the content of the patient's response is *not* related to the treatment focus, the therapist listens politely and looks for an opening to redirect the patient. For instance, if the treatment focus is a role dispute and Ms. G starts the session by telling Dr. E about her recent high school reunion, the therapist may make a general comment about the reunion but then reframe the discussion in terms of the dispute:

Dr. E: It sounds like it was nice to connect with old friends. Did Jeff go to the reunion with you? What's been going on between the two of you?

Usually, patients respond to gentle redirection. On occasion, however, the therapist may need to firmly invoke the treatment contract made in the initial phase.

Dr. E: You and I agreed to focus on your role dispute with Jeff because we both saw that your role dispute with him seemed inextricably connected to your mood symptoms. I think it's important for us to return to this because we still have a lot of work to do in this area. If we have extra time at the end of the session, we can spend a few minutes talking about your high school reunion, as social supports from friends certainly can be helpful when you're feeling depressed. But we should put our energy into figuring out what's been happening between you and Jeff. How does that sound to you?

Communication analysis. Depressed individuals tend not to communicate well. When angry, they make irritable comments and find themselves being short with significant others but rarely feel capable of expressing the anger directly in the service of resolving interpersonal conflict. Anger feels like a "bad" feeling. Alternatively, many depressed individuals are withdrawn or feel slowed down, which also impairs communication. Some individuals' impairment is long-standing; for others, it is acute and clearly related to the current depressive episode. IPT almost always addresses the patient's capacity to communicate more effectively.

Communication analysis, the primary IPT technique used to enhance communication skills, dissects in detail the communication between two individuals. The analysis includes an exploration of the desired outcome of the communication, what was said and not said, how it was said (paraverbal and nonverbal communication), where it was said, and what the other person heard or understood (perspective taking). The therapist also explores changes in the patient's feelings during and following the encounter. The IPT therapist works to clarify the interaction by asking for details:

Dr. E: What did you hope to communicate? Where were the two of you when this discussion took place? Had he been drinking? What exactly did you say? What exactly did he say? How did you feel then? Can you say it to me using the same tone of voice that you used then? What do you think he took from your conversation?

Having obtained a detailed account, the therapist reinforces the patient's successful interventions and/or helps the patient understand maladaptive aspects of the interaction and how to remediate the situation. At first, Dr. E explores with Ms. G the effect of her communication on her partner with questions such as the following:

Dr. E: What impact do you think having the kids in the room had on your ability to speak freely with Jeff?
Dr. E: How did you feel telling Jeff how angry you've been feeling?
Dr. E: How do you think Jeff felt when you said it to him that way?

Dr. E asks these leading questions, hoping that Ms. G will recognize errors herself and spontaneously offer suggestions for improvement. If the patient is too depressed or too interpersonally impaired to "get it," the therapist makes more directive statements, such as the following:

Dr. E: If the kids are in the room with the two of you, you might edit your comments, making it more difficult for you to say to Jeff what you really feel.
Dr. E: It seems like your mood was a little better after telling him how you felt—even though you didn't get the outcome you hoped for.
Dr. E: I wonder if Jeff felt attacked when you started the conversation with a string of insults.

After identifying problems in communication, the dyad works to identify more adaptive means of interacting. Dr. E ascertains the following: "What do you really want to say to him?," then explores options, asking Ms. G for suggestions on how better to get that idea or feeling across. The therapist may also offer the patient general suggestions such as "It's often helpful to make 'I' statements" or "Strike while the iron is cold." This process is usually framed as a rehearsal for an interaction the patient is encouraged to try out with the significant other between sessions.

Role-play. The therapist can use role-play (in the case vignette, the therapist enacts Jeff and Ms. G plays herself) to learn more adaptive means of communicating. Role-play can focus on practicing a future planned discussion or replaying a past problematic exchange. Role-plays allow the patient to practice new communication techniques, with coaching from the therapist. By switching roles (i.e., Ms. G plays Jeff and the therapist plays Ms. G), role-play can encourage perspective taking and empathy.

Exploration of options and decision analysis. It is important to ask *what the patient wants* in any given situation. Depressed patients often neglect their own needs and desires because they lack energy, motivation, or interest or feel that paying attention to their needs is "selfish." Thus, when faced with an interpersonal problem, Dr. E asks Ms. G how she would like to resolve the issue:

Dr. E: Given Jeff's reluctance to take a different kind of job—one that would let him be home more often—what would help you feel less alone? Are there specific changes that you would like him to make? Are there things that you'd like him to do or say when he's home or while he is on the road? Are there other things you might do differently that would help?

Depressed patients may initially have difficulty envisioning solutions. Therefore, therapists may have to be relatively active at first, helping patients generate a list of options (e.g., talking on the phone more often while Jeff travels, engaging other sources of social support, planning a vacation). After generating options, the patient and therapist evaluate the alternatives to assess how realistic they are. They discuss resources the patient needs to achieve the desired outcome and develop a plan to execute necessary changes. If the patient's desire is not feasible (e.g., Jeff getting a new job), the therapist helps the patient mourn the loss of that potential outcome.

Socialization and activity. Socialization and pleasurable activities are inherently antidepressant. Indeed, behavioral activation is a key active ingredient in cognitive-behavioral therapy (Jacobson et al. 2001). In middle phase IPT, the therapist gently encourages the patient to increase interpersonal activity and decrease social isolation, providing emotional support and practical skills to help achieve these goals. Increasing social engagement is graduated so that the patient does not feel overwhelmed. Unlike behavior therapy, in which activities may occur absent human interactions, graded activities in IPT are interpersonal (e.g., meet a friend for coffee, join a like-minded meetup group, email a former colleague). The therapist presents social encounters as providing crucial interpersonal information and as win-win situations: if the patients succeed, they feel better; if the encounter is disappointing, it provides data to discuss in sessions to generate alternative approaches.

Homework. Although IPT therapists do not assign written homework as would be done in cognitive therapy, patients are explicitly instructed to engage in interpersonally focused activities related to their IPT problem area between sessions. This "work at home" may include trying out new communication skills, increasing social engagement, or taking steps to assist with mastering new social roles (e.g., applying for jobs, reaching out to old friends, enrolling in a class).

Techniques and Strategies Associated With Specific Problem Areas

Grief or complicated bereavement. When grief is selected as the IPT problem area, the goals of treatment are to help the patient work through the loss, ultimately helping the patient to reestablish social contacts and activities. Specifically, the therapist relates the depressive symptoms to the loved one's death or to reactivation of emotions around the anniversary of the death. This process takes place through a careful reevaluation of the relationship with the deceased and clarification of the circumstances of the death. In nonjudgmental fashion, the therapist explores the events leading up to the death, the death itself, and the events immediately following the death. The therapist encourages the patient to relate how the death unfolded and the patient's role in the events. Although it may be painful or frightening for the patient to discuss these memories, it is crucial to grief work. The therapist gently elicits the story. Because this can be difficult work, it may be helpful for the therapist to advise the patient that they may feel worse before they feel better. The therapist may offer a brief phone call of support following particularly emotional therapy sessions.

Individuals who experience complicated bereavement often idealize their relationship with the deceased. It may be too painful to remember fights with or shortcomings of the deceased. Although often beginning with positive reminiscences ("What did you love about him?" "What did you love about your relationship?"), the therapist helps the patient reconstruct a more realistic view of the relationship with the deceased, both positive and negative aspects. To accomplish this goal, it is often useful for the patient to visit places that stir memories and to look at photos or mementos of the deceased. These tangible items may spur the patient to remember additional events and forgotten aspects of the relationship.

As patients achieve some catharsis, therapy helps them to accept and move beyond the loss. Therapists encourage actions to advance the mourning process such as visiting the grave, reconnecting with family and friends of the deceased, making a scrapbook, or writing a letter to the deceased. Toward the end of treatment, therapists encourage patients to reestablish interests and relationships.

Role transition. The role transition problem area links the onset or maintenance of the depressive episode to difficulty coping with recent or impending life changes in areas such as relationships, vocational functioning, financial situation, or physical health status. The transition is conceptualized as difficulty moving from one social role to another (e.g., from stay-at-home mother to working mother, from medical student to doctor). Goals of treatment resemble those of bereavement: to establish a more realistic view of the old role (which is typically idealized) and the new role (which is typically devalued) and to help patients acquire skills and resources needed to improve functioning in the new role. Thus, patients mourn the lost status but also gain appreciation for and mastery of the new role.

Therapists initially encourage patients to review the positive and negative aspects of the old social role, to mourn its loss, and to explore the feelings associated with the change (e.g., anger, sadness, fear). As therapy progresses, focus shifts toward greater attention to the new role. Patients are encouraged to think about new opportunities afforded by the new role as well as new skills that will be needed in order to cope more successfully.

Role dispute. The role dispute problem area links onset or maintenance of the depressive episode to an unsatisfying interpersonal relationship characterized by nonreciprocal role expectations. Role disputes arise when two individuals disagree about these expectations and cannot negotiate a compromise. Examples include the following:

- A college student who expects to be treated as an adult by parents who view him as an adolescent requiring guidance and limits
- An employer who expects her employees to work independently with little supervision, whereas her employee wants frequent suggestions and reassurance

The therapist's first task is to determine the stage of the dispute. In IPT parlance, disputes consist of three stages:

1. *Renegotiation*—an active dispute in which the two parties are trying to work things out, albeit unsuccessfully
2. *Impasse*—a stalemate in which the two parties are locked in opposing positions, not actively negotiating their differences
3. *Dissolution*—the end of the dispute, beyond hope of resolution, when the parties are poised to end the relationship

Disputes require objective staging because depressed patients tend to see hopeless impasses even where negotiation is possible.

In renegotiation, the therapist may intervene to calm overt hostilities while encouraging improved communication. If the relationship is at an impasse, the therapist attempts to move the individuals toward renegotiation so that they can begin to work through their differences. It is often helpful to offer the caveat that "things may get worse before they get better" when the dispute moves from impasse to renegotiation. Typically, therapists use communication analysis and role-play to help patients learn new ways of communicating. If the relationship is in the dissolution phase, the therapeutic task becomes a role transition: to help the patient mourn the loss of the relationship and focus on new activities or relationships.

Role dispute work is sometimes likened to *unilateral couple therapy*. In working on this problem area, it may be helpful to bring the other party in the dispute into a session. The purpose of this single couple session is to educate the other person about depression and for the therapist to gain a better understanding of the relationship. Aside from one pilot study (Foley et al. 1989), however, IPT has not been conceptualized as couple therapy.

IPT techniques used to identify and resolve role disputes include expression of affect, relationship appraisal to identify nonreciprocal role expectations, communication analysis, role-play, and problem solving. As in other IPT problem areas, the therapist continually links the patient's mood to the role dispute, expecting to see improvement as the dispute resolves.

Interpersonal deficits. Interpersonal deficits is the poorly named IPT category of last resort. Although many patients seeking IPT treatment have notable deficits in interpersonal functioning, the deficits category is reserved for cases for which no other potential foci exist: that is, for patients who lack life events. Such patients tend to have chronic impairments in relationships and may have comorbid dysthymic disorder (Markowitz 1998), social phobia (Lipsitz et al. 1999), and/or traits of Cluster A or C personality disorders (American Psychiatric Association 1994). Not surprisingly, patients with chronic impairment in social functioning who lack the life events on which IPT focuses fare worse in IPT (Sotsky et al. 1991), and their treatments are more difficult to conduct.

The goals of treatment for acutely depressed individuals in the interpersonal deficits focus include reducing the patient's isolation and encouraging new social relationships. Although this may sound like an agenda for a longer therapy, the IPT therapist focuses on the patient's isolation in the context of the current depressive episode rather than its historical origins. The therapist reviews depressive symptoms and relates these depressive symptoms to the problems of social isolation or unfulfillment. The therapist explores past significant relationships, asking patients to discuss both their positive and their negative aspects. The therapist attempts to determine any evident maladaptive patterns in these relationships and to help the patient understand them. In a departure from the general IPT stance, the therapist may explicitly discuss the patient's feelings about the therapist—using an interpersonal here-and-now focus—and seek parallels in other relationships.

In other problem areas, the therapist uses the IPT label to explain the problem area to the patient (e.g., "We call this a role transition"). Because the word *deficits* has disparaging connotations, the therapist explains the problem using more appropriate terms such as *interpersonal sensitivity* or *social isolation*.

Termination

The final phase comprises the last two to three sessions of treatment. IPT likens termination to a graduation: the patient has usually made meaningful gains, feels better, and is now ready for something different (i.e., a new treatment, maintenance treatment, no treatment). Thus, termination is a role transition from acute therapy. Table 14–3 summarizes termination tasks.

Therapist and patient review the course of treatment, relating improvement in depressive symptoms to interpersonal changes that the patient made in the focal problem area. The therapist credits the patient for making these changes, emphasizing the patient's independent competence as acute therapy draws to a close. The therapist continues psychoeducation by reviewing depressive symptoms and instructing the patient to seek appropriate treatment should these symptoms reemerge in the future. The therapist reminds the patient that depression is often a recurrent illness and that recurrence is treatable and not the patient's fault. If the patient has not improved, the therapist attributes this to IPT (much as one would in an unsuccessful pharmacotherapy trial), gives the patient credit for making the effort, and encourages the patient to consider available alternative treatment options.

In addition to reviewing gains, the dyad explores areas that have not been adequately addressed in IPT. If the depression has not fully remitted, the therapist, following a psychopharmacology model, blames the treatment rather than the patient and suggests alternative or adjunctive treatments that might address remaining symptoms. The therapist also may identify interpersonal issues that have not been adequately addressed in IPT, such as ongoing marital discord or job dissatisfaction, and perhaps recommend follow-up care for them. In the case vignette, the therapist might make the following comments:

Dr. E: You've done a great job, and your depression has remitted. But you and Jeff still have issues to work out. What options do you have to deal with those?

Throughout the termination phase, therapists attend to patients' feelings about ending therapy, encouraging them to verbalize the range of feelings experienced as IPT comes to an end, including anger, relief, worry, or curiosity. Feelings of sadness or loss are normalized in the context of ending a relationship that has been supportive and helpful. It is critical to differentiate normal feelings of sadness on separation from the pathological symptoms of depression the patient experienced at the outset of treatment.

Therapist: We all feel sad at times. Ending therapy is a time when many people feel a little sad. But sadness is a useful signal of social separation and is very different from the numbness and despair that you felt when you were depressed. Remember that depression usually involves changes in sleep and appetite in addition to changes in mood. That may help you figure out whether you are lapsing into depression again or not.

Because the therapeutic relationship in IPT is more collaborative than paternalistic, IPT therapists may acknowledge they will miss working with patients and (if accurate) tell them they have enjoyed working together. They may voice shared regret about breaking up a good team while indicating confidence in patients' ability to continue to do well on their own.

The final component of the termination phase is addressing relapse prevention. Patients are encouraged to continue to monitor mood, perhaps using a depression screen intermittently. Therapists point out new skills patients have acquired, review

TABLE 14–3. **Techniques associated with the termination phase of interpersonal psychotherapy (IPT)**

Goal	Technique
Determine remaining treatment needs	Review depressive symptoms, current interpersonal functioning, and persistent difficulties
Reinforce treatment gains	Review treatment gains and changes in standardized depression assessment over time; explicitly discuss new skills that were acquired
Plan for relapse prevention	Identify potential triggers for recurrence; provide psychoeducation about risk of recurrence; discuss use of IPT strategies to manage stressors; establish plan for seeking treatment in the future, if needed
Manage feelings associated with termination	Normalize feelings of sadness and loss; differentiate sadness from depression; probe for other feelings associated with termination
Confer mastery	Draw analogies with graduation and congratulate the patient on gains made in treatment
Avoid blaming the patient	Blame the therapy rather than the patient for unmet treatment needs and treatment "failures"
Provide for continuity of care	Arrange for follow-up care (maintenance treatment, additional treatment) as needed

opportunities to implement these skills, identify future interpersonal difficulties or high-risk scenarios that might trigger another episode, and discuss strategies to use in those circumstances. Patients should know how to reach a mental health professional in the event of a future episode. When possible, IPT therapists leave the door open for future consultation if needed.

Conclusion

IPT is a time-limited treatment for depression that focuses on the link between mood and interpersonal relationships. Working within the medical model, IPT assumes that the patient has an underlying genetic or biological vulnerability to mood disorders. It also assumes that the environment interacts with biology such that stressful interpersonal relationships or events can precipitate episodes of depression in biologically vulnerable individuals (a diathesis-stress model). By identifying a precipitating interpersonal problem area—grief, role transition, role dispute, or interpersonal deficits—the therapist focuses the treatment on a discrete issue that is directly linked to the current depressive episode, whose resolution is likely to lead to improvement in mood.

As I stated at the outset of this chapter, the individual elements of IPT are not novel. Rather, IPT's innovation rests in the way the elements are organized to provide therapists with a coherent strategy to treat patients who suffer from major depressive disorder. The intuitively reasonable idea that mood is connected to life events appeals to therapists and patients, and the empirical evidence base clearly supports the efficacy of the IPT approach (Ravitz et al. 2019). The International Society of Interpersonal Psychotherapy (www.interpersonalpsychotherapy.org) is an online forum for therapists interested in IPT and provides information about training opportunities for individuals who may be interested in gaining further experience with this modality.

Key Points

- Interpersonal Psychotherapy (IPT) is a time-limited, evidence-based psychotherapy for depression.
- IPT is organized around six concepts: psychotherapy common factors, explicit link between mood and life events, focus on the here and now, selection of an IPT problem area, use of the medical model, and blaming the depression (rather than the patient) for interpersonal difficulties.
- IPT therapists focus on one of four IPT problem areas: role disputes, interpersonal role transitions, grief, and interpersonal deficits/sensitivity.
- IPT's intuitively reasonable idea that mood is connected to life events appeals to therapists and patients.

References

American Psychiatric Association: Diagnostic and Statistical Manual of Mental Disorders, 4th Edition. Washington, DC, American Psychiatric Association, 1994

American Psychiatric Association: Diagnostic and Statistical Manual of Mental Disorders, 5th Edition. Arlington, VA, American Psychiatric Association, 2013

Beck AT, Steer RA: Manual for the Beck Depression Inventory. San Antonio, TX, Psychological Corporation, 1993

Foley SH, Rounsaville BJ, Weissman MM, et al: Individual versus conjoint interpersonal psychotherapy for depressed patients with marital disputes. Int J Fam Psychiatry 10:29–42, 1989

Frank JD: Eleventh Emil A. Gutheil Memorial Conference: therapeutic factors in psychotherapy. Am J Psychother 25(3):350–361, 1971 4936109

Hamilton M: A rating scale for depression. J Neurol Neurosurg Psychiatry 23:56–62, 1960 14399272

Jacobson NS, Martell CR, Dimidjian S: Behavioral activation treatment for depression: returning to contextual roots. Clin Psychol Sci Pract 8(3):255–270, 2001

Lipsitz JD, Markowitz JC: Mechanisms of change in interpersonal therapy (IPT). Clin Psychol Rev 33(8):1134–1147, 2013 24100081

Lipsitz JD, Markowitz JC, Cherry S, et al: Open trial of interpersonal psychotherapy for the treatment of social phobia. Am J Psychiatry 156(11):1814–1816, 1999 10553749

Markowitz JC: Interpersonal Psychotherapy for Dysthymic Disorder. Washington, DC, American Psychiatric Press, 1998

Markowitz JC, Swartz HA: Case formulation in interpersonal psychotherapy of depression, in Handbook of Psychotherapy Case Formulation, 2nd Edition. Edited by Eels TE. New York, Guilford, 2007, pp 192–222

Parsons T: Illness and the role of the physician: a sociological perspective. Am J Orthopsychiatry 21(3):452–460, 1951 14857123

Ravitz P, Watson P, Lawson A, et al: Interpersonal psychotherapy: a scoping review and historical perspective (1974–2017). Harv Rev Psychiatry 27(3):165–180, 2019 30883446

Sotsky SM, Glass DR, Shea MT, et al: Patient predictors of response to psychotherapy and pharmacotherapy: findings in the NIMH Treatment of Depression Collaborative Research Program. Am J Psychiatry 148(8):997–1008, 1991 1853989

Weissman MM, Markowitz JC, Klerman GL: The Guide to Interpersonal Psychotherapy. New York, Oxford University Press, 2018

CHAPTER 15

Efficacy, Indications, and Applications of Individual Interpersonal Psychotherapy

John C. Markowitz, M.D.

Interpersonal psychotherapy (IPT) was developed in the 1970s by the late Gerald L. Klerman, M.D., Myrna M. Weissman, Ph.D., and their colleagues at Harvard and Yale universities (Markowitz and Weissman 2012). From its inception, IPT was a research therapy. Whereas much of psychotherapy research before IPT had studied psychotherapy process, IPT research has focused on outcome. As Klerman said: "Who cares why a therapy works if we don't know *that* it works?" (G.L. Klerman, personal communication, 1989). IPT has been tested in a series of randomized controlled trials, generally with success, now totaling more than 100 (Cuijpers et al. 2011, 2016). Indeed, for many years IPT was essentially *only* a research treatment, with few practitioners in the community. Because of its research success, IPT is now an indicated treatment in guidelines for mood and eating disorders (American Psychiatric Association 2006, 2010; Depression Guideline Panel 1993; Karasu et al. 1993). In the past two decades, clinicians have increasingly been seeking training because of its empirically demonstrated efficacy. A new manual describes how to do IPT (Weiss-

Material for this chapter has been adapted (and revised further for this edition), with permission, from Markowitz JC: "Interpersonal Psychotherapy," in *Psychiatry*, Third Edition. Edited by Tasman A, Kay J, Lieberman JA, et al. Chichester, UK, Wiley, 2008.

man et al. 2018), and an international organization, the International Society for Interpersonal Psychotherapy (https://interpersonalpsychotherapy.org), holds biennial meetings.

In this chapter, I address the efficacy, indications, and applications of IPT as an individual psychotherapy for psychiatric disorders. (For IPT in combination with pharmacotherapy, see Chapter 35, "Combining Medications and Psychotherapy"; for group IPT, see Chapter 21, "Theories and Techniques of Group Therapy.")

Efficacy and Effectiveness

Efficacy research refers to testing a treatment under highly controlled conditions, with participants randomly assigned to different treatments (or no treatment) with experienced therapists, rating instruments, and treatment monitoring. Therapists train by reading the therapy manual, videotaping or audiotaping their treatment sessions, and receiving intensive supervision from expert IPT supervisors during pilot and subsequent study cases (Rounsaville et al. 1986). Patients in these trials meet careful inclusion and exclusion criteria to limit heterogeneity. Demonstrating efficacy answers the question *Does it work?* Efficacy indicates that a treatment is superior to a control condition under these controlled conditions. Once a treatment has demonstrated efficacy for a particular diagnosis, the next step is to test its *effectiveness* under less rigorous monitoring in the community setting. The question becomes *Does it work in a real-life setting?* Both questions are important.

IPT research has demonstrated its efficacy for major depressive disorder across a range of patient ages and contexts; for bulimia nervosa; and, increasingly, for anxiety disorders and PTSD (Table 15–1). Research also indicates the efficacy of IPT (modified as interpersonal social rhythm therapy [IPSRT]) as an adjunctive treatment for bipolar disorder. IPT was never expected to work for all disorders and has shown no advantages over control psychotherapies for dysthymic disorder or substance abuse disorders. For depressed adolescents, IPT has shown not only efficacy (Mufson et al. 1993, 1999) but also effectiveness (Mufson et al. 2004a) in a school-based program.

Because IPT focuses clinically on the social context of the depressive episode, researchers have sometimes adapted IPT when applying it to different treatment populations, developing manuals for different age groups or subpopulations (e.g., Frank 2005; Markowitz 1998, 2016; Mufson et al. 2004b) and occasionally adding focal problem areas. IPT has also been used at different lengths, in different formats, in one pilot couples adaptation (Foley et al. 1989), and as a telephone intervention (Donnelly et al. 2000; Heckman et al. 2017; Miller and Weissman 2002; Neugebauer et al. 2006). Nonetheless, all these adaptations involve the basic principles that constitute IPT: a no-fault definition of the patient's problem as a treatable medical illness, excusing the patient from blame for his or her symptoms, and a continual focus on the relationship between the patient's moods and life situation (Weissman et al. 2018). Thus, IPT remains consistent across conditions and adaptations.

The continuing growth of IPT research precludes an exhaustive description of studies. In this chapter, I present a selection of key research trials of IPT for mood and other disorders.

TABLE 15–1. **Empirically based indications for interpersonal psychotherapy**

Major depression
Acute
Recurrent (prophylaxis)
Geriatric patients
Adolescent patients
HIV-positive patients
Primary care patients
Conjoint therapy for depressed married women
Postpartum and antepartum patients
Bipolar disorder (adjunctive treatment)
Interpersonal counseling (IPC) for **subsyndromal depression**
Bulimia (individual or group format)
Social phobia[a]
Posttraumatic stress disorder[a]

[a]Preliminary results are encouraging.

Major Depressive Disorder

Major depressive disorder was the target diagnosis for which IPT was developed and for which its efficacy remains best demonstrated (Cuijpers et al. 2011).

Acute Treatment of Major Depression

IPT was first tested as an acute antidepressant treatment in a four-cell, 16-week randomized trial (Klerman et al. 1984). This study compared IPT, amitriptyline, combined IPT and amitriptyline, and an unscheduled control treatment for 81 outpatients with major depression (DiMascio et al. 1979; Weissman et al. 1979). Although amitriptyline alleviated symptoms faster, no significant difference appeared between IPT and amitriptyline in symptom reduction at 16 weeks. The active treatments all reduced symptoms significantly more than did the nonscheduled control, and combined amitriptyline plus IPT had greater efficacy than either active monotherapy. Unsurprisingly, IPT did not benefit patients with delusional depression. At 1-year follow-up, many patients sustained improvement from the brief IPT intervention. Moreover, IPT patients had developed significantly better psychosocial functioning, whether or not they received medication. This effect on social function was not found for amitriptyline alone and was not evident for IPT at 16 weeks (Weissman et al. 1981).

A landmark trial in the history of antidepressant psychotherapy was the multisite National Institute of Mental Health Treatment of Depression Collaborative Research Program (NIMH TDCRP; Elkin et al. 1989). Investigators randomly assigned 250 outpatients with major depression to 16 weeks of IPT, cognitive-behavioral therapy (CBT; Beck et al. 1979), or either imipramine or pill placebo with clinical management. This was the first comparison of IPT and CBT, each of which had demonstrated efficacy in separate trials, and the first trial to manualize and monitor the psychotherapeutic input of pharmacotherapists. Most patients completed at least 15 weeks or 12 treatment sessions. Those with milder depression (defined as a score <20 on the 17-item Hamilton Depression Rating Scale [HDRS; Hamilton 1960]) improved equally in all four treatments. For more severely depressed patients (HDRS ≥20), imipramine worked fastest and most consistently better than placebo. IPT and imipramine were comparable on HDRS and several other outcome measures and superior to placebo for more severely depressed patients. CBT was not superior to placebo among the more depressed patients.

A reanalysis of TDCRP data by Klein and Ross using the Johnson-Neyman technique reported an ordering for treatment efficacy, with "medication superior to psychotherapy, [and] the psychotherapies somewhat superior to placebo…particularly among the symptomatic and impaired patients" (Klein and Ross 1993, p. 241), and found "CBT relatively inferior to IPT for patients with Beck Depression Inventory (BDI; Beck 1978) scores greater than approximately 30, generally considered the boundary between moderate and severe depression" (p. 247). The reanalysis sharpens differences among treatments.

In a follow-up of TDCRP subjects 18 months later, Shea et al. (1992) found no significant difference in recovery among remitters (those with minimal or no symptoms when treatment ended, sustained during follow-up) among the four treatments. Thirty percent of CBT, 26% of IPT, 19% of imipramine, and 20% of placebo subjects who had acutely remitted maintained remission during that time span. Among acute remitters, relapse over the 18-month follow-up was 36% for CBT, 33% for IPT, 50% for imipramine (medication having been stopped at 16 weeks), and 33% for placebo. Shea and colleagues concluded that 16 weeks of specific treatments were insufficient to achieve full and lasting recovery for many patients.

Maintenance Treatment

IPT was first tested in an 8-month, six-cell trial (Klerman et al. 1974; Paykel et al. 1975) that today would be considered *continuation* treatment because the concept of long-term maintenance antidepressant treatment has lengthened. In this trial, acutely depressed outpatient women were first treated with amitriptyline for 4–6 weeks. Responders to amitriptyline ($N=150$) were randomly assigned to receive 8 months of weekly IPT, amitriptyline, placebo, combined IPT plus amitriptyline, IPT plus placebo, or no pill. Randomization to IPT or a low-contact psychotherapy condition occurred at entry into the continuation phase, whereas randomization to medication, placebo, or no pill occurred at the end of the second month of continuation. Continuation pharmacotherapy prevented relapse and symptom exacerbation, whereas IPT improved social functioning (Weissman et al. 1974). The effects of IPT on social functioning did not appear for 6–8 months. Combined psychotherapy-pharmacotherapy had the best outcome.

Longer antidepressant maintenance trials of IPT have been conducted in Pittsburgh. Frank et al. (1990, 1991) treated 128 outpatients with multiply and rapidly recurrent depression: a mean six prior episodes of major depression (Frank et al. 1990). These patients initially received combined high-dose (>200 mg/day) imipramine and weekly sessions of IPT. Responders continued high-dosage medication while IPT was tapered to a monthly frequency during a 4-month continuation phase. Patients who remained in remission were then randomly assigned to 3 years of either 1) ongoing high-dose imipramine plus clinical management; 2) high-dose imipramine plus monthly IPT; 3) monthly IPT alone; 4) monthly IPT plus placebo; or 5) placebo plus clinical management. High-dose imipramine (mean dosage >200 mg/day) proved the most efficacious treatment, protecting more than 80% of patients over 3 years. In contrast, most patients receiving placebo relapsed within the first few months. In maintenance IPT, therapists were permitted to switch interpersonal foci in order to deal with patients' current life problems. Once-monthly IPT was less efficacious than medication but statistically and clinically superior to the placebo condition in this high-risk patient population. Reynolds and colleagues (1999) replicated the superiority of IPT over the control condition but found advantages for combined treatment over both monotherapies in a maintenance study comparing IPT, nortriptyline, their combination, and placebo for 187 geriatric patients with recurrent major depression.

In a fascinating analysis, Cyranowski et al. (2004) found that patients who maintained euthymia after 2 years of maintenance IPT tended to lose their apparent Cluster C personality disorders.

The modal depressed patient is a woman of childbearing age. Frank and colleagues' finding of an 82-week survival time without recurrence with IPT would suffice to protect many women with recurrent depression through pregnancy and nursing without medication. Further study is required to determine the efficacy of IPT relative to newer medications (e.g., selective serotonin reuptake inhibitors [Frank et al. 2011]) and the efficacy of dosages other than once-monthly maintenance IPT. A study of differing dosages of maintenance IPT for depressed patients in Pittsburgh has not found differences in outcome on the basis of frequency of sessions (Frank et al. 2007). Perhaps optimal dosing of maintenance IPT depends on individual patients' needs.

Geriatric Depressed Patients

The first study of geriatric depression involving IPT used it as augmentation to a 6-week pharmacotherapy trial to enhance compliance and to provide some treatment for the placebo control group (Rothblum et al. 1982; Sholomskas et al. 1983). The investigators reported that grief and role transition specific to life changes were the prime treatment foci. They suggested modifications of IPT for older patients that included more flexible duration of sessions and greater use of practical advice and support (e.g., arranging transportation, calling the physician), and they noted that with major role changes (e.g., divorce at age 75), IPT may be impractical and detrimental. The 6-week trial compared standard IPT with nortriptyline in 30 geriatric depressed patients. Results showed some advantages for IPT, largely because of higher attrition in the medication group due to nortriptyline side effects (Sloane et al. 1985).

Reynolds et al. (1999) conducted a 3-year maintenance study for geriatric patients with recurrent ajor depression in Pittsburgh using IPT and nortriptyline in a design similar to the Frank et al. (1990) study. The IPT manual was modified to allow more flexible length of sessions, under the assumption that some elderly patients might not tolerate 50-minute sessions. The authors found that older patients needed to address early life relationships in their psychotherapy, a distinction from the typical "here and now" focus of IPT. Like Sholomskas et al. (1983), Reynolds and colleagues felt that therapists needed to help patients solve practical problems and to acknowledge that some problems, such as existential late-life issues or lifelong psychopathology, might not be amenable to resolutions (Rothblum et al. 1982). Elderly depressed patients whose sleep quality normalized by the early continuation phase had an 80% chance of remaining euthymic during the first year of maintenance treatment. Response rates were similar for patients who subsequently received either nortriptyline or IPT.

Reynolds and colleagues (1999) acutely treated 187 geriatric patients (60 years and older) with recurrent major depression using combined IPT and nortriptyline. One hundred seven remitted and then achieved recovery after continuation therapy. The researchers randomly assigned patients to one of four 3-year maintenance conditions: 1) medication clinic with nortriptyline, maintaining steady-state nortriptyline plasma levels within a therapeutic window of 80–120 ng/mL; 2) medication clinic with placebo; 3) monthly maintenance IPT with placebo; or 4) monthly maintenance IPT (IPT-M) plus nortriptyline. Recurrence rates were 20% for combined treatment, 43% for nortriptyline, 64% for maintenance IPT with placebo, and 90% for placebo alone. Each monotherapy was statistically superior to placebo, whereas combined therapy showed superiority to IPT alone and a trend for superiority to medication alone.

In the Reynolds et al. (1999) study, patients in their 70s were more likely to suffer a recurrence and to do so more quickly than patients in their 60s. This study corroborates the maintenance findings of Frank et al. 1990, 1991) with the difference that combined treatment had advantages over pharmacotherapy alone for the geriatric population. In a similar subsequent study, Reynolds and colleagues again found that once-monthly maintenance IPT was not efficacious in preventing relapse in 116 depressed patients 70 years or older who had responded to the combination of IPT and paroxetine (Reynolds et al. 2006).

It is easy to misinterpret the comparison of high-dose tricyclic antidepressants to low-dose IPT-M in the Frank et al. (1999) and Reynolds et al. (1999) studies. These first tests of psychotherapy as a maintenance treatment compared the lowest-ever doses of psychotherapy to the then highest-ever maintenance doses of medication. Had the tricyclics been lowered comparably to the psychotherapy dosage, recurrence in the medication groups might well have been greater; had psychotherapy been more frequent, perhaps relapse would have been lower. This was unprecedented research. Under the circumstances, the choice of monthly dosing for IPT-M, although the lowest ever prescribed in a psychotherapy trial, was reasonable and indeed showed benefit. A subsequent maintenance study by Frank et al. (2007) did not show that varying the maintenance dose of IPT increased its efficacy.

Depressed Adolescents

Mufson et al. (1993) modified IPT to incorporate adolescent developmental issues (IPT-A). First they first conducted an open feasibility and follow-up trial comparing IPT-A with clinical monitoring in 48 clinic-referred adolescents, ages 12–18, who met DSM-III-R (American Psychiatric Association 1987) criteria for major depressive disorder. Then they conducted a controlled 12-week clinical trial with the same patients. Patients were seen fortnightly by blind independent evaluators to assess symptoms, social functioning, and social problem-solving skills. Thirty-two of the 48 patients completed the protocol (21 IPT-A, 11 control).

Patients receiving IPT-A reported significantly greater improvement in depressive symptoms and overall social functioning, including functioning with friends and problem-solving skills. In the intention-to-treat sample, 75% of IPT-A patients met the criterion for remission (HDRS score ≤6), compared with 46% of control patients. These findings support the feasibility, patient acceptance, and efficacy of 12 weeks of IPT-A with acutely depressed adolescents in reducing depressive symptoms and improving social functioning and interpersonal problem-solving skills (Mufson et al. 1999).

Mufson and colleagues (2004b) subsequently tested IPT-A in an effectiveness study of depressed adolescents (N=63) in school-based clinics, a common site for adolescent treatment, yet one where empirically based therapies have been nearly absent. The investigators found IPT-A, delivered by school social workers, to be markedly superior to treatment as usual. The same research group has since studied IPT-A in group format for depressed adolescents (Mufson et al. 2004c) and training therapists in IPT-A in larger health care systems (Mufson et al. 2018).

Roselló, Bernal, and Rivera at the University of Puerto Rico randomly assigned adolescents ages 13–18 who met DSM-III-R criteria for major depression, dysthymia, or both to 12 weeks of IPT (n=22), CBT (n=25), or a waiting list control condition (n=24). The investigators found both IPT (effect size=0.73) and CBT (effect size=0.43) more efficacious than the control condition in reducing adolescents' self-rated depressive symptoms. IPT increased self-esteem and social adaptation more effectively than did CBT (Rosselló and Bernal 1999).

Depressed HIV-Positive Patients

Markowitz and colleagues modified IPT for depressed HIV patients (IPT-HIV), emphasizing issues this population faces, including concerns about illness and death, grief, and role transitions (Markowitz 1998; Markowitz et al. 1992). In a pilot open trial, 21 of 24 depressed patients responded with symptom reduction. In a 16-week study, 101 subjects were randomly assigned to IPT-HIV, CBT, brief supportive psychotherapy (BSP), or imipramine plus BSP (Markowitz et al. 1998). Echoing the outcomes of the more severely depressed subjects in the TDCRP study (Elkin et al. 1989), all treatments were associated with symptom reduction, but IPT and imipramine plus BSP produced symptomatic and functional improvement significantly greater than was observed with CBT or BSP. Many patients reported improvement in depressive physical symptoms that they had mistakenly attributed to HIV infection. Heckman et al. (2017) have since used telephone-IPT to treat depressed rural patients with HIV.

Depressed Primary Care Patients

Schulberg and colleagues compared IPT and nortriptyline for depressed ambulatory medical patients in a primary care setting (Schulberg and Scott 1991; Schulberg et al. 1993). They did not modify the IPT manual but rather integrated IPT into the routine of the primary care center. Nurses took vital signs before each session, and therapists saw patients at the medical clinic. If patients were medically hospitalized, IPT was continued in the hospital when possible.

Patients with current major depression (n=276) were randomly assigned to IPT, nortriptyline, or primary care physicians' usual care. They were seen weekly for 16 weeks and monthly thereafter for 4 months in IPT (Schulberg et al. 1996). Depressive symptom severity declined more rapidly with either nortriptyline or IPT than in usual care. After 8 months, approximately 70% of treatment completers receiving nortriptyline or IPT, but only 20% in usual care, had recovered. Brown et al. (1996) found that patients with a lifetime history of comorbid panic disorder responded more poorly across treatments compared with patients with major depression alone. Frank and colleagues (2000a, 2011) found a similar effect for comorbid panic disorder on depressive outcome.

These studies in depressed medically ill patients suggest that the life event of medical illness may provide a useful focus as a role transition in IPT treatment (cf. Koszycki et al. 2004). On the other hand, a large Canadian study showed no advantage for IPT in treating depressed patients with coronary artery disease (Lespérance et al. 2007).

The Prevention of Suicide in Primary Care Elderly: Collaborative Trial (PROSPECT) study looked at IPT in an effectiveness setting, where IPT was offered as an alternative to or in combination with a serotonin reuptake inhibitor in an intervention to enhance treatment of geriatric patients with major depression in primary care practices. Patients identified by a trained care manager and offered the intervention lowered their depressive symptoms more than did patients in usual care (Alexopoulos et al. 2005) and had reduced rates of suicidal ideation (Bruce et al. 2004). As primary care physicians became acquainted with IPT and its effects, their rate of prescribing IPT over the first study year rose from 11% to 27% (Schulberg et al. 2007).

Conjoint IPT for Depressed Patients With Marital Disputes

Marital conflict can precipitate or complicate depressive episodes (Rounsaville et al. 1979), hence the IPT focus on role disputes. Some clinicians believed that individual psychotherapy for patients in marital disputes may prematurely rupture marriages (Gurman and Kniskern 1978). Therefore, a manual for conjoint IPT of depressed patients with marital disputes (IPT-CM) was developed (Klerman and Weissman 1993) that includes the spouse in all sessions and focuses on the current marital dispute. In a pilot study, 18 patients with major depression linked to the onset or exacerbation of marital disputes were randomly assigned to 16 weeks of either individual IPT or IPT-CM (Foley et al. 1989). Patients in both treatments showed similar reductions in depressive symptoms, but patients receiving IPT-CM reported significantly better marital adjustment, marital affection, and sexual relations, possibly because depressed spouses also benefited. These pilot findings have long required replication in a larger trial using other control groups.

Peripartum Depression

Pregnancy and the postpartum period are times of heightened depressive risk when women may wish to avoid antidepressant medication. Pregnancy and its aftermath also provide natural role transitions as an IPT focus. Exploring these role transitions addresses the depressed pregnant woman's self-evaluation as a parent, the physiological changes of pregnancy, and altered relationships with the spouse or significant other and with other children. Spinelli (1997) used IPT first in an open trial to treat 13 women with antepartum depression and then added "complicated pregnancy" as a fifth interpersonal problem area. Timing and duration of IPT sessions are adjusted in response to bed rest, delivery, obstetrical complications, and childcare. Postpartum mothers may bring children to sessions. As with depressed HIV-positive patients, telephone sessions and hospital visits are sometimes necessary (Spinelli 1997). A controlled clinical trial comparing IPT with a didactic parent education group for 50 depressed pregnant women over 16 weeks of acute treatment showed advantages for IPT (Spinelli and Endicott 2003). A follow-up study largely supported these findings (Spinelli et al. 2016).

O'Hara et al. (2000) randomly assigned 120 women with postpartum depression to IPT or a waiting list control in a 12-week trial with an 18-month follow-up. The investigators assessed both the mothers' symptoms and the mothers' interactions with their infants (Stuart and O'Hara 1995). In the IPT group, 38% met HDRS and 44% met BDI remission criteria, compared with 14% on each measure for the waiting list group. Sixty percent of IPT patients, versus 16% of control subjects, reported more than a 50% reduction on the BDI. Women receiving IPT also showed significant improvement in social adjustment relative to control subjects. Other pregnancy-related trials have included group interventions for postpartum depression (Klier et al. 2001; Zlotnick et al. 2001), a telephone intervention for women with subsyndromal depression postmiscarriage (Neugebauer et al. 2006), and IPT for depressed patients in an infertility clinic (Koszycki et al. 2012).

Persistent Depressive Disorder

In DSM-5 (American Psychiatric Association 2013), chronic depression, formerly termed dysthymic disorder, has been consolidated with major depressive disorder as *persistent depressive disorder (dysthymia)*. Medication benefits roughly half of chronically depressed patients (Kocsis et al. 1988; Thase et al. 1996), but nonresponders may need psychotherapy, and even medication responders may benefit from combined treatment (Markowitz 1994). A modification of IPT for dysthymic disorder (IPT-D) encourages patients to reconceptualize what they have considered their lifelong character flaws as ego-dystonic, chronic mood-dependent symptoms—as a chronic but treatable *state* rather than an immutable *trait*. Therapy itself is defined as an iatrogenic role transition, from believing oneself flawed in personality to recognizing and treating the lingering mood disorder. Markowitz (1994, 1998) openly treated 17 pilot subjects with 16 sessions of IPT-D; none worsened, and 11 remitted.

On the basis of these pilot results, a randomized trial at Cornell Medical College compared 16 weeks of IPT-D alone, BSP, sertraline plus clinical management, and combined IPT plus sertraline for patients with "pure" dysthymia, that is, chronic mild depression without major depression. All groups improved, but IPT showed no greater acute benefits than did BSP, and pharmacotherapy appeared to be more efficacious than either psychotherapy (Markowitz et al. 2005).

Browne and colleagues (2002) at McMaster University in Hamilton, Ontario, Canada treated 707 dysthymic patients in the community with either 12 sessions of standard IPT over 4 months, sertraline (50–200 mg/day) for 2 years, or a combination of both. Patients were followed for 2 years. Using the criterion of a 40% reduction in score on the Montgomery-Åsberg Depression Rating Scale (MADRS) at 1-year follow-up, 51% of IPT-only subjects improved, significantly fewer than the 63% taking sertraline and 62% in combined treatment. On follow-up, however, IPT was associated with significant economic savings in use of family health care and social services. Thus, combined treatment was as efficacious as but less expensive than sertraline alone.

Feijò de Mello and colleagues (2001) randomly assigned 35 dysthymic outpatients to receive moclobemide with or without 16 weekly sessions of IPT. Both groups improved, but there was a nonsignificant trend for greater improvement on the HDRS and the MADRS in the combined treatment group. Similarly, Hellerstein and colleagues (2001) found that combining interpersonal and cognitive elements improved outcome over fluoxetine alone among dysthymic patients responding to fluoxetine.

Chronic depression is by and large more difficult to treat than acute depression, in part because of the ingrained despair that attends its very chronicity. IPT, like other evidence-based antidepressant psychotherapies, has not fared particularly well as a monotherapy for chronically depressed patients, but it may yet have benefit as an adjunct to medication, much as it may for bipolar disorder.

Bipolar Disorder

Frank and colleagues assessed the benefits of adjunctive IPT modified by social zeitgeber theory—behavioral scheduling of daily routines, especially sleep patterns (Ehlers et al. 1988; Malkoff-Schwartz et al. 2000)—as maintenance therapy in a study of 175 medication-treated bipolar patients, comparing IPSRT with medication clinic (Frank et al. 2005). The behavioral component helps to protect sleep patterns and limit the disruptions that may provoke mania; the IPT approach to depression remains largely the same.

In the study by Frank et al. (2005), acutely ill bipolar patients were treated with medication and randomly assigned to IPSRT or clinical management. Once patients achieved 4 weeks of stabilization, they were randomly assigned to either IPSRT or clinical management for 3 years of maintenance treatment with continuing pharmacotherapy. Results of this complicated trial indicated that although treatments did not differ in time to initial stabilization of symptoms, IPSRT with medication was superior to the comparison condition in delaying recurrence of depressive and manic episodes.

A component of the large Systematic Treatment Enhancement Program for Bipolar Disorder (STEP-BD) study compared 9 months of IPSRT with CBT and family-focused psychotherapy for 152 bipolar disorder patients and found all of these treatments more helpful than a collaborative care condition in improving functioning (Miklowitz et al. 2007). Swartz and colleagues (2018) randomly assigned 92 patients with bipolar II disorder to 20 weeks of either IPSRT plus placebo or IPSRT plus quetiapine. Patients receiving combined treatment improved faster, but by end of treatment, response was comparable, and patients receiving quetiapine had greater weight gain, sedation, and other side effects.

In sum, IPT is an efficacious treatment for major depression across the life span, and in adapted form (IPSRT) it benefits patients with bipolar disorder as well.

IPT for Nonmood Disorders

Demonstration of the efficacy of IPT as an antidepressant treatment led to its adaptation as a treatment for other psychiatric disorders. Life events are ubiquitous; when is it useful to focus treatment on them? Research has begun to answer this question.

Bulimia Nervosa

Fairburn et al. (1993) altered IPT for bulimic patients, eliminating the use of the sick role and of role-playing in order to contrast distinct therapeutic strategies in comparing IPT and CBT. In an initial study, 75 patients with bulimia nervosa were randomly assigned to 19 sessions of IPT, CBT, or a behavioral therapy control over 18 weeks. CBT worked faster to relieve bulimic symptoms, but on follow-up IPT had benefits comparable to those of CBT and superior to the control condition. A subsequent multisite trial (N=220) found CBT to be superior to IPT (Agras et al. 2000). Nonetheless, IPT is one of the better-tested treatments for bulimia and is at least a second-line treatment after CBT. Wilfley and colleagues (1993, 2000, 2002) have also demonstrated the efficacy of a group adaptation of IPT for eating disorders (see Chapter 21, "Theories and Techniques of Group Therapy").

A research group in Christchurch, New Zealand, applied IPT to anorexia nervosa (McIntosh et al. 2005). In this trial 56 anorexic women were treated with 20 weekly sessions of IPT, CBT, or a supportive therapy control. Neither IPT nor CBT showed efficacy as an outpatient treatment, faring worse than the control. This finding unfortunately is consonant with anorexia outcome literature generally.

Anxiety Disorders

Long considered the treatment domain of CBT, anxiety disorders have been less studied but increasingly have been shown to respond to IPT. Joshua Lipsitz was an IPT pioneer in this area (Lipsitz et al. 1999, 2006, 2008). My colleagues and I reviewed this literature in 2014 (Markowitz et al. 2014), identifying six open and five controlled trials of IPT for social anxiety disorder, panic disorder, and posttraumatic stress disorder. Although the studies were generally small, underpowered, and sometimes methodologically compromised, IPT yielded positive results in open trials for the three diagnoses. In controlled studies, IPT fared better than waiting list (N=2), was as effective as supportive psychodynamic psychotherapy (N=1)—both worked—but was less efficacious than CBT for social anxiety disorder (N=1) and panic disorder (N=1) in a methodologically complicated study. IPT equaled CBT in a group residential format (N=1). These findings emerged despite minimal adaptation of IPT from its standard depression strategies (in contrast, CBT is quite differently adapted according to diagnosis). We concluded that IPT shows promise for anxiety disorders despite methodological and ecological issues that have complicated its testing but thus far has shown no advantages in controlled trials relative to other therapies.

PTSD is an anxiety disorder defined by a life event, suggesting the utility of IPT in its treatment. Krupnick and colleagues (2008) compared group IPT with a waiting list control in a randomized trial of 48 multiply victimized non-treatment-seeking women with PTSD in public sector gynecology clinics in Virginia. They found that IPT was more effective than the control condition in reducing PTSD and depressive symptoms and in improving interpersonal functioning. In Brazil, Campanini and colleagues (2010) randomly assigned half of a sample of 40 patients with PTSD who had not responded to at least 12 weeks of standard pharmacotherapy to group IPT and found significant improvement, with large effect sizes.

Individual IPT has been adapted for PTSD, focusing on the need for affective attunement in patients whose numbness made it hard for them to connect feelings to life circumstance. A small open pilot trial ($N=14$) found excellent outcomes (Bleiberg and Markowitz 2005). A randomized 14-week trial (Markowitz et al. 2015) then compared IPT with prolonged exposure, the best-tested exposure therapy, and with relaxation therapy, an active control, treating 110 unmedicated patients with chronic PTSD. All treatments showed large effect sizes, with IPT and prolonged exposure having comparable outcomes and being superior to relaxation therapy. Patients preferred IPT to exposure despite its relative lack of supporting evidence (Markowitz et al. 2016). Moreover, IPT had lower dropout than exposure therapy among depressed patients and better outcome than either opposing therapy for patients with sexual trauma (Markowitz et al. 2017). At 3-month follow-up, patients who had responded to or remitted with IPT maintained their gains (Markowitz et al. 2018). These studies, and others awaiting publication, suggest that IPT may provide a tolerable and effective treatment alternative to the exposure-based therapies that have dominated the PTSD literature. IPT has now been added to Department of Defense/Veterans Administration PTSD treatment guidelines (U.S. Department of Veterans Affairs 2017).

Substance Abuse

IPT has not demonstrated efficacy in several clinical trials for patients with substance dependence. Rounsaville and colleagues (1983) studied 72 methadone-maintained opiate users and found that adding adjunctive IPT to standard substance abuse care (which already included a psychotherapy component) had no additional benefit in reducing psychopathology. Both treatment groups improved. The same research group treated 42 subjects with cocaine abuse who were attempting to achieve abstinence and found 12 weeks of IPT to be ineffective and marginally worse than a behavioral control (Carroll et al. 1991). Carroll and colleagues (2004) also treated 121 cocaine-dependent subjects in a 12-week 2×2 cell trial with either IPT or CBT and disulfiram 250 mg or placebo. CBT and disulfiram were superior to IPT and to placebo.

These negative studies suggest limits to the range of utility of IPT but do not necessarily preclude its use for all substance abuse. IPT might be useful, for example, as a treatment for newly abstinent alcohol-dependent patients, who face psychosocial stressors that have been shown to precipitate relapse. A pilot study of patients with chronic depression and secondary alcohol abuse (Markowitz et al. 2008) compared IPT ($n=14$) with brief supportive psychotherapy ($n=12$). Although IPT showed some advantage in reducing depressive symptoms, patients in both groups almost immediately stopped drinking, yielding no difference between treatments.

Other Applications

Research groups have tested the applicability of IPT to depressed cancer patients (Blanco et al. 2019) and to borderline personality disorder (Markowitz et al. 2006b), insomnia, and other disorders (Weissman et al. 2018). The IPT focus on life events suggests its potential applicability to patients with medical illness (Markowitz et al. 1998). Swartz and colleagues (2014, 2016) have found that IPT can be effective in a brief, eight-session form.

Interpersonal Counseling

Many patients present to primary care practices reporting psychiatric symptoms that do not meet threshold criteria for a psychiatric disorder. These symptoms nonetheless can be debilitating and may result in high wasted utilization of medical procedures (Wells et al. 1989). Interpersonal counseling (IPC), based on IPT, was designed to treat distressed primary care patients who do not meet full syndromal criteria for psychiatric disorders. IPC is administered for a maximum of six sessions by health care professionals without formal psychiatric training, usually nurse practitioners. The first session can last up to 30 minutes; subsequent sessions are briefer.

IPC therapists assess the patient's current functioning, recent life events, occupational and familial stressors, and changes in interpersonal relationships. They assume that such events provide the context in which emotional and bodily symptoms occur. Klerman and colleagues (1987) studied 128 patients in a primary care clinic who scored 6 or higher on the Goldberg General Health Questionnaire (GHQ), randomly assigning them to IPC provided by medical nurses without prior psychotherapy training or to usual care without psychological treatment (Klerman et al. 1987). Over an average of 3 months, IPC subjects—often receiving only one or two IPC sessions—showed significantly greater symptom relief, especially mood improvement, on the GHQ than did control subjects. IPC subjects were more likely to subsequently make use of mental health services, suggesting a new awareness of the psychological aspect of their symptoms.

Mossey et al. (1996) noted that even depressive symptoms that do not reach the threshold for major depression impede recovery of hospitalized elderly patients. They conducted a 10-session trial of IPC for elderly hospitalized medical patients with minor depressive symptoms. Nonpsychiatric nurses delivered the treatment. Patients were seen for hour-long sessions on a flexible schedule to accommodate the patient's medical status. Hospitalized patients older than age 60 ($N=76$) who had subsyndromal depressive symptoms on two consecutive assessments were randomly assigned to IPC or to usual care. Researchers also followed an untreated euthymic control group. Patients found IPC feasible and tolerable. Assessment at 3 months showed nonsignificantly greater improvement in depressive symptoms and on all outcome variables for IPC relative to usual care, whereas control subjects showed a slight symptomatic worsening. Rehospitalization was virtually identical in the IPC and euthymic control groups (11%–15%) and significantly less than for the subsyndromally depressed group receiving usual care (50%). Differences between IPC and usual care groups reached statistical significance at 6 months on depressive symptom reduction and self-rated health but not physical or social functioning. The investigators felt that 10 sessions were insufficient for some patients and that a maintenance phase might have been useful.

A dramatic study demonstrating the adaptability of IPT to a very different culture tested a group variant of IPC in randomly assigned villages in a poverty- and AIDS-stricken region of Uganda where depression rates are high. IPT was chosen as an intervention because antidepressant medication was unaffordable and other psychotherapies seemed incompatible with the local outlook. Researchers adjusted for cultural differences but applied the usual IPT paradigm. Local college graduates without mental health experience provided treatment. The group IPC intervention was impressively more effective than treatment as usual (Bolton et al. 2003), and gains persisted at 6-month follow-up (Bass et al. 2006). Indeed, the simplicity and effectiveness of IPC and the universality of recognition of the connection between life events and mood have led to its increasing use in developing countries. Where psychotropic medications can be unaffordable, therapists with limited training have produced impressive results (Bortolotti et al. 2008).

IPT by Telephone

Because many patients avoid or have difficulty reaching an office for face-to-face treatment, IPC is being tested as a telephone treatment. Weissman and Miller at Columbia University conducted a successful pilot feasibility trial comparing IPT by telephone to no treatment for 30 patients with recurrent major depression who had not received regular treatment (Miller and Weissman 2002). Neugebauer and colleagues (2006) found telephone IPC to be a helpful intervention for women with minor depression postmiscarriage. Heckman et al. have found telephone IPT to be effective in treating depression in HIV-positive patients (Heckman et al. 2017; Ransom et al. 2008).

IPT Patient Guide

Weissman (2006) developed an IPT patient guide with worksheets for depressed individuals who want information about or are receiving IPT. Worksheets can be used to facilitate sessions or to monitor problem areas after treatment. The utility of the patient book in enhancing treatment has not been studied.

Summary of Research Findings

IPT has demonstrated efficacy as an acute and as a maintenance monotherapy and as a component of combined treatment for patients with major depressive disorder. It is a second-line treatment for bulimia, less tested and sometimes less effective than CBT. Encouraging research suggests the applicability of IPT to anxiety disorders, particularly to PTSD, although additional randomized controlled trials are necessary to confirm this promise. IPT seems adaptable to different lengths, formats, and cultures.

On the other hand, IPT has not shown benefit for substance use disorders or as a monotherapy for chronic persistent depression. Unlike with some other therapies, IPT researchers have taken a modest, treatment-by-treatment approach to its indications, relying on research to demonstrate efficacy before applying the treatment clinically. It is unsurprising that this treatment, which was never intended for universal application, should have its limits. The unfortunate curtailing of clinical research by the NIMH may constrain such clinically valuable exploration.

Differential Therapeutics

When two or more treatments have demonstrated comparable efficacy for a diagnosis such as major depressive disorder, when is one treatment more likely to yield a better

TABLE 15–2. **Indications for interpersonal psychotherapy (IPT) vs. cognitive-behavioral therapy (CBT)**

Predictor	IPT	CBT
Life events	Present	Absent
Social dysfunction (baseline)	Low	Very high (interpersonal deficits)
Symptom severity (baseline)	Higher	Lower
Personality disorder	Obsessive	Avoidant

outcome than another? Comparative trials have begun to reveal moderating factors or predictors of treatment outcome. Studies such as the NIMH TDCRP, which compared IPT and CBT, have suggested factors that might predict better outcome with either IPT or CBT (Table 15–2).

Sotsky and colleagues (1991) found that depressed patients with a low baseline level of social dysfunction responded well to IPT, whereas those with severe social deficits (probably equivalent to the interpersonal deficits problem area [Weissman et al. 2018]) responded less well. Patients with greater symptom severity and difficulty in concentrating responded poorly to CBT. Greater initial severity of major depression and of impaired functioning predicted superior response to IPT and to imipramine. Imipramine also worked most efficaciously for patients with difficulty functioning at work, likely reflecting its faster onset of action. Patients with atypical depression responded better to either IPT or CBT than to imipramine or placebo (Shea et al. 1999).

Barber and Muenz (1996), looking only at TDCRP completers, found IPT to be more efficacious than CBT for patients with obsessive personality traits, whereas CBT fared better for avoidant personality disorder. Biological factors also play a role: for example, presence of abnormal sleep profiles on electroencephalogram predicted significantly poorer response to IPT than did normal sleep parameters (Thase et al. 1997). Frank and colleagues (1991) found that psychotherapist adherence to a focused IPT approach may enhance outcome. Replication and further elaboration of these predictive factors deserve ongoing study.

Many psychiatrists recognize that medication and psychotherapy each has distinct benefits, making the combination of the two tempting. Yet monotherapy with either IPT or pharmacotherapy is likely to suffice for most patients with major depressive disorder. Hence, combined treatment is probably best reserved for severely or chronically ill patients (Rush and Thase 1999). How best to combine time-limited psychotherapy with pharmacotherapy—for which patients, in what sequence, and so on—is an exciting area for future research.

The Future

The history of IPT has been a succession of outcome trials that have helped to define diagnostic indications for this treatment. Because psychotherapy is underfunded relative to pharmacotherapy, we have fewer studies and know far less about the dosage and indications of IPT than about antidepressant medications. Future outcome trials may continue to define the territory of IPT's utility. These should include both tests for different diagnoses, such as the anxiety disorders, testing of dosage—optimal frequency and duration of IPT sessions—and also studies of the sequencing of IPT with other treatments. For example, when, and for whom, is IPT best combined with pharmacotherapy? Is it best to start with pharmacotherapy and then add IPT? If so, at what interval, and with what frequency? When should IPT be used as augmentation for pharmacotherapy and vice versa? Other research may help to determine the cost-effectiveness and potential cost offset of IPT as a treatment that improves both symptoms and social functioning.

IPT has also been anomalous among psychotherapies in its nearly pure focus to date on outcome studies. Now that it is clear that IPT helps many patients, process research seems warranted to try to identify its active, mediating factors. Little is known about the specific value of many IPT interventions. It is even unclear, for example, whether focusing on a role transition rather than a role dispute makes a difference for patients, or whether particular sorts of life events are helpful or unhelpful foci. It does appear that IPT therapists agree in choosing focal interpersonal problem areas (Markowitz et al. 2000) and that solving an interpersonal problem area correlates with treatment outcome, as IPT theory would predict (Markowitz et al. 2006a). Patient and therapist characteristics may also potentially influence treatment outcome.

Clinical training in IPT is growing. How it spreads will be a function of training programs and of organizations such as the International Society of Interpersonal Psychotherapy. Training now includes formalized accreditation, both to ensure clinical competence and to satisfy managed care organizations. Research is needed on how best to teach and disseminate IPT to ensure that IPT delivered by practitioners in clinical practice (Markowitz 2001) yields results comparable to those of therapists in research trials.

Key Points

- IPT has demonstrated efficacy as an acute treatment for patients with major depressive disorder and bulimia nervosa.
- IPT has demonstrated efficacy as a maintenance treatment for patients with major depressive disorder
- IPT is a time-limited, diagnosis-focused treatment adaptable to multiple diagnoses, formats, durations, and cultures.
- IPT has not demonstrated efficacy in three studies of substance abuse and appears less effective than pharmacotherapy as a monotherapy for dysthymic disorder.

Recommended Readings

Frank E: Treating Bipolar Disorders: A Clinician's Guide to Interpersonal and Social Rhythm Therapy. New York, Guilford, 2005

Frank E, Kupfer DJ, Wagner EF, et al: Efficacy of interpersonal psychotherapy as a maintenance treatment of recurrent depression. Arch Gen Psychiatry 48:1053–1059, 1991

International Society for Interpersonal Psychotherapy: www.interpersonalpsychotherapy.org

Mufson L, Dorta KP, Moreau D, et al: Interpersonal Therapy for Depressed Adolescents, 2nd Edition. New York, Guilford, 2004

Weissman MM, Markowitz JC, Klerman GL: The Guide to Interpersonal Psychotherapy. New York, Oxford University Press, 2018

References

Agras WS, Walsh T, Fairburn CG, et al: A multicenter comparison of cognitive-behavioral therapy and interpersonal psychotherapy for bulimia nervosa. Arch Gen Psychiatry 57(5):459–466, 2000 10807486

Alexopoulos GS, Katz IR, Bruce ML, et al: Remission in depressed geriatric primary care patients: a report from the PROSPECT study. Am J Psychiatry 162(4):718–724, 2005 15800144

American Psychiatric Association: Diagnostic and Statistical Manual of Mental Disorders, 3rd Edition, Revised. Washington, DC, American Psychiatric Association, 1987

American Psychiatric Association: Practice Guidelines for the Treatment of Psychiatric Disorders: Compendium 2006. Washington, DC, American Psychiatric Association, 2006

American Psychiatric Association: Practice Guideline for the Treatment of Patients With Major Depressive Disorder, 3rd Edition. Washington, DC, American Psychiatric Association, 2010

American Psychiatric Association: Diagnostic and Statistical Manual of Mental Disorders, 5th Edition. Arlington, VA, American Psychiatric Association, 2013

Barber JP, Muenz LR: The role of avoidance and obsessiveness in matching patients to cognitive and interpersonal psychotherapy: empirical findings from the Treatment for Depression Collaborative Research Program. J Consult Clin Psychol 64(5):951–958, 1996 8916624

Bass J, Neugebauer R, Clougherty KF, et al: Group interpersonal psychotherapy for depression in rural Uganda: 6-month outcomes: randomised controlled trial. Br J Psychiatry 188:567–573, 2006 16738348

Beck AT: Depression Inventory. Philadelphia, Center for Cognitive Therapy, 1978

Beck AT, Rush AJ, Shaw BF, et al: Cognitive Therapy of Depression. New York, Guilford, 1979

Blanco C, Markowitz JC, Hellerstein DJ, et al: A randomized trial of interpersonal psychotherapy, problem solving therapy, and supportive therapy for major depressive disorder in women with breast cancer. Breast Cancer Res Treat 173(2):353–364, 2019 30343455

Bleiberg KL, Markowitz JC: A pilot study of interpersonal psychotherapy for posttraumatic stress disorder. Am J Psychiatry 162(1):181–183, 2005 15625219

Bolton P, Bass J, Neugebauer R, et al: Group interpersonal psychotherapy for depression in rural Uganda: a randomized controlled trial. JAMA 289(23):3117–3124, 2003 12813117

Bortolotti B, Scocco P, Markowitz JC, et al: Interpersonal counseling: a narrative literature review. J Psychosom Res 64:642, 2008

Bowlby J: Attachment and Loss. New York, Basic Books, 1973

Brown C, Schulberg HC, Madonia MJ, et al: Treatment outcomes for primary care patients with major depression and lifetime anxiety disorders. Am J Psychiatry 153(10):1293–1300, 1996 8831437

Browne G, Steiner M, Roberts J, et al: Sertraline and/or interpersonal psychotherapy for patients with dysthymic disorder in primary care: 6-month comparison with longitudinal 2-year follow-up of effectiveness and costs. J Affect Disord 68(2–3):317–330, 2002 12063159

Bruce ML, Ten Have TR, Reynolds CF III, et al: Reducing suicidal ideation and depressive symptoms in depressed older primary care patients: a randomized controlled trial. JAMA 291(9):1081–1091, 2004 14996777

Campanini RF, Schoedl AF, Pupo MC, et al: Efficacy of interpersonal therapy-group format adapted to post-traumatic stress disorder: an open-label add-on trial. Depress Anxiety 27(1):72–77, 2010 20013958

Carroll KM, Rounsaville BJ, Gawin FH: A comparative trial of psychotherapies for ambulatory cocaine abusers: relapse prevention and interpersonal psychotherapy. Am J Drug Alcohol Abuse 17(3):229–247, 1991 1928019

Carroll KM, Fenton LR, Ball SA, et al: Efficacy of disulfiram and cognitive behavior therapy in cocaine-dependent outpatients: a randomized placebo-controlled trial. Arch Gen Psychiatry 61(3):264–272, 2004 14993114

Cuijpers P, Geraedts AS, van Oppen P, et al: Interpersonal psychotherapy for depression: a meta-analysis. Am J Psychiatry 168(6):581–592, 2011 21362740

Cuijpers P, Donker T, Weissman MM, et al: Interpersonal psychotherapy for mental health problems: a comprehensive meta-analysis. Am J Psychiatry 173(7):680–687, 2016 27032627

Cyranowski JM, Frank E, Winter E, et al: Personality pathology and outcome in recurrently depressed women over 2 years of maintenance interpersonal psychotherapy. Psychol Med 34(4):659–669, 2004 15099420

de Mello MF, Myczcowisk LM, Menezes PR: A randomized controlled trial comparing moclobemide and moclobemide plus interpersonal psychotherapy in the treatment of dysthymic disorder. J Psychother Pract Res 10(2):117–123, 2001 11264335

Depression Guideline Panel: Clinical Practice Guideline. Depression in Primary Care: Volumes 1–4 (AHCPR Publ No 93-0550-0553). Rockville, MD, Agency for Health Care Policy and Research, U.S. Department of Health and Human Services, 1993

DiMascio A, Weissman MM, Prusoff BA, et al: Differential symptom reduction by drugs and psychotherapy in acute depression. Arch Gen Psychiatry 36(13):1450–1456, 1979 518245

Donnelly JM, Kornblith AB, Fleishman S, et al: A pilot study of interpersonal psychotherapy by telephone with cancer patients and their partners. Psychooncology 9(1):44–56, 2000 10668059

Ehlers CL, Frank E, Kupfer DJ: Social zeitgebers and biological rhythms: a unified approach to understanding the etiology of depression. Arch Gen Psychiatry 45(10):948–952, 1988 3048226

Elkin I, Shea MT, Watkins JT, et al: National Institute of Mental Health Treatment of Depression Collaborative Research Program: general effectiveness of treatments. Arch Gen Psychiatry 46(11):971–982, discussion 983, 1989 2684085

Fairburn CG, Jones R, Peveler RC, et al: Psychotherapy and bulimia nervosa: Longer-term effects of interpersonal psychotherapy, behavior therapy, and cognitive behavior therapy. Arch Gen Psychiatry 50(6):419–428, 1993 8498876

Fairburn CG, Norman PA, Welch SL, et al: A prospective study of outcome in bulimia nervosa and the long-term effects of three psychological treatments. Arch Gen Psychiatry 52(4):304–312, 1995 7702447

Foley SH, Rounsaville BJ, Weissman MM, et al: Individual versus conjoint interpersonal psychotherapy for depressed patients with marital disputes. Int J Fam Psychiatry 10:29–42, 1989

Frank E: Interpersonal psychotherapy as a maintenance treatment for patients with recurrent depression. Psychother 28:259–266, 1991

Frank E: Treating Bipolar Disorder: A Clinician's Guide to Interpersonal and Social Rhythm Therapy. New York, Guilford, 2005

Frank E, Kupfer DJ, Perel JM, et al: Three-year outcomes for maintenance therapies in recurrent depression. Arch Gen Psychiatry 47(12):1093–1099, 1990 2244793

Frank E, Kupfer DJ, Wagner EF, et al: Efficacy of interpersonal psychotherapy as a maintenance treatment of recurrent depression: contributing factors. Arch Gen Psychiatry 48(12):1053–1059, 1991 1845438

Frank E, Swartz HA, Mallinger AG, et al: Adjunctive psychotherapy for bipolar disorder: effects of changing treatment modality. J Adnorm Psychol 108(4):579–587, 1999 10609422

Frank E, Shear MK, Rucci P, et al: Influence of panic-agoraphobic spectrum symptoms on treatment response in patients with recurrent major depression. Am J Psychiatry 157(7):1101–1107, 2000a 10873918

Frank E, Kupfer DJ, Thase ME, et al: Two-year outcomes for interpersonal and social rhythm therapy in individuals with bipolar I disorder. Arch Gen Psychiatry 62(9):996–1004, 2005 16143731

Frank E, Kupfer DJ, Buysse DJ, et al: Randomized trial of weekly, twice-monthly, and monthly interpersonal psychotherapy as maintenance treatment for women with recurrent depression. Am J Psychiatry 164(5):761–767, 2007 17475735

Frank E, Cassano GB, Rucci P, et al: Predictors and moderators of time to remission of major depression with interpersonal psychotherapy and SSRI pharmacotherapy. Psychol Med 41(1):151–162, 2011 20380782

Gurman AS, Kniskern DP: Research on marital and family therapy: progress, perspective, and prospect, in Handbook of Psychotherapy and Behavior Change. Edited by Garfield SB, Bergen AB. New York, Wiley, 1978, pp 817–902

Hamilton M: A rating scale for depression. J Neurol Neurosurg Psychiatry 23:56–62, 1960 14399272

Heckman TG, Heckman BD, Anderson T, et al: Tele-interpersonal psychotherapy acutely reduces depressive symptoms in depressed HIV-infected rural persons: a randomized clinical trial. Behav Med 43(4):285–295, 2017 27115565

Hellerstein DJ, Little SAS, Samstag LW, et al: Adding group psychotherapy to medication treatment in dysthymia: a randomized prospective pilot study. J Psychother Pract Res 10(2):93–103, 2001 11264333

Karasu TB, Docherty JP, Gelenberg A, et al: Practice guideline for major depressive disorder in adults. Am J Psychiatry 150(4 suppl):1–26, 1993 8465906

Klein DF, Ross DC: Reanalysis of the National Institute of Mental Health treatment of depression collaborative research program general effectiveness report. Neuropsychopharmacology 8(3):241–251, 1993 8507351

Klerman GL, Weissman MM: New Applications of Interpersonal Psychotherapy. Washington, DC, American Psychiatric Press, 1993

Klerman GL, Dimascio A, Weissman M, et al: Treatment of depression by drugs and psychotherapy. Am J Psychiatry 131(2):186–191, 1974 4587807

Klerman GL, Weissman MM, Rounsaville BJ, et al: Interpersonal Psychotherapy of Depression. New York, Basic Books, 1984

Klerman GL, Budman S, Berwick D, et al: Efficacy of a brief psychosocial intervention for symptoms of stress and distress among patients in primary care. Med Care 25(11):1078–1088, 1987 3695638

Klier CM, Muzik M, Rosenblum KL, et al: Interpersonal psychotherapy adapted for the group setting in the treatment of postpartum depression. J Psychother Pract Res 10(2):124–131, 2001 11264336

Kocsis JH, Frances AJ, Voss C, et al: Imipramine treatment for chronic depression. Arch Gen Psychiatry 45(3):253–257, 1988 3277579

Koszycki D, Lafontaine S, Frasure-Smith N, et al: An open-label trial of interpersonal psychotherapy in depressed patients with coronary disease. Psychosomatics 45(4):319–324, 2004 15232046

Koszycki D, Bisserbe J-C, Blier P, et al: Interpersonal psychotherapy versus brief supportive therapy for depressed infertile women: first pilot randomized controlled trial. Arch Women Ment Health 15(3):193–201, 2012 22526405

Krupnick JL, Green BL, Stockton P, et al: Group interpersonal psychotherapy for low-income women with posttraumatic stress disorder. Psychother Res 18(5):497–507, 2008 18816001

Lespérance F, Frasure-Smith N, Koszycki D, et al: Effects of citalopram and interpersonal psychotherapy on depression in patients with coronary artery disease: the Canadian Cardiac Randomized Evaluation of Antidepressant and Psychotherapy Efficacy (CREATE) trial. JAMA 297(4):367–379, 2007 17244833

Lipsitz JD, Markowitz JC, Cherry S, et al: Open trial of interpersonal psychotherapy for the treatment of social phobia. Am J Psychiatry 156(11):1814–1816, 1999 10553749

Lipsitz JD, Gur M, Miller NL, et al: An open pilot study of interpersonal psychotherapy for panic disorder (IPT-PD). J Nerv Ment Dis 194(6):440–445, 2006 16772862

Lipsitz JD, Gur M, Vermes D, et al: A randomized trial of interpersonal therapy versus supportive therapy for social anxiety disorder. Depress Anxiety 25(6):542–553, 2008 17941096

Malkoff-Schwartz S, Frank E, Anderson BP, et al: Social rhythm disruption and stressful life events in the onset of bipolar and unipolar episodes. Psychol Med 30(5):1005–1016, 2000 12027038

Markowitz JC: Psychotherapy of dysthymia. Am J Psychiatry 151(8):1114–1121, 1994 8037243

Markowitz JC: Teaching interpersonal psychotherapy to psychiatric residents. Acad Psychiatry 19(3):167–173, 1995 24442589

Markowitz JC: Interpersonal Psychotherapy for Dysthymic Disorder. Washington, DC, American Psychiatric Press, 1998

Markowitz JC: Learning the new psychotherapies, in Treatment of Depression: Bridging the 21st Century. Edited by Weissman MM. Washington, DC, American Psychiatric Press, 2001, pp 281–300
Markowitz JC: Interpersonal Psychotherapy for Posttraumatic Stress Disorder. New York, Oxford University Press, 2016
Markowitz JC, Weissman MM: Interpersonal psychotherapy: past, present and future. Clin Psychol Psychother 19(2):99–105, 2012 22331561
Markowitz JC, Klerman GL, Perry SW: Interpersonal psychotherapy of depressed HIV-positive outpatients. Hosp Community Psychiatry 43(9):885–890, 1992 1427695
Markowitz JC, Kocsis JH, Fishman B, et al: Treatment of depressive symptoms in human immunodeficiency virus-positive patients. Arch Gen Psychiatry 55(5):452–457, 1998 9596048
Markowitz JC, Leon AC, Miller NL, et al: Rater agreement on interpersonal psychotherapy problem areas. J Psychother Pract Res 9(3):131–135, 2000 10896737
Markowitz JC, Kocsis JH, Bleiberg KL, et al: A comparative trial of psychotherapy and pharmacotherapy for "pure" dysthymic patients. J Affect Disord 89(1–3):167–175, 2005 16263177
Markowitz JC, Bleiberg KL, Christos P, et al: Solving interpersonal problems correlates with symptom improvement in interpersonal psychotherapy: preliminary findings. J Nerv Ment Dis 194(1):15–20, 2006a 16462550
Markowitz JC, Skodol AE, Bleiberg K: Interpersonal psychotherapy for borderline personality disorder: possible mechanisms of change. J Clin Psychol 62(4):431–444, 2006b 16470711
Markowitz JC, Kocsis JH, Christos P, et al: Pilot study of interpersonal psychotherapy versus supportive psychotherapy for dysthymic patients with secondary alcohol abuse or dependence. J Nerv Ment Dis 196(6):468–474, 2008 18552624
Markowitz JC, Lipsitz J, Milrod BL: Critical review of outcome research on interpersonal psychotherapy for anxiety disorders. Depress Anxiety 31(4):316–325, 2014 24493661
Markowitz JC, Petkova E, Neria Y, et al: Is exposure necessary? A randomized clinical trial of interpersonal psychotherapy for PTSD. Am J Psychiatry 172(5):430–440, 2015 25677355
Markowitz JC, Meehan KB, Petkova E, et al: Treatment preferences of psychotherapy patients with chronic PTSD. J Clin Psychiatry 77(3):363–370, 2016 26115532
Markowitz JC, Neria Y, Lovell K, et al: History of sexual trauma moderates psychotherapy outcome for posttraumatic stress disorder. Depress Anxiety 34(8):692–700, 2017 28376282
Markowitz JC, Choo T, Neria Y: Stability of improvement after psychotherapy of posttraumatic stress disorder. Can J Psychiatry 63:37–43, 2018
McIntosh VV, Jordan J, Carter FA, et al: Three psychotherapies for anorexia nervosa: a randomized, controlled trial. Am J Psychiatry 162(4):741–747, 2005 15800147
Miklowitz DJ, Otto MW, Frank E, et al: Intensive psychosocial intervention enhances functioning in patients with bipolar depression: results from a 9-month randomized controlled trial. Am J Psychiatry 164(9):1340–1347, 2007 17728418
Miller L, Weissman M: Interpersonal psychotherapy delivered over the telephone to recurrent depressives: a pilot study. Depress Anxiety 16(3):114–117, 2002 12415535
Mossey JM, Knott KA, Higgins M, et al: Effectiveness of a psychosocial intervention, interpersonal counseling, for subdysthymic depression in medically ill elderly. J Gerontol A Biol Sci Med Sci 51(4):M172–M178, 1996 8681000
Mufson L, Moreau D, Weissman MM, Klerman GL: Interpersonal Psychotherapy for Depressed Adolescents. New York, Guilford, 1993
Mufson L, Weissman MM, Moreau D, et al: Efficacy of interpersonal psychotherapy for depressed adolescents. Arch Gen Psychiatry 56(6):573–579, 1999 10359475
Mufson L, Dorta KP, Moreau D, et al: Interpersonal Therapy for Depressed Adolescents, 2nd Edition. New York, Guilford, 2004a
Mufson L, Dorta KP, Wickramaratne P, et al: A randomized effectiveness trial of interpersonal psychotherapy for depressed adolescents. Arch Gen Psychiatry 61(6):577–584, 2004b 15184237
Mufson L, Gallagher T, Dorta KP, Young JF: A group adaptation of interpersonal psychotherapy for depressed adolescents. Am J Psychother 58(2):220–237, 2004c 15373283

Mufson L, Rynn M, Yanes-Lukin P, et al: Stepped care interpersonal psychotherapy treatment for depressed adolescents: a pilot study in pediatric clinics. Adm Policy Ment Health 45(3):417–431, 2018 29124527

Neugebauer R, Kline J, Markowitz JC, et al: Pilot randomized controlled trial of interpersonal counseling for subsyndromal depression following miscarriage. J Clin Psychiatry 67(8):1299–1304, 2006 16965211

O'Hara MW, Stuart S, Gorman LL, et al: Efficacy of interpersonal psychotherapy for postpartum depression. Arch Gen Psychiatry 57(11):1039–1045, 2000 11074869

Paykel ES, Dimascio A, Haskell D, et al: Effects of maintenance amitriptyline and psychotherapy on symptoms of depression. Psychol Med 5(1):67–77, 1975 235144

Ransom D, Heckman TG, Anderson T, et al: Telephone-delivered, interpersonal psychotherapy for HIV-infected rural persons with depression: a pilot trial. Psychiatr Serv 59(8):871–877, 2008 18678684

Reynolds CF III, Frank E, Perel JM, et al: Nortriptyline and interpersonal psychotherapy as maintenance therapies for recurrent major depression: a randomized controlled trial in patients older than 59 years. JAMA 281(1):39–45, 1999 9892449

Reynolds CF III, Dew MA, Pollock BG, et al: Maintenance treatment of major depression in old age. N Engl J Med 354(11):1130–1138, 2006 16540613

Rosselló J, Bernal G: The efficacy of cognitive-behavioral and interpersonal treatments for depression in Puerto Rican adolescents. J Consult Clin Psychol 67(5):734–745, 1999 10535240

Rothblum ED, Sholomskas AJ, Berry C, et al: Issues in clinical trials with the depressed elderly. J Am Geriatr Soc 30(11):694–699, 1982 6752250

Rounsaville BJ, Weissman MM, Prusoff BA, et al: Marital disputes and treatment outcome in depressed women. Compr Psychiatry 20(5):483–490, 1979 487804

Rounsaville BJ, Glazer W, Wilber CH, et al: Short-term interpersonal psychotherapy in methadone-maintained opiate addicts. Arch Gen Psychiatry 40(6):629–636, 1983 6342563

Rounsaville BJ, Chevron ES, Weissman MM, et al: Training therapists to perform interpersonal psychotherapy in clinical trials. Compr Psychiatry 27(4):364–371, 1986 3524986

Rush AJ, Thase ME: Psychotherapies for depressive disorders: a review, in Depressive Disorders: World Psychiatric Association Evidence and Experience in Psychiatry Series. Edited by Maj M, Sartorius N. Chichester, UK, Wiley, 1999, pp 161–206

Schulberg HC, Scott CP: Depression in primary care: treating depression with interpersonal psychotherapy, in Psychotherapy in Managed Health Care: The Optimal Use of Time and Resources. Edited by Austad CS, Berman WH. Washington, DC, American Psychological Association, 1991, pp 153–170

Schulberg HC, Scott CP, Madonia MJ, et al: Applications of interpersonal psychotherapy to depression in primary care practice, in New Applications of Interpersonal Psychotherapy. Edited by Klerman GL, Weissman MM. Washington, DC, American Psychiatric Press, 1993, pp 265–291

Schulberg HC, Block MR, Madonia MJ, et al: Treating major depression in primary care practice: eight-month clinical outcomes. Arch Gen Psychiatry 53(10):913–919, 1996 8857868

Schulberg HC, Post EP, Raue PJ, et al: Treating late-life depression with interpersonal psychotherapy in the primary care sector. Int J Geriatr Psychiatry 22(2):106–114, 2007 17096458

Shea MT, Elkin I, Imber SD, et al: Course of depressive symptoms over follow-up. Arch Gen Psychiatry 49(10):782–787, 1992 1417430

Shea MT, Elkin I, Sotsky SM: Patient characteristics associated with successful treatment: outcome findings from the NIMH Treatment of Depression Collaborative Research Program, in Psychotherapy Indications and Outcomes. Edited by Janowsky DS. Washington, DC, American Psychiatric Press, 1999, pp 71–90

Sholomskas AJ, Chevron ES, Prusoff BA, et al: Short-term interpersonal therapy (IPT) with the depressed elderly: case reports and discussion. Am J Psychother 37(4):552–566, 1983 6660341

Sloane RB, Stapes FR, Schneider LS: Interpersonal therapy versus nortriptyline for depression in the elderly, in Clinical and Pharmacological Studies in Psychiatric Disorders. Edited by Burrows GD, Norman TR, Dennerstein L. London, John Libbey, 1985, pp 344–346

Sotsky SM, Glass DR, Shea MT, et al: Patient predictors of response to psychotherapy and pharmacotherapy: findings in the NIMH Treatment of Depression Collaborative Research Program. Am J Psychiatry 148(8):997–1008, 1991 1853989
Spinelli MG: Interpersonal psychotherapy for depressed antepartum women: a pilot study. Am J Psychiatry 154(7):1028–1030, 1997 9210760
Spinelli MG, Endicott J: Controlled clinical trial of interpersonal psychotherapy versus parenting education program for depressed pregnant women. Am J Psychiatry 160(3):555–562, 2003 12611838
Spinelli MG, Endicott J, Goetz RR, et al: Reanalysis of efficacy of interpersonal psychotherapy for antepartum depression versus parenting education program: initial severity of depression as a predictor of treatment outcome. J Clin Psychiatry 77(4):535–540, 2016 27137422
Stuart S, O'Hara MW: Interpersonal psychotherapy for postpartum depression: a treatment program. J Psychother Pract Res 4(1):18–29, 1995 22700210
Swartz HA, Grote NK, Graham P: Brief interpersonal psychotherapy (IPT-B): overview and review of evidence. Am J Psychother 68(4):443–462, 2014 26453346
Swartz HA, Cyranowski JM, Cheng Y, et al: Brief psychotherapy for maternal depression: impact on mothers and children. J Am Acad Child Adolesc Psychiatry 55(6):495–503.e2, 2016 27238068
Swartz HA, Rucci P, Thase ME, et al: Psychotherapy alone and combined with medication as treatments for bipolar II depression: a randomized controlled trial. J Clin Psychiatry 79(2):16m11027, 2018 28703949
Thase ME, Fava M, Halbreich U, et al: A placebo-controlled, randomized clinical trial comparing sertraline and imipramine for the treatment of dysthymia. Arch Gen Psychiatry 53(9):777–784, 1996 8792754
Thase ME, Buysse DJ, Frank E, et al: Which depressed patients will respond to interpersonal psychotherapy? The role of abnormal EEG sleep profiles. Am J Psychiatry 154(4):502–509, 1997 9090337
U.S. Department of Veterans Affairs: VA/DoD Clinical Practice Guideline for the Management of Posttraumatic Stress Disorder and Acute Stress Disorder. Washington, DC, U.S. Department of Veterans Affairs, 2017. Available at: www.healthquality.va.gov/guidelines/MH/ptsd/VADoDPTSDCPGClinicianSummaryFinal.pdf. Accessed February 12, 2022.
Weissman MM: Mastering Depression: A Patient Guide to Interpersonal Psychotherapy. New York, Oxford University Press, 2006
Weissman MM, Klerman GL, Paykel ES, et al: Treatment effects on the social adjustment of depressed patients. Arch Gen Psychiatry 30(6):771–778, 1974 4832185
Weissman MM, Prusoff BA, Dimascio A, et al: The efficacy of drugs and psychotherapy in the treatment of acute depressive episodes. Am J Psychiatry 136(4B):555–558, 1979 371421
Weissman MM, Klerman GL, Prusoff BA, et al: Depressed outpatients: results one year after treatment with drugs and/or interpersonal psychotherapy. Arch Gen Psychiatry 38(1):51–55, 1981 7006558
Weissman MM, Markowitz JC, Klerman GL: The Guide to Interpersonal Psychotherapy, 2nd Edition. New York, Oxford University Press, 2018
Wells KB, Stewart A, Hays RD, et al: The functioning and well-being of depressed patients: results of the Medical Outcomes Study. JAMA 18(7):914–919, 1989 2754791
Wilfley DE, Agras WS, Telch CF, et al: Group cognitive-behavioral therapy and group interpersonal psychotherapy for the nonpurging bulimic individual: a controlled comparison. J Consult Clin Psychol 61(2):296–305, 1993 8473584
Wilfley DE, MacKenzie RK, Welch RR, et al: Interpersonal Psychotherapy for Group. New York, Basic Books, 2000
Wilfley DE, Welch RR, Stein RI, et al: A randomized comparison of group cognitive-behavioral therapy and group interpersonal psychotherapy for the treatment of overweight individuals with binge-eating disorder. Arch Gen Psychiatry 59(8):713–721, 2002 12150647
Zlotnick C, Johnson SL, Miller IW, et al: Postpartum depression in women receiving public assistance: pilot study of an interpersonal-therapy-oriented group intervention. Am J Psychiatry 158(4):638–640, 2001 11282702

PART V

Supportive Psychotherapy

Section Editor: Arnold Winston, M.D.

Supportive psychotherapy is the most widely practiced treatment approach because it is applicable for patients with most psychiatric diagnoses. In addition, it is focused on the patient-therapist relationship and promoting the therapeutic alliance, which is the best predictor of therapeutic success (Horvath and Symonds 1991). The Residency Review Committee for Psychiatry has emphasized the importance of training in supportive psychotherapy. This committee now mandates that all psychiatry residents receive training and become certified as competent by their training program in three types of psychotherapy, one of which must be supportive psychotherapy.

The three chapters on supportive psychotherapy in this book summarize most of the important information about supportive psychotherapy, including theory, techniques, and the research on outcome. In Chapter 16, "Theory of Individual Supportive Psychotherapy," Lippert, Roberts, Winston, and Goldstein describe the important theoretical foundations of this psychotherapy, including psychoanalytic (psychodynamic) theory, cognitive-behavioral theory, and learning theory. The psychotherapy continuum, ranging from supportive to expressive, is elucidated and connected to the psychopathology continuum, ranging from fairly healthy individuals to severely impaired people, so that patients can be matched to the appropriate treatment approach. Case formulation is explained and broken down into structural, genetic, dynamic, and cognitive-behavioral formulations.

In Chapter 17, "Techniques of Individual Supportive Psychotherapy," Rosenthal, Urmanche, and Muran describe the various techniques or interventions used in supportive psychotherapy. These techniques fall within the following categories: alliance building, esteem building, skills building, enhancing ego function, and expanding awareness. Alliance building can be characterized by such things as expressing empathy, understanding, and interest, and esteem building encompasses praise, reassurance, and encouragement. Skills building includes advice, teaching, and anticipatory guidance. Enhancing ego function can be addressed with reframing, normalizing, supporting defenses, and rationalizing. Clarification, confrontation, and interpretation help to expand awareness.

In Chapter 18, "Applications of Individual Supportive Psychotherapy to Specific Disorders," Winston and Punko summarize outcome research and indications for supportive psychotherapy in psychotic, depressive, anxiety, and personality disorders. In addition, outcome studies for addictive, medical, and other disorders are presented. These studies indicate that supportive psychotherapy produces positive results for all of these disorders. However, when outcome studies compare supportive psychotherapy with other forms of psychotherapy, the results indicate that essentially all recognized psychotherapies produce similar results and no psychotherapy is superior to any other psychotherapy. It appears that the best explanation for these findings is that common factors present in all psychotherapies may be responsible for this outcome. The major common factor is likely a caring, empathic therapeutic relationship. All common factors are discussed in this chapter.

Reference

Horvath AO, Symonds BD: Relation between working alliance and outcome in psychotherapy: a meta-analysis. J Couns Psychol 38(2):139–149, 1991

CHAPTER 16

Theory of Individual Supportive Psychotherapy

Csilla Nani Lippert, M.D., Ph.D.
Laura Weiss Roberts, M.D., M.A.
Arnold Winston, M.D.
Michael Goldstein, M.D.

Individual supportive psychotherapy "is a treatment approach focused on patients' overall health and well-being and their abilities to adapt constructively to their life circumstances" (Winston et al. 2020, p. 1) in an individual care setting. The first iterations of what we currently understand as supportive psychotherapy developed in the twentieth century as a therapeutic approach for individuals who could not be treated with insight-oriented psychoanalysis. Therapy providers needed a helpful treatment approach for individuals with a wide range of issues, including relationship problems, personal crises, time-limited transitions, or severely impairing psychopathology. Although supportive psychotherapy framed in this way developed as a reaction or alternative to psychoanalysis, the earliest elements of supportive psychotherapy date back more than 2,000 years to the Ancient Greeks (Novalis et al. 2020), and modern versions continue to have wide applicability.

Supportive psychotherapy has been at times defined by the elements of psychoanalysis and other expressive therapies that it does not include, such as the absence of an insight-oriented approach or that instead of focusing on unconscious conflicts, the therapist and patient directly and actively address conscious conflicts (Dewald 1971, 1994). Views of supportive psychotherapy vary, with some people considering it a distinctive therapy, a branch of psychodynamic therapy, or a compilation of other therapy approaches. Winston et al. (2020, p. 3) summarize the commonalities that emerge in descriptions of supportive psychotherapy (Table 16–1) as the following themes:

TABLE 16–1. **Commonalities in descriptions of supportive psychotherapy**

Theme	Description
Objectives	What the therapist hopes to achieve:
	Maintain or improve self-esteem
	Maintain or improve ego functions
	Minimize or prevent symptom recurrence
	Maximize adaptive capacities
Goals	What the patient wants to achieve:
	Maintain or improve function
Technique	What the therapist does:
	Encourage
	Reassure
	Educate
	Advise

1. What the therapist hopes to achieve (objectives)—for example, to maintain or improve the patient's self-esteem and ego function, to minimize or prevent recurrence of symptoms, and to maximize the patient's adaptive capacities (Pinsker et al. 1991)
2. What the patient wants to achieve (goals)—for example, to maintain or reestablish the patient's best possible level of functioning given the limitations of his or her personality, inherent ability, and life circumstances (Ursano and Silberman 1996)
3. What the therapist does (technique)—for example, provide encouragement, reassurance, education, and advice

Some features of the therapist objectives in supportive psychotherapy are helpful to define in further detail. Self-esteem encompasses "the patient's sense of efficacy, confidence, hope, and self-regard" (Pinsker 1997, p. 1). Ego functions, also called psychological functions, include relation to reality, object relations, defenses, regulation of impulses and affects, and thinking (Bellak 1958; Beres 1956; Winston et al. 2004). Adaptive capacities "are actions associated with effective functioning" (Pinsker 1997, p. 2) and are often responses to the ego function or assessment of events.

To accomplish supportive psychotherapy objectives and patient goals, treatment involves an examination of symptoms, relationships, everyday functioning, and patterns of emotional responses and behaviors. The therapist takes information gleaned from this examination to choose goal-oriented interventions, such as psychoeducation and encouragement, within a supportive therapeutic alliance (Novalis et al. 2020).

Describing the theory of supportive psychotherapy presents several challenges. As with definitions of supportive psychotherapy, descriptions of its theory were framed initially according to how supportive psychotherapy theory differed from psychoanalytic theories. Furthermore, "[a]lthough supportive psychotherapy is the most widely practiced form of psychodynamically oriented psychotherapy…[s]upportive psychotherapy is not based on rigorous and internally consistent or appealing theory" (Winston et al. 2020, p. 10). Supportive psychotherapy "differs from most other psychotherapies in its epistemological basis to the extent that it does not require a deeply theoretical concept or theory of mind"; it is "empirically based and patient driven" and thus "can draw as needed from particular schools of psychotherapy, including psychodynamic, cognitive-behavioral, interpersonal, and experiential" (Novalis et al. 2020, pp. 10–11). In discussing supportive psychotherapy theory here, we focus on a couple of the most relevant theoretical frameworks.

The theory of supportive psychotherapy is based on several approaches, including psychoanalytic, cognitive-behavioral, and learning theories (summarized in Table 16–2). These theoretical approaches help to guide the clinician regarding the indications, strategies, goals, and types of interventions used in supportive psychotherapy. These theoretical approaches also help the clinician understand the nature and configuration of the patient-therapist relationship, which can strengthen the supportive therapeutic alliance. Supportive psychotherapists must be able to integrate various theoretical approaches into a cohesive and well-organized psychotherapy that addresses the needs of the patient.

The Impairment-Psychotherapy Continuum

An important concept in understanding both the indications for supportive psychotherapy and how supportive psychotherapy relates to expressive or exploratory psychotherapy is the impairment-psychotherapy continuum, as shown in Figure 16–1 (Dewald 1971, 1994; Winston et al. 2004, 2020). Individuals function along an impairment continuum according to their level of psychopathology, adaptive capacity, self-concept, and ability to relate to others. The continuum extends from the most impaired patients to the least impaired individuals. Impairments consist of symptoms and behaviors that interfere with function. Function comprises an individual's ability to think clearly and realistically, complete tasks of everyday life, form relationships, and act in an adaptive and mature manner. Individuals on the least impaired side of the continuum tend to function well; for example, they have healthy relationships, lead productive lives, enjoy a wide range of activities, and effectively handle conflict. Moving toward the impaired side of the continuum, patients have increasing difficulty maintaining consistent functioning on the basis of limitations in their adaptation and behavior.

A psychiatric diagnosis cannot be given without some form of disability or impairment, and the nature of the psychiatric condition may influence the placement of individuals on the impairment-psychotherapy continuum. Patients with schizophrenia, bipolar disorder, or borderline personality disorder are generally located on the more impaired side of the continuum. By contrast, patients with dysthymia, adjustment disorder, or obsessive-compulsive personality disorder are generally located on the less impaired side of the continuum. Although diagnosis can provide a general idea of where a person might reside on the continuum, actual placement will depend on the combination of the individual's psychopathology and degree of adaptation (Winston and Winston 2002). For example, a patient with well-controlled schizophrenia who is fully employed, lives independently, and enjoys meaningful relationships would be on a less impaired region of the continuum than an age-matched patient with obsessive-compulsive disorder who cannot maintain a job, lives with their parents, and lacks friends as a result of uncontrolled contamination fears.

TABLE 16–2. Theories contributing to supportive psychotherapy

Approach	Component	Details
Psychoanalytic theory	Ego psychology and ego functions	Relation to reality (reality testing, sense of reality, adaptation to reality)
		Object relations (capacity to meaningfully, consistently relate to others)
		Affects, impulse control, and defenses
		Thought processes
		Autonomous functions (perception, intention, intelligence, language, motor development)
		Synthetic function
		Conscience, morals, and ideals
	Object relations	"Good enough" mother (or parent)
		Attachment
		Corrective emotional experience
	Self psychology	Promote development through accurate and empathic understanding
	Therapeutic relationship	Transference and countertransference
		Real relationship
		Therapeutic alliance
Cognitive-behavioral theory	Targets	Schemas
		Dysfunctional attitudes
		Automatic thoughts
		Cognitive distortions
Learning theory	Basic concepts	Learning as part of therapy
	Strategies	Therapeutic alliance
		Standards and expectations
		Resource identification
		Techniques (interpretation, generation, interleaving, critical reflection)

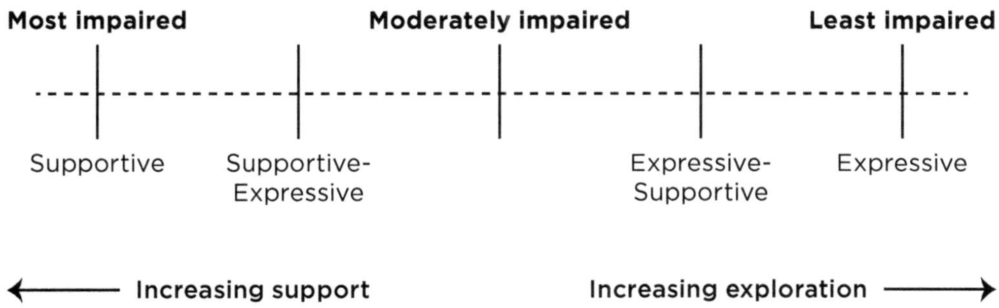

FIGURE 16–1. Impairment-psychotherapy continuum.

Matching the psychotherapy technique to the patient locus on the impairment continuum is of crucial importance. On the left side of the continuum are supportive approaches that aim to enhance strengths; coping skills; and capacity to use environmental supports to feel better, reduce distress, and improve behavior (Novalis et al. 2020). More concretely, supportive approaches consist of building psychological structure, stability, self-esteem, a cohesive sense of self, and interpersonal relationships, which are especially helpful in more impaired patients who have significant psychopathology or limitations in adaptation.

At the less impaired end of the continuum are expressive therapies, which focus more on achieving self-understanding. Expressive therapy is a collective term for a variety of approaches that seek personality change through both analysis of the patient-therapist relationship and insight into previously unrecognized feelings, thoughts, needs, and conflicts. In expressive therapy, the patient attempts to consciously resolve and better integrate such feelings, thoughts, needs, and conflicts.

In reality, neither end of the impairment-psychotherapy continuum accurately describes patients. Instead, most patients have both conflicts and structural problems and will thus require a supportive-expressive combination treatment. Of note, even the most exploratory therapies include supportive components, and supportive therapy includes elements of exploratory therapy (de Jonghe et al. 1992; Dewald 1994; Luborsky 1994).

Psychoanalytic Theory

Psychoanalytic theory is a theoretical background with important fundamental contributions to supportive therapy. Psychoanalytic theory extends from traditional drive/conflict theory, ego psychology, object relations theory, self-experience, and interpersonal/relational models. Pine (1989) argues that all analytic approaches are connected and inform our understanding of adult functioning. Although drive/conflict models are foundational for all psychoanalytic approaches, patients with higher levels of impairment typically benefit more from models that focus less on conflicts and drives. In the following sections, we concentrate more on ego psychology, object relations theory, and the therapeutic relationship, which are more applicable to supportive psychotherapy.

Ego Psychology

Ego psychology, which encompasses developmental theory, offers insight into patients with high levels of impairment. Ego functions, as outlined by Freud's (1923/1961) structural approach of the ego, id, and superego, are at the theoretical core of ego psychology. A structural approach like Freud's attempts to capture the relatively fixed characteristics of an individual's personality and symptoms as understood within a functional context. In general, the greater the disturbance in ego functions, the more a supportive approach is indicated. The following description of psychological or ego functions is based on the work of Beres (1956) and Bellak (1958), including an abridged list inspired by Bellak's 12 major ego functions, with a focus on the ego functions that are most relevant to consider in supportive psychotherapy.

Relation to Reality

Relation to reality comprises reality testing, sense of reality, and adaptation to reality. Reality testing reflects an individual's ability to accurately differentiate between the external world and internal experiences. An extreme example of impaired reality testing is in patients with limited insight who experience delusions and hallucinations. Reality testing is also impaired when an individual has limitations in judgment. Sense of reality describes an individual's ability to distinguish between self and other; an intact sense of reality generally indicates that an individual has a stable, cohesive body image (Mahler et al. 1975). Adaptation to reality describes how an individual functions in everyday life, including work, school, social situations, and relationships. Patients with impaired relation to reality require a supportive, reality-based approach that emphasizes their current functioning and daily life instead of the exploration of dreams and fantasies or extensive examination of past issues.

Object Relations

In the context of ego psychology, object relations considers a person's capacity to meaningfully and consistently relate to significant individuals. Object relations includes the ability to form intimate relationships, tolerate separation and loss, and maintain independence and autonomy. This capacity also involves the sense of self, knowing what is within versus outside the self, and development of a cohesive and stable self-image (Mahler et al. 1975) without diminishing or overidealizing the self or others (Mitchell and Black 1995). Patients with significant impairment in interpersonal relationships, such as chaotic relationships, withdrawal from others, and/or self-centered or highly dependent needs, generally require a supportive approach framed within an empathic relationship.

Affects, Impulse Control, and Defenses

Affects are complex psychophysiological states that consist of subjective feelings and physiological expressions, such as crying, sweating, facial expression, and tone of voice. The nine primary affects (some with low- or high-intensity labels) described by Tomkins (1962) are enjoyment/joy, interest/excitement, surprise/startle, anger/rage, disgust, dissmell, distress/anguish, fear/terror, and shame/humiliation. Affective impairments can include difficulties experiencing, identifying, and modulating affects.

The capacity to control impulses and modulate affect in an adaptive manner, such as through delayed gratification and frustration tolerance, indicates a well-functioning defensive structure. When impulse control is impaired, individuals may engage in socially unacceptable behavior, such as physically or verbally lashing out at others or making unreasonable demands.

Defenses mediate between a person's wishes, needs, feelings, and both internal and external prohibitions (Freud 1936/1966). Individuals tend to have patterned behavioral responses in reaction to perceived danger, difficult situations, or painful affects. Defenses range from primitive (less constructive) to mature (more constructive).

Primitive defenses, poor impulse control, severe affective instability, and shallow affect are indicators of structural deficits, suggesting the need for a more supportive psychotherapeutic approach. For example, a supportive approach can provide concrete practice for people who are unable to experience a wide range of affects at some depth or to differentiate between affects (Jacobson 1964). Supportive psychotherapy also may include directed practice that promotes impulse control. Furthermore, defenses, especially adaptive defenses, are strengthened in supportive psychotherapy instead of analyzed; this approach promotes stability and adaptive functioning (Pinsker 1997). By contrast, expressive psychotherapy includes examining—and sometimes challenging—affects, impulses, and defenses, which requires that patients tolerate deep exploration of their psyche. For patients with more impairing psychopathology, deep exploration would be too disruptive and anxiety provoking.

Thought Processes

Successful thought processing incorporates the ability to think clearly, logically, and abstractly. Automatic thoughts and negative self-schemas, as defined by cognitive-behavioral theorists and discussed in greater detail in the section "Cognitive-Behavioral Theory," can further influence thought processes. An individual with persecutory automatic thoughts (e.g., "I experience misfortune because others want to harm me") and negative self-schemas (e.g., "I am weak and useless") would likely struggle more to work and maintain relationships than an individual with balanced automatic thoughts (e.g., "I experience misfortune because sometimes things go my way and sometimes they don't") and a positive self-schema (e.g., "I am competent and determined"). Impaired adaptive skills and poor interpersonal functioning often result from problematic automatic thoughts and negative self-schemas, which may need to be addressed in supportive psychotherapy.

Autonomous Functions

Perception, intention, intelligence, language, and motor development are autonomous functions that are thought to develop in a relatively conflict-free manner (Hartmann 1939/1958). Impairments may be observed in individuals with severe psychopathology, such as those suffering from untreated or treatment-resistant psychotic illnesses, who are more likely to have abnormal perceptions, struggle with language, and experience cognitive decline. When these autonomous functions are impaired, a supportive approach may be indicated.

Synthetic Function

Synthetic function includes an individual's ability to organize the self and world in a productive fashion to form a cohesive whole or gestalt (Nunberg 1931). This function involves putting together the other ego functions and organizing them so that the individual can function in an integrated manner. Individuals with inadequate synthetic function may find that exploratory psychotherapeutic approaches further disrupt their sense of cohesion; they would thus benefit more from supportive psychotherapy.

Conscience, Morals, and Ideals

Internalized aspects of parental figures and societal mores contribute to conscience, morals, and ideals. Beyond being an indication for supportive psychotherapy, impairments in these superego functions may interfere with the patient-therapist relationship. For instance, if a patient threatens to physically harm the therapist, achieving success in psychotherapy may be difficult.

The ego or psychological functions can be used as the foundation for case formulations that summarize patient strengths and impairments. The following clinical example has several structural impairments that are conceptualized in a case formulation.

Case Vignette 1

A 28-year-old man seeks therapy to "feel better—to be in a better mood every day." On intake, he reports distress from frequent difficulties distinguishing between when people are and are not talking to him on the street. He shares some examples of thinking that other people were saying derogatory things about him even though their lips were not moving. He says he has no friends and that his parents would describe him as "needy and demanding," especially because he has broken pieces of furniture after his mother lost one of his socks in the laundry or served dinner slightly late. He returned to live with his parents at age 20, after dropping out of college. He has not worked in the past 6 years, saying about prospective employers, "It's not my fault that they ask mean questions about college and don't like when I answer, 'It's none of your business.'"

Helping this patient will involve addressing multiple issues and concerns and, to the extent possible, should use his framework of "feeling better" and finding a path toward his being "in a better mood." The therapist will provide reassurance, accurate information, and an emotionally stable relationship and, in this case, will need to work with the patient on several fronts in order to help strengthen his daily life functioning and mood. The patient has an impaired sense of reality, particularly his reality testing, on the basis of his description of likely auditory hallucinations. His object relations center on his needs, and he has notable difficulties both connecting with others and maintaining independence. The patient's adaptation to reality is severely impaired on the basis of his inability to finish school, maintain a job, and form meaningful relationships. He exhibits impaired impulse control. He uses immature defenses, such as projection, acting out, and denial. Given these structural deficits, supportive psychotherapy, with clear and concrete goals related to everyday functioning and mood, is more likely than expressive psychotherapy to be helpful for this patient.

Object Relations Theory

A part of psychoanalytic theory that was already introduced but is valuable to further expand on is object relations and its role in supportive psychotherapy. In object relations, children are posited to seek satisfying relationships with their parents. The theory suggests that many individuals have inadequate or faulty parenting skills, and, according to Fairbairn (1952, 1994), their children absorb pathological traits of their parents to remain connected to them. Although these prototypes of past relationships are reenacted in the therapeutic relationship, the patient must be able to experience the therapist in a new, more positive manner. Winnicott (1965, 1971) describes this process as the therapist becoming the *good enough mother* (or parent) by providing a *holding environment* in which content and interpretations are relatively unimportant and support is more important. The patient is encouraged to experience the self in relation to the therapist, and the therapist becomes a new object for the patient. Fairbairn and Winnicott believed that change, instead of developing from insight, develops from the capacity for relatedness that grows out of connecting to the therapist in a new manner. Therapists can employ supportive techniques to foster a new kind of connection for patients.

Bowlby (1969, 1988) added yet another important dimension to the patient-therapist relationship: the concept of attachment. He proposed that the nature of an infant's attachment to a parent will become internalized as a working model of attachment. In this model, children develop secure or insecure attachments on the basis of their parents' sensitivity to the signals the children make as infants. Responsive parents can help reduce uncomfortable emotions in their children, such as fear, anxiety, and sadness. In patients with insecure attachments, uncomfortable emotions in childhood and resultant relationship ruptures were inadequately followed by repair and reconnection. The therapist's skilled ability to repair ruptures in the therapeutic alliance contrasts with the limited ability that parents of insecurely attached children possess to sustain connection and heal relationship breaches. This process of repair in therapy is related to the *corrective emotional experience*, a concept described by Alexander and French (1946). The corrective emotional experience occurs when the therapist helps the patient repeatedly face and overcome previously insurmountable emotional situations within the patient-therapist relationship, providing practice for a new way of being.

The following dialogue illustrates how the therapist may facilitate a corrective emotional experience.

Patient: You kept me waiting! I'm furious! Once I get angry and start not trusting someone…I write them off.

Therapist: I'm sorry to have kept you waiting. It makes sense that you got angry with me for being late.

Patient: I didn't think you were coming.

Therapist: I disappointed you. I know that's hard.

In this example, the therapist does not confront or react to the highly vulnerable patient's anger and lack of trust. Instead, the therapist facilitates a corrective emotional experience by responding in an accepting and empathic manner. Additionally, the therapist focuses on the current situation and does not explore symbolic or transference issues such as "Does this remind you of times your parents were not there for you?" In supportive psychotherapy, corrective experiences are more relevant than insight.

Self Psychology

Early object relations are of crucial importance in the development of the self, which is also relevant to supportive psychotherapy. When parents' empathic responsiveness to their children is repeatedly distorted or inappropriate, developmental problems of the self may occur. According to Kohut (1971, 1977), the therapist offers this kind of patient a new experience—an empathic/introspective stance. The goal of Kohut's psychoanalytic approach is to promote patient development through accurately and empathically understanding the patient's needs and then interpreting these needs to the patient. However, the therapist will inevitably fail to meet the patient's needs. In supportive psychotherapy, the therapist does not interpret the patient's needs; instead, the therapist acknowledges failures in meeting the patient's needs and uses supportive techniques to reestablish the patient-therapist alliance. This approach to repairing alliance ruptures will generally strengthen self-structures and help the patient internalize the therapist's good qualities. The following dialogue illustrates this process.

Patient: I have been really upset with you since we last met. You didn't understand me. You defended Jeff [the patient's boyfriend], who was being horrible to me.

Therapist: Yes, I see what you mean. I suggested you try to make peace with Jeff instead of focusing on your hurt feelings. It is helpful that you let me know you have been upset and that it feels like I didn't understand you.

In this example, the therapist acknowledges the mistake and immediately attempts to repair the misalliance. If a misalliance or rupture is not attended to in a timely fashion, the possibility of the patient leaving treatment increases. To protect ongoing patient engagement in therapy, the supportive psychotherapist readily acknowledges and repairs alliance ruptures.

Therapeutic Relationship

The therapeutic relationship, or patient-therapist relationship, is likely the most important variable in producing a positive psychotherapy outcome, as noted more than three decades ago (Gaston 1990; Horvath and Symonds 1991). The therapeutic relationship consists of the following components: the transference-countertransference configuration, the real relationship, and the therapeutic alliance (Greenson 1967, 1971). Transference and real relationship issues play a role in every transaction within the therapeutic relationship. Sometimes, the real relationship predominates; at other times, transference may be more important.

Transference is a special type of object relationship consisting of behaviors, thoughts, feelings, wishes, and attitudes directed at the therapist that are related to important people in the patient's past (Greenson 1967). The real relationship exists in the here and now of the therapeutic interaction between the patient and therapist, encompassing a genuine liking for each other without the distortions that are characteristic of transference (Greenson 1967, 1971). The real relationship includes the patient's hopes and aspirations for help, care, understanding, and love, as well as the everyday interactions that take place on a social level between individuals. Supportive psychotherapy may be especially helpful in multicultural settings because of the immediacy of the real relationship between the patient and therapist and the specificity of goals of treatment.

In supportive psychotherapy, the real relationship is paramount and a major source of support. Importantly, in supportive psychotherapy and in contrast with other therapeutic approaches, transference issues are minimized. Although supportive psychotherapists are mindful of transference, they generally do not explore it unless the transference is negative. Negative transference must be discussed with the patient because it can disrupt or threaten the psychotherapy and often results in the patient dropping out of treatment (Samstag et al. 1998).

The following two dialogues illustrate how positive and negative transference reactions are managed in supportive psychotherapy.

Patient: Work is going much better. I'm getting along with my boss now, and I can't remember the last time I had an anxiety dream about losing my job. Thank you so much for your help. Your expert understanding has made all of this possible.

Therapist: I'm pleased you are doing better at work and that our work together has helped.

In this example, the therapist readily accepts what the patient has said instead of exploring the compliment. At the same time, the therapist indicates that this positive outcome resulted from a joint effort of both the patient and the therapist.

Patient: I've really been struggling since Ted [the patient's son] went to college. He hasn't been responding to my calls or messages, except to say he would rather talk to my ex [the father of the patient's son]. Oh, and that talking to me reminds him of how abusive and clingy I was in his childhood.

Therapist: It might be helpful to give Ted some space. I wonder if he would start responding to your messages and calls if you take a break from sending them.

Patient: Have you been talking to my ex? I mean, you're sounding just like him. It's so easy for you to just tell me to stop reaching out to Ted. Your kids probably wish you, busy therapist, would reach out to them more.

Therapist: I am starting to understand how hard this is for you and how much anguish you feel. I was so eager to repair your relationship with Ted that I neglected to respond to your needs.

In this example, the patient becomes angry with the therapist, who immediately addresses the negative transference and attempts to repair it through an empathic intervention and taking responsibility for an error.

From a classical point of view, countertransference is the therapist's transference to the patient (Gabbard 2001; Greenson 1967). A broader definition of countertransference includes the real relationship, which consists of reactions most people would have to the patient within moment-to-moment interactions in the therapeutic relationship. In this sense, countertransference is affected by what the therapist brings to the situation, what the patient projects, and how the therapist and patient interact (Gabbard 2001; Kiesler 2001). A therapist who is unknowingly biased by countertransference reactions can misunderstand the patient and may even behave inappropriately toward the patient. However, countertransference reactions that a therapist is aware of can be a powerful tool for understanding and empathizing with the patient. Empathy facilitates countertransference awareness (Wolf 1983), and the ability to empathize by accurately sensing and understanding what a patient is experiencing will enable the therapist to attend to countertransference reactions.

The following is an example of the use of countertransference in supportive psychotherapy.

Case Vignette 2

A parent of two young children speaks about being angry with a 3-year-old daughter and yelling at her. The therapist begins to feel upset, anxious, and angry and then quickly recognizes strong feelings about what the patient did to the daughter. The therapist realizes that the patient shared this behavior as a way of asking for help and testing to see if the therapist would get angry and retaliate or reject the patient. The therapist is then able to respond in a helpful manner by saying, "I'm glad you told me about what happened with your daughter. Let's try to understand what you were experiencing and see if we can come up with an alternative way of dealing with your daughter when she acts up." In this way, the therapist's awareness of and reflection on countertransference allows the therapist to be more attuned to the patient's needs.

The therapeutic alliance is part of the real relationship and is necessary to support the work of psychotherapy (Zetzel 1956, 1966), and a positive therapeutic alliance early in supportive psychotherapy is predictive of positive outcome (Hellerstein et al. 1998; Luborsky 1984). Freud recognized the importance of a positive patient-therapist relationship, which he called the "friendly or affectionate feelings" that were "unobjectionable" and "the vehicle of success in psychoanalysis" (Freud 1912/1958). Greenson (1967) emphasized the collaborative nature of the alliance in which patient and therapist work together to promote therapeutic change. Bordin (1979) and Gaston (1990) further clarified and broadened the concept of the therapeutic alliance to include the following components: the affectionate bond between patient and therapist, agreement on the goals and tasks of therapy, the patient's capacity to perform the work of therapy, and the therapist's empathic relatedness and involvement. All of these components of the alliance are important in supportive psychotherapy.

Alliance ruptures occur less often in supportive psychotherapy than in expressive psychotherapy. The lower frequency of ruptures is likely due to a number of different factors. First, the alliance in supportive psychotherapy is not threatened by challenging confrontations or interpretations that may in turn heighten patient anxiety (Hellerstein et al. 1998). Furthermore, when a misalliance does occur in supportive psychotherapy, the use of supportive measures is the initial approach to repair the misalliance (Bond et al. 1998). The therapist addresses the rupture in a practical manner, within the context of the current situation, before examining transference issues (Pinsker 1997).

Cognitive-Behavioral Theory

Cognitive-behavioral techniques are an indispensable part of supportive psychotherapy and can be applied to targeted problems, such as panic, depression, obsessive-compulsive symptoms, and dysfunctional thinking. Cognition refers to the content of thought (what we think), the processes involved in thinking (how we think), and self-schemas (what structures our thinking). Cognitive-behavioral techniques focus on how individuals make use of information to understand the meaning of events in their lives. In this framework, behavior and feelings are thought to derive from the nature and characteristics of thinking. Maladaptive behavior is believed to result from idiosyncratic dysfunctional thinking.

The key concepts of cognitive-behavioral therapy include schemas, dysfunctional attitudes, automatic thoughts, and cognitive distortions or errors. Schemas, or cognitive structures, are relatively enduring beliefs and attitudes that reflect experientially derived abstractions about an individual's self-view or identity (Kovacs and Beck 1978). These beliefs and attitudes are based on early learning experiences, and they are thought to account for problems in screening and encoding new information. Examples of self-schemas include the view of oneself as extroverted versus introverted, athletic versus nonathletic, or detail-oriented versus a "big picture" thinker. Self-schemas influence automatic thoughts and cognitive errors, which are activated by events that are similar in content to the self-schemas. Automatic thoughts and cognitive errors involve arbitrary inference, overgeneralization, magnification, personalization, selective abstraction, and absolute thinking. Examples of automatic thoughts include the following: "If I am not wealthy, then I am a failure"; "If my children are not successful, then I am a terrible parent"; and "If I have an illness, then I did something wrong and deserve it."

Drawing on cognitive-behavioral theory, the supportive psychotherapeutic process involves identifying and challenging automatic thoughts, including subjecting them to empirical testing. Patients are taught to monitor automatic thoughts, test their validity, and develop alternative ways of thinking. Reframing is another commonly used cognitive technique to correct cognitive distortions. A clinical example of reframing is as follows:

Patient: My toddler keeps running away from me and laughing every time I enter his room. He hates me!

Therapist: He doesn't hate you. He can run off and laugh because you helped him develop the independence and playfulness to do so.

In this way, the therapist offers a supportive challenge—via reframing—to a patient's distorted thinking pattern. The therapist and patient may choose to design experiments to challenge the patient's automatic thought that "If my son runs away from me, then it means he hates me."

Learning Theory

Basic Concepts

Many therapeutic interventions used in supportive psychotherapy can be viewed as a form of teaching via imparting knowledge. Encoding the information taught by the therapist constitutes the other half of the therapeutic process. In general, learning is the cognitive process of acquiring skills or knowledge, and memory is the retention of learned information. Given that psychotherapy can be considered a controlled form of learning (Etkin et al. 2005), incorporating research on adult learning into supportive psychotherapy may enhance its effectiveness.

Learning theory has been applied primarily to adult education, and the studies in this area have tended to focus on how to enhance learning. The history of learning theory began with Socrates and Plato, and it evolved with contributions from Piaget (1937/1999), Skinner (1938), Thorndike (1932), and Bandura (1974). The work of Knowles et al. (1998), Brookfield (1995), and Geake and Cooper (2003), including adult learning theory and brain-based learning, has been applied to the practice of adult education, corporate functioning, and marketing.

Research studies in the cognitive and affective neurosciences have made major contributions to understanding learning and learning impairments, which could strengthen work in supportive psychotherapy. This research has expanded our knowledge of the molecular and neural bases of learning (Kandel et al. 2000), cognition (Gazzaniga 2004), and emotion (Panskeep 1998), providing the basis for understanding how impairments in neural functioning may impede psychotherapy and how neural growth may enhance psychotherapy. Patients with schizophrenia (Ongür et al. 2006), major depressive disorder (Bremner et al. 2004), bipolar disorder (Thompson et al. 2005), borderline personality disorder (Judd 2005; Monarch et al. 2004), and attention-deficit hyperactivity disorder (Doyle et al. 2005; Fuggetta 2006) and individuals who have encountered significant psychological trauma (Bremner 2006; Navalta et al. 2006) have observable learning impairments. Furthermore, transient mood shifts and stress can affect encoding and the ability to process information (Buchanan et al. 2006; Dreisbach 2006; Dreisbach and Goschke 2004; Lewis et al. 2005; Liston et al. 2006), and altered neural processing with cognitive deficits may be present in these patients. Although the use of learning theory techniques may help patients process information, little has been written about considering learning impairments when applying supportive psychotherapy to these populations. Historically, learning deficits have been viewed within the context of traumatic brain injury, pervasive developmental disorder, intellectual disability, and other developmental disabilities. However, neuroscience research such as that mentioned above suggests that learning styles should be assessed and the presence of learning deficits should be considered when evaluating all patients with psychiatric disorders for psychotherapy. This type of evaluation involves monitoring a patient's ability to encode information from one session to the next or even within a session.

Learning extends beyond a simple recording process. Learning requires active processing and interpretation during the psychotherapy session in which new information is stored by relating that information to what is already known. In this way, new information is stored in relation to its meaning, associations, and relationships to existing knowledge. It is thus important for the therapist to facilitate effective processing during psychotherapy sessions using the techniques of interpretation, elaboration, and generation (deWinstanley and Bjork 2002; Richland et al. 2005), which are discussed in greater detail in the learning theory techniques section. It is important to note that interpretation in learning theory consists of linkage to preexisting knowledge and differs from the classical understanding of interpretation in dynamic psychotherapy. Interpretation in learning theory avoids mention of the unconscious, whereas interpretation in dynamic psychotherapy is often more inclusive of the unconscious.

Strategies

Therapeutic Alliance

A positive learning experience takes place in a supportive relationship through which the patient's assumptions, conclusions, and habitual responses can be challenged, which facilitates change (Caine and Caine 1994). Patients need to understand that learning may involve taking risks, including embracing uncertainty and change, which often requires that the therapist be dialectical in their stance, occasionally modeling and providing reassurance for the need to consider change. On the other hand, a threatening environment may inhibit learning. Patients should be involved in mutual, collaborative planning with the therapist to set relevant goals and objectives (Knowles et al. 1998). When patients help determine their goals and objectives, they have higher motivation and control over their learning.

Standards and Expectations

In a learning theory-informed approach to supportive psychotherapy, patients participate in an educational process. They may occasionally feel puzzled and make mistakes, requiring support, empathy, and reassurance from the therapist. Patients should understand that learning is an important part of supportive psychotherapy and that preparation and homework may be required to enhance the learning process.

Resource Identification

Patients should be encouraged to identify and use resources to achieve their objectives. Resources include libraries, the internet, books, journals, videos, and more. The use of resources could perhaps be offered as a homework assignment if conducive to the patient's learning style. At the same time, patients should be involved in evaluating their own learning, which promotes the skill of critical reflection (Brookfield 1995). This skill is described in more detail in the following subsection. Patients should also practice self-assessment to help identify their strengths, weaknesses, and problems.

Techniques

A major approach that facilitates learning is effective processing (deWinstanley and Bjork 2002). Processing involves interpretation that is focused and accurate and, importantly, that is accompanied by thorough elaboration. Information that can be interpreted (linked) through associations with preexisting knowledge will be easier to learn than information that is not interpreted (unlinked). In elaborative processing, information is thought of in several different ways and connected with other, previously known information. This can be viewed as looking at an issue from many different sides and angles. Generation and interleaving are also important components of the learning process (Richland et al. 2005). Generation is defined as the production of new conclusions or information during learning; this contrasts with information that a teacher or therapist directly presents to the patient. Interleaving is the method of learning two or more sets of information wherein instruction or focus alternates between the sets; this contrasts with learning in which each set is considered separately. An example of interleaving is discussing interpersonal problems at work, then switching to working on a negative self-image, and then making the point that incomplete assumptions are being made in both cases. Interleaving needs to be performed with skill to avoid a session consisting of psychotherapy multitasking. In supportive psychotherapy, these techniques can be used by asking questions that help patients think about their problems in several different ways without supplying the answers. This process encourages the patient to process information in collaboration with the therapist.

Critical reflection (Mezirow 1998) is the process by which a patient questions and then replaces or reframes an assumption. Alternative perspectives are formed on ideas, actions, and forms of reasoning that were previously taken for granted. Supportive psychotherapy incorporates critical reflection through attempting to provide patients with alternative ways of thinking about the world, relating to others, and solving problems.

The following dialogue is a clinical example illustrating the use of processing with a patient who has bipolar disorder and a history of medication nonadherence. The patient was recently discharged from an inpatient hospital stay for acute mania.

Patient: My sleep has been terrible.
Therapist: Tell me more about that.
Patient: Most nights, I struggle to fall asleep. Then, almost as soon as I fall asleep, I wake up again. I'm probably averaging 5 hours a night.
Therapist: How many days a week are you taking your medications?
Patient: It's hard to say—sort of on and off.
Therapist: I wonder if there is any link between your sleeping difficulty and missing doses of your medication.
Patient: Maybe. I don't know.
Therapist: How do you decide whether to take or not take your medications?
Patient: Taking the medications is cumbersome. I don't like the reminder that something is wrong with me.
Therapist: That sounds important.
Patient: Yes. It scares me that if I have to take medication, it means I'm crazy.

The therapist potentially feels concerned and irritated that the patient is again becoming nonadherent with medication; however, instead of admonishing the patient, the therapist explores that patient's experience with taking medication.

Therapist: What is your understanding of your illness?
Patient: You know I have bipolar.
Therapist: Go on.
Patient: Sometimes I have super high energy, which feels amazing, but then I take risks that I regret later. Other times, I am too depressed to get out of bed and need help remembering to eat and drink.
Therapist: What have you found helpful for treating your bipolar?
Patient: They always give me medications in the hospital. I think it won't help at first, but then I start sleeping around 8 hours a night. I feel better for a bit…until I stop taking my medication consistently.

Here, the therapist is engaging the patient in generation, wherein the therapist provides space for the patient to make learning connections instead of telling the patient about bipolar disorder and treatments for bipolar disorder.

Therapist: Do you mind if we talk for a moment about your brother with diabetes?
Patient: Sure. It's such a pain for him to take insulin every day.

Therapist: Right. What would happen if he stopped taking insulin?
Patient: He would end up in the hospital and they would restart his insulin.
Therapist: Does that remind you of anyone else?
Patient: Oh geez, that's exactly what happened with me, isn't it? I stopped taking my medication and ended up in the hospital. And now that I'm not taking it as regularly, I might end up back in the hospital.

Here, the therapist is facilitating interleaving by helping the patient compare medication adherence in bipolar disorder to medication adherence in a brother with diabetes. Exploration of this type promotes encoding and processing of information, including through generation, elaboration, interleaving, and linkage to preexisting knowledge. Using these teaching techniques to address medication adherence can have a deeper impact than reviewing the risks and benefits of adherence in the usual manner.

Conclusion

Individual supportive psychotherapy focuses on patient health; well-being; and ability to constructively adapt to life circumstances, including crises, transitions, and impairing psychopathology. Therapy objectives include maintaining or improving self-esteem, ego function, and adaptive capacities while bolstering against symptom recurrence; these objectives are achieved in a reassuring, educational alliance. The theory of supportive psychotherapy incorporates multiple approaches, including psychoanalytic, cognitive-behavioral, and learning theories, which are applied according to patient needs. A useful tool for determining patient needs in therapy is the impairment-psychotherapy continuum; supportive psychotherapy may be highly suited for patients with greater functional impairment who have clear and specific goals for whom other therapeutic approaches may not be appropriate. Psychoanalytic concepts of ego psychology, object relations, self psychology, and the therapeutic relationship are helpful to consider in supportive psychotherapy. Application of psychoanalytic concepts can be further enriched with emphases on bolstering structural function, promoting internalization of good objects and corrective emotional experiences, performing rupture repairs, and sustaining the therapeutic relationship. In addition, combining and integrating approaches from cognitive-behavioral and learning theories, particularly reframing and processing, can enhance the effectiveness of supportive psychotherapy.

Key Points

- The theory of supportive psychotherapy is based on a number of approaches, including psychoanalytic, cognitive-behavioral, and learning theories.
- Matching the psychotherapy technique to patient locus on the psychopathology continuum is of crucial importance.
- Psychoanalytic models (ego psychology, object relations theory, attachment theory, and self psychology) that focus less on conflicts and drives have greater utility in patients with higher levels of psychopathology.

- Prototypes of past relationships, which are present in internal object relationships, appear within the patient-therapist relationship.
- In supportive psychotherapy, the therapist offers the patient a new kind of experience, namely, an empathic/introspective stance, so that the therapist is experienced in a new and positive manner.
- Generally, positive transference reactions are not addressed in supportive psychotherapy, whereas negative transference reactions are always examined to help prevent major alliance ruptures.
- Cognitive-behavioral concepts underlie many of the techniques of supportive psychotherapy.
- Psychotherapy can be considered as a controlled form of learning.
- Learning during psychotherapy requires active processing so that new information is stored by relating it to what is already known.

Recommended Readings

Dewald PA: Principles of supportive psychotherapy. Am J Psychother 48(4):505–518, 1994 7872414

Knowles MS, Holton EF, Swanson RA: The Adult Learner: The Definitive Classic in Adult Education and Human Resource Development. Burglinton, MA, Gulf Professional Publishing, 1998

Novalis PN, Singer V, Peele R: Clinical Manual of Supportive Psychotherapy, 2nd Edition. Washington, DC, American Psychiatric Publishing, 2020

Pinsker H: A Primer of Supportive Psychotherapy. Hillsdale, NJ, Analytic Press, 1997

Rockland LH: Supportive Psychotherapy: A Psychodynamic Approach. New York, Basic Books, 1989

Winston A, Winston B: Handbook of Short-Term Psychotherapy. Washington, DC, American Psychiatric Publishing, 2002

Winston A, Rosenthal RN, Roberts LR: Learning Supportive Psychotherapy: An Illustrated Guide, 2nd Edition. Washington, DC, American Psychiatric Publishing, 2020

References

Alexander F, French TM: Psychoanalytic Psychotherapy. New York, Ronald Press, 1946

Bandura A: Behavior theory and the models of man. Am Psychol 29(12):849–869, 1974

Bellak L: The schizophrenic syndrome: a further elaboration of the unified theory of schizophrenia, in Schizophrenia: A Review of the Syndrome. New York, Logos, 1958, pp 3–63

Beres D: Ego deviation and the concept of schizophrenia. Psychoanal Stud Child 11:164–235, 1956

Bond M, Banon E, Grenier M: Differential effects of interventions on the therapeutic alliance with patients with personality disorders. J Psychother Pract Res 7(4):301–318, 1998 9752641

Bordin E: The generalizability of the psycho-analytic concept of the working alliance. Psychotherapy (Chic) 16(3):252–260, 1979

Bowlby J: Attachment and Loss, Vol 1: Attachment. New York, Basic Books, 1969

Bowlby J: A Secure Base: Parent-Child Attachment and Healthy Human Development. New York, Basic Books, 1988

Bremner JD: The relationship between cognitive and brain changes in posttraumatic stress disorder. Ann N Y Acad Sci 1071:80–86, 2006 16891564

Bremner JD, Vythilingam M, Vermetten E, et al: Deficits in hippocampal and anterior cingulate functioning during verbal declarative memory encoding in midlife major depressionn. Am J Psychiatry 161(4):637-645, 2004 15056509

Brookfield S: Adult learning: an overview, in International Encyclopedia of Education. Edited by Tuinjman A. Oxford, UK, Pergamon, 1995, pp 175–380

Buchanan TW, Tranel D, Adolphs R: Impaired memory retrieval correlates with individual differences in cortisol response but not autonomic response. Learn Mem 13(3):382–387, 2006 16741288

Caine RN, Caine G: Making Connections: Teaching and the Human Brain. Lebanon, IN, Dale Segmore, 1994

de Jonghe F, Rijnierse P, Janssen R: The role of support in psychoanalysis. J Am Psychoanal Assoc 40(2):475–499, 1992 1593081

deWinstanley PA, Bjork RA: Successful lecturing: presenting information in ways that engage effective processing. New Directions for Teaching and Learning 2002(89):19–31, 2002

Dewald PA: Psychotherapy: A Dynamic Approach, 2nd Edition. New York, Basic Books, 1971

Dewald PA: Principles of supportive psychotherapy. Am J Psychother 48(4):505–518, 1994 7872414

Doyle AE, Biederman J, Seidman LJ, et al: Neuropsychological functioning in relatives of girls with and without ADHD. Psychol Med 35(8):1121–1132, 2005 16116938

Dreisbach G: How positive affect modulates cognitive control: the costs and benefits of reduced maintenance capability. Brain Cogn 60(1):11–19, 2006 16216400

Dreisbach G, Goschke T: How positive affect modulates cognitive control: reduced perseveration at the cost of increased distractibility. J Exp Psychol Learn Mem Cogn 30(2):343–353, 2004 14979809

Etkin A, Pittenger C, Polan HJ, et al: Toward a neurobiology of psychotherapy: basic science and clinical applications. J Neuropsychiatry Clin Neurosci 17(2):145–158, 2005 15939967

Fairbairn WRD: An Object-Relations Theory of the Personality. New York, Basic Books, 1952

Fairbairn WRD: From Instinct to Self: Selected Papers of WRD Fairbairn, Vols 1–2. Edited by Birtles, ED, Sharff DE. Northvale, NJ, Aronson, 1994

Freud A: The Writings of Anna Freud, Vol 2 (1936): The Ego and the Mechanisms of Defense. New York, International Universities Press, 1966

Freud S: The dynamics of transference (1912), in Standard Edition of the Complete Psychological Works of Sigmund Freud, Vol 12. Translated and edited by Strachey J. London, Hogarth Press, 1958, pp 99–108

Freud S: The ego and the id (1923), in Standard Edition of the Complete Psychological Works of Sigmund Freud, Vol 19. Translated and edited by Strachey J. London, Hogarth Press, 1961, pp 12–66

Fuggetta GP: Impairment of executive functions in boys with attention deficit/hyperactivity disorder. Child Neuropsychol 12(1):1–21, 2006 16484099

Gabbard GO: A contemporary psychoanalytic model of countertransference. J Clin Psychol 57(8):983–991, 2001 11449380

Gaston L: The concept of the alliance and its role in psychotherapy: theoretical and empirical consideration. Psychotherapy (Chic) 27(2):143–153, 1990

Gazzaniga MS: The Cognitive Neurosciences III. Cambridge, MA, MIT Press, 2004

Geake J, Cooper P: Cognitive neuroscience: implications for education? Westminster Studies in Education 26(1):7–20, 2003

Greenson RR: The Technique and Practice of Psychoanalysis. New York, International Universities Press, 1967

Greenson RR: The real relationship between the patient and the psychoanalyst, in The Unconscious Today. Edited by Kanzer M. New York, International Universities Press, 1971, pp 213–232

Hartmann H: Ego Psychology and the Problem of Adaptation (1939). Translated by Rapaport D. New York, International Universities Press, 1958

Hellerstein DJ, Rosenthal RN, Pinsker H, et al: A randomized prospective study comparing supportive and dynamic therapies: outcome and alliance. J Psychother Pract Res 7(4):261–271, 1998 9752637

Horvath AO, Symonds BD: Relation between working alliance and outcome in psychotherapy: a meta-analysis. J Couns Psychol 38(2):139–149, 1991
Jacobson E: The Self and the Object World. New York, International Universities Press, 1964
Judd PH: Neurocognitive impairment as a moderator in the development of borderline personality disorder. Dev Psychopathol 17(4):1173–1196, 2005 16613436
Kandel ER, Schwartz JH, Jessell TM: Principles of Neural Science. Maidenhead, UK, McGraw-Hill, 2000
Kiesler DJ: Therapist countertransference: in search of common themes and empirical referents. J Clin Psychol 57(8):1053–1063, 2001 11449388
Kohut H: The Analysis of the Self. New York, International Universities Press, 1971
Kohut H: The Restoration of the Self. New York, International Press, 1977
Kovacs M, Beck AT: Maladaptive cognitive structures in depression. Am J Psychiatry 135(5):525–533, 1978 645943
Knowles MS, Holton EF, Swanson RA: The Adult Learner: The Definitive Classic in Adult Education and Human Resource Development. Burlington, MA, Gulf Professional Publishing, 1998
Lewis PA, Critchley HD, Smith AP, et al: Brain mechanisms for mood congruent memory facilitation. Neuroimage 25(4):1214–1223, 2005 15850739
Liston C, Miller MM, Goldwater DS, et al: Stress-induced alterations in prefrontal cortical dendritic morphology predict selective impairments in perceptual attentional set-shifting. J Neurosci 26(30):7870–7874, 2006 16870732
Luborsky L: Principles of Psychoanalytic Psychotherapy: A Manual for Supportive-Expressive Treatment. New York, Basic Books, 1984
Luborsky L: Therapeutic alliances as predictors of psychotherapy outcomes: factors explaining the predictive success, in The Working Alliance: Theory, Research, and Practice. Edited by Horvath AO, Greenberg LS. New York, Wiley, 1994, pp 38–50
Mahler MS, Pine F, Bergman A: The Psychological Birth of the Human Infant. New York, Basic Books, 1975
Mezirow J: On critical reflection. Adult Education Quearterly 48:185–198, 1998
Mitchell SA, Black MJ: Freud and Beyond. New York, Basic Books, 1995
Monarch ES, Saykin AJ, Flashman LA: Neuropsychological impairment in borderline personality disorder. Psychiatr Clin North Am 27(1):67–82, viii–ix, 2004 15062631
Navalta CP, Polcari A, Webster DM, et al: Effects of childhood sexual abuse on neuropsychological and cognitive function in college women. J Neuropsychiatry Clin Neurosci 18(1):45–53, 2006 16525070
Novalis PN, Singer V, Peele R: Clinical Manual of Supportive Psychotherapy, 2nd Edition. Washington, DC, American Psychiatric Association Publishing, 2020
Nunberg H: The synthetic function of the ego. Int J Psychoanal 12:123–140, 1931
Ongür D, Cullen TJ, Wolf DH, et al: The neural basis of relational memory deficits in schizophrenia. Arch Gen Psychiatry 63(4):356–365, 2006 16585464
Panskeep J: Affective Neuroscience: The Foundations of Human and Animal Emotion. New York, Oxford University Press, 1998
Piaget J: The Construction of Reality in the Child (1937). London, Routledge, 1999
Pine F: Motivation, personality organization, and the four psychologies of psychoanalysis. J Am Psychoanal Assoc 37(1):31–64, 1989 2708777
Pinsker H: A Primer of Supportive Psychotherapy. Hilldale, NJ, Analytic Press, 1997
Pinsker H, Rosenthal R, McCullough L: Dynamic supportive psychotherapy, in Handbook of Short-Term Dynamic Psychotherapy. Edited by Crits-Christoph P, Barber JP. New York, Basic Books, 1991, pp 220–247
Richland LE, Bjork RA, Finley JR, et al: Linking cognitive science to education: generation and interleaving effects, in Proceedings of the 27th Annual Conference of the Cognitive Science Society, Mattwah, NJ, 2005, pp 1850–1855
Samstag LW, Batchelder ST, Muran JC, et al: Early identification of treatment failures in short-term psychotherapy: an assessment of therapeutic alliance and interpersonal behavior. J Psychother Pract Res 7(2):126–143, 1998 9527957

Skinner BF: The Behavior of Organisms: An Experimental Analysis. New York, Appleton-Century, 1938
Thompson JM, Gallagher P, Hughes JH, et al: Neurocognitive impairment in euthymic patients with bipolar affective disorder. Br J Psychiatry 186:32–40, 2005 15630121
Thorndike E: The Fundamentals of Learning. New York, Teachers College Press, 1932
Tomkins SS: Affect Imagery Consciousness. New York, Springer, 1962
Ursano RJ, Silberman EK: Psychoanalysis, psychoanalytic psychotherapy, and supportive psychotherapy, in The American Psychiatric Press Synopsis of Psychiatry. Edited by Hales RE, Yudofsky SC. Washington, DC, American Psychiatric Press, 1996, pp 969–989
Winnicott DW: The Maturational Process and the Facilitating Environment: Studies in the Theory of Emotional Development. London, Hogarth Press, 1965
Winnicott DW: Playing and Reality. Middlesex, UK, Penguin, 1971
Winston A, Winston B: Handbook of Integrated Short-Term Psychotherapy. Arlington, VA, American Psychiatric Publishing, 2002
Winston A, Rosenthal RN, Pinsker H: Introduction to Supportive Psychotherapy, Washington, DC, American Psychiatric Publishing, 2004
Winston A, Rosenthal RN, Roberts LR: Learning Supportive Psychotherapy: An Illustrated Guide, 2nd Edition. Washington, DC, American Psychiatric Association Publishing, 2020
Wolf ES: Empathy and countertransference, in The Future of Psychoanalysis. Edited by Goldberg A. New York, International Universities Press, 1983, pp 309–326
Zetzel ER: Current concepts of transference. Int J Psychoanal 37(4–5):369–376, 1956 13366506
Zetzel E: The analytic situation, in Psychoanalysis in America. New York, International Universities Press, 1966, pp 86–106

CHAPTER 17

Techniques of Individual Supportive Psychotherapy

Richard N. Rosenthal, M.D.
Adelya A. Urmanche, M.A., Ph.D.
J. Christopher Muran, Ph.D.

The goal of supportive psychotherapy is to ameliorate symptoms and to maintain, restore, or improve self-esteem, adaptive skills, and psychological function (Pinsker and Rosenthal 1988, p. 1). These objectives often can be accomplished with specific and direct supportive techniques, delivered in a conversational style, that are responsive to the patient's identified goals and that are targeted to specific reparative tasks that the clinician has identified—such as examination of relationships and patterns of emotional response or behavior.

Within the supportive psychotherapy framework, the role of the therapist fundamentally differs from that of insight-oriented psychotherapy, where the focus is on the identification and working through of unconscious conflicts. Rather, supportive treatment may resemble a more social relationship; as such, it requires a deliberate balancing of appropriate social disclosure with a direct focus on therapeutic tasks and goals.

Historically, many clinicians saw the benefits of supportive techniques only while working with severely mentally ill patients, arguing that healthier individuals could be helped by more expressive techniques. However, the existing literature consistently suggests that healthier patients can also benefit from supportive psychotherapy (Hellerstein et al. 1998; Rosenthal et al. 1999). This is particularly evident when discussing a patient's psychological development operationalized by defensive operations. Defensive operations can range from primitive (e.g., projection, splitting, denial) to more advanced (e.g., rationalization, displacement, suppression), with the former typically being more globally maladaptive. If a patient is presenting with more primitive defenses, it is likely that the therapist will need to use more awareness-expanding interventions. As in other therapeutic approaches, typical interventions used with a healthier patient may differ from those used with a patient demonstrating more severe psychopathology. In supportive psychotherapy, defenses are rarely addressed directly; however, they are respected, and more adaptive defenses are generally and specifically supported.

Techniques of conducting supportive psychotherapy can be broken down into two levels: contextual and tactical. Contextual techniques can be thought of as the groundwork of treatment, to be used with all patients in all settings. Tactical techniques, on the other hand, are more targeted and can be used accordingly on the basis of patient characteristics, therapeutic goals, and communication content.

Contextual Techniques

Recognize the Relational Context

In an attempt to better understand and conceptualize the patient, clinicians are often very focused on the patient and what the patient brings into the sessions (e.g., symptoms). In supportive therapy, patterns of relationships are as important as behavioral patterns and symptoms. The patient and therapist collaborate to understand interpersonal and other patterns in order to discover what can be changed, not to discover reasons for the existence of the behavior or feelings that should be changed (Rosenthal et al. 1999). As such, an increased focus on the relational context—the way patient and clinician communicate and interact—can provide an important insight for both parties and does not suggest that what the patient does in other relationships is a complete mirror of the patient-clinician relationship. In conducting supportive psychotherapy, the therapist is not technically neutral because the therapist is an active proponent of the patient's ego functioning and self-esteem.

Although it is not part of supportive psychotherapy to explicitly analyze the patient-therapist relationship, it is important to recognize that during a session, clinicians are continuously making decisions. These decisions (e.g., how to phrase something, how to position themselves) are often informed by the patient's anxiety as well as their own. For example, sometimes the therapist will make bridging comments simply to keep the flow of the conversation going because awkward silences can raise a patient's anxiety. At other times, the therapist can wait with interest and concern for the patient to finish formulating their thoughts or to get a handle on a difficult feeling before responding. Through their interventions, clinicians have the power to either increase or decrease their patients' anxiety. Therefore, it is in the interest of being supportive and effective that the therapist is encouraged to pay attention to their own reactions to the patient and how those reactions may unwittingly affect their use of interventions, the therapeutic alliance, or the treatment as a whole. Muran and Eubanks (2020) discuss this as the concept of affect coregulation—that is, the ability of the therapist to model appropriate affect regulation for the patient, thereby empowering the patient to do the same.

In sum, the therapist can maintain the focus on relationships that are in the here and now, including the therapist relationship when appropriate, and may make connections to genetic figures, when appropriate, especially to describe a current maladaptive pattern in a rationalized and practical way or if the patient is demonstrating real insight and driving a more expressive process. Although supportive psychotherapy is not a transference-focused treatment, the therapist must still be mindful of transference material and object relationship patterning (Westen and Gabbard 2002).

Adopt a Conversational Style

Psychotherapy depends largely on verbal communication, so the therapist's language becomes an important instrument. Within supportive psychotherapy, an active, conversational style emulates familiar social interaction and thus tends not to raise anxiety such as that seen with the therapist's more abstaining, exploratory stance when conducting an expressive treatment.

The therapist tends to be more active than in traditional expressive therapies, in which, even if not abstinent in the classical sense, the therapist practices restraint as the default position (Gabbard 2004). The therapist's language should be as clear and concise as possible to ensure patient understanding. Werman (1984) highlights the difference between statements such as "Your behavior tends to be self-destructive" and "You often spit in your own soup" to demonstrate the impact of more vivid language. Moreover, patients and therapists alike often use abstract language (e.g., "psychobabble") to obscure their thoughts and feelings. This can often deter the process of psychotherapy; therefore, a therapist who is not sure what the patient is saying is encouraged to tactfully ask them to explain or clarify.

At the same time, the therapist should be wary of asking too many questions. An interrogatory style consistent with medical student history taking peppers the patient with "why" questions that may be perceived as accusatory or attacking, so the supportive therapist uses a more conversational, nonchallenging approach to gather information (Pinsker 1997).

The therapist is charged with the responsibility of keeping the conversation going in a balanced way. Free association, a fundamental process of psychoanalysis and related expressive therapies that uncovers defenses in the form of resistances, is not germane to the objectives of supportive psychotherapy and is thus neither expected nor promoted. Similarly, the patient may proceed to expand on a narrative with much affect, which reduces tension, provides relief, and may support self-esteem but leaves no room for dialogue.

Should the therapist allow the patient to continue to ventilate or attempt to have a conversation? The therapist should determine what purpose the ventilation serves. Cutting off the ventilation prematurely may be unsupportive. However, unless the therapist sees that the patient is benefiting from ventilation, it is best to redirect it after a time in order to move the treatment in the direction of improving ego functioning and adaptive skills. Through the use of clarification, humor, and other tactical techniques described in more detail later in this chapter, the therapist should be able to practice and model flexibility and empathy, doing what they believe would further the therapeutic process—in short, be of help to the patient.

Maintain the Frame of Treatment

The frame of treatment entails common components and processes such as the office setting, the therapist's role, and expected interactions. The frame also includes explaining the rules of therapy: the patient's role, setting fees, scheduling, beginning and ending sessions, and how missed sessions are handled. The therapist conducts these discussions, in addition to history taking, setting of goals, and discussing the length of treatment, much in the same way as the rest of the supportive treatment. Sometime during the first session, the therapist covers the rules of treatment. With overly anxious patients, this discussion can take place at the beginning of the session as a way of structuring the session and to reduce anxiety with a relatively benign protocol. Similarly, toward the end, the clinician conducting supportive therapy will anticipate the end of a session and clue in the patient by remarking about the time left, as well as making concluding or summarizing statements at the end.

The broad context in which therapy takes place should be structured, predictable, and reliable. The *holding environment* as described by Winnicott (1960, 1971) and others is the optimized interpersonal space that offers nurture, relatedness, organizing feedback, and mirroring to the developing ego. Through creation of a holding environment, the frame of treatment in supportive psychotherapy lowers anxiety by providing consistency and structure while offering and augmenting this environment (Pine 1984). Moreover, the advantage of having a stricter frame around psychotherapy is that if, at any point, the frame is broken or questioned, both patient and therapist are less likely to perceive it as a personal rejection. Obviously, the patient abruptly terminating therapy destroys the frame of treatment. Therefore, the frame of treatment also includes therapist interventions that address a potential rift in the therapeutic alliance or frank evidence that the patient may terminate prematurely because of psychopathology and/or a rupture in the therapeutic alliance. Positive transference is allowed to build because it tends to strengthen and deepen the therapeutic alliance. Similarly, negative transference is not addressed explicitly unless the continuity of the treatment is threatened, in which case it is typically confronted and distortions are corrected because a buildup of negative transference threatens the therapeutic alliance and, thus, the frame of treatment.

Be Like a Good Parent

The clinician conducting supportive psychotherapy needs to continually reevaluate the developmental strengths and weaknesses of the patient (Misch 2000). Using expectations about what responsibilities are age-appropriate and empathic and experiential feedback about a child's current functioning, a good parent balances the wish to protect the child from harm against the child's need to develop autonomy. That balance moves toward autonomy as the child matures and their procedural knowledge and capacity to exercise judgment improve. However, it may swing back toward needing adult intervention in times of crisis, novelty associated with risk, or other situations requiring the parent to comfort, protect, or set limits. In a manner analogous to good parenting, the supportive therapist's goal is to increase the individuation and autonomous functioning of the patient. At times, this means dealing with developmental immaturity in a mentoring and reassuring manner (e.g., giving expert advice or leading anticipatory guidance so that the patient has a clearer understanding of the potential positive and negative consequences of their choices). At others, it means backing off (in spite of a wish to "fix it") and witnessing as the patient makes their own choices and faces the consequences. Regardless of the parenting-like roles of the therapist, we do not substitute our own wishes or values for those of the patient, and although we may have strong reactions, we never punish the patient for negative attitudes, thoughts, or behavior.

John Bowlby, Mary Ainsworth, and other trailblazers of attachment theory (see Bretherton 1992) described a fundamental and evidence-based account of relationships (i.e., attachments) on which survival, developmental progress, and psychological flourishing depend. The basic principles include a need and desire for a *secure base* (e.g., parent, friend, or, arguably, therapist) that provides support and emotional availability and facilitates affect regulation and exploration of the inner and outer worlds. Holmes (2015), a self-identified "attachment-informed psychodynamic psychotherapist with relational tendencies," extensively discussed the potential of the therapist as a secure base. Enlisting supportive techniques, Holmes suggested a number of key features of secure or safe relationships, including acceptance and non-shame-inducing processing of negative affect, positive encouragement and celebration of achievements, promotion of autonomy, and an overall "you can do it, but I am here if you need me" attitude (p. 4).

Tactical Techniques

The tactical techniques of supportive psychotherapy can be organized into four general categories that correspond to the establishment and maintenance of a working relationship in order to effectively conduct treatment: 1) alliance building and the three core objectives of supportive psychotherapy, 2) esteem building, 3) enhancing ego functioning, and 4) skills building. Alliance building aligns with the contextual technique of recognizing the relational context, and the goal is to support the development of a strong working alliance within which to conduct the treatment. However, because the techniques that fall under the rubric of alliance building also have tactical utility in that they are responsive to patients' statements, they are included in this section. Esteem building might otherwise be included under ego functioning, but because it is a primary objective of supportive psychotherapy and has many core techniques specifically associated with it, it is given its own category. In addition, many of the interventions could be placed in more than one category because effects are often multimodal. For example, expression of empathy is often reassuring depending on the context and thus could support self-esteem, but the primary intent is to strengthen the therapeutic alliance. Similarly, encouragement is esteem building but also allays anxiety. For simplicity, each technique is organized in relation to its main effect.

Alliance Building

General principles of supportive psychotherapy related to the patient-therapist relationship are described by Winston et al. (2020), building on the work of Pinsker (1997), Misch (2000), and Novalis et al. (1993). According to Bordin (1979), the therapeutic alliance is composed of an affective therapist-patient bond and agreement on therapy tasks and goals. It continues to be one of the most robust predictors of successful therapy outcome, across various treatment approaches and patient pathology (Flückiger et al. 2018). Barber et al. (2001) argued that a positive therapeutic alliance is not in itself a technique, offering support for various supportive techniques used across different treatment modalities. That stated, supportive psychotherapy focuses on the development of a strong therapeutic alliance as a *purposive* core strategy and thus offers several proactive techniques that can be used to support that goal. Establishing agreement on tasks and goals can be quite technical, and fostering a strong positive bond is more complex; although therapist authenticity and flexibility can certainly facilitate the process, more discernable techniques include therapist genuineness and expression of curiosity and empathy.

Establishing Agreement on Tasks and Goals

Agreement on tasks and goals includes both a general agreement about the goals of therapy and ongoing agreement about the tasks and interventions within sessions. Setting realistic expectations for the treatment in a collaborative manner not only assists in fostering a healthy therapeutic alliance but also facilitates a holding environment of structure and safety. Sometimes, patients come into therapy with goals such as "to get married" or "for my son to shape up"; at such times, it is crucial to recognize that those are significant life wishes and distinguish more concrete goals for therapy specifically. Accepting grand, longer-term, or potentially unachievable goals can be a setup for patient failure and would go against the broader goals of supportive treatment, whereas shorter-term, more concrete, achievable goals (e.g., signing up for a dating app) can potentially result in the patient gaining a sense of achievement and autonomy. At the same time, collaboration is key, and therapists should be wary of trying to fulfill their own wishes and goals for their patients.

Similarly, during a session, the therapist and patient might get "stuck" if the patient suddenly states something along the lines of "I don't want to talk about that." Within the supportive framework, the therapist would respect the patient's wishes; however, supportive psychotherapy is not nondirective (Rogers 1957). The therapist may consider an opportunity to revisit the function of such an abrupt statement and whether the supportive approach would include dropping the topic completely because it increases the patient's anxiety or gently inquiring about the difficulties of discussing it.

Expression of Genuineness

Therapist genuineness is a condition of therapy first introduced by Carl Rogers (1957). By genuineness, he suggested that the therapist "is freely and deeply himself, with his actual experience accurately represented by his awareness of himself. It is the opposite of presenting a façade, either knowingly or unknowingly" (p. 97). In supportive psychotherapy, this merely suggests that therapists are promoting a self-awareness in relation to themselves and their patient. Certainly, no one could reasonably maintain the ideal state of complete self-awareness all the time, nor is that the expectation. However, if, for example, a therapist *consistently* finds themself bored or distracted when with a particular patient, it may point to a more significant matter concerning the patient's pathology, the therapeutic alliance, or even the treatment approach. These patterns do not need to be explicitly shared with the patient or become the focus of therapy; however, the therapist's own curiosity and, perhaps, acceptance of the patterns may facilitate a more genuine approach toward the patient. Moreover, if the patient experiences the therapist as being inauthentic, it will likely damage the therapist's credibility and thus the alliance.

Expression of Curiosity and Interest

Deliberately reiterating material from past sessions is a way to deliver the message that the patient is important to the therapist (self-esteem), and it is also directive. Whenever the therapist forgets specifics of a patient's experience or recalls them incorrectly and casually reveals this to the patient, this is nonsupportive. Although the patient might express interest in the therapist's questions, some patients experience being asked too many questions, particularly "why" questions, as an intrusion or an attack.

Communication should never be taken for granted, and the risk that the therapist might miss the point of a patient's statements and say something incorrect necessitates that the therapist solicit the patient's feedback to determine whether the therapist is on target. Tentative statements such as "It sounds like..." or "Am I getting that right?" can go a long way in not only showing the patient that the therapist is listening but also fundamentally ensuring that the patient and therapist are on the same page. Cultural differences, for example, may influence expressive style and inadvertently result in misattunements. In line with the conversational nature of supportive therapy, certain expressions or "street talk" could have different meanings for the therapist and patient. At other times, the statements by the patient may be generally vague or otherwise unclear. Therefore, as a basic therapeutic strategy, the therapist always wants to know more about unclear communications and asks for clarification.

Moreover, a growing body of literature points to the utility of facilitative nonverbal behaviors, such as eye contact and the "forward lean." These behaviors help patients feel supported, and clinicians who provide this kind of support are more likely to be viewed as likable and credible (see Leierer et al. 1996; Toriello and Strohmer 2004). Even simple nods can send the message that the therapist is attentive and engaged with the patient. The function of witnessing and feeding back clinician understanding tends to support the development of a strong working alliance, even when what the patient communicates is painful or problematic.

Expression of Empathy

Empathic relatedness underscores a core relational aspect of positive regard and so forms part of the patient's experience of the therapist that the therapist cares in a meaningful way. Empathic relating goes beyond simple caring and concern. Being known by the therapist in this way is intrinsically supportive and provides the patient a sense of recognition and connection, strengthening the self and influencing the unconscious affective bonds often described as *implicit relational knowing* (Lyons-Ruth et al. 1998). When the opportunity presents itself in treatment, the therapist gives feedback in the form of relating their own internal emotional experience to corroborate that of the patient (e.g., "You must have felt humiliated when he treated you that way"). This empathic validation demonstrates the "therapist's empathic attunement with the patient's internal state" (Gabbard 2005) and serves to deepen the patient's experience of being understood in an essential way.

Repairing of a Misalliance or Alliance Rupture

On the basis of the previous definition of the therapeutic alliance, an alliance rupture is a deterioration in the alliance, manifested in a disagreement on treatment goals or therapeutic tasks, or a strain in the emotional bond between patient and therapist (see Safran and Muran 2000). Such ruptures can be marked by confrontation behaviors (attempts to challenge the other by controlling or criticizing) or by withdrawal behaviors (attempts to move away from another or from an uncomfortable experience) (see Muran 2019; Muran and Eubanks 2020). Ruptures are a natural occurrence in psychotherapy across different approaches and patient populations. Accordingly, rupture repair can involve the reestablishment of agreement on tasks and goals or of trust in the emotional bond. Eubanks et al. (2018) found that rupture resolution correlates significantly with positive patient outcome. As such, it is important for therapists to 1) recognize when a rupture is occurring and 2) address it in a timely and effective manner.

Supportive measures have historically been the first line of repair for alliance ruptures (see Bond et al. 1998), primarily because repair fits well into the overarching goals of supportive psychotherapy. First, any successfully repaired rupture can provide the patient with a new interpersonal experience. Sometimes called a *corrective emotional experience* (see Alexander and French 1946), it can build esteem and foster patient agency. Second, the therapist engages in skills building by modeling adaptive behavior. Because one of the hypothesized mechanisms of change in supportive psychotherapy is through identification with a well-compensated and effective therapist, the therapist must consistently demonstrate adaptive, reasonable, and organized thinking and behavior to the patient (Pinsker et al. 1991). However, at times in therapy, as in any human relationship, the therapist is going to get it wrong—as manifested in an incorrect understanding, assumption, statement, or action. How the therapist is able to address these moments with honesty, grace, humility, and resilience can impart an important message to the patient and offer a more interpersonally flexible and adaptive model of character with which the patient can identify. Third, the therapist demonstrates curiosity and interest in the patient's experience rather than prioritizing their own comfort level. Last, the nature of rupture repair is inherently supportive; by attempting repair, the therapist invites collaboration and sends the message "This is uncomfortable, but I'm with you and we can figure this out together."

Muran and Eubanks (2020) described repair strategies that range from supportive (what they called *immediate*) to expressive. Immediate or supportive strategies include 1) acknowledging one's own contribution, 2) clarifying a misunderstanding, 3) changing tasks or goals, and 4) illustrating a task or rationale for therapeutic intervention. Expressive strategies essentially use the rupture marker as an opportunity to explore core relational themes for the patient. These strategies tend to evoke anxiety, although supportive techniques are applied to manage the anxiety. (For more detail on the more expressive approach to rupture repair, see Muran and Eubanks 2020; for the beneficial effect of training in rupture repair, see Muran et al. 2018.)

Any repair strategy can begin with the acknowledgment of a rupture. Sometimes, a rupture or potential rupture can be easily identified by the therapist, especially if the therapist has contributed to it. Mere acknowledgment can hold reparative power and demonstrate to the patient that the therapist is paying attention and can reflect on their actions.

Therapist: Oof, I really screwed it up by missing our session last week, huh? [*Approach to acknowledging own contribution*]

At other times, the patient could show signs suggesting that a rupture may have occurred or is under way. The following three dialogues show some ways in which patients may signal a potential rupture, with differing therapist responses.

Therapist 1: How is it going today?
Patient 1 (*few minutes of silence*): Fine. [*Minimal response, very unlike the patient*]
Therapist 1: Well, I was reflecting on what you said last time about our sessions being too late in the day. I'm wondering if we can figure out another time that works better for us. [*The therapist lets the patient know they have been on the therapist's mind, approaches changing parameters of the therapy on the basis of the patient's desire, and uses "we" to suggest collaboration.*]

Patient 2: I hate when you ask me so many questions.
Therapist 2: Yes, I imagine that must be frustrating. I suppose I was so interested in this new relationship of yours, I got a little carried away. [*Validates anxiety and illustrates rationale for questioning; acknowledges own contribution*]

Therapist 3: It sounds like playing in this game was a huge win!
Patient 3: No, not at all. We didn't win. What are you talking about?
Therapist 3: Sure. But I guess I meant for you, personally. You really stepped outside of your comfort zone by not sitting on the bench this time. [*Clarifies misunderstanding*]
Patient 3: Oh. Yeah, I definitely did.

Supportive therapy makes use of more practical ways to address a rupture. With lower-functioning patients, the therapist may need to alter his or her stance, as one does in normal social discourse when the person is becoming distant or more obviously angry (Pinsker et al. 1991).

Self-Disclosure

Although it is not inappropriate for the patient to know something about the therapist as a person in the real world, in general, the information should be that which might be available in the public record, such as the internet or other media. When the therapist chooses to reveal less obvious personal information, it should be for a clearly therapeutic purpose. In expressive therapies, one buys out of the direct question about what the therapist's experience is by asking why the patient is interested or by interpreting. In supportive psychotherapy, if it seems reasonable, the therapist may self-disclose, being careful not to be seductive, competitive, or unnecessarily gratifying or otherwise exploit the patient. As a contrast, it may be useful to state here that some of the best self-disclosure occurs through a process wherein the therapist reveals themself by modeling appropriate behavior—thinking through a problem collaboratively, being steadfast and compassionate in a crisis, manifesting patience and emotional strength, demonstrating flexibility when necessary, exercising both wisdom and humility, and teaching the patient how to emulate these qualities when possible. Three therapist responses demonstrating different levels of self-disclosure are provided in the following example.

Patient: I don't think you like me.
Therapist 1: It's important for you to know how I feel. [*Traditional clarification does not reveal the therapist's feelings but is responsive.*]

Therapist 2: I hear a question in your statement, and I will answer it, but first, I'd like to know what it means to you. [*One can answer with a question as long as it is not off-putting or avoiding answering and it is combined with anticipatory guidance.*]

Therapist 3: Sure, I like you. What makes you think differently? [*This response is used with a fragile, lower-functioning patient.*]

Sometimes a patient will ask for an opinion that draws on the therapist's subjective experience and that may have direct impact on the patient's self-esteem. The therapist is best off responding with a teaching moment based on principle, reflecting back on the framework of psychotherapy.

Patient: I brought in some of my drawings. What do you think of them?

Therapist: It's important that you've been putting your creative impulses into action, and I'd like to see your work. However, it's generally unwise for psychotherapists to make comments on things that they are not expert in, so I'm not going to comment as if I were. It's one of those unwritten rules of psychotherapy. [*Sets limits in a nonpunitive way, softens potential rejection through praise and generalization, and frames expected patient behavior through declaration of a principle*]

Self-Esteem Building

Self-esteem is the collection of beliefs and experiences that a person has of their inherent value and includes the individual's actual competence or self-efficacy. Interventions that augment psychological functioning or adaptive skills raise the patient's capacity to function appropriately in the world and support increased self-esteem. However, some supportive interventions are intended to directly restore or improve self-esteem.

Praise

Praise, along with the other esteem-building interventions, is used proactively and liberally in supportive treatment. In one sense, praise is a clarification that raises self-esteem by raising the patient's awareness about their accomplishments. However, in order for praise to be effective, it must be data based, that is, grounded in the therapist's understanding of the patient's values and experience. Thus, the therapist must be careful not to impose their values on the patient. If the patient does not experience the therapist's statements as praise because what has been identified is not felt by the patient to be praiseworthy, then the therapist has not been supportive. Praise that is empty or undeserved is likely to be experienced negatively. One is better off not saying anything in that situation because praise for something the patient does not feel is praiseworthy belittles the patient. Similarly, it is important that the therapist choose words that do not deliver a subtly denigrating, dismissive, or patronizing message or tone (Pinsker 1997).

Honest praise can be given for positive movement in the usual objectives of supportive therapy—an accomplishment of a stated task, use of a more adaptive skill, or demonstration of a more mature emotional strategy.

Patient: So I walked into his office and decided I had to put my cards on the table. Like usual, he started to put up a fuss, but I said he needed to hear me out because I'd had other offers, which wasn't true (*grins*). Inside, I was sort of watching myself deal with him. Some part of me couldn't believe I was doing that. But he listened to me and then he gave me the raise!

Therapist: That's great! [*Smiles, mirroring the patient.*] You knew the right way to deal with your boss. In contrast to your statements that you're a pushover, here you demonstrated real initiative and got what you wanted. Are there other times when you act so self-assured? [*The therapist praises the patient's successful bargaining and attempts to broaden the role in the patient's self-concept.*]

The therapist can praise the patient's ability to negotiate (i.e., the patient's adaptive skills), an intervention firmly in the realm of the supportive approach, and here we are the experts. Patients are often unaware of the gains they have made, so the therapist can build self-esteem by making strengths explicit.

In the following example, the patient is able to talk about his experiences of failure, but in a balance because he has other things of value in his life.

Patient: I've screwed up plenty of relationships over the years—we've talked about that. Also, my attempt at law school was a bust. I kept trying and trying but just couldn't cut it. I've also blown through a bunch of jobs since then, especially 2 years ago when I had that billing supervisor job at the medical clinic. Boy, was I in way over my head! I tried to ride it out, figuring I'd get the hang of it, but it didn't work out. I like the numbers, but I don't like the pressure. But now I'm doing pretty well at this new place. I track their inventory on a computer, and I've been there 8 months with no major upheaval. It suits me better. And of course, now I have Lisa in my life.

Therapist: So now your confidence is much more realistic. [*Clarifies the patient's statement*]

Patient: I just get myself into these situations and then find out I'm not prepared or it's too stressful.

Therapist: But I'm struck by your ability to go round after round and see things through. You always land on your feet. [*Self-esteem building by making strengths explicit*]

Reassurance

Reassurance is used as a supportive intervention within supportive psychotherapy as well as in other situations in which one person allays the fears of another by delivering truthful information in a caring way. In general medical practice, reassurance is used frequently to dispel patients' negative expectations about the course of an illness or sequelae of a treatment or surgery and thus to alleviate patients' anxieties. When supportive psychotherapy is being conducted, reassurance is best when it is data based or based on principle. It usually is not good to reassure without knowledge of the patient's life and expectations. Similarly, the therapist should first let the patient voice their concerns before attempting to be reassuring, lest such reassurance be perceived as hollow or nonspecific to the patient's needs.

Normalizing is a particular form of reassurance that relies on comparisons with others whom the patient is likely to deem "normal" or "regular." The therapist's message that "other people do it too" normalizes by recategorizing the patient's beliefs about their own or others' experience or behavior.

Patient: It's really difficult. I know I have to move forward with my plan, but I'm really scared about what could happen. There must be something wrong with me. I should be able to "just do it" (*anxious smile*). I feel guilty, too, 'cause I see Dad in my head saying, "Feeling scared is just so ridiculous. Look at your opportunity!"

Therapist: Anyone would be afraid and proceed with caution in your situation. [*Depathologizes and empathizes*]

The therapist's comments when normalizing must be targeted, specific, and helpful. Empty comments are not supportive, even if accurate:

Patient: I'm the weirdest person there is. I'm all alone—isolated and no friends, no interests, and no prospects (*frowns, stares into space*).
Therapist: Many people feel this way. [*Gives a fatuous response*]

Encouragement

When a patient is discouraged in the face of difficult external obstacles or their own incapacities, the therapist may provide encouragement. Frequently, patients present in therapy in a demoralized state—they experience distress at an inability to rectify a problem against what is experienced as great odds, combined with subjective incompetence and decreased self-esteem (de Figueiredo 1993; Frank 1974). When patients are demoralized, they do not try new things to improve their quality of life because they presume that they have no power to effect change (Pinsker et al. 1991). Patients can be demoralized because of moral beliefs they have about their own behavior, externalizing defenses that promote the experience of powerlessness, disempowering responses of others to their maladaptive behavior, or their experience of treatment systems that communicate their low expectation of real change (Rosenthal 2002). With the patient faced with problems that appear to loom large, the therapist can provide encouragement by assisting the patient in taking one step at a time. This means that the therapist acts to spur on or to instill hope, an elemental factor that may contribute to therapeutic change (Yalom 1995). Many common adages (e.g., "Rome wasn't built in a day"; "Every cloud has a silver lining") are available to present an encouraging or hopeful message that can be used in therapy.

Exhortation

Exhortation is a more insistent form of encouragement in which the clinician urges or spurs the patient to pursue a goal. Typically, this is done with a more impaired patient, who, though reluctant, must have a high likelihood of accomplishing the task (Pinsker 1997). Because of the risk of overwhelming or disempowering the patient, caution must be used in tempering the manner and the message so that the patient feels the strong alliance with and conviction of the therapist that what the therapist is suggesting is the right course of action. The following example presents different responses to a patient's statement, from highly definitive to more layered and nuanced, based on the therapist's current appraisal of the patient.

Patient: I'm not sure I have what it takes to get through this.... I have to tell them whether I'll take their offer in the next week.
Therapist 1: I've seen what you are capable of. You can do this! [*Frank cheerleading*]
Therapist 2: You've spent many weeks convincing me that this is the goal you want to pursue, and you were quite eloquent in laying out the arguments as to why it was appropriate for you. It's not unusual to have some doubts along the way, especially before you commit yourself, but I think you have a great rationale for making this choice. [*Reiterates the patient's own arguments to counter the patient's*

ambivalence, normalizes doubts, and adds the weight of the therapist's reasoning to the decisional process]

Inspiration

The aim of inspiration is to support the patient's experience of self-esteem and self-efficacy through self-transcendence, a powerfully validating experience. Inspiration is seen more commonly in the context of religious or spiritual guidance or participation or when spontaneously experiencing a noble or heroic action by another. However, as a purposive technique in supportive psychotherapy, inspiration is difficult to use and is used infrequently because it requires a situation in which the therapist experiences an opportunity both to self-transcend and to communicate their authentic experiences or beliefs or those of another in a manner that the patient experiences as elevating. Inspiration goes beyond reassurance and encouragement because in this highly motivated state the patient's fear and the experienced need for small steps are supervened. When one is inspired, there is an increase in motivation for self-actualizing behavior.

Enhancement of Ego Functioning

The domain of ego functioning includes the various functions of the mental operations of the self, including reality testing, sense of reality, affect regulation, defensive functions, synthetic function, object relations, thought processes, and superego (conscience, morals, ideals) (Bellak 1958; Beres 1956). Because anxiety tends to exacerbate impairments in ego functioning, as well as amplifying symptoms of major mental disorders, supportive psychotherapy offers several interventions that directly address it.

Anxiety-Reducing Interventions

Interventions that reduce anxiety are fundamental to the repertoire of supportive psychotherapy. The rationale of many of the contextual techniques is that they reduce anxiety or prevent its exacerbation. Anxiety in supportive psychotherapy generally is framed as psychopathological or at least as contributing to the patient's sense of dysphoria and maladaptation. When anxiety or fear is experienced as overwhelming, people have difficulty trying new things and as a result may not master important adaptive skills, such as asking someone out for a date, driving a car, or learning to swim. Thus, in supportive treatment, anxiety is usually reduced through direct means except when the therapist is purposefully titrating it (e.g., through exposure) or is working with skills to help the patient cope more adaptively. In contrast, in expressive therapies, unless anxiety is at the disorder level, it is seen as a motivator of the psychotherapeutic work or as a signal to the participants that conflictual unconscious content is emergent (Freud 1936/1966).

Structuring the environment. When the patient has more severe psychopathology and is relatively low functioning, the therapist acts to increase the amount of structure available to the patient through therapeutic interventions and interactions with the patient's environment. These mechanisms may include interaction with such individuals as case managers, family members, and employers (Rockland 1989). With higher-functioning patients, the clinical necessity to intervene directly in the patient's life or environment is greatly reduced and, with respect to the patient's actual functional autonomy, becomes intrusive or otherwise inappropriate.

Maintaining a protected environment. Although maintaining a protected environment is not supportive psychotherapy proper, at times the most supportive activity is to provide a holding environment that literally contains the patient. Clearly, for safety reasons, as when a patient cannot be relied on to contain self-destructive or other destructive impulses and there is insufficient community support, hospitalization can provide respite and containment.

Setting limits. At times, the therapist will choose to exercise professional and relational power to set limits when the patient is behaving in a way that is maladaptive in that the patient is not following the rules of therapy. A patient's transgression can take the form of behaviors that are unresponsive to therapist's cueing and feedback, such as being threatening or seductive, arriving intoxicated, not leaving the session when the time is up, or acting in an otherwise inappropriate manner. Assuming that the intoxicated patient can leave the session safely, they must do so with the clear message to come back in a nonintoxicated state. Otherwise, if the patient is able to pull back on the behavior and discuss it in session after being made aware of it, many such behaviors are amenable to discussion in the context of supporting ego function and adaptive skills.

The therapist decides when to alter the structure of the session. For example, with a patient in crisis and also under other circumstances, it may be therapeutically appropriate to extend the time of a session. The therapist pays proper attention to not gratuitously satisfying the patient's infantile wishes but tempers this with reasonableness, which is the therapist modeling reasonable behavior and judgment (Winston et al. 2020). At other times, such as with a patient who has a pattern of continuing to engage and speak after the end of a session, the therapist can choose not to extend the session because it would enable maladaptive, regressive behavior without reasonable clinical or environmental justification. In this case, the therapist gets up and shows the patient the door.

Designating the topic explicitly. Because of the inherent power imbalance in the therapeutic relationship, the therapist attempts to empower the patient by involving them as a decision-making participant in what is discussed. Compared with free association, which is anxiety provoking, agenda setting gives the patient a structured topic on which to focus and reduces anxiety by putting the patient into the position of acceding or refusing to discuss the topic.

Modulating affect. Modulating affect pertains to how people manage emotions—their own and their responses to the feelings of others or to an emotionally charged situation. When patients have impairments in this area of ego functioning, they may respond disproportionately to the situation with an overly intense, overly constricted, dysphoric, or otherwise maladaptive manner. The patient's loss of control of affect is typically maladaptive. For patients with an inability to contain their expression of affect, continuing to focus on what is making the person angry only escalates the problem, so often it is best to change the subject (Pinsker 1997). Gaining emotional competence improves self-esteem, so in the context of a good therapeutic alliance the therapist focuses the patient on how to better contain affects and intervenes in ways that help the patient develop their capacity for affective regulation. Reducing the patient's reactions to environmental or intrapsychic stress or altering the inclination toward negative emotional states and misinterpretations of their physical states can improve self-efficacy (Bandura 1994).

Supporting defenses. Defenses usually are not confronted unless they are clearly maladaptive (e.g., primitive denial, regression, projection, splitting) or threaten the frame of treatment. Adaptive defenses such as repression, rationalization, intellectualization, and reaction formation are generally and specifically supported, as in the following dialogue.

> **Patient:** I spend too much time thinking about everything. [*Bemoans obsessional style*]
> **Therapist:** Standing in front of the closet deciding what to wear helps you stall some and put off what would be very anxiety provoking. [*Notes the patient's difficulty with having to make a decision and supports obsessional defenses.*

Universalizing. Rather than personalizing a comment to the patient, an approach that may be received as an attack or a criticism, the supportive therapist can cloak the comment in an impersonal remark, as distinguished between the two following therapist responses:

> **Therapist 1:** You heard what you wanted to hear. [*Confronts directly*]
> **Therapist 2:** The mind has a tendency to hear what it wants to hear. [*Declares a general principle*]

Naming the problem. Identifying and naming a problem helps the patient to conceptualize it and thus to better understand and cope with it. For example, with a patient who is overly digressive, making the pattern of communication with the therapist the exemplar for a more general pattern can focus the patient on working to be better understood, if it is the patient's desire to do so.

> **Therapist:** I notice that when you are explaining something, you tend to use a lot of extra words and refer to subjects that are not necessary to get the point across. I'm finding it hard to understand. Has anyone ever brought that up as an issue?
> **Patient:** People always seem to get huffy and impatient with me when I talk about things.
> **Therapist:** So, that I'm having some difficulty following your train of thought is not something unusual for you?
> **Patient:** I don't think so.
> **Therapist:** Maybe your experience of people's negative responses is related to their having trouble with easily understanding you, too. Should we put this pattern of speaking to others on the problem list? [*Connects people's responses to the patient's style and offers it as something that can be worked on*]

The patient can answer the therapist's question and still have his autonomy supported.

Rationalizing. Rationalization allows a patient to explain unacceptable attitudes, beliefs, or behaviors so as to make them bearable (Gabbard 2004). When the therapist offers a rationalizing comment, they are shoring up a healthier defensive mode for the patient that is adaptive in that it aids the patient in coping with realities that tend to reduce the patient's self-esteem.

Reframing. Reframing is a rationalization strategy in which the therapist offers a different point of view given the same information, with the intended effect of interfering with the patient's maladaptive beliefs about their thoughts or behavior.

> **Patient:** I really want to talk to him, but then I get tongue-tied and I walk away. Then I try again and end up somewhere else, like at the front desk, or one time right out the door. Last time, I actually walked right by him, but all I could manage was a weak smile. I'm sure it looked goofy because I was so anxious. I'm so inept; I'll never connect with him this way.
>
> **Therapist:** Being shy around someone you are really attracted to is pretty common, so in this you are definitely not alone. [*Normalizes*] Sometimes it takes a bunch of tries in order to be successful. It's like testing the shallow part before you go out to the deep end of the water. [*Relabels approach-avoidance behavior as "getting used to"*]

Reframing can soften the impact of an unpleasant reality on the patient's self-esteem, as in the following example:

> **Patient:** Ugh, sometimes I'd get through the voir dire, but by the end of it they'd rejected me from five juries. Five juries! I couldn't believe it (*scowls*).
>
> **Therapist:** You can be rejected for being too well educated. [*Esteem building by reframing and rationalizing*]

At times, reframing can be used in a more traditional way within the context of supportive psychotherapy. Pointing out maladaptive behavior as part of an illness is reframing it to make it ego-dystonic, a standard psychotherapeutic technique to increase motivation for change. Given the rationale of supportive psychotherapy, the delivery must be couched in a reassuring and hopeful manner that minimizes anxiety, reduces potential blows to self-esteem, and outlines an achievable pathway for change. In the following example, the patient recognizes the pattern that his life is unstable and blames himself for its damaging his interpersonal relationships.

> **Patient:** I've been really down since Tuesday, when Beth broke up with me. I screwed it up because my life isn't together. But I know it's my fault…it happens with every relationship. When I was going out with Sandi, the same thing happened. Same with Leslie. I should have acted like I was more in charge. I'm such a loser.
>
> **Therapist:** Is there a utility in your rehashing old relationships? Let's make a distinction between the use of analyzing interpersonal patterns and self-punishing. It seems that each time you bring it up, rather than looking objectively for ways to be more successful in going forward, you use it to underscore your failures and beat yourself up. This has a direct negative effect on your self-esteem, so it's not adaptive for you. Maybe we can use the patterns you recognize to be more successful? [*Reframing, which proposes that the patient change his perspective on the same information*]

Minimization. Another form of rationalization is one in which the therapist substitutes minimization for the patient's denial of affect in order to make the affect more palatable for the patient to accept. For example, the therapist might say, "So, there was *some* resentment?"

Awareness-Expanding Interventions

The aim of expanding awareness is contrasted with development of insight, which in psychodynamic terms is emotional awareness based on genetic material, usually via the transference. Clarification, confrontation, and, more rarely, interpretation are useful techniques in supportive psychotherapy, but there is no requirement that the unconscious be made conscious or that full linkage of impulses, wishes, or affects be made with early important figures. In supportive psychotherapy, the therapist clarifies frequently and confronts periodically but interprets infrequently.

Clarification. Without elaboration, the therapist using clarification reduces cognitive distortion or points out patterns by restating, acknowledging, summarizing, paraphrasing, or organizing a patient's statements.

Patient: I'm so mad Beth dumped me. Maybe if she told me earlier that she was getting unhappy and frustrated, I could've changed things (*frowns*). I was really trying to be a good partner. It's so painful—I don't understand why she did this. Things were going pretty well. I miss her and want her back.

Therapist: Can we look at what happened?

Patient: I took her out for dinners and always had to fit everything to her schedule. I even went to plenty of events with her and did lots of other stuff that I didn't really want to do. And then, nothing. When's it my turn? It's just not fair (*reddens*)!

Therapist: Did you tell her what you were dissatisfied about?

Patient: Not so much.

Therapist: So, your experience is that you made a lot of adjustments to sustain the relationship with her, but it makes you angry that she didn't reciprocate the effort before she broke up with you. [*Clarifies*]

Using humor. Sometimes, framing a clarification in a humorous wrapper softens the potential esteem-lowering impact of finding out that what one is doing is getting in one's own way.

Patient: I'm still so lonely. I think a lot about how it would be to meet someone and have a relationship, but it doesn't happen.

Therapist [*sees issue of procrastinating*]: It's difficult for you to meet men. [*Clarification*]

Patient: I've been getting things done, but I have so much to do: I'm busy at work, then there's dating, answering personals, going online, and so on....

Therapist: If you can use your creativity to find ways of doing what you say is your intention instead of making creative excuses, you'll probably be successful. [*Avuncular encouragement*]

The content in this case might be the same as what a friend or family member would tell the patient, but a therapist saying it might give it more power.

Confrontation. Confrontation is an intervention that brings to the patient's awareness something they are avoiding or suppressing or an unrecognized maladaptive pattern of behavior. If the therapist in the previous interaction went further and elaborated on the information in a way that brought into awareness the maladaptive pattern of behavior the patient is avoiding looking at, it would be a confrontation.

Therapist: I notice that you tend to say "I don't understand" about things you actually do understand. [*Confronts without giving rationale*]

Therapist: I'm going to point out something I think will help you to better get your needs met in relationships. It seems that you expect that people should know what you need. Then when you don't get it, you get angry. [*Gives rationale for confronting, then confronts*]

When the therapist chooses to confront in supportive psychotherapy, they put the confronting into a specific context and give a clear rationale for it (e.g., to increase adaptive skills), making sure there is ample feedback that the patient understands the therapist's intent. For example, "I'm bringing this to your awareness so that the next time you get into a dispute with your father that makes you angry, you can respond in a way that makes you feel more competent." This is especially useful in working with a patient's more primitive defenses.

Patient: It made me so angry and jealous when I caught him looking at another woman. Then he has the nerve to claim that he wasn't looking at her.

Therapist: Is that not possible? Did you actually see him looking at her? [*Continues to reality test the basis of her assessment*]

Patient: I could sense that he was looking, but, well, no, I didn't actually see him looking. You think he might be doing it on purpose?

Therapist: I'm thinking maybe that question is a little far-fetched. Is it offensive to you that I point this out? [*In dealing with a paranoid style, the therapist encourages the patient to "consider the alternatives."*]

Patient: No, it's OK. I just get angry when he's checking out another woman. I've told him about that.

Therapist: I understand, but since you didn't actually see him, is it possible that he really didn't look at her? It seems that you assume that if a woman you think he thinks is attractive walks by, he will look at her, even though you've made it clear that it upsets you.

Patient: Don't know. Maybe I do that. There have been times I've accused people of stuff and they denied it—they even had what looked like proof—so I backed off. But I get the feeling anyway that somehow they got away with it.

Therapist: So, you've described a pattern where people disagree with your take on things, and even with some evidence they are speaking honestly, you have this vexing sense they are not. Is it a possibility that somehow things may be at times a little different from how you experience them? [*The therapist clarifies, then points out that this is not an isolated experience for her but part of a pattern (confrontation) and, finally, softens and minimizes the observation that the patient is distorting.*]

Patient: I guess it's possible. It just doesn't seem that way, but I see your point about the pattern—I do that a lot, and not just with him. [*Responds to the confrontation with increased awareness*]

Denial is a common defense that can be adaptive or maladaptive. The supportive task here is how to improve the patient's reality testing without damaging their self-esteem, as in the following dialogue about the end of a relationship.

Therapist: I see that it is difficult or maybe painful for you to look at, but this may help you to think about moving forward. You are acting toward these women as if you still had a relationship so you don't have to let go. [*Confronts pattern of denial that relationships are in the past*]

Patient: I still think about Beth. She should call me so we could discuss things.

Therapist: However, you are no longer in a relationship with her. [*Reiterates confrontation more specifically*]

Patient: But I still care for her (*long silence*). She's out having a wonderful time. I think it's bad for me to think she didn't have any genuine feelings for me.

Therapist: That's an assumption. Why would she have feelings for you now since the relationship is over? That's probably why she hasn't called. But that doesn't mean that she was not genuine when you were together. [*Confronts distortion*]

Patients will at times talk in a vague manner. This manner can be due to a vague style, which may be the result of cognitive, interpersonal, or cultural factors or a situational vagueness caused by obsessional defenses that are aroused in response to a conflictual feeling, wish, or impulse. In the following example, three possible therapist responses are given, ranging from direct and potentially anxiety-provoking to a more softened and overtly supportive delivery.

Therapist: How did you feel when, again, she didn't give you what you had clearly asked for?

Patient: Oh, this happens all the time (*shrugs*). We ended up going out to the movies instead. [*Uninformative*]

Therapist 1: You are being vague. [*Confronts the defense without contextual support, potentially raising anxiety*]

Therapist 2: Could you be more specific? I'm not sure what you are getting at, but I hear you aren't getting what you want from her. [*Confronts in a more diluted and empathic fashion, lowering the risk of raising anxiety*]

Therapist 3: People often talk around a topic when they are uncomfortable about how they feel or how they may be perceived. I hope you understand that I've pretty much heard it all and am comfortable with the issues people are most uncomfortable with. [*Confronts in a softened and normalized fashion, balancing with alliance building and reassurance, thus lowering anxiety*]

The patient then continues:

Patient: Well, I get upset when she does this. She does this all the time (*reddens and clenches hands together*).

Therapist 3: How upset?

Patient: I was disappointed. It makes me feel wimpy and hopeless.

Therapist 3: Did you communicate your feelings to her so that she might address your concerns?

Patient: We went to the movies like nothing happened.

Therapist 3: So we can see that although you are able to initially ask her for what you want, she frequently dismisses this, and you get dejected and feel a loss of self-esteem because you feel ineffective in getting your needs met. Maybe we can work on a way for you to more effectively address getting your needs met. [*Confronts, then encourages by offering a path toward increased self-efficacy*]

Similarly, patients may have a digressive style or become digressive only as a defensive posture. Should the therapist intervene when the patient digresses, or should the therapist let the patient move toward the point? Focusing too early with confrontation may cut off the final point, but letting the patient digress too much may avoid the adaptive context. The therapist must make a data-based intervention based on the patient's goals and the objectives of supportive psychotherapy.

Indirect or impersonal suggestion is a confrontive technique that does not engage defenses directly, in order to raise awareness. Rather than asking something that the patient must answer such as "Are you angry?" one can embed the query in the conversation.

Patient: And then he said he was sorry I was mad he didn't pick me up, and I wasn't even mad. He's just a jerk sometimes (*loudly and emphatically*)!

Therapist: When people raise their voices, sometimes they're angry. [*Sidesteps defenses and doesn't arouse anxiety*]

Interpretation. Interpretation focuses awareness on a thought, behavior, affect, defense, or symptom by connecting it to its unconscious origin or meaning. Transference interpretation is used infrequently in supportive psychotherapy, although it may be used provided it is aimed toward adaptive functioning or to maintain the frame of treatment. Interpretive ideas can be offered in a variety of more supportive configurations (Winston et al. 1986). Linkages can be made at times even to genetic figures, but waiting to make the interpretation until the patient is not in the grip of the affect or impulse ("striking while the iron is cold") decreases the likelihood of anxiety generation (Pine 1984). One can also structure an interpretation by removing or reducing key elements in order to reduce the interpretation's potential to arouse anxiety or dysphoria.

Intellectualized interpretation. Intellectualized interpretation ignores specific dynamic referents, transferential aspects, and nonverbal communication and gives a rationale connecting phenomena about which the patient is already conscious. No connection is made to a purported unconscious fantasy or mechanism (Rockland 1989, p. 96).

Inexact interpretation. Inexact interpretation (Glover 1931) protects the fragile patient by offering an explanation about impulses or behavior that is plausible but not the whole truth about infantile fears. This is related to what Langs (1973) would call *interpretation upward*, in which, as a means of reducing anxiety and supporting ego function, the conflictual affect or impulse is tied to a more mature (and ego-syntonic) or triadic conflict rather than to the actual pre-oedipal, dyadic construct.

Patient: I'm so mad I want to make a fat hamburger out of him.
Therapist: It makes you angry that he asked her out when you wanted to see her—so you want your rival out of the way, so you can get the girl. [*Focuses the affect on rivalry; sidesteps exploring or interpreting primitive incorporative aspects of fantasy*]

Incomplete interpretation. Incomplete interpretation (Pinsker et al. 1991), an intervention formulated within the supportive psychotherapy frame, leaves out the genetic references in an interpretation and generalizes the subject in order to decrease the generation of anxiety while increasing the patient's awareness of avoided material.

Patient: They hold the meetings at inconvenient times, so I'm usually a few minutes late. My boss gets a little annoyed at waiting, but nothing comes of it.
Therapist: So, habitually coming a few minutes late to the meeting is a way for you to show people that you resent conforming to expected behavior that doesn't take your needs into account and that you can do things your way and exert some control. [*Makes a connection to the angry feeling, supports self-esteem, and contrasts the patient's behavior with a real-world expectation*]

Skills Building

The intention of skills building is to impart factual or procedural knowledge the patient can use to increase adaptive functioning.

Giving Advice

Giving advice is a mainstay of supportive psychotherapy. Within the context of "being like a good parent," advice is given when needed but is tempered against the patient's developmental needs. The therapist judges whether a patient needs to be told what to do (with an eye toward the behavior being learned), will benefit from being pointed in the direction of information, or can simply be reassured that they already have what is needed to make a decision. Advice needs to be specific and individualized and should come from the therapist's expertise in such areas as mental illness, adjustment, and reasonable living in society (Winston et al. 2020). Advice is usually not helpful when not asked for—as with most supportive interventions, advice that is perceived as not relevant to the patient's issues is not helpful, even if it is reasonable advice.

Teaching

Teaching is the imparting of information as an expert or as a wise, adaptive person. Moreover, teaching is the realm in which patients can be given principles that they may internalize so as to be able to make more adaptive judgments and decisions. Teaching principles tends to be a more powerful tactic than giving advice about a particular issue because principles are more easily generalized and used adaptively over time in different situations.

Therapist: The mind tends to lump unconnected problems together to make sense of chaos. The result is we fear a scary monster outside the house, when the truth is that it is the wind that is howling, it is the window shutter banging in the wind, and the lights are flickering because a tree fell on the power lines a few blocks away.

Providing Anticipatory Guidance

Rehearsing before the actual need to perform a task or decision allows the patient to consider what problems might arise and to come up with coping strategies in advance. In addition to building up the patient's behavioral repertoire, working through a task in advance can reduce performance-related or decisional anxiety.

Patient: When I'm in school, I get flustered about things I know don't really matter. I know it's about dealing with her. I end up clamming up or focusing on minutiae and not getting my ideas across.

Therapist: Who?

Patient: The school principal.

Therapist: So talking to her is anxiety provoking for you, and you find yourself getting upset over stuff you think is trivial. [*Clarifies*]

Patient: Yeah, I've never been good around powerful people, but I used what we talked about before—I go over what the play of the hand is going to be before I go into the meeting. I know better now what she's going to ask, and I rehearse my responses. Last meeting, I was OK, and I noticed that I didn't get all twisted up. I was still nervous, but not so much (*smiles*).

Therapist: So, because you rehearsed it, you were able to interact with the principal in a way that was more effective. The old adage "practice makes perfect" comes to mind. [*Clarifies and adds a confirmatory slogan*]

In sessions focused on an upcoming termination of treatment, anticipatory guidance can play a major role. The therapist, in addition to reviewing the accomplishments achieved, can use anticipatory guidance to outline issues for the patient to explore in the future. Further, because it is typical for patients to have a range of feelings about the end of treatment, and about the therapist after treatment, it is useful to help the patient anticipate how they will deal with these feelings.

Therapist: Later when you wish to talk about something, you might be angry at feeling cut off. What might you do?
Patient: Well, I wouldn't be able to talk it out with you.
Therapist: Not exactly, but when things come up, you can remember similar things that would come up in treatment and how we would deal with it then. [*Helps the patient model his own holding environment*]

Redirecting

Steering the patient away from painful affects through distraction is a strategy that the patient can learn to do. The therapist works with the patient to identify alternatives that are more adaptive when they are anxious or dysphoric. The patient's attention can be diverted to either increased activity (cleaning, distraction) or decreased activity (relaxation tape, good old memories). For example, a patient with a substance or behavioral addiction can learn to better tolerate episodes of craving through instituting distracting or differently rewarding activities. Remembering good things when things are bad adds perspective and may temper dysphoria or hopelessness.

Patient: Often when it's getting late, I feel sad and afraid, like I need to eat something to calm myself down. So I chow down comfort food from the pantry or the freezer. Now I'm gaining weight because of it.
Therapist: Maybe there are other things you can do that can help you cope with those feelings in a healthier way. You've spoken about how you are so busy with work and your other responsibilities you can't seem to get the time to get things put away and clean up.
Patient: What does that have to do with feeling bad and then eating too much?
Therapist: Perhaps rather than overeating, which you also feel bad about, you can distract yourself from the uncomfortable feelings by using that time to focus on putting things away and cleaning up.

Promoting Autonomy

Despite its supportive nature, the supportive therapeutic relationship is different from other supportive relationships (e.g., friendships) in that it should include a development of new skills or new ways of looking at problems. Pinsker (1997) compared the two, highlighting the therapy's goal of promoting autonomy, by stating, "To some extent, the supportive relationship is a crutch. Take it away and there is risk that the patient may fall. Supportive therapy has the objective of teaching the patient to walk alone" (p. 191).

Conclusion

Supportive psychotherapy has a long history and a wide platform of techniques with a broad range of applicability. It continues to change with advances in the field, and in this chapter we broaden the contextual technique of focusing on the real relationship to a more modern, relational orientation. As with other psychotherapy interventions, supportive techniques have an intrinsic logic but must have an appropriate rationale for being implemented. These techniques can be mastered over time with proper attention, supervision, and practice.

Key Points

- Supportive psychotherapy objectives of maintaining or increasing self-esteem, ego functioning, and adaptive skills are promoted through the use of contextual and tactical interventions.
- The main contextual techniques applicable in all treatments are the use of a conversational style; the maintenance of the frame of treatment, including the purposive establishment of a strong therapeutic alliance; relating to the developmental needs of the patient as would a good parent; and focusing generally on here-and-now relationships.
- Tactical techniques based on the content of current communication, patient characteristics and goals, and therapist objectives are therapist responses that address the therapeutic alliance or aim to bolster self-esteem, ego functioning, or adaptive skills.

Recommended Readings

Barber JP, Stratt R, Halperin G, et al: Supportive techniques: are they found in different therapies? J Psychother Pract Res 10(3):165–172, 2001 11402079

De Jonghe F, Rijnierse P, Janssen R: Psychoanalytic supportive psychotherapy. J Am Psychoanal Assoc 42(2):421–446, 1994 8040550

Hellerstein DJ, Pinsker H, Rosenthal RN, et al: Supportive therapy as the treatment model of choice. J Psychother Pract Res 3(4):300–306, 1994 22700197

Novalis PN, Rojcewicz SJ, Peele R: Clinical Manual of Supportive Psychotherapy. Washington, DC, American Psychiatric Press, 1993

Pinsker H: A Primer of Supportive Psychotherapy. Hillsdale, NJ, Analytic Press, 1997

Rosenthal RN: Group treatments for schizophrenic substance abusers, in The Group Psychotherapy of Substance Abuse. Edited by Brook DW, Spitz HI. New York, Haworth, 2002, pp 327–349

Winston A, Rosenthal RN, Muran JC: Supportive psychotherapy, in Handbook of Personality Disorders. Edited by Livesley WJ. New York, Guilford, 2001, pp 344–358

Winston A, Rosenthal RN, Roberts LR: Learning Supportive Psychotherapy: An Illustrated Guide, 2nd Edition. Washington, DC, American Psychiatric Association Publishing, 2020

References

Alexander F, French TM: Psychoanalytic Therapy: Principles and Application. New York, Ronald, 1946

Bandura A: Self-efficacy, in Encyclopedia of Human Behavior, Vol 4. Edited by Ramachaudran VS. New York, Academic Press, 1994, pp 71–81

Barber JP, Stratt R, Halperin G, et al: Supportive techniques: are they found in different therapies? J Psychother Pract Res 10(3):165–172, 2001 11402079

Bellak L: The schizophrenic syndrome: a further elaboration of the unified theory of schizophrenia, in Schizophrenia: A Review of the Syndrome. New York, Logos, 1958, pp 3–63

Beres D: Ego deviation and the concept of schizophrenia. Psychoanal Study Child 11:164–235, 1956

Bond M, Banon E, Grenier M: Differential effects of interventions on the therapeutic alliance with patients with personality disorders. J Psychother Pract Res 7(4):301–318, 1998 9752641
Bordin ES: The generalizability of the psychoanalytic concept of the working alliance. Psychotherapy (Chic) 16(3):252–260, 1979
Bretherton I: The origins of attachment theory: John Bowlby and Mary Ainsworth. Dev Psychol 28(5):759–775, 1992
de Figueiredo JM: Depression and demoralization: phenomenologic differences and research perspectives. Compr Psychiatry 34(5):308–311, 1993 8306640
Eubanks CF, Muran JC, Safran JD: Alliance rupture repair: a meta-analysis. Psychotherapy (Chic) 55(4):508–519, 2018 30335462
Flückiger C, Del Re AC, Wampold BE, et al: The alliance in adult psychotherapy: a meta-analytic synthesis. Psychotherapy (Chic) 55(4):316–340, 2018 29792475
Frank JD: Psychotherapy: the restoration of morale. Am J Psychiatry 131(3):271–274, 1974 4812687
Freud A: The Writings of Anna Freud, Vol 2, The Ego and the Mechanisms of Defense (1936). New York, International Universities Press, 1966
Gabbard GO: Long-Term Psychodynamic Psychotherapy: A Basic Text. Washington, DC, American Psychiatric Publishing, 2004
Gabbard GO: Psychodynamic Psychiatry in Clinical Practice, 4th Edition. Washington, DC, American Psychiatric Publishing, 2005
Glover E: The therapeutic effect of inexact interpretation: a contribution to the theory of suggestion. Int J Psychoanal 12:397–411, 1931
Hellerstein DJ, Rosenthal RN, Pinsker H, et al: A randomized prospective study comparing supportive and dynamic therapies: outcome and alliance. J Psychother Pract Res 7(4):261–271, 1998 9752637
Holmes J: Attachment theory in clinical practice: a personal account. Br J Psychother 31(2):1–20, 2015
Langs R: The Technique of Psychoanalytic Psychotherapy, Vol 1. New York, Jason Aronson, 1973
Leierer SJ, Strohmer DC, Leclere WA, et al: The effect of counselor disability, attending behavior, and client problem on counseling. Rehabil Couns Bull 40:82–93, 1996
Lyons-Ruth K; Members of the Change Process Study Group: Implicit relational knowing: its role in development and psychoanalytic treatment. Infant Ment Health J 19:282–289, 1998
Misch DA: Basic strategies of dynamic supportive therapy. J Psychother Pract Res 9(4):173–189, 2000 11069130
Muran JC: Confessions of a New York rupture researcher: an insider's guide and critique. Psychother Res 29(1):1–14, 2019 29254460
Muran JC, Eubanks CF: Therapist Performance Under Pressure: Negotiating Emotions, Difference, and Rupture. Washington, DC, American Psychological Association, 2020
Muran JC, Safran JD, Eubanks CF, et al: The effect of alliance-focused training on a cognitive-behavioral therapy for personality disorders. J Consult Clin Psychol 86(4):384–397, 2018 29648858
Novalis PN, Rojcewicz SJ, Peele R: Clinical Manual of Supportive Psychotherapy. Washington, DC, American Psychiatric Press, 1993
Pine F: The interpretive moment: variations on classical themes. Bull Menninger Clin 48(1):54–71, 1984 6692050
Pinsker H: A Primer of Supportive Psychotherapy. Hillsdale, NJ, Analytic Press, 1997
Pinsker H, Rosenthal RN: Beth Israel Medical Center Supportive Psychotherapy Manual, in Social and Behavioral Sciences Documents Abstracts, Vol 18, No 2, 2886. Washington, DC, American Psychological Association, 1988
Pinsker H, Rosenthal R, McCullough L: Dynamic supportive psychotherapy, in Handbook of Short-Term Dynamic Psychotherapy. Edited by Crits-Christoph P, Barber JP. New York, Basic Books, 1991, pp 220–247
Rockland LH: Supportive Therapy: A Psychodynamic Approach. New York, Basic Books, 1989
Rogers CR: The necessary and sufficient conditions of therapeutic personality change. J Consult Psychol 21(2):95–103, 1957 13416422

Rosenthal RN: Group treatments for schizophrenic substance abusers, in The Group Psychotherapy of Substance Abuse. Edited by Brook DW, Spitz HI. New York, Haworth Press, 2002, pp 327–349

Rosenthal RN, Muran JC, Pinsker H, et al: Interpersonal change in brief supportive psychotherapy. J Psychother Pract Res 8(1):55–63, 1999 9888107

Safran JD, Muran JC: Negotiating the Therapeutic Alliance: A Relational Treatment Guide. New York, Guilford, 2000

Toriello PJ, Strohmer DC: Addiction counselors' credibility: the impact of interactional style, recovery status, and nonverbal behavior. J Addict Offender Couns 25(1):43–57, 2004

Werman DS: Practice of Supportive Psychotherapy. Abingdon, UK, Routledge, 1984

Westen D, Gabbard GO: Developments in cognitive neuroscience II: implications for theories of transference. J Am Psychoanal Assoc 50(1):99–134, 2002 12018876

Winnicott DW: The theory of the parent-infant relationship. Int J Psychoanal 41:585–595, 1960 13785877

Winnicott DW: Playing and Reality. New York, Basic Books, 1971

Winston A, Pinsker H, McCullough L: A review of supportive psychotherapy. Hosp Community Psychiatry 37(11):1105–1114, 1986 3781499

Winston A, Rosenthal RN, Roberts LR: Learning Supportive Psychotherapy: An Illustrated Guide, 2nd Edition. Washington, DC, American Psychiatric Association Publishing, 2020

Yalom ID: The Theory and Practice of Group Psychotherapy, 4th Edition. New York, Basic Books, 1995

CHAPTER 18

Applications of Individual Supportive Psychotherapy to Specific Disorders

Efficacy and Indications

Arnold Winston, M.D.
Diana Punko, M.D., M.S.

Supportive psychotherapy, with its focus on a genuine, caring, and empathic patient-therapist relationship, has been increasingly recognized as a significant contributor to successful psychotherapy outcomes. It is likely that the supportive elements in all psychotherapies are the critical factors that produce positive patient change in psychotherapy. In fact in 1992, de Jonghe, Rijnierse, and Janssen identified the *support-experience factor* as one of two curative factors in classical psychoanalysis (its counterpart being the *interpretation-insight factor*):

> [A]dequate support given by the analyst and the resulting specific experience occurring in the analysand together contribute significantly to the power of psychoanalysis… [which] applies not only to treatment of severely disturbed patients by "modified psychoanalysis" or "psychoanalytically oriented psychotherapy," but is valid even for "ordinary analysis" in the treatment of "ordinary neurosis." Without minimizing the importance of the interpretation-insight factor, we contend that the support-experience factor is the mute and underestimated power of psychoanalysis; it is its "silent force." (de Jonghe et al. 1992, p. 476)

In this chapter we report on a number of clinical trials of supportive psychotherapy in the treatment of various disorders. Review of the efficacy and outcome research of supportive psychotherapy indicates that supportive treatment can be useful across a broad spectrum of psychiatric and medical conditions. In fact, it has even been described as the treatment model of choice for most people with mental illness (Hellerstein et al. 1994). Of note, many of the following studies included medication management ancillary to the experimental psychotherapy condition.

Menninger Psychotherapy Research Project

First described by Wallerstein et al. (1956), the Menninger Foundation's Psychotherapy Research Project was a naturalistic study comparing psychoanalysis versus expressive or exploratory psychotherapy versus supportive psychotherapy on measures of outcome and process over a period of an average of 2–3 years (and, in some cases, 30 years) of follow-up. The study population included 42 psychiatric inpatients with a wide range of disorders, including severe neuroses, addictions and sexual disorders, and narcissistic and borderline disorders. Numerous writings have been published on this project, but the major relevant findings were that all treatments, including psychoanalysis, became more supportive during the course of therapy and that noninterpretive, supportive mechanisms across all groups accounted for substantially more of the achieved changes than expected (Wallerstein 1989). Of note, this study did not include control subjects or random assignment of subjects, but the following more recent controlled trials provide better evidence on the efficacy of supportive psychotherapy for a number of specific indications.

Schizophrenia Spectrum and Other Psychotic Disorder Studies

Many psychosocial treatments (e.g., cognitive-behavioral therapy, social skills training, family therapy) are available for persons with schizophrenia, and no single treatment is considered to be definitive. When evaluating efficacy in this population, many target outcomes can be considered, including positive symptoms, negative symptoms, neurocognitive deficits, and global functioning. Most studies suffer from methodological issues: participant withdrawal or attrition, lack of fidelity to treatment condition, inconsistency in skill and technique of therapists, confounding by alcohol or drug misuse, and using supportive psychotherapy as a comparator rather than the main treatment arm. The best evidence for the use of individual supportive psychotherapy in schizophrenia follows.

The first major well-designed trial on effects of psychotherapy in schizophrenia came from a National Institute of Mental Health multisite study comparing exploratory, insight-oriented psychotherapy versus reality-adaptive, supportive psychotherapy over 2 years (Gunderson et al. 1984; Stanton et al. 1984). The results overall showed minimal outcome differences between the two groups aside from clear positive effects on recidivism and role performance for supportive psychotherapy compared with the insight-oriented approach. This result is especially impressive given that the insight-oriented psychotherapy met thrice weekly, whereas the supportive psychotherapy met only once weekly. This study produced similar results to those of the Menninger Psychotherapy Research Project (which excluded participants with "open psychoses") in that the exploratory, insight-oriented psychotherapy contained major supportive elements, and thus the two treatments were not as distinct as had been intended.

It should be noted that most modern psychotherapy efficacy studies in schizophrenia involve participants who are concomitantly receiving antipsychotic medications in addition to the experimental or control psychotherapy condition. The Danish National Schizophrenia Project was a prospective, comparative, longitudinal naturalistic treatment study of psychosocial interventions in first-episode psychosis (Rosenbaum et al. 2005). Patients were allocated to treatment as usual (TAU); individual and/or group supportive psychodynamic psychotherapy as a supplement to TAU; or an integrated, assertive psychosocial and educational 2-year treatment program. Compared with the TAU group, both experimental conditions showed a nonsignificant tendency toward greater improvement in social functioning. A more recent prospective, comparative, longitudinal multisite study of consecutively referred patients offered a contemporary supportive psychodynamic psychotherapy for up to 3 years as a supplement to standard treatment or standard treatment alone (Rosenbaum et al. 2012). The intervention group improved significantly on social functioning, overall symptomatology, and positive psychotic symptoms during the period of active intervention and at the 2-year follow-up. However, the improvement found was not sustained at a subsequent 5-year follow-up, during which time standard treatment continued for both groups (Harder et al. 2014). This likely reflects the chronicity of the symptomatology and deficits seen in schizophrenia and the resulting need for long-term (perhaps even lifelong) treatment.

Multiple studies have evaluated the efficacy of family therapy in schizophrenia. Rea et al. (1991) found that in comparing individual supportive psychotherapy to family therapy for 33 randomly assigned patients with schizophrenia who resided, or had daily contact, with one or both biological parents, both treatment groups demonstrated a systematic change toward a more neutral coping style with relatives after 3 months of treatment. Interestingly, but perhaps unsurprisingly, psychotherapy efficacy outcomes can be tied to residential status. Hogarty et al. (1997) compared personal therapy (described as a definitive psychosocial intervention designed to forestall late relapse in patients with schizophrenia) versus family therapy versus supportive therapy on measures of psychotic relapse in schizophrenic patients. In patients living with family, personal therapy showed benefit over family and supportive therapies; however, in patients living independently, those who received personal therapy had significantly more psychotic decompensations than did those who received supportive therapy. This differential response may reflect lack of stability or a containing environment for schizophrenic patients living independently relative to those living with family.

Other alternative forms of psychotherapy, such as social skills training, show benefit in independent living skills and everyday community functioning for individuals with schizophrenia (Glynn et al. 2002; Liberman et al. 1998), although few direct comparisons to supportive psychotherapy are available. Marder et al. (1996) compared social skills training and supportive group psychotherapy for outpatients with schizophrenia over a 2-year period and found that social skills training resulted in greater improvement in certain measures of social adjustment (Marder et al. 1996). It is important to note that this was group therapy, not individual supportive psychotherapy, and that difference may have had an impact on the efficacy of the intervention. Hogarty et al. (2004) studied the benefits of cognitive enhancement therapy for schizophrenia relative to control comparator enriched supportive psychotherapy and found that both treatment groups demonstrated improvements, suggesting that supportive psychotherapy can also have positive effects on cognitive deficits (Hogarty et al. 2004).

In a Cochrane review on supportive therapy for schizophrenia, Buckley et al. (2015) concluded that insufficient data exist to identify a difference in outcome between supportive therapy and standard care and that the available evidence suggesting that other psychological therapies are superior to supportive therapy is rated as very low quality. However, it is noted that this review defined the scope of supportive therapy as "any intervention from a single person aimed at maintaining a person's existing situation or assisting in people's coping abilities" (Buckley et al. 2015, p. 2) and included such interventions as "befriending" and peer social support as opposed to the individual supportive psychotherapy that requires a trained therapist and is the focus of this chapter.

In addition to benefiting patients with diagnosed schizophrenia, supportive psychotherapy may carry benefit for individuals who are prepsychotic. McGorry et al. (2013) provided evidence that supportive psychotherapy may be considered an effective and less risky intervention than antipsychotic medication for preventing transition to psychosis in individuals at ultrahigh risk of psychosis.

Overall, these results indicate that supportive psychotherapy is both applicable to and beneficial for individuals with schizophrenia and related psychotic disorders. The supportive modality is conducive to incorporating additional psychosocial therapies such as skills training and vocational therapy that are particularly useful in schizophrenia. More research is clearly needed to fully elucidate the ideal frequency and duration of supportive psychotherapy for optimal sustained long-term outcomes as well as its role in other psychotic disorders such as schizoaffective disorder and delusional disorder.

Depressive Disorder Studies

In the National Institute of Mental Health Treatment of Depression Collaborative Research Program, two psychotherapies (cognitive-behavioral therapy [CBT] and interpersonal psychotherapy [IPT]) were compared with an antidepressant (imipramine) clinical management condition and a control condition consisting of drug placebo and clinical management (Elkin 1994; Elkin et al. 1989; Imber et al. 1990). The clinical management was a low-level supportive psychotherapy approach. The two psychotherapies were found to be efficacious but not significantly different from the placebo–clinical management condition on measures of depressive symptoms and overall functioning. In other words, the low-level supportive psychotherapy was just as effective as cognitive-behavioral and interpersonal psychotherapies.

Thompson and Gallagher (1985) studied 30 outpatients ranging in age from 60 to 81 years. Patients were randomly assigned to a 16-week treatment with cognitive therapy, behavioral treatment, or supportive psychotherapy. Improvement was similar across the three treatment conditions at termination, but at 1-year follow-up, more of the patients in the supportive psychotherapy group received a diagnosis of depression. Unfortunately, the small number of patients in each treatment group and the type of supportive psychotherapy used make these findings of limited value.

In a randomized clinical trial involving 100 adolescents with depression, Renaud et al. (1998) compared cognitive, family, and supportive psychotherapies and found that rapid responders to therapy had better outcomes at 1-year follow-up and better scores on some measures at 2-year follow-up. The investigators concluded that their findings suggest that patients with milder forms of depression may benefit from initial supportive psychotherapy or short trials of more specialized types of psychotherapy.

Maina et al. (2005) completed a randomized controlled trial comparing brief dynamic psychotherapy with supportive psychotherapy in treating patients with minor depressive disorder. Both psychotherapies resulted in significant improvement in comparison with untreated control subjects, but brief dynamic psychotherapy was found to be more effective at follow-up evaluation.

Kocsis et al. (2009) compared a cognitive-behavioral analysis system of psychotherapy with brief supportive psychotherapy (BSP) in their ability to augment treatment for patients with chronic depression who did not respond to antidepressant treatment. Although 37.5% of subjects experienced partial response or remission, neither form of adjunctive psychotherapy improved outcome as much as did a flexible, individualized pharmacotherapy regimen alone.

In a study comparing supportive psychotherapy and CBT for treatment of depression following traumatic brain injury, Ashman et al. (2014) found that both forms of psychotherapy were efficacious in improving diagnoses of depression and anxiety and reducing depressive symptoms.

In a study of mothers with major depressive disorder, Swartz et al. (2016) randomly assigned patients to nine sessions of either brief IPT or BSP. Both treatments demonstrated comparable beneficial effects on maternal depression. Of note is the finding that improvement in mothers' depressive symptoms was associated with improvement in child functioning 3–6 months after the mothers improved.

Tompson et al. (2017) performed a study of 134 children with depression with a mean age of 11 years. The children were treated with either family-focused treatment or individual supportive psychotherapy. Results indicated that both treatments demonstrated high rates of adequate clinical depression response, but family-focused treatment had a higher rate of response.

Schramm et al. (2017) found that a specific form of cognitive-behavioral analysis system of psychotherapy (CBASP) for chronic depression had somewhat better outcome results than a nonspecific supportive psychotherapy. However, both forms of psychotherapy produced good results, and the supportive psychotherapy was not specific for depression. In a 2-year follow-up of this study, Schramm et al. found that after 1 year, CBASP had significantly more remission rates, but by the second year, CBASP lost its superiority over supportive psychotherapy (Schramm et al. 2019).

The results of these studies suggest that psychotherapy is applicable in most depressive disorders, with the possible exception of chronic depression. Additionally, there is evidence (Parikh et al. 2019) that mild depression can be treated with either psychotherapy or medication, whereas severe depression should be treated with antidepressant medication. However, combined treatment with both medication and psychotherapy can often provide a better outcome. In addition, treatment professionals should discuss treatment effects, adverse effect profiles, cost, accessibility, and preferences with the patient (Qaseem et al. 2016). Finally, it should be noted that cognitive-behavioral techniques for depression can be incorporated easily into supportive psychotherapy, especially cognitive approaches such as eliciting and testing negative cognitions (i.e., automatic thoughts) (Winston and Winston 2002).

Anxiety Disorder Studies

CBT has been well established in the effective treatment of anxiety disorders across the diagnostic category; however, as the studies in this section indicate, there is a clear role for supportive psychotherapy as well. Supportive psychotherapy can incorporate CBT principles while adding an empathic approach to reliably achieve anxiety remission. In addition, supportive psychotherapy tends to be more accessible in the community than other specialized therapies such as CBT. This is based on the finding that individuals with anxiety disorders report more often receiving nonspecific treatments, such as supportive psychotherapy, rather than CBT (Stein et al. 2004).

Specific Phobias

Zitrin et al. (1978) randomly assigned 111 participants with phobias to one of three treatment modalities: behavioral therapy plus imipramine, behavioral therapy plus placebo, and supportive therapy plus imipramine. The participants were divided into three groups depending on the features of their phobias—agoraphobia, simple phobia, and mixed phobia (having characteristics of both)—and were treated with 26 weekly sessions of their assigned condition. In contrast to the authors' expectations, behavioral therapy failed to show any benefit over supportive psychotherapy for any of the diagnostic groups. Interestingly, the behavioral therapy intervention included supportive therapy as part of treatment sessions, suggesting that the supportive element may in fact be the active ingredient.

The same group published results of a similar study 5 years later (Klein et al. 1983). In this study, systematic hierarchical desensitization was compared with nondirective supportive psychotherapy in a 26-week treatment trial involving patients classified into the three phobia categories described above. They found essentially no difference in effectiveness and attributed the finding not to the inefficacy of the behavioral intervention but rather to the efficacy of the supportive intervention. The authors identified some common elements between the two interventions, including the psychotherapeutic relationship, persuasiveness, and generation of hopeful expectancies, that may account for the improvement. Similarly, a large project on evaluation of psychotherapy in phobic disorders in Sweden showed that psychodynamically oriented supportive therapy and therapist-directed prolonged exposure in vivo were equally effective for the treatment of women with agoraphobia who were deemed not suitable for dynamic insight-oriented psychotherapy (Alström et al. 1984a). In fact, by the end of the 9-month follow-up period, supportive therapy showed superiority over all treatments tested.

Social Anxiety Disorder (Social Phobia)

Another study from the Swedish research project found different results when testing the same interventions in patients with social phobia who were deemed not suitable for dynamic insight-oriented psychotherapy (Alström et al. 1984b). Supportive psychotherapy was associated with improvement in several respects but to a lesser degree than with prolonged exposure. The authors postulated that the discrepancy may be because circumscribed phobias (as opposed to the more general agoraphobia) are better treated with behavioral therapies.

More recent studies have shown mixed results for social anxiety disorder. In a randomized controlled trial evaluating two psychotherapies administered over 14 weekly sessions for the treatment of 70 patients with social anxiety disorder, improvement with IPT (the experimental condition) was not superior to that with supportive psychotherapy (Lipsitz et al. 2008). Both treatments produced improvement in many patients; however, IPT did not provide greater benefit than supportive psychotherapy as was hypothesized by the authors.

Panic Disorder

Shear et al. (1994) compared 15 weekly sessions of CBT versus a nonprescriptive treatment similar to supportive psychotherapy for the treatment of 65 subjects with panic disorder. Contrary to the authors' predictions, both treatment groups showed improvement in symptoms, raising questions about the necessity of using CBT techniques for the relief of symptoms of panic disorder. In a subsequent replication and expansion study, Shear et al. (2001) used emotion-focused psychotherapy, a form of supportive psychotherapy, as the active comparator for treatment of 112 participants with panic disorder in addition to imipramine and placebo treatment groups. The results showed that emotion-focused psychotherapy had low efficacy for the treatment of panic disorder, with responses similar to those found in the placebo group.

In a Cochrane network meta-analysis on psychological therapies for panic disorder with or without agoraphobia in adults (Pompoli et al. 2016), nonspecific supportive psychotherapy was found to be noninferior relative to eight different forms of psychological therapy and three forms of a control condition. However, the authors stated that the results should be interpreted cautiously because of the sparsity of evidence regarding this treatment.

Together, these studies suggest that nonspecific factors may play a more important role than expected in the treatment of panic disorder. Available evidence indicates that for treatment of anxiety disorders, supportive psychotherapy may be especially effective in panic disorder and agoraphobia. Supportive psychotherapy easily lends itself to an integrative psychotherapy approach and can incorporate elements of exposure therapy and cognitive restructuring along with anxiety-reducing techniques of progressive muscle relaxation and meditation.

It is important to note that no studies are available showing efficacy of supportive psychotherapy in the treatment of obsessive-compulsive disorder (OCD), which is now classified in the diagnostic class obsessive-compulsive and related disorders in the *Diagnostic and Statistical Manual of Mental Disorders*, 5th Edition (DSM-5; American Psychiatric Association 2013). OCD in general does not respond to therapy alone and requires medication management (typically with high-dose selective serotonin reuptake inhibitors) for adequate treatment.

Trauma- and Stressor-Related Disorder Studies

Previously classified as an anxiety disorder in DSM-IV-TR (American Psychiatric Association 2000), posttraumatic stress disorder (PTSD) is now classified as a trauma- and stressor-related disorder in DSM-5. Bryant et al. (1999) tested the efficacy of CBT versus supportive counseling techniques to prevent development of PTSD among 45 civilian trauma survivors with acute stress disorder who were randomly assigned to treatment. The study revealed that prolonged exposure, with or without anxiety management, was superior to supportive counseling in reducing intensity of symptoms and preventing PTSD. A systematic review and meta-analysis by Cusack et al. (2016) assessed the comparative efficacy of a number of therapies used for the treatment of PTSD and found that exposure therapy had the greatest strength of evidence for effectiveness (Cusack et al. 2016). Similarly, Lee et al. (2016) conducted a systematic review and meta-analysis comparing various forms of psychotherapy versus pharmacotherapy for PTSD. They found that trauma-focused psychotherapy (including trauma-focused CBT, eye movement desensitization and reprocessing, prolonged exposure, cognitive processing therapy, and imaginal exposure) was superior to medication management and to the other psychotherapies. In this study, supportive psychotherapy was considered to be an active control condition. Future PTSD psychotherapy studies incorporating effects of demographic variables or trauma type on treatment efficacy would be useful for targeting specific populations.

Although studies show that trauma-focused psychological treatment is most effective for PTSD, there are certain situations for which supportive psychotherapy may prove to be more appropriate. These include when trauma-focused psychotherapy may induce retraumatization in susceptible patients or practical considerations such as the lack of broad availability of the treatment. In addition, supportive psychotherapy can easily incorporate exposure therapy as part of the supportive psychotherapy approach (Winston et al. 2020).

Personality Disorder Studies

In a study comparing supportive with interpretive psychotherapy, Piper et al. (1998) found no outcome differences between the two treatments. Patients presented with anxiety or depressive disorders, and 60.4% of subjects had a comorbid personality disorder. Hellerstein et al. (1998) compared BSP with short-term dynamic psychotherapy in treating patients with primarily Cluster C and not-otherwise-specified personality disorders, as well as comorbid disorders such as depression and anxiety disorders. The authors reported positive changes on measures of symptomatology, presenting complaints, and interpersonal functioning with both psychotherapies. These changes were found not only at termination but also at 6-month follow-up. In substudies of the Hellerstein et al. study, the authors used the Inventory of Interpersonal Problems mapped to an interpersonal circumplex model and graphically demonstrated lasting positive change in interpersonal functioning in the subjects treated with supportive psychotherapy (Rosenthal et al. 1999; Winston et al. 2001).

Clarkin et al. (2007) compared transference-focused psychotherapy, dialectical behavior therapy, and supportive psychotherapy in patients with borderline personality disorder and found significant positive changes in multiple domains after 1 year of treatment with all three psychotherapies. They suggested that these structured treatments for borderline personality disorder are generally equivalent with respect to broad positive change in these patients. Jørgensen et al. (2013) compared mentalization-based psychotherapy with supportive psychotherapy in patients with borderline personality disorder and found significant positive changes in both treatment groups on general functioning, depression, and social functioning.

Two meta-analyses on the effectiveness of psychotherapy for personality disorder have been conducted. The first one, by Perry et al. (1999), included 15 studies consisting of psychodynamic interpersonal, cognitive-behavioral, mixed, and supportive psychotherapies. All studies demonstrated improvement in personality disorders with psychotherapy, and psychotherapy may be associated with up to a sevenfold faster rate of recovery in comparison with the natural history of these disorders. The second study by Bateman and Fonagy (2000), found overall evidence for the effectiveness of psychotherapy for personality disorders. However, this study had problems with case identification, comorbidity, randomization, specificity of treatment, and outcomes measures. Evidence from both meta-analyses did not suggest the superiority of one type of psychotherapy over another.

Eating Disorder Studies

Although specialized treatments such as CBT and IPT tend to be more effective than supportive psychotherapy on primary eating disorder outcome measures in the treatment of bulimia nervosa, comparison studies have shown noninferiority or superiority of supportive psychotherapy on secondary outcome measures such as mood symptoms (e.g., Walsh et al. 1997). In an evaluation of the efficacy of family-based treatment compared with supportive psychotherapy for adolescent bulimia nervosa (le Grange et al. 2007), family-based treatment was found to have a clinical and statistical benefit over supportive psychotherapy on eating disorder symptomatology, but no differences were found between groups in self-esteem and depression.

In contrast, studies show better efficacy of supportive psychotherapy on primary outcome measures in the treatment of anorexia nervosa. Originally designed as a control treatment, specialist supportive clinical management (SSCM) for anorexia nervosa combines features of clinical management and supportive psychotherapy, including education, care, support, fostering of a therapeutic relationship, praise, reassurance, and advice. McIntosh et al. (2005) found that, contrary to their original hypothesis, SSCM was superior to specialized psychotherapies (i.e., CBT and IPT) in a randomized controlled trial comparing treatments for anorexia nervosa. In a study examining long-term efficacy, with a mean follow-up of 6.7 years, Carter et al. (2011) found no significant differences on outcome measures among the three aforementioned psychotherapies, although supportive psychotherapy was associated with a more rapid response than was IPT.

Since this study, additional specialized psychotherapies have been developed. The Maudsley Model of Anorexia Nervosa Treatment for Adults (MANTRA) targets factors specific to the cognitive-interpersonal theory of the maintenance of anorexia nervosa. Two randomized controlled trials comparing MANTRA with SSCM showed that MANTRA was no more effective than SSCM in terms of eating disorder and other outcomes (Schmidt et al. 2012, 2015). CBT-E is an enhanced form of CBT that has been adapted to treat eating disorders across the diagnostic class (i.e., bulimia nervosa, binge-eating disorder, and anorexia nervosa). A multicenter randomized controlled trial of SSCM, MANTRA, and CBT-E for 120 individuals with anorexia nervosa found no significant differences in weight gain or eating disorder psychopathology between treatment groups (Byrne et al. 2017). All treatment conditions resulted in clinically significant improvements in body mass index and other measures that were well maintained over 12-month follow-up.

Although SSCM was originally designed as a control treatment, it is now considered to be a valuable first-line intervention for adults with anorexia nervosa and has practical advantages over specialized treatments in terms of costs and availability. Regardless of treatment condition, overall recovery and remission rates in these eating disorder treatment studies tended to be poor, ranging from only about one-third to one-half of participants, indicating that more progress needs to be made. Disappointingly, a novel treatment approach targeting disturbances in self-concept called the identity intervention program, which sounded promising, was no more effective than supportive psychotherapy in reducing eating disorder symptoms (Stein et al. 2013).

Medical Disorder Studies

Few controlled studies of the efficacy of supportive psychotherapy in the ancillary treatment of medical conditions have been conducted. Mumford et al. (1982) found increased compliance and speed of recovery and fewer complications and hospital days in patients recovering from myocardial infarction and surgical procedures when they received supportive psychotherapy as opposed to patients who did not receive supportive psychotherapy.

Sjödin et al. (1986) randomly assigned 103 outpatients with chronic peptic ulcer disease to receive either medical treatment only or the same medical treatment plus supportive psychotherapy. Follow-up indicated significant positive differences in favor of those assigned to medical treatment plus supportive psychotherapy.

A study by Mukherjee et al. (2017) found that cancer patients receiving chemotherapy for recurrent disease often report the presence of anxiety and depression. On the basis of this finding, they decided to investigate the use of supportive psychotherapy in 40 such patients. They found that supportive psychotherapy helps to reduce levels of anxiety and depression and increase quality of life.

Rutledge et al. (2018) studied 66 patients with chronic back pain. Fifty of the 66 patients completed the 8 weeks of treatment, which consisted of either CBT or supportive psychotherapy conducted by telephone. Both treatments produced reductions in pain severity and back disability but did not differ in overall outcome.

Blanco et al. (2019) conducted a randomized trial of IPT problem-solving therapy, and supportive psychotherapy for major depressive disorder in women with breast cancer. They found that among patients who completed treatment, all three psychotherapies were associated with meaningful improvements in depression.

The results of these studies of patients with medical disorders treated with supportive psychotherapy suggest that supportive psychotherapy can enhance medical treatments as well as reduce psychiatric symptoms such as anxiety and depression and improve quality of life. Of interest is the number of findings reported by many studies indicating that different therapies produce similar outcome results.

Other Disorders: Body Dysmorphic Disorder

A study by Wilhelm et al. (2019) compared CBT with supportive psychotherapy for treatment of body dysmorphic disorder. CBT was enhanced with psychoeducation, case formulation, setting valued goals, motivational enhancement, cognitive restructuring, exposure and ritual prevention, mindfulness advice, and attentional retraining. Additional enhancements included advanced strategies to modify self-defeating assumptions about the importance of appearance and to enhance self-acceptance, self-esteem, and self-compassion. All patients in CBT received relapse prevention in the final two sessions. Supportive psychotherapy focused on improving self-esteem and adaptive coping skills while emphasizing the therapeutic relationship. Supportive psychotherapy was enhanced with body dysmorphic disorder–specific psychoeducation and treatment rationale. The two sites used for this study produced somewhat different results. At one site both psychotherapies produced consistent improvement in symptom severity and quality of life, whereas at the other site improvement in symptom severity was better with CBT. However, it should be noted that CBT was greatly enhanced compared with supportive psychotherapy.

Substance Use Disorder Studies

In the National Institute on Drug Abuse Collaborative Cocaine Treatment Study, a large multisite psychotherapy clinical trial for outpatients who met DSM-IV criteria for cocaine dependence (American Psychiatric Association 1994), Crits-Christoph et al. (1997, 1999) compared four treatment groups: 1) individual drug counseling (IDC) plus group drug counseling (GDC), 2) cognitive therapy plus GDC, 3) supportive-expressive (SE) psychodynamic psychotherapy plus GDC, and 4) GDC alone. All groups showed substantial reductions in cocaine use, but patients receiving IDC and GDC had the best results. In a more recent article, the researchers took a closer look at the SE condition (Crits-Christoph et al. 2018). For patients who achieved abstinence earlier in treatment, SE produced comparable drug use outcomes to those of IDC. Additionally, the researchers found evidence that SE was superior to IDC on change in family or social problems at the 12-month follow-up assessment.

A 2008 pilot study of IPT versus BSP for dysthymic disorder and alcohol abuse revealed that although IPT was superior on depression, BSP was more effective on percentage of days abstinent from alcohol (Markowitz et al. 2008). In a Cochrane review of psychological interventions for co-occurring depression and substance use disorders, which cited the Markowitz study among others, Hides et al. (2019) concluded that in terms of differences between psychotherapies, although some significant effects were found, the effects were too inconsistent and small, and the evidence of too poor quality, to be of relevance to practice.

Indications and Applications

Common Factors

As described in the previous sections, most psychotherapy studies indicate that supportive psychotherapy has positive outcomes with virtually all psychiatric disorders. In addition, these studies report similar results when comparing different psychotherapies. Luborsky et al. (1975) have called these similar results the Dodo bird effect or verdict. This refers to Lewis Carroll's *Alice's Adventures in Wonderland* (Carroll 1865), in which, after a race, the Dodo bird proclaims, "*Everybody* has won, and all must have prizes." In his landmark paper, Rosenzweig (1936) used the Dodo bird verdict to explore the common factors present in all forms of psychotherapy.

Many papers and books (e.g., Frank and Frank 1991) have been written about the common factors, which include the relational aspects of psychotherapy (therapeutic alliance), considered the most important common factor. The therapeutic alliance includes the bond between therapist and patient and agreement on the goals and procedures of the psychotherapy. Additionally, other common factors are expectation of help, a rationale or conceptual scheme that explains the given symptoms and prescribes a given ritual or procedure for resolving them, the active participation of both patient and therapist in carrying out that ritual or procedure, and promoting mastery over the patient's problems or symptoms.

Supportive psychotherapy clearly promotes and uses all the common factors, which makes it appropriate to use for almost all psychiatric disorders. For highly pathological disorders, supportive psychotherapy is generally combined with medication. These disorders include schizophrenia and other psychotic disorders, bipolar spectrum disorders, moderate to severe depression, anxiety disorders such as panic disorder, PTSD, and borderline personality disorder.

Severe Mental Illness, Personality Disorders, and Substance Use Disorders

Supportive psychotherapy is particularly useful for severe mental illness as described earlier in this chapter in the section "Schizophrenia Spectrum and Other Psychotic Disorder Studies." It improves deficient ego functions, reduces anxiety, and prevents downward social drift due to loss of adaptive skills and increasing isolation. It can be easily combined with social skills training and family psychoeducation (Liberman et al. 1998; Vaughn and Leff 1976).

Individuals with personality disorders, especially those who are extremely angry, demanding, suspicious, or overly dependent, can be particularly difficult to treat (Horowitz and Marmar 1985). Therapists treating patients with personality disorders must be able to deal with strong countertransference issues to avoid reacting in a negative manner. That being said, most patients with personality disorders can be treated successfully with supportive psychotherapy (Hellerstein et al. 1998), with the possible exception of patients with antisocial personality disorder. These patients tend to be highly manipulative, are often untruthful, and deny problems, which makes them very difficult to treat. However, if they have comorbid depression and are suffering, they may become amenable to psychotherapy.

In individuals with substance use disorders, supportive psychotherapy can be quite helpful in developing effective coping strategies to control or reduce substance use. In addition, therapists can use supportive psychotherapy to prevent relapse by working with the patient to avoid high-risk situations and to manage anxiety and dysphoria (Rosenthal and Westreich 1999; Winston et al. 2020). Supportive psychotherapy's focus on the development of a positive and active therapeutic alliance helps to maintain the patient in psychotherapy and to focus on problematic issues.

Motivational interviewing (Rollnick and Miller 1995) can be a useful addition to supportive psychotherapy for patients with substance use disorder. It is a directive, patient-centered intervention that helps patients to explore and resolve their ambivalence about changing. The main principles of motivational interviewing include understanding the patient's view accurately, avoiding and de-escalating resistance, and increasing the patient's self-efficacy and perception of the discrepancy between actual and ideal behavior. The respectful, collaborative, and empathic style of both motivational interviewing and supportive psychotherapy supports the development of a positive and healthy relationship that can reinforce reduction or cessation of substance use (Miller and Rose 2010).

Finally, it should be noted that patients with severe dementia or delirium are not amenable to supportive psychotherapy or, for that matter, any psychotherapy.

Conclusion

The outcome studies and clinical reports suggest that supportive psychotherapy can be useful for a wide variety of psychiatric disorders as well as medical disorders. The theoretical basis and techniques of supportive psychotherapy have been well described in Chapter 16 ("Theory of Individual Supportive Psychotherapy") and Chapter 17 ("Techniques of Individual Supportive Psychotherapy") and are central in producing successful outcomes. The primary factor in helping patients to improve in all psychotherapies is the patient-therapist alliance, which has been shown to be the best predictor of a successful psychotherapy (Horvath and Symonds 1991). Supportive psychotherapy therapists consistently strive to maintain a positive alliance based on the therapist's empathic-introspective stance and to repair ruptures in the alliance through the use of supportive interventions.

Key Points

- Outcome studies of the efficacy of supportive psychotherapy indicate that it is an effective treatment for virtually all psychiatric disorders. Additional outcome studies are needed to better define the indications and essential elements of supportive psychotherapy.
- Supportive psychotherapy is a useful treatment for psychosis, depression and anxiety disorders, personality disorders, substance use disorders, and medical disorders.

- Maintaining and enhancing the therapeutic alliance through the therapist's use of an empathic-introspective stance, as well as the appropriate employment of the wide variety of supportive techniques, helps to produce positive outcomes.

References

Alström JE, Nordlund CL, Persson G, et al: Effects of four treatment methods on agoraphobic women not suitable for insight-oriented psychotherapy. Acta Psychiatr Scand 70(1):1–17, 1984a 6147066

Alström JE, Nordlund CL, Persson G, et al: Effects of four treatment methods on social phobic patients not suitable for insight-oriented psychotherapy. Acta Psychiatr Scand 70(2):97–110, 1984b 6148843

American Psychiatric Association: Diagnostic and Statistical Manual of Mental Disorders, 4th Edition. Washington, DC, American Psychiatric Association, 1994

American Psychiatric Association: Diagnostic and Statistical Manual of Mental Disorders, 4th Edition, Text Revision. Washington, DC, American Psychiatric Association, 2000

American Psychiatric Association: Diagnostic and Statistical Manual of Mental Disorders, 5th Edition. Arlington, VA, American Psychiatric Association, 2013

Ashman T, Cantor JB, Tsaousides T, et al: Comparison of cognitive behavioral therapy and supportive psychotherapy for the treatment of depression following traumatic brain injury: a randomized controlled trial. J Head Trauma Rehabil 29(6):467–478, 2014 25370439

Bateman AW, Fonagy P: Effectiveness of psychotherapeutic treatment of personality disorder. Br J Psychiatry 177:138–143, 2000 11026953

Blanco C, Markowitz JC, Hellerstein DJ, et al: A randomized trial of interpersonal psychotherapy, problem solving therapy, and supportive therapy for major depressive disorder in women with breast cancer. Breast Cancer Res Treat 173(2):353–364, 2019 30343455

Bryant RA, Sackville T, Dang ST, et al: Treating acute stress disorder: an evaluation of cognitive behavior therapy and supportive counseling techniques. Am J Psychiatry 156(11):1780–1786, 1999 10553743

Buckley LA, Maayan N, Soares-Weiser K, et al: Supportive therapy for schizophrenia. Cochrane Database Syst Rev (4):CD004716, 2015 25871462

Byrne S, Wade T, Hay P, et al: A randomised controlled trial of three psychological treatments for anorexia nervosa. Psychol Med 47(16):2823–2833, 2017 28552083

Carroll L: Alice's Adventures in Wonderland. London, Macmillan, 1865

Carter FA, Jordan J, McIntosh VVW, et al: The long-term efficacy of three psychotherapies for anorexia nervosa: a randomized, controlled trial. Int J Eat Disord 44(7):647–654, 2011 21997429

Clarkin JF, Levy KN, Lenzenweger MF, et al: Evaluating three treatments for borderline personality disorder: a multiwave study. Am J Psychiatry 164(6):922–928, 2007 17541052

Crits-Christoph P, Siqueland L, Blaine J, et al: The National Institute on Drug Abuse Collaborative Cocaine Treatment Study: rationale and methods. Arch Gen Psychiatry 54(8):721–726, 1997 9283507

Crits-Christoph P, Siqueland L, Blaine J, et al: Psychosocial treatments for cocaine dependence: National Institute on Drug Abuse Collaborative Cocaine Treatment Study. Arch Gen Psychiatry 56(6):493–502, 1999 10359461

Crits-Christoph P, Wadden S, Gaines A, et al: Symptoms of anhedonia, not depression, predict the outcome of treatment of cocaine dependence. J Subst Abuse Treat 92:46–50, 2018 30032944

Cusack K, Jonas DE, Forneris CA, et al: Psychological treatments for adults with posttraumatic stress disorder: a systematic review and meta-analysis. Clin Psychol Rev 43:128–141, 2016 26574151

de Jonghe F, Rijnierse P, Janissen R: The role of support in psychoanalysis. J Am Psychoanal Assoc 40(2):475–499, 1992 1593081

Elkin I: The NIMH Treatment of Depression Collaborative Research Program: where we began and where we are, in Handbook of Psychotherapy and Behavior Change, 4th Edition. Oxford, UK, Wiley, 1994, pp 114–139

Elkin I, Shea MT, Watkins JT, et al: National Institute of Mental Health Treatment of Depression Collaborative Research Program: general effectiveness of treatments. Arch Gen Psychiatry 46(11):971–982, discussion 983, 1989 2684085

Frank JB, Frank JD: Persuasion and Healing: A Comparative Study of Psychotherapy, 3rd Edition. Baltimore, MD, Johns Hopkins University Press, 1991

Glynn SM, Marder SR, Liberman RP, et al: Supplementing clinic-based skills training with manual-based community support sessions: effects on social adjustment of patients with schizophrenia. Am J Psychiatry 159(5):829–837, 2002 11986138

Gunderson JG, Frank AF, Katz HM, et al: Effects of psychotherapy in schizophrenia II: comparative outcome of two forms of treatment. Schizophr Bull 10(4):564–598, 1984 6151246

Harder S, Koester A, Valbak K, et al: Five-year follow-up of supportive psychodynamic psychotherapy in first-episode psychosis: long-term outcome in social functioning. Psychiatry 77(2):155–168, 2014 24865198

Hellerstein DJ, Pinsker H, Rosenthal RN, et al: Supportive therapy as the treatment model of choice. J Psychother Pract Res 3(4):300–306, 1994 22700197

Hellerstein DJ, Rosenthal RN, Pinsker H, et al: A randomized prospective study comparing supportive and dynamic therapies: outcome and alliance. J Psychother Pract Res 7(4):261–271, 1998 9752637

Hides L, Quinn C, Stoyanov S, et al: Psychological interventions for co-occurring depression and substance use disorders. Cochrane Database Syst Rev 2019(11):CD009501, 2019 31769015

Hogarty GE, Kornblith SJ, Greenwald D, et al: Three-year trials of personal therapy among schizophrenic patients living with or independent of family, I: description of study and effects on relapse rates. Am J Psychiatry 154(11):1504–1513, 1997 9356557

Hogarty GE, Flesher S, Ulrich R, et al: Cognitive enhancement therapy for schizophrenia: effects of a 2-year randomized trial on cognition and behavior. Arch Gen Psychiatry 61(9):866–876, 2004 15351765

Horowitz M, Marmar C: The therapeutic alliance with difficult patients, in Psychiatry Update: The American Psychiatric Association Annual Review, Vol 4. Edited by Hales RE, Frances AJ. Washington, DC, American Psychiatric Press, 1985, pp 573–585

Horvath AO, Symonds BD: Relation between working alliance and outcome in psychotherapy: a meta-analysis. J Couns Psychol 38(2):139–149, 1991

Imber SD, Pilkonis PA, Sotsky SM, et al: Mode-specific effects among three treatments for depression. J Consult Clin Psychol 58(3):352–359, 1990 2195085

Jørgensen CR, Freund C, Bøye R, et al: Outcome of mentalization-based and supportive psychotherapy in patients with borderline personality disorder: a randomized trial. Acta Psychiatr Scand 127(4):305–317, 2013 22897123

Klein DF, Zitrin CM, Woerner MG, et al: Treatment of phobias II: behavior therapy and supportive psychotherapy: are there any specific ingredients? Arch Gen Psychiatry 40(2):139–145, 1983 6130751

Kocsis JH, Gelenberg AJ, Rothbaum BO, et al: Cognitive behavioral analysis system of psychotherapy and brief supportive psychotherapy for augmentation of antidepressant nonresponse in chronic depression: the REVAMP Trial. Arch Gen Psychiatry 66(11):1178–1188, 2009 19884606

Lee DJ, Schnitzlein CW, Wolf JP, et al: Psychotherapy versus pharmacotherapy for posttraumatic stress disorder: systemic review and meta-analyses to determine first-line treatments. Depress Anxiety 33(9):792–806, 2016 27126398

le Grange D, Crosby RD, Rathouz PJ, et al: A randomized controlled comparison of family based treatment and supportive psychotherapy for adolescent bulimia nervosa. Arch Gen Psychiatry 64(9):1049–1056, 2007 17768270

Liberman RP, Wallace CJ, Blackwell G, et al: Skills training versus psychosocial occupational therapy for persons with persistent schizophrenia. Am J Psychiatry 155(8):1087–1091, 1998 9699698

Lipsitz JD, Gur M, Vermes D, et al: A randomized trial of interpersonal therapy versus supportive therapy for social anxiety disorder. Depress Anxiety 25(6):542–553, 2008 17941096

Luborsky L, Singer B, Luborsky L: Comparative studies of psychotherapies: is it true that "everywon has one and all must have prizes"? Arch Gen Psychiatry 32(8):995–1008, 1975 239666

Maina G, Forner F, Bogetto F: Randomized controlled trial comparing brief dynamic and supportive therapy with waiting list condition in minor depressive disorders. Psychother Psychosom 74(1):43–50, 2005 15627856

Marder SR, Wirshing WC, Mintz J, et al: Two-year outcome of social skills training and group psychotherapy for outpatients with schizophrenia. Am J Psychiatry 153(12):1585–1592, 1996 8942455

Markowitz JC, Kocsis JH, Christos P, et al: Pilot study of interpersonal psychotherapy versus supportive psychotherapy for dysthymic patients with secondary alcohol abuse or dependence. J Nerv Ment Dis 196(6):468–474, 2008 18552624

McGorry PD, Nelson B, Phillips LJ, et al: Randomized controlled trial of interventions for young people at ultra-high risk of psychosis: twelve-month outcome. J Clin Psychiatry 74(4):349–356, 2013 23218022

McIntosh VVW, Jordan J, Carter FA, et al: Three psychotherapies for anorexia nervosa: a randomized, controlled trial. Am J Psychiatry 162(4):741–747, 2005 15800147

Miller WR, Rose GS: Motivational interviewing in relational context. Am Psychol 65(4):298–299, 2010

Mukherjee A, Mazumder K, Kaushal V, et al: Effect of supportive psychotherapy on mental health status and quality of life of female cancer patients receiving chemotherapy for recurrent disease. Indian J Palliat Care 23(4):399–402, 2017 29123345

Mumford E, Schlesinger HJ, Glass GV: The effect of psychological intervention on recovery from surgery and heart attacks: an analysis of the literature. Am J Public Health 72(2):141–151, 1982 7055315

Parikh SV, Riba MB, Greden JF: Depressive disorders, in The American Psychiatric Association Publishing Textbook of Psychiatry. Edited by Roberts LW. Washington, DC, American Psychiatric Association Publishing, 2019, pp 307–340

Perry JC, Banon E, Ianni F: Effectiveness of psychotherapy for personality disorders. Am J Psychiatry 156(9):1312–1321, 1999 10484939

Piper WE, Joyce AS, McCallum M, et al: Interpretive and supportive forms of psychotherapy and patient personality variables. J Consult Clin Psychol 66(3):558–567, 1998 9642895

Pompoli A, Furukawa TA, Imai H, et al: Psychological therapies for panic disorder with or without agoraphobia in adults: a network meta-analysis. Cochrane Database Syst Rev 4(4):CD011004, 2016 27071857

Qaseem A, Barry MJ, Kansagara D: Nonpharmacologic versus pharmacologic treatment of adult patients with major depressive disorder: a clinical practice guideline from the American College of Physicians. Ann Intern Med 164(5):350–359, 2016 26857948

Rea MM, Strachan AM, Goldstein MJ, et al: Changes in patient coping style following individual and family treatment for schizophrenia. Br J Psychiatry 158:642–647, 1991 1860018

Renaud J, Brent DA, Baugher M, et al: Rapid response to psychosocial treatment for adolescent depression: a two-year follow-up. J Am Acad Child Adolesc Psychiatry 37(11):1184–1190, 1998 9808930

Rollnick S, Miller WR: What is motivational interviewing? Behav Cogn Psychother 23(4):325–334, 1995

Rosenbaum B, Valbak K, Harder S, et al: The Danish National Schizophrenia Project: prospective, comparative longitudinal treatment study of first-episode psychosis. Br J Psychiatry 186:394–399, 2005 15863743

Rosenbaum B, Harder S, Knudsen P, et al: Supportive psychodynamic psychotherapy versus treatment as usual for first-episode psychosis: two-year outcome. Psychiatry 75(4):331–341, 2012 23244011

Rosenthal RN, Westreich L: Treatment of persons with dual diagnoses of substance use disorder and other psychological problems, in Addictions: A Comprehensive Guidebook. Edited by McCrady BS, Epstein EE. New York, Oxford University Press, 1999, pp 439–476

Rosenthal RN, Muran JC, Pinsker H, et al: Interpersonal change in brief supportive psychotherapy. J Psychother Pract Res 8(1):55–63, 1999 9888107
Rosenzweig S: Some implicit common factors in diverse methods of psychotherapy. Am J Orthopsychiatry 6(3):412–415, 1936
Rutledge T, Atkinson JH, Chircop-Rollick T, et al: Randomized controlled trial of telephone-delivered cognitive behavioral therapy versus supportive care for chronic back pain. Clin J Pain 34(4):322–327, 2018 28877139
Schmidt U, Oldershaw A, Jichi F, et al: Out-patient psychological therapies for adults with anorexia nervosa: randomised controlled trial. Br J Psychiatry 201(5):392–399, 2012 22995632
Schmidt U, Magill N, Renwick B, et al: The Maudsley Outpatient Study of Treatments for Anorexia Nervosa and Related Conditions (MOSAIC): comparison of the Maudsley Model of Anorexia Nervosa Treatment for Adults (MANTRA) with specialist supportive clinical management (SSCM) in outpatients with broadly defined anorexia nervosa: a randomized controlled trial. J Consult Clin Psychol 83(4):796–807, 2015 25984803
Schramm E, Kriston L, Zobel I, et al: Effect of disorder-specific vs nonspecific psychotherapy for chronic depression: a randomized clinical trial. JAMA Psychiatry 74(3):233–242, 2017 28146251
Schramm E, Kriston L, Elsaesser M, et al: Two-year follow-up after treatment with the cognitive-behavioral analysis system of psychotherapy versus supportive psychotherapy for early onset chronic depression. Psychother Psychosom 88(3):154–164, 2019 31121581
Shear MK, Pilkonis PA, Cloitre M, et al: Cognitive behavioral treatment compared with nonprescriptive treatment of panic disorder. Arch Gen Psychiatry 51(5):395–401, 1994 8179463
Shear MK, Houck P, Greeno C, et al: Emotion-focused psychotherapy for patients with panic disorder. Am J Psychiatry 158(12):1993–1998, 2001 11729015
Sjödin I, Svedlund J, Ottosson J-O, et al: Controlled study of psychotherapy in chronic peptic ulcer disease. Psychosomatics 27(3):187–191, 195–196, 200, 1986 3961091
Stanton AH, Gunderson JG, Knapp PH, et al: Effects of psychotherapy in schizophrenia: I. Design and implementation of a controlled study. Schizophr Bull 10(4):520–563, 1984 6151245
Stein KF, Corte C, Chen D-GD, et al: A randomized clinical trial of an identity intervention programme for women with eating disorders. Eur Eat Disord Rev 21(2):130–142, 2013 23015537
Stein MB, Sherbourne CD, Craske MG, et al: Quality of care for primary care patients with anxiety disorders. Am J Psychiatry 161(12):2230–2237, 2004 15569894
Swartz HA, Cyranowski JM, Cheng Y, et al: Brief psychotherapy for maternal depression: impact on mothers and children. J Am Acad Child Adolesc Psychiatry 55(6):495–503.e2, 2016 27238068
Thompson LW, Gallagher D: Depression and its treatment in the elderly. Aging 348:14–18, 1985
Tompson MC, Sugar CA, Langer DA, et al: A randomized clinical trial comparing family focused treatment and individual supportive therapy for depression in childhood and early adolescence. J Am Acad Child Adolesc Psychiatry 56(6):515–523, 2017 28545757
Vaughn CE, Leff JP: The influence of family and social factors on the course of psychiatric illness: a comparison of schizophrenic and depressed neurotic patients. Br J Psychiatry 129:125–137, 1976 963348
Wallerstein RS: The Psychotherapy Research Project of the Menninger Foundation: an overview. J Consult Clin Psychol 57(2):195–205, 1989 2708605
Wallerstein RS, Robbins LL, Sargent HD, et al: The psychotherapy research project of the Menninger Foundation. Bull Menninger Clin 20(5):221–278, 1956 13364559
Walsh BT, Wilson GT, Loeb KL, et al: Medication and psychotherapy in the treatment of bulimia nervosa. Am J Psychiatry 154(4):523–531, 1997 9090340
Wilhelm S, Phillips KA, Greenberg JL, et al: Efficacy and posttreatment effects of therapist-delivered cognitive behavioral therapy vs supportive psychotherapy for adults with body dysmorphic disorder: a randomized clinical trial. JAMA Psychiatry 76(4):363–373, 2019 30785624
Winston A, Winston B: Handbook of Integrated Short-Term Psychotherapy. Washington, DC, American Psychiatric Publishing, 2002

Winston A, Rosenthal RN, Muran JC: Supportive psychotherapy, in Handbook of Personality Disorders: Theory, Research, and Treatment. Edited by Livesley WJ. New York, Guilford, 2001, pp 344–358

Winston A, Rosenthal RN, Roberts LW: Learning Supportive Psychotherapy: An Illustrated Guide. 2nd Edition. Washington, DC, American Psychiatric Association Publishing, 2020

Zitrin CM, Klein DF, Woerner MG: Behavior therapy, supportive psychotherapy, imipramine, and phobias. Arch Gen Psychiatry 35(3):307–316, 1978 31847

PART VI

Family, Couple, and Group Psychotherapy

Section Editor: Alison Heru, M.D.

Healthy relationships are a strong protective factor for illness outcome and contribute to the quality of our lives. The science of relationships, our concepts, assessments, and interventions, are the basis for family, couple, and group psychotherapies. Advances in neuroscience show resting state connectomes synchronizing with daily emotional connections between a parent and their child, leading Lee et al. (2017) to conclude that "families that fire together smile together" (p. 31). Cultural norms influence the expression of emotion and the meaning of expressed emotion, necessitating cultural adaptation of our interventions (Heru 2020).

Despite the science and evidence base, relational work has not been well implemented, although it can be done with planning and forethought (Heru 2015). Simply involving the family as part of the team with the attitude of "Come on in and let's work together to help the patient" improves patient outcome. This requires no formal training, just an openness to meeting with the family. Family psychoeducation is the most highly researched and successful family intervention, but it requires clinic organization and a minimum of 6 hours of training in the basic techniques of group dynamics. Complex health care systems can benefit from this type of streamlined care. For example, in a hospital-based clinic for the assessment and management of patients with nonepileptic seizures described by Libbon et al. (2019a), group and family psychoeducations form the basis of care. Family systemic therapy is the only family intervention that requires intensive supervision and training. The Group for the Advancement of Psychiatry (GAP) Committee on the Family developed a model curriculum outlining didactic material for understanding and working with systems and systemic therapies in psychiatry residency programs (Berman et al. 2006).

The chapters in Part 6 reflect years of research and experience in family, couple, and group psychotherapies. John Rolland, Froma Walsh, Seamus Bhatt-Mackin, Molyn Leszcz, and Jay Lebow, are our authoritative voices. Additionally, several early career psychiatrists are creating new ways of understanding and working systemically. Allen and colleagues (2016) created an innovative systems curriculum containing individual modules customized for specific needs, such as the financial aspects of health care, interagency issues, and cultural influences. Nguyen focused on how to conceptualize and understand the interpersonal contexts in the workplace, using a genogram to understand systemic patterns (S. Nguyen, "Family Matters: Using Genograms to Unlock Organizational Systems," grand rounds, Middlesex Hospital, Middletown, Connecticut, 2019). Libbon and colleagues (2019b) modernized the use of the genogram and the ecomap. J. Zik (personal communication, December 2020) has provided guidelines for telehealth, such as increasing structure by announcing all parties present (even if off camera) and ensuring careful use of one screen or multiple screens to see as many nonverbal cues as possible, and recommends that we "don't fall into the trap of only looking at one face at a time." Zik suggests a mutual viewing of rooms to establish safety, a frank discussion with families about how to manage in-session conflict, and designation of a cool-down time postsession. Our field has the science and the evidence base; we need to be more aggressive about the implementation of our approach in our complex health care systems.

References

Allen N, Knowles A, Patterson D, et al: Transforming frustration into possibility: a model for understanding and navigating complex systems in a changing landscape. Acad Psychiatry 40(6):887–892, 2016 27044408

Berman EM, Heru AM, Grunebaum H, et al; Group for the Advancement of Psychiatry Committee on the Family: Family skills for general psychiatry residents: meeting ACGME core competency requirements. Acad Psychiatry 30(1):69–78, 2006 16473998

Heru AM: Family-centered care in the outpatient general psychiatry clinic. J Psychiatr Pract 21(5):381–388, 2015 26352224

Heru AM: Cultural research deconstructs the psychosocial construct "expressed emotion." Br J Psychiatry 219(4): 565–568, 2020 32778202

Lee TH, Miernicki ME, Telzer EH: Families that fire together smile together: resting state connectome similarity and daily emotional synchrony in parent-child dyads. Neuroimage 152:31–37, 2017 28254510

Libbon R, Gadbaw J, Watson M, et al: The feasibility of a multidisciplinary group therapy clinic for the treatment of nonepileptic seizures. Epilepsy Behav 98 (Pt A):117–123, 2019a

Libbon R, Triana J, Heru A, Berman E: Family skills for the resident toolbox: the 10-min genogram, ecomap, and prescribing homework. Acad Psychiatry 43(4):435–439, 2019b 30905028

CHAPTER 19

Family Therapy

Systemic Concepts and Methods

John S. Rolland, M.D., M.P.H.
Froma Walsh, Ph.D.

Family Systems Theory and Practice

Family systems theory and research have advanced our understanding and treatment of individual and relational distress (Heru 2006; Lebow 2013). Practice approaches are guided by a developmental, multilevel systems orientation to human functioning and processes of change, attending to the family and social context of dysfunction and well-being. In this chapter we provide an overview of family systems assessment and intervention in psychiatry. We first describe basic principles of a systems orientation to practice and a framework for family assessment. We offer a brief outline of major family therapy approaches, core concepts, and methods. Next, we describe their practice utility, including family or couple assessment, consultation, brief interventions, multisystemic approaches, multifamily groups, and more intensive therapy. We consider how to apply family systems principles with varied therapeutic approaches, in a range of behavioral health care and practice settings, and with severe mental health conditions. Emphasis is given to initial consultations, family psychoeducation, and brief interventions.

Family Systems Orientation

A family systems orientation is distinguished by its view of the family as a transactional system. Stressful events and problems of an individual member affect the whole family as a functional unit, with ripple effects for all members and their relationships.

In turn, the family response—how the family handles problems—contributes significantly to positive adaptation or to individual and relational dysfunction. Thus, individual problems are assessed and addressed in the context of the family, with attention to socioeconomic and other environmental stressors. Relational problems are addressed directly in couple and family sessions or between individual sessions in contacts with those involved.

Biopsychosocial Orientation

The practice of family therapy is grounded in a biopsychosocial orientation, recognizing the complex interplay of individual, family, and social processes (Bertalanffy 1969; Engel 1980). The family is viewed as an open system that functions in relation to its broader sociocultural context and evolves over the life cycle (Minuchin 1974). Family systems theory advanced conceptualization of human functioning and dysfunction from a linear, dyadic, deterministic view of causality in traditional psychoanalytic theory to the recognition of multiple recursive influences within and beyond the family that affect both individual and family functioning over the life course.

In the evolution of the field over recent decades, an ecological view considers the family's interface with larger systems, such as school, workplace, and health care systems. With a broad biopsychosocial systemic perspective, greater attention is given to biological and sociocultural influences, including the impact of race, class, gender, and sexual orientation. Racism, income and health care disparities, and other forms of discrimination that disadvantage low-income families, racial minorities, and other marginalized groups are addressed (Boyd-Franklin, in press; McGoldrick and Hardy 2019). Regardless of the origin of problems or genetic influence in mental health conditions, the family is regarded as an essential partner in treatment, fostering optimal adaptation and resilience (Walsh 2003, 2016).

Multigenerational Family Life Cycle Perspective

In a systemic model of human development, individual and family development are seen to coevolve over the life course and across the generations (McGoldrick et al. 2015). Relationships grow and change, boundaries shift, roles are redefined, and new members and losses require adaptation. Each developmental phase presents salient challenges; distress often occurs around major transitions, such as the birth of the first child, entry into adolescence, launching young adults, or needs for eldercare. All families must cope with stressful events, including both the predictable, normative stresses, as with child-rearing, and unexpected, disruptive circumstances, such as raising a child with disabilities (Walsh, in press). Divorce, single parenting, and stepfamily integration pose additional challenges for many families (Hetherington and Kelly 2002). Over an expanded life course, family members may transition in and out of single status, couple bonds, and varied family configurations, adding complexity to all relationships. The diversity of family forms, lifestyle options, and timing of nodal events makes it imperative that no single model or life trajectory be deemed as essential for healthy child development (Walsh 2012).

Systemic Lens: Patterns That Connect

Including Family Members

Family therapy is not simply a therapeutic modality in which all members are treated conjointly. In fact, individuals may be seen separately or brought together for some sessions in different combinations. A family systems approach is distinguished less by who is in the room and more by the clinician's attention to relationship systems in assessment and treatment planning. The clinician considers how family members may contribute to—and are affected by—problem situations. Most importantly, regardless of the source of difficulties, the clinician involves key family members who can contribute to needed changes. Therapy may focus on strengthening a couple's relationship; it might combine individual sessions with an adolescent and sessions with parents or caregivers, or it might include siblings or extended kin. Members unavailable to meet or living at a distance may participate through telehealth. Interventions are aimed at modifying dysfunctional patterns, tapping family resources, and strengthening both individual and family functioning.

Mutual Influences

Family members are interrelated such that each individual affects all others and the group as a whole, in turn, affects the first member in recursive influences. Even for psychiatric conditions that are strongly biologically influenced, such as depression, it is important to understand how depression affects family interaction, how those transactions contribute to or reinforce symptoms, and how changes can reduce stress and improve individual—and family—functioning and well-being. A circular tracking process is a key element in a systems-oriented assessment of biological and relational influences to guide interventions.

In a chain of influence, every action is also a reaction: a mother's overly harsh response to a child's tantrum may exacerbate the child's out-of-control behavior. In tracking the *sequence of interactions* around a presenting problem, we often find repetitive patterns involving other family members. For example, if the other parent then berates the mother and sides with the child, it can make matters worse. Regardless of how a sequence began, co-parents can be helped to pull together as a team to handle challenges more effectively. Skilled intervention involves interrupting vicious cycles to promote "virtuous cycles" and problem resolution.

Although processes may be recursive, not all participants have equal power or influence. Clinicians are cautioned not to take a neutral stance or a "no-fault" position in cases in which an abusive spouse or parent must be held accountable for any harmful behavior. Moreover, therapist neutrality tends to support the status quo and can perpetuate destructive patterns.

Clinicians should not reflexively type a family by the diagnosis of a member, such as an "alcoholic family." Such labels carry faulty attributions of blame. Family distress should not be presumed to have caused individual symptoms; family distress may *result* from unsuccessful attempts to cope with an overwhelming situation. For instance, marital conflict between parents of an adolescent with bipolar disorder may have been fueled by repeated unsuccessful attempts to deal with their youth's emotional outbursts. With multiple influences, the impact of external stressors and socioeconomic conditions should be taken into account. For instance, a son's plummeting school grades must be seen in the context of his father's recent job loss and related family financial strains. Sensitive family therapy intervention acknowledges family stress and frustrations and helps members find more effective ways to approach challenges and prevent problematic behavior.

Assessment of Family Functioning

Mapping the Family System

A broad and flexible conception of *family* is needed to encompass the wide range of family structures, relationship options, and cultural diversity in contemporary society (Walsh 2012). Attention to multigenerational relationships is especially important in elder caregiving, in the role of the extended family for single parents, and in kinship care for children (Engstrom 2012). The idealized mid-twentieth-century nuclear family model, with gendered breadwinner/homemaker roles, is out of touch with contemporary family life. Yet social expectations can compound a sense of deficiency for those who do not fit that model, especially single parents.

Those who do not conform to certain cultural or religious standards for marriage and family, such as gender-variant couples and LGBTQ+ parents, are gaining wider acceptance yet still face stigma, inequalities, and legal challenges (Green 2012). Studies over two decades have found abundant evidence that children can thrive in a variety of family arrangements, including gay parenting (Walsh 2012). What matters most are stable, caring, and committed relationships and effective family processes for nurturing, guidance, and protection.

In an initial meeting, it is important to learn who is important in the family system. This may include all household members, nonresidential parents, step relations, and the extended kin network, as well as other significant relationships (e.g., intimate partner, informal kin, godparents, caregivers). The *genogram* and *time line* (McGoldrick et al. 2020) are essential tools for mapping family relationships, key information, and system patterns to guide intervention. A diagram is valuable for the clinician—and family members—to be able to visualize and explore family patterns. Seeing all key members and how they are related can bring coherence to complex family constellations for intervention planning, such as with families with remarried parents and children from present and former partners across households.

Family therapy theory and practice have become increasingly attentive to the challenges many families face in their social environment, particularly those who confront economic and racial barriers and larger systemic or structural disparities. Falicov's (2013) multidimensional framework with immigrant families considers each family within a complex ecological niche, sharing borders and common ground with other families, as well as differing positions with the intersection of such variables as gender, economic status, life stage, ethnicity, and location in the dominant society. A holistic assessment includes the varied contexts to understand the constraints and possibilities in each family's situation.

A resilience-oriented assessment searches for positive relational influences and potential resources, as well as problematic patterns and troubled relationships. Inquiry about a family's organizational shifts and coping strategies in response to past stressors can help to illuminate the family's meaning-making efforts, coping strategies, and adaptation with current challenges, such as a threatened separation. It is important to identify strengths, such as courage and perseverance, in the midst of ongoing and past struggles and to draw out positive stories and experiences in overcoming adversity (Walsh 2016).

Family functioning is assessed in the context of the multigenerational system moving forward over time (McGoldrick et al. 2015). A time line can be sketched to note the timing and sequence of critical events or a pile-up of stressors and family tensions. Frequently, symptoms coincide with stressful events, such as a business failure; disruptive transitions, such as postdivorce relocation; and relationship changes, as with a new stepparent (Greene et al. 2012; Walsh 2022). Because family members may not initially mention such connections, the genogram and time line can guide inquiry for further exploration.

Change and Conflict

Although all change is stressful, strain increases exponentially when current stressors intersect with sensitive multigenerational issues. Nodal events are likely to reactivate past conflicts, particularly when similar developmental challenges are confronted. An impending separation may reactivate past losses. Clinicians should routinely note family histories of traumatic loss that can contribute to depression, substance abuse, and self-destructive behavior (Walsh 2007; Walsh and McGoldrick 2013). Families may conflate current situations with past adverse experience, generating catastrophic fears. In one case, a husband's avoidance of intimacy and conflict over his wife's desire to have a second child became more understandable in learning that his mother had died in childbirth with his younger sibling. Families can explore such linkages and untold stories, helping them to draw lessons from their past as they approach their current situation.

Components of Family Functioning

Family process research over the past three decades has provided considerable empirical grounding for assessment of family functioning (Lebow and Stroud 2012). The Family Resilience Framework (Walsh 2003, 2016) was developed as a conceptual map to guide clinical assessment and to target and strengthen key processes that foster positive adaptation. This framework, informed by social science and clinical research, identifies nine core beliefs and practices for effective family functioning in three domains: 1) shared belief systems, 2) organizational processes, and 3) communication/problem-solving processes (Table 19–1). Family functioning is assessed in context, relative to cultural and situational differences and each family's values, resources, and life challenges.

Family Belief Systems

Shared belief systems are at the core of family functioning, providing a set of explanations and expectations that make sense of adverse experience and guide members'

TABLE 19–1. **Key processes in family resilience**

Shared belief systems

1. Making meaning of adversity
   - Take a relational view of resilience
   - Normalize and contextualize distress
   - Gain sense of coherence
   - Engage in facilitative appraisal and active agency
2. Positive outlook
   - Have hope, an optimistic bias, and confidence
   - Provide encouragement; affirm strengths and potential
   - Encourage active initiative and perseverance
   - Master the possible; accept what cannot be changed
3. Transcendence and spirituality
   - Larger values, purpose
   - Spirituality: faith, practices, congregation; nature
   - Inspiration: aspirations, creativity, social action
   - Transformation: learning, positive growth

Organizational processes

4. Flexibility
   - Rebound; adaptive change to meet challenges
   - Reorganize, restabilize: be dependable, predictable
   - Provide authoritative leadership: nurture, guide, protect
   - Establish cooperative parenting/caregiving teams
5. Connectedness
   - Encourage mutual support, teamwork, and commitment
   - Respect individual needs and differences
   - Seek reconnection and repair grievances
6. Mobilization of social and economic resources
   - Extended kin; social and community supports
   - Financial security: navigate work and family stresses
   - Larger systems: institutional, structural supports

Communication/problem-solving processes

7. Clarity
   - Provide clear, consistent information
   - Clarify ambiguous situation; facilitate truth seeking
8. Open emotional sharing
   - Painful (sorrow, suffering, anger, fear)
   - Positive (appreciation, humor, joy, respite)
9. Collaborative problem solving
   - Creative brainstorming; resourcefulness
   - Shared decision-making
   - Steps toward goals; learning from setbacks
   - Proactive mode: preparedness, prevention

approaches to their challenges about roles, actions, and consequences that guide family life and members' behaviors. Shared values and assumptions are constructed through transactions with significant others and the larger social world and are strongly influenced by cultural beliefs transmitted across generations. Clinicians should routinely explore a family's beliefs concerning their problematic situation: the meaning it holds for them, how it came about, and how it might be improved (Wright and Bell 2009). Patients from immigrant families might not mention traditional faith beliefs and healing practices unless the therapist inquires respectfully about them (Falicov 2013).

Family history and patterns of relating are transmitted across the generations, influencing current and future expectations, hopes, and dreams. Multigenerational stories, secrets, and taboos become encoded into family scripts that can rally efforts or fuel catastrophic fears when facing a threatening situation. Some families become stuck in the past; others cut off emotionally from painful memories and contacts. Well-functioning families are better able to balance intergenerational continuity and change and to maintain links between their past, present, and future directions.

Family identity and beliefs are conveyed through family rituals, including celebrations of holidays, rites of passage, and routine interactions (e.g., family dinner). Rituals provide stabilization and continuity over time and facilitate difficult transitions. Family therapists often encourage rituals in therapeutic intervention to foster healing and adaptation (Imber-Black et al. 2003), as in cases of suicide or stillbirth.

Therapists aim to understand constraining beliefs and narratives and to expand those that facilitate positive change. Research suggests that clinicians can foster resilience by helping distressed families to 1) make meaning of their crisis situation and their options; 2) regain a hopeful, positive outlook, active efforts, and perseverance and focus on mastering what is possible; and 3) forge larger transcendent or spiritual values, purpose, and bonds in their lives, inspiring creativity and positive growth (Walsh 2003, 2016).

Family Organizational Patterns

Family functioning requires effective organization to maintain integration, foster healthy development of members, and master life challenges that arise. Varying family structures, such as a two-earner two-parent family, a single-parent family, a divorced joint custody family, a stepfamily, and a three-generation household, need to organize workable roles and relationship patterns that fit their situation.

Flexibility

Flexibility is necessary for effective family functioning and resilience to adapt to changing conditions. In times of crisis, such as a medical emergency, or disruptive transitions, such as family separation, flexibility must be counterbalanced by efforts to restabilize, reorganize, and reestablish patterns and role functioning in daily living.

Role relations may need to be negotiated. For dual-earner couples navigating job, child-rearing, and household responsibilities, an equitable sharing of authority, responsibility, and privilege fosters more satisfying relationships. Of note, same-sex couples tend to have more equitable role relations than do heterosexual couples. In kinship care, when grandparents step in to raise grandchildren, renegotiation of roles, relationships, and households is needed (Engstrom 2012). The complexity of divorce and stepfamilies poses challenges to sustaining workable parenting coalitions across households and to knitting together biological relations and step-relations (Papernow 2018).

Family boundaries need to be clear and firm yet permeable to promote differentiation, autonomous functioning, and generational authority (Minuchin 1974). Children can gain competencies by assisting parents with responsibilities, and their role may be vital in single-parent and large families and in cases of parental illness or disability. When boundaries are breached destructively, as in sexual abuse, it is imperative to strengthen family structure for clear leadership and protection.

Connectedness

Strong connected bonds (cohesion) are essential for stable, nurturing, committed attachments and for collaboration in teamwork to resolve problems. With varying cultural norms, personal preferences, and situational demands, clinicians must be cautious not to reflexively label a highly cohesive family style as enmeshed or presume it is necessarily dysfunctional.

Mobilizing Social and Economic Resources

Extended kin and social networks are lifelines for family functioning and support through hard times, especially for multistressed, under-resourced families. Friendship networks are important for adults living alone and are often chosen families formed in LGBTQ+ communities to counter stigma and nonacceptance. Faith communities offer valued resources to many families through congregational support, spiritual practices, clergy guidance, and involvement in a range of programs and services. Clinicians are encouraged to become acquainted with faith-based resources in their communities. In working with immigrant and refugee families, adaptation and resilience are facilitated by finding ways to sustain kinship and cultural connections with loved ones and the community left behind (Falicov 2007; Walsh 2007).

Communication Processes

Clear Information

Open communication facilitates meaning making and problem solving in facing serious life challenges. Anxiety is heightened in ambiguous situations, such as an unclear medical prognosis or the threat of divorce. When communication is blocked, children may imagine the worst and express fears through somatic or behavioral symptoms. However, clinicians should be mindful of varied cultural norms regarding directness and expressivity of information and feelings. For instance, in traditional Chinese culture, physicians and families do not tell an ill patient that they have a fatal prognosis, believing that the bad news would upset them and could hasten their death.

Open Emotional Sharing

Open communication, supported by a climate of mutual trust, empathy, and tolerance for differences, enables family members to share a wide range of feelings that can be aroused by crisis situations and chronic stress. Members need to feel safe in *expressing painful emotions*, such as sadness, yearning, frustration, remorse, outrage, or anxiety, which may fluctuate over time and vary depending on different personalities, ages, relationships, and implications of an adverse situation. A parent may suppress painful feelings in order to keep functioning; a child might do so to avoid burdening others. Members may be out of sync over time; some may feel ready to move on before others.

It is important to address constraints of gender-based assumptions. Expectations that men should be tough problem solvers and not reveal vulnerability, fear, or "soft" emotions can block their ability to address significant emotionally laden issues and to give and receive emotional support. It is useful to reframe vulnerability as inherent in the human condition and the expression of difficult feelings as a strength rather than a shameful weakness.

Collaborative Problem Solving and Proactive Approach

Creative brainstorming opens new possibilities in problematic situations. Shared decision-making and conflict management involve negotiation skills encouraging fairness, respect for differences, and reciprocity over time. Families need to tackle practical problems and also meet the emotional needs of members, such as comforting anxious children. Families strengthen competence and confidence by building on small successes, anticipating setbacks, and viewing mistakes as learning experiences. The family becomes more resourceful when therapy shifts from crisis reaction to a proactive approach to anticipate, prepare for, and avert future problems. Families forge varied pathways in coping, adaptation, and resilience.

Whether patterns are functional depends on the *fit* between the patient and family and the psychosocial demands of their problematic situation. For example, when a serious health crisis requiring close teamwork strikes a family with low cohesion, in which members fend for themselves, family sessions would be useful to build more collaboration and support to meet the overwhelming challenges (Rolland 2018).

Evolution in the Field of Family Therapy: From Deficits to Strengths

The field of family therapy has evolved and expanded focus since its beginnings in the 1960s. Reflecting the mental health field's pathology focus, early foundational family therapy models focused on changing dysfunctional family patterns that were thought to maintain individual symptoms. Since the mid-1980s, the field of family therapy reformulated theory and application of systems interventions, refocusing from family deficits to family strengths. For an in-depth description and comparison of models, see Goldenberg and Stanton (2016). In the following subsections, we highlight major models, principles, and techniques.

Foundational Models of Family Therapy

Intergenerational Approaches

Growth-oriented intergenerational approaches to family therapy bridge psychodynamic, object relations, and family systems theories. In *psychodynamically oriented approaches*, therapists attend to the web of dynamic processes in the family network of relationships. The therapeutic aim is for family members to deal with one another directly in order to work through unresolved conflicts and losses (Byng-Hall 1995;

Framo 1976). The *contextual approach* of Boszormenyi-Nagy (1987) emphasizes the importance of powerful, covert family-of-origin loyalty patterns with the aim of reconstruction and healing of wounded relationships.

The *Bowen model* (Bowen 1978) attends to the family emotional system, viewing functioning as impaired by poor differentiation, high anxiety, and emotional reactivity, producing conflict or cutoffs in highly charged relationships. In *triangulation*, two conflicting members (e.g., parents) draw in a third member (e.g., a child), who may distract, serve as a go-between, or side with one in loyalty against the other. Therapists use a *coaching process* (McGoldrick and Carter 2001), often in individual therapy sessions, to help patients change their own behavior and reactivity with other family members, in or between sessions. Opportunities are pursued in visits and family gatherings, as well as letters and phone calls. Experiential approaches to family therapy were developed by Virginia Satir (1972), who blended a communication approach with a humanistic orientation, and by Carl Whitaker (1992), who practiced an idiosyncratic style of intervention.

Structural and Strategic-Systemic Approaches

Structural family therapy was developed by Minuchin (1974) and colleagues at the Philadelphia Child Guidance Center working with multistressed, largely ethnic/racial minority, inner city families. This approach focuses on the patterning of transactions in which symptoms are embedded, and problems are viewed as an indication of imbalance in family organization, particularly a malfunctioning hierarchy. Brief therapy—through processes of *joining*, *enactment*, and *restructuring*—aims to strengthen the family structural foundation for better functioning and coping with life stresses.

Early strategic and systemic approaches were developed by the Palo Alto Mental Research Institute group (Weakland et al. 1974) and by Haley (1976). These problem-solving models view presenting problems as both a symptom of and a response to current stresses, a communicative act within a repetitive sequence of interactions. The therapeutic task is to interrupt ways of handling the problem that are not working. Widely used techniques—*relabeling*, *reframing*, and *positive connotation*—involve strategic redefinition of a problem situation to cast it in a new light. The Milan Approach (Boscolo et al. 1987) stresses the importance of learning a family's language and beliefs, seeing the problem through various members' eyes and appreciating the values and expectations that guide their handling of problems and their inability to change. This approach employs *working hypotheses, circular questioning, and a stance of respectful curiosity.*

Behavioral Approaches

Behavioral approaches to family therapy, notably *functional family therapy* (Robbins et al. 2016) with adolescent conduct disorders, were developed from behavior modification and social learning traditions. In these approaches, families are viewed as critical learning contexts, created and responded to by members. Therapy attends to transactional rules, behaviors, and conditions under which social behavior is learned, influenced, and changed. The therapist guides family members to learn more effective modes of dealing with one another by changing the interpersonal consequences of behavior—to give each other approval and acknowledgment for desired behavior instead of reinforcing maladaptive behavior through attention or punishment. The therapist builds communication skills in negotiation and problem solving, increasing adaptability.

Strengths-Based Collaborative Approaches

The field of family therapy has shifted increasingly from a deficit to a strengths perspective and a respectful collaboration with family members. Assessment and intervention are redirected from problems and how they are maintained to solutions and how they can be attained. Therapeutic efforts aim to identify and mobilize competencies and resources. Therapist and patients work in partnership to see new possibilities in a problem-saturated situation and to overcome impasses to change and growth. This positive, future-focused stance shifts the emphasis of therapy from what went wrong to what can be done for enhanced functioning and well-being.

These approaches oppose assumptions that symptoms serve ulterior functions for the family. Therapists attribute benign intent to all members, assume that they want positive change, and strive to overcome constraints. The therapeutic relationship eschews the hierarchical power-based position of earlier models and rejects the use of clever techniques to battle family resistance. Instead, it is built on respect of families, appreciating their lived experience, and amplifying their positive strengths, resources, and untapped potential.

Postmodern Approaches

Postmodern perspectives recognize that views of normality, health, and pathology are socially constructed (Hoffman 1990; Walsh 2012), influencing therapeutic assessment and objectives. Clinicians and researchers cannot be neutral: inadvertently, they bring their own values and biases and thus co-construct the patterns they "discover" in families. Awareness is needed of implicit assumptions embedded in cultural norms, gender and social location, professional orientations, and personal experience. Postmodern practice approaches are based in constructivist and social constructionist views. When patients are constrained by narrow, pessimistic views of problems limiting the range of alternatives, therapy refocuses from problems and the patterns that maintain them to positive future visions and the steps to attain them (Madsen 2011).

Narrative approaches emphasize the therapeutic conversation (Anderson 1997) and processes of *"restory-ing"* and *externalizing* a problematic experience (Freedman and Combs 1996; White and Epston 1990). A basic premise is that people strive to make meaning of their experience. Through appreciative inquiry, therapists listen well to patient narratives, are curious about their stories, ask questions to thicken descriptions, and consider alternative constructions to expand possibilities. Therapy attends to the ways language and meaning reflect cultural values and the larger social context, supporting patient efforts to construct new narratives that are less constraining and more empowering and satisfying.

Solution-focused approaches (de Shazer 1988) search for exceptions to immediate problems: solutions that have worked in other situations and might work now. Techniques such as *scaling*, in which patients rate themselves to concretize aims and progress, are used to refocus from complaints to desired outcomes and the steps to reach them.

Evidence-Based Intervention Models

Family Psychoeducation

Family psychoeducational approaches have been empirically demonstrated to be an essential component of effective treatment for schizophrenia (McFarlane 2016) and have been usefully applied with a range of chronic mental and physical conditions (Lucksted et al. 2012; Lyman et al. 2014; Miklowitz 2010; Rolland 2018). This approach addresses the interaction of environmental stresses with a core biological vulnerability in producing disturbed cognitions and behaviors. In controlled studies, family intervention combined with medication maintenance and social skills training dramatically reduced relapse rates and improved functioning of individuals with schizophrenia and also reduced family distress. Family psychoeducation has been successfully adapted for Mexican Americans who have a family member with schizophrenia (Kopelowicz et al. 2012).

Therapists engage families as valued collaborators in the treatment process, with respect for their challenges, unlike the marginalization and blaming attributions many families have previously experienced. Families are viewed as vital caregiving resources for the long-term management of the condition. Family-oriented programs aim to avoid treatment dropout, to sustain functioning in the community, and to decrease family stress and relapse rates. This approach focuses on solving immediate problems, measuring success in small increments, and maintaining family morale.

Psychoeducational family interventions have been adapted to a variety of formats, including one-time or periodic family consultations, brief time-limited groups, and ongoing multifamily groups. Intervention modules can be timed with critical phases or transitions in a condition. This encourages families to accept and digest manageable portions of a long-term coping process. Examples of manageable portions of the process include the initial crisis; the chronic, terminal, or bereavement phases of a chronic or life-threatening illness; and community reentry postdiagnosis or after hospital discharge (Rolland 2018).

Psychoeducation is of value with challenges such as teen pregnancy, family separation and divorce, single parenting, and planned remarriage and stepfamily integration. It provides a cost-effective preventive approach and can identify families at high risk of maladaptation or relapse who may require more intensive services.

Multisystemic Approaches With Adolescent Behavior Problems

Several evidence-based multisystemic and multidimensional intervention models offer highly effective approaches with high-risk, substance-abusing, and seriously troubled youth by involving families and larger community systems (Henggeler and Schaeffer 2016; Liddle 2016; Robbins et al. 2016; Santisteban et al. 2003; Szapocznik and Williams 2000). These approaches also yield improvements in family functioning, including increased cohesion, improved communication, and improved parenting practices, and are linked to more positive youth behavioral outcomes than in standard youth services. Multisystemic interventions may involve school counselors, teachers, coaches, and peer groups; these individuals may work with police officials, probation officers, and judges to address legal issues. They might help a youth and family access vocational services, youth development organizations, social support networks, and religious resources.

With families that are often prejudged as too dysfunctional or unmotivated for therapy, these approaches engage family members in a strengths-oriented, collaborative alliance. Family members develop a shared atmosphere of hope, expectation for change, sense of responsibility, and empowerment. Rather than seeing troubled youths and their families as "resistant" to change, attempts are made to identify and overcome barriers to success in family and social contexts. Therapeutic contacts emphasize the positive and draw out systemic strengths and competencies for change. Clinicians communicate an optimistic perspective throughout the assessment and intervention processes.

Integrative Practice Approaches

Most clinicians with a family systems orientation increasingly integrate elements of various practice approaches (Lebow 2013; Scheinkman 2008). Examples include the evidence-based multidimensional, multisystemic approach with troubled adolescents (Liddle 2016) and emotionally focused therapy (Johnson 2019), which combines attachment theory and behavioral approaches to foster secure relationships.

A *family resilience* practice approach builds on strengths-based developments to build family capacities to deal with adversity (Walsh 2003, 2016). It links symptoms of distress with highly stressful events, disruptive transitions, and chronic conditions. Families most often come for help in crisis but may not initially connect presenting problems with relevant stressors. A family resilience framework serves as a conceptual map to guide intervention efforts to target and strengthen key processes as presenting problems are addressed. This approach changes the deficit-based view of distressed families as *damaged* and beyond repair to see them as *challenged* by life's adversities, with potential for healing and growth. As families become more resourceful, risk and vulnerability are reduced and they are better able to meet future challenges. Thus, building resilience is also a preventive measure.

Value of Systems Approaches in Psychiatry

A systemic perspective is valuable in all clinical practice, whether in individual, family, couple, or multifamily group intervention approaches. It includes attention to the following:

- Individuals, problems, and resources in family and sociocultural context
- Transactional processes in the couple relationship, family unit, and extended relational network
- Multiple ongoing mutual biopsychosocial influences
- Patterns, critical events, phases, and transitions across the multigenerational family life cycle

Despite differences in particular strategies and techniques, all approaches focus on direct assessment and change to improve functioning, adaptation, and relationships.

A systemic lens enriches all forms of psychiatric intervention, from a biomedical model to psychodynamic and cognitive-behavioral approaches. A systems viewpoint can be used to understand family processes regardless of how many people are in the room. It broadens the focus from intrapersonal and dyadic influences to larger systemic patterns in problems and positive change. From this clinical stance, inquiry includes the social and temporal context of a problem, relevant multigenerational patterns, interactional processes that contribute to problems, and relational resources that can be tapped for problem resolution and well-being.

When working primarily with an individual patient, direct contact with significant family members facilitates their engagement, collaboration, and building of family resources. Conjoint sessions, when feasible, enable therapists to observe interactions, encourage discussion of multiple perspectives, and facilitate shared problem solving and conflict resolution. Telehealth options expand possibilities for involvement of significant family members, separately or together.

Systemic Approaches in Clinical Practice

Family Consultation and Assessment

A common question, "When is family consultation/therapy indicated?," requires reframing from a systems perspective. Relational support and positive changes in stressful transactions facilitate individual change and growth. Thus, the question of indications becomes a question of "What is the symptom-maintaining context of a problem; how can it most effectively be altered; and how can key family members support therapeutic objectives?"

The assessment of most problems therefore includes evaluation of the couple or family system, preferably in most cases by convening both spouses/partners and/or significant family members for a conjoint session, or consultation. It is important to consider all key relationships in the evaluation, to clarify treatment objectives, and to decide whom to include in subsequent sessions. This approach will clarify diagnostic questions, treatment objectives, and the choice of therapeutic intervention. With such conditions as schizophrenia, acute mania, neurocognitive disorders (Rolland 2017), and substance abuse, family members can provide more accurate information regarding symptoms and behavior. When feasible, patients taking medication or who are in danger of crises should routinely be seen with their partner or family early in treatment to develop a treatment plan. This should include education about the course of the illness, the role and side effects of medication, an agreement on what constitutes a relapse or crisis, when the physician or hospital should be contacted, and whether or not the family has a role in medication monitoring.

The clinical advantages of meeting with family members far outweigh drawbacks. Family members are less likely to interfere with subsequent individual treatment, as with an adolescent, when they feel the therapist understands and respects their positions. Multiple perspectives more fully inform the clinician to make sound intervention decisions. Because a clinician's request for a family session may arouse concerns by parents or a spouse that they will be blamed or shamed for their loved one's problem, it is important to explicitly convey the conviction that families are essential partners in all treatment, that they can make valuable contributions to patient gains, and that their stressors and concerns will be addressed. The invitation should convey respect for the family and interest in their experience.

An initial family assessment can lay the groundwork for timely conjoint sessions even if the therapy remains primarily individual. Systems-oriented therapy can use such sessions to share information, facilitate communication and change, consolidate new behaviors, or set the stage for the next phase of an individual treatment. An initial conjoint meeting tends to balance the alliance with an individual patient, permitting the therapist more latitude to bring in other members comfortably later, if helpful.

At times, some therapists may be reluctant to convene a large family or include small children when concerned that it might be overwhelming or upset a child or vulnerable family member. Providing structure and ground rules is helpful. It is valuable to form a working alliance, observe how family members relate, and invite different perspectives in discussion of stressful issues. In an assessment session, a therapist can observe how parents handle a child's upset or misbehavior.

For *child- and adolescent-focused problems,* an initial family assessment places the identified patient's behavior in context. This is particularly true for a variety of conduct, eating, and separation anxiety disorders. Often, problematic behavior is connected to family dynamics, such as when a child is triangled into conflict between warring parents. A boy's angry, oppositional behavior toward his mother, a single parent, may be, in part, a deflection of anger and sense of abandonment with a nonresidential father's lack of contact, interest, or support. For problems that have biological and/or social influences, it is especially important to reduce parental guilt and blame, which sometimes has been stoked by prior contacts with school or other authorities. The therapist should join with parents to empower their authority and competence to handle child-focused problems. If the therapist takes an expert position in "fixing" or rescuing a child, it can communicate the idea that "I am a better parent than you are," giving parents a sense of deficiency and shame.

Many *inpatient programs* include a family orientation and assessment as part of their standard intake or initial evaluation process (Heru 2004). When family consultation is seen as integral to inpatient evaluation and treatment, it serves a number of functions. It promotes a joining process with the family and helps in identifying and reducing family stresses and resistances to treatment. It familiarizes families with the structure and functioning of the treatment unit. It ensures opportunities for family psychoeducation related to the mental health challenges of the patient, pharmacological and psychosocial treatment options, and expected treatment and prognosis. It facilitates family members' linkages for social support, respite, and self-care and to family support organizations, such as the National Alliance on Mental Illness (NAMI) and online resources. Additionally, the treatment team can be alerted to dysfunctional transactional patterns that may be replicated within the treatment system, such as triangular conflicts involving the patient and two clinicians. With brief hospitalization and reentry to the community, assessment of the family as a support system is critical.

With diagnosis or progression of *serious illness* or *disability*, a prevention-oriented family consultation is extremely useful. Most families lack a psychosocial map for their experience. In the *consultation-liaison* or *outpatient* context, families benefit from information and support to cope with and adapt to a family member's major illness. Family processes can influence adherence, disease course, and the well-being of the patient and key family caregivers (Campbell 2003; Shields et al. 2012). Therefore, brief consultation with key family members near the time of initial diagnosis and at major nodal points over the course of the illness (e.g., rehospitalization, recurrence or progression of the illness, transfer to rehabilitation or hospice) facilitates the treatment process and supports the family unit in a time of crisis (Rolland 2018). With the new era of genomics, family consultation increasingly will be needed in the context of genetic testing and living with risk information for a broad spectrum of medical and psychiatric conditions (Miller et al. 2006; Rolland and Williams 2005).

Research has demonstrated that a family-centered collaborative team approach that includes health and mental health care providers, patients, and their families fosters optimal biopsychosocial care (McDaniel et al. 2014; Shields et al. 2012). Convening the family early on in an illness promotes this integrated, collaborative model of care. The rationale is more than crisis management: it is prevention oriented and psychoeducational, counteracting marginalization of family members. It encourages an ongoing relationship with a mental health care provider as the family proceeds with living with a serious illness. The Family Systems Illness model, developed by Rolland (2018), provides a useful framework for consultation with families facing chronic illness, disability, and loss. Convening families in the consultation-liaison context is not difficult because family members typically visit their hospitalized member.

The goals of a *family-oriented mental health consultation* include the following:

- Emphasize that all family members are affected by the strains and challenges of living with a major illness and address the immediate emotional and practical needs of the patient and family members such as helplessness and the reactivation of old family conflicts around illness decision-making
- Provide information about the illness and treatment and ways family members can be helpful
- Provide family psychoeducation regarding a psychosocial understanding of the particular illness over time in relation to family expectations, offering practical management guidelines; this includes helping the family understand the illness in longitudinal and developmental terms: how different phases of the illness might affect plans and dreams for the patient, family members, and the family unit
- Elicit history and information that may be vital to diagnosis and treatment decisions, including the family's multigenerational experience with illness and loss that may hinder or facilitate current coping and adaptation
- Facilitate communication about the illness and treatment-related and caregiving issues and decisions
- Understand the cultural and spiritual beliefs that guide the family; this is essential to fostering culturally sensitive collaborative care and helping the family make meaning of the illness experience
- Identify high-risk, multistressed patients and families needing more intensive follow-up care
- Educate the family about the usefulness of periodic family-centered consultations (psychosocial checkups) and brief interventions at nodal points and transitions in the illness course and in the patient's, other family members', or the family's development

Brief Family Therapy

Brief family therapy is particularly useful with a focal chief complaint, such as a problematic behavior, conflict, situation, life transition, or major life challenge. A consultation-oriented preventive, early-intervention approach with a family can avert a major crisis or spiraling of distress. Problematic behaviors can be helped by attention to the web of surrounding interactions. Frequently, with focal problems, the therapist and family contract for a certain number of sessions, in which the goals are clearly delineated and progress is objectively monitored. This approach is similar to individual brief treatment models. At completion, the therapist and family can renegotiate a new contract or, in complicated cases, shift to more intensive longer-term therapy. Some families learn to use family consultations and treatment in a periodic time- and cost-effective way when family strains emerge over time. This approach is particularly useful for families coping with recurrence or exacerbation of psychiatric or physical conditions who simply want to go on with their lives during periods of remission.

Intensive Family Therapy

More intensive family therapy may be needed in cases of multiple and persistent difficulties. There is a myth that working with family members together is inherently more "superficial" than one-to-one treatment. In fact, profound and lasting change can occur, often more rapidly. In attending to the system, the therapist can anticipate others' reactivity to change and can alter symptom-maintaining patterns. Intrapsychic issues are also interpersonal; the systems therapist understands that behavioral change in the system is easier to bring about by facilitating interpersonal change, regardless of the problem origin or chronicity. Last, direct intervention and change with significant family members, whether planned in sessions or between sessions, has potential therapeutic benefit for all members, not only the current symptom bearer.

Therapy may selectively focus on specific problems and planfully bring in those members most critically involved for problem solving at different phases of intervention. Conjoint sessions with a family presenting with a child- or adolescent-focused problem might include parents, siblings, and any significant members. Marital problems identified during the assessment are best approached by first strengthening the co-parental alliance in resolving the presenting problem. After the child-focused issues are improved, the couple has established a working therapeutic alliance with the clinician, and there is a greater likelihood they will work on their couple relationship. With child- or adolescent-focused issues, it is often preferable to have the same therapist meet individually with the youth and conjointly with the family.

Family therapy is useful for a range of clinical situations, such as the following:

- Crisis events (e.g., child or adolescent behavior problems; death and loss of a child or parent/caregiver; critical situations involving substance use, violence, or sexual abuse)
- Disruptive life transitions (e.g., separation, divorce, remarriage and stepfamily formation)
- Serious and persistent psychiatric and medical conditions
- Problems strongly connected to family-of-origin issues

Couple Therapy

Couple therapy can be highly successful with a range of presenting problems (see Chapter 20, "Theories and Techniques of Couple Therapy"). When individuals present with problems of intimacy and they are currently in a primary relationship, a couple evaluation and at least some couple sessions are generally indicated. Individual therapy for couple relationship issues, lacking a systemic lens, may negatively impact the marriage. Without engaging the partner and directly assessing the relationship, the therapist may gain a one-sided view of problems and an overly negative impression of the partner. The therapist risks being triangled on the side of the patient in scapegoating the spouse or in futile attempts to change them. A prevention-oriented family consultation is extremely useful with the diagnosis or progression of a serious illness or disability when relationship imbalances and ongoing support or caregiving are likely (Rolland 2018).

Individual Systemic Therapy

Individual systemic therapy involves a conceptual stance incorporating systems-based thinking into individual treatment. This method is particularly useful for helping young adults and older adults to understand and repair wounded, conflictual, or estranged family relationships, to gain perspective and compassion for a parent's limitations, or to work on unresolved issues with a deceased parent. Coaching methods are used for individuals to become less anxious and reactive and more differentiated in order to change their own part in "stuck" relational patterns (McGoldrick and Carter 2001). The individual can be encouraged to gather information and broader perspectives from other key persons to enlarge their own subjective view. With the aid of a genogram to note systemic patterns and their context, the clinician and patient carefully plan meetings for change with key family members outside sessions and later process those meetings. Rather than attacking, blaming, or trying to change others, this approach focuses on changing oneself in interactions, which interrupts old patterns and is more likely to generate positive response and patient empowerment.

Multifamily Groups

Multifamily group interventions, usually with a psychoeducational component, have been expanded to a range of psychiatric and medical populations in inpatient, outpatient, and day treatment settings (Fristad et al. 2003; McFarlane 2002; Steinglass et al. 2011). Groups are typically composed of four or more patients with their spouse or with families, including parents, siblings, and significant kin or friends. Objectives include practical guidelines for crisis management and the improvement of communication and structural patterns to reduce interactional stress and to facilitate optimal functioning, coping, and problem solving.

The group context provides opportunities for families to learn from each other and to try new adaptive patterns of relating and handling problems. Family members can relate to the experience of their counterparts in other families, gain perspective on their own stressful situation, reduce guilt and blame, and feel less stigma and isolation. Family relationship change is less threatening with the mutual supportive network the group provides.

Multifamily interventions tend to have a short-term structure, varying from a single daylong workshop (McFarlane 2002) to four to eight weekly meetings. They may include monthly or occasional follow-up sessions. Psychoeducational groups have a strong informational component (e.g., teaching families about schizophrenia as a chronic biologically based illness and addressing related management and medication issues). Guidelines are offered for what to expect, common stressors, and ways to reduce tensions and support optimal functioning. This modular, time-limited format is particularly useful for a wide range of chronic psychiatric and physical disorders and life cycle challenges, such as divorce and remarriage, single parenthood, and bereavement.

Ongoing multifamily groups, often meeting monthly, are useful and cost-effective alternatives or adjuncts to other modalities, particularly for situations of persistent biopsychosocial strain, as with chronic conditions. They establish support networks that extend well beyond the group sessions with families facing similar kinds of challenges.

Combined Interventions

With the recognition that complex biopsychosocial issues are often not resolved by a single approach, combined modalities are increasingly common. For chronic conditions, such as schizophrenia or serious physical conditions, research documents the combined effectiveness of psychotropic interventions with individual, family, and group approaches (Dixon et al. 2001; Lucksted et al. 2012). Treatment models for substance abuse or for physical or sexual abuse also typically require a multimodality approach. For the safety of other family members, it is essential for addiction and abusive behavior to be under control before couple or family intervention.

One question concerns the advisability of combining individual and conjoint sessions with family members or relational partners. Many family therapists include individual sessions in their conjoint approach. During an evaluation, this allows the clinician to gain a fuller picture, particularly when communication is guarded or volatile. Sometimes, in the course of treatment, individual sessions can help overcome reluctance to dialogue with other family members. Likewise, systems-oriented therapists may include one or more conjoint sessions in the course of an individual therapy. Careful planning, timing, and focus are important. Inpatient or partial hospitalization programs with built-in time limits of treatment may make it advantageous for the same therapist to conduct a number of treatment modalities. Family treatments that are intended for supportive or psychoeducational purposes can more easily be carried out by the individual therapist.

A family consultation or treatment component enhances collaboration with complex treatment plans. For example, adherence to pharmacotherapy is facilitated by discussing the treatment plan with the patient and family together. This approach encourages support for multimodality treatments, thereby reducing treatment resistance.

Conclusion

In this chapter, we have provided an overview of family systems concepts and methods. In recent decades, the theory and practice of family therapy have expanded to respond to increasing cultural diversity, challenging socioeconomic conditions, varied family forms, changing gender roles, and the variable and extended life course. As the very definition of the family has broadened, so too has the practice of family therapy to encompass a wide variety of approaches and formats, including family consultation and brief therapy; intensive family therapy; family psychoeducation; individual coaching approaches; multifamily groups and workshops; and collaboration with school, workplace, health care, and other larger systems. In all direct practice, a developmental, systemic orientation is valuable as an integrative framework, fostering an understanding of each person in family and sociocultural contexts and facilitating respectful collaboration with families in clinical and community-based interventions for optimal functioning, well-being, and resilience.

Finally, our knowledge base and practice approaches are informed and enriched through the contributions of both quantitative and qualitative research on family processes and the therapeutic process (Lebow and Stroud 2012; Sprenkle et al. 2009; Walsh 2012). Given the broad diversity of families and their challenges, no single model fits all. Most important, at the heart of the therapeutic endeavor is our common humanity and compassionate alliance with the families we serve, supporting their best potential and positive strivings.

Key Points

- A family systems approach is a conceptual orientation to practice that can be used with individuals, couples, and families.
- Contemporary approaches are strength-based and collaborative, seeing the family as a resource in treatment.
- Evidence-based practices are used with serious mental and physical illness and adolescent substance use and conduct disorders.
- Systemic approaches include consultation, brief or intensive therapy, and multifamily group modalities.

References

Anderson H: Conversation, Language, and Possibility: A Postmodern Approach to Therapy. New York, Basic Books, 1997

Bertalanffy L: The history and status of general systems theory, in General System Theory and Psychiatry. Edited by Gray W, Duhl FJ, Rizzo N. Boston, MA, Little, Brown, 1969, pp 33–50

Boscolo L, Cecchin G, Hoffman L, et al: Milan Systemic Family Therapy: Conversations in Theory and Practice. New York, Basic Books, 1987

Boszormenyi-Nagy I: Foundations of Contextual Family Therapy. New York, Brunner/Mazel, 1987

Bowen M: Family Therapy in Clinical Practice. New York, Jason Aronson, 1978

Boyd-Franklin N: Black Families in Therapy: Understanding the African American Experience, 3rd Edition. New York, Guilford (in press)

Byng-Hall J: Rewriting Family Scripts: Improvisation and Systems Change. New York, Guilford, 1995

Campbell TL: The effectiveness of family interventions for physical disorders. J Marital Fam Ther 29(2):263–281, 2003 12728782
de Shazer S: Clues: Investigating Solutions in Brief Therapy. New York, WW Norton, 1988
Dixon L, McFarlane WR, Lefley H, et al: Evidence-based practices for services to families of people with psychiatric disabilities. Psychiatr Serv 52(7):903–910, 2001 11433107
Engel GL: The clinical application of the biopsychosocial model. Am J Psychiatry 137(5):535–544, 1980 7369396
Engstrom M: Family processes in kinship care, in Normal Family Processes, 4th Edition. Edited by Walsh F. New York, Guilford, 2012, pp 196–221
Falicov CJ: Working with transnational immigrants: expanding meanings of family, community, and culture. Fam Process 46(2):157–171, 2007 17593882
Falicov CJ: Latino Families in Therapy: A Guide to Multicultural Practice, 2nd Edition. New York, Guilford, 2013
Framo JL: Family of origin as a therapeutic resource for adults in marital and family therapy: you can and should go home again. Fam Process 15(2):193–210, 1976 1026439
Freedman J, Combs G: Narrative Therapy: The Social Construction of Preferred Realities. New York, Norton, 1996
Fristad MA, Goldberg-Arnold JS, Gavazzi SM: Multi-family psychoeducation groups in the treatment of children with mood disorders. J Marital Fam Ther 29(4):491–504, 2003 14593691
Goldenberg I, Stanton M: Family Therapy: An Overview, 9th Edition. Pacific Grove, CA, Brooks/Cole, 2016
Green RJ: Gay and lesbian family life: risk, resilience, and rising expectations, in Normal Family Processes, 4th Edition. Edited by Walsh F. New York, Guilford, 2012, pp 172–195
Greene S, Anderson E, Forgatch MS, et al: Risk and resilience after divorce, in Normal Family Processes, 4th Edition. Edited by Walsh F. New York, Guilford, 2012, pp 102–127
Haley J: Problem-Solving Therapy. San Francisco, CA, Jossey-Bass, 1976
Henggeler SW, Schaeffer CM: Multisystemic therapy: clinical overview, outcomes, and implementation research. Fam Process 55(3):514–528, 2016 27370172
Heru A: Basic family skills for an inpatient psychiatrist: meeting ACGME core competency requirements. Fam Syst Health 22:216–227, 2004
Heru AM: Family psychiatry: from research to practice. Am J Psychiatry 163(6):962–968, 2006 16741194
Hetherington M, Kelly J: For Better or for Worse: Divorce Reconsidered. New York, WW Norton, 2002
Hoffman L: Constructing realities: an art of lenses. Fam Process 29(1):1–12, 1990 2178969
Imber-Black E, Roberts J, Whiting R (eds): Rituals in Families and Family Therapy, 2nd Edition. New York, Norton, 2003
Johnson S: The Practice of Emotionally Focused Couple Therapy: Creating Connection, 3rd Edition. New York, Routledge, 2019
Kopelowicz A, Zarate R, Wallace CJ, et al: The ability of multifamily groups to improve treatment adherence in Mexican Americans with schizophrenia. Arch Gen Psychiatry 69(3):265–273, 2012 22393219
Lebow J: Couple and Family Therapy: An Integrative Map of the Territory. New York, Routledge, 2013
Lebow J, Stroud C: Assessment of couple and family functioning: prevailing models and instruments, in Normal Family Processes, 4th Edition. Edited by Walsh F. New York, Guilford, 2012, pp 501–528
Liddle HA: Multidimensional family therapy: evidence base for transdiagnostic treatment outcomes, change mechanisms, and implementation in community settings. Fam Process 55(3):558–576, 2016 27565445
Lucksted A, McFarlane W, Downing D, et al: Recent developments in family psychoeducation as an evidence-based practice. J Marital Fam Ther 38(1):101–121, 2012 22283383
Lyman DR, Braude L, George P, et al: Consumer and family psychoeducation: assessing the evidence. Psychiatr Serv 65(4):416–428, 2014 24445678

Madsen WC: Collaborative helping maps: a tool to guide thinking and action in family centered services. Fam Process 50(4):529–543, 2011 22145724
McDaniel S, Doherty H, Hepworth J: Medical Family Therapy and Integrated Care, 2nd Edition. New York, Basic Books, 2014
McFarlane W (ed): Multifamily Groups in the Treatment of Severe Psychiatric Disorders. New York, Guilford, 2002
McFarlane WR: Family interventions for schizophrenia and the psychoses: a review. Fam Process 55(3):460–482, 2016 27411376
McGoldrick M, Carter B: Advances in coaching: family therapy with one person. J Marital Fam Ther 27(3):281–300, 2001 11436422
McGoldrick M, Hardy K (eds): Re-Visioning Family Therapy: Addressing Diversity in Clinical Practice, 3rd Edition. New York, Guilford, 2019
McGoldrick M, Garcia Preto N, Carter B (eds): The Expanding Family Life Cycle: Individual, Family, and Social Perspectives, 4th Edition. New York, Pearson, 2015
McGoldrick M, Gerson R, Petry S: Genograms: Assessment and Treatment, 4th Edition. New York, Norton, 2020
Miklowitz D: Bipolar Disorder: A Family Focused Treatment Approach, 2nd Edition. New York, Guilford, 2010
Miller S, McDaniel S, Rolland J, et al (eds): Individuals, Families, and the New Era of Genetics: Biopsychosocial Perspectives. New York, WW Norton, 2006
Minuchin S: Families and Family Therapy. Cambridge, MA, Harvard University Press, 1974
Papernow PL: Clinical guidelines for working with stepfamilies: what family, couple, individual, and child therapists need to know. Fam Process 57(1):25–51, 2018 29057461
Robbins MS, Alexander JF, Turner CW, et al: Evolution of functional family therapy as an evidence-based practice for adolescents with disruptive behavior problems. Fam Process 55(3):543–557, 2016 27329051
Rolland JS: Neurocognitive impairment: addressing couple and family challenges. Fam Process 56(4):799–818, 2017 28887888
Rolland JS: Helping Couples and Families Navigate Illness and Disability: An Integrated Approach. New York, Guilford, 2018
Rolland JS, Williams JK: Toward a biopsychosocial model for 21st-century genetics. Fam Process 44(1):3–24, 2005 15807075
Santisteban DA, Coatsworth JD, Perez-Vidal A, et al: Efficacy of brief strategic family therapy in modifying Hispanic adolescent behavior problems and substance use. J Fam Psychol 17(1):121–133, 2003 12666468
Satir V: Peoplemaking. Palo Alto, CA, Science and Behavior Books, 1972
Scheinkman M: The multi-level approach: a road map for couples therapy. Fam Process 47(2):197–213, 2008 18605121
Shields CG, Finley MA, Chawla N, et al: Couple and family interventions in health problems. J Marital Fam Ther 38(1):265–280, 2012 22283390
Sprenkle D, Davis S, Lebow J: Common Factors in Couple and Family Therapy. New York, Guilford, 2009
Steinglass P, Ostroff JS, Steinglass AS: Multiple family groups for adult cancer survivors and their families: a 1-day workshop model. Fam Process 50(3):393–409, 2011 21884077
Szapocznik J, Williams RA: Brief strategic family therapy: twenty-five years of interplay among theory, research and practice in adolescent behavior problems and drug abuse. Clin Child Fam Psychol Rev 3(2):117–134, 2000 11227062
Walsh F: Family resilience: a framework for clinical practice. Fam Process 42(1):1–18, 2003 12698595
Walsh F: Traumatic loss and major disasters: strengthening family and community resilience. Fam Process 46(2):207–227, 2007 17593886
Walsh F (ed): Normal Family Processes: Growing Diversity and Complexity, 4th Edition. New York, Guilford, 2012
Walsh F: Strengthening Family Resilience, 3rd Edition. New York, Guilford, 2016

Walsh F: Family transitions: challenges and resilience, in Textbook of Child and Adolescent Psychiatry, 3rd Edition. Edited by Dulcan M. Washington, DC, American Psychiatric Association Press, 2022, pp 637–652
Walsh F: Complicated Loss, Healing, and Resilience: A Family Systems Approach. New York, Guilford (in press)
Walsh F, McGoldrick M: Bereavement: a family life cycle perspective. Family Science 4(1):20–27, 2013
Weakland J, Fisch R, Watzlawick P, et al: Brief therapy: focused problem resolution. Fam Process 13(2):141–168, 1974
Whitaker C: Symbolic experiential family therapy: model and methodology, in The Evolution of Psychotherapy. Edited by Zeig JK. Philadelphia, PA, Brunner/Mazel, 1992, pp 13–23
White M, Epston D: Narrative Means to Therapeutic Ends. New York, WW Norton, 1990
Wright L, Bell JM: Beliefs and Illness: A Model for Healing. Calgary, AB, Canada, 4th Floor Press, 2009

CHAPTER 20

Theories and Techniques of Couple Therapy

Jay L. Lebow, Ph.D., ABPP
Rosa Garcia, M.S.

Couple therapy has evolved in recent years to become a crucial intervention modality in mental health treatment. The words *couple* and *marital* are both employed to describe the full range of committed couple relationships, and thus the terms *marital therapy* and *couple therapy* are used interchangeably in this chapter.

Numerous sources contribute to the development of couple therapy. Foremost of these sources is the epidemic of relationship difficulties in couples. Epidemiological studies show that 20% of the population has significant couple distress at any particular moment in time (Lavner and Bradbury 2019). In addition, about half of all marriages end in divorce; 70% of marriages last a decade, and 10%–15% of couples separate within the first 4 years of marriage (Emery and Dinescu 2016).

These epidemiological data translate into a high level of demand for couple therapy to alleviate prevalent couple distress amid increased efforts at last-chance therapy to avoid divorce (Doherty and Harris 2017; Fraenkel 2019). The most frequent reason that people seek mental health treatment is relationship difficulties, typically so identified in 40% of patients (Gurman and Fraenkel 2002). When couples do seek therapy, it is principally for communication issues, problems in affection, and infidelity (Doss et al. 2004). Although once stigmatized, couple therapy has become widely accepted as *the* viable treatment for people experiencing problems in their relationships. The times have changed so much that there often is now a stigma when people choose to end their marriages *without* seeking couple therapy. In an international survey of psychotherapists, Orlinsky and Ronnestad found that 70% of therapists treat at least some couples (Orlinsky and Ronnestad 2005; Ronnestad and Orlinsky 2005). Although most couple therapy is aimed at distress, couple therapy also has substantial derivatives focused on prevention and enrichment in satisfied couples (Markman et al. 2019).

Another important basis for couple therapy lies in the individual and family comorbidities associated with couple distress. Higher level of work difficulty, increased health problems, and increased distress in children occur in the context of relationship distress, especially when high conflict is present (Whisman 2019). Research has established that the causal pathways involved are circular: psychopathology leads to higher rates of couple difficulty, *and* couple distress leads to higher rates of psychopathology (Whisman 2019). People who are relationally distressed have twice the rate of a DSM disorder (American Psychiatric Association 2013) compared with those who are not (Fiese et al. 2019; Whisman 2007, 2019). Whisman (2007) found that among individuals with significant levels of couple distress, 15% had concurrent mood disorders, 28% had anxiety disorders, and 15% had alcohol or substance use disorders. Furthermore, studies highlight the negative consequences of couple distress on physical health and work performance as well as in children (Whisman 2019). Given such well-established associations, couple therapy has also become an evidence-based treatment for people with individual disorders such as depression, anxiety, and substance abuse (Baucom et al. 2014, 2018).

As the need for intervention in couples developed and became more salient, couple researchers and clinicians have responded. Over the past 20 years, couple therapy moved from a backwater in psychotherapy to a field in which numerous well-articulated approaches have a strong evidence base for their efficacy (Gurman et al. 2015).

In this chapter, we provide an overview of the field of couple therapy today. First, we briefly review the history of couple therapy. Second, we explore current research on couples' processes that serve as the underpinning for today's couple therapy. A brief section on couple assessment is followed by a summary of today's most widely circulated couple therapies. In the final section, we summarize the evidence for the impact of couple therapy.

History of Couple Therapy

Gurman and Fraenkel (2002) described four stages in the history of couple therapy. Phase 1 began in 1929 and was characterized by practical advice giving. During this period, most clinicians did not label themselves as psychotherapists or even see couples conjointly. Phase II, psychoanalytic experimentation, began with both spouses in therapy treated by the same therapist concurrently but segued into spouses participating in conjoint sessions (Gurman and Fraenkel 2002). The interventions used were psychoanalytic and included free association, dream analysis, and introspection of defenses and unconsciousness. Phase III was marked by the family systems revolution, in which models of systemic therapy emerged, with subvariations focused on couple therapy. In its current phase, couple therapies has emerged as a distinct area of practice and expanded to include feminism, multiculturalism, integrative methods, and evidence-based practices.

Research on Couples' Process

Couple therapy has a crucial foundation in the science of couple relationships. Numerous findings from relational science inform couple therapy (Finkel et al. 2017). In this section we accentuate a very few of the most essential findings.

John Gottman studied the differences between satisfied and unsatisfied couples and how couples move toward dissatisfaction and divorce (Gottman 1999; Gottman and Gottman 2015). In Gottman's work, satisfied couples manifested higher rates of positive to negative behaviors in their exchanges when compared with the dissatisfied couples. Satisfied couples maintained a ratio of 5 positive behaviors to 1 negative behavior, whereas dissatisfied couples manifested a ratio of about 0.8 positive to 1 negative behavior. Gottman also found high levels of certain special behaviors in couples who were distressed: defensiveness, criticism, contempt, and stonewalling (which he called *the four horsemen*). The four horsemen often displayed nonverbally, manifested early within the relationship, and predicted subsequent divorce and relationship distress (Gottman and Levenson 1992).

Gottman's research also indicated that both unhappy and happy relationships have problems in the marriage that tend to be irreconcilable and stable over time (Gottman 1999). Gottman found that whereas satisfied couples learned to employ direct communication as a way to problem solve and navigate differences, dissatisfied couples became stuck in a repetitive cycle of conflict. Contrary to popular belief, this research showed that satisfied couples also argued but were able to resolve differences successfully. They also did not engage as frequently as distressed couples in rapid start-ups in which one partner aggressively began the conversation, followed by flooding and withdrawal on the part of the other partner.

Another important concept articulated by Gottman is *positive sentiment override* (Gottman 1999). This cognitive-emotional nexus describes the tendency to hold a positive view of one's partner and to override problematic views with good thoughts and feelings about one's partner. Again, satisfied couples tend to have high levels of positive sentiment override, whereas highly distressed couples show its parallel in negative sentiment override, in which even positive behavior can be viewed negatively (e.g., "you are just being nice to me today because you know I am angry with you").

Other research has demonstrated that unhappy couples are frequently stuck in a sequence of demand and withdrawal (Finkel et al. 2017). The sequence manifests as one partner tries to engage the other in problem solving, communication, or affection, and the other partner distances. Studies indicate that in heterosexual couples it is often the male partner who withdraws and the female partner who pursues (Eldridge et al. 2002). Distressed couples also have much higher rates of mutual coercion and violent behavior was than earlier thought (O'Leary 2008).

Such findings have led to a set of fairly universal process goals for couple therapy. Many quite different ways of approaching couples exist, but shared goals include ameliorating crises, providing a calm environment (where one can communicate and negotiate), increasing mutual acceptance, improving communication, improving problem solving, building attachment, enhancing marital friendship, and working with sexuality (Lebow 2014).

Assessment

Numerous foci exist for assessment in couples. Most obviously, there are the specific complaints that are the concrete focus of attention. The most common concerns clients bring to couple therapy are communication, problem solving, affective connection, sexuality, conflict resolution, violence, parenting, finances, and relationships with extended family. Clinical assessment moves beyond this level of problem assessment to examine the behavioral exchanges, cognitions, affect, attachment, and internal dynamics that become part of the formulation of what is at issue, leading to plans for intervention based in that formulation. As we describe here, different methods of couple therapy accentuate different key aspects in such formulations.

Several assessment tools are available to track couple process. Self-report instruments include the Marital Satisfaction Inventory-R (MSI-R; Snyder and Aikman 1999), which assesses marital satisfaction; the Weiss-Cerreto Marital Status Inventory (Weiss and Cerreto 1980), which assesses thoughts about terminating the relationship; the Dyadic Adjustment Scale (Spanier 1988), which assesses relationship satisfaction; the Conflict Tactics Scale (Straus and Douglas 2004), which assesses violent and controlling behaviors; and the Positive and Negative Quality in Marriage Scale (Fincham and Linfield 1997), which assesses the positives and negatives each partner feels toward each other and the relationship. More complex measures used in the laboratory focus on the observation of behavior. These include Gottman's Rapid Couples Interaction Scoring System (Krokoff et al. 1989) and the Marital Interaction Coding System (Weiss and Tolman 1990).

Treatments

Numerous couple therapies have been developed. In this section we summarize the most widely disseminated treatments and those with the strongest empirical support.

Behavioral Couple Therapy

Behavioral couple therapy (BCT) is a treatment with a basis in social exchange theory (Jacobson and Margolin 1979). The primary goal of BCT is to increase the frequency of positive behaviors by both partners on the basis of the principle that one person's positive behaviors influence the other, creating a circular and reciprocal sequence of positive reinforcers. BCT consists of two main components: 1) behavior exchange and 2) communication or problem-solving training. The goal of behavioral exchange interventions is to increase positive behaviors and decrease negative behaviors in the couple's daily life. Communication or problem-solving interventions help couples learn skills to help them resolve future problems. One communication intervention is the speaker-listener technique, a skill in which one partner expresses a thought, feeling, or emotion and the other partner restates what the person said before giving their own response. BCT has been widely investigated, and its efficacy has been demonstrated in many studies (Lebow et al. 2012).

Cognitive-Behavioral Couple Therapy

Cognitive-behavioral couple therapy (CBCT) adds a cognitive emphasis to BCT (Baucom et al. 2015). CBCT was developed in accordance with the belief that relationship dysfunction occurs in part because of how partners process information and how partners frame their thoughts about one another. The assumption is that in combination with changing exchanges as in BCT, once partners' distorted appraisals of events are altered, shifts in emotional connection ensue. CBCT distinguishes two different types of stress that occur in a relationship. Primary distress arises from unmet needs in the relationship such as autonomy, intimacy, achievement, and affiliation. Secondary distress describes the behaviors or maladaptive strategies that occur in relationships in which there is primary distress, such as ignoring one another and verbally or physically attacking one another (Epstein and Baucom 2002). CBCT targets both the exchanges that occur and partners' feelings in relation to those exchanges. Intervention targets are clear and direct.

Typically, CBCT occurs over 8–25 sessions of weekly therapy, but numerous successful randomized clinical trials assessing CBCT use fewer sessions (Baucom et al. 2015). Assessment occurs over the first two or three sessions, typically followed by a feedback session about the assessment. The therapist and couple then collaborate to define treatment goals. CBCT includes the full range of interventions from BCT such as the behavioral exchange techniques and teaching and practicing communication or problem-solving skills. Cognitive interventions include Socratic questioning and guided discovery. Socratic questioning centers on using questions to help clients understand their beliefs and assess those beliefs against some rational standard. Guided discovery creates experiences intended to shift each partner's perspective about the relationship. This can include role-playing or exploring the pros and cons of conducting the relationship according to each partner's standards.

CBCT has been demonstrated to be an effective treatment in numerous studies, both in improving relationship satisfaction (Lebow et al. 2012) and in the amelioration of individual psychopathology such as depression, anxiety, obsessive-compulsive disorder, and eating disorder (Fischer et al. 2016). This latter body of research has established CBCT as a treatment of choice for several individual disorders; the effects are most pronounced when there is co-occurring relationship distress (Baucom et al. 2014).

Integrative Behavioral Couple Therapy

Highlighting the limits of BCT and CBCT in achieving durable change, Jacobson and Christensen developed integrative behavioral couple therapy (IBCT; Christensen et al. 2014), a treatment that adds the concept of emotional acceptance to the framework of BCT. IBCT promotes mutual acceptance. Jacobson and Christensen theorized that in the early stages of a relationship, couples appreciate the differences in personality and functioning between them as the source of their attraction to one another. However, as time goes on, these differences can become sources of concern, even of discontent, and distressed couples may respond with mutual coercion, vilification, and polarization. IBCT helps couples navigate their differences by focusing on both the agent of behavior and the recipients of behavior. Increased acceptance is viewed not only as reducing conflict but also as a catalyst for positive change. Change techniques are directed to alter behaviors in the couple system. Acceptance techniques are directed to help soften the adversarial stance that partners can take toward one another. IBCT acceptance work attempts to turn areas of conflict into sources of intimacy and closeness (Jacobson 1992) instead of having resolution of all conflict as the end goal. This work has a foundation in Gottman's findings that many problems simply cannot be solved (Gottman 1999). Instead of aiming to resolve the conflict, IBCT "attempts to turn areas of conflict into sources of intimacy and closeness" (Jacobson 1992, p. 497).

IBCT therapists identify one central theme for each couple they treat, a summary of the main issue the couple faces in their relationship. From the IBCT viewpoint, as couples make efforts to change one another, a polarization process occurs, which serves to exacerbate the conflict between partners. IBCT therapists call the result the *mutual trap*, the hopelessness and frustration the couple experiences as a result of the defeat they face on trying to change one another. As part of their formulation, IBCT therapists are interested in the history of the relationship, the family-of-origin story of the individuals, and the romantic history of both partners.

IBCT provides four broad methods for increasing emotional acceptance: 1) empathic joining around a problem (creating intimacy by examining the problem together), 2) unified detachment in examining a problem ("taking a step back" to examine the problem as objectively as possible), 3) increasing tolerance of an aversive problem (e.g., by presenting the positive aspects of a negative behavior), and 4) increasing self care until the problem is ameliorated or alleviated (Doss et al. 2002). IBCT has a few state-of-the-art randomized clinical trials in support of the efficacy of this approach, and the therapy has been widely disseminated (Christensen et al. 2020; Lebow et al. 2012; Roddy et al. 2016).

Emotionally Focused Couple Therapy

Susan Johnson and Les Greenberg developed an experiential approach called emotionally focused couple therapy (EFCT; Greenberg and Johnson 1988). There are now two variations on this method. Johnson's (2015) EFCT emphasizes attachment in addition to emotion, whereas Greenberg and Goldman's (2008) emotion-focused therapy for couples emphasizes identity in addition to emotion. In this discussion, we focus on the Johnson variation, which is the more widely disseminated of the two.

EFCT focuses not on understanding the past but on shifting bonds in couples by restructuring and expanding their emotional responses to each other (Johnson 2015). The new secure bond helps couples experience a more satisfying way of interacting with each other and cope better with life transitions. Couples are encouraged to find opportunities to help soothe each other and heal through their attachment. Couples are also encouraged to explore their vulnerabilities together to increase their attachment to each other.

The EFCT therapist seeks to accomplish three main tasks. The first is to create a safe and collaborative alliance; the second is to gain access to and expand the emotional responses in the couple system; and the third is to shift the interactions through accessibility and responsiveness. The therapist uses techniques derived from humanistic or experiential therapy that focus on acceptance, empathy, and authenticity. The therapist serves as a secure base helping the couple shift to see the negative cycle as the common enemy rather than placing the blame on each other. A variety of intervention techniques are used to achieve the goal of exploring and reformulating emotion within the couple. The therapist may use heightening techniques, such as repetition, images, or metaphors, to help the couple engage in a constructive emotional experience. Examples include "So could you say that again, directly to her, that you do shut her out?" and "It seems like this is so difficult for you, like climbing a cliff, so scary." Couples also are encouraged to engage in the softening process, in which "hard" emotions such as anger are explored and shifted into exploring "softer" emotions such as fear, sadness, and shame that may lie behind the hard emotion. Interactions experienced in the therapy serve as the base to help couples be more open and vulnerable and, in turn, develop a more secure attachment to each other.

EFCT is usually delivered in about 10–12 sessions. Many research studies show EFCT to be effective (Lebow et al. 2012; Wiebe and Johnson 2016).

Object Relations Couple Therapy

Object relations couple therapy (Siegel 2015) is an offshoot of individual object relations–based treatment. In object relations theory the infant is seen as driven primarily by a desire to have a relationship with a nurturing figure. As the infant bonds, attachment develops. However, the attachment experience is inherently unsatisfying because the infant's needs cannot be met before they cause discomfort. In turn, the infant self is viewed as splitting into three distinct parts: 1) the central self, whose needs are satisfied and met by the mother, 2) the craving self, which is attached longingly and unsatisfyingly to an unavailable figure, and 3) the rejecting self, who is angrily attached to the rejecting figure. Object relations theory holds that couples seek lost parts of themselves in their spouses and that through committed relationships unacceptable parts of the self can be expressed vicariously. From this perspective, the success of the marriage depends on the spouses' ability to receive and return these projections to one another, as well as contain and modify each other's views of the self and the other (the object).

Object relations couple therapy provides a safe holding environment in which the couple is enabled to better understand their own defenses and anxieties and ultimately free themselves from the confining pattern of projection and identification. The holding environment provided by the therapist and interpretation of the mutual transferences that emerge between the couple are the major agents of change. Object relations couple therapy is typically delivered as long as necessary and may last years. Sessions often are longer than 50 minutes and may occur once or twice weekly. There is little empirical support for this approach to couple therapy, mostly because few studies of its efficacy exist.

Affective Reconstruction

Affective reconstruction (Snyder et al. 2008) is a pluralistic, developmental approach. It is centered in the notion that injuries from previous relationships follow the person into their current relationship and result in stress for the couple system. Partners develop defensive strategies in response to those injuries that interfere with intimacy.

Affective reconstruction is the interpretation of persistent maladaptive relationship patterns as having their source in previous developmental experiences. This process occurs in the context of a pluralistic model that incorporates structural, behavioral, and cognitive interventions. This therapy includes six fundamental tasks: developing a collaborative alliance, containing disabling relationship crises, strengthening the marital dyad, promoting relevant relationship skills, challenging the cognitive components of relationship distress, and examining developmental sources of relationship distress. Affective reconstruction affords the therapist flexibility to move in a nonlinear way among these six tasks according to the couple's needs and level of functioning. The average treatment length is 25 sessions, with each session lasting about 50 minutes. A randomized clinical trial of affective reconstruction (then called insight-oriented marital therapy) found the treatment to be efficacious, with couples maintaining change at 5-year follow-up (Snyder and Wills 1989).

Narrative Couple Therapy

Narrative couple therapy (Freedman and Combs 1996, 2015) is a treatment grounded in the belief that change happens when couples shift their view of themselves and others. This therapy is based in poststructural theory, which suggests people define themselves with the stories they tell themselves. Narrative couple therapy seeks to help couples create stories that better reflect the lives they want to live and the relationship they want to experience. Narrative couple therapists are not typically interested in the assessment of problems in a relationship, nor do they see people as having stable characteristics. Instead they are interested in helping people generate new stories about themselves and their relationships that invite the possibility for change and growth. These new stories help the clients empower themselves, spurring change and growth. Problems in a relationship are thought of as plots, and the problems are tackled by developing what narrative therapists call "projects" that serve as counterplots. Couples may identify joint projects involving both partners, individual projects to be addressed by one person, or both.

There is no specified treatment length for narrative therapy; some couples may take a few sessions to redefine their stories, and others may take years to explore and reauthor their own stories. The time, duration, and dates of the therapy sessions are also not rigidly defined. Rather, these structures unfold over time and are decided by the couple in treatment on the basis of their perceived needs at the end of each session. Although narrative therapies have become among the most widely disseminated couple therapies (Lebow et al. 2012), no studies of their efficacy have been conducted.

Integrative Systemic Therapy

Integrative systemic therapy (IST; Pinsof et al. 2015, 2018) is a psychotherapeutic framework that approaches problem solving by integrating individual, couple, and family models. Developed with the belief that each psychotherapeutic approach has its domain of expertise and that no single psychotherapeutic approach is sufficient to treat all presenting problems, IST offers a hierarchical approach to therapy whereby specific psychotherapeutic techniques are used sequentially. Therapy begins with the most direct and least expensive form of treatment and progresses to more complex, indirect, and extensive strategies if the previous methods have failed.

One of the key concepts of IST lies in uncovering a solution sequence that stems from an understanding of the problem sequence. The approach highlights six categories of constraints to problem solving that may need to be addressed: social organization constraints, biological constraints, meaning constraints, family-of-origin constraints, object relations constraints, and self-psychological constraints. IST also highlights the web of human experience, which includes social location and the influence of other systems.

IST progresses from the simplest to more complex therapist operations, from outside in, and from the present (behavioral interventions) to the past (analysis of childhood events and attachments). Movement from one set of interventions to the next one is triggered mostly by the failure of the earlier method to fully address the problem. Such progressions between intervention strategies are not always strictly linear;

instead, the therapist may move back and forth as the problem sequence reveals itself during therapy.

Just as the intervention strategies in IST are flexible, so too are the formats in which the therapy is delivered. IST can include individual and family sessions as well as couple sessions, and the length of therapy varies with the problem and goals of the clients. To date, only effectiveness studies (e.g., Knobloch-Fedders et al. 2015) have been conducted in support of IST, although IST is predicated on drawing primarily from interventions that already have a strong evidence base.

Feminist Couple Therapy

Feminist couple therapy has brought into focus issues of gender in couple therapy (Goldner 1989). Rampage (2002) states, "Although there is no monolithic feminist method of couple therapy, all feminist-informed approaches carefully attend to the ways in which power differences are manifested in the couple relationship" (p. 535). Feminist couple therapists believe that intimacy cannot be achieved without equality. The feminist approach considers power and autonomy within the relationship and aims to balance them in the system.

Other Couple Therapies

Numerous other couple therapies exist. Many have an integrative focus, combining ingredients of various approaches (Fraenkel 2019; Lebow 2014). Others focus on intergenerational processes (Baker 2015; Fishbane 2015) or mentalization (Asen and Fonagy 2017).

Therapy for Specific Relational Problems

Specialized interventions are needed when couples present with specific relational problems. Therefore, specific therapies have been developed for such problems. For distressed couples facing issues that involve sexuality, sex therapy is the treatment of choice (McCarthy and Wald 2016). Couples who suffer from the trauma and mistrust resulting from infidelity benefit from specific therapies aimed at addressing trust and forgiveness (Gordon et al. 2015). Special strategies are also crucial in treating couples experiencing significant couple violence (Epstein et al. 2015). The presence of violence in a relationship requires careful planning around safety, as well as an ongoing evaluation of whether couple therapy might place women at greater risk. Still other specific strategies are indicated to address couples struggling with one partner's individual psychopathology or personality disorder (see the subsection "Cognitive-Behavioral Couple Therapy"). Evidence-based treatments are beginning to emerge for each of these specific populations (Lebow et al. 2012).

Importance of Culture

In the past couple of decades, increased attention has been paid to the importance of various intersectionalities with relationships. These include racial identities, ethnic identities, sexual identities, and gender identities. Couples live in the context of belief systems and attitudes shaped by their communities and the world around them. Multicultural therapy considers how the intersecting identities influence their behavior (Rastogi and Thomas 2009).

One very important intersectionality in couple therapy focuses on gender orientation and sexual preference. Assumptions are often made in the transferability from opposite-sex couples to sexual minority couples that may be appropriate at times, but such generalizations may not apply in other instances. Important literatures have begun to accrue about helping both sexual minority couples (Green and Mitchell 2015) and couples from diverse cultures (Chambers 2019).

Ethical Issues

Ethical considerations are essential aspects of couple therapy (Barnett and Jacobson 2019). Couple therapy poses special ethical issues beyond those in individual therapies. Guidelines for confidentiality and record keeping must be directly communicated to each member of the system. It also essential to clarify at the onset of treatment who is considered the client in the therapy: the couple, each partner, or the whole family. A particularly vexing issue concerns secrets between one partner and the therapist. It is generally suggested that couple therapists refrain from harboring major individual secrets affecting a marriage.

The couple therapist must deal endlessly with interface issues in couple therapy and the impact of personal values in the therapy. One common example of such a challenge lies in creating therapeutic goals when partners have very different goals for their relationship, such as when one partner wants to divorce and the other wants to work on the marriage (Lebow 2015). Most couple therapists agree that it is a goal of therapy to try to maintain and build better relationships rather than to save them at all costs. However, there are therapists whose unyielding purpose is to save marriages; in contrast, other therapists place a greater value on personal rather than relational happiness.

Research Assessing Couple Therapy

Meta-analyses have demonstrated that couple therapy is an effective method of intervention (Roddy et al. 2020). Rates of success are essentially the same as for individual therapy, with three out of four couples improving their relationship in therapy. As already noted, more specifically, traditional BCT, CBCT, IBCT, and EFCT have a strong evidence base for their efficacy. Additionally, BCT and CBCT have strong records of positive impacts on depression, anxiety, obsessive-compulsive disorder, eating disorder, and bipolar disorder. Couple therapies targeted at individual disorders are of two types. In the first, called partner-assisted therapy, partners assist in the delivery of the cognitive-behavioral treatment for the specific disorder. In the second, called disorder-specific therapy, the relationship is primarily in focus, with the goal being for changes in the relationship to help in the process of change in the individual (Baucom et al. 2014).

One of the greatest challenges that couple therapists face concerns the high rates of recidivism in problems that emerge in research over the long term. The vicissitudes of life and the many transitions couples face throughout their life span often create conditions ripe for problems. A common approach is for clients to approach their couple therapy in an open-ended fashion and return to therapy if their problems resurface. Clearly, couple therapies must address the maintenance of problem resolution. Additionally, even when therapy is effective, many clients still experience some distress in their relationships. For example, Jacobson and Addis (1993) found in their quite successful behavioral couple therapy that only 35% of couples were without any distress at the end of treatment.

Conclusion

Recent decades have seen tremendous growth in the field of couple therapy. It remains an area in which researchers and clinicians continue to strive for greater understanding of the complexities found in human relationships. The goals of couple therapy include providing treatment to improve relational functioning and providing relief to those experiencing distress. It is a propitious time in the field of couple therapy, with research on couple processes relevant to practice blossoming and evidence-based treatments that point to effective pathways for change beginning to emerge.

Key Points

- As the need for intervention in couples has developed and become more salient, couple therapy has blossomed into a substantial field.
- Recently, there has been a movement toward integration of various treatment modalities for couples and use of couple therapy as part of multiformat therapies for treating individual disorders.
- Numerous couple interventions have been developed, many of which are now strongly supported by empirical evidence.
- Couple therapists have a unique set of ethical considerations to address as they strive to create therapy that is equally supportive of both partners.

Recommended Readings

Christensen A, Doss BD, Jacobson NS: Reconcilable Differences: Rebuild Your Relationship by Rediscovering the Partner You Love—Without Losing Yourself, 2nd Edition. New York, Guilford, 2014

Gottman JM: The Marriage Clinic: A Scientifically Based Marital Therapy. New York, WW Norton, 1999

Gottman JM, Silver N: The Seven Principles for Making Marriage Work. New York, Three Rivers Press, 1999

Gurman AS, Lebow J, Snyder DK: Clinical Handbook of Couple Therapy, 5th Edition. New York, Guilford, 2015

Johnson SM: Emotionally focused couple therapy, in Clinical Handbook of Couple Therapy, 5th Edition. Edited by Gurman AS, Lebow JL, Snyder DK. New York, Guilford, 2015
Lebow JL: Couple and Family Therapy: An Integrative Map of the Territory. Washington, DC, American Psychological Association, 2014
Lebow JL, Chambers AL, Christensen A, et al: Research on the Treatment of Couple Distress. J Marital Fam Ther 38(1):145–168, 2012
Snyder DK, Baucom DH, Gordon KC: Getting Past the Affair: A Program to Help You Cope, Heal, and Move On—Together or Apart. New York, Guilford, 2007

References

American Psychiatric Association: Diagnostic and Statistical Manual of Mental Disorders, 5th Edition. Arlington, VA, American Psychiatric Association, 2013
Asen E, Fonagy P: Mentalizing family violence part 1: conceptual framework. Fam Process 56(1):6–21, 2017 27861799
Baker KG: Bowen family systems couple coaching, in Clinical Handbook of Couple Therapy, 5th Edition. Edited by Gurman AS, Lebow JL, Snyder DK. New York, Guilford, 2015, pp 246–267
Barnett JE, Jacobson CH: Ethical and legal issues in family and couple therapy, in APA Handbook of Contemporary Family Psychology: Family Therapy and Training, Vol 3. Edited by Fiese BH, Celano M, Deater-Deckard K, et al. Washington, DC, American Psychological Association, 2019, pp 53–68
Baucom DH, Belus JM, Adelman CB, et al: Couple-based interventions for psychopathology: a renewed direction for the field. Fam Process 53(3):445–461, 2014 24773298
Baucom DH, Epstein NB, Kirby JS, et al: Cognitive-behavioral couple therapy, in Clinical Handbook of Couple Therapy, 5th Edition. Edited by Gurman AS, Lebow JL, Snyder DK. New York, Guilford, 2015, pp 23–60
Baucom DH, Fischer MS, Worrell M, et al: Couple-based intervention for depression: an effectiveness study in the National Health Service in England. Fam Process 57(2):275–292, 2018 29205325
Chambers AL: African American couples in the 21st century: using integrative systemic therapy (IST) to translate science into practice. Fam Process 58(3):595–609, 2019 31381844
Christensen A, Doss BD, Jacobson NS: Reconcilable Differences: Rebuild Your Relationship by Rediscovering the Partner You Love—Without Losing Yourself, 2nd Edition. New York, Guilford. 2014
Christensen A, Doss BD, Jacobson NS: Integrative Behavioral Couple Therapy: A Therapist's Guide to Creating Acceptance and Change. WW Norton, 2020
Doherty WJ, Harris SM: Helping Couples on the Brink of Divorce: Discernment Counseling for Troubled Relationships. Washington, DC, American Psychological Association, 2017
Doss BD, Jones JT, Christensen A: Integrative behavioral couples therapy, in Comprehensive Handbook of Psychotherapy, Vol 4: Integrative/Eclectic. Edited by Kaslow FW. Hoboken, NJ, Wiley, 2002, pp 387–410
Doss BD, Simpson LE, Christensen A: Why do couples seek marital therapy? Prof Psychol Res Pract 35(6):608–614, 2004
Eldridge KA, Christensen A, Noller P, Feeney JA: Demand-withdraw communication during couple conflict: a review and analysis, in Understanding Marriage: Developments in the Study of Couple Interaction. Edited by Noller P, Feeney J. Cambridge, UK, Cambridge University Press, 2002, pp 289–322
Emery RE, Dinescu D: Separating, divorced, and remarried families, in Handbook of Family Therapy. Edited by Sexton TL, Lebow J, Sexton TL, et al. New York, Routledge/Taylor & Francis, 2016, pp 484–499
Epstein NB, Baucom DH: Enhanced Cognitive-Behavioral Therapy for Couples: A Contextual Approach. Washington, DC, American Psychological Association, 2002

Epstein NB, Werlinich CA, LaTaillade JJ: Couple therapy for partner aggression, in Clinical Handbook of Couple Therapy, 5th Edition. Edited by Gurman AS, Lebow JL, Snyder DK. New York, Guilford, 2015, pp 389–411

Fiese BH, Celano M, Deater-Deckard K, et al: APA Handbook of Contemporary Family Psychology: Applications and Broad Impact of Family Psychology, Vol 2. Washington, DC, American Psychological Association, 2019

Fincham FD, Linfield KJ: A new look at marital quality: can spouses feel positive and negative about their marriage? J Fam Psychol 11(4):489–502, 1997

Finkel EJ, Simpson JA, Eastwick PW: The psychology of close relationships: fourteen core principles. Annu Rev Psychol 68(1):383–411, 2017 27618945

Fischer MS, Baucom DH, Cohen MJ: Cognitive-behavioral couple therapies: review of the evidence for the treatment of relationship distress, psychopathology, and chronic health conditions. Fam Process 55(3):423–442, 2016 27226429

Fishbane MD: Couple therapy and interpersonal neurobiology, in Clinical Handbook of Couple Therapy, 5th Edition. Edited by Gurman AS, Lebow JL, Snyder DK. New York, Guilford, 2015, pp 681–701

Fraenkel P: Love in action: an integrative approach to last chance couple therapy. Fam Process 58(3):569–594, 2019 31334852

Freedman J, Combs G: Narrative Therapy: The Social Construction of Preferred Realities. New York, Norton, 1996

Freedman J, Combs G: Narrative couple therapy, in Clinical Handbook of Couple Therapy, 5th Edition. Edited by Gurman AS, Lebow JL, Snyder DK. New York, Guilford, 2015, pp 271–299

Goldner V: Sex, power, and gender: the politics of passion, in Intimate Environments: Sex, Intimacy, and Gender in Families. New York, Guilford, 1989, pp 28–53

Gordon KC, Khaddouma A, Baucom DH, et al: Couple therapy and the treatment of affairs, in Clinical Handbook of Couple Therapy, 5th Edition. Edited by Gurman AS, Lebow JL, Snyder DK. New York, Guilford, 2015, pp 412–444

Gottman JM: The Marriage Clinic: A Scientifically Based Marital Therapy. New York, WW Norton, 1999

Gottman JM, Gottman JS: Gottman couple therapy, in Clinical Handbook of Couple Therapy, 5th Edition. Edited by Gurman AS, Lebow JL, Snyder DK. New York, Guilford, 2015, pp 129–157

Gottman JM, Levenson RW: Marital processes predictive of later dissolution: behavior, physiology, and health. J Pers Soc Psychol 63(2):221–233, 1992 1403613

Green R-J, Mitchell V: Gay, lesbian, and bisexual issues in couple therapy, in Clinical Handbook of Couple Therapy, 5th Edition. Edited by Gurman AS, Lebow JL, Snyder DK. New York, Guilford, 2015, pp 489–511

Greenberg LS, Goldman RN: Emotion-Focused Couples Therapy: The Dynamics of Emotion, Love, and Power. Washington, DC, American Psychological Association, 2008

Greenberg LS, Johnson SM: Emotionally Focused Therapy for Couples. New York, Guilford, 1988

Gurman AS, Fraenkel P: The history of couple therapy: a millennial review. Fam Process 41(2):199–260, 2002 12140960

Gurman AS, Lebow J, Snyder DK: Clinical Handbook of Couple Therapy, 5th Edition. New York, Guilford, 2015

Jacobson NS: Behavioral couple therapy: a new beginning. Behav Ther 23(4):493–506, 1992

Jacobson NS, Addis ME: Research on couples and couple therapy: what do we know? Where are we going? J Consult Clin Psychol 61(1):85–93, 1993 8450112

Jacobson NS, Margolin G: Marital Therapy: Strategies Based on Social Learning and Behavior Exchange Principles. Larchmont, NY, Brunner/Mazel, 1979

Johnson SM: Emotionally focused couple therapy, in Clinical Handbook of Couple Therapy, 5th Edition. Edited by Gurman AS, Lebow JL, Snyder DK. New York, Guilford, 2015, pp 97–128

Knobloch-Fedders LM, Pinsof WM, Haase CM: Treatment response in couple therapy: relationship adjustment and individual functioning change processes. J Fam Psychol 29(5):657–666, 2015 26376428

Krokoff LJ, Gottman JM, Hass SD: Validation of a global rapid couples interaction scoring system. Behav Assess 11(1):65–79, 1989
Lavner JA, Bradbury TN: Marriage and committed partnerships, in APA Handbook of Contemporary Family Psychology: Foundations, Methods, and Contemporary Issues Across the Lifespan, Vol 1. Edited by Fiese BH, Celano M, Deater-Deckard K, et al. Washington, DC, American Psychological Association, 2019, pp 445–461
Lebow JL: Couple and Family Therapy: An Integrative Map of the Territory. Washington, DC, American Psychological Association, 2014
Lebow JL: Separation and divorce issues in couple therapy, in Clinical Handbook of Couple Therapy, 5th Edition. Edited by Gurman AS, Lebow JL, Snyder DK. New York, Guilford, 2015, pp 445–463
Lebow JL, Chambers AL, Christensen A, et al: Research on the treatment of couple distress. J Marital Fam Ther 38(1):145–168, 2012 22283385
Markman HJ, Halford WK, Hawkins AJ: Couple and relationship education, in APA Handbook of Contemporary Family Psychology: Family Therapy and Training, Vol 3. Edited by Fiese BH, Celano M, Deater-Deckard K, et al. Washington, DC, American Psychological Association, 2019, pp 307–324
McCarthy B, Wald LM: Sexual dysfunction and couple dysfunction, in Oxford Library of Psychology. Edited by Sullivan KT, Lawrence E. New York, Oxford University Press, 2016, pp 83–95
O'Leary KD: Couple therapy and physical aggression, in in Clinical Handbook of Couple Therapy, 5=4th Edition. Edited by Gurman AS. New York, Guilford, 2008, pp 478–498
Orlinsky DE, Ronnestad MH: Current development: growth and depletion, in How Psychotherapists Develop: A Study of Therapeutic Work and Professional Growth. Edited by Orlinsky DE, Ronnestad MH. Washington, DC, American Psychological Association, 2005, pp 117–129
Pinsof WM, Breunlin DC, Chambers AL, et al: Integrative problem-centered metaframeworks approach, in Clinical Handbook of Couple Therapy, 5th Edition. Edited by Gurman AS, Lebow JL, Snyder DK. New York, Guilford, 2015, pp 161–191
Pinsof WM, Breunlin DC, Russell WP, et al: Integrative Systemic Therapy: Metaframeworks for Problem Solving With Individuals, Couples, and Families. Washington, DC, American Psychological Association, 2018
Rampage C: Marriage in the 20th century: a feminist perspective. Fam Process 41(2):261–268, 2002 12140961
Rastogi M, Thomas V: Introduction to multicultural couple therapy, in Multicultural Couple Therapy. Thousand Oaks, CA, Sage, 2009, pp 3–8
Roddy MK, Nowlan KM, Doss BD, et al: Integrative behavioral couple therapy: theoretical background, empirical research, and dissemination. Fam Process 55(3):408–422, 2016 27226235
Roddy MK, Walsh LM, Rothman K, et al: Meta-analysis of couple therapy: effects across outcomes, designs, timeframes, and other moderators. J Consult Clin Psychol 88(7):583–596, 2020 32551734
Ronnestad MH, Orlinsky DE: Comparative cohort development: novice to senior therapists, in How Psychotherapists Develop: A Study of Therapeutic Work and Professional Growth. Edited by Orlinsky DE, Ronnestad MH. Washington, DC, American Psychological Association, 2005, pp 143–157
Siegel JP: Object relations couple therapy, in Clinical Handbook of Couple Therapy, 5th Edition. Edited by Gurman AS, Lebow JL, Snyder DK. New York, Guilford, 2015, pp 224–245
Snyder DK, Aikman GG: Marital Satisfaction Inventory—revised, in The Use of Psychological Testing for Treatment Planning and Outcomes Assessment, 2nd Edition. Edited by Maruish ME. Mahwah, NJ, Erlbaum, 1999, pp 1173–1210
Snyder DK, Wills RM: Behavioral versus insight-oriented marital therapy: effects on individual and interspousal functioning. J Consult Clin Psychol 57(1):39–46, 1989 2925973

Snyder DK, Mitchell AE, Gurman AS: Affective-reconstructive couple therapy: a pluralistic, developmental approach, in Clinical Handbook of Couple Therapy, 4th Edition. New York, Guilford, 2008, pp 353–382
Spanier GB: Assessing the strengths of the Dyadic Adjustment Scale. J Fam Psychol 2(1):92–94, 1988
Straus MA, Douglas EM: A short form of the Revised Conflict Tactics Scales, and typologies for severity and mutuality. Violence Vict 19(5):507–520, 2004 15844722
Weiss RL, Cerreto MC: The Marital Status Inventory: development of a measure of dissolution potential. Am J Fam Ther 8(2):80–85, 1980
Weiss RL, Tolman AO: The Marital Interaction Coding System—Global (MICS–G): a global companion to the MICS. Behav Assess 12(3):271–294, 1990
Whisman MA: Marital distress and DSM-IV psychiatric disorders in a population-based national survey. J Abnorm Psychol 116(3):638–643, 2007 17696721
Whisman MA: Psychopathology and couple and family functioning, in APA Handbook of Contemporary Family Psychology: Applications and Broad Impact of Family Psychology, Vol 2. Edited by Fiese BH, Celano M, Deater-Deckard K, et al. Washington, DC, American Psychological Association, 2019, pp 3–20
Wiebe SA, Johnson SM: A review of the research in emotionally focused therapy for couples. Fam Process 55(3):390–407, 2016 27273169

CHAPTER 21

Theories and Techniques of Group Therapy

Seamus Bhatt-Mackin, M.D.
Molyn Leszcz, M.D.

What is referred to as *group therapy* is much more than one entity. Hence, an overview of the theories and techniques of the group therapies requires focus. A similarly intentional effort is necessary for the practice of group psychotherapy because, in comparison with dyadic work, there is more of everything in human groups. There are more interactions between members, more anxieties to investigate, and more difficulties to navigate. There is more content and more process. There is more affect to track. In addition, there are situations unique to this multipatient treatment format. For the clinician training as a group therapist, there is more knowledge to integrate and more skills to acquire. It is a complex therapeutic undertaking.

However, when a therapist can make use of the group, more collective resources are available. There are more points of view on any particular problem. There are more sources for giving and receiving kindness, more chances for therapeutic conflict, and more pathways toward a deeper understanding of self. In sum, there are simply more people to consider, and, as a result, more of the complexity that we generate in our interactions with one another becomes accessible in groups (Forsyth 2018).

Five questions focus our attention in this chapter. What clinical opportunities are available to group therapists and their patients? What are some core concepts of group psychology? What are best practices for group therapy? Which patients with what problems are best to refer to therapy groups? And how does one get the necessary training?

Opportunities for Patients and Therapists in Clinical Groups

For both patients and therapists, group therapy presents clinical opportunities that are similar to and different from dyadic treatment, as well as clinical opportunities that are unavailable in dyadic treatment. Seven key opportunities exist. Universality helps patients counter stigmatizing and isolating beliefs (Yalom and Leszcz 2020). Diversity allows for the investigation of similarities and differences (Agazarian 1997). The group's social context deepens self-understanding (Schlapobersky 2016). Giving and receiving peer feedback integrates interpersonal learning (Leszcz and Malat 2012). Imparting information and broadening knowledge about specific psychiatric and medical disorders and human psychology in general occur (Brown 2018), and experience giving and receiving support through altruism elevates self-esteem while helping others (Motherwell 2012). Therapists can capitalize on the efficiency of the group format (Kaklauskas and Greene 2020) and make use of peer consultation groups for emotional support, professional growth, and clinical accountability (Kassan 2010; Sayrs and Linehan 2019). These therapeutic opportunities are described with reference to common group psychotherapy models, illustrating the theoretical range available in the group format and giving life to the concepts.

Universality

"I am not the only one. There are other people like me."

Some therapy groups focus on the treatment of a specific disorder such as depression (Simmonds-Buckley et al. 2019), social anxiety (Barkowski et al. 2020), or borderline personality disorder (McLaughlin et al. 2019) and teach cognitive or behavioral skills (Bieling et al. 2009), which have been empirically shown to ameliorate symptoms (Linehan 2015) in the service of decreasing suffering and promoting well-being.

For these groups, the referral indication is narrow, sometimes even homogeneous with regard to diagnosis. When patients in these groups witness the participation of other group members and *see themselves and their problems in the other group members' problems*, they recognize that they have much in common with other people. This fact that we share a common humanity is referred to as *universality* (Yalom and Leszcz 2020), and the experience is qualitatively different from watching a major motion picture about mental illness, reading about epidemiology on a National Institute of Mental Health blog post, or getting the same information from a trusted therapist. It decreases stigma and feelings of social isolation.

Diversity

"I am different in this way. Anybody else?"

Some therapy groups focus on discriminating and integrating difference (Gantt 2012) in the process of moving from simple to more complex group work. Among multiple benefits, this creates the possibility that ambivalence can be held by the group—instead of being contained only within each group member—as described by the founder of systems-centered therapy (Agazarian 1997) and her colleagues (O'Neill et al. 2012).

More generally, by including in the therapeutic endeavor more people who have distinct aspects to their histories, their social identities, their cultures, and their points of view, therapy groups afford the opportunity to explore and learn from the social and cultural issues as they occur in vivo. We continue to learn more empirically and relationally about the complexity of cultural dynamics that occur in therapy groups

(Kivlighan et al. 2019) and the human systems in which they are embedded (McRae and Short 2009).

Social Context for Understanding and Change

"We can help each other to understand and change ourselves."

Some therapy groups make use of the social context and balance focusing on the individual member and focusing on the group as a whole. An example of this approach is called group analysis (Foulkes and Anthony 1957/2014), which combines psychoanalytic insights with an understanding of social and interpersonal functioning. Group analysis is the most commonly used psychodynamic approach to group psychotherapy outside the United States and Canada.

In this approach, the *group-as-a-whole* (see section "Core Concepts in Group Psychology") is viewed as an entity worthy of explicit focus alongside each member. The group therapist, called the *conductor*, contributes fewer explicit verbal interpretations and aims to address individual concerns through exploration of the dynamics of the *group as a whole* and each member's relationship to it, embedded in the larger social milieu and shaped by both conscious and unconscious forces. Many other theoretical and practice considerations have been developed in this rich method (Schlapobersky 2016).

Giving and Receiving Peer Interpersonal Feedback

"I can understand others. I can understand myself."

Some therapy groups focus on the content and dynamics of interpersonal exchange (Leszcz 1992). We know that feedback from a therapist is received differently than feedback from peers. The former can be dismissed or discounted. However, when the group member has an established relationship in an ongoing psychotherapy group with a peer group member, it is often possible to accept the very same feedback in a different way, even if it is identical in content.

Interpersonal feedback works best when it emerges from the patient's treatment goals, involves a self-disclosure risk on the part of the sender, centers on observable behavior in the relevant here and now in lieu of inferences to childhood, and occurs at the appropriate developmental stage of group life (Leszcz 2018).

Imparting Information

"I can learn that which I don't yet know."

Some therapy groups focus on imparting information through psychoeducation (Brown 2018). Content may be related to specific psychiatric conditions such as bipolar disorder (Buizza et al. 2019; Colom and Vieta 2010) and posttraumatic stress disorder (Herman et al. 2018), or it may also be on broader topics such as parenting, coping with chronic medical conditions, and bereavement. Psychoeducation is also often an integral part of group work that focuses on cognitive or behavioral skills. Even in a skills training session, patients benefit from the clinician's attention to group process and group dynamics in order to deepen support and engagement without attempting deeper emotional exploration.

Economy and Amplification in the Use of Resources

"We can do more with more."

For more than a century, clinicians have turned to group interventions when treatment need is greater than clinician availability (Burlingame and Baldwin 2011). In this way, the U.S. Department of Veterans Affairs health system has a long-standing commitment to group therapy (Greene et al. 2013; Powdermaker and Frank 1953). In our modern era of value-based care, in which health care systems seek to maximize quality of care and minimize cost, group therapy contributes to both goals, with improvements in quality and decreases in cost (Johnson et al. 2019; Olmstead et al. 2019). A major health system in the Midwest, when actively focused on effectiveness in their delivery of group treatment, reported improved clinical outcomes, fewer critical incidents, and improved staff morale (Whittingham and Graham 2018).

Psychotherapy Consultation Groups

"We all need support with our challenging work."

Effective and meaningful clinical group work is also helpful to practicing therapists (Kassan 2010). Consultation groups provide a range of functions, including emotional support, validation, connection with other therapists, and clinical consultation, and they support ethical practice and accountability to our patients and our profession. In addition, consultation groups offer a deeper promise (Hawkins 1998) in the opportunity to join together in difficulty, to deepen one's understanding of self, and to work on personal goals with regard to knowledge, attitudes, and skills, as well as making clinical work meaningful (Kassan 2010). These aspects of group work have been discovered and forgotten over time, only to be rediscovered (Herman 2015). For example, the dialectical behavior therapy (DBT) treatment team was originally developed as a means to maintain therapist fidelity in a clinical research program (Sayrs and Linehan 2019) but soon became valued as an intrinsic treatment component. This has evolved into an established set of principles, including group agreements (see section "Best Practices in Group Psychotherapy"), and one is not "doing DBT" if one is not participating in a DBT treatment team in the spirit of "therapy for the therapist." Other treatment models, such as psychodynamic psychotherapy (Counselman and Weber 2004) and acceptance and commitment therapy (Thompson et al. 2015), have their own approaches to psychotherapy consultation groups.

In presenting this collection of clinical opportunities, a few clarifications are necessary. First, some of the clinical opportunities described are also the therapeutic factors (*universality, interpersonal feedback, imparting information*) noted originally by Irvin Yalom, whereas other clinical opportunities (*diversity, social context, resource economy and amplification, psychotherapy consultation groups*) are not.

Second, we have chosen to use the term *group therapy* broadly to include skills groups, psychoeducational groups, and support groups. Some theorists, researchers, and clinicians embrace the use of the term group therapy, some avoid it, and some authorities in the field use it differently. However, we emphasize the importance of training in the core concepts of group psychology and the best practices of group psychotherapy for all practitioners who lead groups.

Third, this list is not exhaustive; psychotherapy groups vary in design (e.g., formal change theory, duration, size, time limited vs. open ended) and in practice (e.g., indication, member selection, group composition, interventions). Pluralism in the field is illustrated by a recent special issue of the *International Journal of Group Psychotherapy* in which 18 leading group therapists responded to the same clinical vignette (Shay 2017). Last, there is overlap in that these opportunities can be leveraged in multiple different treatment models.

Core Concepts in Group Psychology

Barlow (2013) has outlined specialty competencies in group psychology in the areas of assessment strategies, group formulation, therapeutic factors, leader interventions, and other areas. She recommends three basic questions that can help a group therapist generate a group formulation to guide intervention:

1. What is going on in the group?
2. What is going on in each individual in the group? (How are 1 and 2 related?)
3. Given 1 and 2, what do I need to do to be an effective leader?

In this method, the general principle that assessment precedes treatment planning in psychotherapy is expanded to include the level of the whole group. For this assessment to occur and to be communicated to others, we need access to core concepts to be able to speak to each other in a common language.

Imposed and Emergent Structure

Effective and meaningful therapy groups require enough psychological safety (Edmondson and Lei 2014) to engage with emotionally vulnerable psychological territory. In such groups, it is not possible to declare by fiat what will happen. Burlingame et al. (2004) have illustrated this fact by outlining two types of structure in therapy groups: 1) structure that can be *imposed* by the group leader and 2) structure that is necessarily *emergent* through interactions during the life of the group. In therapy groups, examples of imposed structure include selection of the leader, selection of the membership, location of the meetings, frequency of the meetings, and time boundaries. Examples of emergent structure include group process, group cohesion, group culture, and group development.

Group Process

Group process has been described simply as "what happens inside the group" (Beck and Lewis 2000); this is accurate but not instructive to the novice group therapist. Brown (2003) reviewed the use of the terms *process* and *group process* across 14 different textbooks on group counseling, therapy, and psychotherapy and found substantial heterogeneity in their presence and description. Brown offered a group process definition as "the here-and-now experience in the group that describes how the group is functioning, the quality of the relationships between and among group members and with the leader, the emotional experiences and reactions of the group, and the group's strongest desires and fears" (Brown 2003, p. 228).

Individual therapists are well acquainted with here-and-now experience, in contrast to "there-and-then" experience (sometimes called *outside the room*). Individual therapists are also experienced with the quality of relationships. However, the functioning of the group and its strongest desires and fears are not found in individual work. One way to conceive of the group as a whole is to imagine that *every communication from each group member belongs to every member*, as if one is overhearing a dialogue through the wall of another room, unable to discern who said what. When listening in this way, we can hear that each group member is speaking simultaneously for themselves and for the group as a whole.

Although some group therapists and treatment approaches focus on the group as a whole (Eisold 1985; Rioch 1970; Schlapobersky 2016), most group therapists learn to listen and communicate across multiple process levels. These process levels have been called the *intrapsychic* level, the *interpersonal* level, the *subgroup* level, and the *group-as-a-whole* level (Rutan et al. 2014; Tasca et al. 2014). Attending to group process involves shifting awareness across levels and choosing to focus on one or more of them in a particular treatment frame at any particular time with regard to intervention. Attending to the group as a whole is invaluable in identifying a potentially harmful group-level process, such as scapegoating.

Example of Group-as-a-Whole Process: Scapegoating

A group member arrives late repeatedly, skips sessions, or does not complete homework without explicitly taking responsibility. There are many ways to make sense of their behavior and many ways to respond. Other members may grumble about this form of participation and choose to not direct their frustration directly. *Scapegoating* can develop if the whole group comes to believe that "if only" that group member were "fixed" (or expelled), then the work of the group could "really begin" (or meaningfully continue).

In the psychodynamic frame, the scapegoating process is a form of collective projective identification whereby the denied and split-off aspects of self are projected onto the scapegoat. In this case, "what is disliked most about the scapegoat is also what group members dislike most about themselves" (Gemmill 1989, p. 409). As long as the scapegoat can be blamed, the group dynamics of that social system remain unexamined and unchanged.

Scapegoating can happen in therapy groups because it is the group leader who has the gatekeeping function; it is the leader who decides who can stay and who must go. It may be that frustration with the group leader is misdirected at a group member. The group leader's avoidance of aggression can increase the risk of its displacement onto other group members.

When scapegoating occurs, it is important to note that it is not something "done" to one person by the other members. Rather, it is a whole-group process that involves all of the members and the leader(s) (Scheidlinger 1982). From this standpoint, it is incumbent on the group leader to try to notice the existence of scapegoating as quickly as possible and to intervene and turn the group participants' attention onto their behavior, fears, and wishes (Clark 2002).

Group Cohesion

Similar to group process, little consensus on defining group cohesion exists; this is ironic given that group cohesion is the factor in group therapy that is most robustly correlated with positive outcomes (Burlingame et al. 2011, 2018). Group cohesion is highest when group members believe that they are "in it together." It is a construct with multiple dimensions (Johnson et al. 2005) that involve both emotional connection and the sense of task effectiveness. It is the force that keeps the group members engaged through interpersonally and emotionally challenging times (Yalom and Leszcz 2020).

Consider the following different settings where groups of people meet regularly to engage in a variety of activities: a morning commuter train, a homeroom in a secondary school, an office coffee break room, the operating room in a small hospital. Also consider some different groups of people: a study group in a school that is new to all the members, a cohort of psychiatric residents in their final year of training, a special forces military unit with a history of multiple combat deployments together. Each of these examples has different levels of emotional connection, sense of belonging, and task effectiveness.

Group cohesion is often described as the analogue of the therapeutic alliance in individual therapy (Malat and Leszcz 2015). In line with discussion of other psychotherapy common factors (Cuijpers et al. 2019), group cohesion functions both as a *therapeutic factor* unto itself through its comforting and valuing presence for its members and as a *mediator* that facilitates the impact of other factors.

Group cohesion should be distinguished from two other constructs—psychological safety and group climate—because they can covary together. *Psychological safety* is described by Edmondson and Lei (2014) as *the perception of the consequences of taking interpersonal risks in a particular context*. In some settings where competence is prized, it is interpersonally risky to ask questions. In other settings, it may be interpersonally risky to engage in disagreement or argument. It is possible to have high group cohesion—where the members have a strong sense of belonging to the group—and low psychological safety. *Group climate* refers to the atmosphere that is both created and experienced by a group of people (Kivlighan and Paquin 2014); it is a broader term that can involve either low group cohesion or high group cohesion.

Finally, it is important to note that the potential for adverse effects or harm is understudied in psychotherapy research in general (Scott and Young 2016), and this is true in clinical groups as well. High group cohesion can lead to adverse effects if the pressure to belong and fit in is oppressive and constraining (Janis 1982; Rovio et al. 2009). For this reason, it is vital to cultivate a health-promoting group culture.

Group Culture

Group culture refers to the explicit and implicit behavioral norms and conscious and unconscious core beliefs of a particular group (Yalom and Leszcz 2020). Once established, these norms and beliefs are durable and resistant to change. With regard to behavioral norms, consider different staff meetings that you attend. In some meetings, people are allowed to bring food and eat; in other meetings, this is forbidden. This is true with regard to, for example, time boundaries (e.g., it is permissible, forbidden, or forgiven to arrive after the agreed-on start time), attendance (regular vs. drop-in), and content. Beliefs and attitudes regarding authority, power, and conflict also vary across groups (Yalom and Leszcz 2020). Multiple strategies are used by group therapists to shape the therapy group culture (see the section "Best Practices in Group Psychotherapy," particularly the subsection "Consider Member Selection and Group Composition").

Group Size

Group researchers and writers have described three group sizes: small, median, and large. *Small groups* are groups in which face-to-face interactions are possible (e.g., the size of a reading group). *Large groups* are groups in which face-to-face interactions are difficult or impossible (e.g., the size of an audience in an auditorium). *Median groups* are between small groups and large groups (Lenn and Stefano 2012). Roughly, small groups are 5–10 members; large groups include more than 50 members; and median groups fall somewhere between. Similar and unique dynamics are present in each of these group sizes.

Group cohesion is affected by group size. Forsyth (2018) contrasts a 5-person group, in which 10 relationships are needed to connect every single member to every other member, with a 20-person group, in which that number of relationships rises to 190. Group psychotherapy is rarely conducted in large groups; it is much more common for large groups to be used for a deeper understanding of broader group process generally, providing a window into the impacts of larger societal forces at psychological levels, as occurs in the Group Relations and Tavistock traditions (see the section "Training in Group Psychotherapy"). Empirical support exists for a smaller group size in order to leverage small group dynamics. For example, a study of 329 work groups showed that groups containing 3–8 members were significantly more productive and more developmentally advanced than groups with 9 members or more (Wheelan 2009). The most effective psychotherapy groups meet with 7–9 members (Burlingame et al. 2018). Despite the temptation to maximize efficiency, health care systems cannot expect good results by increasing the numbers of group participants.

Group Development

It is clear to a casual observer that the dynamics that occur in the first meeting of a human group differ from the dynamics of a mature group. This phenomenon is called *group development* (a term that has its own set of associations through analogy to human development). Social psychologists and group therapists have chopped up these dynamics into different stages of group development, falling into one of three categories: progressive-linear models, life cycle models, and recurring cycle models. The most widely cited model, reported by Tuckman, was developed through a consensus of group therapists and likely persists because of its rhyming scheme and its kernels of truth (Tuckman 1965; Tuckman and Jensen 1977).

In Tuckman's first stage of development, called *forming*, the group members and leader(s) must address inclusion and exclusion, answering the question "In this group, who will be in and who will be out?" *Storming* occurs when the group members and leader(s) address role authority: "In this group, who will take charge and what will they take charge of?" In a subsequent stage, called *norming*, the group members and leader(s) address methods: "In this group, how will we work together?" After the work of forming, storming, and norming, the group attends to what the group members and leader will do together in *performing*. After the work is done, the ending is referred to as *adjourning*.

Adding to the complexity of group development, recent group therapy clinical research suggests that it is not always necessary to move through these developmental stages in the order described (Johnson 2013). However, understanding the stages is useful for group therapists to track unfolding group process. Any change in the membership is a new group. Given the complexity of interactions in small groups, this makes sense because in the new group, the stages of development occur anew.

Best Practices in Group Psychotherapy

Even before the group begins, the group therapist implements strategies to influence behavioral norms in the direction of a therapeutic culture.

Attend to the Larger System

Psychotherapy groups need support from larger systems to survive and thrive. Group therapists must provide education to colleagues about referrals (indication, inclusion and exclusion criteria, availability, meeting time and day of the week), must obtain and maintain support from influential decision-makers, and must evaluate the impact of their work on an ongoing basis. Without effort in these areas, it is unlikely the endeavor will succeed.

Make Use of Practice-Based Evidence

Support has accumulated for the use of selection, process, and outcome measures (Jensen et al. 2012) as a source of clinical guidance to supplement clinician judgment. Examples include the Group Therapy Questionnaire (MacNair-Semands 2002) for selection; the Group Questionnaire (Griner et al. 2018) for process; and the Inventory of Interpersonal Problems (Horowitz 1999) for outcome. Accessible reviews are recommended (Barlow 2013; Jensen et al. 2012).

Develop Proficiency in Diversity, Equity, and Inclusion

Conformity, unfairness, and systematic exclusion will persist without the therapist's active effort to counter them (Comas-Diaz 2012). It is the ethical duty of all clinicians to address gaps in awareness and understanding. For these reasons, it is vital for group therapists to become proficient at understanding the concepts of cultural humility, intersectionality, unconscious bias, social privilege, and microaggressions at both the theoretical and the practical level and know how to work with them in their groups (Barlow 2013; Kaklauskas and Nettles 2020).

Consider Member Selection and Group Composition

Individual assessment and case formulation are completed before any potential group member is *selected* to participate in a therapy group (Barlow 2013). This assessment bolsters the therapeutic alliance and helps the group leader to identify core clinical foci. In addition to decision-making about each individual member, a group therapist considers the *composition* of the group as a whole. This consideration will be influenced by the model of treatment and the imposed structure of the therapy group, including such factors as frequency of meetings, open versus closed membership, time-limited versus open-ended course of treatment, and homogeneous versus heterogenous membership (Kaklauskas and Greene 2020). In general, it is preferable to not have singletons along major demographic variables (e.g., gender, age, race). Even with careful assessment, it is not always possible to identify a "good enough fit" ahead of time, such that group therapists must feel empowered in their role to remove a member if this is indicated (Tasca et al. 2016).

Establish Group Agreements

Group agreements are the foundation of group relationships. Whereas the group culture is co-created and emergent over the life of the group, the *group agreements* shape group culture in the early stages. A primary task of the leader is to establish and attend to these group agreements.

Agreements can exist in many areas relevant to the group's functioning, including confidentiality, permissible and forbidden content, permissible and forbidden behaviors, nature of participation (drop-in, no miss), and the role of the leader. For open-ended groups, the group agreements need to be reviewed with each change in membership—even if the addition or removal consists of only one member—because the new collection of people is considered a newly forming group. For open-ended groups, guidelines about termination should be included in the group agreements.

Implement Pregroup Preparation

Pregroup preparation decreases unilateral premature discontinuation (dropouts) and increases the likelihood of a good fit between the patient and the therapy group. Pregroup preparation involves conducting a clinical assessment to determine if the formulation of the patient's problems fits with the therapy group that they will join. It also involves outlining the rationale for the group work and reviewing expectations about participation, such as a review of group agreements. If the patient is unwilling from the outset to state an intention to hold to the basic group agreements, it is unwise to include that patient in the group (Tasca et al. 2016). Meta-analytic reviews (Swift and Greenberg 2012; Wierzbicki and Pekarik 1993) show that patients drop out of therapy groups at a similar rate to individual treatment dropout. However, because dropouts from therapy groups occur with an audience, they have an impact on the remaining members that can be profound and demoralizing.

Consider and Monitor for Iatrogenic Harm

The potential for adverse effects from psychological treatments must be considered (Scott and Young 2016). There are no clear guidelines regarding whether a treatment is harmful, but this possibility must be considered by the group therapist. Outcome and process monitoring, such as formal measures to supplement patient verbal report and therapist clinical assessment (Jensen et al. 2012), can alert group therapists to struggling patients whose difficulties are outside the therapist's awareness (Yalom and Leszcz 2020). This area has been relatively neglected by psychotherapy researchers (Cuijpers 2019).

Integrating Group Psychology Core Concepts With Best Practices in Group Psychotherapy

In summary, imposed and emergent structures in small groups are relevant to building and maintaining effective and meaningful psychotherapy groups. Starting and maintaining a therapy group requires attention to the larger systems involved. Skilled group therapists use thoughtful member selection, deliberate group composition, pregroup preparation, and group agreements to build and shape the therapy group culture. Attention to group process at the group-as-a-whole level and to group development can facilitate group cohesion and assist early identification of scapegoating.

Indications, Efficacy, and Effectiveness

Who can benefit from group psychotherapy? This depends on factors related to both the therapy group and the patient. As reviewed at the beginning of this chapter, there is a rich diversity of group psychotherapy approaches (Shay 2017) that vary in design and practice. As examples of this variety, clinical indications can be framed narrowly (e.g., by DSM diagnosis, problem, or difficulty [American Psychiatric Association 2013]) with a more homogenous membership or broadly (e.g., "difficulties in interpersonal relationships" or "emotional dysregulation") with a more heterogeneous membership. Groups can be designed to be short-term and problem or theme focused.

Unsurprisingly, the narrow indications and homogeneous membership are more easily studied in scientifically rigorous randomized controlled trials, and, as a result, efficacy and effectiveness research is more available for these groups than for groups with broad indications and heterogeneous membership. Recent meta-analytic reviews support the use of group psychotherapy for the treatment of social anxiety disorder (Barkowski et al. 2016), borderline personality disorder (McLaughlin et al. 2019), depression (Simmonds-Buckley et al. 2019), substance use disorders (Lo Coco et al. 2019), posttraumatic stress disorder (Schwartze et al. 2019), and eating disorders (Grenon et al. 2017).

The authors of these studies universally recommend increased attention to group psychotherapy research. Group therapy is generally undervalued and underutilized (Piper 2008), although group therapy is valued and frequently used in substance use disorders. Wendt and Gone (2017) noted that although "clinical trial and EBT [evidence-based treatment] implementation research has focused nearly exclusively on interventions for individual clients, a large majority of real-world SUD [substance use disorder] treatment is in group format" (pp. 233–234). Similar to trends in psychotherapy research, the preponderance of research studies uses the cognitive-behavioral approach and is focused on specific disorders and outcomes. A small literature is focused on process-oriented group psychotherapy research—studying the how and the why of therapeutic change (Greene 2012). This is an opportunity for psychotherapy research in general (Greene 2017).

Training in Group Psychotherapy

Comprehensive training in group psychotherapy requires acquisition of interpersonal skills, conceptual knowledge, and therapeutic attitudes. It traditionally involves formal didactics, observation of an experienced group therapist, a personal group experience, and a period of clinically supervised practice in a professional program (Malat and Leszcz 2015). It is optimal to follow this foundational experience with ongoing peer consultation (Counselman and Weber 2004).

The practice of group psychotherapy is conducted by a range of mental health professionals, and each discipline has a distinct training pathway. For example, psychiatrists tend to start with a larger number of patients seen for a shorter duration of time, whereas psychologists tend to start with a smaller number of patients with a longer duration of time. Although these early experiences contribute to each therapist's learning history, the practice of group psychotherapy itself is also formative. Prominent group therapy organizations, such as the American Group Psychotherapy Association, are intentionally and consciously multidisciplinary in membership, leadership, and focus. Diversity of experience and different points of view are a strength of the multidisciplinary training environment.

Analogous to engaging in personal therapy during training (Habl et al. 2010), the personal group experience is a time-honored tradition with a range of available options. In psychiatry residency training programs, *T-groups* are process groups that study their own behavior in the here and now with a goal of increasing knowledge and understanding of interpersonal and group dynamics (Gans et al. 1995; Swiller 2011). Professional organizations (e.g., the American Group Psychotherapy Association and its regional affiliates) facilitate training through experientially oriented small groups led by a senior group leader; this form of training has been invaluable for many group therapists—both as a member and as a leader—to find their voice as a therapist (Gans 2015). Group therapy workshops sometimes include demonstration groups (called *fishbowls* or *bubble groups*) in which workshop members volunteer to participate in an observed group session in front of their peers as a means to better understand a new approach or to establish an approach to leading groups by an experienced group therapist (Gans et al. 2002). In some DBT programs, trainees attend the DBT skills group as a participant-observer to learn the skills and get an introduction to common practices (Sayrs and Linehan 2019). Finally, some group therapists participate as members in psychotherapy groups.

In addition to the group dynamics of small groups, group therapists must navigate larger social systems such as clinics, hospitals, health care organizations, and community agencies. The group relations tradition of experiential learning—as exemplified by the Tavistock Institute and the A.K. Rice Institute—investigates the dynamics of boundary, authority, role, and task (Green and Molenkamp 2005) in experiential small-group and large-group settings. In this method, group conferences are considered *temporary educational institutions* that are co-created by all participants.

Psychotherapy Groups in Residential Settings and Organizations and Online

Group psychotherapy is not restricted to outpatient face-to-face settings. In fact, despite the decreased length of stay, group work continues to be part of inpatient psychiatric wards (Cook et al. 2014; Deering 2014; Snyder et al. 2012), intensive outpatient programs (Schaffner and Buchanan 2008; Shaffer et al. 2019; Zalta et al. 2018), and residential treatment facilities (Hale et al. 2019; Magliano et al. 2016; Watkins et al. 2012). In addition, some leaders have made use of the large group for ongoing work with organizations at the level of the hospital (Peleg and Milstein 2018). Some empirical work (Falkenström et al. 2018) suggests a relationship between organizational culture and positive treatment outcomes; however, this area is underexamined empirically given the face validity of its importance (Shapiro 2019).

Although online forms of group psychotherapy have been available for decades, the worldwide coronavirus SARS-CoV-2 disease (COVID-19) pandemic has increased the delivery of mental health services online in general, including individual psychotherapy (Békés et al. 2020; Waller et al. 2020) and group psychotherapy. The enterprising group therapist learns from the established knowledge, skills, and attitudes of experienced colleagues (Weinberg and Rolnick 2020) and will develop new knowledge, skills, and attitudes to work further in this area. The use of video teleconferencing improves access to care and brings treatment right into patients' homes. Although teleconferencing provides less access to nonverbal communication and eye contact is lost on the screen, this mode of service delivery also provides more access to the fuller context of the patient's world.

Future of Group Psychotherapy

Group psychotherapy has a long history (Burlingame and Baldwin 2011; Malat and Leszcz 2015), with access to rich traditions (Eisold 1985), new knowledge (Kaklauskas and Greene 2020; Yalom and Leszcz 2020), and evidence-based strategies (Marmarosh 2018). The format of group psychotherapy is uniquely poised to interrogate and address in vivo the social aspects of mental disorder and relational difficulty at a time when the social impacts on cognition, health, and general well-being are abundantly clear.

Researchers describe the benefits of group work in the clinical and research literature with optimism. In addition to the therapeutic opportunities, real work is involved in building and maintaining psychotherapy groups. The American Psychological Association has recognized group therapy as a specialty that requires specific training and skill, and group psychology is recognized as a specialty by the American Board of Professional Psychology.

Engaged readers are encouraged to embrace two streams of writing that influenced the construction of this chapter: principles of practice developed by experienced group therapists (Gans 2010; Motherwell and Shay 2015) and empirical outcomes research on group psychotherapy (Burlingame et al. 2016). Both of these streams guide the novice group therapist in their development (Gans 2015; Klein et al. 2011), inform the experienced and evidence-based group therapist in their practice (Leszcz 2018), and move the field forward (Greene 2017). It is also recommended that group psychotherapists join a peer consultation group (Kassan 2010; Sayrs and Linehan 2019) or a training group (Hawkins 2000).

Key Points

- A wide range of treatment frames and therapeutic opportunities are available to the group therapist. Some of these therapeutic opportunities are uniquely available in group work.
- Group therapy makes efficient use of therapist time and economy of resources.
- Effectively facilitated consultation groups are invaluable for psychotherapists.
- Core concepts specific to group psychology include group process, scapegoating, group cohesion, group climate, group size, and group development.
- Best practices in clinical group work include attention to the larger system, use of practice-based evidence, proficiency in multiculturalism and diversity, thoughtful member selection and group composition, clear group agreements, consistent pregroup preparation, and monitoring for harm.
- Training in group psychotherapy has traditionally included formal didactics, observation, clinical practice, foundational supervision, personal group experiences, and ongoing clinical consultation.
- The treatment of most mental health problems is as effective in the group format as in the individual format.
- Group psychotherapy is filled with opportunities for clinicians, for researchers, and—most importantly—for patients.

Recommended Readings

Barlow S: Specialty Competencies in Group Psychology. New York, Oxford University Press, 2013

Bieling PJ, McCabe RE, Antony MM: Cognitive-Behavioral Therapy in Groups. New York, Guilford, 2009

DeLucia-Waack JL, Kalodner CR, Riva MT: Handbook of Group Counseling and Psychotherapy, 2nd Edition. London, SAGE, 2013

Gans JS: Difficult Topics in Group Psychotherapy: My Journal From Shame to Courage. London, Karnac, 2010

Jensen DR, Abbott MK, Beecher ME, et al: Taking the pulse of the group: the utilization of practice-based evidence in group psychotherapy. Prof Psychol Res Pract 43(4):388–394, 2012

Kaklauskas FJ, Greene LR: Core Principles of Group Psychotherapy: An Integrated Theory, Research and Practice Training Manual. New York, Routledge, 2020

Klein RH, Bernard HS, Schermer VL: On Becoming a Psychotherapist: The Personal and Professional Journey. New York, Oxford University Press, 2011

Kleinberg JL: The Wiley-Blackwell Handbook of Group Psychotherapy. Malden, MA, Wiley-Blackwell, 2012

Linehan MM: DBT Skills Training Manual, 2nd Edition. New York, Guilford, 2015

McCrae MB, Short EL: Racial and Cultural Dynamics in Group and Organizational Life: Crossing Boundaries. London, SAGE, 2009
Motherwell L, Shay JJ: Complex Dilemmas in Group Therapy: Pathways to Resolution, 2nd Edition. New York, Routledge, 2015
Ormont LR: The Group Therapy Experience: From Theory to Practice. New York, St Martin's Press, 1992
Rutan JS, Stone WN, Shay JJ: Psychodynamic Group Psychotherapy, 5th Edition. New York, Guilford, 2014
Schlapobersky J: From the Couch to the Circle: Group-Analytic Psychotherapy in Practice. New York, Routledge, 2016
Yalom ID, Leszcz M: The Theory and Practice of Group Psychotherapy, 6th Edition. New York, Basic Books, 2020

References

Agazarian YM: Systems-Centered Therapy for Groups. New York, Guilford, 1997
American Psychiatric Association: Diagnostic and Statistical Manual of Mental Disorders, 5th Edition. Arlington, VA, American Psychiatric Association, 2013
Barkowski S, Schwartze D, Strauss B, et al: Efficacy of group psychotherapy for social anxiety disorder: a meta-analysis of randomized-controlled trials. J Anxiety Disord 39:44–64, 2016 26953823
Barkowski S, Schwartze D, Strauss B, et al: Efficacy of group psychotherapy for anxiety disorders: a systematic review and meta-analysis. Psychother Res 30(8):965–982, 2020 32093586
Barlow S: Specialty Competencies in Group Psychology. New York, Oxford University Press, 2013
Beck AP, Lewis CM: The Process of Group Psychotherapy: Systems for Analyzing Change. Washington, DC, American Psychological Association, 2000
Békés V, Aafjes-van Doorn K, Prout TA, et al: Stretching the analytic frame: analytic therapists' experiences with remote therapy during COVID-19. J Am Psychoanal Assoc 68(3):437–446, 2020 32589042
Bieling PJ, McCabe RE, Antony MM: Cognitive-Behavioral Therapy in Group. New York, Guilford, 2009
Brown NW: Conceptualizing process. Int J Group Psychother 53(2):225–244, 2003 12712590
Brown NW: Psychoeducational Groups: Process and Practice, 4th Edition. New York, Routledge, 2018
Buizza C, Candini V, Ferrari C, et al: The long-term effectiveness of psychoeducation for bipolar disorders in mental health services: a 4-year follow-up study. Front Psychiatry 10:873, 2019 31849726
Burlingame GM, MacKenzie D, Strauss B: Small group treatment: evidence for effectiveness and mechanisms of change, in Bergin and Garfield's Handbook of Psychotherapy and Behavioral Change, 5th Edition. Edited by Lambert, ML. New York, Wiley, 2004, pp 647-696
Burlingame GM, Baldwin S: Group therapy, in History of Psychotherapy: Continuity and Change, 2nd Edition. Edited by Norcross JC, Vandenbos GR, Freedheim DK. Washington, DC, American Psychological Association, 2011, pp 505–515
Burlingame GM, McClendon DT, Alonso J: Cohesion in group therapy. Psychotherapy (Chic) 48(1):34–42, 2011 21401272
Burlingame GM, Seebeck JD, Janis RA, et al: Outcome differences between individual and group formats when identical and nonidentical treatments, patients, and doses are compared: a 25-year meta-analytic perspective. Psychotherapy (Chic) 53(4):446–461, 2016 27918191
Burlingame GM, McClendon DT, Yang C: Cohesion in group therapy: a meta-analysis. Psychotherapy (Chic) 55(4):384–398, 2018 30335452
Clark AJ: Scapegoating: dynamics and interventions in group counseling. J Couns Dev 80:271–276, 2002

Colom F, Vieta E: Psychoeducation Manual for Bipolar Disorder. Cambridge, UK, Cambridge University Press, 2010
Comas-Diaz L: Psychotherapy as a healing practice, scientific endeavor, and social justice action. Psychotherapy (Chic) 49(4):473–474, 2012 23205834
Cook WG, Arechiga A, Dobson LA, et al: Brief heterogeneous inpatient psychotherapy groups: a process-oriented psychoeducational (POP) model. Int J Group Psychother 64(2):180–206, 2014 24611701
Counselman EF, Weber RL: Organizing and maintaining peer supervision groups. Int J Group Psychother 54(2):125–143, 2004 15103999
Cuijpers P: Targets and outcomes of psychotherapies for mental disorders: an overview. World Psychiatry 18(3):276–285, 2019 31496102
Cuijpers P, Reijnders M, Huibers MJH: The role of common factors in psychotherapy outcomes. Annu Rev Clin Psychol 15:207–231, 2019 30550721
Deering CG: Process-oriented inpatient groups: alive and well? Int J Group Psychother 64(2):164–179, 2014 24611700
Edmondson AC, Lei Z: Psychological safety: the history, renaissance, and future of an interpersonal construct. Annu Rev Organ Psychol Organ Behav 1:23–43, 2014
Eisold K: Recovering Bion's contributions to group analysis. Am J Psychoanal 45(4):327–347, 1985 4083361
Falkenström F, Grant J, Holmqvist R: Review of organizational effects on the outcome of mental health treatments. Psychother Res 28(1):76–90, 2018 27012962
Forsyth DR: Group Dynamics, 7th Edition. Boston, MA, Cengage, 2018
Foulkes SH, Anthony EJ: Group Psychotherapy: The Psychoanalytical Approach (1957). London, Karnac, 2014
Gans JS: Difficult Topics in Group Psychotherapy: My Journal from Shame to Courage. London, Karnac, 2010
Gans JS: The insufficiency of theory: gaining one's voice as a group therapist. Int J Group Psychother 65(2):317–325, 2015 25760791
Gans JS, Rutan JS, Wilcox N: T-groups (training groups) in psychiatric residency programs: facts and possible implications. Int J Group Psychother 45(2):169–183, 1995 7759178
Gans JS, Rutan JS, Lape E: The demonstration group: a tool for observing group process and leadership style. Int J Group Psychother 52(2):233–252, 2002 11928201
Gantt SP: Functional subgrouping and the systems-centered approach to group therapy, in The Wiley-Blackwell Handbook of Group Psychotherapy. Edited by Kleinberg JL. Malden, MA, Wiley-Blackwell, 2012, pp 113–138
Gemmill G: The dynamics of scapegoating in small groups. Small Group Behavior 20(4):406–418, 1989
Green ZG, Molenkamp RJ: The BART System of Group and Organizational Analysis: Boundary, Authority, Role and Task. Unpublished manuscript, 1–10, 2005
Greene LR: Studying the how and why of therapeutic change: the increasingly prominent role of mediators in group psychotherapy research. Int J Group Psychother 62(2):325–331, 2012 22468578
Greene LR: Group psychotherapy research studies that therapists might actually read: my top 10 list. Int J Group Psychother 67(1):1–26, 2017
Greene LR, Harpaz-Rotem I, Sanders KA, et al: Group treatments within the Department of Veterans Affairs, in Handbook of Group Counseling and Psychotherapy, 2nd Edition. Edited by DeLucia-Waack JL, Kalodner CR, Riva MT. Thousand Oaks, CA, SAGE, 2013, pp 351–364
Grenon R, Schwartze D, Hammond N, et al: Group psychotherapy for eating disorders: a meta-analysis. Int J Eat Disord 50(9):997–1013, 2017 28771758
Griner D, Beecher ME, Brown LB, et al: Practice-based evidence can help! Using the Group Questionnaire to enhance clinical practice. Psychotherapy (Chic) 55(2):196–202, 2018 29863401
Habl S, Mintz DL, Bailey A: The role of personal therapy in psychiatric residency training: a survey of psychiatry training directors. Acad Psychiatry 34(1):21–26, 2010 20071719

Hale AC, Rodriguez JL, Wright TP, et al: Predictors of change in cognitive processing therapy for veterans in a residential PTSD treatment program. J Clin Psychol 75(3):364–379, 2019 30485430

Hawkins DM: An invitation to join in difficulty: realizing the deeper promise of group psychotherapy. Int J Group Psychother 48(4):423–438, 1998 9766087

Hawkins DM: Will the mother group have a face? The future of the facilitating environment. Group 24(2/3):193–201, 2000

Herman JL: Trauma and Recovery: The Aftermath of Violence From Domestic Abuse to Political Terror, 2nd Edition. New York, Basic Books, 2015

Herman JL, Kallivayali D; Members of the Victims of Violence Program: Group Trauma Treatment in Early Recovery: Promoting Safety and Self-Care. New York, Guilford, 2018

Horowitz LM: Manual for the Inventory of Interpersonal Problems. San Antonio, TX, Psychological Corporation, 1999

Janis IL: Groupthink: Psychological Studies of Policy Decisions and Fiascos, 2nd Edition. Boston, MA, Cengage, 1982

Jensen DR, Abbott MK, Beecher ME, et al: The utilization of practice-based evidence in group psychotherapy. Prof Psychol Res Pract 43(4):388–394, 2012

Johnson JE, Burlingame GM, Olsen JA, et al: Group climate, cohesion, alliance, and empathy in group psychotherapy: multilevel structural equation models. J Couns Psychol 52(3):310–321, 2005

Johnson JE: Beware of storming: research implications for interpreting group climate questionnaire scores over time. Int J Group Psychother 63(3):433–446, 2013 23734923

Johnson JE, Stout RL, Miller TR, et al: Randomized cost-effectiveness trial of group interpersonal psychotherapy (IPT) for prisoners with major depression. J Consult Clin Psychol 87(4):392–406, 2019 30714749

Kaklauskas JF Greene LR: Core Principles of Group Psychotherapy: An Integrated Theory, Research and Practice Training Manual. New York, Routledge, 2020

Kaklauskas JF, Nettles R: Towards multicultural and diversity proficiency as a group psychotherapist, in Core Principles of Group Psychotherapy: An Integrated Theory, Research and Practice Training Manual. Edited by Kaklauskas FJ, Greene LR. New York, Routledge, 2020, pp 25–46

Kassan LD: Peer Supervision Groups: How They Work and Why You Need One. Northvale, NJ, Jason Aronson, 2010

Kivlighan DM, Paquin JD: Whose perceptions matter more: mine or my group's? An actor-partner interdependence analysis disaggregating between-person and between-session effects of group climate perceptions on intimate behaviors. J Couns Psychol 61(3):333–339, 2014 25019537

Kivlighan DM, Drinane JM, Tao KW, et al: The detrimental effect of fragile groups: examining the role of cultural comfort for group therapy members of color. J Couns Psychol 66(6):763–770, 2019 31144844

Klein RH, Bernard HS, Schermer VL: On Becoming a Psychotherapist: The Personal and Professional Journey. New York, Oxford University Press, 2011

Lenn R, Stefano K: Small, Large and Median Groups: The Work of Patrick De Maré. New York, Routledge, 2012

Leszcz M: The interpersonal approach to group psychotherapy. Int J Group Psychother 42(1):37–62, 1992 1563903

Leszcz M: The evidence-based group psychotherapist. Psychoanal Inq 38(4):285–298, 2018

Leszcz M, Malat J: The interpersonal model of group psychotherapy, in The Wiley-Blackwell Handbook of Group Psychotherapy. Edited by Kleinberg JL. Malden, MA, Wiley-Blackwell, 2012, pp 33–58

Linehan MM: DBT Skills Training Manual, 2nd Edition. New York, Guilford, 2015

Lo Coco G, Melchiori F, Oieni V, et al: Group treatment for substance use disorder in adults: a systematic review and meta-analysis of randomized-controlled trials. J Subst Abuse Treat 99:104–116, 2019 30797382

MacNair-Semands RR: Predicting attendance and expectations for group therapy. Group Dyn 6(3):219–228, 2002
Magliano L, Puviani M, Rega S, et al: Feasibility and effectiveness of a combined individual and psychoeducational group intervention in psychiatric residential facilities: a controlled, non-randomized study. Psychiatry Res 235(235):19–28, 2016 26723137
Malat J, Leszcz M: Group Psychotherapy, in Psychiatry, 4th Edition. Edited by Tasman A, Kay J, Lieberman JA, et al. New York, Wiley, 2015
Marmarosh CL: Introduction to special issue: feedback in group psychotherapy. Psychotherapy (Chic) 55(2):101–104, 2018 29863390
McLaughlin SPB, Barkowski S, Burlingame GM, et al: Group psychotherapy for borderline personality disorder: a meta-analysis of randomized-controlled trials. Psychotherapy (Chic) 56(2):260–273, 2019 30869973
McRae MB, Short EL: Racial and Cultural Dynamics in Group and Organizational Life: Crossing Boundaries. London, Sage, 2009
Motherwell L: Support and process-oriented therapy groups, in The Wiley-Blackwell Handbook of Group Psychotherapy, 1st Edition. Edited by Kleinberg JL. West Sussex, UK, Wiley-Blackwell, 2012, pp 275–298
Motherwell L, Shay JJ: Complex Dilemmas in Group Therapy: Pathways to Resolution, 2nd Edition. New York, Routledge, 2015
Olmstead TA, Graff FS, Ames-Sikora A, et al: Cost-effectiveness of individual versus group female-specific cognitive behavioral therapy for alcohol use disorder. J Subst Abuse Treat 100:1–7, 2019 30898323
O'Neill RM, Constantino MJ, Mogle J: Does Agazarian's systems-centered functional subgrouping improve mood, learning and goal achievement? A study in large groups. Group Analysis 45(3):375–390, 2012
Peleg I, Milstein MJ: On conducting an ongoing large staff group in a psychiatric hospital. Group Analysis 52(1):65–81, 2018
Piper WE: Underutilization of short-term group therapy: enigmatic or understandable? Psychother Res 18(2):127–138, 2008 18815970
Powdermaker FB, Frank JD: Group Psychotherapy Studies in Methodology of Research and Therapy: A Report of the Group Psychotherapy Research Project of the U.S. Veterans Administration. Cambridge, MA, Harvard University Press, 1953
Rioch MJ: The work of Wilfred Bion on groups. Psychiatry 33(1):56–66, 1970 4906171
Rovio E, Eskola J, Kozub SA, et al: Can high group cohesion be harmful? A case study of a junior ice-hockey team. Small Group Research 40(4):421–435, 2009
Rutan JS, Stone WN, Shay JJ: Psychodynamic Group Psychotherapy, 5th Edition. New York, Guilford, 2014
Sayrs JHR, Linehan MM: DBT Teams: Development and Practice. New York, Guilford, 2019
Schaffner AD, Buchanan LP: Integrating evidence-based treatments with individual needs in an outpatient facility for eating disorders. Eat Disord 16(5):378–392, 2008 18821362
Scheidlinger S: Presidential address: on scapegoating in group psychotherapy. Int J Group Psychother 32(2):131–143, 1982 7095934
Schlapobersky J: From the Couch to the Circle: Group-Analytic Psychotherapy in Practice. New York, Routledge, 2016
Schwartze D, Barkowski S, Strauss B, et al: Efficacy of group psychotherapy for posttraumatic stress disorder: systematic review and meta-analysis of randomized controlled trials. Psychother Res 29(4):415–431, 2019 29179647
Scott J, Young AH: Psychotherapies should be assessed for both benefit and harm. Br J Psychiatry 208(3):208–209, 2016 26932480
Shaffer RC, Wink LK, Ruberg J, et al: Emotion regulation intensive outpatient programming: development, feasibility, and acceptability. J Autism Dev Disord 49(2):495–508, 2019 30143951
Shapiro ER: Finding a Place to Stand: Developing Self-Reflective Institutions, Leaders, and Citizens. London, Phoenix, 2019

Shay JJ: Contemporary models of group therapy: where are we today? Int J Group Psychother 67(S1):S7–S12, 2017
Simmonds-Buckley M, Kellett S, Waller G: Acceptability and efficacy of group behavioral activation for depression among adults: a meta-analysis. Behav Ther 50(5):864–885, 2019 31422844
Snyder JA, Clark LM, Jones NT: Provision and adaptation of group treatment in state psychiatric hospitals. Prof Psychol Res Pr 43(4):395–402, 2012
Swift JK, Greenberg RP: Premature discontinuation in adult psychotherapy: a meta-analysis. J Consult Clin Psychol 80(4):547–559, 2012 22506792
Swiller HI: Process groups. Int J Group Psychother 61(2):262–273, 2011 21463097
Tasca GA, Francis K, Balfour L: Group psychotherapy levels of interventions: a clinical process commentary. Psychotherapy (Chic) 51(1):25–29, 2014 24059738
Tasca GA, Mcquaid N, Balfour L: Complex contexts and relationships affect clinical decisions in group therapy. Psychotherapy (Chic) 53(3):314–319, 2016 27631861
Thompson BL, Luomo JB, Terry C, et al: Creating a peer-led acceptance and commitment therapy consultation group: the Portland model. J Contextual Behav Sci 4(3):144–150, 2015
Tuckman BW: Development sequence in small groups. Psychol Bull 63:384–399, 1965 14314073
Tuckman BW, Jensen M: Stages of small-group development revisited. Group and Organization Studies 2(4):419–427, 1977
Waller G, Pugh M, Mulkens S, et al: Cognitive-behavioral therapy in the time of coronavirus: clinician tips for working with eating disorders via telehealth when face-to-face meetings are not possible. Int J Eat Disord 53(7):1132–1141, 2020 32383530
Watkins KE, Hunter S, Hepner K, et al: Group cognitive-behavioral therapy for clients with major depression in residential substance abuse treatment. Psychiatr Serv 63(6):608–611, 2012 22638007
Weinberg H, Rolnick A: Theory and Practice of Online Therapy. New York, Routledge, 2020
Wendt DC, Gone JP: Group therapy for substance use disorders: a survey of clinician practices. J Groups Addict Recovery 12(4):243–259, 2017 30546274
Wheelan S: Group size, group development, and group productivity. Small Group Res 40(2):247–262, 2009
Whittingham M, Graham L: The impact of providing group performance feedback on a large mental health system. Psychotherapy (Chic) 55(2):203–206, 2018 29863402
Wierzbicki M, Pekarik G: A Meta-analysis of psychotherapy dropout. Prof Psychol Res Pract 24(2):190–195, 1993
Yalom ID, Leszcz M: The Theory and Practice of Group Psychotherapy, 6th Edition. New York, Basic Books, 2020
Zalta AK, Held P, Smith DL, et al: Evaluating patterns and predictors of symptom change during a three-week intensive outpatient treatment for veterans with PTSD. BMC Psychiatry 18(1):242, 2018 30053860

PART VII

Racial and Ethnic Diversities in Psychotherapy

Section Editor: Dionne R. Powell, M.D.

Throughout the history of psychotherapy a panoply of treatment options have been available for clinicians, from psychodynamic treatments to cognitive-behavioral therapy; interpersonal, dialectical, and transference-focused psychotherapy; and supportive therapies, to name a few. Although the treatment options are rich and varied, mental health clinicians have paid less attention to the cultural, ethnic, and racial variables of their patients as essential to clinical understanding and therapeutic success. (A list of those who have written from various disciplines can be found throughout this section). It is as if one psychotherapeutic treatment is applicable to a specific generic population without regard to the cultural, ethnic, and racial makeup of the patient. However, clinicians should be asking several questions related to the diversity of their patients. How do patients from marginalized or nonmajority populations experience mental health care? How can clinicians address differences in the patient populations they treat? Individuals who decide to train to become psychiatrists, psychologists, social workers, and mental health professionals should be aware of the impacts that cultural, ethnic, and racial sensitivity on the part of the clinician can have on the patient's inclination to pursue and participate in mental health treatment. The therapeutic fit between patient and clinician is potentially affected by the cultural, ethnic, and racial identities of the participants. This section is an attempt to articulate and integrate cultural and ethnic diversities into the psychotherapeutic milieu.

In this section, the chapter authors refute the notion of "cultural competence" because it narrows and provides a superficial lens through which people are viewed as being "other," devoid of the rich cultural and ethnic challenges and signifiers, including one's community of origin, that shape us all. For instance, mental health trainees (psychologists, social workers, psychiatrists) are not taught "white competence," thus enforcing the systemic institutionalized racism that has adversely affected the field, suggesting that a diversity course or seminar is sufficient for "competency" when it comes to the other. There is an embedded notion that white trainees and clinicians have attained competence in treatment of white patients, and that it is only the other, the racial stranger, that requires explication. The trouble and tensions involved in this approach are part of the challenges of modern society (Gladwell 2019; Metzl 2019). In each chapter in this section, the authors implicitly or explicitly highlight the common theme of "whiteness" as an impediment to acceptance within American society for people of color. What we consider commonplace—whiteness, Blackness, otherness—is an American narrative fiction created for societal divisiveness as power is held within narrow, primarily European male descendant, groups. Attacks on Asian Americans during the coronavirus SARS-CoV-2 disease (COVID-19) pandemic; Black and brown congresswomen shouted at to return to their native country; and Blacks who call the police for their mentally ill family member, only for them to be killed, are all examples of the projective use of nonwhiteness in the United States to defensively justify prejudice, discrimination, supremacy, and—too many times—death (Asian Pacific Policy and Planning Council 2020; Rogers and Fandos 2019; Tessler et al. 2020; Wilson et al. 2020).

Sociologist Eduardo Bonilla-Silva provides the following clarification: "Racism is the product of racial domination projects (e.g., colonialism, slavery, labor migration, etc.)," and once this form of social organization emerged in human history, it became embedded in societies (Bonilla-Silva 2015, p. 2). Therefore, he argues, "racism creates race" in that the structuralizing institutions of colonialism and slavery promoted societal categorization based on one's closeness to a white ideal (Bonilla-Silva 2015, p. 2). Beverly Stoute in her chapter within this section provides the important distinction: "The term *race*, to be clear, refers to a social, political, and cultural identification that, although phenotypically correlated with skin color, has no clear biological correlate" (Chapter 26, "How Our Mind Becomes Racialized: Implications for the Therapeutic Encounter, p. 597).

Every aspect of mental health training is affected by systemic institutionalized racism and the racist states of mind that we all inhabit (Keval 2016). In the twenty-first century, to be a competent clinician requires cultural humility, informed inquiry, and open curiosity about one's internalized views about the familiar and the other and how these views shape the therapeutic alliance, countertransference, and one's affective states. This type of exploration can occur within the clinician's own treatment or in a racial and cultural experiential group (e.g., workshop on white fragility) or study groups on race, culture, and whiteness. Some authors emphasize the value of mentalization and the development of racial reflective functioning as an effective approach to remain present with one's patient and not be subsumed by one's prejudices, biases, and assumptions about the racial other (Fonagy et al. 2002). It is this cultural and ethnic milieu of our patients and of mental health trainees that we seek to address in this section, which should serve as an invitation to engage and improve the depth of the therapeutic process for all our patients and to create welcoming environments for all trainees.

Unfortunately, for people of color, the history of mental health treatment has not been an open and welcoming one. Numerous historical falsehoods about people of color—that their mental capacities were inferior, that they had poor intelligence, that they lacked reflective functioning—and overdiagnoses in the psychotic sphere were promulgated by psychologists and psychiatrists in society and training institutions. This has had lasting effects on the relationship between mental health services and communities of color. Many potential patients of color (close to 50%) drop out of treatment after one session (Sue and Sue 1999). And increasingly, clinicians of color are leaving academic institutions as a result of lack of advancement in an arena of unmitigated racial and sexual microaggressions (Anushri Anandaraja 2020; Lee 2019; Shim 2020; Wadman 2019). This fact suggests that there is a lack of cultural attunement and humility on the part of clinicians when engaged with patients, trainees, and faculty of color. As long as whites continue to remain homogeneous in their social groupings and there is a paucity of clinicians of color in the mental health field, a treatment gap will remain for those people and communities of color who seek care with a clinician from their own racial or cultural group (Chang 2018).

In addition, for clinicians who enter the mental health field, there is an absence of integrated knowledge on how to approach patients of diverse cultural, ethnic, and racial backgrounds. This absence is particularly devastating for the clinician of color and others who recognize that patients seek mental health care on the basis of their unique history, which includes race, ethnicity, and culture. Clinicians need education regarding this vital component of patients' lives.

Mental health services are in increasingly short supply, which occurs simultaneously with an increasingly diverse population in need. To place the need for improved representation in the mental health field in context, we provide the following grim statistics: African Americans make up 13% of the U.S. population yet only 2% of the psychiatrists in the American Psychiatric Association (2020 data) and 5.3% of active psychologists; Asian Americans (both East and South Asians) represent 5.6% of the U.S. population and 4.3% of the active psychology workforce (2013 data); and Latinx individuals represent 18% of the U.S. population but only 5% of active clinical psychologists and psychiatrists. This is far less diverse than the U.S. population (Luona et al. 2018; Shim 2021; Warner 2021).

How can we cover the diversity of three-fourths of the planet in five chapters? We start by acknowledging that we cannot. Rather, we have asked our writers to think deeply about the collective cultural and ethnic experiences within the United States that would be of benefit to clinicians attempting to enhance their understanding of the identities, unique cultural signifiers, and features that may enhance the therapeutic encounter and clinicians' ability to practice cultural humility, therefore improving the therapeutic experience. We have also asked them to consider the challenges for clinicians wanting to enter the field that continue throughout their training. We are fortunate to have eight clinician-scholars who have thought and written about people of color as part of their academic lives. Each brings their unique perspective to the training and treatment of people of color. Each chapter serves as a cultural, racial, and ethnic metaphor for the diversity within specific groupings. For instance, the authors of each chapter convey the context of otherness as specific to their voice and theoretical position: Other as a racialized self, unique and specific from gender, the sexualities, or religion, emphasizing that within a racist society Other connotes an immediate pejorative difference of exclusion. Some authors in this section do not use an uppercase O for other and have their unique perspective when thinking and writing about race and ethnicities. In both content and context we are attempting to convey the diversity of thoughtfulness when considering such complex and emotionally charged subjects as the racial ethnic and hope that stimulates readers' thinking as well.

The section begins with Anton Hart and my writing about the psychotherapeutic treatment of African Americans. For the African American population, acknowledging the diversities inherent within each cultural and ethnic grouping includes the profound effects of the slave trade and individuals who immigrated to the United States, including those from Africa, the Caribbean, and South America. Jasmine Ueng-McHale and Calvin R. Chin consider the Asian American experience, which includes individuals from China, Korea, Japan, Vietnam, the Philippines, Malaysia, and Thailand and the silent consequences of being considered the model minority (Eng and Han 2018). Pratyusha Tummala-Narra and Gurmeet Kanwal consider the South Asian American experience, which includes individuals from India, Pakistan, Bangladesh, Sri Lanka, Nepal, Maldives, Bhutan, and Afghanistan, for whom issues around immigration and discrimination are front of mind (Inman et al. 2015). Daniel Gaztambide has written extensively on the Latinx experience from the perspectives of psychoanalysis, critical race theory, and psychosocial justice, evident in his 2019 book *A People's History of Psychoanalysis* (Gaztambide 2019). In his chapter, he focuses on the rich diversity of what is described as Latin, including the Caribbean, Puerto Rico, Cuba, Mexico, and South and Central America, along with generational challenges, immigration, and the complexities of colorism and how it is incorporated into identity. Gaztambide emphasizes the fluidity and subtleties of these concepts, which are dependent on one's psychic location, whether within one's country of origin or within the United States. Finally, Beverly Stoute provides a unique perspective on racial identity development and formation. She posits that working with children and adolescents of color is crucial to our understanding of adult persons of color who increasingly will be seeking treatment (Stoute 2019; Vaughans and Harris 2016).

Each author brings their expertise to this section, but all of us have been impacted by the seismic events of 2020 that accelerated long-standing inequities that are increasingly impossible to ignore or deny: discriminatory immigration policies, voting discrimination, inequitable distribution of health care, mass incarceration of brown and Black people, and families separated at the border with unsupervised children in cages. In addition, over the course of months, we have observed COVID-19 affecting millions around the world, with accelerated, disproportionate rates of infection and death of brown and Black people; the move to distance learning, treatments, and supervision; anti-Asian attacks due to racist messaging; massive unemployment; a country in lockdown; recent videotaped murders of two Black men, Ahmaud Arbery and George Floyd, and the death of a Black woman, Breonna Taylor, who was murdered while she slept (a possible case of mistaken location by the police); and the video recording by a white woman, Amy Cooper, in Central Park using the language of lynching in making a false allegation against a Black man, Christian Cooper (Closson, 2020). All of these events have galvanized people's attention, which has been the spark to the current outrage. The resulting protests have been fueled by persistent discriminatory traumas and systemic institutional racism; individuals affected by these traumas now refuse to be silenced and demand equity for all Americans, regardless of ethnicity, religion, or whom they love. All of the authors of this section have been affected, both personally and professionally, by these events, and the magnitude of the impact on people and communities of color cannot be overstated. The need for mental health care for people of color is essential because of the long-term consequences of these cumulative events, thus speaking to the importance and potential challenges of this section.

This section was born out of a labor of love for our fellow Americans, many of whom have been ignored, silenced, marginalized, and discriminated against for too long, and for those other Americans who recognize, acknowledge, and react from a position of equity and inclusion toward their fellow citizens, whether patient or colleague.

Terminology

Because immigration is so prominent within this section, we want to provide readers with the following information that may benefit them in engagement with patients. This information is provided courtesy of one of our contributors, Dr. Gurmeet Kanwal.

- *Acculturation* is a complex and variably defined term. It has to do with taking on the characteristics of the host culture but also includes the notion of preserving elements of the home culture.
- *Assimilation* is a process that involves loss of one's original cultural traits.
- An *asylum seeker*, as defined by the United Nations, is someone whose request for sanctuary has yet to be processed. Every year, about one million people seek asylum.
- *Displaced people* are individuals who have fled their homes to avoid violence, human rights violations, or natural or human-made disasters. Displacement can be internal or to other countries. Some individuals are forcibly displaced, others are not. According to the United Nations (UN) High Commissioner for Refugees, there were 82.4 million forcibly displaced individuals at the end of 2020; approximately 1% of the world's population is displaced, 42% of the displaced population are children, and 85% are being hosted in developing countries (UNHCR 2022).
- *Immigration* means traveling to a country other than one's own with the intention of residing there permanently. On the other hand, to emigrate means to leave one's country or region of residence and move to another. Emigration is about leaving, and immigration is about arriving and settling in a new place.
- *Migration* refers to movement across an international border or within a state away from the migrant's habitual place of residence, regardless of 1) the person's legal status, 2) whether the movement is voluntary or involuntary, 3) the causes for the movement, and 4) the length of the stay. According to the UN Migration Agency, the number of migrants globally reached an estimated 281 million in 2020, 60 million more than in 2010. International migrants comprise 3.6% of the global population (International Organization for Migration, www.iom.int/data-and-research, 2022).
- A *permanent resident alien* is an alien admitted to the United States as a lawful permanent resident. Permanent residents are also commonly referred to as immigrants. However, according to the Office of Immigration Statistics, an illegal alien who entered the United States without inspection would be defined as an immigrant under the Immigration and Nationality Act of 1952 but is not a permanent resident alien.

- A *refugee*, as defined by the 1951 Refugee Convention, a key legal document, is "someone who is unable or unwilling to return to their country of origin owing to a well-founded fear of being persecuted for reasons of race, religion, nationality, membership of a particular social group, or political opinion" (United Nations High Commissioner for Refugees 2010, p. 3). By the end of 2017, 25.4 million refugee men, women, and children were registered globally (United Nations High Commissioner for Refugees 2001–2021). According to the Immigration and Nationality Act of 1952, the term refugee refers to

> (A) any person who is outside any country of such person's nationality or, in the case of a person having no nationality, is outside any country in which such person last habitually resided, and who is unable or unwilling to return to, and is unable or unwilling to avail himself or herself of the protection of, that country because of persecution or a well-founded fear of persecution on account of race, religion, nationality, membership in a particular social group, or political opinion, or (B) in such special circumstances as the President after appropriate consultation (as defined in section 1157(e) of this title) may specify, any person who is within the country of such person's nationality or, in the case of a person having no nationality, within the country in which such person is habitually residing, and who is persecuted or who has a well-founded fear of persecution on account of race, religion, nationality, membership in a particular social group, or political opinion. (Immigration and Nationality Act of 1952, 8 USC 1101, sec. 1101)

References

Anushri Anandaraja N: Leaving Mount Sinai. Equity Now, October 14, 2020

Asian Pacific Policy and Planning Council: Stop AAPI Hate Report 3.19.20 - 5.13.20. Stop AAPI Hate, 2020. Available at: https://secureservercdn.net/104.238.69.231/a1w.90d.myftpupload.com/wp-content/uploads/2020/10/Stop_AAPI_Hate_Report_200513.pdf. Accessed March 31, 2022.

Bonilla-Silva E: The structure of racism in color-blind, "post-racial" America. Am Behav Sci 59:1358–1376, 2015

Chang A: White America is quietly self segregating. Vox, August 31, 2018

Closson T: Amy Cooper falsely accused Black bird-watcher in 2nd 911 conversation. The New York Times. Article updated on October 16, 2020, from original reporting on October 14, 2020

Eng DL, Han S: Racial Melancholia, Racial Dissociation: On the Social and Psychic Lives of Asian Americans. Durham, NC, Duke University Press, 2018

Fonagy P, Gergely G, Jurist EL, Target M: Affect Regulation, Mentalization, and the Development of the Self. New York, Other Press, 2002

Gaztambide DJ: A People's History of Psychoanalysis. New York, Roman & Littlefield, 2019

Gladwell M: Talking to Strangers: What We Should Know About the People We Don't Know. Lanham, MD, Little, Brown, 2019

Inman AG, Tummala-Narra P, Kaduvettor-Davidson A, et al: Perceptions of race-based discrimination among first-generation Asian Indians in the United States. Couns Psychol 41(2):217–247, 2015

Keval N: Racist States of Mind: Understanding the Perversion of Curiosity and Concern. London, Karnac, 2016

Lee BY: Lawsuit alleges age, race, sex discrimination at Mount Sinai Med School. Forbes, May 12, 2019

Luona L, Stamm K, Christidis P: How diverse is the psychology workforce? News from APA's Center for Workforce Studies. Monitor on Psychology 49(2):19, 2018

Metzl JM: Dying of Whiteness: How the Politics of Racial Resentment Is Killing America's Heartland. New York, Basic Books, 2019
O'Malley L: Addressing the lack of Black mental health professionals. St Louis, MO, Insight into Mental Health Diversity, November 2021
Rogers K, Fandos N: Trump tells Congresswomen to "go back" to the countries they came from. The New York Times, July 14, 2019
Shim RS: Structural racism is why I'm leaving organized psychiatry. STAT, July 1, 2020
Shim RS: Dismantling structural racism in psychiatry: a path to mental health equity. Am J Psychiatry 278(7):592–598 2021 34270343
Stoute BJ: Racial socialization and thwarted mentalization: psychoanalytic reflections from the lived experience of James Baldwin's America. Am Imago 76(3):335–357, 2019
Sue DW, Sue D: Counseling the Culturally Different, 3rd Edition. New York, Wiley, 1999
Tessler H, Choi M, Kao G: The anxiety of being Asian American: hate crimes and negative biases during the COVID-19 pandemic. Am J Crim Justice 45(4):636–646, 2020 32837158
United Nations High Commissioner for Refugees: Convention and Protocol Relating to the Status of Refugees. Geneva, Switzerland, United Nations High Commissioner for Refugees, 2010. Available at: www.unhcr.org/3b66c2aa10.html. Accessed March 14, 2022.
United Nations High Commissioner for Refugees: What is a refugee? Geneva, Switzerland, United Nations High Commissioner for Refugees, 2001–2021. Available at: www.unhcr.org/afr/what-is-a-refugee.html. Accessed March 14, 2022.
United Nations High Commissioner for Refugees: Global trends: forced displacement in 2020. UNHCR Flagship Reports. Geneva, Switzerland, United Nations High Commissioner for Refugees, 2020. Available at: www.unhcr.org/flagship-reports/globaltrends. Accessed March 14, 2022.
Vaughans KC, Harris L: The police, Black and Hispanic boys: a dangerous inability to mentalize. J Infant Child Adolesc Psychother 15(3):171–178, 2016
Wadman M: Update: Mount Sinai institute director facing discrimination allegations leaves post. Science, July 3, 2019
Warner J: Psychiatry tries to confront its racist past and tries to make amends. The New York Times, April 30/May 21, 2021
Wilson M, McKinley J, Ferre-Saurni L, et al: Daniel Pride's death: police silence and accusations of a cover-up. The New York Times, September 4, 2020

CHAPTER 22

African Americans and Psychotherapeutic Treatment

Challenges and Opportunities

Dionne R. Powell, M.D.
Anton Hart, Ph.D.

Not everything that is faced can be changed; but nothing can be changed until it is faced.

—James Baldwin (1962a)

In this chapter, we attempt to explore and provide useful insights into the experience of African American people for anyone working clinically with this population or, more broadly, communities made up of people from the African Diaspora. Our goal is to capture this experience through the histories of the African American people to explore how psychology and psychiatry, in particular, have been primary contributors to systemic racist practices that keep Black people from seeking mental health care and discourage those considering training in the mental health field (Baquet and Corbett 2020). The field of social work, while also historically embedded in racist viewpoints and practices (e.g., Dominelli 1997), has tended toward an orientation that is more explicitly attentive to issues of race and discrimination than its other mental health counterparts, although it is not devoid of discriminatory and exclusionary practices (Bobo 2001, 2004; Bonilla-Silva 2015).

After this background review, we explore the theoretical implications of this history on the practice of psychotherapy, followed by a section on breaking down common stereotypes. Next, we provide notes for the African American considering pursuit of clinical mental health training, a section on the ways that race impacts supervisory and curricular issues, and clinical considerations. We conclude the chapter with suggestions on how to fight racism within every therapist and training center, corresponding to the inherently subversive emancipatory endeavor of psychodynamic psychotherapy.

The Future Has a Past: The American Dream as Perpetual Nightmare for Black People—A Brief History

> *We keep loving this country, and this country doesn't love us back.*
>
> —Doc Rivers, head coach of the Philadelphia 76ers, in the aftermath of the murder of George Floyd by Minneapolis policemen (Memorial Day, May 25, 2020)

The history of the African in the United States has an origin story that is concurrent with, although intentionally separated from, the republic's beginning and is cloaked in silence and misinformation. This history remains foundational to the ongoing systemic problems of race and racism that have had devastating impacts on modern society. The United States, except for its Native people, is a country of immigrants, those who chose America in pursuit of freedom and opportunity for themselves and future generations. Not so the slave. Slaves were stolen and separated from their families and communities; forced onto packed slave ships, where more than a million died through disease, suicide, and revolt in the middle passage (Sharpe 2016); and auctioned and enslaved in North and South America and the Caribbean. From 1619 onward, these human captives in America were not considered "Americans" and lived without human rights, legal rights, voting rights, property rights, the ability to marry, and opportunity to make an independent living. Their entire fate was controlled by their white masters (Hannah-Jones 2019). Although there were a few free Black men, their potential bondage was a constant threat without legal recourse (as illustrated in the 2013 film *12 Years a Slave,* based on a memoir by Solomon Northrup). Thus, the African in America has undergone 400 years of trauma, rape (nonconsensual sex by white property owners or anyone else as designated by such owners), physical and psychological abuse, lynching, and systematic denial of human rights (Anderson 2016).

Simultaneously, the United States was founded on the principal that all men are created equal. As evident from the republic's inception, equality was meant for white men of financial means. Thus, a hierarchical system was created whereby advantage (i.e., privilege) was ascribed to those who most approximated white cisgender men with wealth. These dual facts—equality and advantage afforded to white men of means and abject subjugation as owned property deemed less than human for the African slave—formed the social-political-economic DNA, the racial double helix, of the foundational underpinnings of the republic and were the source of institutional racism, white supremacy, and America's unique caste system (Powell 2020; Wilkerson 2020).

This interconnection between history, slavery, and democracy has formed stable hierarchies over time based on one's closeness to or distance from a white ideal that also included women and immigrants who arrived in the mid to late nineteenth and twentieth centuries. From Crispus Attucks, who on March 5, 1770 was the first to be killed fighting the British for American independence, throughout all major wars, including the Civil War, African Americans have fought both physically and psychologically to integrate as equals, prove their citizenry, and hold Americans to task that all men, and women, are actually created equal. The history of African American patriotism on the battlefield and rights denied once home speaks to the harsh injustices, along with the notion of service without recognition, that result from a caste system, described by Wilkerson (2020) as "the urgent necessity of a bottom rung" (pp. 224–228).

For instance, white consensus considers the actions by NFL players taking a knee for injustices inflicted on Black people by whites as unpatriotic, but within the African American community, military service far exceeds the proportions of Blacks in America: African Americans comprise 30% of all women in the military and 17% of all men despite making up only 13% of the U.S. population (Statista 2020). If the lack of patriotism ascribed to these athletes' actions were true, it would actively disavow the contributions of their fathers, uncles, grandfathers, sisters, brothers, and mothers who have served their country valiantly. On a more personal note (D. R. P.), my great uncle, a Purple Heart recipient in World War II, chose to remain in Germany rather than return to the States, where the Ku Klux Klan were specifically targeting and murdering Black veterans. It is this ongoing American tragedy—Black deaths by white hands—that the NFL players are protesting. Questioning the capacity of Blacks, on and off the playing field, to serve this country and protest its discriminatory tactics belies our fundamental democratic tenets.

Hampering the efforts of African Americans to prove their patriotism and obtain equal rights has been an intergenerational disregard by the majority of society, a conscious and unconscious lack of acknowledgment of these complicated racial truths. The majority of whites are *innocently ignorant* of this history and thus do not assume responsibility for the fate of their Black and brown fellow citizens. They are unaware that the notion of whiteness, originating in America, transformed what was once the vilified stranger, the late nineteenth- and twentieth-century European immigrant, and created a caste system that allowed entry to the highest standards that America has to offer solely based on skin color (Wilkerson 2020).

As Wilkerson persuasively articulates in her book *Caste: The Origins of Our Discontents*, "Slavery in this land was not merely an unfortunate thing that happened to Black people. It was an American innovation, an American institution created by and for the benefit of the elites of the dominant caste and enforced by poorer members of the dominant caste who tied their lot to the caste system rather than their consciences (Wilkerson 2020, p. 44)." The disjunction for the African American is captured poignantly in "My Dungeon Shook: Letter to My Nephew on the One Hundredth Anniversary of the Emancipation" by James Baldwin in his book *The Fire Next Time*: "The details and symbols of your life have been deliberately constructed to make you believe what white people say about you. Please try to remember that what they believe, as well as what they do and cause you to endure, does not testify to your inferiority but to their inhumanity and fear" (Baldwin 1962b, p. 8).

The consequences of institutional racism and white supremacy are numerous, from the landmark legal case of *Plessy v. Ferguson*, which marked anyone with a drop of Black blood as Colored and thus able to be discriminated against, through the Thirteenth Amendment; from slavery to sharecropping (a system of perpetual indebtedness) and the destruction of independent Black communities in Wilmington, North Carolina; Rosewood, Florida; and Tulsa, Oklahoma (Staples 2020); to laws and procedures that guarantee that equal access and opportunities for voting, housing, employment, education, and medical care remain systematically denied to African Americans. Normalized over time as a consequence of slavery and its aftermath, African Americans' property, civil, and human rights are systematically denied with impunity on the basis of hierarchy, division, and caste (Alexander 2010; Anderson 2016). Recent incidents speak to the overt remnants of being enslaved on a manifest level that are daily aspects of African American lives: Blacks being assaulted (Jacob Blake) or killed by police; Blacks killed in their communities while jogging (Amaund Avery), walking (Trayvon Martin, Elijah McClain), or sleeping in their homes (Breonna Taylor); Blacks arrested for not signaling a lane change (Sandra Bland) or killed for having a mental illness (Walter Wallace Jr., Daniel Prude) or leaving a convenience store (George Floyd). The only common factor is that all of these individuals were African Americans not charged with a crime. As a society we are not accustomed to hearing similar narratives about white people, requiring us all to form justifications, typically of criminality, in order to explain away the deaths; otherwise, it would be too horrific to accept that this *is* America (Alexander 2010).

Beneath this cruel reality is the subtle entrenched discrimination in all aspects of society. The lack of recognition, acknowledgment, and attempts at repair of this complicated American story of race, both past and present, suggests that the truth about race and America continues to be an untold one. The effects on individuals immigrating to the United States or being born and raised in a society that continues to promote discrimination and caste make us all victims of, or benefiting from, an unjust system based solely on race. Even the revolutionary 2015 musical *Hamilton*, in which slavery is presented as a South (slavery) versus North (no slavery) divide, continues to perpetuate a fantasy in the collective American imagination. In reality, slavery did not end in New York State until 1827, and Philip Schuyler and Alexander Hamilton both purportedly were slave owners. Ignorance surrounding these facts makes one defensive, increasing the challenges for acknowledgment and psychic repair. Understanding these issues is essential for anyone contemplating working with African American patients or providing mental health education for African American people.

This chapter explicitly concerns African Americans in the aggregate, but we write from the perspective of the larger African Diaspora that represents those Americans of African descent who immigrated or were forced by kidnapping and slavery to the United States from Europe, Africa, the Caribbean, and Central and South America (Fanon 1952/2008). This perspective acknowledges both the historical migration patterns of *Homo sapiens* originating from Africa beginning 70,000–80,000 years ago and the effects of colonialism and slavery, which have left a malevolent imprint on Black communities (Fanon 1952/2008; Hammonds and Herzig 2008; Roberts 2011).

These multifactorial aspects of race as a sociopolitical construct without genetic, scientific proof are a means to categorize on the basis of colorism (prejudice or discrimination based on skin tone, favoring lighter skin over darker skin) stratified by white supremacist hierarchical structures that result in our unconscious mapping of the other on the basis of race and class (Moss 2019, 2006; Powell 2018). These stratifications result in an unconscious labeling of others who are different on the basis of their presumed caste or placement in society. The collective work of scientists, sociologists, psychiatrists, psychologists, and clinical and laboratory researchers are beginning to show the cumulative generational response to stress and trauma, including racial trauma, found in epigenetic phenomena across generations where stress and trauma, *our environment*, impact gene expression in second- and third-generation offspring (Carcea et al. 2021; DeGruy 2005; Hammonds and Herzig 2008; Heijmans et al. 2008; Jones Marlin 2020; Stein et al. 2004).

This work is beginning to enhance our understanding of how externally derived racial trauma, whether experienced transgenerationally or personally, can have lasting effects on self-esteem, stress mitigation, and other health outcomes throughout generations. For 12 generations, slavery had impacted African Americans and the rest of America. As Wilkerson (2020) states, "the country cannot become whole until it confronts what was not a chapter in its history, but the basis of its economic and social order. For a quarter millennium slavery *was* the country" (p. 43). Thus, racial trauma can create *dis-eased* communities of color, enhancing health disparities. The argument that there are genetic differences to these health disparities has been debunked, yet clinicians and scientists alike continue to focus on genetics instead of fully addressing the fixable health disparities caused by the consequences of systemic racism (Hammonds and Herzig 2008; Hoffman et al. 2016; Roberts 2011; Skloot 2010). The reality for too many African Americans is shaped by persistent discrimination in safe housing, toxic and criminalized communities, and anti-Black injustices in which invisible structural forces and individual biases and prejudices guarantee inequities in health care and education from cradle (the adverse childhood events that disproportionately affect brown and Black children, including the disproportionate Black maternal death rate; Pagán et al. 2020) to grave (the increased mortality rate of African Americans as a result of chronic illnesses).

This chapter does not allow us sufficient space to fully address the contributions of American psychiatrists, psychologists, and scientists to the fraught history of racism, but this history is worth extensive study, especially by clinicians treating people of color and/or aspiring to increase the admission and retention of Black and brown trainees in the mental health field (Grier and Cobbs 1968; Guthrie 1976; Powell 2018; Thomas and Sillen 1972; Washington 2006). Society has heavily relied on religion and science as primary defenders of slavery and its aftermath. From the scientific perspective, slavery was "good" for the slave because it prevented the idolatry or insanity that was expected to result if the individual were freed. Persistent notions that Africans had very little brain capacity and were less than human and therefore benefited from the domestication provided by slavery furthered attempts, by any and all means, to control their movements and freedom. Samuel A. Carthwright, M.D. (1793–1863), was one of the chief advocates favoring slavery and the inherent inferiority of slaves. Draeptomania, a disease causing Negros to run away, and *dysaesthesia aethiopis*, a condition causing rascality, are both attributable to Carthwright (Thomas and Sillen 1972; Washington 2006). Postslavery, the twentieth-century Negro continued to be denied basic human rights of education, voting, employment, housing, and health care, concurrent with the rise of eugenics in the early 1920s as African Americans continued to be labeled inferior on the basis genetics (Roberts 2011). These "scientific" conclusions served as justifications for further discrimination of Black and brown people.

After the formal end of slavery following emancipation and the Reconstruction Era (1863–1877), laws including the Thirteenth Amendment in 1865; the Civil Rights Act of 1866; and the Fourteenth Amendment, which afforded freedom, citizenship, and protections and privileges similar to those of other Americans, were rarely, if ever, enforced (Meacham 2020). Scientific, political, and sociological barriers were maintained and justified to keep the newly freed African Americans subjugated under white supremacy and Black disenfranchisement. The rise of the Ku Klux Klan (1865) and the Black codes, in which Southern state legislatures enacted laws intended to deny and control the newly freed African American, ensuring white supremacy post–Civil War, served as signifiers of state-sanctioned terror based on the perpetual goal of keeping Blacks in bondage (Briggs and Krakauer 2020).

These impediments to true African American emancipation were buttressed later by eugenics, which promoted "race betterment" that included state-sanctioned sterilization for those subgroups furthest from the white heteronormative Christian standard, also referred to as "Mississippi appendectomies." Indiana was the first state to enact laws for sterilization in 1907. By 1945, two-thirds of the United States had laws sanctioning sterilization, with more than 44,000 sterilization procedures performed. Forced sterilizations continued past the 1960s, especially for poor and minority women. As Robert Guthrie expressed in his book *Even the Rat Was White: A Historical View of Psychology*, "Eugenicists most often appeared to be white supremacists using the concept of genetics as their weaponry" (Guthrie 1976, p. 94). The atrocities committed on the Black mind and body during the Tuskegee syphilis experiment, in which approximately 600 men were falsely told that their syphilis was being treated so the scientists could use the *feeble, primitive brains* of Blacks to prove that the disease had more of a cardiovascular versus neurological outcome, have become the metaphor for the egregious inhumane treatment of African Americans; other atrocities included radiation treatment without consent and testing of medicines and vaccinations without consent (Washington 2006). All of this contributed to the greatest migration of people in recorded history from the South to the North and West, with new threatening challenges for African Americans (Wilkerson 2010).

In modern times, Black men, protesting for equal justice under the law during the peak of the Civil Rights Era, were overly diagnosed with schizophrenia at record rates as the general population and the white public's imagination were instilled with fear about African Americans' alleged paranoia and criminality (Bell 2011; Luhrmann 2010; Metzl 2010). Today, government leaders and media organizations attribute violent, psychotic, and paranoid behavior to the participants of the Black Lives Matter movement in attempts to suppress the Black body and mind that refer to the 400-year history of slavery, dating back to the arrival of the first slaves in Jamestown, Virginia (Hannah-Jones 2019). Every generation of African Americans—from Frederick Douglass, Harriet Tubman, Sojourner Truth, W.E.B. Du Bois, Marcus Garvey, Booker T. Washington, writers from the Harlem Renaissance, and James Baldwin to Martin Luther

King Jr., Malcolm X, Fannie Lou Hamer, Medgar Evers, Huey P. Newton, Bobby Seale, Shirley Chisholm, Angela Davis, Elijah Cummings, John Lewis, President Barack Obama, the founders of the Black Lives Matter movement, and countless others—has attempted to reconcile this disjunction between American freedom and racial subjugation. The inextricable tension of the American experiment of democracy and freedom interwoven with racial subjugation of Black and brown people is the racial DNA, America's double helix that without sufficient reckoning, explanation, and integration will continue to limit much-needed national reconciliation and prevent articulation of the true capabilities of an equal American society. Where clinicians fall within this polarity of democracy and subjugation will determine their ability to work with people of color.

Finally, although the topic of this chapter is African Americans in the aggregate, we would be remiss if we did not articulate that racism has effects on the non–African American majority as well, although this is frequently denied. Centuries of silence about the effects of racism without acknowledgment and attempts to repair can reduce one's empathic capacities and lead to a type of psychic numbing (Lifton 1982) as a form of denial and isolation of affect (Bonilla-Silva 2015; Powell 2020). The recent American presidential election revealed the tenacity of today's racial pandemic and xenophobia, showing that racism often results in whites' behavior that is against their best interests. For instance, Metzl (2019) described in detail how the softening of restrictions on gun ownership, the refusal of states to accept and adopt the Patient Protection and Affordable Care Act (Obamacare), and state-imposed limitations on education and social services and states' refusal to accept federal government help have created drastic decreases in life expectancy and health outcomes and poorer education for whites. Thus, whiteness reduces the unique complexity and nuance of the human spirit, leading to a groupthink that can have profound deleterious effects for our democracy and the entire nation.

The opioid epidemic, in which 450,000 people died between 1999 and 2018, highlighted disparities in health care, with a disproportionate number of white deaths due to different perceptions of pain: when Blacks complained of pain, their needs were met with denial and their believability was challenged, whereas when whites complained of pain, they were medicated in excess, contributing to dependence and addiction (Hoffman et al. 2016; Metzl 2019; Washington 2006). Similarly, we would not be surprised if the soaring rates of illness outside urban areas during the coronavirus SARS-CoV-2 disease (COVID-19) pandemic could be attributed in part to the disproportionate rates of illness in Black and brown communities, which provided a false sense of security for white Americans that resulted in far riskier behavior and potential exposure to contagion in non-urban settings. When science and medicine are broken down along racial lines, we all suffer.

Theoretical Implications

Institutionalized racism is present throughout American society, although discussion of this issue has been silenced by white supremacy and national complacency. More recent attempts to silence discussions about institutional racism and diversity, equity, and inclusion for institutions of higher learning that receive federal monetary support include a September 2020 executive order by President Donald Trump (https://trumpwhitehouse.archives.gov/presidential-actions/executive-order-combating-race-sex-stereotyping) and challenges of factually based attempts to address health care disparities (Hoffman et al. 2016; Roberts 2011; Skloot 2010; Washington 2006). Excavation and remediation of this influence in the mental health field require ongoing efforts from leaders, teachers, and supervisors, starting with the understanding that we all have conscious and unconscious "racists states of mind" (Keval 2016). Relevant to the clinical or supervisory experience, this realization allows for active engagement with our biases and stereotypes that may impede understanding of our patients and supervisees, especially if they are persons of color. It requires an awareness of projective mechanisms operating on an individual and societal level that become activated when experiencing the other, especially in moments of tension.

Although appropriate usage of the term *the other* has been debated, we believe that it refers to more than just a stranger and includes the negative stigmata that are placed both unconsciously and consciously on someone who is different on the basis of race, religion, country of origin, ability level, or gender. These stigmata influence one's subsequent beliefs and interactions. Implied in this discussion is the importance of placing race, racism, bias, and privilege as integral areas of exploration in one's own self-reflections and personal therapy and/or analysis. This apparently revolutionary notion extends the idea of a racialized self, with its inherent fears, defenses, and manifestations, as an inherent component of identity formation. Particularly in our polarized American society, we are emphasizing that the racial self is worth the same focus and attention as the sexual and aggressive self. Clinically, this would speak to same-race treatment pairs as much as biracial treatment pairs, thus allowing for an affirmative exploration of the placement of race in the psychic mind.

Opening up this area for exploration regardless of the race of the treatment pair mitigates the notion that race is clinically relevant only when the treatment pair is racially different. For example, in the midphase of my own treatment, I (D.R.P.) confronted my analyst, accusing her of "talking like a white woman," a defensive retreat from intimacy on a racial level (Powell 2020). Analysts and psychotherapists have had African American patients attempt to defensively bypass the underpinnings of rage, shame, and guilt by an apparent partnership on racial lines, with the suggestion that race, bias, privilege, and supremacy would not be explored because of shared race, especially when whiteness, through a discriminatory slight or gesture (Hart 2019a), was the subject of exploration. Such moments of collusion, in which race can potentially be bypassed or ignored, have been shared with us by our white colleagues as well, especially when race becomes a topic of exploration with their white patients. However, in these explorations, the presumed shared, often false, racial narrative of collusion around whiteness is rarely explored (Goldberger 1993).

From a clinical, supervisory, and pedagogical standpoint, it is more useful to presume the existence of prejudice in us all. In this sense, the psychopathology of racism is ubiquitous. We all tend toward the self-securing shortcuts and avoidances of knowing things about others before we can possibly know them. We curtail our own curiosity, and starting from very early in our lives we learn to shape our experiences on the basis of unfounded familiarity. This knowing what to expect prior to encountering it directly and immediately, in our own experience, represents a way of being that is self-protective and defensive in nature. People ward off the anxieties associated with uncertainty and unknownness by deploying personal illusions of having foreknowledge (Gadamer 2004) about others, securing themselves from the vulnerabilities associated with states of curiosity and discovery. Being prejudiced or having prejudice involves a presumed knowing before you actually have a direct experiential basis for knowing someone. Knowing what a person is like on the basis of the color of their skin or their ethnicity rather than on the basis of interacting and dialoguing with that person represents a way of avoiding an encounter with someone (presumably someone unknown) solely on the basis of appearances. This experience is fraught with anxieties, both conscious and unconscious, about foundational matters such as personal continuity of being. A psychodynamic perspective offers insight into why curiosity requires such vulnerability and why people universally tend to reduce their own curiosity in the service of protecting themselves from being open to novel, emergent, and unpredictable experiences (Hart 2017). This is no less true for the mental health clinician.

From birth, a child's inherent curiosity is present. Yet curiosity is a force to be reckoned with. It is not simply benign; it is also shaped and influenced by anxieties, especially from our earliest caretakers. What is determinative of an individual's background of safety is heavily influenced by the sociocultural milieu within which that person is reared. Although all of us have had similar basic needs attended to that are pivotal for our survival to adulthood, how race and culture are experienced and shaped informs our development. What we are curious about and what we are blinded to are determined to a great degree by our caretakers and are reinforced through education and experience. The baby's, the child's, the adolescent's, and the adult's curiosities inherently raise questions not just for the developing person but for those with whom that developing person comes into contact. For further discussion of this process, see Chapter 26, "How Our Mind Becomes Racialized."

White people remain the most segregated group in the country, rarely having friends or family from other ethnic groups (Chang 2018). Much of this is because of societal segregation, the lack of direct exposure to African Americans in their community, or forming superficial friendships that do not extend beyond work or professional relationships (Bonilla-Silva 2015). Whites hold a monolithic opinion of Black people that tends to concentrate them into particular categories relating to depictions on social media focused on entertainment, athletics, and criminality. What is increasingly apparent for all Americans is the whitewashing of American history within our educational system, which suggests that any teaching of the racial history of America, in its multicultural manifestations, is anti-American. These myths and stereotypes require active, conscious dismantling (Holmes 2019).

What this implies for white therapists, who often receive their training in an urban setting, is a series of misaligned perceptions that can directly affect the therapeutic alliance with people of color (Altman 2006; DiAngelo 2018). With curiosity, questions arise, raising uncertainties, and those uncertainties are imbued with anxiety. "Who is this person?" "How will they act?" "What do they want?" "Will they be reliable?" "Will their ways of being be familiar or foreign?" "Will they respond to me with affection or with disdain?" Everything unfamiliar is a source of tension and, thus, a potential existential threat. The threat is derived not just from the potential for actual physical or emotional attack but also from the sense of mental discontinuity that coming to know each new other represents. If I construe life in a certain way on the basis of my experience in the world, both of myself and of others, then each new situation with each new person presents the possibility that I will have an experience, awareness, or insight that will demand a revision or reorganization of the things I thought I knew. I am potentially unsettled, or even disoriented, by a disequilibrium that may come up between me and the strange, foreign other in any given instance.

Although such mental disequilibrium represents an opportunity, both for the satisfaction of my ever-present, recurrent curiosity and also for personal growth and expansion, it also presents a threat to the stability and reliability of my life-acquired ways of understanding the world and others in that world. I thought I knew what was dangerous and what was safe; I felt I had acquired a familiarity with my own senses of personal goodness and badness; I thought I knew how to act, how to get what I might want and avoid getting what I do not want. Yet the other who is unknown to me has other ideas, beliefs, customs, manners, morals, and aesthetics. Even if we speak a common (verbal) language, it may be that we have very different expectations and desires. And these potentially different expectations and desires may collide in ways that are minor or major. Part of this challenge, especially for the clinician or trainee, is that the foreignness of the other regardless of categorization precludes acknowledgment of core human beliefs and tendencies, thus making empathy, as opposed to sympathy or pity, harder to experience.

Prejudice solves the problem of unknownness by proceeding as if that which is undiscovered and unknown is already discovered and known. If I already know you, then I do not have to experience the anxieties associated with opening myself up to you and to the mutual discoveries that may ensue. However, although it is true that there may be anxieties associated with the prejudices I hold, such as "You are dangerous because you are part of the racial group that I know is dangerous," and I may spend time fretting about the danger that I already know you pose, such anxieties are nothing compared with the anxieties associated with the prospect of personal disorientation and destabilization that come with my making myself available for contact and being open to where that contact might lead me (and us) (Hart 2019b). A prejudiced orientation, held either consciously (in the form of attitudes and beliefs), unconsciously (in the form of biases), or both, represents a person's curtailment of their own original curiosity—a curiosity that, at the beginning of life, orients itself toward everything and everyone new and unknown. One can begin to understand how built-up prejudices and biases can limit the capabilities of human interactions and therefore curtail the imaginative capacities of mind.

Being prejudiced as a primary form of self-protection is very human. The psychoanalyst Joseph Sandler has written about how the child builds an intrapsychic background of safety, based on the earliest interactions with caregivers that give shape to one's self-identity, and object representations based on affective experiences that become defined over time (Sandler 1960; Sandler and Rosenblatt 1962). In America, race is shaped in mind as well. You see young children playing innocently regardless of race or religion, then incrementally devolving into strangers who need to be feared and misunderstood at every interaction. Racism and other forms of prejudice and discrimination have all the characteristics of what we refer to as *mental defenses*: the distortion of experience in order to protect against mental or emotional threat by bending experience to fit with what can be tolerated. But, also common with all defenses, there is a cost, both to the individual deploying the defense and to those whom the individual might use in the process of such deployment. A racist orientation harms both the racist—in its sacrificing of the experience of reality perception in favor of proceeding on the basis of convenient fantasy about how things surely must be—and those who are the subjects of the racist's defensive-destructive fantasy.

Doing psychotherapy in a racialized world, a world filled with racial prejudices and the distortions of authentic relatedness that are invariably part of the picture, means working with the fallout from the renouncement of open relatedness used by so many. And when it comes to working with African American patients, it also involves working with the perhaps acute, and cumulative, trauma of being targeted and victimized by racial discrimination and hatred.

Prejudice relies on complicity in silence. So does the dissociative minimization of racial trauma. Thus, from the beginning of any psychotherapeutic dialogue in which issues of race and racism may be features (which is, in our view, virtually *every* psychotherapeutic endeavor regardless of the homogeneity or heterogeneity of the psychotherapeutic dyad), a primary resistance to be overcome is the unwillingness to speak openly about matters of prejudice, race, and racism. Simply engaging in open discussion of prejudice and discrimination interferes with patients' ability to perpetuate themselves, just as talking about any form of trauma, including racial trauma, threatens to unseat the mental space that such trauma has held.

Originally coined by Pierce (1974), the term *microaggression* has become widely used as a way of describing the pervasiveness of discriminatory acts that have a cumulatively damaging effect on the minds and, demonstrably, the bodies of Black people. However, although the microaggression concept has been of profound importance in our attempts to recognize the corrosive effects on Black people of living in a white supremacist society, there is a sense in which the prefix *micro-* can sometimes be misleading. As in the metaphor of "death by a thousand cuts," the terms microaggression and microtrauma refer to the way that relatively minor, sometimes even imperceptible, negative experiences can cumulatively lead to quite pronounced negative effects. And this is indisputably so in many instances. What we need to remember, however, is that sometimes experiences are not as "micro" as they may seem on the surface. From a psychodynamic perspective, we must attend not only to conscious experience but also to that which is unconscious, to trauma that is concrete and obvious and to trauma that is symbolic and evident only in the context of its symbolic meanings and resonances.

One of the authors of this chapter (A.H.) coined the term *the discriminatory gesture* to refer to forms of treatment that are, on the surface, relatively benign but that, through their symbolic connection to slavery and the violent persecution and oppression of Black people, can have traumatic impact equal to or even surpassing overtly observable, violent acts directed toward the subject (Hart 2019a). That human beings have minds that are partly conscious and largely unconscious and that we have the capacity for the formation and interpretation of symbols means that mental suffering is, invariably, multiply determined, including by factors that have to do with the meaning of things for the particular individual. This is why experiences of trauma, both micro and macro, take different tolls on people. It is the psychotherapist's task not to objectively determine the nature and intensity of the patient's experience but, instead, to inquire with the patient into what the patient has experienced on both overt and symbolic levels.

Breaking Stereotypes

Relying on stereotypes is a form of prejudice. Instead of remaining open to learning about each new, different person, proceeding on the basis of a stereotype represents a way of preempting contact and dialogue, substituting what is already "known" for what could potentially be discovered. Proceeding on the basis of stereotypes serves as a defensive adoption of a shorthand manner for knowing other people. If I already know what Asian or Black or Latin or white people are like, I do not have to engage in the emotionally risky process of making contact with someone who is different from me. I do not have to bother with the process of mentally accommodating someone new, someone who might challenge the stereotyped categories that I have already taken in and/or created for myself. Stereotyping, like all forms of prejudice, protects people from the unsettling feelings associated with encountering situations and interactions that are unfamiliar; it provides the illusion that the world, and other people in it (including those who are different from us, and thus "other"), are already known. However, although stereotyping provides an immediate sense of security ("I know what they are like," "I know what is going on," "I know what to expect"), it invariably has a long-term cost due to its reliance on oversimplification and distortion of the existing complexities of reality. It is this form of stereotyping that requires constant undoing when it comes to African Americans because the history of racism in the United States has sanctioned death to the Black populace on the basis of trumped-up charges that rarely have basis in fact. The deaths of Emmett Till and George Floyd are poignant examples of the lethality associated with such stereotypes.

It is crucial that psychotherapists working with diverse populations engage in an ongoing process of self-inquiry and self-education in order to transcend their own, quite human, tendency toward stereotyping. Psychotherapists must understand not just that stereotyping and other forms of prejudice are wrong but also how they connect to each person's way of maintaining emotional equilibrium and security. The psychodynamic psychotherapeutic process involves, most centrally, the cultivation of curiosity. When patients manifest various forms of curtailed or absent curiosity, the psychotherapeutic task must necessarily involve the anxieties associated with being curious and open, starting with those that emerge in the psychotherapeutic situation itself. In a sense, analysis of the patient's transference experience—the inquiry into the patient's experience of the therapist and how this may be connected to the patient's earlier life experiences in relation to their caretakers and significant others—represents the addressing of the patient's tendency toward prejudiced, stereotypical perception and thought.

By engaging in the psychotherapeutic conversation in a manner that refrains from resorting to presumption, the psychoanalytic psychotherapist sets a tone of curiosity and inquiry, encouraging the patient to be curious and inquiring in kind. The cultivation of such curiosity paves the way for the reflective, dialogic scrutiny of multiple presumptions, including stereotypes and prejudices, that patients have regularly deployed as features of their emotional security operations.

One of the most pernicious stereotypes that directly affects treatment engagement and outcome is the notion that all Black people are alike. The challenge for the clinician is to look at each patient or client through the lens of cultural humility (Watkins and Hook 2016) and radical curiosity, promoting the ability to stand in a position of unknowing and cultural neutrality while also listening for nuances in tone, affect, and language to pursue further with openness and respect. For example, when a white male patient in psychodynamic psychotherapy inquired about whether my ancestors were slaves, my (D.L.P.) nonjudgmental and curious stance led to him revealing his envy and unconscious longing for me to be dependent on him in an enslaved position (Gay 2016; Powell 2020).

For African American clinicians in training, the stereotype that "all Blacks are alike" becomes most egregious when two trainees of color are frequently confused by name or achievements. In my 30 years of experience, I have not seen this confusion of identity between white trainees. It speaks to one of the vestiges of slavery (along with colonial and caste societies), where slaves were identified solely by gender, with the "N word" as prefix (Desmond 2019; Gay 2016). Appreciating the subjectivity and humanity of all patients, but in particular African American patients and trainees, is essential as the country continues to work through the denial that Black lives matter. This has been especially highlighted recently by the disproportionate deaths of Black and brown people from COVID-19.

Another stereotypical trope, dating from the Civil Rights movement and continuing through the 2020 presidential election, surrounds white perceptions of Black folks and *anger*. Black women have been pivotal contributors to recent elections, but African American women are often labeled as being "angry" at the slightest hint of authority and passion. In many instances, the backbone of the African American home is the African American woman, whether in partnership or as a single parent. Lacking the privilege of gender, African American women have fought and struggled for their families and communities, often with minimal support aside from each other. Most Black women can ill afford to be demure. That being said, African American patients seeking treatment are not opposed to dynamic interventions, but they do not want to be patronized or offered pitying support either. This is what we have regularly heard from our combined 60 years of practice. African American women, and also men, want to be heard, listened to, and understood as individuals, just like all patients. For the non–African American clinician this entails seeing beyond preconceived, often sociological, notions and shows the value of a psychodynamic approach in meeting the patient where they are.

For the African American man, his "anger" is enfolded in the narrative fiction of paranoia and criminality and in the historical realities of not being able to protect and often provide for his family. African Americans have healthy suspiciousness due to the legacy of discrimination and ill treatment by the law, education, employment, housing, and health (Washington 2006). In addition, the stigma of being labeled as mentally ill, especially in African American men, is so profound that, as discussed by psychiatrist and academician William Lawson, for Black men it is "better to be bad (i.e., angry) than mad" (Lawson 2020). Lawson speaks to the need for more mental health care and services for people of color during the COVID-19 pandemic and afterward because the typical outlets for stress reduction for Black people—the church or mosque, barbershop, beauty shop, and fraternities and sororities—have not been available options. As Black people continue to speak up and out regarding the ubiquity of racism's impact, the stigma against mental illness gives way to acknowledgment of the trauma of racism and reparations, which must include mental health care and services.

The events highlighted in 2020 starting with the death and/or injury of Jared Polis (in 2019), Ahmaud Arbery, George Floyd, Jacob Blake, Breonna Taylor, and Daniel Prude illustrate the precarious risks of being African American in modern society (Alexander 2010; Anderson 2016; Noah 2020). From cradle to grave, the African American boy-child-man is subjected to injustices. For instance, studies reveal that Black male children are perceived as being 3 years older than their actual age, whereas white children of similar age are perceived as younger by 2 years; this misperception often leads to African American children being tried and imprisoned by adult standards (Stevenson 2014; Vaughans 2015). Children of color are disproportionately assigned to special education, providing additional financial resources to school districts but pigeonholing the child away from their fellow students, decreasing their ability to perform in general education and advanced course work. These practices can permanently disadvantage African American children. African American parents in both urban and suburban communities have described reflexive attempts by the school district to place their children in special education that were not supported by IQ tests but were summarily suggested on the basis of their race.

When working with African American patients, clinicians must appreciate the inherent accumulative trauma and posttraumatic stress resulting from daily microaggressions and the macroaggressions of living in a society where unequal justice and discrimination are tolerated and, depending on leadership by the government or in the workplace, even encouraged. Most of this occurs on an unconscious and not overt level, but it is the idea of unawareness or "unknowing" that promulgates institutional racism. African Americans insisting on the literal removal of "your knee from my neck" is a demand for moving away from unconscious or ignorant unknowing to full awareness of people's participation in the process of discrimination, with attempts at remediation.

The final stereotype comes from the paucity of media attention toward the plight of transgender men and women of color. Kimberlé Crenshaw has highlighted that by attending to the intersectional aspects of gender, race, and class we can draw attention to marginalized communities *within* minority communities (Crenshaw 1989, 2016; Follins and Lassiter 2017). Transgender people of color experience high rates of violent attacks, and suicide rates are especially high among members of this population because they are frequently rejected by their families and communities and are subject to continued abuse as they attempt to survive with minimal support. This bias against transgender people is unyielding despite inroads in popular culture (e.g., *RuPaul's Drag Race*, *Pose*), and particular sensitivity is required to prevent further violations within the clinical setting.

Considerations for the African American Psychotherapist

African Americans are poorly represented in the clinical mental health profession (i.e., social workers, psychologists, and psychiatrists). African Americans represent 13% of all U.S. citizens, but Black psychiatrists comprise less than 2% of all American psychiatrists, 5% of clinical psychologists, and 7% of clinical social workers (O'Malley 2021; Powell 2012; U.S. Census Bureau 2015). These low numbers have a multifactorial explanation that speaks to the influences of family and communities of color that many African Americans come from, the perceptual disjunctions between the church and mental health care, and the high degree of subjectivity and therefore discrimination in a field that often is viewed as more of an art than a science. In terms of family and community influence, because of the troubled history of psychiatry and race, African Americans have a natural aversion to seeking mental health care or to pursuing a career as a mental health care practitioner (Thomas and Sillen 1972). I (D.L.P.) have often heard younger African American medical and graduate students speak of opposition to this professional pursuit from family members, who expect that if they are going to medical school, they should become a "real doctor," and I personally experienced the same.

Many clinicians of color are reluctant to pursue a field that appears too aligned with Western ideas of the individual over the community or collective; others are opposed to pursuing mental health specialties because doing so opposes their religious beliefs. In more than 25 years of clinical practice, only my (D.L.P.) African American patients have asked about my religious beliefs, suggesting an apparent contradiction to my chosen profession and the power of prayer. I imagine that my African American colleagues in other medical specialties are not questioned about whether their competence as a medical specialist has any connection to their religion. If African American patients express this level of suspiciousness toward me as an African American clinician, what types of suspiciousness (both stated and unstated) are affecting the therapeutic relationship between white clinicians and their African American patients?

For those of us African Americans who choose a career in mental health clinical services, navigating the hierarchical white supremacist institutions, often in the midst of major urban communities of color, can be tortuous without guides or safety or even an acknowledgment of potential dangers for the trainee of color (e.g., Stoute 2017). For example, African American trainees have described not being assigned patients of color for their long-term psychotherapy cases, with the implication that the African American patient is not psychologically minded enough. African American trainees also describe being nudged away from independent psychodynamic psychotherapy practice and instead guided toward research, inpatient psychiatry, or work in a clinic or administrative roles; the corresponding bias is that African American clinicians are not psychodynamic enough in their outlook or clinical acumen to have a successful practice or that there are too many nonwhite patients in need, and therefore the Black clinician would better serve the community if they worked in clinics and hospitals. Although this also represents a nod toward the realistic need for clinicians of color, the intersection of going against the grain of familial pressure to pursue psychiatric or graduate-level psychological training and the pressures from the training centers mentioned above represents specific challenges for African Americans that may discourage the pursuit of psychodynamic training or clinical practice. We emphasize that psychodynamic training is of benefit regardless of one's ultimate career path.

Supervision and Curriculum Issues

What is taught and how one is supervised are the most pertinent aspects of the development of clinical psychotherapists. Our experiences with patients shape us; however, the pedagogical shape of experiential learning is based on the extent of the faculties' biopsychosocial orientation. Nothing about the patient is subject to tacit exclusion. Race and ethnicity, therefore, are pivotal in understanding how the self is composed. Although one might argue that we are specifically addressing the needs of racial and ethnic minorities, this is furthest from our intent. Our interest is in challenging hegemonic notions of "whiteness" as we simultaneously attempt to explicate the "other," with a goal of moving away from the unconsciously supremacist notion that there is one group, the white one, and everything else is other and, implicitly, secondary. The subtle unconscious tendency to assume whiteness as the exemplar of our working model has an untoward impact particularly, although not exclusively, for the trainee of color. Faculty, both supervisors and teachers, must familiarize themselves with their own bias toward a white cultural monolith, educate themselves about the multicultural milieu that makes up modern psychotherapy practice, and actively and nondefensively explore their racist states of mind that impede these efforts (Blechner 2020; DiAngelo 2018; Keval 2016).

A word about whiteness: in our experience, whiteness is a nondynamic, defensive cover that reveals a minimal amount about the person and their ethnicity/ethnicities or cultural roots. As European immigrants came to the United States in the twentieth century, they often were greeted by great opposition and discrimination by the current citizenry, and their ability to enfold themselves into whiteness has been a source of maintaining white supremacist systems of institutional racism. However, this form of whitewashing has a cost (Holmes 2016, 2019): withdrawal from the cultural and ethnic signifiers that privilege the uniqueness of a multicultural society. These factors, along with the hierarchical structure of training, where power and position can make or break a training experience, deserve thoughtful reconsideration as those who train as clinicians of color remain underrepresented compared with the diverse population.

As psychotherapists, we are interested in cultural and ethnic milestones as part and parcel with the development of the self and how that might simultaneously be in conflict and in conversation with what the patient is struggling with in treatment. For these reasons, it is essential that these faculty and supervisors bring race and ethnicity into the conversation with their trainees. Openness, including a nondefensive, respectful curiosity, promotes an environment that is potentially safe enough for learning. Although many psychotherapists speak of the importance of creating a "safe space" in psychotherapy, we believe that any notion of psychotherapeutic safety is not fully attainable and ultimately can be only aspirational.

The most reliable way to increase safety during the course of a psychotherapeutic process is not by pronouncing the therapeutic space a "safe" one but rather by having a psychotherapist who is willing to attend to and explore with the patient the ways in which safety may be lacking or promoted. Training centers should consider using outside consultants on race and ethnicity to better prepare faculty and supervisors, along with other outside sources and reading materials on these issues (e.g., materials from the Association of Black Psychologists [https://abpsi.org], writings from African Studies departments, guest lecturers) to support a multicultural curriculum and prepare trainees, faculty, and supervisors to expand their knowledge of the importance of culture and ethnicity in the training of mental health professionals.

Although it is important for clinicians conducting psychotherapy with diverse populations to think, read, and engage in the Black experience, particularly because it has largely been neglected in the literature on psychotherapy, we believe that it is important to articulate the caveat that the notion of *the* Black experience is problematic in that Black people's lives and identities are hardly monolithic. It is certainly true that Black people, as a group, are almost universally the subject of racism and discrimination, but wide variations exist within the Black community regarding racial identity and racial experience. Often, these differences are determined by skin complexion, with darker-skinned people being more regularly targeted with discriminatory treatment than those with lighter skin. However, lighter skin does not provide immunity to racist treatment (Tummala-Narra 2007). And race and racism always manifest themselves intersectionally, with dimensions of social class, gender, and sexuality (among other categories) regularly codetermining the ways in which racial identity and racial discrimination manifest themselves (Hart 2019b).

It is important for psychotherapists to examine their own "benign" prejudices deriving from their sense of what traumas, injuries, and other features of Black experience must be like for all African Americans. Psychotherapists should, ideally, aspire to an informed yet open approach to each new patient with whom they work. They should avoid presumptions and instead judiciously draw from an awareness of the context from which a given patient comes—what that patient has had to deal with and what their forbears have come through. Such an approach, characterized by openness, curiosity, and discovery, is not the same as aspiring toward color-blindness. It is entirely worthwhile learning about African Americans' experience by reading (both professional and literary writing), studying all manner of artistic and social phenomena, and engaging in dialogue with people of diverse backgrounds in order to acquire a level of awareness of those aspects of life that may not be familiar to a given clinician. In this manner, certain basic levels of cultural competence may be attained (Tummala-Narra 2013; Tummala-Narra et al. 2017). However, there are limitations to where such competence efforts may take the clinician. And, indeed, "competence" may often serve as a form of defensiveness on the clinician's or supervisor's part: instead of approaching the clinical or supervisory encounter with openness (with its attendant vulnerability), acquiring competence can serve as a way for the clinician to feel oriented, knowledgeable, and secure in advance of the emergent encounter (Constantine and Sue 2007).

Clinical Considerations and Examples of Working With African Americans

The numerous examples of African American patients and trainees who have been scared off by their experiences working with white therapists could easily fill the rest of this chapter. Two clear scenarios have been described multiple times to one author (D.L.P.). The first is that white therapists look to their nonwhite patients to educate them about race, with the therapist bringing up and even focusing the treatment on racial issues even if that is not the patient's agenda. This overindulgence in all things racial can impede the formation of a working relationship in which the patient's clinical needs are intentionally placed as the highest priority. The therapist in this racial enactment feels that they are being "woke" because of this type of engagement, but in reality they are not awake (i.e., mindful, reflective) toward their actual patient, leaving the patient feeling unheard and merely the vehicle for the therapist's interests.

Case Vignette 1

Shortly after the death of Michael Brown in Ferguson, Missouri, in 2014, Jason, an African American male student preparing to go to law school, presented to me (D.L.P.) for a consultation on whether he should switch his therapist. From the first session with his therapist, a single white woman, Jason, self-described as "a big teddy bear," experienced her desires to talk about Michael Brown, Black Lives Matter, or any other current racial incident instead of what happened to lead him to arrive at her door. When he attempted to redirect his therapist, she became visibly upset, looking to him for comfort. When Jason attempted to point this out to her, she became defensive and suddenly concerned about her safety. After several months, Jason found my name and came in initially for a consultation, but in short time he began intensive psychodynamic treatment focused on the suicide of his brother and his traumatic past, including a mother who was a tough "functional alcoholic," which may have contributed to his brother's death and his own ambivalence about how to proceed in his life (Holmes 2006). Jason actively pursued treatment because he wanted to work through his grief over the loss of his brother and work on his rage toward his mother due to her treatment of both his brother and himself. He did not want to carry over these complicated emotions toward his fiancée, whom he loved and cherished, but for inexplicable reasons he would fly into rages with her at the slightest provocation.

Even though Jason's relationship with his previous therapist did not work out, he came to understand that a maternal transference had developed in which he was doing everything for his mother/therapist with little in return. This led him to get in touch with his rage, which we were able to connect with both maternal and paternal abandonment, reinforced by the loss of his older brother, who was a paternal substitute. When Jason attempted to redirect his former therapist, she demonstrated her fragility (DiAngelo 2018; Irving 2014) through her countertransference response in which Jason became an object to be feared. Correspondingly, later in treatment, Jason revealed to me that during any discussion about his fiancée, his former therapist would attempt to focus on feelings he must be having toward her. We speculated that the imaginary fantasy of Black men lusting over white women may have unconsciously been at play in the therapist's mind, yet what was most available to Jason was that the therapist's need to be the center of his attention was more closely aligned with his mother's narcissistic needs, exemplified by her alcoholism and the fact that every man in her life either abandoned her or died. This dynamic contributed to Jason's choosing to change therapists and getting in touch with me.

The other challenge for white therapists is to be dynamic and exploratory with African American patients and not solely supportive in a manner that borders on pitying. Some of these dynamics result from how African Americans have been depicted in history and through the media and the continued struggle to experience African Americans in their full humanity (Gay 2016). The works of Toni Morrison, Alice Walker, James Baldwin, Jordan Peele (2017) and Ta-Nehisi Coates (2015) bring the interior life of African people into sharper focus. The reason this is so important for clinicians who work with Black people is because of the experiential lack of this type of involvement by most white people, especially and including psychotherapists. Stated another way by the poet Claudia Rankine, "Blackness in the white imagination has nothing to do with Black people" (Kellaway 2015). Closing that experiential gap between what the white clinician imagines and the actual Black person seeking treatment should be the goal of all clinicians and all training centers. One of the vestiges of slavery and institutional racism is the misguided notion that Black people have too many real-life issues and are not capable of doing insight-oriented work and therefore are not appropriate candidates for dynamic treatments. Therefore, it is best to be supportive. We have worked in some of the most liberal areas of the country, and the continuing absence of dynamic care and training for African Americans that we have witnessed is a modern-day tragedy.

Case Vignette 2

Ms. L, an African American woman recently discharged from the hospital to me (D.L.P.) for follow-up care, described with much pain and sorrow the inpatient treatment she received from white clinicians that felt retraumatizing. She was hospitalized for depression with passive suicidal ideation on the 1-year anniversary of the death of her only child, a son, who was stabbed on the playground of his middle school. During her stay, Ms. L actively reported speaking to her son while on the unit. This was a source of comfort to her. On several occasions, various members of the treatment team reminded her that speaking to her son was impossible because he was dead, and the team gave active consideration to whether a psychotic process was complicating her grief and depression. Although it was a fact that her son was dead, these statements by Ms. L's clinicians only deepened her hurt and grief. Some of the team suggested that she was delusional, but her treatment both within the hospital and with me did not reach that conclusion, and her care did not include a neuroleptic. However, the hospital clinicians could not understand her continued sense of loss. The emphasis during her hospital stay was on possible use of antipsychotics instead of or in addition to ongoing dynamic grief work.

Most clinicians are aware of culturally attuned methods for honoring the dead, but what about the African American who exists in a past and present environment where the loss of loved ones can be violently abrupt and unaddressed? There is an unconscious notion that when Black people experience a loss, it does not hold the same magnitude as other Americans' losses. This, again, has vestiges of slavery, in which one's child, wife, or husband could be sold off, be accused falsely of a crime, or be lynched or killed without explanation or further knowledge of their whereabouts. For the slave owner, any recognition of the loss felt by individuals resulting from a slave being sold would mean coming face to face with their humanity and the cruelty and injustice inflicted. Therefore, what was sanctioned was a return to work for those left behind. Further cruelty would result if bereaved slaves expressed sorrow or mourning.

As the vestiges of terror and trauma have become part of our daily media menu, we have to question how we psychically contain, withdraw from, or become numb to these experiences that are more in our conscious awareness. This was exemplified by the disproportionate loss of persons of color at the beginning of the COVID-19 pandemic. For many people, the early pandemic losses were a "not me" experience, which developed unconsciously in the white mind as a false form of protection from COVID-19. In my (D.L.P.) opinion, as the pandemic ravaged all areas of the United States, from urban to rural, this false belief contributed to the spread of the disease.

Reflecting on how these unconscious feelings may be operating in the clinician's mind is the type of self-inventory required to move away from racist ways of thinking, and we believe that such self-examination is a task required of every psychodynamic psychotherapist. Again, this is best achieved by practicing *cultural humility,* which entails openness about race and culture similar to the clinician's approach toward sex and aggression. It cannot be overstated how important the clinician's own treatment can be in exploring and confronting issues of racism, privilege, bias, and difference. In previous writing, I have addressed the benefits of such exploration even when the treatment pair is of a similar race (Powell 2018). African American patients have described preferring to have the clinician speak up and pick up on the racial issues that appear on the surface than to remain silent, which communicates to the patient that not everything is available to explore in therapy.

We are speaking here about the receptivity of the clinician to hear what the patient wants to bring into treatment. This includes the experiential knowledge that what is silenced is typically shaped by trauma, shame, and guilt. The practice of psychodynamic psychotherapy is an inherently subversive emancipatory endeavor with the intent to free the individual from psychic, mental bondage (mitigating old patterns and perceptions about one's self and others) to allow for the lessening of conflict and to have adaptive options available for one's psychic use. From a racial perspective, we are also speaking to the deep familial identifications that shaped us in our youth and, depending on the depth of these internalizations, may continue to actively determine whom we love and whom we hate.

Therefore, when we speak of *racial matters* within psychodynamic psychotherapy, it is imperative that we are clear about whose agenda is being addressed. Why are we here? How should we listen to the racial "unthought known" (Bollas 1987)? I (D.L.P.) recall early in my career, postresidency, pre-analytic training, treating an older white man from the Depression era who was having great difficulties in his marriage. He was referred to me with a diagnosis of mild depression and narcissistic personality disorder. His wife, who had been hospitalized for symptoms of borderline personality disorder with multiple suicide attempts, was considered the most challenging member of the couple, but as the treatment advanced, this distinction became more difficult to discern. Issues of race never came up in the treatment; however, during the course of the work I became pregnant. With most of my patients, issues related to my pregnancy would emerge through dreams, expressed fantasies of abandonment, envious rage, or enactments, leaving us plenty of opportunity to discuss. However, with this particular patient, I could discern no indication that he was responding to my advancing pregnancy. Knowing that I had already planned my maternity leave and had made provisions of dates and coverage known to all of my other patients, I began questioning how long should I wait to inform him. For whom was this information intended? Why hadn't he noticed what was completely available to anyone who saw me (I had almost literally become the "elephant in the room")? Eventually, in my thirty-ninth week of pregnancy, I had to directly inform my patient of my upcoming leave, deciding that to continue in silence would be malpractice and acceding to a chronic enactment. His response stays with me to this day: "I have seen so many Black women prostitutes throughout my tortuous marriage; I decided when I began working with you to never look at you below your neck." My patient was actually blind to my pregnancy. The intersection of race, gender, treatment, and his narcissistic obsession to be the sole focus of attention had created this moment of psychic blindness. Exploring my patient's need to split off my sexuality in order to work with me while he was also dependent on me as his deepest vulnerabilities were expressed revealed the power of displacement and defensive compromise, particularly when it came to race, and his lingering dependency on me as his mistress/prostitute/therapist. This example reinforced the importance of considering race in all treatments and to have humility, empathy, and an ability to play (allowing a type of flexibility with consideration of the developmental regressive components that race engenders) and lean into the discomfort, including being open to being surprised, that often arises when issues of race reveal our shared humanity (Powell 2020).

It is important to reinforce that the obstacle, in our opinion, for most therapists attempting to work with race within the treatment setting is their ongoing investment in perceiving themselves as being "personally good." We embark on becoming experts at the talking cure through our individual traumas and a desire to help. Race, racism, bias, and privilege complicate this image, serving as a narcissistic injury with shame and guilt for not adhering to that stated goodness. The societal silence about these issues only promotes their toxicity. The events of 2020 have exposed the complicated reality of the American story in ways that cannot be ignored. Acknowledgment of the epidemic of racism can lead toward a path of remediation. As clinicians, when we experience ourselves being more supportive or silent about these issues, we are part of the problem and not its resolution. This includes white fear of Black anger: therapists reflexively turn to a more supportive stance instead of addressing what is behind Black anger, which is the fear of further trauma to their loved ones or themselves, who just want acknowledgment of a shared humanity and the ability to live their lives and contribute to this country without a knee on their neck. Black people are not asking for special treatment; unflinchingly, they are unapologetically demanding equal treatment. Neutrality is asked of our profession, but a detached analysis is easier to maintain when one is not likely to be a victim of racism. Empathic striving to embrace, resonate with, and contain our patients' experiences and affects is the work of good enough psychotherapeutic practices.

"Good Trouble": Toward the Dismantling of Racism in Mental Health Pedagogy and Practice

> *Get in good trouble, necessary trouble, and redeem the soul of America.*
>
> —John Lewis on Edmund Pettus Bridge,
> March 1, 2020, in Selma, Alabama,
> commemorating Bloody Sunday on March 7, 1965,
> when Lewis and other peaceful protesters
> were brutally beaten by law enforcement (Meacham 2020)

If our collective goal is to dismantle racism, we would do well to recognize that such dismantling will inevitably involve engagement in a long-term process. We recognize the utility of the term *antiracist* as a statement of intention and aspiration. However, we are concerned that, psychodynamically, identifying oneself as antiracist might narrow openness to addressing and mitigating racism that is ever present, both consciously and unconsciously, on both personal and organizational levels. Addressing such matters is, inherently, a work in progress and is never fully resolved (Kendi 2019).

Similar to the sexual and aggressive drives that are with us throughout life, racism has unconscious roots that, in our opinion, make its extinction—becoming nonracist—impossible. What we are advocating is the value of working through one's racist states of mind within dynamic treatments that reduce the deleterious effects of racism, lessening its impact as the foreign other, both within and outside therapeutic sessions, becomes more known as a projected part of the self. Racism is ubiquitous and is most harmful when unacknowledged or actively denied. Thus, addressing racism requires a particular mindfulness and, also, an unusual openness, especially in the mental health field within therapeutic situations and the training setting.

Especially for African American patients, recognizing the legacy and ongoing challenges of institutional racism, injustice, and discrimination in every aspect of life is an important empathic step for the clinician to ameliorate the effects of this unique American tragedy. Thus, to get into "good trouble" as a therapist is to be good enough in acknowledging the potential traumas and the resiliencies of people who have been systematically abused and discriminated against as American citizens. When we think of reparation, it is the unacknowledged psychic and physical trauma inflicted on Blacks by whites, both consciously and unconsciously, that needs continuous recognition and remediation. Thus, we consider being antiracist to be a verb, a behavior, not a noun or a destination. To become antiracist requires ongoing practice and mindfulness in our thinking and actions.

Important steps to mitigate prejudice, bias, and privilege in mental health training institutions include the following:

1. Recruit trainees of color and actively work on retention.
2. Provide development opportunities and promote faculty of color to administrative and clinical positions with high visibility.
3. Integrate issues of race and diversity in curricular and supervisory experiences, including faculty development, and make this instruction available to all trainees.
4. Consider outside nonpsychiatric/nonpsychological sources on issues related to race and ethnicity, appreciating the intersection of the biopsychosocial model that includes culture, race, and ethnicity.
5. Engage outside consultants to assist faculty's understanding of white fragility, privilege, and supremacy to mitigate their effects at every level of training.
6. Offer supervision and mentoring by people of color, even if the mentor is in another discipline (e.g., African American Studies, literature, film, poetry, critical theory, history) or outside the formal structure of training. Recognize the intersection of race, culture, history, and the mind.
7. When applicable, provide financial support for trainees of color and others in financial need.
8. Create organizational cultures that allow people at all hierarchical levels the security to speak up about the biases and discriminatory practices that they are encountering.
9. Encourage self-examination and interpersonal dialogue on the part of both individuals and groups within the organization.

Psychoanalytic/Psychodynamic Psychotherapy as an Inherently Subversive Emancipatory Endeavor

Psychoanalytic psychotherapy seeks to cultivate curiosity, in every direction possible. When the patient is invited to say whatever comes to mind—the fundamental rule—the patient is being beckoned toward a way of engaging their own mind that runs counter to dissociation-based social convention. The psychotherapist refrains from engaging in "ordinary" social discourse such as small talk in order to promote a psychotherapeutic climate in which each emergent thought and feeling may be regarded as worthy of interest, curiosity, inquiry, and association. In this manner, the status quo, including, most particularly, the oppressive and discriminatory aspects of self, other, and society, is subversively brought to light (Hymer 2005).

For all psychotherapeutic contexts, but particularly for the psychotherapist who is working with African American patients, all aspects of the psychotherapeutic dialogue should be permitted to be subject to curiosity and inquiry, including aspects of the therapy itself, the therapist, and the therapist's attitudes and beliefs. The more that the patient can feel authorized to look into everything that is said or comes to mind, including any and all aspects of the therapy itself, the more curious and usefully inquiring the patient will be able to be. It is important for the psychotherapist to be dedicated to considering and reflecting on their own personal thoughts, feelings, attitudes, and beliefs (i.e., self-analysis and analysis of the countertransference), but it is never possible for the therapist to be aware of those mental contents and processes that are unconscious. For this reason, the therapist's openness to the *patient's* observations and assertions about all of the things that emerge in the psychotherapeutic conversation is crucial to ensuring the fullest examination possible of oppressive, authoritarian, or supremacist forces that are likely to be embedded in both partners in the psychotherapeutic dialogue, regardless of their respective racial or ethnic identities. Patients should be encouraged to speak up and speak out, even at those times when what they might think of saying would question the social order as it is presently constituted or might be uncomfortable for or unflattering to the therapist (Hart 2017).

Within therapy, one's curiosity is allowed to expand away from the narrower strictures developed through defensive or identificatory mechanisms. However, such expansion of curiosity is also dependent on the clinician's willingness to recognize their countertransference and to consider, acknowledge the existence of, and work through their own biases, prejudices, and racist or supremacist points of view. The hierarchical nature of training and therapy makes the above an ongoing challenge, never leading to a definitive resolution. Training and therapy are best thought of as foundations requiring a form of ongoing work and investment from the clinician. This is particularly the case because for too long, issues of race, prejudice, and bias have been systematically denied and ignored by the vast majority of theorists and practitioners.

Key Points

- The major mental health disciplines, particularly psychiatry and psychology, have been primary contributors to systemic racist structures and practices, which has discouraged Black people from seeking treatment.
- The American history of the enslavement of Black people and the subsequent continuous violence and social and institutional discriminatory treatment of them have led to profound traumatization and the transgenerational transmission of trauma in Black communities. It is not just Black people, but all people, who have suffered, and continue to suffer, the effects of anti-Black racism, discrimination, and oppression.

- In the United States, the tortuous history of democracy simultaneous with slavery has resulted in unconscious racial symbolization of children from birth that, without active mitigation, enforces fear, prejudice, and discrimination against the racial other.
- Prejudice and discrimination are universal and universally pernicious and are derived from self-protective defenses. They involve profoundly destructive dissociative defensive uses of one group by another group or of one person by another person who is othered for the purposes of evacuating that which is unwanted and, indeed, intolerable in the racist's own mind.
- Black experience is not monolithic, and clinicians must be careful to be curious about and open to the details of experience of patients. The impact of any given instance of the experience of racism, be it an overt attack or a "discriminatory gesture," will depend on the person's history and identity and the actual and symbolic meanings of the aggression directed toward them, be it micro or macro.
- Racial hazards exist at every level and in every context of the mental health field. Patients and practitioners alike are subject to the prevailing white supremacist attitudes and traditions that exist in broader culture. These cannot be eliminated by wishing or pronouncing them so. Instead, matters of unsafety must be listened for and explored when and wherever they may arise. Especially for African American patients, recognizing the legacy and ongoing challenges of institutional racism, injustice, and discrimination in every aspect of life is an important empathic step for the clinician to ameliorate the effects of this unique American tragedy.
- Multicultural and racial competency should be considered as a starting, rather than an ending, point. A receptive, respectful, open orientation characterized by persistent humility on the clinician's part is essential for the fostering of building necessary trust and willingness to be open on the part of the patient.

References

Alexander M: The New Jim Crow: Mass Incarceration in the Age of Colorblindness. New York, The New Press, 2010

Altman N: Whiteness. Psychoanal Q 75(1):45–72, 2006 16482960

Anderson C: White Rage: The Unspoken Truth of our Racial Divide. New York, Bloomsbury, 2016

Baldwin J: As much truth as one can bear: to speak out about the world as it is, says James Baldwin, is the writer's job. The New York Times, January 14, 1962a. Available at: www.nytimes.com/1962/01/14/archives/as-much-truth-as-one-can-bear-to-speak-out-about-the-world-as-it-is.html. Accessed January 1, 2021.

Baldwin J: The Fire Next Time. New York, Vintage Books, Random House, 1962b

Baquet D, Corbett P: Uppercasing "Black." The New York Times, June 30, 2020. Available at: www.nytco.com/press/uppercasing-black. Accessed January 1, 2021.

Bell C: The protest psychosis: how schizophrenia became a Black disease. Psychiatr Serv 62(8):979–980, 2011

Blechner M. Racism and psychoanalysis: how they affect one another. Contemp Psychoanal 56(2–3):245–254, 2020

Bobo LD: Racial attitudes and relations at the close of the twentieth century, in America Becoming: Racial Trends and Their Consequences. Edited by Smelser N, Wilson WJ, Mitchell F. Washington, DC, National Academy Press, 2001, pp 262–299
Bobo LD: Inequalities that endure? Racial ideology, American politics, and the peculiar role of the social sciences, in The Changing Terrain of Race and Ethnicity. Edited by Krysan M, Lewis AE. New York, Russell Sage Foundation, 2004, pp 13–42
Bollas C: The Shadow of the Object: Psychoanalysis of the Unthought Known. New York. Columbia University Press, 1987
Bonilla-Silva E: The structure of racism in color-blind, "post-racial" America. Am Behav Sci 59(11):1–19, 2015
Briggs W, Krakauer J: The massacre that emboldened white supremacists. The New York Times, August 28, 2020. Available at: www.nytimes.com/2020/08/28/opinion/black-lives-civil-rights.html. Accessed January 1, 2021.
Carcea I, Lopez Carabllo N, Marlin BJ, et al: Oxytocin neurons enable social transmission of maternal behavior. Nature 596(7873):553–557, 2021 34381215
Chang A: White America is quietly self-segregating. Vox, August 31, 2018. Available at: www.vox.com/2017/1/18/14296126/white-segregated-suburb-neighborhood-cartoon. Accessed January 11, 2021.
Coates T-N: Between the World and Me. New York, Penguin Random House, 2015
Constantine MG, Sue DW: Perceptions of racial microaggressions among Black supervisees in cross-racial dyads. J Couns Psychol 54(2):142–153, 2007
Crenshaw K: Demarginalizing the intersection of race and sex: a Black feminist critique of antidiscrimination doctrine, feminist theory and antiracist politics. University of Chicago Legal Forum 1989(1):139–168, 1989
Crenshaw K: The urgency of intersectionality. TED Talk, October 2016. Available at: www.ted.com/talks/kimberle_crenshaw_the_urgency_of_intersectionality?utm_campaign=tedspread&utm_medium=referral&utm_source=tedcomshare. Accessed January 11, 2021.
DeGruy J: Post Traumatic Slave Syndrome: America's Legacy of Enduring Injury and Healing. Portland, OR, Uptone Press, 2005
Desmond M: In order to understand the brutality of American capitalism, you have to start on the plantation. The New York Times Magazine, August 14, 2019. Available at: nyti.ms/2uXTBPA. Accessed September 23, 2021.
DiAngelo R: White Fragility: Why It's So Hard for White People to Talk About Racism. Boston, MA, Beacon Press, 2018
Dominelli L: Racism permeates social work ideology and practice, in Anti-Racist Social Work. Practical Social Work Series. London, Palgrave, 1997, pp 23–41
Fanon F: Black Skin, White Masks (1952). Translated by Philcox R. New York, Grove, 2008
Follins LD, Lassiter JM (eds): Black LGBT Health in the United States: The Intersection of Race, Gender and Sexual Orientation. Lanham, MD, Lexington, 2017
Gadamer H-G: Truth and Method. Translated by Weinsheimar J, Marshall DG. New York, Continuum, 1975
Gay V: On the Pleasures of Owning Persons: The Hidden Face of American Slavery. New York, International Psychoanalytic Books, 2016
Goldberger M: "Bright spot," a variant of "blind spot." Psychoanal Q 62(2):270–273, 1993 8502731
Grier WH, Cobbs PM: Black Rage. New York, Basic Books, 1968
Guthrie RV: Even the Rat Was White: A Historical View of Psychology. Boston, MA, Pearson, 1976
Hammonds EM, Herzig RM: The Nature of Difference: Sciences of Race in the United States From Jefferson to Genomics. Cambridge, MA, MIT Press, 2008
Hannah-Jones N: The 1619 project. The New York Times Magazine, August 2019. Available at: nyti.ms/37JLWkZ. Accessed January 1, 2021.
Hart AH: From multicultural competence to radical openness: a psychoanalytic engagement of otherness. The American Psychoanalyst 51(1):12–27, 2017
Hart AH: The discriminatory gesture: a psychoanalytic consideration of posttraumatic reactions to incidents of racial discrimination. Psychoanalytic Social Work 26(1):5–24, 2019a

Hart AH: Why diversities? The American Psychoanalyst 53(3):8–10, 2019b
Heijmans BT, Tobi EW, Stein AD, et al: Persistent epigenetic differences associated with prenatal exposure to famine in humans. Proc Natl Acad Sci USA 105(44):17,046–17,049, 2008 18955703
Hoffman KM, Trawalter S, Axt JR, et al: Racial bias in pain assessment and treatment recommendations, and false beliefs about biological differences between Blacks and whites. Proc Natl Acad Sci USA 113(16):4296–4301, 2016 27044069
Holmes DE: The wrecking effects of race and social class on self and success. Psychoanal Q 75(1):215–235, 2006 16482966
Holmes D: Culturally imposed trauma: the sleeping dog has awakened: will psychoanalysis take heed? Psychoanal Dialogues 26(6):641–654, 2016
Holmes D: Our country 'tis of we and them: psychoanalytic perspectives on our fractured American identity. Am Imago 76(3):359–379, 2019
Hymer S: Subversive redemption in psychoanalysis. Am J Psychoanal 65(3):207–217, 2005 16142526
Irving D: Waking Up White, and Finding Myself in the Story of Race. Cambridge, MA, Elephant Room, 2014
Jones Marlin B: Breakthrough: the trauma tracer [video]. SciFri, October 2, 2020. Available at: www.youtube.com/watch?v=pBkVx12yc2M. Accessed January 1, 2021.
Kellaway K: Interview: Claudia Rankine: Blackness in the white imagination has nothing to do with Black people. The Guardian, December 27, 2015. Available at: www.theguardian.com/books/2015/dec/27/claudia-rankine-poet-citizen-american-lyric-feature. Accessed August 15, 2019.
Kendi IX: How to Be an Antiracist. New York, Random House, 2019
Keval N: Racist States of Mind: Understanding the Perversion of Curiosity and Concern. London, Karnac, 2016
Lawson W: Black Psychiatrists are few. They've never been more needed. The Washington Post, August 11, 2020. Available at: www.washingtonpost.com/local/black-psychiatrists-are-few-theyve-never-been-more-needed/2020/08/11/7df9eeea-dbeb-11ea-8051-d5f887d73381_story.html. Accessed January 1, 2021.
Lifton RJ: Beyond psychic numbing: a call to awareness. Am J Orthopsychiatry 52(4):619–629, 1982 7148983
Luhrmann TM: The Protest Psychosis: How Schizophrenia Became a Black disease. Am J Psychiatry 167(4):479–480, 2010
Meacham J: The South's fight for white supremacy. The New York Times, August 23, 2020. Available at: www.nytimes.com/2020/08/23/books/review/lost-cause-meacham.html?smid=url-share. Accessed January 1, 2021.
Metzl JM: The Protest Psychosis: How Schizophrenia Became a Black Disease. Boston, MA, Beacon, 2010
Metzl JM: Dying of Whiteness: How the Politics of Racial Resentment Is Killing America's Heartland. New York, Basic Books, 2019
Moss DB: Mapping racism. Psychoanal Q 75(1):271–294, 2006 16482968
Moss D: Free speech, love speech, hate speech, and neutrality: in and out of the consulting room. J Am Psychoanal Assoc 67(2):313–327, 2019 31088135
Noah T: George Floyd, Minneapolis protests, Ahmaud Arbery & Amy Cooper. The Daily Show With Trevor Noah, May 29, 2020. Available at: www.youtube.com/watch?v=v4amCfVbA_c. Accessed July 4, 2020.
O'Malley L: Addressing the lack of Black mental health professionals. St Louis, MO, Insight into Mental Health Diversity, November 2021
Pagán AM, Quintana V, Spotnitz J: Mitigating Black maternal mortality. Berkeley Public Policy Journal, Spring 2020. Available at: https://bppj.berkeley.edu/2020/04/13/spring-2020-journal-mitigating-black-maternal-mortality. Accessed January 1, 2021.
Peele J (dir): Get Out. Blumhouse Productions, Monkey Paw Productions, QC Entertainment, 2017
Pierce C: Psychiatric problems of the black minority, in American Handbook of Psychiatry. Edited by Arieta S. New York, Basic Books, 1974, pp 512–523

Powell D: Psychoanalysis and African Americans: past, present, and future, in The African American Experience: Psychoanalytic Perspectives. Edited by Akhtar S. New York, Rowman & Littlefield, 2012, pp 59–84
Powell D: Race, African Americans, and psychoanalysis: collective silence in the therapeutic situation. J Am Psychoanal Assoc 66(6):1021–1049, 2018
Powell D: From the sunken place to the shitty place: the film Get Out, psychic emancipation and modern race relations from a psychodynamic clinical perspective. Psychoanal Q 89(3):415–445, 2020
Roberts D: Fatal Invention: How Science, Politics, and Big Business Re-create Race in the Twenty-First Century. New York, The New Press, 2011
Sandler J: The background of safety. Int J Psychoanal 41:352–356, 1960 13746183
Sandler J, Rosenblatt B: The concept of the representational world. Psychoanal Study Child 17:128–145, 1962
Sharpe C: In the Wake: On Blackness and Being. Durham, NC, Duke University Press, 2016
Skloot R: The Immortal Life of Henrietta Lacks. New York, Crown, 2010
Staples B: The burning of Black Wall Street, revisited. The New York Times, June 19, 2020. Available at: www.nytimes.com/2020/06/19/opinion/tulsa-race-riot-massacre-graves.html?smid=url-share. Accessed January 1, 2021.
Statista: Distribution of active-duty enlisted women and men in the U.S. Military in 2019, by race and ethnicity. New York, Statista, 2020. Available at: www.statista.com/statistics/214869/share-of-active-duty-enlisted-women-and-men-in-the-us-military/. Accessed January 21, 2020.
Stein AD, Zybert PA, van de Bor M, Lumey LH: Intrauterine famine exposure and body proportions at birth: the Dutch Hunger Winter. Int J Epidemiol 33(4):831–836, 2004 15166208
Stevenson B: Just Mercy: A Story of Justice and Redemption. New York, Spiegel & Grau, 2014
Stoute B: Race and racism in psychoanalytic thought: the ghosts in our nursery. The American Psychoanalyst 51(1):10–29, 2017
Thomas A, Sillen S: Racism and Psychiatry. Secaucus, NJ, Citadel, 1972
Tummala-Narra P: Skin color and the therapeutic relationship. Psychoanal Psychol 24(2):255–270, 2007
Tummala-Narra P: Psychoanalytic applications in a diverse society. Psychoanal Psychol 30(3):471–487, 2013
Tummala-Narra P, Claudius M, Letendre PJ, et al: Psychoanalytic psychologists' conceptualizations of cultural competence in psychotherapy. Psychoanal Psychol 35(1):46–59, 2017
U.S. Census Bureau: American Community Survey 1-Year PUMS file. Suitland, MD, U.S. Census Bureau, 2015. Available at www.census.gov/programs-surveys/acs/data/pums.html. Accessed April 1, 2022.
Vaughans K: To unchain haunting blood memories: intergenerational trauma among African Americans, in Fragments of Trauma and the Social Production of Suffering. Edited by O'Loughlin M, Charles M. London, Rowman & Littlefield, 2015, pp 277–290
Washington HA: Medical Apartheid: The Dark History of Medical Experimentation on Black Americans From Colonial Times to the Present. New York, Anchor, 2006
Watkins CE, Hook JN: On a culturally humble psychoanalytic supervision perspective: creating the cultural third. Psychoanal Psychol 33(3):487–517, 2016
Wilkerson I: The Warmth of Other Suns: The Epic Story of America's Great Migration. New York, Random House, 2010
Wilkerson I: Caste: The Origins of Our Discontents. New York, Random House, 2020

CHAPTER 23

Contextualizing Psychodynamic Psychotherapy With Asian Americans

Integration of Transnational and Intergenerational Histories and Asian American Racialization

Jasmine Ueng-McHale, Ph.D.
Calvin R. Chin, Ph.D.

We are what we are because we have been what we have been.

—Sigmund Freud (2016, p. 179)

[W]e did not simply live in two cultures, as celebrants of the great American melting pot imagined. Displaced people also lived in two time zones, the here and the there, the present and the past, being as we were reluctant time travelers. But while science fiction imagined time travelers as moving forward or backward in time, this timepiece demonstrated a different chronology. The open secret of the clock, naked for all to see, was that we were only going in circles.

—Viet Thanh Nguyen (2015)

When considering psychotherapeutic issues within Asian American communities, it is important to first recognize the diversity of Asian Americans. Asian Americans comprise more than 40 different ethnic groups and speak more than 800 languages. Each subgroup has its own traditions, values, and history that affect the psychology of individual members. Moreover, generational status, immigration status, and intergenerational family history all intersect in shaping an individual's psychology. Both authors of this chapter identify as Asian American: Calvin Chin is a first-generation Chinese American gay man, and Jasmine Ueng-McHale is a second-generation Taiwanese American heterosexual woman. In planning for this chapter, we were struck by the similarities in our experiences in graduate training regarding the psychology of Asian Americans. The approaches taught were often grounded in a discussion of cultural norms and the process of assimilation in the absence of a racialized historical context in America—approaches that reinforce the idea of Asians as "other" with fixed cultural identities, overemphasizing East-West dichotomies and the role of cultural differences (Hung 2016). It was not until after graduate training that we began to integrate an understanding of our own racial identity, racialization, and Asian American and transnational histories into our work.

Asian American racialization changes throughout American history, with a "friend today, foe tomorrow" or "foe today, friend tomorrow" treatment that is contingent on domestic and international American interests (Zia 2000). In this chapter, we summarize some of the stereotypes and dominant narratives that continue to affect Asian Americans today, and we illustrate some ways these narratives have been constructed and reconstructed in American history. We then present clinical approaches to working with Asian American clients through building racial reflective functioning, interrogating dominant narratives, maintaining a stance of informed inquiry, and contextualizing one's experiences in transnational and intergenerational histories.

History and Its Discontents

Anti-Asian racism and stereotypes have deep roots in American history, institutions, laws, and culture. American racialization of Asians is embedded in intersecting forms of oppression (Collins 2000) across interpersonal, systemic, and cultural contexts. From the time significant numbers of Asians first stepped foot on American soil in the mid-1800s, they experienced the profound impacts of Anti-Asian racism in concrete ways through violent harm to their bodies; exclusion of their presence in white spaces; expulsion; forced migration; limitations to their social and legal status; and restrictions on their freedom of movement, freedom to work, and freedom to marry (Lee 2015; Lew-Williams 2018). Over time, they also experienced the fickleness of American sentiment toward Asian ethnic groups in the changing representations of Asian communities: primitive, subservient coolies; people who threaten national security with their foreign allegiances; hard-working wartime allies; competitors to white American interests; refugees unfairly "freeloading" off of American resources; or a people to be tolerated as a means to American economic and political power in Asia. Whatever the rhetoric of the day, they were perceived as "foreign" and "other" compared with white Americans. Throughout American history, these narratives have continued to shape policies and practices, directly affecting the lives of Asian Americans.

In addition to the concrete impact on people's daily lives, anti-Asian racism and stereotypes also have profound effects on the psychological formation and well-being of Asian Americans. There are explicit and implicit meanings within the racialization of Asians interpersonally and culturally and through national policies—meanings about belonging and its limits, what is acceptable and valued, the precariousness of social and legal status and protections, and the limits to being seen and valued in ways that are congruent with how one knows oneself to be. Narratives of racialization of Asians can come to inform one's sense of self and one's racial identity, including parts of the self that express resistance to and internalization of racism. These narratives also inform Asian American activism and community advocacy.

For all of these reasons, it is important to understand the origins of anti-Asian racism and how the representations of Asians in America have been constructed and reconstructed over time. An understanding of racialization makes it possible to integrate the meanings about belonging and value and where the trauma and psychic dangers lie within the contexts of national and transnational histories and within intergenerational family and attachment histories. This situates and tethers the individual's development within an intricate contextual web stretching between the Americas and Asia across multiple generations.

Orientalism, Yellow Peril, and Asian Exclusion

One of the oldest racist tropes predicated on the East-West binary, Orientalism is a patronizing Western view of Asian people that essentializes "the East" or "the Orient," including Asian, Middle Eastern, and North African societies, as static, undeveloped, less rational, primitive, and uncivilized; driven by bodily impulses; and exotic and mystical as compared with Western societies (Said 1978). Dating back to Hippocrates and European travel logs (Okihiro 2001), Orientalism has been used to justify European and American imperialism, as well as restriction and exclusion of Asian immigration to the United Sates. Foundational to anti-Asian racism, the Orientalist view has persisted for centuries within the United States.

The early history of Orientalism in the racialization of Asians in America beginning in the 1850s is important because from that time forward, these events powerfully shaped racialization of Asians and anti-Asianist rhetoric and exclusionary policies, as well as adaptation and activism in Asian American communities. An Orientalist view dominated anti-Asian sentiment in the mid-nineteenth century, when large numbers of Chinese, mostly men, began to arrive in the United States, first to join the gold rush in California and later to work on the transcontinental railroad. Chinese people were portrayed as inferior, dishonest, heathen "coolies" who were servile, dirty, and unhygienic and spread disease; they were people with strange foods and customs who were foreign and "other" compared with white Americans. Unlike European migrants, Chinese were seen as unassimilable to American values, with traditional customs and loyalties that would always lie with China (Lew-Williams 2018; Okihiro 2001).

Paradoxically, although Anti-Asianists viewed coolies as servile, they also portrayed them as cunning, resilient, and indomitable in their perseverance and capacity in work and business—presenting a "yellow peril" that threatened white American values and opportunities. Anti-Asianist perspectives such as these assert that Asian migrants pose a threat to the interests of the United States and advocate for the separation, exclusion, and expulsion of Asians (Okihiro 2001), often under the justification of protecting jobs for white workers. This fear grew as Chinese workers, having completed work on the transcontinental railroad, began to enter many other industries. Chinese were seen as a unique threat to white interests, despite the fact that many other immigrant groups such as Irish and German migrants were also taking on work in the same industries (Lew-Williams 2018). Competing portrayals of compliant, servile Asians and threatening, cunning Asians were also used to compare and contrast different Asian ethnic groups as the demand for labor attracted workers to the United States from across Asia. For example, Chinese were depicted as servile in contrast to Japanese, who were depicted as competitive threats (Cox 2011).

Beyond rhetoric and attitudes, these anti-Asian perspectives have been used to justify expulsion, exclusion, and white Americans' racial political violence toward Asians at different points in U.S. history, shaping local and federal policies—expressions of anti-Asian racism routinely left out of historical accounts and collective memory (Lew-Williams 2018). As described by Lew-Williams (2018), between 1885 and 1886, white Americans escalated violence to the point that at least 168 communities across the Western United States drove out their Chinese residents in violent purges targeting all Chinese people. The intent of the anti-Chinese movement was exclusion across multiple spheres: at the local level, excluding Chinese from public spaces and work reserved for white Americans; at the national level, barring entry and denying citizenship to those already in the United States; and at the international level, excluding China from conversations about immigration in which policies were set unilaterally by the United States (Lew-Williams 2018).

The Chinese were caught in racist rhetoric that was exploited by both political parties—a racial conflict that was used to distract from other inequities among white workers. The "Chinese question" was used "to inflame and distract white workers, frustrated by rising unemployment and economic depression" (Zia 2000, p. 28). Racist narratives about Asians have continued to be used through current times as a wedge between racial and ethnic groups or as a distraction to suppress political movements that might otherwise focus attention on addressing injustices. One example of this triangulation is seen in the 1982 murder of Vincent Chin, a 27-year-old of Chinese descent who was killed with a baseball bat by autoworkers who blamed Japanese people for taking their jobs amid the oil crisis. The trial prompted outrage in Detroit because the judge sympathized with the defendants, who pleaded guilty, and sentenced them to a mere 3 years of probation and fines (Zia 2000). In another example, anti-Asian rhetoric, policies, and violence increased from 2016 through 2022, causing significant anxiety about discrimination and hate crimes among Asian Americans (American Psychological Association 2016; National Asian Pacific American Women's Forum 2022; Yellow Horse et al. 2021). This occurred as white anxieties rose amid polarizing census talk of the shifting demographic of the United States toward a "majority-minority" in which whites will comprise less than 50% of the population, an ever-widening income gap, increasing geopolitical tensions between the United States and China, and hundreds of thousands of American deaths and job losses in the winter of 2020 during the coronavirus SARS-CoV-2 disease (COVID-19) pandemic. All of this occurred as white anxieties rose amid polarizing Census talk of the demographics of the United States shifting toward a "majority minority" in which whites will comprise less than 50% of the population, an ever-widening income gap, and the more than 300,000 American deaths and the unemployment of 30 million people as of December 2020 during the SARS-CoV-2 disease (COVID-19) pandemic.

Lew-Williams (2018) noted that Anti-Chinese violence is routinely left out of our national narrative of racial violence in America. She suggested that "When we use black oppression and Indian extermination to define racial violence in nineteenth-century America, Chinese expulsions seem insignificant. Or, even more inaccurately, they appear not to be violent at all" (p. 3). The harmful impact of Orientalism and "yellow peril" narratives in the racialization of Asians and the connections between anti-Asian rhetoric, exclusionary policies, and racial violence against Asians continue to be minimized and dissociated in collective memory and awareness. Many people do not acknowledge that racism against Asians persists over time, and even if they do, they see it as insignificant compared with racism against other groups.

Border Control, Immigration Status, Surveillance, and the Making of the Perpetual Foreigner

Anti-Chinese rhetoric and violence led to border control and exclusion of Asians from a path to citizenship, which in turn have further reinforced the stereotype of Asians as "perpetual foreigners" in the national imaginary. These racialized narratives leave Asians more vulnerable to surveillance, civil rights violations, and insecurity as the tide of anti-Asian sentiments shifts and reshapes policies. In response to Anti-Chinese rhetoric and violence in the late 1800s, immigration laws were created to bar Chinese migration, full participation, and residency in U.S. communities, ending a policy of open migration for all (Lew-Williams 2018). This was the first time that immigration and citizenship policies came into use as a tool for maintaining white economic and political power in the United States. The U.S. government created a border control system and introduced the term *alien* as a descriptor of legal and social status for individuals who were not naturalized.

Following other federal restrictions, the Chinese Exclusion Act was passed in 1882, explicitly prohibiting all Chinese from becoming naturalized citizens and banning migration of Chinese laborers for 10 years, allowing entry only to teachers, students, merchants, diplomats, and travelers. Because few women fit these categories at the time, this legislation effectively prevented the migration of Chinese women (Lee 2015). This created obstacles for marriage for Chinese men because between 1850 and 1950, 15 states passed anti-miscegenation laws prohibiting Chinese men from marrying white women, in effect creating a bachelor society of Chinese men. The Chinese Exclusion Act would not be lifted for more than 50 years (Lew-Williams 2018). Immigration from Asia would not be opened in a significant way until the Hart-Cellar Immigration Act of 1965, corresponding to the height of the Civil Rights Era (Lee 2015).

The perpetual foreigner and yellow peril narratives make Asian Americans vulnerable to state-sanctioned surveillance and violations of civil rights as U.S. foreign policy shifts, resulting in perceptions of threat from one "bad" ethnic group of Asian enemies, in contrast to perceptions of another "good" ethnic group of Asian allies (Lee 2015). At the same time that the Chinese Exclusion Act was repealed to strengthen the World War II allyship between China and the United States, narratives of Asian threat and foreign loyalties were leveraged to justify the unlawful internment of Japanese Americans from the West Coast of the United States, of all ages, including children, through President Franklin D. Roosevelt's 1942 Executive Order 9066, which established the War Relocation Authority (Lee 2015). Despite failure to find evidence of espionage, Americans of Japanese descent were forced to relinquish almost all of their possessions and to leave their homes and businesses to relocate to internment camps, separating families across the country and subjecting them to live in poor conditions in camps, some of which were converted from animal stables. The internment of Japanese Americans traumatized Japanese communities and divided them in their responses to the federal government, resulting in both the intergenerational transmission of trauma and a tradition of civil rights activism in generations to come.

Asian racialization has also made other Asian American communities vulnerable to civil rights violations and surveillance with the vicissitudes of U.S. foreign policy. The U.S. government targeted Chinese communities for surveillance after China became communist in 1949 (Lee 2015). There is also the surveillance of Asian American scientists such as Wen Ho Lee, a Taiwanese American scientist at the University of California at Los Alamos National Laboratory, who was falsely accused of stealing secrets for the Chinese government in 1999 and was jailed and placed in solitary confinement for 278 days in federal custody without bail. Similarly, after the 9/11 attacks in 2001, Muslim communities were surveilled, and suspected terrorists were held at detention centers without due process and civil rights protections, affecting not only Middle Eastern communities but also South Asian Muslim communities (Lee 2015).

Anti-Asian racism has continued to be expressed through U.S. immigration and border control policies. In the early twentieth century, border control policies and anti-Asian rhetoric, which first specifically targeted Chinese people, were used as a blueprint for Asian exclusion applied to Japanese, Korean, South Asian, and Filipino migrants (Lew-Williams 2018). For Filipino migrants (for a review, see Lee 2015), the rhetoric about Filipinos and immigration policies shifted with the American colonization of the Philippines beginning in 1898 and the later recognition of Philippine independence in 1946, changing the status of Filipinos from U.S. nationals to "aliens." In more recent years, during the Trump administration (2016–2020), travel and migration from Muslim countries was banned, affecting Asian American Muslims, including Indonesian, Pakistani, Indian, Malaysian, and Bangladeshi communities. The administration also issued executive orders revoking long-term residential status such as Temporary Protected Status for hundreds of thousands of Southeast Asians who had migrated under protected refugee status and then suspended visas, specifically targeting Chinese international students and researchers amid escalation of anti-Chinese rhetoric and Anti-Asian racism during the COVID-19 pandemic. People in Southeast Asian American communities were already three to four times more likely to be deported for old convictions compared with other immigrant communities because of the specifics of immigration policies enacted in 1996. The retroactive nature of those policies resulted in individuals being sentenced for deportation decades after they had already served their sentences and rebuilt lives in their communities (Dinh et al. 2021).

Border control systems continue to affect a large number of Asian Americans and their families. From 2016 to 2020, the federal government escalated immigration enforcement and border control, including the construction of immigration detention facilities, affecting 1.7 million undocumented Asians in the United States. In 2019, it was estimated that about one out of every seven Asian immigrants was undocumented (Asian Americans Advancing Justice 2019). This included childhood arrivals of about 29,000 South Koreans, 25,000 Filipinos, 20,000 Indians, and 23,000 Chinese with no clear path to citizenship or legal residency.

The changes in immigration policies and enforcement leave individuals in a chronic state of insecurity with the ground shifting beneath them—insecurity both in the risk of having lives uprooted with little notice and in feeling criminalized, restricted, and judged as a person of lower status, despite the fact that immigration status has been seen legally as a civil matter, not a criminal one. American propaganda overseas overwhelmingly "sells" the American dream, extolling the virtues of freedom and inclusion in the American "melting pot," particularly in countries with histories of American military interventions. Furthermore, universities and businesses market to potential workers and students overseas, with little acknowledgment of the hardships presented by the U.S. immigration system. Therefore, for people who immigrate to the United States, when tides turn against them, there can be a sense of having been peddled a misrepresentation of life in the United States, with resulting feelings of betrayal and bitterness.

Expulsion and exclusion through immigration and citizenship policies have further reinforced the stereotype of Asians as "perpetual foreigners" without political power or civic relevance because these policies denied Asian immigrants a path to citizenship and thus voting rights until 1952. This rhetoric not only leaves Asian Americans vulnerable to surveillance, civil rights violations, and insecurity in immigration status, but it also contributes to common racial microaggressions based on the perpetual foreigner stereotype. Asian Americans are commonly asked, "Where are you from? No, where are you really from?" with the implication that they must be from an Asian country as opposed to an American town. It is often assumed that their native language is not English and that they speak an Asian language or that they have familiarity with an Asian country and customs. People habitually approach Asian Americans to try out the words they know in Asian languages. Hearing from others that "Your English is so good" is a common microaggression, as well as being asked how to cook Asian foods and where to get "authentic" Asian cuisine.

Model Minority Myth: Orientalism and Yellow Peril Repackaged

Erika Lee (2015) writes that during the Cold War era, "Good Asian Americans were assimilated Americans whose cultural heritage and ties to noncommunist Asia were assets to the United States. Bad Asian Americans were unassimilated aliens whose ties to communist Asian countries were threats to U.S. national security. The lines between good and bad, however, were not always clear and could shift without warning" (p. 276). Sometimes, Asians' "otherness" and cultural ties to their ethnic Chinese or Japanese culture was seen as evidence of disloyal, treasonous tendencies. When the narrative flipped, Asian ethnic culture was held up as a traditional family model used to negatively judge other groups in America who were engaging in civil unrest or inciting societal change. Emerging out of the Cold War in the late 1950s, as the country witnessed white youth increasingly exhibit rebellious and delinquent behavior, a narrative emerged of Asian Americans, particularly Chinese and Japanese families, as model minorities who "supposedly respected authority, had high moral values, adhered to strict gender roles, and enjoyed strong, stable nuclear families. Confucian traditions, social scientists said, led to upstanding youth and model families and communities" (Lee 2015, p. 277).

In the 1960s, the Asian American model minority myth was perpetuated into a new stereotype leveraged against the Civil Rights Movement as "evidence" to disprove the existence of systemic racial discrimination against African Americans (Lee 2015; Zia 2000). As riots and civil unrest arose in American cities, news stories suddenly began portraying Asian Americans, particularly Chinese Americans and Japanese Americans, as the one racial minority achieving success, specifically in contrast to African Americans. The model minority narrative was used to uphold the myth of American meritocracy—the belief that in America anyone can achieve economic success if only they are willing to work hard enough (Zia 2000). As Lee (2015) writes, "Social scientists and journalists argued that Asian Americans were able to succeed both in spite of their racial difference and because the allegedly Asian traits that they possessed—family values, traditional virtues of hard work, thrift, morality, respect for authority, and persistence—were perfectly suited to the U.S.'s meritocracy" (p. 279). The model minority narrative contrasted Asian Americans to those Americans who eschewed hard work and chose instead a welfare check, completely omitting the significance of social context such as social networks (Wailoo 2020). Despite its supposed basis in Asian ethnic cultural values, the model minority stereotype is applied to anyone of Asian descent regardless of their cultural background, including mixed-race individuals or transnational Asian adoptees who have grown up in non-Asian families.

In the 1980s, news sources continued to write about the model minority narrative, focusing on Asian American "whiz kids" and their high-achieving school performances, including Southeast Asians whose families had immigrated to the United States under refugee status, fleeing wartime persecution (Lee et al. 2009). This resurgence of the model minority narrative coincided with policies aimed at rolling back gains in civil rights legislation, including affirmative action, redistricting and desegregation appeals, and social welfare programs, once again racially triangulating Asian Americans vis-à-vis white and Black Americans (Kim 1999). This approach enlisted Asian Americans in racial entrenchment through organizing conservative Asian Americans to oppose programs such as affirmative action. As Claire Jean Kim (1999) writes, "The valorization of Asian Americans as a model minority who have made it on their own cultural steam only to be victimized by the 'reverse discrimination' of race-conscious programs allows White opinionmakers to lambast such programs without appearing racist—or to reassert their racial privileges while abiding by the norms of color blindness" (p. 117). In a more recent example of this strategy, conservative Chinese Americans who immigrated during the 1990s organized against affirmative action and use of racial data in admissions to competitive institutions of higher education. Recruited to file lawsuits against universities, they unsuccessfully sued Harvard in 2019, accusing the institution of unconstitutionally using racial quotas, after similar lawsuits had been attempted without success with white students as plaintiffs, as in the case of *Fisher v. University of Texas at Austin* (2016).

In 2011, amid anxieties about an Asian invasion in higher education, Amy Chua's book *Battle Hymn of the Tiger Mother* capitalized on the model minority myth, further inflaming fears and stereotypes of successful Chinese children and the Asian values of parents who put enormous, even emotionally abusive, pressure on their children to forge their success (Chua 2011). When Asian Americans are asked about their parenting, it is not unusual to hear them preface their remarks with "I'm not the typical Asian parent" as a way to distance themselves from that stereotype.

Inherently part of anti-Black racism, the model minority narrative also suppresses attention to anti-Asian discrimination. Eng and Han (2019) describe how the model minority myth "persistently represents Asian Americans as nerdy automatons, technically gifted in math and sciences, continuously working, compliant, wealthy, and exempt from discrimination.... More often than not, racism against Asian Americans occurs without recognition and without provoking any serious outcry or protest" (p. 2). This myth persisted in the 1960s despite the facts that Japanese American men had a lower median income compared with white males; the upward mobility of Chinese and Japanese Americans trailed behind that of white Americans; and racial discrimination in housing, employment, and social life continued (Lee 2015). The model minority myth has persisted in recent years even as the gains in income for lower-income Asians lagged behind those in other racial and ethnic groups between 1970 and 2016 (Kochhar and Cilluffo 2018). These narratives also obscure the inequities that exist in the workplace, the "bamboo ceiling" that excludes Asian Americans from advancing to middle management (a problem for all racial minority groups) and to leadership positions, as Asian American men lag behind men of all other races and Asian American women lag behind women of all races in reaching executive roles (Gee and Peck 2017; Gee and Wong 2016). In an American Psychological Association (2016) study of the impact of discrimination, 25% of Asian American participants reported being unfairly denied promotions

The model minority myth also obscures the disparities of economic and social privilege between different Asian ethnic communities. In 2018 the Pew Research Center found that Asians had displaced African Americans as the most economically divided racial or ethnic group in the United States (Kochhar and Cilluffo 2018). As a result, many Asian Americans advocate for disaggregating the data collected on Asian Americans so that the extreme economic and social disparities between different Asian American communities can be revealed.

Even "positive" racial stereotypes create psychological harm. The model minority myth creates psychological distress in the "never enough-ness" that many Asian Americans carry inside them whether or not they are high achievers. Many Asian Americans experience microaggressions based on this stereotype. One Asian American teenager confided in session that white students were always asking her for the answers to questions during class—answers they assumed she knew but that she often did not know. Painfully, she confessed, "I'm the dumb Asian." The myth compels Asian Americans to meet expectations of high achievement, but that very same achievement can engender envy and anti-Asian resentment. The model minority myth also contributes to exclusion from opportunities in the workplace based on these stereotypes. For example, Asian Americans are more likely to be perceived as having more quantitative and less relational skills or to be seen as timid, cooperative, and compliant, making them highly qualified workers rather than leadership material—valued hires, but not worthy of promotion.

Furthermore, religion scholar Jonathan Tran (2002) links Asian American racialization to the early construction of race in America as a construct that protects power and property for white Americans and maintains the commodification of people as a source of cheap labor. In this way, the construct of race and the model minority myth are intertwined with concepts of labor and productivity and the linking of one's worth to one's productivity. This reinforces a social and intrapsychic mandate to be productive and to work all the time. For example, in a discussion with a college student about feeling the constant pressure to be productive even in leisure activities, Dr. Ueng-McHale suggested that he was a person, not a robot, to which he replied, "I wish I were a robot." There is a feeling of one's value being so tightly tied to one's productivity that it is perhaps a little threatening to claim one's humanity. Because of and in the face of racism, it may feel like a more protected position to work "like a machine."

Refugees and the Effects of American Anticommunist Military Action in Asia

U.S. residents of Cambodian, Vietnamese, Lao, and Hmong descent; recent immigrants from Myanmar; and other Asian Americans in the late twentieth century and early twenty-first century who entered the United States through refugee programs encountered some differences in the ways they were racialized. Aggressive anticommunist foreign policy after World War II led to American military campaigns in Vietnam, Laos, and Cambodia and the formation of a Secret Army of Hmong soldiers inside Laos allied with the United States, involving the entire Hmong population (Lee 2015). The defeat of the United States and anticommunist Vietnamese, Laotian, Hmong, and Cambodian forces and the rise of communist governments in all three countries resulted in the migration of 1.2 million Vietnamese, Lao, Hmong, and Cambodian people to the United States between 1975 and 2010 (Lee 2015). Many who arrived under protected refugee status received both humanitarian aid and hostility when entering the United States, despite the fact that they were allied with the United States in these wars. For example, South Vietnamese refugees, many of whom fought as allies with the United States in the Vietnam War, were sometimes met with hostility in the United States stemming from how Vietnamese were maligned as enemies during the war. Many Southeast Asian refugees experienced significant trauma throughout their journey to the United States. Some were escaping genocide or military conflicts in their countries of origin, and many bore witness to extreme violence as they escaped their countries. Their experiences of trauma continued in the refugee camps, where they were often held from months to years while awaiting eventual placement in the United States.

While demonstrating immense resilience in their escape and resettlement in the United States, many Southeast Asian immigrants faced significant challenges as a result of experiences of trauma and racism and their limited financial resources. In resettlement programs, many were placed in public housing complexes in poor, urban neighborhoods (Lee 2015). Resentment toward the refugees grew with the cost of resettlement and backlash against the number of new immigrants. Some Americans saw the newcomers as unassimilated "freeloaders" given an "unfair advantage" over other Americans for access to aid "despite regulations that offered Southeast Asian refugees the same level of federal assistance as others in the same income bracket" (Lee 2015, p. 339).

Asian Americans who fail to achieve the model minority stereotype are sometimes perceived as "failed Asians" (Lee 2005; Lee et al. 2009). Ong (2003) argues that nonwhite immigrants are either ideologically "Whitened" or ideologically "Blackened" depending on their economic status. Although many Southeast Asian Americans have found economic success, others are ideologically Blackened when they fail to perform model minority identities. S.J. Lee (2005) found that teachers tried to make sense of their Hmong students by comparing them with both their middle-class East Asian American students and the working-class African American students in their school. The Hmong students were blamed for their academic struggles, in much the same way that African Americans are blamed instead of taking into account the racist structures that perpetuate differences in achievement. Similarly, Chhuon and Hudley (2010) found that teachers assumed Cambodian high school students in California to be low achieving, gang involved, and "ghetto." Reyes (2007) also found that Southeast Asians were often stereotyped as being gang members, welfare-dependent, and criminal, similar to ways that African Americans were stereotyped.

Racialization of Gender and Sexuality

Gender and sexuality are intersecting aspects of identity that have a large impact on the experience of Asians and Asian Americans. Asian American lesbians are frequently fetishized and stereotyped in white culture as being passive, sexually exotic, asexual, or nonexistent. For gay Asian men, racism within the gay community is quite explicit. For example, in online dating platforms it is not uncommon to see profiles that specifically exclude "fats, femmes, and Asians." As a result, many gay Asian American men internalize these negative racial representations and idealize white bodies. Some choose to date white men exclusively, disavowing interest in other Asian men. Gay Asian men are often racially and sexually stereotyped (Wilson and Yoshikawa 2004) as passive or even feminine as the same fetishized stereotypes of Asian women as submissive geishas are subverted and applied to gay and bisexual Asian men. White men who seek out gay Asian men are often referred to as "rice queens." Discrimination and prejudice against Asian gay men are associated with a host of negative physical, mental, and behavioral health outcomes (e.g., Jackson et al. 1996; Krieger 2000; Krieger and Sidney 1997; Martin et al. 2003; Mays and Cochran 2001; Noh and Kaspar 2003; Williams et al. 1997), including greater mental health distress and higher rates of HIV-risk behavior (Chae and Yoshikawa 2008; Yoshikawa et al. 2004).

In addition to experiencing racism in the gay community, Asian gay men and lesbians also experience homophobia in the Asian community (Chan 1989; Sung et al. 2015). Chan (1989) notes that some traditional Asian values, such as the strong emphasis on family as the primary social unit, familial obligations to continue the family line through marriage and children, and rigid socialized gender roles, may result in Asian gay men and lesbian women being cast as rejecting the importance of family and Asian cultural values. In some families, being gay or lesbian can be seen as bringing shame to the family. As a result, many gay Asian men do not feel that they can disclose their sexuality to their families, which leads to situations in which gay Asian men may be very out in their communities while remaining in the closet with their families. As a gay Asian psychologist, Dr. Chin has observed how difficult it can be to inhabit these intersecting identities and to feel affirmed and recognized. In professional circles, he has witnessed both how marginalized sexual identity can be in communities of Asian mental health professionals and how marginalized racial identities can be in LGBTQ+ professional spaces.

The gendered and sexualized racialization of Asian people in American culture and white masculine hegemony inform these intersectional dynamics. Many Asian American women must deal with others' racial fetish—a person's preference for sexual intimacy with others belonging to a specific racial out-group—popularly known as "yellow fever" (Zheng 2016). This fetishization places psychological burdens on Asian Americans "to fulfill, resist, or otherwise negotiate those stereotypes" (Zheng 2016, p. 405) and can feel uncomfortable, objectifying, and violating (Chou et al. 2015). Rather than being loved for the particulars of who they are as individuals, women can feel depersonalized and fungible, as though they are a love object interchangeable with other women as long as they are Asian (Zheng 2016). Asian women are represented either as the mysterious, seductive, "Dragon Lady" on the one hand or as the docile, domestic "Lotus Blossom" whose primary worth and desirability stem from serving a man's every need on the other (Chou et al. 2015; Zheng 2016). The latter can be seen as a mash-up of Asian racial stereotypes—a sexual model minority in its combination of "exotic," obedient sexual appeal and hardworking, family-centered values (Cho 2003; Zheng 2016). For women, stereotypes extend to specifics of genitalia, with myths that Asian women have "sideways" vaginas or that they have "tighter" vaginas than other women because they are smaller in stature. Asian American women are infantilized as small and obedient, often described as "cute" or "adorable," which is even more disturbing when these words are applied to women's bodies in men's desire for their tight, small genitalia. These stereotypes lead to increased risk for Asian American women to be subjected to sexual harassment and assault (Cho 2003).

In contrast to the "yellow fever" for Asian women, many Asian American men feel that they are seen as less attractive and emasculated compared with white men, stereotypes that have historical roots. Reinforced by anti-miscegenation laws that created Chinese bachelor communities and laws that limited Chinese men to jobs traditionally performed by women (e.g., laundry, housekeeping, cooking) from the late 1800s onward, Orientalist racial stereotypes emasculated Asian men, representing them as either effeminate and weak or sexually deviant and threatening. In one study, many Asian American males struggled with portrayals of Asian American men as not attractive and effeminate as compared with white men, as well as the stereotype that Asian men have small penises (Chou et al. 2015). These internalized attributions contribute to feelings of negative self-worth and painful feelings about themselves as unattractive, "nerdy" Asian guys in the eyes of others. These stereotypes play out in the marginalization of both straight and gay Asian men in dating and marriage; for example, increased earnings and education do not increase Asian American men's dating and marriage prospects as they do for other men (Kao et al. 2018).

Transgender and gender-nonconforming Asian and Pacific Islander Americans navigate high levels of discrimination and heavily underresourced living conditions. Like other queer and transgender people of color, they experience microaggressions from their families, from other racial/ethnic communities, from white LGBTQ+ communities, and from society in general (Nadal 2013). In a national study (Grant et al. 2011; Harrison-Quintana et al. 2011), transgender and gender-nonconforming Asian Americans and Pacific Islanders (AAPIs) reported facing pervasive discrimination, anti-transgender bias, and persistent structural and interpersonal acts of racism. This included 18% living in extreme poverty, compared with 15% of respondents of all races combined, and high rates of employment and housing discrimination, negative effects of social and economic marginalization on health outcomes, and harassment and assault in school and by police. More than half (56%) had attempted suicide, compared with 41% of all study participants and 2.5% of the general Asian American population. Acceptance by their families (44%) was an important protective factor, and significant efforts have been made in AAPI communities to counteract discrimination and foster acceptance and trans pride in families (e.g., see the Asian American Psychological Association's LGBTQ resources page, https://aapaonline.org/resources/lgbtq-aapi-resources).

Yellow Peril, Anti-Asian Racism, and Disease Scapegoating During the COVID-19 Pandemic

Asian racialization persists and evolves with a past, present, and future. During the COVID-19 pandemic, which began in 2020, there was a rise in the already elevated incidences of anti-Asian and specifically anti-Chinese sentiment and violence. Misinformation about the origins of the virus played on Orientalist stereotypes, with one theory identifying the virus's origin as contaminated bat meat and another claiming that the virus originated in a biotech medical research facility within Wuhan. The biotech laboratory narrative is an example of techno-Orientalism (Roh et al. 2015), an extension of Orientalist stereotypes capturing Western anxieties about Asia's scientific dominance, playing on tropes of the Asian evil genius (e.g., the evil scientist Dr. Fu Manchu in films and television shows) or Asians as mindless tech automatons. Both of these stereotypes of the uncouth Oriental and the industrious high-tech coolie play on North American and European fears of Asian threats (Zia 2020). Yellow peril was evoked by President Trump as he stoked anti-Asian violence by repeatedly blaming China and using racist, inflammatory language in his references to the "Chinese virus" and "kung flu." Following his lead, campaigns blaming the Chinese for the virus spread across social media.

Asian Americans responded to these rising racist incidents with antiracism activism. The Asian Pacific Policy and Planning Council formed a Stop AAPI Hate Reporting Center to record and tally reports of anti-Asian racist attacks. During the first 8 weeks of data collection between March 19, 2020, and May 13, 2020, Stop AAPI Hate tallied nearly 1,900 incidents of anti-Asian discrimination across the United States (Asian Pacific Policy and Planning Council and Chinese for Affirmative Action 2020); by September 30, 2021, that tally would increase to 10,370 (Yellow Horse et al. 2021). Asian American women were disproportionately targeted. In a tragic example of the ways in which the sexualization and racialization of Asian women makes them more vulnerable to racial and gendered violence, on March 16, 2021, Robert Aaron Long killed eight people, six of whom were Asian women, in a shooting spree at three spas in Atlanta, Georgia. One year later, in a national survey conducted by the National Asian Pacific American Women's Forum (National Asian Pacific American Women's Forum 2022), 74% of AAPI women reported experiencing racism or discrimination, 38% reported experiencing sexual harassment, and 12% reported experiencing gender- or race-based physical violence within the previous year.

New York City established a Commission on Human Rights to respond to COVID-19-related discrimination. Many of the estimated 2 million Asian American frontline workers in health care reported incidences of racism in the hospitals where they were risking their own lives to provide care to COVID-19 patients. They also reported treating Asian American victims of racial violence. Asian Americans reported boycotts and vandalism of Asian businesses, as well as being blamed for the coronavirus, looked at with contempt when "coughing while Asian," spat on, threatened, and assaulted. These events caused increased anxiety and fear, self-consciousness of how one is seen, and attempts to hide one's Asian identity or to assert American status or patriotism, as well as antiracist activism (Tessler et al. 2020).

Clinical Considerations

We have outlined the myriad ways that history shapes the creation of stereotypes and how these stereotypes can then impact the individual. In this section, we review several important clinical considerations to keep in mind when working with Asian Americans. These include increasing the capacity for racial reflective functioning, the importance of social and historical context, and a consideration of intersectionality in racial melancholia and racial dissociation, the utility of adopting a clinical stance of informed inquiry, and the power of challenging dominant narratives. We consider supervision and training, and finally, we present a clinical case that illustrates these points, as well as the importance of holding the dialectic between self-determination and the impact of historical and sociocultural forces.

Racial Reflective Functioning and Working With Microaggressions

To address racialized dynamics in psychotherapy, we have developed the concept of *racial reflective functioning*, expanding on Fonagy and colleagues' (2002) theory of mentalization. In their original conceptualization, mentalization, or reflective functioning, is the reflexive ability to envision mental states in oneself and others and to interpret one's own and others' behavior in terms of these underlying mental states (for an overview, see Slade 2005). Reflective functioning involves "thinking about feeling and feeling about thinking" (Mary Target, personal communication, 2005, quoted in Wallin 2007), all within a broader theory of mind. Racial reflective functioning expands mentalization theory to address the sociohistorical context of racism, transnational histories, white supremacy, and the privilege of whiteness and the racialization of people of color in interpersonal interactions. In this way, a theory of racial reflective functioning ties and weaves together new connections to our broader social contexts and explores how these dynamics influence the expression of our most basic relational needs as social beings. To be effective in supporting clients, therapists must work to develop their own racial reflective functioning.

In his research on microaggressions, Derald Wing Sue (2010) describes how we occupy different racial realities; exposure to one kind of oppression does not ensure a greater understanding of the oppression that others experience. Depending on the level of racial consciousness of our social network, we may then find ourselves very much alone in our racial realities. This may be particularly true for Asian Americans because a number of factors deny and suppress discussion of Asian American racialization. Race is often constructed as a Black and white conflict. There is also a reluctance to "take up space" in a social system that assumes a scarcity of attention for any one oppressed group, creating pressure to triage attention to focus on the most oppressed. The triangulation of Asian Americans vis-à-vis Black and white Americans is another factor: Asian Americans are racialized along different dimensions (e.g., superior/inferior, insider/foreigner)—portrayed as superior to African Americans and inferior to whites but foreign and excluded from political power (Kim 1999). There is also the model minority myth and the problematic rhetoric that places Asian Americans as "honorary whites" or white-adjacent in privilege.

In order to build racial reflective functioning, as therapists we need to develop an ear for hearing microaggressions and macroaggressions. We also need to become practiced at listening to racialized experiences, inviting discussion of them, centering the client's experience (as opposed to the microaggressor's), and mirroring and validating the client's responses. It is important that we enact this process from the perspective of our own positionality, including our institutional privilege in the role of the therapist and our personal identity in relation to the client's positionality (Hung 2016). The practice of reflexivity, situating our knowledge and inquiry within our social and historical context rather than assuming the objectivity and universality of our knowledge, is also important (Hung 2016).

Derald Wing Sue (2010) defines racial microaggressions as everyday verbal or nonverbal slights, insults, devaluations, invalidations, and misinterpretations or mistaken assumptions that marginalized people experience in their daily interactions with well-intentioned people who may be unaware that they have been behaving in a racially demeaning way toward an individual from a marginalized racial group. Racial macroaggressions are systemic and institutional forms of racism that are manifested in the philosophy, programs, policies, and structures of organizations and institutions (Huber and Solorzano 2014; Sue et al. 2019). Sue and colleagues (2016) list common themes in racial microaggressions reported by Asian Americans, including the following: 1) being treated as an alien in one's own country, 2) ascriptions of intelligence, 3) denial of racial reality, 4) exoticization of Asian women, 5) invalidation of interethnic differences, 6) pathologizing cultural values or communication styles, 7) second-class citizenship (receiving poorer treatment), and 8) invisibility (being unheard, unseen, or not remembered).

People of Asian descent are sometimes in the position of repeatedly suffering devaluations and denigrations that are dismissed and denied by the people in their social world and by friends and family who may also be Asian American or people of color, as well as by the initial microaggressors. Suppressing discussion of an individual's experiences of racism can incur psychological trauma, leaving the person isolated in their own racial reality—a reality that includes the experiences of racialization that often go unnoticed or denied by others. Building racial reflective functioning can mitigate some of this trauma by tethering the person to the broader social world when they feel exiled to a reality that no one else can see.

When Asian Americans bring up microaggressions, others commonly respond defensively, communicating verbally or nonverbally that they are responding in an overly sensitive or crazy way and that their communication is hurtful, discomforting, or confusing to the microaggressor. When people hear this criticism repeatedly, they may internalize some of these distortions. They can develop insecurity about their own competencies and perceptions, sometimes invalidating and criticizing themselves. They may also compare themselves to other people of color, including other Asian Americans, who say that they are not bothered by these experiences. They can become preoccupied with incidents of microaggressions and experience decreased motivation and concentration at work. It is not uncommon for people to respond to racialized interactions by limiting self-expression and withdrawing from relationships, prioritizing self-protection and conservation of energy over relational needs. It requires time and energy to detox from these experiences—processing a kind of social toxin packed with implicit racialized meanings. When a person has their racialized experiences mirrored back to them in an attuned way, it helps them process these racialized interactions, and the individual can "find themselves in the other" (Fonagy et al. 1995) in a shared racial reality.

In processing these experiences, it can be helpful to expand racial reflective functioning to understand the ways that the assessment of power and centering of white privilege limit and direct our attention: whose perspective we attend to; whom we identify with in a racialized interaction; whom we empathize with; whose pain we assuage or coddle, validate or minimize; whom we remember; and whom we even register as visible and audible. Power and privilege shape our attention, learning, and memory in significant ways, with a tendency to attend to those of greater power and privilege. For example, it is common for people to be preoccupied with the intentionality of a white microaggressor, to take the perspective of the dominant group, and to minimize the pain of people who are members of a marginalized group. These impairments in attention function both to protect our relational needs and also to direct attention away from tabooed discussion of systemic injustices. In discussions about racialization with Asian Americans, Dr. Ueng-McHale often hears a qualifying lead-up, such as "I'm sure he didn't mean it this way," "I know she meant well," or "He is a good person." These may be ways for Asian Americans to mitigate the blame and criticism that often come their way.

Raising the issue of racism is a vigorously enforced taboo because race talk raises both representations of disavowed racist states and a challenge to the meritocracy, another powerful taboo. Questioning the fairness of the system can be judged as an indication of envy, laziness, or even deceitfulness. Because of the connection between racialization, productivity, and commodification of labor, defensive reactions to racialization can include judgments about one's relationship to work and equal opportunity.

As Eng and Han (2019) write, "Simultaneously, the social contract for Asian Americans demands acquiescence to the ideology of colorblindness—to the idea of the level playing field" (p. 124). Race talk is triggering because people tend to disavow these aspects of our racialized history, making us hostile to racial reflective functioning and leaving us with terrible stamina for tolerating the emotions triggered by discussions of race or systemic oppression. Furthermore, contact with disavowed, dissociated "not me" parts trigger defenses and a psychic equivalence mode of thinking in which one's own subjective experience is seen as the only psychological reality (Fonagy et al. 2002), leading individuals to become dysregulated and to blame and attack others. They defend against disavowed "not me" states of racist, exploiter, and colonizer or internalized racist states of "unassimilable Asian automaton" or "uncouth Oriental."

In developing racial reflective functioning, we as therapists must move historical and systemic contexts to the forefront of our attention. The background of social and racial history in which the individual lives must become the foreground of our understanding. In a common path to invalidating others, many people try to identify with the person who is reporting the microaggression by relating it to their own personal experience or by putting themselves in the person's shoes. Instead, we need to see distress as both a response to a single incident and as the cumulative effect of multiple racist experiences with historically racialized meanings, directing our attention to the greater context of the society in which we live. As therapists, we can ask ourselves, "How can we link this pain to the collective history of oppression and to the transnational and transgenerational experiences of this person?" We can then facilitate the process of grieving and the integration of the parts of the client that have previously been repressed, dissociated, and disavowed.

Finally, therapists can support clients in beginning to predict and plan for potential exposure to microaggressions, as well as their responses and needs. How would the client like to respond to microaggressions? (For microintervention strategies, see, e.g., Sue et al. 2019.) When can clients limit their exposure? How can they identify and spend time with people who can understand their racialized experiences? How can they allot time to recovering? How can clients confront the values that devalue, commodify, and silence them? What counternarratives and values do they want to cultivate instead? In this planning, it can be helpful to affirm the ways people protect and navigate multiple attachment needs in relation to groups as they consider racialized experiences—ways of maintaining the security of connection, proximity, and access to social groups. These methods include the following: 1) assessing the power relations between group members to maintain one's standing or power; 2) minimizing risk of being othered, excluded, ostracized, or physically attacked; and 3) maintaining relationships.

Validating all the parts of one's experience and mentalizing interconnections provides a sense of wholeness and rootedness. Doing so has interstitial integrity, as described by feminist Asian American theologian Rita Nakashima Brock (1998), and locates us in a place that is bound and situated intergenerationally, historically, and transnationally, relieving us of self-criticism and shame. Linking-weaving-validating their responses allows our clients to give up the idea that there is a "right" way to navigate, making room for their agency and pragmatism to discern what is right for them given all their relational needs and risks.

Considerations of Context and Intersectionality: Racial Melancholia and Racial Dissociation

As emphasized throughout this chapter, context (transnational and family history, immigration, racialization) is critical in understanding any single Asian American's experience. Spurred by their discussions with students following suicides at the university where they both worked, David Eng and Shinhee Han began a 20-year interdisciplinary collaboration that is integrated into their groundbreaking work *Racial Melancholia, Racial Dissociation: On the Social and Psychic Lives of Asian Americans* (Eng and Han 2019), offering a compelling framework to understand how the social realities of Asians in America impact the psychic experiences of individual Asian Americans. In their framework, Eng and Han describe racial melancholia and racial dissociation, two psychic mechanisms used by Asian Americans in Generation X (born between 1965 and 1980) and Generation Y (born in the early 1980s and early 1990s; also known as Millennials), respectively, to adapt to their experiences of racialization, exclusion, loss, and grief. These two contextualized psychodynamic formulations are foundational for anyone working with Asian American clients.

In their theory of *racial melancholia*, Eng and Han (2019) have reconceptualized processes of mourning and melancholia to help clarify the experience and predicament of many second-generation immigrant Asian Americans in Generation X. As they write, "To the extent that ideals of whiteness for Asian Americans and other people of color remain unattainable, processes of assimilation are suspended, conflicted, and unresolved" (Eng and Han 2019, p. 36). In response to racialization and the limits of belonging, many second-generation Asian Americans in Generation X experience conflictual identification with their Asian ethnic culture. In order to claim a sense of belonging and group identity, individuals who experience racial melancholia can adhere to and invest in the model minority stereotype as a form of mimicry, developing a "false self" in order to achieve a certain level of social acceptance and protection. Eng and Han challenge the narrative of Asian immigrant parents who sacrifice everything for their child's opportunities in the United States and the resulting sense of indebtedness and responsibility children feel to their parents. They reframe the narrative to make visible the role of Asian immigrant parents' unresolved traumas and losses (e.g., of family, community, language, culture, social legibility) as their experiences of immigration and racialization presented barriers to their ability to attain the American dream. These painful failed aspirations and unresolved traumas are then enacted in their relationship with their children through pressures placed on their children and sometimes through misattuned or even abusive parenting behavior. In this formulation, second-generation children, who carry both the pressures to succeed and their parents' unconscious, unresolved grief, suffer under depression, unresolved mourning, and sometimes suicidality, carrying a sense of their own deficiency. Racial melancholia, or perpetual mourning, is depathologized as a response to intergenerational transmission of racial trauma and the profound losses and disappointments that can be part of immigrants' experiences, with mimicry of the model minority role as a form of adaptation or coping for Asian Americans.

The second psychic mechanism formulated by Eng and Han (2019) is *racial dissociation*, a mechanism they explore in the first-generation immigrant "parachute children" of Generation Y. These are individuals who as young as age 8 were "parachuted" by themselves or with a relative or caregiver to attend schools in Western, English-speaking countries in hopes of improving their chances of attending a reputable American college. For these individuals, it was unclear whether they would remain in the United States, return home, or move elsewhere following their college or graduate school years. As children, adolescents, or young adults, they experienced the trauma of being dropped all by themselves into the social complexities of immigration, assimilation, and racialization while living far away from their families. This occurred within the sociopolitical context of American neoliberal "colorblindness" and queer liberalism, which created a devastating absence of language or concepts to represent and make sense of their racialized or homophobic experiences.

In contrast to adaptive dissociation, in which one can move flexibly and playfully to "stand" in different psychic "spaces," racial dissociation reflects a rigid, defensive dissociation into a "psychic nowhere" in which racialized and homophobic experiences overwhelming to a child all alone are walled off from consciousness, and unbearable or unprocessable experiences can remain inaccessible to the self. These clients do not talk about immigration, racism, or discrimination toward LGBTQ+ people in session. Instead, clients can present a "false self" in "psychic limbo" who on the one hand is compliant with family expectations or the hyperproductive model minority demands of society, while on the other hand is experiencing high levels of psychological distress in depression, anxiety, panic attacks, eating disorders, addiction and substance abuse, or acting out through illegal activity. Eng and Han (2019) have observed that gay Asian parachute children can also experience splitting between intellectual activity and the body, which is subjugated and sacrificed to meet the demands of high achievement, while the starvation of their unmet basic bodily needs is expressed in panic attacks. In a sense, they attempt to "pass" in American society not as an honorary white, or as a straight person, but as a hyperproductive "robot."

Maintaining a Stance of Informed Inquiry

It is useful to maintain a stance of informed inquiry when working with clients, regardless of their identity markers. The experience of Asian Americans is not monolithic, even when they share similar backgrounds. How dominant racialized narratives affect each individual will vary widely. That being said, it is important for clinicians to do their own work in learning about the culture of their client. Awareness of common intersectional, racialized experiences of people from the client's background is essential; thus, the therapist assumes responsibility for some of the labor of multicultural education that is often placed on clients who are people of color. Taking a stance of informed inquiry flows naturally from this research, followed by more specific questions to delve into an individual's particular experience from a place of knowledge, allowing the therapist to deepen discussion more quickly.

For instance, if you are treating a second-generation Vietnamese American, knowing about the trauma experienced by refugees in escaping the ravages of the Vietnam War may allow you to ask more pointed questions about the experience of the client's parents. Or understanding the dynamics that may be at play for parachute children from Asia may help you in identifying some themes that may emerge clinically when working with these clients. It is important not to assume too much. It can be helpful to proceed with cultural humility and a practiced, but informed, hesitancy as you introduce a broader theme when it comes up in an individual's material in the session. Particularly with dissociated experiences, this can be a way of dipping your toes in the water together while not stirring up strong defenses. You should also avoid the appearance of demonstrating your knowledge to the client in a performative way or imposing that knowledge on the client. For example, you might say, "Many Asian Americans who came to the U.S. as young as you did for school really missed having parents who were physically there to talk through their experiences in America. For some it was also hard for their parents to understand what they were going through here. I wonder if these kinds of experiences came up for you? Your experiences may also have been very different from that." Again, the dialectic becomes important to hold. Knowledge about historical racialized themes is important, but rather than being used as a source for heavy interpretation, it can provide broader Asian American experiences for the client to relate to, as a starting place for reflection and inquiry into the individual client's experiences.

Challenging Dominant Narratives

It can be very powerful to cocreate narratives that challenge dominant racialized narratives. Even just holding in mind that an individual's experience may be partially shaped by larger social determinants can be a helpful therapeutic stance for shifting a client's sense of self in the social world. For example, it can be freeing for Asian Americans to be able to see their perfectionism and feelings of never being enough or not doing enough as part of societal demands to fulfill model minority expectations—racialization that also commodifies Asian Americans, making their self-worth and belonging contingent on the quality of their labor. We can then support the cocreation of a new narrative with the client by asking questions such as the following: "What do you think about that idea?" "On what basis would you like to feel worthy? How would it be to feel your own inherent worth separate from what you do? Is that possible? Who sees you this way?"

Another example of a dominant narrative that may be helpful to challenge that many second-generation Asian Americans internalize is the belief that their parents sacrificed everything just for the betterment of the next generation's lives. Certainly, Asian immigrants to America suffer considerable losses of family, friends, country, language, food, customs, status, and so on. The enormity of these losses can drive a process of racial melancholia as described earlier. However, it is often a myth that the parents of these second-generation Asian Americans were totally selfless in their pursuit of the American dream. For many of these parents, the decision to come to America was made out of self-interest, often to pursue opportunity or to escape dire circumstances. Articulating this reality can free individuals from the mandate to fulfill all of their parents' wishes out of respect for and indebtedness to their parents' sacrifices, creating space to make different choices.

Knowing that their individual experience may be a product of a history of racism and transnational/intergenerational traumas can be freeing and can help clients feel less pathologized. This understanding can also increase empathy among Asian Americans for their parents' experiences and attitudes. Of course, holding the dialectic between acknowledging that historical forces may have contributed to an individual's harmful behavior and not excusing that person's behavior becomes crucial. For example, although it can be helpful to understand an abusive parent's anger as stemming from a history of encounters with racism, it does not mean that the parent should not be held accountable for their behavior.

Supervision and Training

There is a dearth of Asian mental health professionals in the United States. According to the 2015 report by the American Psychological Association Center for Workforce Studies, only 4.3% of the active psychology workforce identified as Asian in the U.S. Census Bureau's 2013 American Community Survey (American Psychological Association 2015). According to the Medscape Psychiatrist Lifestyle Report (Peckham 2021), only 8% of active psychiatrists identify as Asian. Recruiting and supporting early career mental health professionals of color is essential if we are to diversify our field and better serve our patients.

The same racial dynamics that exist in the world exist in our training programs and supervision relationships. It is essential that the power differentials between supervisor and supervisee be attended to for all supervision relationships, but especially in cross-racial dyads. It is also important that supervisors become familiar with racialization of Asian Americans and Asian American history and skilled at the practices such as those recommended in this chapter, including positionality and reflexivity. Lack of attention to these power differentials can result in racial enactments in supervisory relationships (Burkard et al. 2006; Constantine and Sue 2007).

Supervisors can commit microaggressions against their supervisees of color. In a study of Black supervisees, Constantine and Sue (2007) described seven microaggression themes that emerged in cross-racial supervision dyads. These themes included invalidating racial-cultural issues, making stereotypical assumptions about clients, making stereotypical assumptions about supervisees, reluctance to give performance feedback for fear of being viewed as racist, focusing primarily on clinical weaknesses, blaming clients of color for problems stemming from oppression, and offering culturally insensitive treatment recommendations. These findings are also relevant to Asian American supervisees. Both Dr. Chin and Dr. Ueng-McHale have been in countless supervision meetings where supervisors have made disparaging remarks about Asian patients or committed microaggressions toward the supervisee. Such microaggressions can take the form of Asian mothers being stereotyped as "Tiger Moms" or instances in which the supervisor consistently sides with the white member of a white-Asian biracial couple. In supervision groups, Asian supervisees sometimes are called on to speak for all Asians—often about Asian groups to which the supervisee does not even belong.

Supervisors also may try to downplay the impact of social factors such as race, national origin, and immigration history on the patient's emotional experience. However, not only does such an approach represent a clinical misstep, it also negates the lived experience of the supervisee of color. Given the power differentials that exist, it may be difficult for supervisees of color to voice disagreement when they feel that the impacts of these sociocultural factors are being downplayed by their supervisors. These missteps may also represent a repetition of negative experiences supervisees may have had in their own psychotherapy treatments, serving to further undermine their relationship to the field.

Supervisors have several ways to ensure a more positive relationship with their supervisees. The first is for supervisors to commit to being antiracist. As Ibram X. Kendi 2019) states, "being antiracist requires persistent self-awareness, constant self-criticism, and regular self-examination" (p. 34). Supervisors need to make sure they educate themselves around multicultural issues and diversity. Constantine and Sue (2007) found that whereas more than 70% of supervisees had received training in multicultural counseling in graduate school, only 30% of supervisors had received training in multicultural counseling in their academic programs. This discrepancy can result in supervisees feeling further marginalized as their competence around multicultural issues is minimized or ignored.

Second, supervisors can make explicit the fact that power differentials exist in the supervisory relationship and try to establish a more collaborative stance. For example, supervisors can be explicit about inviting disagreement, especially around issues of diversity, and can seek training to be able to appropriately engage in these discussions. Traditional psychoanalytic supervision positions the supervisor as expert and the supervisee as trainee. We ask supervisors to challenge this frame and consider whether a more collaborative stance would be more helpful. Such a stance also models what the therapeutic encounter should be, where the therapist is not considered the all-knowing expert but a facilitator of meaning making in a collaborative relationship with the client. This kind of feminist social justice frame around psychotherapy may be especially meaningful to new clinicians of color who may have had experiences of feeling marginalized in patriarchal and traditional frameworks.

The third recommendation is to engage in culturally responsive supervision. Culturally responsive supervision is marked by an appreciation for, awareness of, and respect for the client and supervisee's culture and ethnicity and the positionality of the client's and supervisee's problems within a cultural context (Burkard et al. 2006). Burkard and colleagues (2006) found that in culturally responsive supervision, supervisees felt supported in exploring cultural issues, which positively affected the supervisee, the supervision relationship, and client outcomes, in contrast to the results of culturally unresponsive supervision. These differences were even more stark for supervisees of color. Compared with white supervisees, supervisees of color reported more instances of culturally unresponsive supervision and more negative outcomes.

Finally, we encourage Asian Americans in training to consider forming study groups together or to seek out a senior Asian American therapist for individual or group supervision. The authors of this chapter experienced a lack of Asian American role models and supervisors as we pursued our graduate educations, and this made it difficult to fully understand the impact of our Asian American identities on our clinical work. Finding connections with peers who share a similar background can be helpful in expanding racial reflective functioning among therapists in training. It can be powerful for Asian American trainees to be supervised by Asian American supervisors, who may provide a safer space to explore aspects of identity that may be disenfranchised by the dominant culture.

Case Vignette

Dr. Chin treated Ellen, a second-generation cisgender Asian American woman who was attending a prestigious university. Ellen's presenting complaints were depression and a tendency to self-injure in superficial ways when she felt overwhelmed by academics. From the outside, Ellen appeared to be thriving. She excelled academically, had many friends and acquaintances, and was successful in her job applications. However, she also reported feeling empty and dissatisfied with her life much of the time. Although she was on track for a lucrative career, she was uncertain about what her true passions were professionally. She also felt trapped and locked into her professional career without permission to explore, perhaps unconsciously internalizing and embodying the stereotype of Asians as unfeeling, successful automatons. She reported a great deal of shame about the fact that she struggled, and she was invested in being perceived as a happy person who did not have any problems. She often came to sessions smiling brightly but became tearful when describing painful moments in her childhood. She would then apologize profusely for becoming upset and joke and smile through her tears as she quickly tried to reconsolidate.

As she discussed her family history, Ellen revealed how her father, who emigrated from China in his 20s, was physically and emotionally abusive toward her as she was growing up. She was punished severely if she did not live up to his very high expectations (e.g., receiving less than 100% on a test). He hit and slapped her, and he often berated her. The physical abuse stopped as she got older, and she described her current relationship with her father as characterized by benign neglect. Her mother lavished attention on her when she returned home and cooked all of her favorite foods, but her father remained largely silent and stoic. Ellen maintained that she loved both of her parents despite her experience of abuse, only hinting at more ambivalent feelings. On the one hand, she recognized that her father's punishments were uncalled for and represented abuse. But on the other hand, she often wondered if his abusive parenting was the secret to her success—that his strict and brutal approach may have actually led to her achieving as much as she did in her life.

It was helpful to contextualize Ellen's family experience historically in terms of the social and political realities that she and her parents had to negotiate. Ellen's father chased the elusive American dream. He worked in information technology (IT) and was able to achieve some success, although he often got the family into financial trouble through ill-advised investments in the pursuit of a financial windfall that never came to pass. There were periods when the family did very well, but inevitably, her father would take a big risk that put them in financially perilous positions. His rage toward Ellen often coincided with these times of financial instability. While he was trying to achieve success through his entrepreneurship, he also experienced considerable racism and discrimination at his regular job in IT. He was passed over for promotions several times in his career because his English "wasn't good enough." However, being passed over for promotions likely had very little to do with his English proficiency and more to do with the larger historical context of Asian immigrants never being fully considered American. His sense of impotence around not being able to achieve the success that he longed for translated into rage toward his daughter for her perceived failings. Ellen then internalized her father's harsh and judgmental attitude into the way she treated herself, perpetuating her depression and leading her to feel that she was never good enough. The dynamics of racial melancholia as described by Eng and Han (2019) were thus embodied in Ellen as she internalized the losses of her father in a way that could never truly be resolved.

Helping Ellen understand this dynamic was useful in making sense of her father and his behavior toward her, while also holding the dialectic of what she appreciated as positive outcomes of her experiences in childhood. Knowing that his treatment of her may have been caused not by her failings but instead by his own feelings of impotence and disappointment as racial discrimination limited his pursuits helped Ellen to question whether she was indeed deserving of such scorn. At the same time, it was also important that her father be held accountable for his actions. The context was an explanation and not an excuse. Holding this dialectic between autonomy and social determinism was crucial.

This dialectic was also helpful to hold with Ellen herself. It was important for Ellen to recognize the ways she may have been unconsciously perpetuating her own suffering. For example, during this time she was in a relationship with a man that was often unsatisfying. She spoke about the ways their relationship felt superficial and how she knew on a certain level that they would never end up together. Yet she remained. Ellen explained that it was just easier to stay together because the relationship made her less lonely. Ellen's boyfriend was not violent, like her father, but he was also not loving. Staying with someone who ultimately was invalidating was a pattern she found herself caught in. The connection to Ellen's familial dynamics was outside her awareness.

Another essential component of the treatment was helping Ellen to build racial reflective functioning in understanding not only her father's experiences of racism but also her own. Ellen's investment in appearing "happy" and "carefree" was in part a result of her need to deny the reality of racism and the microaggressions she was forced to endure in many aspects of her life. Creating a space for her to freely express ways in which she was the target of microaggressions, Dr. Chin validated her anger, sadness, and disappointment with the racist encounters she experienced. It was powerful for her to be able to share these experiences with an Asian American therapist and to feel validated that this "race talk" was not only allowed but valued. As an Asian American man, Dr. Chin found himself acutely aware of wanting to embody the role of "good father" who would accept Ellen unconditionally and provide her with a corrective emotional experience.

Conclusion

Working with Asian American clients requires an appreciation of the ways in which culture, intergenerational family traumas and attachment patterns, as well as transnational historical events and racial narratives, intersect to shape the psychology of Asians in America. An understanding of these narratives makes it possible to meet the client as an individual in relationship with the therapist in this social and historical milieu, going beyond the fixity of well-meaning, but limiting, "rules" about what one should do, say, or feel about racialized situations. The ability to hold the whole of our clients' experiences—individually, within their families, and in society—reclaims the dissociated links within our national and transnational family narratives. It allows for acknowledgment, mourning, and coconstruction of new narratives, therefore liberating Asian American clients from the intersectional oppressions that withhold their belonging and reduce their worthiness to the value of their productivity within the American experiment. As therapists, our mentalization of our own racial experiences linking to this broader familial, historical, and social webbing can allow for a fierce and compassionate stance as we and our clients walk this racial tightrope.

Key Points

- Stereotypes and dominant narratives about Asians and Asian Americans have been constructed and reconstructed throughout American history and continue to affect the psychology of Asian Americans today.

- American racialization of Asians is embedded in intersecting forms of oppression across interpersonal, systemic, and cultural contexts and has directly affected the lives of Asian Americans as well the psychological formation and well-being of Asian Americans.
- Orientalism, as well as the narratives of Asians as "perpetual foreigners" and representing "yellow peril" have been used to create exclusionary anti-Asian policies and laws, which have contributed to prejudice against Asians.
- The model minority myth suppresses attention to anti-Asian discrimination, obscures the disparities of economic and social privilege between different Asian ethnic communities, and creates psychological distress in the "never enoughness" that many Asian Americans carry inside them.
- Southeast Asians who entered the United States through refugee programs often experienced significant trauma throughout their journey and were met with hostility once they arrived.
- Racialization of gender and sexuality are intersecting aspects of identity that have a large impact on the experience of Asians and Asian Americans.
- Yellow peril, anti-Asian racism, and disease scapegoating saw a resurgence during the COVID-19 pandemic, illustrating how Asian racialization persists and evolves.
- Racial reflective functioning is the ability to reflect on the feelings, thoughts, behavior and power dynamics, as well as social and historical contexts involved in racialized interactions. Developing racial reflective functioning in psychotherapy is an important mechanism for treating and mitigating racial trauma.
- In order to build racial reflective functioning in clients, therapists need to develop their own racial reflective functioning to develop an ear for hearing microaggressions and macroaggressions and to build stamina for tolerating the states that come up in "race talk."
- Racial melancholia and racial dissociation are two psychic mechanisms that are helpful to consider when working with Asian Americans across Generations X and Y.
- Maintaining a stance of informed inquiry requires an awareness of common intersectional and racialized experiences of people of color paired with an appreciation for the uniqueness of any client's specific experience.
- Holding the dialectic between the power of social determinants and individual agency and accountability is important.
- Challenging dominant narratives can be a helpful therapeutic stance in shifting a client's sense of self in the social world.
- Asian therapists in training should seek out peer support and mentorship from other Asian mental health professionals. Supervisors should invest time in their own antiracist work to increase awareness of power differentials, microaggressions, racialized enactments.

Suggested Readings and Films

Eng DL, Han S: Racial Melancholia, Racial Dissociation: On the Social and Psychic Lives of Asian Americans. Durham, NC, Duke University Press, 2019

Lee E: The Making of Asian America. New York, Simon & Schuster, 2015

Sue DW: Microaggressions in Everyday Life. Hoboken, NJ, Wiley, 2010

WETA-TV and the Center for Asian American Media: Asian Americans. PBS, May 1, 2020. Available at: www.pbs.org/weta/asian-americans. Accessed September 23, 2021.

Zia H: Asian American Dreams: The Emergence of an American People. New York, Farrar, Straus & Giroux, 2000

References

American Psychological Association: Demographics of the U.S. psychology workforce: findings from the American Community Survey. Washington, DC, American Psychological Association, 2015. Available at: www.apa.org/workforce/publications/13-demographics/report.pdf. Accessed February 7, 2020.

American Psychological Association: Stress in America™: the impact of discrimination. Washington, DC American Psychological Association, 2016. Available at: www.apa.org/news/press/releases/stress/2015/impact-of-discrimination.pdf. Accessed March 20, 2022.

Asian Americans Advancing Justice: Inside the Numbers: How immigration shapes Asian American and Pacific Islander communities. Washington, DC, Asian Americans Advancing Justice, June 12, 2019. Available at: www.advancingjustice-aajc.org/publication/inside-numbers-how-immigration-shapes-asian-american-and-pacific-islander-communities. Accessed March 20, 2022.

Asian Pacific Policy and Planning Council; Chinese for Affirmative Action: Stop AAPI hate report 3.19.20-5.13.20. San Francisco, CA, Asian Pacific Policy and Planning Council and Chinese for Affirmative Action, 2020. Available at: https://stopaapihate.org/wp-content/uploads/2021/04/Stop-AAPI-Hate-Report-3Month-200513.pdf. Accessed April 20, 2022.

Burkard AW, Johnson AJ, Madson MB, et al: Supervisor cultural responsiveness and unresponsiveness in cross-cultural supervision. J Couns Psychol 53:288–301, 2006

Chae DH, Yoshikawa H: Perceived group devaluation, depression, and HIV-risk behavior among Asian gay men. Health Psychol 27(2):140–148, 2008 18377132

Chan CS: Issues of identity development among Asian-American lesbians and gay men. J Couns Dev 68(1):16–20, 1989

Chhuon V, Hudley C: Asian American ethnic options: how Cambodian students negotiate ethnic identities in a U.S. urban school. Anthropol Educ Q 41(4):341–359, 2010

Cho SK: Converging stereotypes in racialized sexual harassment: where the model minority meets Suzy Wong, in Critical Race Feminism: A Reader, 2nd Edition. Edited by Wing AK. New York, New York University Press, 2003, pp 349–366

Chou R, Lee K, Ho S: Love is (color)blind: Asian Americans and white institutional space at the elite university. Sociol Race Ethn (Thousand Oaks) 1(2):302–316, 2015

Chua A: Battle Hymn of the Tiger Mother. New York, Penguin, 2011

Collins PH: Black Feminist Thought: Knowledge, Consciousness, and the Politics of Empowerment. New York, Routledge, 2000

Constantine M, Sue DW: Perceptions of racial microaggressions among Black supervisees in cross-racial supervision dyads. J Couns Psychol 54:142–153, 2007

Cox OC: Race, prejudice, class conflict, and nationalism. Race/Ethnicity: Multidisciplinary Global Contexts 4(2):169–182, 2011

Dinh Q, McDavid J, Mariategue KD: Southeast Asian Americans in 2020: 45 years of resilience and resistance. Asian American Policy Review 31, April 16, 2021. Available at: https://

aapr.hkspublications.org/2021/04/16/southeast-asian-americans-in-2020-45-years-of-resilience-and-resistance. Accessed on March 25, 2022.
Eng DL, Han S: Racial Melancholia, Racial Dissociation: On the Social and Psychic Lives of Asian Americans. Durham, NC, Duke University Press, 2019
Fisher v University of Texas at Austin, 136 S. Ct. 2198 (2016)
Fonagy P, Steele M, Steele H, et al: Attachment, the reflective self, and borderline states: the predictive specificity of the Adult Attachment Interview and pathological emotional development, in Attachment Theory: Social Developmental and Clinical Perspectives. Edited by Goldberg S, Muir R, Kerr J. Hillsdale, NJ, Analytic Press, 1995, pp 223–279
Fonagy P, Gergely G, Jurist EL, et al: Affect Regulation, Mentalization, and the Development of the Self. New York, Other Press, 2002
Freud S: Dream Psychology: Psychoanalysis for Beginners (Annotated). Translated by Elder MD. Scotts Valley, CA, CreateSpace Independent Publishing, 2016, p. 25
Gee B, Peck D: The illusion of Asian success: scant progress for minorities in cracking the glass ceiling from 2007–2015. New York, Ascend Foundation, 2017. Available at: www.ascendleadershipfoundation.org/research/the-illusion-of-asian-success. Accessed March 20, 2022.
Gee B, Wong J: Lost in aggregation: the Asian reflection in the glass ceiling. New York, Ascend Foundation, 2016. Available at: www.ascendleadershipfoundation.org/research/lost-in-aggregation. Accessed March 20, 2022.
Grant JM, Mottet LA, Tanis J, et al: Injustice at every turn: a report of the National Transgender Discrimination Survey. Washington, DC, National Center for Transgender Equality and National Gay and Lesbian Task Force, 2011. Available at: https://transequality.org/sites/default/files/docs/resources/NTDS_Report.pdf. Accessed March 19, 2022.
Harrison-Quintana J, De Guzman B, Chaudhry A, Grant J: Injustice at every turn: a look at Asian American, South Asian, Southeast Asian and Pacific Islander respondents in the National Transgender Discrimination Survey. Washington, DC, National Center for Transgender Equality and National Gay and Lesbian Task Force, 2011. Available at: https://transequality.org/sites/default/files/docs/resources/ntds_asianamerican_api_english.pdf. Accessed March 19, 2022.
Huber LP, Solorzano DG: Racial microaggressions as a tool for critical race research. Race Ethn Educ 18(3):297–320, 2014
Hung N: Boundaries and belonging: Asian America, psychology, and psychoanalysis. Unpublished doctoral dissertation, New York, City University of New York, 2016
Jackson JS, Brown TN, Williams DR, et al: Racism and the physical and mental health status of African Americans: A thirteen year national panel study. Ethn Dis 6(1–2):132–147, 1996 8882842
Kao G, Stamper Balistreri K, Joyner K: Asian American men in romantic dating markets. Contexts 17(4):48–53, 2018
Kendi IX: How to Be an Antiracist. New York, One World, 2019
Kim CJ: The racial triangulation of Asian Americans. Polit Soc 27(1):105–138, 1999
Kochhar R, Cilluffo A: Income inequality in the U.S. is rising most rapidly among Asians: Asians displace Blacks as the most economically divided group in the U.S. Washington, DC, Pew Research Center, July 7, 2018. Available at: www.pewresearch.org/social-trends/2018/07/12/income-inequality-in-the-u-s-is-rising-most-rapidly-among-asians. Accessed March 19, 2022.
Krieger N: Discrimination and health, in Social Epidemiology. Edited by Berkman L, Kawachi I. New York, Oxford University Press, 2000, pp 36–75
Krieger N, Sidney S: Prevalence and health implications of anti-gay discrimination: a study of Black and white women and men in the CARDIA cohort: coronary artery risk development in young adults. Int J Health Serv 27(1):157–176, 1997 9031018
Lee E: The Making of Asian America. New York, Simon & Schuster, 2015
Lee SJ: Up Against Whiteness: Race, School, and Immigrant Youth. New York, Teachers College Press, 2005
Lee SJ, Wong N-WA, Alvarez AN: The model minority and the perpetual foreigner: stereotypes of Asian Americans, in Asian American Psychology: Current Perspectives. Edited by Tewari N, Alvarez AN. New York, Routledge, 2009, pp 69–84

Lew-Williams B: The Chinese Must Go: Violence, Exclusion, and the Making of the Alien in America. Cambridge, MA, Harvard University Press, 2018
Martin JK, Tuch SA, Roman PM: Problem drinking patterns among African Americans: the impacts of reports of discrimination, perceptions of prejudice, and "risky" coping strategies. J Health Soc Behav 44(3):408–425, 2003 14582316
Mays VM, Cochran SD: Mental health correlates of perceived discrimination among lesbian, gay, and bisexual adults in the United States. Am J Public Health 91(11):1869–1876, 2001 11684618
Nadal KL: That's So Gay! Microaggressions and the Lesbian, Gay, Bisexual, and Transgender Community. Washington, DC, American Psychological Association, 2013
Nakashima Brock R: Interstitial integrity: reflections toward an Asian American woman's theology, in Introduction to Christian Theology: Contemporary North American Perspectives. Edited by Badham RA. Louisville, KY, Westminster John Knox Press, 1998, pp 183–196
National Asian Pacific American Women's Forum: The state of safety for Asian American and Pacific Islander women in the U.S. Washington, DC, National Asian Pacific American Women's Forum, March 2022. Available at: www.napawf.org/assets/download/napawf-state-of-safety-report.pdf. Accessed March 19, 2022.
Nguyen VT: The Sympathizer: A Novel. New York, Grove Press, 2015
Noh S, Kaspar V: Perceived discrimination and depression: moderating effects of coping, acculturation, and ethnic support. Am J Public Health 93(2):232–238, 2003 12554575
Okihiro GY: The Columbia Guide to Asian American History. New York, Columbia University Press, 2001
Ong A: Buddha Is Hiding: Refugees, Citizenship, the New America. 1st Edition, Berkeley, University of California Press, 2003
Peckham C: Medscape psychiatrist lifestyle report 2017: race and ethnicity, bias and burnout. Medscape, January 11, 2017. Available at: www.medscape.com/features/slideshow/lifestyle/2017/psychiatry. Accessed February 7, 2021.
Reyes A: Language, Identity, and Stereotype Among Southeast Asian American Youth: The Other Asian. New York, Routledge, 2007
Roh DS, Huang B, Niu GA: Technologizing Orientalism: an introduction, in Techno-Orientalism: Imagining Asia in Speculative Fiction, History, and Media. Edited by Roh DS, Huang B, Niu GA. New Brunswick, NJ, Rutgers University Press, 2015, pp 1–20
Said EW: Orientalism. New York, Pantheon, 1978
Slade A: Parental reflective functioning: an introduction. Attach Hum Dev 7(3):269–281, 2005 16210239
Sue DW: Microaggressions in Everyday Life. Hoboken, NJ, Wiley, 2010
Sue DW, Bucceri J, Lin AI, et al: Racial microaggressions and the Asian American experience, in Contemporary Asian America: Multidisciplinary Reader, 3rd Edition. Edited by Zhou M, Ocampo AC. New York, New York University Press, 2016, pp 464–484
Sue DW, Alsaidi S, Awad MN, et al: Disarming racial microaggressions: microintervention strategies for targets, white allies, and bystanders. Am Psychol 74(1):128–142, 2019 30652905
Sung MR, Syzmanski DM, Henricks-Beck C: Challenges, coping, and benefits of being an Asian American lesbian or bisexual woman. Psychol Sex Orientat Gend Divers 2(1):52–64, 2015
Tessler H, Choi M, Kao G: The anxiety of being Asian American: hate crimes and negative biases during the COVID-19 pandemic. Am J Crim Justice 45(4):63–646 2020 32837158
Tran J: Asian Americans and the Spirit of Racial Capitalism. New York, Oxford University Press, 2022
Wailoo K: Remarks at Race in the COVID Era: What America's History of Racism and Xenophobia Means for Today. Panel discussion, Equity, Inclusion and COVID-19 Series, Princeton, NJ, Princeton University, June 8, 2020
Wallin DJW: Attachment in Psychotherapy. New York, Guilford, 2007
Williams DR, Yan Y, Jackson JS, Anderson NB: Racial differences in physical and mental health: socio-economic status, stress and discrimination. J Health Psychol 2(3):335–351, 1997 22013026

Wilson PA, Yoshikawa H: Experiences of and responses to social discrimination among Asian and Pacific Islander gay men: their relationship to HIV risk. AIDS Educ Prev 16(1):68–83, 2004 15058712

Yellow Horse AJ, Jeung R, Matriano R: Stop AAPI Hate National Report 3/19/20 9/30/21. Stop AAPI Hate, November 21, 2021. Available at https://stopaapihate.org/wp-content/uploads/2021/11/21-SAH-NationalReport2-v2.pdf. Accessed March 19, 2022.

Yoshikawa H, Wilson PA, Chae DH, et al: Do family and friendship networks protect against the influence of discrimination on mental health and HIV risk among Asian and Pacific Islander gay men? AIDS Educ Prev 16(1):84–100, 2004 15058713

Zheng R: Why yellow fever isn't flattering: a case against racial fetishes. Journal of the American Philosophical Association 2(3):400–419, 2016

Zia H: Asian American Dreams: The Emergence of an American People. New York, Farrar, Straus & Giroux, 2000

Zia H: Remarks at Race in the COVID Era: What America's History of Racism and Xenophobia Means for Today. Panel discussion, Equity, Inclusion and COVID-19 Series, Princeton, NJ, Princeton University, 2020

CHAPTER 24

South Asian Americans

Pratyusha Tummala-Narra, Ph.D.
Gurmeet Kanwal, M.D.

The term *South Asia* refers to a geographic region known during British colonization as the *Indian subcontinent*. The region of South Asia is most commonly thought to include Bangladesh, Bhutan, India, Nepal, Maldives, Pakistan, and Sri Lanka. The South Asian diaspora consists of a diverse group of people reflecting a multitude of ethnicities, languages, religions, cultural traditions and practices, national origins, and historical experiences of colonization. Within India alone, more than 22 major languages with hundreds of dialects are spoken, and a number of major religious traditions are practiced, including Hinduism, Islam, Sikhism, Buddhism, Jainism, Christianity, Zoroastrianism, and Judaism. Additionally, the South Asian diaspora is wide spanning, including migration from South Asia to such regions as Southeast Asia, East Asia, Oceania, Africa, the Middle East, Europe, North America, South America, and the Caribbean.

As of 2017, approximately 5.4 million South Asian Americans, including those who migrated from South Asian countries and across the diaspora, live in the United States (South Asian Americans Leading Together 2019). People of Indian descent compose 80% of the total South Asian American population, followed by people of Pakistani, Bangladeshi, Nepali, Sri Lankan, and Bhutanese descent. Notably, the South Asian American population grew by approximately 40% between 2010 and 2017, with the most significant growth among Nepali immigrants (South Asian Americans Leading Together 2019). In addition, the numbers of 1.5-generation and second-generation South Asian Americans, referring to those individuals who arrived in the United States as children and those who were born and raised in the United States, respectively, are increasing (Inman et al. 2015; Tummala-Narra and Deshpande 2018). It is worth noting that although South Asian Americans are often included in a broader categorization of Asian Americans, there is growing recognition of the distinct position of South Asians within the broader umbrella group of Asian Americans.

When considering the diversity of South Asians in the United States, it is important that we, as the authors of this chapter, situate our distinct South Asian backgrounds. Pratyusha Tummala-Narra is a 1.5-generation Indian American Hindu woman who was born in Hyderabad and immigrated to the United States at age 7. Gurmeet Kanwal is a first-generation Indian American Sikh man who grew up in New Delhi and immigrated to the United States at age 23. As Indian immigrants, we share some common experiences of cultural norms and traditions and at the same time have unique experiences with language, religion, immigration journeys, and postmigration adjustment and acculturation. We underscore that this chapter cannot capture a comprehensive view of the psychological experiences or the mental health concerns of South Asian Americans. Rather, we provide an exploration of critical areas relevant to the immigration and acculturation process, including the negotiation of identity, traumatic stress, and mental health issues among South Asians. After providing a brief overview of South Asian immigration to the United States, we discuss these various dimensions of psychological experience and how they inform access to mental health services and psychotherapy practice. Although the majority of existing literature related to mental health issues among South Asians has centered on Indian Americans, we explore concerns that are shared across South Asian families and communities more broadly.

South Asian Immigration to the United States

The first visitors from South Asia to the United States were cultural ambassadors, such as Swami Vivekananda in 1893, during an era of growing interest in Eastern mysticism, which still influences mainstream American culture today. The first sizable group of immigrants from South Asia to permanently settle in the United States arrived between 1905 and 1912 and consisted of men who worked in railroad construction and lumber mills on the West Coast (e.g., Washington State). These men, most of whom were Sikhs from the region of Punjab, had served in the British army during colonization of the Indian subcontinent (Bhatia and Ram 2018). This initial wave was followed by subsequent migrations of Sikh farmers to California and Arizona. Sikhs in each of these waves of migrants faced discrimination, being termed as "Hindu undesirables" and "ragheads" (Bhatia and Ram 2018). Many of these men married Mexican women who worked in cotton fields in California, and over time, Punjabi-Mexican marriages became commonplace on the West Coast.

In the 1880s, Muslim traders from Bengal arrived in New York in the context of growing demand for silk and other products. Other early immigrants to the East Coast, who arrived during World War I, were Indian maritime workers who had worked as indentured laborers under the British. These Bengali immigrants married women of various ethnic and racial backgrounds, such as Creole, Puerto Rican, and African American. Shortly after these migrations, South Asians were restricted from entering the United States under the Immigration Act of 1917 (also known as the Asiatic Barred Zone Act), and in 1924, labor migration from Asia was ended by the Oriental Exclusion Act. Further, people of Asian descent were denied citizenship between 1924 and 1943 (Bhatia and Ram 2018).

With the passage of the Immigration and Nationality Act of 1965, a growing number of South Asians migrated to the United States. This wave of immigrants consisted primarily of students and professionals in medicine, engineering, science, and other professions, such as business (Inman and Tummala-Narra 2014). These individuals were highly educated and were fluent or proficient in the English language. As immigration policies gradually allowed for reunification of families, spouses, siblings, and children migrated to the United States, and in the 1980s, the numbers of South Asian immigrants who worked in family-run businesses and in the service industry grew (Bhatia and Ram 2018). By the 1990s, South Asian immigrants were increasingly diverse with respect to educational and socioeconomic backgrounds and national origins. Since the early 2000s, there has been a surge in South Asian Americans employed in information technology, and the numbers of older adults migrating to join their families have grown (Tummala-Narra 2013).

Today, South Asian Americans comprise diverse demographics with regard to income, education, and immigration status. Approximately 10% of South Asians in the United States live in poverty (South Asian Americans Leading Together 2019). With regard to immigration status, at least 630,000 Indians in the United States as of 2017 are undocumented, reflecting a 72% increase since 2010, and at least 4,300 South Asians have Deferred Action for Childhood Arrivals (DACA) status (South Asian Americans Leading Together 2019). The tremendous variations in religion, language, ethnicity, and traditions within and across different South Asian communities in the United States, along with distinct reasons for and circumstances of migration, are important to consider as clinicians approach the psychological experiences of acculturation.

Psychological Experience of Immigration and Acculturation

We live in a world where larger and larger numbers of people are on the move every day. Many different terms are used in describing the population on the move. For clinicians who may find themselves working with this part of the world's population, it is important to understand the various distinctions between these terms as noted in the introduction to Part 7, "Racial and Ethnic Diversities in Psychotherapy," section "Terminology." For simplicity, we use the term *immigrant* most of the time in this chapter, but it is not to erase the distinctions. When working with immigrants, refugees, and displaced people (i.e., those living in a country and culture other than their own, especially when the host culture is vastly different from the home culture), engaging clinically with all the facets of the immigration experience is absolutely essential.

Acculturation Process

Immigration is not an event that happens at a moment in time. It is a psychological, social, legal, financial, and pragmatic process that begins long before the immigrant arrives in the new country and continues for the rest of the immigrant's life in one form or another. Thus, it is important for clinicians to keep in mind that when a patient says, "I immigrated 30 years ago," it does not make the issue irrelevant or noncurrent.

Prelude

Acculturation may begin prior to immigration, especially in the current state of information flow occurring via social media and other online platforms, in addition to the older television and radio media. Individuals who are immigrating with planning may begin to create familiarity with, and even adopt attitudes of, the host culture long before actually getting there. As a result of their British colonial history, South Asians immigrating to the United States are very often already carrying representations of the host culture in their identity before arriving. For example, many speak English to a greater or lesser degree. Kumar and Nevid, using 2004 U.S. Census Bureau data, observed that when compared with other South Asian American groups, "Asian Indians have the greatest percentage of individuals who speak English 'very well' (76.9%), the highest educational attainment (63.9% of Asian Indians have a bachelor's degree or more), and the greatest percentage of employment in management, professional, and related occupations (59.9%)" (Kumar and Nevid 2010, p. 274).

Increased international student exchange possibilities have also provided opportunities for immigrants to become familiar with the new culture and even create cross-cultural identities (Hoersting and Jenkins 2011). However, these familiarities can be deceiving as well. What one learns from social media, radio and television, or even short visits can often create unrealistic expectations or misunderstandings that may make the reality encountered after immigration harder to deal with. Akhtar (1999) lists many different factors that can influence the outcome of immigration and acculturation. These include the ease with which the immigrant can go back and forth, age at migration, preexisting personality dynamics, nature of the home culture, the degree of difference between the home and host cultures (which is very great in the case of South Asians immigrating to the United States), the nature of the host culture's response (e.g., think about a South Asian Muslim vs. a non-Muslim immigrating after 9/11), the experience of competency in the host culture, and the experience of having children and parenting in the host culture.

Loss and Mourning

One of the most important aspects of immigration and acculturation has to do with the negotiation of loss and the processes of mourning. Without some degree of successful mourning it is unlikely that one can acculturate effectively. Of course what successful mourning looks like will vary from person to person and from culture to culture. For South Asians immigrating to the United States, for example, what is lost often has to do with the experience of being a part of an extended family, the quality of emotional warmth and engagement with relatives and friends, and the experience of the inanimate (but emotionally animated) elements of the cultural environment such as cuisine, smells, and places of worship (Akhtar 2011). Immigrating from a South Asian culture to the United States, or to another Western culture, inevitably calls for an identity adjustment for most immigrants because of the great difference in the two cultures and can often create an identity crisis that may take years to resolve.

Tummala-Narra (2016b) describes the struggle of conflicting loyalties and the intersectionality that needs to be appreciated. It is good to keep in mind that intersectionality is not only about multiple dimensions of identity in the present; it is also about the intersectionality of identity elements that belong to the past with identity elements that belong to the present. For example, one of my (G.K.) patients described his mother as "all-American." What he meant was that she had adopted certain American mores such as wearing Western-style clothes instead of the traditional Indian sari and that she had many American friends and was deeply involved with

American politics. However, I later learned that when it came to whom her son should marry, there was no question that it should be someone of Indian origin and preferably from the same subculture. Thus, the old identity elements were just as significant to recognize as the new ones. One way to think about it is in Boulanger's (2015) terms of "seeing double and being double." Using the visual phenomenon as metaphor, Boulanger highlighted the constant flux that immigrant identity has to learn to accommodate. This means holding different self-states in one's subjectivity. Kanwal (2018) discussed the "activation/inactivation, emergence/withdrawal and preservation/extinction" of these self-states that can become a deep kind of loss for immigrants. The core need for immigrants is so often a need to be seen. Tummala-Narra and colleagues (2016) noted that adolescents wish for others to see and recognize their cultures and families and, more broadly, their psychological experiences. Boulanger (2015) emphasized how "belonging is the condition of being understood" (p. 301). This experience of being seen can also become lost to the immigrant in the new country.

How one is seen and how one sees oneself can shift significantly as a result of immigration. Akhtar (2011) made the point that as long as he lived in India he was "never conscious of living in India." After immigrating to the United States, he could not help but periodically register that he was living in the United States. Tummala-Narra (2016a) discussed how significant the issue of names can be for immigrants. Not only are names representations of subjective identity, but they can also determine how others respond. That can vary from a sense of familiarity and affiliation to prejudice and racism. In the South Asian context, names can also be extremely informative about place of birth, religious affiliation, subculture of origin, and caste. However, such information is known only to people who have familiarity with the culture. Therefore, sometimes being in a new culture that knows nothing about one's name can help to avoid the shame one might feel by being seen a certain way within one's own culture. At other times, mispronunciation of names by individuals in the host culture can become a constant source of alienation.

Akhtar (1999) described four tracks that identity changes can follow during the process of acculturation, encompassing losses: from love or hate to ambivalence, from near or far to optimal distance, from yesterday or tomorrow to today, and from yours or mine to ours. Akhtar (1995) described immigration as a *third individuation* with some phenomenological similarities to the individuation processes of childhood and adolescence. The losses can be real ones, such as the ones described above, but they can also be losses in fantasy. For example, South Asian immigrants, especially as parents, often will mourn the loss of traditional values of the "old country," even though some of those values may no longer be relevant in current Indian culture. Eng and Han (2000) similarly described these losses in the context of Asian Americans: "one must mourn a host of losses both concrete and abstract. These include homeland, family, language, identity, property, status in community—the list goes on" (p. 680). Eng and Han also pointed to another important element that influences the acculturation process: racism. For South Asians, immigration after 9/11 has been a much more complicated process than it was before 9/11. The receptivity of the host culture, as mentioned in the subsection "Prelude," is an important factor. Post-9/11, the perception of South Asians by Americans has been deeply influenced by racial profiling. Many South Asians are easily perceived as being of Middle Eastern origin. The large population of South Asian Muslims has been particularly targeted, as have Sikhs because many of them wear turbans and have beards. Such racism encountered by immigrants is deeply traumatizing, creating a sudden and harsh shift in their acculturated identity. For those who may have recently immigrated, such experiences are disruptive to the acculturation process, creating shifts in loyalties, identifications, and interpersonal relations.

Class and social power are also important determinants in the processes of acculturation and assimilation. The greater the power differential in favor of the host culture, the greater the pressure to assimilate. It is also important to consider gender differences and familial roles in South Asian immigrants' adaptation processes because these vary so greatly between South Asian and American cultures.

Family Context and Developmental Issues

A major task of acculturation for South Asians involves the shift from being a part of an extended and joint family system to having to negotiate priorities and parenting as part of a culture of nuclear family structures. This has been described by many psychoanalytic authors as the most important developmental context of Indian as well as the larger South Asian culture. The expectations, obligations, priorities, and conditions involved in living in a joint family system become deeply ingrained as one grows to adulthood. Depending on the age at which one immigrates, these values and expectations may be more or less open to modification by the conditions of the host culture (Akhtar 2011). Children of South Asian immigrants often experience their most significant conflicts from being caught between the obligations and requirements that come from a joint family system, as well as its implications for the larger social group, and the individualistic expectations that emerge out of a Western nuclear family system. These conflicts often become most acute for children of immigrants who come into adolescence in American society. This is partly because adolescence, besides being biologically and psychologically a time of transition, is such a culturally determined rite of passage in American society and a time that is experienced and handled quite differently in South Asian cultures. Time and time again one encounters South Asian parents who are completely confused and bewildered by the demands and needs of their children who have grown up in the United States. As an example from personal experience, I (G.K.) could never understand how my kids could have friends whose families were unknown to me. In India it is natural for families of children's friends to be friends or acquaintances as well. The notion of adolescence being the second separation-individuation (Blos 1979) is just not relevant within the Indian context. However, for Indian immigrants, it becomes another being-double experience. At home it is not relevant, but outside the house it is.

Relational and Marital Issues

South Asian American marriages are diverse with regard to how couples meet (Dupree et al. 2013). Arranged marriages in the diaspora take unique forms in different families, with some resembling traditional introductions by parents or extended family and others involving a less formal introduction by family or friends followed by the couple dating. Many couples also meet via online dating and marital sites specific to South Asians. A common concern is the involvement of parents and extended family in the choice of a marital partner. Connection with family continues to be a value cherished by most South Asian Americans, regardless of immigrant generation. Akhtar (2011) writes, "Pressure for an arranged marriage can suffocate a child's efforts to date in the host country. Some children succumb to such pressures. Others express their independence defiantly when making spousal choices" (p. 65).

Children of immigrants can take one of three paths when it comes to dating. The first is the compliant path, that is, approval seeking and wanting to belong to one's culture of origin. This involves accepting arranged marriage (or some modification of it). The second is the rebellious path, or wanting to belong to the host culture. This involves avoiding South Asian partners at all cost. The third path is the getting stuck path. This involves being paralyzed by conflict between the two cultures, leading to no or little dating or sexual experience into one's late 20s or early 30s.

As an example of the getting stuck path, a patient in his early 30s had no trouble functioning professionally. He went to an ivy league school, became a highly valued professional, and had good social and friend relationships. Yet he found himself feeling completely inhibited from dating seriously or letting his parents arrange a match. It was not a matter of sexual inhibition. He did have some sexual experiences that he could enjoy. He simply could not bring himself to consider looking for a long-term relationship or thinking of marriage. The choice of a life partner had become for him a choice between two cultural identities, between remaining in a "we-self" cultural orientation versus taking on a more individualistic approach. He felt conflicted regarding loyalties to his family, his extended family, and the South Asian community and the expectations of his U.S. peers and community. The relational choice had become way too overburdened with other existential and identity choices.

Interracial and intercultural marriages often are a source of contention among family members. In particular, parents may not be open to their children marrying outside their cultural, racial, and religious backgrounds because of anxiety about losing continuity with their heritage culture, religion, and community and about the lack of familiarity with the cultural and/or religious backgrounds of the prospective in-laws. Interracial, intercultural, and interfaith couples who seek psychotherapy further cope with the impact of systemic differences and inequalities on their relationships. Smelson-Kanwal (2019) aptly noted the experience of being an outsider within one's family or community and how one may project unintegrated feelings about being an outsider to a partner who is othered in broader society (e.g., a racial minority partner). These shared and distinct feelings of otherness are critical to explore in interracial, intercultural, and interfaith relationships as couples negotiate intimacy with each other and their relationships with children and other family members (Smelson-Kanwal 2019). As such, therapists should engage couples in exploring the ways in which factors such as immigration, losses, relationships with extended family, and social location shape intimacy.

Role of Ethnic and Religious Communities

Developing friendships with people of a similar ethnicity, religion, or national origin "stirs up powerful affects of belonging and kinship," involving "a sense of deep and instantaneous mutual recognition" (Akhtar 2011, p. 86). Conversely, developing friendships with people of different ethnicities can help to foster a sense of belonging because heteroethnic friends can become a "bridge to acculturation" (Akhtar 2011, p. 91). However, cultural unfamiliarity and the anxiety of losing connection to one's heritage culture can produce ambivalence in heteroethnic friendships. Further, as Kanwal (2019) aptly noted that in an explicitly xenophobic nation, an individual's friendliness and friendships across different ethnic and religious groups become especially challenging.

For South Asian American immigrants and their children, challenges of negotiating friendships and intimacy are often influenced by interactions within their ethnic and religious communities, which are important spaces of connecting with one's heritage language, culture, food, traditions, and festivals. These communities can help to diminish loneliness and alienation within the broader U.S. context, particularly under xenophobic and racist conditions. The growing population of South Asians in the United States has culminated in communities based on common national origins, such as Indian American, Bangladeshi, and Pakistani cultural associations as well as subgroups within these broader communities, such as the Gujarati Samaj and the Telugu Association of North America among Indian Americans. It is worth noting that South Asians in the United States have differential access to such communities depending on their geographic location and their specific wave of immigration. For example, many South Asians who arrived in the United States in the 1970s and 1980s, particularly in rural areas, had little access to connecting with other South Asian individuals or communities.

Ethnic and religious communities can be important sources of "refueling" (Akhtar 2011) and provide a sense of cultural continuity and socialization to younger generations, and they are experienced in unique ways by South Asian immigrants and their children. For example, Mona, a second-generation Pakistani American woman in her early 20s who is deeply connected with her mosque community, finds it difficult to be fully herself within this community because she identifies as queer, an identity that she keeps private because of her fear that she and her family will be ostracized. Mona faces an impossible dilemma of remaining connected with a community that allows her to feel a sense of intimacy with extended family, friends, and heritage culture and religion while burying aspects of her identity and psychological experience. In psychotherapy, she contemplates how to reconcile her wish to introduce her partner to her family and friends in the mosque and her fear of losing her faith community both physically and psychically.

Identity Issues Across First and Second Generations

Mona's experiences within her community in part reflect conflicts in worldviews and experiences across different immigrant generations. Intergenerational conflicts are common among immigrant families and communities as younger and older members navigate the acculturation process. Prathikanti (1997) used the term *acculturation gap* to refer to the contrast in cultural worldviews between immigrant parents and their children. As parents and children are engaged in a distinct and shared acculturation process, conflicting perspectives emerge that contribute to familial stress (Khaleque et al. 2015). Differences in worldviews may concern appropriate or desired forms of expressing affection, choice of friendships and romantic partners and spouses, and choice of career. For example, parents may be opposed to the idea of their children dating someone from a different racial, cultural, religious, or caste background, whereas the children may espouse a belief that these differences bear less relevance in their lives as they negotiate a bicultural or multicultural identity. Acculturation gaps between older and younger family members are shaped by the stress that each individual faces outside the home, such as coping with language barriers, discrimination, and bullying at school.

Acculturation Gaps

Importantly, parents and children often do not explicitly speak of acculturative stresses, such as experiences of race-based bullying or teasing at school, because the children tend to be concerned about burdening their parents with additional stress or believe that their parents cannot relate to their struggles to belong in mainstream contexts. Further, studies indicate that South Asian American adolescents are often in the position of translating culturally and linguistically for their parents and caregivers, which the adolescents can experience as being both valuable and stressful (Tummala-Narra et al. 2016). The divergent acculturative experiences of parents and children often contribute to communication challenges and psychological distance within the family, even while parents and children have great affection for each other. Such conflicts related to acculturation and acculturative stress are also met with parental expectations of high academic achievement and professional success in many families, with implications for significant levels of stress among adolescents and young adults (Kaduvettoor-Davidson and Inman 2012; Tummala-Narra et al. 2016).

These acculturation gaps shape the development of bicultural and/or multicultural identity among 1.5- and second-generation South Asian Americans. The term *dual sense of self* was described by Alan Roland (2006) to refer to how immigrants and their children can form compartmentalized self-states that contain certain aspects of their cultural experience. As a person shifts across different cultural contexts, such as the mainstream U.S. context and an ethnic community context, only certain partial experiences of the self are revealed to others (e.g., friends, family members, partners, teachers, coworkers). The ability to interact effectively with others across contexts is a source of survival and resilience for many South Asian Americans, but the shifting between contexts occurs primarily on an unconscious level and can produce significant distress as one experiences a sense of invisibility in multiple contexts. Additionally, shifting can shape how one idealizes and/or devalues the heritage context and the mainstream context at different points, contributing to split identifications in which significant experiences within each context remain dissociated from one another (Akhtar 2011; Tummala-Narra 2016b).

An example of such a split is the case of Chirag, a 30-year-old second-generation Indian American man, who cannot imagine introducing his multiracial (Black and white) girlfriend to his parents or grandparents, who have planned for him to marry an Indian American woman. The prospect of disappointing his family is unbearable, as is disconnecting from his American self that he associates with his girlfriend. Rather than bearing this tension, Chirag maintains separate, unintegrated relationships with his family and his girlfriend in ways that leave him feeling despair.

In another example, Susan, a 19-year-old Christian Indian American woman, copes with feeling alienated from her church and from her Indian American peers at her college. She is the only Indian American at her church and typically the only Christian among her Indian American social circles. Although she is frustrated with not being seen fully in either context, she attempts to hide aspects of herself both at church and at gatherings with her Indian American friends. She describes her experience in the following way: "I feel lonely even though I'm with people most of the time." Such loneliness or the feeling that no one can truly understand the psychic experience of living in multiple contexts with divergent and sometimes dissociated sociocultural expectations and demands is a part of bicultural identity development for many South Asian Americans.

Another important aspect of bicultural identity involves intersectionality. The concept of intersectionality was developed by Kimberlé Crenshaw (1989), who described both the subjective experience of multiple social locations and the ways in which structural inequality shapes these social locations with respect to privilege and marginalization. South Asian Americans' interactions within multiple sociocultural contexts reflect both intersectional marginalization and privilege (Shin et al. 2017; Tummala-Narra 2016b). Race, ethnicity, gender, sexual orientation, social class, caste, religion, disability, education level, immigration status, and skin color all play a role in securing power within South Asian American communities and within mainstream U.S. society. For example, a woman with darker skin color and a lower caste background may be perceived as less attractive, competent, and desirable, and a gay man may be perceived as defying religious and cultural norms. On the other hand, a person from a higher social class and educational background may be regarded as a role model or authority figure within a family or broader community. These experiences of privilege and marginalization create the groundwork for intersectional identity as individuals negotiate where and with whom they can secure a sense of acceptance and belonging.

It is also important to consider that bicultural identity, similar to acculturation, involves a dynamic process of change throughout the life span for both first- and second-generation South Asian Americans (Akhtar 2011). For many South Asian Americans, each developmental transition can elicit either a longing for the country of origin or a wish to further acculturate to mainstream society. For instance, becoming a mother or father may bring forth nostalgia for a deeper connection with extended family in the country of origin. On the other hand, coping with conflict and dysfunction within one's family can produce a desire to separate from family and engage with others outside one's family and community.

Another issue relevant to cultural identity among South Asian Americans relates to their relationship with and access to travel to their heritage countries. Conceptions of home can vary among South Asian Americans as a function of this relationship to a heritage country. For example, a first-generation South Asian American who travels once or twice a year to the country of origin typically maintains close ties with extended family and with the heritage culture in a way that reifies a sense of continuity of the country of origin as home. However, a second-generation South Asian American less apt to travel regularly to the parents' country of origin is more likely to view the United States as their only home. South Asians in the United States also consist of international students in high schools, colleges, and universities who form unique psychological connections with their countries of origin and the United States. Older adults arriving in the United States to care for their grandchildren are another unique subgroup who experience distinct connections with the heritage and adopted cultures. For this latter group, the heritage country may be experienced as offering more autonomy, and the U.S. context can be experienced as restrictive because of language barriers and dependency on their adult children and grandchildren (Mukherjee and Diwan 2016; Tummala-Narra et al. 2013). These variations in relationships with the country of origin and heritage culture make for complex and diverse outlooks regarding a sense of home, with important implications for identity. In fact, some South Asian Americans carry transnational identities in which home rests in multiple places and in relationships that are situated in distinct national and cultural contexts.

As Kanwal (2015) noted, notions of separateness that signify transition to adulthood in the United States and other parts of North America and Europe diverge from the traditional South Asian cultural emphasis on lifelong connection to a collective self. Kanwal pointed out that the experience of separation and nonseparation in development is not dichotomous but rather should be understood as existing along a continuum at different periods in life. The navigation of how separate one should be in relation to one's family, ethnic and/or religious community, and heritage culture and language can be a key question to explore with regard to identity and psychological well-being.

Gender and Sexuality

Traditional gender-based ideologies of men and women in South Asian cultures contain defined and sometimes rigid attributes and roles (Methikalam et al. 2016; Patel 2007). Specifically, perceptions of men as providers and women as caretakers are prevalent among South Asian Americans, even though the roles of men and women have become increasingly fluid across immigrant generations (Guzder and Krishna 2005; Joseph et al. 2020; Tummala-Narra 2013). Many women are expected to carry out the primary caretaking responsibilities of children and older family members even when their work responsibilities match or exceed those of their spouses. For some women who immigrate to the United States to join a spouse, these caretaking responsibilities can be especially challenging when facing language or cultural barriers. It is also common within South Asian cultures for women, particularly mothers, to transmit cultural and religious traditions to their children and to uphold the family's reputation and sense of unity (Mehrotra and Calasanti 2010). It is worth noting that the location of power and authority that women carry within and outside their homes (e.g., workplaces) is highly variable; some women hold authority primarily in their homes and others primarily in the workplace or community settings (e.g., place of worship, cultural organization) (Tummala-Narra 2013). These individual variations reflect contradictory messages about women in South Asian cultures, where women may be both idealized and devalued, depending on the context. For example, in Hinduism, mother goddesses are revered, while women of lower caste and class privilege are among the most vulnerable to violence, abuse, and marginalization.

Variations concerning gender roles are important to consider in the context of immigrant generations in the United States. For instance, Devna, a 35-year-old second-generation Nepali American woman, shares her distress in psychotherapy about watching her mother being "put down" by the men in her family. In making deliberate efforts to avoid being devalued by others, she struggles with securing emotional intimacy with her partner as she worries that she will be overpowered by him. In another example, Sahan, a 25-year-old second-generation Sri Lankan American man, copes with the pressure of choosing a career that meets the expectations of his parents as connected with his masculine role as a future provider for his family. He is anxious that he will not be perceived as desirable to a partner unless he earns a higher income than she does. In fact, his father has told him, "No Sri Lankan girl will be interested in you if you become an artist." These types of conflicts surrounding gender role ideologies and the pressure to adhere to cultural norms contribute to psychological distress. Research indicates the importance of connecting with one's heritage culture and community (including collective roles and responsibilities) as critical to psychological well-being among many 1.5- and second-generation South Asian Americans (Inman et al. 2014; Joseph et al. 2020; Tummala-Narra et al. 2016). Yet familial pressure to adhere rigidly to heritage cultural worldviews and traditions can produce intense distress.

One of the most conflict-laden and complicated areas of life for South Asian immigrant families centers on the exploration of sexuality. Across South Asian countries, mores around sexuality can vary a great deal. Even in very socially liberal and permissive households, concerns about social shaming, honor, and reputation place strict limits on what is or is not allowed. It is important for clinicians to keep in mind that the Indian subcontinent is a place of strange contradictions when it comes to sexuality. For instance, a wide range of religiosity and traditionalism exists across different religious traditions in South Asian countries. One can find ancient Hindu temples with scenes of sexual intercourse (including same-sex sexual behavior), yet modern South Asians often exhibit extremes of sexual inhibition. Indian (Bollywood) cinema spends millions of dollars every year producing fantastical romantic movies, yet romance in real life has to be conducted within strict bounds and mostly in secret, hidden from parents and extended family, and has little to no place in the typical Indian marriage.

When South Asian families immigrate and attempt to acculturate to the customs of their host culture, while still needing to maintain good standing in their South Asian communities, tensions are set up, especially between parents and children but also between more and less permissive spouses. When these families immigrate to a generally more permissive and bodily revealing culture such as the United States, an inevitable conflict is set up between the past and the present, the home and the outside, and the South Asian community environment and the host culture environment. Children of South Asian immigrants often complain that their parents are bringing them up according to customs and rules that even the kids in South Asia are not following anymore. Akhtar (2011) makes the point that cross-cultural differences in handling sexuality are also evident in the language. He observed that there is no "neutral way to discuss sex, even between a physician and patient" because of lack of commonly usable "non-obscene words for the male and female genitals or the act of sex" (Akhtar 2011, p. 56)

Similar to the range of attitudes toward sexuality, a wide variation in attitudes toward same-sex relationships exists. As Akhtar writes, depending on the subculture, attitudes can "range from being hostile to the homosexual lifestyle to quietly 'tolerating' homosexuality as long as one's role as parent and spouse are fulfilled" (Akhtar 2011, p. 59). Schaffner (2001) addressed the interesting issue of androgyny in Indian culture:

> In India, androgyny is not thought of as an odd mixture of sexual organs but is usually viewed as a fortunate combination of male and female qualities. Indians stress that men and women are painfully incomplete without each other, that both masculine and feminine traits are needed to be a complete person. Indeed these traits are joined in superior human beings and gods." (p. 115)

Kalra et al. (2010, p. 267) observed that "a large proportion of MSM (men who have sex with men) in India are married, unlike in the West." The authors note that same-sex sexual behavior has been around in India for millennia, and in fact male same-sex relationships became illegal only through the colonization by the British. Only in 2018 was the law (Section 377 of the Indian Penal Code) finally repealed by the Indian Supreme Court, thus decriminalizing consensual same-sex intercourse. Nevertheless, significant homophobia and prejudice (often leading to violence) against the LGBTQ+ community continue to exist in South Asia.

In immigrating to the United States, LGBTQ+ individuals are often in a position to have an opportunity to come out with community support that they may have a hard time finding in India. Nevertheless, this does not mean there are no challenges. Coming out can be complicated for second-generation immigrants because they have to face the dilemma of possible alienation from their families and home culture community even though they may be able to find support in the host culture community. In these situations, family interventions, including psychoeducation, gender and sexual orientation education, and cultural education, are often very important to help the immigrant family adjust to their family member's identity. In working with a South Asian transgender person who came to the United States as an adolescent and began transitioning a couple of years later, I (G.K.) found it necessary to see the patient and her father in sessions together for a considerable period of time to deal with various cultural and personal adjustment issues. In cultures with strong family and community bonds and a we-self orientation (Roland 2006), shifts in gender identity or sexual orientation are always a shift for the entire family in a much more intense way than it might be for patients from more individualistically oriented cultures.

Traumatic Experiences

Racial Trauma and Ethnic- and Religious-Based Discrimination and Violence

Racial discrimination, profiling, and violence have been a part of South Asian Americans' experiences since the earliest waves of immigration in the United States. In recent history, since the terrorist attacks of 9/11, South Asian Americans, alongside Middle Eastern Americans, have been profiled and targeted for verbal harassment and physical violence. The severe violent backlash against South Asians in the United States after 9/11 was evident in the murder of Balbir Singh Sodhi, a Sikh American man in Arizona, just a few days following the terrorist attacks. Since 9/11, profiling of South Asians and anyone who is perceived to be Muslim in airports has become normalized in the United States, and verbal and physical assaults on South Asian American youth and adults have largely remained unknown to those outside South

Asian communities. In February 2017, in the aftermath of Donald Trump's election, Srinivas Kuchibotla, an Indian American man in Kansas, was murdered by a white man who yelled, "Get out of my country!" prior to killing him (Mudambi 2019). Incidents of racial violence and racist attitudes against South Asian Americans continued to increase during the Trump administration, with growing numbers of children and adolescents facing verbal and physical abuse.

Research examining racial and ethnic discrimination experienced by South Asian Americans indicates both the deleterious effects of discrimination on mental health (e.g., depression) and the invisibility of discrimination against South Asians in mainstream U.S. society (Inman et al. 2015; Tummala-Narra et al. 2012). When examining the effects of discrimination on mental health, it is important to consider its specific impact on the development of children and adolescents whose identities and relationships are formed in the context of sociocultural oppression. In a study exploring South Asian adolescents' (ages 14–18) experiences of acculturative stress (Tummala-Narra et al. 2016), participants reported both subtle and blatant forms of discrimination directed toward them and their families. One 18-year-old male participant stated, "I was walking home and all I hear is, 'You f----desi.' And then right in the back of my head, I felt a crack and I went crashing down. And then they start pounding the daylights out of me." These incidents were typically not reported to school officials, and therefore there was little to no protection for these adolescents. In addition to their own experiences of discrimination, South Asian American youth witness their parents and other family members experiencing discrimination within their neighborhoods, where they are teased for their accents, dress, or other cultural markers, and in workplaces, where they are devalued (e.g., passed up for promotions or raises). The impact of discrimination and violence is profound, and youth and adults struggle with sadness, frustration, helplessness, embarrassment, and anger (Tummala-Narra et al. 2016).

Racial trauma encompasses not only harassment and violence but also stereotyping, which often manifests in microaggressions. South Asian Americans are targeted with contradictory stereotypes that are often normalized across different contexts, including schools, neighborhoods, workplaces, online dating sites, and social media. In particular, the model minority stereotype portrays Asian Americans, including South Asian Americans, as innately successful with regard to academic and career achievements. Despite being considered a "positive" stereotype, the model minority stereotype diminishes the struggles faced by South Asian Americans in the acculturation process, including experiences of discrimination. The internalization of this stereotype among South Asian Americans also contributes to psychological distress, particularly when an individual cannot meet expectations of achievement (Gupta et al. 2011). Additionally, the model minority stereotype serves to dismiss or ignore mental health concerns within South Asian American communities, impeding access to appropriate help and resources. In direct contrast to this "positive" stereotype, perceptions of South Asian Americans include negative attributes such as lack of social competence or attractiveness. These latter stereotypes reflect gendered racism in which South Asian men are on one hand viewed as desexualized and weak and on the other hand seen as dangerous terrorists. Relatedly, South Asian women are viewed as submissive, exotic, or asexual, depending on the context (Patel 2007; Tummala-Narra 2013).

The experience of being stereotyped across the life span has significant implications for one's sense of belonging and identity within a mainstream U.S. context as the subjectivity of a person is continually removed or ignored (Akhtar 2014; Davids 2009; Tummala-Narra 2016b). As Kanwal (2018) noted, every immigrant "has a dream that never comes true. It is the dream of a perfect integration, of a seamless acceptance, of an unequivocal belonging" (p. 426). Experiences of racial, religious, and ethnic oppression disrupt this dream and create melancholic states reflecting either a loss of or a lack of a sense of home (Eng and Han 2000; Kanwal 2018; Tummala-Narra 2020).

Marginalization Within Communities: Caste and Colorism

In addition to sociocultural trauma in the mainstream context, many South Asian Americans experience social marginalization within their families and communities. Specifically, bias and discrimination based on caste, region of origin, religion, social class, and education are prevalent in the South Asian diaspora. Caste, which originated in ancient Hinduism, continues to have a stronghold on the mindset of many South Asians regardless of religious background. The caste system, which includes four major social status distinctions, became a rigid system of oppression over the course of centuries in South Asia and was further exploited by the British during colonization (Vallabhaneni 2015). The most extreme violence and oppression has been directed against those considered to fall outside the traditional caste system, the Dalits, formerly called "untouchables" (Roy 2017; Tummala-Narra 2020).

Paralleling race in the United States, caste assumes the inferiority and superiority of different groups, permeating the psyche with regard to one's social position and decisions about whom one socializes with and whom one marries (Roy 2017; Wilkerson 2020). Although caste may carry little social significance in the mainstream American context, it remains a relevant problem contributing to marginalization of people of lower castes and Dalits within South Asian American communities. At the same time, caste may carry less social and interpersonal relevance to South Asian Americans who are raised primarily in the United States. Nevertheless, the issue of caste is a legacy of South Asian history and culture that can be important to explore in psychotherapy because it can provide a framework for understanding experiences of racism and other forms of oppression in the United States (Inman et al. 2015; Tummala-Narra 2020). It is important to consider that casteism and racism intersect in the experience of many South Asian Americans, who carry prejudiced views of others and/or face marginalization within their ethnic and religious communities and in mainstream U.S. society. However, these issues often are not discussed openly outside one's family (Tummala-Narra 2020).

Another prominent feature of marginalization within South Asian American communities entails the problem of colorism. Dark skin color has traditionally been associated with less attractiveness and desirability and with lower social status in the South Asian diaspora. Colorism, although relevant to both men's and women's experiences, is especially directed toward girls and women, many of whom are encouraged to stay out of the sun and use skin-lightening creams and other products in order to "improve" their complexion.

The psychological impact of colorism on self-esteem, identity, and belonging can be profound, especially when it occurs within the family context (Tummala-Narra 2007). For example, Mira, a 32-year-old Indian American woman who is considered in her family to have dark complexion, shared that "I don't think that Indian guys would be interested in me. They're all looking to marry up, you know, someone lighter." Mira's perception of Indian American men is reified in online dating sites, where she finds numerous profiles of Indian American men desiring to meet someone with lighter skin tone. In other instances, for many multiracial or multiethnic South Asian Americans, lighter skin tone can indicate a lack of authenticity or belonging within their South Asian families or communities. In each of these cases, skin color remains a significant intrapsychic, interpersonal, and systemic issue.

Interpersonal Violence

Research indicates relatively high rates of intimate partner violence (IPV) within South Asian American communities, with estimates as high as 77% (Inman et al. 2014; Mahapatra 2012). In a study by Robertson and colleagues (2016), 25.2% of South Asian American participants had experienced childhood sexual abuse. Little attention has been directed toward the experience of childhood sexual and physical abuse, neglect, and sexual assault occurring outside the context of IPV. Further, few studies have been conducted with 1.5 and later generations of women, and no studies have been conducted with South Asian American male survivors of IPV or sexual violence or specifically with LGBTQ+ survivors. Interpersonal violence continues to be a highly stigmatized issue within South Asian American communities, where sex, sexuality, and sexual violence remain taboo topics. For many first-generation survivors, barriers such as patriarchal family systems, limited English language proficiency, lack of knowledge concerning resources, limited economic resources, and documentation status all contribute to problems in accessing help in coping with traumatic stress (Rai and Choi 2018). Additionally, research into the impact of IPV on children, such as the role of multiple cultural contexts in the experience of traumatic stress, has been emerging. In a study conducted with staff from South Asian domestic violence agencies in the United States, the researchers noted the impact of domestic violence on children, including the pressure to maintain an image of a perfect family, experiences of shame within their communities, and challenges in identifying with two cultural contexts (Ragavan et al. 2018).

Increasingly, there has been a call to better understand interpersonal violence from the perspectives of South Asian American survivors rather than adopting white, Euro-American feminist conceptualizations of violence and trauma. A recent qualitative study with 1.5- and second-generation Indian American women indicated that conceptualizations of and responses to sexual violence are formed through an interaction of various individual and contextual factors (Tummala-Narra et al. 2019). For example, one participant described how she experienced her family's cultural practice of genital cutting as traumatic, whereas her sister experienced the practice as a nontraumatic cultural ritual. This is only one example among many in which individual and cultural factors must be examined closely in order to respond effectively to complex experiences of trauma and violence among South Asian Americans. It is also important to note that although ongoing silence is maintained regarding interpersonal violence, a growing number of South Asian women's collectives and groups are actively engaged in advocacy for survivors and in raising awareness of the impact of interpersonal violence on women and families (Kanukollu and Mahalingam 2011; Tummala-Narra et al. 2019).

Mental Health Issues

Mental health issues tend to be underrecognized and underreported among South Asian Americans (Roberts et al. 2016). Although no clear prevalence estimates of specific mental health problems among different South Asian American groups are available, evidence exists that South Asian American youth and adults cope with a range of different mental health issues, including depression, suicidality, anxiety, psychosis, traumatic stress, substance abuse, eating disorders, and relational stress (Chandra et al. 2016).

Suffering in South Asian Culture

It is well documented that psychological distress takes different forms in different parts of the world. In his book *Crazy Like Us: The Globalization of the American Psyche,* Watters (2010) documents how American forms of illness and diagnoses have been exported to many parts of the world and how quickly that can change the way mental illness is expressed in those cultures. One can think about a new form of psychic colonialism that determines the legitimization of certain forms of suffering over others. When working with immigrants of South Asian origin, it is very important to recognize and respect these differences in how suffering and healing are experienced (Shweder 2003, 2008).

Shweder (2008) described the Indian experience of illness and healing as involving three worlds: the world of gods, the world of spirits, and the world of human beings. I would add a fourth one—the world of nature. In order to understand the Indian (and to a great extent, South Asian) experience of suffering, illness, and healing, interactions between all four worlds need to be appreciated. These notions are also deeply intertwined with the Indian system of medicine known as Ayurveda (specifically for Hindu India, although these principles have seeped into most other religious communities as well in some form). Ayurvedic principles that underlie much of the way Indians think about health and well-being have to do with contextuality, individuality, and a holistic approach. Contextuality implies that one always has to understand illness in a particular context—which can range from individual to cosmic. The same illness in two different individuals may require a completely different medicine or intervention. And the holistic approach implies that there is no separation between mind and body, between individual and community, or between the human and the natural worlds. Anything can cause any illness, and anything can function as a medicine. Thus, when Indian patients seek therapy, it is very natural for them to engage in other forms of healing and help as well, without feeling any sense of competition or disloyalty with regard to the therapist.

On a more phenomenological level, psychological distress is more likely to be expressed through physical symptoms and metaphors in South Asian individuals (Chandra et al. 2016). For example, Kumar and Nevid (2010) found that Indian men were more likely than Indian women to attribute mental distress to biological factors. This was seen as reflecting the need for men to hide their vulnerability behind more culturally acceptable somatic explanations. Also, it has been interestingly, and perhaps counterintuitively, noted that "Social support may protect against elevated symptoms of depression in South Asian immigrants with lower levels of integration into US culture" (Needham et al. 2018, p. 792). In other words, those individuals who are more integrated into U.S. culture are more vulnerable than those who are still embedded in and supported by their host culture community.

Suicide

Among the consequences of immigration and acculturation, it is important to consider the particular factors related to suicidal thoughts and behaviors among immigrants of South Asian origin. Although the research specifically on South Asian immigrants' suicide rates in the United States is not very robust, a general myth exists that Asian American immigrants are overall at higher risk. In fact, according to an American Psychological Association (2012) fact sheet, "The suicide rate for Asian-Americans (6.10 per 10,000) is about half that of the national rate (11.5 per 10,000)."

Given that the South Asian diaspora is not a homogeneous one, it is also important to consider the differences between groups from different countries and different religious backgrounds. In one study, Lane and colleagues (2016) found that South Asian immigrants (college undergraduates) of Islamic background had a lower rate of suicidal thoughts and behavior than South Asians of Hindu background. Clearly, both protective factors and challenging pressures are present for any immigrant group. When working with patients of South Asian origin, clinicians should keep in mind some key social and psychodynamic factors: 1) the presence or absence of social support, given the family- and community-oriented cultural context; 2) the emphasis placed on family honor, family reputation, and avoidance of shame; and 3) the intense level of competitive pressure placed on children of immigrants not only to succeed but to outshine both their American peers and their South Asian peers.

When these factors are combined with the strong family bonds that must not be broken, the pressure, especially on second-generation immigrants, can reach a boiling point. A supervisee reported the suicide of a young man of South Asian origin who had struggled to fulfill his father's vision of him becoming a doctor. The father's expectations and the son's sense of self were deeply connected, and the son could not find a way either to disappoint his father and fall from his own ideal of being a good son (with dynamics that included shame, honor, and his family's reputation) or to comply with his father and lose all sense of his own desires and his own existence. In the end, after repeated failed attempts to satisfy his father's vision, it came down to killing himself or killing his father (in fantasy), and he chose to kill himself. It is also important to keep in mind that in South Asian cultures, girls are seen as being much more liable to bring shame to the family than boys. Their behavior is therefore often guarded with greater vigilance, and the pressure can become stifling.

Theoretical and Technical Issues in Psychoanalysis and Psychodynamic Psychotherapy

For most South Asian Americans, the notion of seeking psychotherapy is both unfamiliar and undesirable. Stigma and a sense of shame are associated with seeking mental health care. There is also an assumption that a person has to be mentally ill or in crisis in order to seek help from a therapist. In addition to having language and economic barriers to psychotherapy, patients often have concerns about whether a therapist would be able to understand their cultural and religious background, worldviews, and experiences of discrimination. Patients also may have concerns about whether the therapist will pathologize their family and heritage culture. Unfortunately, these cultural and social barriers to seeking help leave many South Asian Americans without access to adequate, culturally informed psychotherapy.

The concerns surrounding psychotherapy are met with the real gaps in culturally informed training and practice that exist in mental health care settings in the United States. It is not uncommon to find that South Asian American patients are misdiagnosed because of their symptom presentations (e.g., somatic symptoms) or the therapist's unconscious cultural or racial bias. It is also not unusual for therapists to struggle with conceptualizing patients' relational conflicts when their training has not included an understanding of the impact of sociocultural issues on psychological health, identity, and relationships.

The losses incurred in immigration, acculturative stress, identity conflicts, and trauma all contribute to relational conflicts (Kaduvettoor-Davidson and Inman 2012; Kanwal 2017; Tummala-Narra 2016b). Acculturation gaps between parents and children are often compounded by traumatic stress. As such, it is often the case that when parents seek help from a therapist, conflicts with their child(ren) have reached crisis levels. First-generation parents often are reluctant to disclose mental health concerns to anyone outside their family because of stigma and shame. Parents may seek the help of a therapist hoping for the therapist to "fix" the child's disobedience or emotional distress, locating the problem within the child rather than dysfunctional communication or dynamics among family members. Parent-child conflicts are best addressed with a combination of individual and family therapy in which each member of the family has the opportunity to explore their own acculturative process and can discover new, more effective ways of communicating with each other.

No single theoretical paradigm is best suited to working with South Asian Americans in psychotherapy. Rather, a deep examination and consideration of South Asian Americans' experiences, including the role of intersecting individual, interpersonal, sociocultural, and systemic factors, is critical for psychotherapy from any particular theoretical orientation. As psychoanalytically oriented therapists, we highlight the importance of conscious and unconscious dynamics in exploring mental health issues with South Asian American patients. In the following subsections, we describe four specific areas of consideration in theory and practice with South Asian Americans: attachment patterns, religious/spiritual perspectives, family conflict, and sociocultural oppression.

Attachment Patterns

Separation Versus Integration

A clinician who was working with Prajwal, a man of Indian (Hindu) origin who was married to a white American woman, approached me (G.K.) for a consultation because she found herself having great trouble with Prajwal's inability to see why his wife could not agree to the presence of his parents in their home for a month or more, starting before the birth of their first child. The clinician then found herself having strong countertransferential reactions of anger and frustration. Her stance became one of pathologizing Prajwal's "enmeshed" relationship with his parents, especially his mother. The therapeutic goal in her mind was to help him separate from his mother so that he could focus on his nuclear family and his child who was about to be born. That goal, however, assumes a notion of an adult individuated self that is a construction from a Western cultural tradition (Cushman 1995). Kakar and Kakar (2007), Kurtz (1992), and Roland (2006) have described the different self structure one finds in South Asian cultures. G. Kanwal (unpublished manuscript, November 2021) has referred to the developmental pathway that leads to this different outcome as *integrative individuation* to distinguish it from Mahler's *separation-individuation.*

Roland (2006) described the significance of conceptualizing three kinds of self in Indian culture: the familial self (which he also refers to as the *we-self*), the individual self (which is emphasized less than and structured differently from the Western individual self, with more permeable boundaries), and the transcendent or spiritual self (linked to the idea of *atman*, or cosmic self). One has to be mindful, however, of not lumping together the nature of the spiritual self across the many religious traditions found in South Asia. For example, there is no notion of reincarnation in Islam, including the Sufi tradition. Similarly, notwithstanding resurrection, there is not a tradition of believing in reincarnation in Christianity, although one can encounter many Christians in India who carry an amalgam of Christian and Hindu beliefs. Although the terminology used in Roland's descriptions, such as atman and moksha (liberation through enlightenment), is specific to Hindu culture, the significance of a spiritual self does pervade the identity of most South Asians across many religious traditions.

Attachment and Allomothering

Another way of understanding the difference in the developmental and self experience of South Asians is through the lens of attachment. Many scholars (see Quinn and Mageo 2013) have critiqued attachment paradigms as being culturally biased toward one-to-one mother-infant bonding. Allomothering, when someone other than the biological mother performs the functions of mothering, is a commonly occurring nurturing pattern in joint family households. Kurtz (1992) emphasized the importance of various women figures in South Asian homes: mother-in-law, sisters-in-law, visiting aunts, grandmothers, and women hired to do housework who are often also live-in nannies in more affluent homes. In the case of Prajwal, the patient who had difficulty saying no to his parents, the nature of the familial self, constructed in growing up within a joint family system, needs to be considered. Prajwal's case also involves issues having to do with the spiritual self, based on notions of dharma (the law according to which Hindu Indian society measures its conduct) and karma (the idea of actions in one life having an impact on the conditions of the next incarnation). Saying no to his parents may violate his deeply embedded feelings about his dharma and karma, which could shake his identity and self-esteem to the core.

Therapist-Patient Relationship

For clinicians working with patients of South Asian origin, the structure of the self and such dimensions as emotionality, intimacy, closeness, warmth, and interdependency demand modifications in both theory and technique if the therapist is to work more successfully with and understand more accurately the experience of South

Asians. Roland (2006), p. 457) described one of the differences in the kind of relationship Indian (and other South Asian) patients are likely to form with their therapist, stating that "the subordinate, or patient, by displaying deference and respect, expects the superior, the psychoanalytic therapist, to be responsible and nurturing, and that each should maintain and enhance the esteem of the other."

Kanwal (2017) describes a similar dynamic, referring to it as *benevolent transformation*, as contrasted with Sullivan's (1953) concept of *malevolent transformation*. Many Western therapists can find themselves feeling uncomfortable with that kind of idealization. Trying to interpret this dynamic in terms of narcissism is not very useful and can often leave the South Asian patient feeling misunderstood.

Akhtar (1999) described eight guidelines to be kept in mind in therapy with immigrant patients, all of which are relevant to South Asian patients:

1. Maintain cultural neutrality.
2. Accommodate the therapeutic framework to cultural differences.
3. Adopt a developmental stance.
4. Unmask the cultural rationalizations of intrapsychic conflict and transference reactions.
5. Validate feelings of dislocation and facilitate mourning.
6. Interpret defensive functions of nostalgia as well as defenses against emergence of nostalgia.
7. Accept seemingly nonoptimal individuation and involvement of relatives in treatment.
8. Face the challenge posed by a patient's polyglottism and polylingualism.

Similarly, Kanwal (2015) discussed various parameters and goals that might need to be understood differently with South Asian patients in treatment. These relate to money and fees (because wisdom is valued most when it is free), privacy and loyalty (because family ties determine what can or cannot be discussed with outsiders), individual fulfillment versus social fulfillment (because social obligations are the primary determinant of conduct), and difficulties with as-if intimacy (because emotional reciprocity is a fundamental assumption).

Religious and Spiritual Perspectives

Psychoanalysis and psychotherapy have a long history of a deep skepticism about religious and spiritual experience and preoccupation, which are traditionally seen as reflecting more psychologically primitive or early modes of experience connected with Freud's (1911/1958) notions of "primary process thinking." However, this orientation creates an obstacle when one is working with patients of South Asian origin whose lives and psychic structure may be deeply permeated by religious and spiritual experience, thought, and practice. Roland (2006), as mentioned earlier, has emphasized the need to be aware of the spiritual self of South Asian patients. Clinicians working with South Asian patients need to be able to question the cultural bias involved in Freud's formulations about the place of spirituality in human psychology. The clinical issue is not whether the clinician shares the patient's beliefs but whether the patient can feel the presence of a nonjudgmental space where spirituality or religiosity is not automatically pathologized or demeaned.

South Asian patients are also very eclectic in their search for a cure to suffering. They tend to try everything—astrologers, palm readers, Muslim peers (Sufi master), Hindu fakirs (wandering ascetic), homeopathy, Ayurveda, exorcism—and they will expect their psychotherapist to consider that a natural and legitimate perspective. One of my (G.K.) analytic patients regularly consulted her favorite astrologer and shared the updates with me. It was important for me to not see that as competition or regression or magical thinking but to take it as a cultural given and include those astrological insights as part of the patient's creativity and self-healing.

The South Asian worldview is basically one of unity, cyclicity, and contextuality. Ramanujan (1989) described the two kinds of cultural orientation that differentiate Western from Indian thinking styles: context-free and context-sensitive. South Asian cultures tend to be much more context-sensitive. This context-sensitive style allows South Asians to express different kinds of beliefs and relationships to reality in different contexts.

Family Tensions and Conflicts

Conflicts occurring within families can be addressed in a number of ways. Family conflicts among South Asian Americans often are constructed as cultural value conflicts (Inman 2006. It is important to bear in mind that cultural value conflicts that contribute to disconnection among family members are determined by an interplay of various factors (Dupree et al. 2013). Some conflicts between parents and children reflect the interplay between the parents' experiences of immigration and the expectations of their children.

Case Vignette

Asha, a 20-year-old 1.5-generation Bengali American woman, struggles with an eating disorder and depressed mood. In psychotherapy, she compares herself to other South Asian women at her college campus, who she thinks are perceived by others to be more attractive than she is. She also recalls the pressure that she has always felt from her parents and other Bengalis to excel in all aspects of her life, including academics, her musical interests, and her physical appearance. In fact, her mother has told her on multiple occasions that she expects her to be "a perfect Bengali girl." Her parents further emphasize that they emigrated to the United States and sacrificed living with their extended family in order to provide a better life for her. Her parents work long hours and have few economic resources. Asha has internalized the message that she is responsible for justifying her parents' decision to emigrate from Bangladesh and for securing financial stability for her family. In psychotherapy, she says, "I feel so guilty for being sad or complaining. They [my parents] work so hard and sent me to a good school so that I can have it easier than them." In other instances, she shares her frustration with her parents for not understanding the immense pressure that she feels in college. She states, "How will they possibly understand my body image issues? To them, it's nothing. It's trivial compared to everything they went through." Asha has trouble imagining that she can communicate with her parents about her concerns and, at the same time, expresses a deep desire for them to understand her stress. Despite her conflicts with her parents, she shares how much she loves and admires them. In psychotherapy, Asha struggles with feeling guilty for sharing her negative feelings toward her parents and worries that her Indian American therapist will view her as an ungrateful daughter.

Asha's conflicts illustrate a common pattern of family dynamics among South Asian Americans, in which 1.5 and second generations contend with a pressure to fulfill their parents' dreams in the United States. It is important that therapists attend to transferential and countertransferential reactions to avoid pathologizing the parents. At the same time, therapists must help the patient explore a more expansive experience of the self in relation to the patient's family and peers. This requires that therapists engage in their own self-reflection and in dialogue with colleagues in order to address their countertransference effectively.

In some cases, it is appropriate to include family members in working with a patient in individual psychotherapy. For example, an adolescent patient coping with traumatic stress rooted in bullying at school can benefit from the therapist meeting with his parents. The therapist can provide psychoeducation about the impact of bullying on adolescents and develop strategies with the parents to advocate for their child in school. Involving family members in psychotherapy under these types of circumstances can help to relieve the stigma of seeking help, provide empathy and support to family members, and empower families. In other cases, when family members are unlikely to be supportive of the patient, such as in the case of a patient who has experienced childhood trauma by a family member, it is not recommended that the therapist include family members in treatment, even though family connections may be significant for the patient. In each of these cases, the therapist must pay close attention to the role and meaning of family members and the heritage community in the patient's life as well as to transferential and countertransferential responses shaped by the therapist's sociocultural background.

Exploring Sociocultural Oppression

The impact of sociocultural oppression is an important aspect of psychotherapy with South Asian Americans. Therapists can initiate discussions regarding discrimination rooted in racism, xenophobia, religious bias, sexism, homophobia, transphobia, classism, and ableism early in psychotherapy, such as when learning about the patient's developmental history. Early life experiences of microaggressions, bias, verbal harassment and bullying, and physical violence are often left unspoken and unprocessed. In fact, patients may even report early memories of discrimination without recognizing that these experiences have had any psychological impact. For example, Mr. N, a 35-year-old second-generation Pakistani American man, recalled several incidents of being called a terrorist in his teens. Although he recognized that these incidents were racially motivated, he thought that they should not have affected him emotionally. He stated, "These are things that we are just supposed to put up with so that we can live in this country." Mr. N proceeded to share that although discrimination against South Asians is not as bad as that directed against African Americans, he often feels frustrated that his experiences are largely invisible in American society. Mr. N's assessment regarding the right to feel angry or sad about discrimination is shared by many South Asian Americans who believe that putting up with racism is the price that they and their children pay in order to secure a better life in the United States. In such cases, therapists can help patients develop an understanding of the impact of discrimination and sociocultural oppression on their lives and explore ways to cope with discrimination-related stress without further marginalization.

In other instances, South Asian Americans feel empowered to speak out against racism and other forms of discrimination but feel marginalized within their ethnic and religious communities. For example, a South Asian American queer woman may struggle with coming out to her family members who have heterosexist beliefs. In psychotherapy, it is critical for the therapist to be aware of the challenges that this patient faces in multiple contexts, to help her with securing safe spaces where she is able to talk about her sexuality openly, and, when possible, to find ways to secure her connection to her family. Further, it is not always desirable to encourage a Western, Euro-American psychological approach to coming out. Rather, the therapist should consider the intersection of family, contextual, and individual issues that shape the patient's decision-making.

Concluding Thoughts

When considering psychotherapy with South Asian Americans, closer attention to sociocultural context is needed because this context shapes intrapsychic and interpersonal experiences. Psychoanalytic and psychotherapy training in the United States remains, by and large, geared toward working with people from a Western cultural perspective. Clinicians in training are not taught anything about why, or what kind, of modifications may be required in one's theoretical framework or technical stance when working with patients from other cultural backgrounds, including the large South Asian population in the United States. Clinicians who run into trouble with grasping other cultural modes of being are left to seek consultations or supervision with clinicians who might know more about the patient's culture in order to resolve those impasses.

In recent years, psychoanalytic scholars have written about the inextricable connection between the psychic and the social. They have detailed the importance of exploring transference and countertransference rooted in social context and dynamics and the specific issues that arise in working with patients with ethnic, religious, and racial backgrounds similar to or different from those of the therapist (Akhtar 2011; Holmes 2016; Kanwal 2015; Layton and Leavy-Sperounis 2020; Shah 2020; Tummala-Narra 2016b, 2020). In culturally informed psychoanalytic psychotherapy, the therapist attends to the cultural or indigenous narrative of the patient, including language and culturally embedded expressions of affect and distress; explores the impact of sociocultural oppression on the patient's and therapist's lives; recognizes the complexity of cultural identifications; and engages in self-examination (Tummala-Narra 2016b). It is also important for therapists to examine cultural biases inherent in the theoretical paradigms in which they were trained and to navigate contrasting worldviews regarding stress, trauma, mental health, and recovery. Finally, in working with South Asian Americans, it is of paramount importance that therapists recognize the heterogeneity of experiences within South Asian communities, as evidenced in different waves of immigration, and variations in acculturation, family dynamics, social locations, trauma, and discrimination.

Key Points

- It is important to recognize cultural values and practices related to attachment in the family system, such as a value placed on integrative individuation rather than only separation-individuation.
- Therapists' attention to how the therapeutic frame is conceptualized and experienced by the patient is critical because cultural expectations may vary significantly within and across South Asian communities.
- For many South Asian Americans, religion and spirituality play a central role in their understandings of self and self in relationship to others and the external world. As such, therapists can explore religious and spiritual beliefs and practices significant to the patient and the patient's family and community.
- Because the stress of migration and acculturation affects family structure and dynamics, it is important that conflicts related to acculturation and acculturative stress be explored in psychotherapy.
- South Asian Americans have faced racism throughout the history of migration to the United States and other nations, and therefore, experiences of racism and stereotyping are key areas of exploration in psychotherapy.

References

Akhtar S: A third individuation: immigration, identity, and the psychoanalytic process. J Am Psychoanal Assoc 43(4):1051–1084, 1995 8926325

Akhtar S: Immigration and Identity: Turmoil, Treatment, and Transformation. Northvale, NJ, Jason Aronson, 1999

Akhtar S: Immigration and Acculturation: Mourning, Adaptation, and the Next Generation. New York, Jason Aronson, 2011

Akhtar S: The mental pain of minorities. Br J Psychother 30(2):136–153, 2014

American Psychological Association: Suicide among Asian Americans. Washington, DC, American Psychological Association, 2012. Available at: www.apa.org/pi/oema/resources/ethnicity-health/asian-american/suicide. Accessed May 1, 2021.

Bhatia S, Ram A: South Asian immigration to the United States: a brief history within the context of race, politics, and identity, in Biopsychosocial Approaches to Understanding Health in South Asian Americans. Edited by Perera MJ, Chang EC. New York, Springer, 2018, pp 15–32

Blos P: The Adolescent Passage: Developmental Issues. Madison, CT, International Universities Press, 1979

Boulanger G: Seeing double, being double: longing, belonging, recognition, and evasion in psychodynamic work with immigrants. Am J Psychoanal 75(3):287–303, 2015 26356775

Chandra RM, Arora L, Mehta UM, et al: Asian Indians in America: the influence of values and culture on mental health. Asian J Psychiatr 22:202–209, 2016 26442987

Crenshaw K: Demarginalizing the intersection of race and sex: a Black feminist critique of antidiscrimination doctrine, feminist theory and antiracist politics. University of Chicago Legal Forum 1989(1):139–168, 1989

Cushman P: Constructing the Self, Constructing America: A Cultural History. Reading, MA, Addison-Wesley, 1995

Davids MF: The impact of Islamophobia. Psychoanal Hist 11(2):175–191, 2009 19795546
Dupree WJ, Bhakta KA, Patel PS, et al: Developing culturally competent marriage and family therapists: guidelines for working with Asian Indian American couples. Am J Fam Ther 41(4):311–329, 2013
Eng DL, Han S: A dialogue on racial melancholia. Psychoanal Dialogues 10(4):667–700, 2000
Freud S: Formulations on the two principles of mental functioning (1911), in The Standard Edition of the Complete Psychological Works of Sigmund Freud, Vol 12. Translated and edited by Strachey J. London, Hogarth Press, 1958, pp 213–26
Gupta A, Szymanski DM, Leong F: The "model minority myth": internalized racialism of positive stereotypes as correlates of psychological distress, and attitudes toward help-seeking. Asian Am J Psychol 2(2):101–114, 2011
Guzder J, Krishna M: Mind the gap: diaspora issues of Indian origin women in psychotherapy. Psychol Dev Soc J 17(2):121–138, 2005
Hoersting RC, Jenkins SR: No place to call home: cultural homelessness, self-esteem and cross-cultural identities. International Journal of Intercultural Relations 35(1):17–30, 2011
Holmes DE: Culturally imposed trauma: the sleeping dog has awakened. Will psychoanalysis take heed? Psychoanal Dialogues 26(6):641–654, 2016
Inman AG: South Asian women: identities and conflicts. Cultur Divers Ethnic Minor Psychol 12(2)306–319, 2006 16719579
Inman AG, Tummala-Narra P: Immigration and human rights, in The Handbook of Race-Ethnicity and Gender in Psychology. Edited by Miville M, Ferguson A. New York, Springer, 2014, pp 87–109
Inman AG, Devdas L, Spektor V, et al: Psychological research on South Asian Americans: a three-decade content analysis. Asian Am J Psychol 5(4):364–372, 2014
Inman AG, Tummala-Narra P, Kaduvettoor-Davidson A, et al: Perceptions of race-based discrimination among first-generation Asian Indians in the United States. Couns Psychol 43(2):217–247, 2015
Joseph A, Jenkins SR, Wright B, et al: Acculturation processes and mental health of Asian Indian women in the United States: a mixed-methods study. Am J Orthopsychiatry 90(4):510–522, 2020 32614212
Kaduvettoor-Davidson A, Inman AG: Predictors of cultural values conflict for Asian Indian women. J Multicult Couns Devel 40(1):2–10, 2012
Kakar S, Kakar K: The Indians: Portrait of a People. New Delhi, Viking, 2007
Kalra G, Gupta S, Bhugra D: Sexual variation in India: a view from the west. Indian J Psychiatry 52 (suppl 1):S264–S268, 2010 21836691
Kanukollu SN, Mahalingam R: The idealized cultural identities model on help-seeking and child sexual abuse: a conceptual model for contextualizing perceptions and experiences of South Asian Americans. J Child Sex Abuse 20(2):218–243, 2011 21442534
Kanwal GS: Indian culture and the experience of psychoanalytic treatment. Psychoanal Rev 102(6):843–872, 2015 26653061
Kanwal G: "Benevolent transformation" and the centrality of idealization dynamics in Indian culture. Psychoanalytic Discourse 3, 2017
Kanwal G: Loss, self-states, and the immigrant analyst: exploring the "analytic fourth." J Psychoanal Cult Soc 23(4):419–436, 2018
Kanwal G: Friendship, friendliness and intimacy, in Intimacy: Clinical, Cultural, Digital, and Developmental Perspectives. Edited by Kanwal G, Akhtar S. New York, Routledge, 2019, pp 66–79
Khaleque A, Malik F, Rohner RP: Differential acculturation among Pakistani American immigrant parents and children. Psychol Stud (Mysore) 60(4):407–411, 2015
Kumar A, Nevid J: Acculturation, enculturation, and perceptions of mental disorders in Asian Indian immigrants. Cultur Divers Ethnic Minor Psychol 16(2):274–283, 2010 20438166
Kurtz S: All the Mothers Are One: Hindu India and the Cultural Reshaping of Psychoanalysis. New York, Columbia University Press, 1992
Lane R, Cheref S, Miranda R: Ethnic differences in suicidal ideation and its correlates among South Asian American emerging adults. Asian Am J Psychol 7(2):120–128, 2016 27525054

Layton L, Leavy-Sperounis M (ed): Toward a Social Psychoanalysis: Culture, Character, and Normative Unconscious Processes. New York, Routledge, 2020

Mahapatra N: South Asian women in the U.S. and their experience of domestic violence. J Fam Violence 27(5):381–390, 2012

Mehrotra M, Calasanti TM: The family as a site for gendered ethnic identity work among Asian Indian immigrants. J Fam Issues 31(6):778–807, 2010

Methikalam B, Sandhu S, McClincey S: Implementing a psychodynamic approach with South Asian women, in From Research to Action. Edited by Littleford LN, Alexander CA. Muncie, IN, Ball State University Scholar, 2016, pp 112–137

Mudambi A: South Asian American discourses: engaging the yellow peril–model minority dialectic. Howard J Commun 30(3):284–298, 2019

Mukherjee AJ, Diwan S: Late life immigration and quality of life among Asian Indian older adults. J Cross Cult Gerontol 31(3):237–253, 2016 27245988

Needham BL, Mukherjee B, Bagchi P, et al: Acculturation strategies and symptoms of depression: the mediators of atherosclerosis in South Asians Living in America (MASALA) study. J Immigr Minor Health 20(4):792–798, 2018 28748299

Patel NR: The construction of South-Asian-American womanhood: implications for counseling and psychotherapy. Women Ther 30(3–4):51–61, 2007

Prathikanti S: East Indian American families, in Working With Asian Americans: A Guide for Clinicians. Edited by Lee E. New York, Guilford, 1997, pp 79–100

Quinn N, Mageo JM (Eds): Attachment Reconsidered: Cultural Perspectives on a Western Theory. New York, Palgrave Macmillan, 2013

Ragavan MI, Fikre T, Millner U, et al: The impact of domestic violence exposure on South Asian children in the United States: perspectives of domestic violence agency staff. Child Abuse Negl 76:250–260, 2018 29161645

Rai A, Choi YJ: Socio-cultural risk factors impacting domestic violence among South Asian immigrant women: a scoping review. Aggress Violent Behav 38:76–85, 2018

Ramanujan AK: Is there an Indian way of thinking? An informal essay. Contrib Indian Sociol 23(1):41–58, 1989

Roberts LR, Mann SK, Montgomery SB: Mental health and sociocultural determinants in an Asian Indian community. Fam Community Health 39(1):31–39, 2016 26605953

Robertson HA, Chaudhary Nagaraj N, Vyas AN: Family violence and child sexual abuse among South Asians in the US. J Immigr Minor Health 18(4):921–927, 2016 26032775

Roland A: Across civilizations: psychoanalytic therapy with Asians and Asian Americans. Psychotherapy (Chic) 43(4):454–463, 2006 22122136

Roy A: The Doctor and the Saint: Caste, Race, and Annihilation of Caste—The Debate Between B.R. Ambedkar and M.K. Gandhi. Chicago, IL, Haymarket Books, 2017

Schaffner B: Androgyny in Indian art and culture: psychoanalytic implications. J Am Acad Psychoanal 29(1):113–125, 2001 11490672

Shah D: Dangerous territory: racist moments in the psychoanalytic space. Psychoanal Q 89(3):399–413, 2020

Shin RQ, Welch JC, Kaya AE, et al: The intersectionality framework and identity intersections in the Journal of Counseling Psychology and The Counseling Psychologist: a content analysis. J Couns Psychol 64(5):458–474, 2017 29048193

Shweder RA: Why Do Men Barbecue? Recipes for Cultural Psychology. Cambridge, MA, Harvard University Press, 2003

Shweder RA: The cultural psychology of suffering: the many meanings of health in Orissa, India (and elsewhere). Ethos 36(1):60–77, 2008

Smelson-Kanwal B: Intimacy and otherness in multicultural/interracial/interfaith couples, in Intimacy: Clinical, Cultural, Digital, and Developmental Perspectives. Edited by Kanwal G, Akhtar S. New York, Routledge, 2019, pp 80–95

South Asian Americans Leading Together: Demographic snapshot of South Asians in the United States. Silver Spring, MD, South Asian Americans Leading Together, April 2019. Available at: https://saalt.org/wp-content/uploads/2019/04/SAALT-Demographic-Snapshot-2019.pdf. Accessed May 1, 2021.

Sullivan HS: The Interpersonal Theory of Psychiatry. WW Norton, 1953
Tummala-Narra P: Skin color and the therapeutic relationship. Psychoanal Psychol 24(2):255–270, 2007
Tummala-Narra P: Psychotherapy with South Asian women: dilemmas of the immigrant and first generations. Women Ther 36(3–4):176–197, 2013
Tummala-Narra P: Names, name changes, and identity in the context of immigration, in Immigration in Psychoanalysis: Locating Ourselves. Edited by Beltsiou J. New York, Routledge, 2016a, pp 151–165
Tummala-Narra P: Psychoanalytic Theory and Cultural Competence in Psychotherapy. Washington, DC, American Psychological Association, 2016b
Tummala-Narra P: The fear of immigrants. Psychoanal Psychol 37(1):50–61, 2020
Tummala-Narra P, Deshpande A: Mental health conditions among South Asians in the United States, in Biopsychosocial Approaches to Understanding Health in South Asian Americans. Edited by Perera MJ, Chang E. New York, Springer, 2018, pp 171–192
Tummala-Narra P, Alegría M, Chen C: Perceived discrimination, acculturative stress, and depression among South Asians: mixed findings. Asian Am J Psychol 3(1):3–16, 2012
Tummala-Narra P, Sathasivam-Rueckert N, Sundaram S: Voices of older Asian Indian immigrants: mental health implications. Prof Psychol Res Pr 44(1):1–10, 2013
Tummala-Narra P, Deshpande A, Kaur J: South Asian adolescents' experiences of acculturative stress and coping. Am J Orthopsychiatry 86(2):194–211, 2016 26765547
Tummala-Narra P, Gordon J, Gonzalez LD, et al: Breaking the silence: perspectives on sexual violence among Indian American women. Asian Am J Psychol 10(4):293–306, 2019
Vallabhaneni MR: Indian caste system: historical and psychoanalytic views. Am J Psychoanal 75(4):361–381, 2015 26611129
Watters E: Crazy Like Us: The Globalization of the American Psyche. New York, Free Press, 2010
Wilkerson I: Caste: The Origins of our Discontents. New York, Random House, 2020

CHAPTER 25

There Is No Such Thing as Latinx

Race, Intersectionality, and Immigration in Clinical Work and Supervision With Latin American Communities

Daniel Gaztambide, Psy.D.

British psychoanalyst D.W. Winnicott (1965/2018) is often quoted as stating that "there is no such thing as a baby" outside the context of a caregiving relationship. More broadly, there is no parent-infant relationship and no family outside their constitutive social, cultural, economic, and political power relations (Dalal 2013). It is in that spirit that I approach the issue of clinical work with Latinx populations—and the question of the term Latinx itself—through a critical lens that raises questions and highlights context. Chapters of this kind often aim to serve as a "handbook" on working with a specific racial/ethnic group, an "alien other" who must be rendered intelligible to a clinical audience (Brown 2009). Although well intentioned, this approach risks homogenizing the diversity of specific groups in a way that masks not only cultural differences but also underlying power relations, commodifying that population in a manner that can be "consumed" by the mental health disciplines, with no complexity or interiority (Viego 2007). Although cultural competence is multidimensional (Sue 2001), in practice clinicians often interpret it as implying that one lacks specific skills, knowledge, and awareness related to specific cultures that, *once acquired*, lead to "competence," a discourse that masks white supremacist ideologies of mastery and control (Fisher-Borne et al. 2015; Moncayo 1998; Tascon and Gatwiri 2020).

Hence, in this chapter I stress the diversity and complexity of the populations grouped under the terms *Latinx*, *Hispanic*, and *Latin American*, with a focus on race, intersectionality, and immigration. I begin by positioning myself theoretically and culturally in the writing of this chapter, followed by a brief unpacking of the term Latinx to underscore the cultural, racial, and linguistic diversity of Latin American people. I then provide an abbreviated history of race and Latin America, with an emphasis on the forces of colonialism, *mestizaje*, and, in particular, anti-Blackness. Given the more in-depth discussion of immigration in Chapter 24, "South Asian Americans," in this chapter I go against type—rather than an exclusive focus on immigration issues as central to the Latin American experience, I focus on immigration in the context of anti-Blackness and racial hierarchy across North and Latin America. With this approach, I am inviting us to think critically and dynamically about diversity *within* panethnic groups. Relatedly, given a robust discussion of the psychodynamics of racism in psychotherapy with African Americans in Chapter 22, "African Americans and Psychotherapeutic Treatment," this chapter serves as a companion piece illustrating the internalization of anti-Blackness (and anti-Indigeneity) in a global context.

After providing a brief review of the history of Latin America and race, I present themes relevant to clinical work with Latin American populations, followed by 1) clinical questions clinicians might pose to themselves and their patients and 2) vignettes illustrating the implications of these questions in clinical practice. For the sake of space, the vignettes have been abbreviated to highlight illustrations of the preceding questions and themes. Last, I address these themes in the training and supervision of Latinx trainee therapists. In sum, I do not aim to provide the reader a "primer" on Latin American populations and mental health but rather to raise a series of clinically relevant questions with which to begin the process of developing not cultural competence but cultural humility.

Positionality and Theoretical Background

It is critical for both scholars and clinicians to "map" their social identities and the impacts they have on the production of knowledge, the valuing of different modes of knowledge, and how knowledge itself reflects intersecting relations of power (Crenshaw 1990). In the case of the chapter author, I am a white island-born Puerto Rican cisgender male who migrated to the United States mainland, living in New York City during the coronavirus SARS-CoV-2 disease (COVID-19) crisis, and as a clinical psychologist I have achieved middle-class status as a member of the professional-managerial class. Each of these terms is relevant to my approach in this chapter.

Although I am Puerto Rican, born in what continues to be the world's oldest colony (Denis 2015) and defined as a "person of color" in the United States (Lloréns 2018), I am phenotypically white. Depending on context, I am read as ambiguously white and thus a recipient of white privilege or read as a racial other and thus subject to discrimination and violence. Although Puerto Ricans are racially diverse, comprising people who could be read as phenotypically white, Brown, and Black, the question of race itself was silenced in Puerto Rico—one could self-identify as white, at most multiracial, with Black an abject term to be avoided. Whiteness represented a desired ideal, whereas the possibility of a Black identity needed to be erased (Godreau 2015; Rodríguez-Silva 2012). I name my whiteness not out of a desire to "be white" or as a repudiation of my family's and community's heritage but out of recognition of how power, love, and resources are unequally distributed across skin lines, even among members of one's own family. Thus, the complex history of anti-Blackness and colonialism in Latin America is a central theme of this chapter.

The approach to psychotherapy that informs my thinking is grounded in an integration of cultural humility, liberation psychology and critical race theory, and psychoanalytic approaches (Gaztambide 2019a). Research on cultural humility in psychotherapy emerged out of the limitations of the cultural competence approach, leading to an approach to difference centered not on competence but on the therapist's "not-knowing" stance. Cultural humility is defined as an openness to the other that holds one's knowledge lightly and expresses curiosity for the other person's cultural worldview in terms of the identities that are most salient and important to *them* (Mosher et al. 2017). In the therapeutic process, cultural humility includes 1) the therapist's critical self-examination and awareness of their intersecting identities, values, and biases; 2) building a culturally congruent therapeutic alliance; 3) attending to and repairing ruptures due to cultural and racial difference; and 4) navigating value differences between patient and therapist (Mosher et al. 2017). Research on cultural humility—more broadly called a *multicultural orientation*—shows that a culturally humble stance, attending to opportunities for exploring cultural themes and displaying comfort (e.g., maintaining emotional regulation) in discussing cultural differences, leads to better psychotherapy outcomes, in part by strengthening the social bond between patient and therapist, a bond in which identity differences, conflicts, and ruptures can be negotiated and repaired (Davis et al. 2018).

Liberation psychology is a framework originally developed by the revolutionary Jesuit priest and psychologist Ignacio Martín-Baró (1994), who synthesized decolonial theory, critical theory, liberation theology, and psychoanalytic perspectives to ground psychology in a social justice perspective (Gaztambide 2019b). Contemporary scholars and clinicians have critiqued and integrated cultural humility within a race-conscious liberation psychology framework, emphasizing critical reflection not only on intersecting identities but on oppressive structures, negotiating power differences between patient and therapist alongside cultural differences, and developing narratives that integrate personal and collective experiences (Abe 2020; Gaztambide 2019a; Moon and Sandage 2019). To orient the reader to the perspective of this chapter, I offer the following reflection questions:

- What is *my* positionality with respect to race/ethnicity, gender, sexuality, culture, class, and immigration status?
- In what ways do I feel disempowered in my life on the basis of these identities? In what ways am I privileged and empowered by them?
- What does it mean for me to *not know* or have expertise about a given topic as a clinician, especially with regard to race and culture?
- What anxieties might I have about practicing from a not-knowing stance? How can I be curious and open toward the patient's cultural frame of reference?
- What biases, prejudices, or misconceptions do I have about specific cultural, ethnic, and racial groups? What about Latin American populations in particular?
- If I were to have a conflict due to cultural differences with my patient, how would that make me feel? What kind of conflicts makes it hard for me to stay curious and open?

What Is Latinx?

The term *Latinx* is a relatively recent phenomenon in Latin American diasporic identity within the United States (for a review, see Salinas and Lozano 2019). Populations of Latin American descent—whether first, second, or third generation—have used different terms to self-identify, including their country of origin in both singular (e.g., Cuban, Mexican, Argentinian) and hyphenated forms (e.g., Cuban American), culture-specific terms (e.g., Chicano for Mexican Americans, Boricua for Puerto Ricans), and broader terms (e.g., Latin, Hispanic, Latina/Latino, and, more recently, Latinx). The term *Hispanic* generally refers to people from Latin American countries that were formerly colonies of Spain whose primary language is Spanish. Latina/Latino and South/Latin American are terms that include Spanish-speaking countries as well as those countries whose primary language is not Spanish that were former colonies of other European powers, such as Brazil (Portuguese), Suriname (Dutch), French Guiana (French), and Guyana (English).

The term Latinx itself seems to have evolved from U.S.-based queer Latin American communities on social media and later was adopted in higher education institutions (Salinas and Lozano 2019). The terms Latina/Latino, and even the rarely used Latin@, reflect the gendered nature of the Spanish language with feminine (-a) and masculine (-o) forms; hence, Latinx is an attempt to construct identities outside the gender binary and patriarchal scripts of sex and gender (Trujillo-Pagán 2018). However, use of the term Latinx is troubled not only for gender and sexual categories but for racial ones as well through its "queering" of the Black-white binary in the United States, proposing notions of hybridity or racial *mestizaje* (mixture) that complexify racial narratives while also making space for identities all too often erased within Hispanic spaces, such as Indigenous and Afro-Latinx peoples (Morales 2019; Salinas 2020). Because Hispanic, Latina/Latino, or Latinx identities raise important questions about race, ethnicity, and culture, I take a more critical perspective on notions of hybridity and *mestizaje* here.

Despite public discourse around the term Latinx, including its adoption by major organizations such as the National Latinx Psychological Association (formerly the National Latina/o Psychological Association; see Cardemil et al. 2019), only about 25% of Latin Americans in the United States have heard of the term, and only 3% use it as part of their identity (Noe-Bustamante et al. 2020). Some Latin American students in university settings, where the term has the most currency, may identify with the term, with few ever using it among their families and home communities (Salinas 2020). The use and meaning of the term can be inconsistent, reflecting either sincere attempts at inclusion of LGBTQ+ people within the broader pan–Latin American community or policing by academic elites seeking to exert discursive power in institutional contexts—what Salinas (2020) refers to as *voces perdidas* (lost voices) and *voces de poder* (voices of power), respectively.

From a culturally humble and critical point of view, it becomes important to 1) make room for and convey understanding of the idiosyncratic and contingent ways Latin American peoples self-identify and 2) be mindful of how modes of identification reflect underlying power relations. Keeping in mind these complexities, I use the term Latinx as an inclusive term representing the gender, sexual orientation, racial, and cultural diversity of Latin American peoples in the United States. I do not assume that most Latin American people in the United States identify with the term nor that it should be imposed on them. Cultural humility does not consign an identity to the patient but creates space for the patient to articulate their identity on their own terms. At the same time, I also employ the term because of the importance of making room for lost and marginalized voices.

Practice Questions

- How does my patient identify culturally? As Hispanic? Latin American? A specific national identity (e.g., Mexican, Nicaraguan, Puerto Rican, Uruguayan)? A hybrid identity (e.g., Mexican American)? A culturally specific term (e.g., Chicano, Boricua)? Latina/Latino/Latin@? Latinx? All or none of the above?
- What does this cultural, ethnic, or national identity mean to my patient? How did they develop this identity in the context of their family and community? What relationship does this identity have to their presenting problem?
- How does my patient's cultural identity interact with other dimensions of identity such as class, gender, gender identity, and sexuality? To what extent are these identities salient to the patient's experience?

Case Vignette 1

Mr. C is a cisheterosexual Latinx man in middle adulthood presenting for treatment for bipolar I disorder. Over the course of the initial interview, the clinician inquired as to Mr. C's living situation. Mr. C described living with his 70-year-old mother, whom he described as "very controlling," adding, "Spanish moms are like that, you know." The clinician expressed curiosity about this remark, asking Mr. C for more detail about "Spanish moms" and how he himself identified. "Well, not Spanish Spanish," he said, clarifying, "we're Puerto Rican, *de pura cepa* (full-blooded)." Mr. C also identifies as Latino but made a distinction between Puerto Ricans and other Latinos because of Puerto Rico's specific relationship with the United States. This led to an exploration of how Mr. C's mother brought him stateside as a child following his father's death and how she was affected by the lack of employment opportunities, leading the clinician to reframe Mr. C's mother as being "very protective." Mr. C accepted this reframing, noting that his mother became even more protective following his bipolar I diagnosis when he was in his early 20s. This opened up an exploration of how he sometimes discontinued his medication as a form of protest toward his mother.

A Brief History of Race in Latin America

Space does not allow for a full account of the history of Latin America. The following is provided as a way of contextualizing contemporary racial tensions in Latin America and the United States. The first peoples to arrive in "the Americas" came from northeast Asia 15,000 years ago, or about 30,000–70,000 years later than people who settled on other continents (Moya 2018). This led the population density of Indigenous peoples across the Americas to be much lower than that of other continents—it is estimated that about two-thirds of Latin America's population today descend from people who arrived after 1492 (Moya 2018). Population density and different methods for adapting to the environment, alongside mere historical contingency, led to a serious technological divide between Amerindian peoples and the Europeans who arrived post-1492, alongside different immunological profiles—the colonizers literally brought the plague in the form of diseases to which Amerindian peoples were vulnerable. (It must be noted, however, that most of the technological advances that gave advantage to European powers over Amerindian peoples were developed not in Europe but in the Middle Eastern/North African world [Moya 2014].) A combination of lower population density among Amerindian peoples, their genocide by European colonizers, and the advent of the trans-Atlantic slave trade would not so much discover but *create* a "new world" and a new category of people—Latin Americans.

This was not without incident, and Amerindian and African revolts against enslavement were rampant, a regular occurrence stemming the efforts of colonizers—especially when European indentured servants joined them in allegiances against the wealthy landed classes. Whereas England and later colonial America developed a "whiteness project" (Horne 2020) that helped consolidate the diverse—and warring—peoples of Europe within the category *white*, with Blackness as its opposite representing the unfree and nonhuman (Wilderson 2010), Spanish and Portuguese colonizers and their descendants among the elite developed notions of race that stressed racial mixture. This ideology, known as *mestizaje*, posits a "harmonious" society in which national identity supersedes issues of race, albeit in different forms depending on the specific Latin American country, its history of Indigenous genocide or survival, patterns of African slave trade and abolition, and immigration from European countries. For example, Mexico, Brazil, and Puerto Rico represent different permutations of *mestizaje* acknowledging white European, Indigenous, and African heritage so long as the resulting "blend" produces whiteness, erases Blackness, and "manages" Indigenous populations (Miller 2009).

Don't Judge a Book by Its Cover: Implications of *Mestizaje* Ideology for Latinx Racial Identity and Mental Health

The essence of *mestizaje* ideology is that Latin American peoples are a mixture of African, Indigenous, and European peoples, with the implicit social contract that whiteness represents progress, development, and humanity, and African heritage is something progressively "overcome" and erased—with Indigenous heritage and peoples either representing an in-between Brown category or being erased altogether in popular cultural narratives (Wade 2017). This ideology has real-world psychological and material implications, requiring a distinction between national, cultural, and ethnic identity on the one hand and skin and racial identity on the other. In both the United States and Latin America, having darker skin is predictive of discrimination, worse medical and mental health outcomes, reduced economic opportunities, and reduced ability to integrate into the labor force post–U.S. immigration, over and above class dynamics alone (Bozo et al. 2018; Garcia et al. 2015). These outcomes, however, are *separate* from racial self-identification (Perreira and Telles 2014).

Racial classification systems in Latin America have evolved to regulate and manage the twin anxieties of 1) reaching the "top," identified with whiteness, while 2) avoiding and dissociating from the "bottom," identified with Blackness (Silva and Saldivar 2018). For example, across contexts as diverse as Argentina, Colombia, and the Latinx Caribbean, multiple overlapping and contradictory terms for racial classification exist that function to simultaneously point both *toward* Blackness and Indigeneity and *away* from it—one might say, "I'm not *Black (negro)*, I'm *mixed (pardo)*." These anxieties produce not only a cacophony of terms meant to avoid association with Blackness (Godreau 2015) but also the imperative to *mejorar la raza*, or "improve the race." One might physically "look Brown" but have light skin and therefore identify as white. Similarly, one might have wavy or curly hair, but as long as it is not dense or Afro-textured hair, it may be redefined as *pelo lacio*, or straight hair, which in the hair hierarchy (whether Latin or North American) is seen as being *pelo bueno*—"good hair." The desire for a partner with lighter skin and children with lighter skin and *pelo bueno* becomes both an explicit and an implicit imperative across the Americas (Muro and Martinez 2018). Precisely because of these complex dynamics, the literature reflects the existence of a skin color paradox: although skin color predicts psychosocial outcomes, it is distinct from racial self-identification, which may not.

Skin color may not necessarily inform Latinx identity, culture, and values, especially for recent immigrants, in the ways it does for minority individuals who identify as Black, such as African Americans in the United States (Faught and Hunter 2012). How first and subsequent generations of Latinx immigrants *experience* the color line in the United States, and how it challenges or reinforces Latin American racial hierarchies, may then lead to renewed narratives of racial self-identification or may silence them. For example, one study of acculturation among Puerto Ricans found that whereas skin color (whether one was white, Black, or Brown) had no relationship to their identity, perceived discrimination from whites led to greater disaffiliation from whiteness and white culture (Capielo Rosario et al. 2019). It is because of these complexities that Bonilla-Silva (2004) argued that as the United States becomes "Latin Americanized," it will adapt its existing racial hierarchy, with Latinx communities falling into one of three categories—white, honorary white, or collective Black (including displaced Afro-descendant and Indigenous peoples).

Subjective Experience of Race Among Black, Indigenous, and White or Racially Ambiguous Latinx People

The Latin American racial hierarchy, with its whiteness-Blackness continuum, often leaves Indigenous communities in the position of adapting themselves into a middle position of being mestizo or Brown that passes for honorary white, facing erasure outside mainstream social and political participation, or experiencing victimization through ongoing cultural and literal genocide (Pedersen 2006). Indeed, the marginalization of Indigenous cultures, languages, and healing practices is deepened through medical and psychiatric discourses seeking to discipline or control Indigenous communities (Flood and Rohloff 2018; Lucana and Elfers 2020). It may be assumed that Spanish or Portuguese (in the case of Brazil) is the primary language of all Latinx immigrants, whereas for Latinx immigrants from Indigenous communities, Spanish or

Portuguese may actually be their second or third spoken language—their first language might be Quechua (Peru), Zapotec (Mexico), or Guarani (Paraguay), among others (Durston and Mannheim 2018). Providing mental health services in the patient's first language must account for both pre-Columbian and post-Columbian languages in treatment delivery, including the use of interpreter services (Frandsen et al. 2019).

Another dimension that is important to consider is the development of Black or Afro-Latinx consciousness—Latinx people who are phenotypically Black or Afro-descendant and self-identify as Black—in the United States (Hordge-Freeman and Loblack 2020). Afro-Latinx identity may lead to identification with other Black communities such as the African American community on the basis of shared histories of enslavement, social struggle, and resilience. Conversely, some individuals may experience marginalization from other Black communities on the basis of 1) anti-Blackness in the broader Latinx community and/or 2) a perception that Afro-Latinx people are appropriating Blackness or are not "Black enough" (Hordge-Freeman and Loblack 2020). Negotiating Blackness in North America thus adds another layer of complexity to the effects of Latin American anti-Blackness (Adames et al. 2018). Internalized anti-Blackness—whether in its Latin or North American varieties—may lead some Afro-Latinx people to disaffiliate from other Black communities on the basis of negative associations between socialism and Black identity (Hordge-Freeman and Loblack 2020).

As stated in the previous subsection, lighter skin has been associated with better outcomes under anti-Black, white supremacist structures across the Americas, yet evidence suggests that Latinx individuals with lighter skin are not more likely to endorse racial hierarchy ideologies despite these privileges (Vargas 2018). White and racially ambiguous Latinx people may experience spillover effects of North American racism in ways they could not in their home countries (Aranda et al. 2014; Garcia 2009). Hence, white and racially ambiguous Latinx may benefit from white Latinx privilege while also being subject to discrimination in the United States, which then leads to disaffiliation from white values (Capielo Rosario et al. 2019) and identification with the broader Latinx community (Vargas 2018). Conversely, notions of *mestizaje* transmitted intergenerationally postimmigration and reinforced by U.S. racism might predispose white and racially ambiguous Latinx people toward identifying with white supremacist, anti-Black discourses. Consider the example of white, lighter-skin, cis male Latinx who participated in the 2017 "Unite the Right" rally in Charlottesville, Virginia (Soto Vega and Chávez 2018).

Keeping in mind the complexities of Latinx racial identity, *mestizaje* ideologies, and the patient's specific experience and their family's national origin (and their nation's history of colonialism and race) is critical to culturally and social justice–centered assessment and treatment (Adames et al. 2016). At the same time, per a cultural humility perspective, these relationships are not necessarily linear or self-evident for all Latinx patients—as reviewed earlier, although skin color affects economic, medical, and mental health outcomes, it does not necessarily lead to a reflective, conscious, or transparent racial identity. Engaging in *dynamic sizing* by switching organically between 1) minding historical, sociopolitical, and cultural trends and 2) minding the specific experience of the individual patient becomes important for joining the patient's world while avoiding stereotyping (Sue 2006).

Questions for Mental Health Practitioners to Ask Themselves

- Alongside my patient's cultural, ethnic, and national identity, how do they understand their identity in terms of race? Do they identify as white, Brown, Indigenous, Black or Afro-descendant (e.g., Afro-Latinx)—or none of the above? How do they narrativize the relationship between their cultural/ethnic/national identity and their racial identity? How did they learn these scripts and relationships within their family, local community, and culture?
- What is my patient's preferred or primary language? Is their primary language something *other* than English, Spanish, or Portuguese, such as an Indigenous pre-Columbian language? If I do not speak my client's preferred or primary language, are interpreter services or a referral called for?
- How does my client's racial narrative relate (or not) to their presenting problem? How might anti-Blackness and anti-Indigeneity structure my client's experience of race?

Case Vignette 2

Ms. Y is a cisheterosexual young adult female (preferred pronouns she/her) who self-identified as Afro-Dominicana when presenting for treatment at a counseling center because of difficulties concentrating in her undergraduate studies. During exploration of Ms. Y's experience of her attentional difficulties, she stressed the difficulty with transitioning back and forth between her home life with her intergenerational family and going to school. The therapist, an African American woman, expressed how difficult it must be moving back and forth between home and school and asked more questions about Ms. Y's family background. As Ms. Y expanded on her family history, she shared that her grandparents were "very old school," and so were her parents. They expected her to both be successful in school and fulfill traditional gender norms as a caretaker for her younger siblings. "Even though I'm the oldest," Ms. Y said, "it always felt like I wasn't wanted." The therapist inquired further about these feelings, and Ms. Y disclosed that her father regularly made denigrating comments about her weight, her *pelo malo* ("bad hair"), and her dark skin.

Ms. Y's family reflected a three-tiered hierarchy valuing whiteness at the top (with her paternal grandfather perceived as the exemplar), brown skin and self-identification as Indio (Taino or Indigenous, which was how her father identified) in the middle, and Blackness at the bottom. Ms. Y's siblings were lighter skin, and because she and her mother were both darker skin, she was often made to feel it was her fault the family was "going backward" instead of *mejorando la raza* ("improving the race"). Her mother was often quiet during her father's tirades about Ms. Y's body, making Ms. Y feel alone in navigating her family's anti-Blackness. In ongoing treatment, she and her therapist engaged in skills training and behavior modification to develop coping skills around concentration issues, alongside exploration of anti-Blackness in herself and her family and across both the United States and the Dominican Republic. In the therapeutic relationship, they discussed how colorism is both similar and different across African American and Afro-Latinx communities. The therapist disclosed how in her community the image of a strong Black woman who is expected to sacrifice herself for others without receiving care kept coming to mind when listening to Ms. Y's experience. Across cultural differences, Ms. Y was able to explore her Blackness in a safe, welcoming space, develop new skills for navigating the transition between home life and school, and renegotiate boundaries with her family.

Case Vignette 3

Mr. V is a male-presenting individual (preferred pronouns he/him/they/them, used interchangeably) who identifies as queer. He is from Mexico and is in middle adulthood and presents to a community mental health clinic for treatment for depression following a legal complication related to their immigration status. Mr. V was originally assigned to a bilingual treatment team, which included a white male Puerto Rican therapist and an Afro-Dominican male psychiatrist, with sessions conducted in Spanish. After an initial assessment, the treatment team developed concern that Mr. V's depression might be complicated by his immigration status, but the tempo of his speech might also reflect an underlying neurocognitive disorder. The team agreed to withhold a diagnostic impression and to conduct an ongoing assessment.

In their initial sessions, Mr. V and his therapist explored his experience of his sexuality and gender identity within his family and community and the struggles associated with the U.S. immigration system. Noting the nature of Mr. V's speech—he often paused midsentence, slowing down—the therapist expressed curiosity about those moments in which he "seemed stuck" *(como que se trababa).* Mr. V became embarrassed, stating that sometimes the words "don't come to me" *(no me llegan las palabras).* The therapist reflected back, "Don't come to you?" *(No le llegan?)* Mr. V disclosed that his first language is actually Zapotec, the language of his Indigenous community in the state of Oaxaca, Mexico.

Realizing that Mr. V had not disclosed this fact during the initial intake (which asked about preferred language), the therapist wondered aloud if asking about language made them uncomfortable. Mr. V shared how as he reached adolescence, his parents stressed that he should speak Spanish in the home—when he struggled or became anxious speaking Spanish, this would lead to ridicule. "*Imaginate*" (Just imagine), he exclaimed, "If I get put down for not speaking Spanish, how will my family react for not speaking hetero [i.e., not being heterosexual]!" Mr. V and his providers organized a team session with a Zapotec medical interpreter to allow him to be heard in his first language, lessening his anxiety by allowing him to express himself fluidly and freely. Being able to alternate between Spanish and Zapotec in psychotherapy allowed him to access different parts of himself—across race, gender identity, and sexuality—contextualizing his family's emphasis on learning Spanish in the history of Indigenous erasure on both sides of the border.

Case Vignette 4

Ms. I is a young adult white Argentinian bisexual woman (preferred pronouns she/her) of Italian descent presenting for treatment because of difficulties with her family over her sexuality and her current relationship. In her initial sessions Ms. I shared that her family had immigrated from Argentina in the 1980s and still held on to "old world" values around family and status. She rebelled against these values while attending college, when she came out as bisexual to her family. This led to a rift with her parents, which resulted in a tacit agreement to a shared silence around her personal life. In graduate school, when she began dating her current partner, an Afro-Bolivian woman who identifies as a lesbian, both her bisexual identity and her interracial relationship became a source of conflict. The renewed tension with her family raised numerous questions about Ms. I's identity—she thought of herself as "a typical Italian girl," but in the United States she was racialized as Latinx and tacitly as being Brown despite her white skin. At the same time, she sensed her family's perception of other Latinx groups as "lesser," with Argentinians seen as "more refined."

Ms. I felt uncomfortable being identified as a "person of color" because that terminology "didn't quite fit" her and her family's experience, especially given her father's racial resentment. During heated arguments, he would remind Ms. I how he and her mother waited to have children until they came to the United States. He saw the rise in

Black and Indigenous immigrants from nearby Bolivia, Peru, and Paraguay as "corrupting" Argentine society, and to him the United States symbolized the "last bastion of civilization." And Ms. I had now crossed multiple gender, sex, and racial boundaries. Ms. I and her therapist, a white Latinx male, explored the complexities of being white in Latin America, "off-white" or Brown in the United States, and a perpetual other because of her bisexuality—judged both by her family and at times by her partner. She recognized that although her whiteness afforded her privilege and others might hold biphobic anxieties, she valued being part of the LGBTQ+ community and felt solidarity with other Latinx and ethnic minority groups. Reflecting on how culture, race, and sexuality intersect in her life allowed Ms. I more room to accept herself and tolerate difficult conversations with her family and her partner.

Training and Supervision of Latinx Psychotherapists

It is important to consider the complexities of Latinx experience on both sides of the couch—not only as potential patients but as clinicians and psychotherapists in training as well. The experience must also be understood contextually in relation to graduate training in psychotherapy-related fields such as social work, clinical and counseling psychology, and psychiatric and professional counseling. Although comprising 16% of the U.S. population, Hispanic or Latino-identifying people make up only 7.1% of those who earn advanced graduate degrees (National Science Foundation 2017). Given their underrepresentation in graduate school and related psychotherapy training contexts, Latinx psychotherapy trainees may often feel that they do not belong, feel that they are not valued in their training programs, or experience the tacit and explicit message that they are not a good fit within their training settings, factors that may impact academic achievement and emotional distress (Miller and Orsillo 2020).

Latinx Trainee Clinicians in Graduate School: Structural and Institutional Considerations

The sense of impostor syndrome, disconnect, and not feeling welcomed or valued must be seen in the context of local, national, and international adversities, such as ongoing xenophobia toward Latinx and other immigrants; the continued violence against Black, Indigenous, and other people of color; and, as of this writing, the ravages of coronavirus SARS-CoV-2 disease (COVID-19). Regarding COVID-19 specifically, research has shown a surge in emotional distress and mental health symptoms across undergraduate and graduate settings, along with a greater sense of disconnection from school and remote instruction, commensurate with the global mental health impact of the pandemic (Chirikov et al. 2020). Similarly, news reports of racialized violence against Black, Latinx, Asian, and Native American peoples likely will exacerbate stressors that students of color experience in their training programs—especially if faculty and administration take no action to acknowledge this impact (Jones et al. 2018). This relates to a broader issue in most institutions and academic departments, whereby questions of equity, diversity, and inclusion are rarely discussed in the curriculum except in moments of crisis or to focus on the need for more recruitment of ethnic minority students and faculty (Perez et al. 2020). Such silences may lead students of color and Latinx students in particular to feel unseen and unprepared on how to tackle issues of culture and difference in their clinical work.

Indeed, graduate school culture and climate may lead Latinx students to feel "othered" in the mental health field, essentialized into rigid conceptions of who Latinx individuals are, and socialized into the discipline in ways that pull them away from their own communities and ways of relating and being in the world (Ayala and Ramirez 2019). It is important to consider the role of individual and communal trauma because Latinx students may seek graduate school in a psychotherapy-related field to pursue self-growth and gain tools to bring back to their families and communities. Such trauma can both be exacerbated by graduate training and serve as a source of resilience in the face of institutional adversity (Montero-Hernandez and Drouin 2020). Supervisors, instructors, and program administrators should be mindful of how Latinx students may feel pressured to "code switch" (move back and forth between cultures) to cope with the acculturative demands of predominantly white institutions. In line with this chapter's perspective, recruiting and retaining *diverse* Latinx faculty (e.g., from different racial, linguistic, cultural backgrounds); developing or connecting to a Latinx resource center; developing cultural affinity groups; and considering how Latinx students negotiate identity across professional, communal, and familial domains can help trainees "hold" and process these tensions in a facilitative training environment (Limas 2019).

Access to funding, culturally congruent mentorship, and developing one's "extended professional family" (N. Boyd-Franklin, personal communication, September 2009) are critical components of success for Latinx and other students of color. Minority fellowship programs (MFPs) funded by the Substance Abuse and Mental Health Services Administration provide full-tuition scholarships and stipends alongside ongoing mentoring for trainees of color across nursing, clinical and counseling psychology, social work, and psychiatry. MFPs have been found to reliably support and increase numbers of culturally competent ethnic minority clinicians capable of providing clinical services in underserved communities, in part by helping ensure graduate program completion, connecting students to a network of scholars of color as well as a supportive cohort of MFP fellows, and professional development mentoring (Branco and Davis 2020). MFP fellows in turn report that involvement in the program helped heighten their clinical and multicultural competence, inculcated a desire to "pay it forward" to future generations of ethnic minority candidates, and empowered them to engage in leadership roles in their local institutions and national professional organizations (Branco and Davis 2020). (In the interest of full disclosure: I was a recipient of an MFP in graduate school. It is not an exaggeration that I could not have finished my studies without its culturally mindful financial support and mentorship.)

Cultural Humility and Critical-Decolonial Approaches in Supervision

Much like in psychotherapy, considerations of relatedness, power, and humility are integral to good supervision. Humility in supervision implies an other-centered stance and openness on the part of the supervisor to the supervisee's background, feelings, and perspectives (Watkins and Mosher 2020). Watkins and Mosher (2020) distinguish between relational, cultural, and intellectual humility. Relational humility involves being open in one's personal relationship and evaluative judgments with the supervisee. Cultural humility is similar to relational humility but with regard to the supervisee's cultural beliefs, viewpoints, and differences with the supervisor. Last, intellectual humility means being open to and valuing different ideas, opinions, and intellectual perspectives between supervisor and supervisee. Being able to sustain these different modes of humility increases supervisor-supervisee multicultural competence; strengthens the supervisory alliance; helps *both* supervisor and supervisee become receptive to feedback; and facilitates repair of relational, cultural, and intellectual ruptures in supervision.

It is important to underscore how all psychotherapy trainees, but *especially* trainees of color, operate under unique challenges (Watkins and Mosher 2020). Trainees are challenged by the amorphous and nonlinear nature of their development as a therapist, operating with an urgency to "do" something in treatment with patients and feeling ineffective and "less than" as a budding clinician. These anxieties are further deepened by being in the role of learner in relation to patients, often reinforcing impostor syndrome feelings—"How can I possibly help this patient when I'm learning psychotherapy?" Last, the disproportionate power relation inherent in the supervisory relationship and the experience of being evaluated may lead trainees to engage in overly submissive, avoidant, or challenging behavior, which can impair humility on the part of both supervisor and supervisee.

Given the importance of cultural humility in psychotherapy outcome, multidimensional aspects of humility can be fostered in the curriculum by providing instruction about the benefits of humility, assigning experiential exercises to heighten humility awareness (e.g., developing a cultural and family genogram), developing a supervisee bill of rights as part of the supervisory process, modeling humility in supervision, and encouraging deliberate practice and awareness building (Watkins and Mosher 2020). The importance of such recommendations notwithstanding, issues of power and race require cultural humility to be further nuanced. The traumatic effects of racism, intergenerational trauma, and pressure to assimilate to whiteness render the practice of cultural humility fraught for trainee therapists of color (Moon and Sandage 2019). What would it mean to be culturally humble as a queer Latinx trainee-therapist working with a white patient who regularly expresses racist and queerphobic beliefs? In such a therapeutic context, the call to practice an *other-oriented* stance—say, by a white male supervisor—might compromise the trainee's well-being through a demand to accommodate to racist, cisheteropatriarchal discourses. This is not to imply that cultural humility or relational attunement is not important, only that the capacity to reflect on self and others—whether relationally or socioculturally—is itself a function of the surrounding social system (Twemlow et al. 2005).

Although relational safety is stressed as a component of culturally humble supervision in a general sense, it is integral to the supervision of Latinx and other trainees of color from a critical decolonial supervision framework (Ramírez Stege et al. 2020). A critical decolonial approach would stress not only the diversity of cultural perspectives one can be open to but also how these perspectives are both valued and loaded on the basis of power hierarchies and social structures. Identities, privilege, and underprivilege are seen as being contextual rather than a function of discrete monadic traits. This allows for a more complex understanding of 1) how an inherent power relation exists between patient and therapist and between supervisor and supervisee;

2) how this power relation can be heightened, dampened, or problematized dynamically on the basis of the intersecting identities of patient/supervisee and therapist/supervisor; and 3) how to negotiate and redefine those relationships through critical dialogue. A critical decolonial approach to supervision thus takes the cultural humility perspective deeper by helping trainees explore intercultural *and* intracultural transferences with patients, build greater self-efficacy by understanding relational and sociopolitical dynamics flexibly, and be more culturally responsive to patients' needs (Ramírez Stege et al. 2020).

Existing literature suggests that the process of negotiating and brokering between different linguistic and cultural worlds continues throughout training and postgraduation (Delgado-Romero et al. 2018). Hence, a culturally congruent *facilitative environment* is imperative for buffering against these stressors during training. It cannot just be assumed that because a trainee is Latinx that automatically means they can speak Spanish, Portuguese, or another Latin American language. Further, even if a trainee has conversational or first-language Spanish skills, this does not mean that they are prepared to practice psychotherapy in Spanish "out of the box." Just as it cannot be assumed that being a person of color means *by default* that one is already culturally competent, so too is linguistic competency something that must be trained and developed in the curriculum. For example, a Latinx student whose first language is Spanish may struggle with finding the right word in English to deliver an intervention in an English-speaking treatment. Conversely, another Latinx student conducting a session in Spanish may similarly struggle with finding the right words to express something formulated in English to their client. In both cases, the student may have difficulty finding the words not because they may not know them, but because they may not have been trained to think clinically in both English and Spanish. This is all the more egregious when one considers that clinical courses, supervision, readings, and training videos *are almost entirely in English.* Culturally congruent training, then, should support Latinx students in navigating both cultural and (for those who speak a Latin American language) linguistic worlds.

Valencia-Garcia and Montoya (2018) point to the American Psychological Association–accredited Psychological Services for Spanish Speaking Populations program as a promising training model that combines language proficiency training by a Spanish language instructor with cultural competency and application taught by a psychology instructor. Their general recommendations include recruiting and retaining faculty with language-specific competence; teaching the distinction between cultural and linguistic competence; and providing language-specific training tracks (e.g., Bellevue's inpatient Bilingual Treatment Program in New York City), formal coursework, and supervision on linguistic competency. In regard to clinical supervision, the practice of expecting—even demanding—trainees to provide services in Spanish without a Spanish-speaking supervisor should be terminated. When there is immediate clinical need, providing services in Spanish should be explored with the trainee as a possibility, but ultimately it should be undertaken at the trainee's discretion. Last, on the basis of faculty and peer availability, formal consultation and theory reading groups in Spanish would enhance the training experience (Valencia-Garcia and Montoya 2018).

Although limited research exists on the developmental trajectories of Latinx mental health professionals, some studies suggest that Latinx professionals often leverage their cultural assets in treatment with patients, often using self-disclosure of their cultural and spiritual values to connect with Latinx patients, negotiate the balance between professional and cultural selves, and stress the value of "giving back" and supporting future generations of Latinx clinicians (Airhart-Larraga et al. 2021; Nadathur 2019). Institutional structures alongside clinical supervision can help develop these capacities among Latinx and other trainees of color by enhancing psychological and cultural flexibility—increasing acceptance of internal experiences while empowering the trainees to engage in values-based living, which is predictive of outcomes over and above the negative effects of racial-ethnic microaggressions and low perceived belongingness in school (Miller and Orsillo 2020). The mutative value of individual or collective resilience notwithstanding, I would underscore the importance of creating institutional structures that *reduce* the incidence of racial-ethnic microaggressions and increase the felt sense of belongingness.

Institutional and Supervisory Case Vignette

The Graduate and Advanced Program for Psychology (GAPP), a doctoral-level scientist-practitioner program in clinical psychology, is grounded in values of social justice, scientific inquiry, and applied practice. GAPP has over time recruited, retained, and developed a diverse cohort of senior and junior faculty of color. This includes faculty of color whose primary interests are in social justice, equity, and multicultural competence, as well as faculty of color whose primary areas involve other issues in clinical psychology (e.g., evidence-based treatments for depression, couple therapy, trauma treatment) examined through a culture- and justice-informed lens. In addition, white faculty at GAPP have similarly made a commitment to research and practice using a culture-informed lens, even if that is not their primary area of study and inquiry. The full faculty collaborate on developing curricula, courses, and training opportunities in line with these values. Alongside clinical and research training in line with American Psychological Association guidelines, GAPP's programming includes 1) an orientation to psychology, social justice, and the public interest; 2) student affinity groups based on identity and language; and 3) a diverse roster of clinical supervisors. GAPP's in-home clinic, based in a racially diverse metropolitan area, also offers language-specific treatment and supervision teams, along with the opportunity to train in culturally and linguistically congruent assessments.

Ms. S is a bilingual Afro-Honduran cisheterosexual young adult female who is a second-year doctoral candidate at GAPP. She is the first in her family to work toward earning a doctoral degree and has found in that a source of cultural and familial pride. Ms. S was excited to begin her studies at GAPP, where she found a sense of being "at home." She attended a weekly Spanish-language consultation group led by a Spanish-speaking Latinx faculty member and was a member of her faculty adviser's lab on substance use and racial health disparities. Ms. S's adviser was a second-generation Filipina American queer woman who allowed a space for her to explore their cultural and linguistic similarities while also expressing curiosity and humility toward their differences.

As part of her training through GAPP's in-house clinic, Ms. S was assigned a psychodynamic case and an external supervisor. The supervisor, Dr. R, was an older cisheterosexual white male from South Africa with an interest in critical race theory. He was assigned to Ms. S by the clinic director on the basis of the needs of the case as well as their mutual interest in decolonial and critical studies. A Spanish-speaking supervisor was sought, but unfortunately, none of the clinicians on their roster was available at the time. Because Ms. S was interested in delivering psychotherapy in Spanish, she agreed to receive a Spanish-speaking Latinx client who had immigrated from South America, and she began supervision with Dr. R.

In the beginning of their work together, Ms. S and Dr. R built rapport over their shared interests and negotiated the frame of their supervision together. They agreed to watch video recordings of sessions together, and Ms. S would periodically pause the video to translate both the clinical process and the actual words spoken for Dr. R. Although this was a challenging process at first, Dr. R and Ms. S entered a flow working together on her client's treatment. Over time, however, they became embroiled in an enactment in which Ms. S would try to both translate the clinical exchange and also engage as a "cultural broker" trying to explain certain Spanish idioms and sayings as well as culture-specific understandings of the presenting problem. Although Dr. R was mindful of issues related to race, immigration, and identity, he found himself concerned that Ms. S was too identified with her client and unable to pull back into a therapeutic as opposed to supportive role. Ms. S, in turn, felt that if only Dr. R had a better sense of her and the client's cultural world, he would better understand the dilemmas emerging in treatment. Sensing the push and pull emerging between them, Dr. R reflected on how he may not have been sufficiently humble culturally, relationally, and intellectually. In disclosing his sense of the power play coming up between them, Dr. R acknowledged that the power differential inherent in the supervisory relationship was further heightened by his positionality as an older white male.

Ms. S was appreciative of Dr. R's acknowledgment of the enactment playing out between them, disclosing her fears of being negatively evaluated and having such an evaluation impact her journey as a young woman of color pursuing her degree. In addition, she worried she was doing something wrong by insisting on a cultural frame through which to examine her work with her client. This anxiety also triggered feelings of impostor syndrome and doubt about whether she belonged in this field. Exploring the stimulus value Dr. R and Ms. S had for one another opened up room in supervision for her to reflect on how *she* may not have been sufficiently culturally humble with her client, assuming a cultural congruence when in fact there were deep national, linguistic, and cultural differences not being acknowledged between them. In a related way, Dr. R reflected on how he had let his seemingly progressive bona fides blind him to the possibility he could enact a microaggressive "(white) father knows best" stance toward Ms. S as a Black Latinx woman and that he had not allowed enough space for her to feel safe articulating how much she connected with her client, *in order to then* appreciate their cultural differences. Renegotiating space for cultural similarities and differences reflected a parallel process with Ms. S and her client, empowering her to own her own cultural biases and assumptions toward her client. Dr. R and Ms. S's supervisory relationship took on a more open ambience. However, the language difference remained.

After a year in supervision, Ms. S was both appreciative of Dr. R's mentorship and guidance and also mindful that an important aspect of her training, which she deeply yearned for, was still missing. She consulted with her faculty adviser about her dilemma. They explored the pros and cons of continuing to work with Dr. R versus returning to the clinic director and seeking reassignment to a Spanish-speaking clinician (and how to process termination with Dr. R). Ms. S decided that as a third-year student she wished to deepen her training as a Spanish-speaking clinician. With her adviser's encouragement, she broached the subject with Dr. R, who shared that he had similarly wondered if they had reached a comfortable but limited phase in their work together. After exploring what an ending of their supervisory relationship meant for both of them, they agreed to begin a termination process. Ms. S returned to her clinic director, who informed her that one of the Spanish-speaking Latinx supervisors had become available for supervision. Ms. S was enthused at the opportunity to have both her Spanish-speaking consultation group and a Spanish-speaking Latinx supervisor but felt guilty about terminating with Dr. R given the journey they had been on together. In processing the termination, Ms. S and Dr. R explored how they had been able to survive a cultural rupture together in a way that supported Ms. S's growth as a clinician while acknowledging that she had professional and training needs he could not meet as a supervisor. Grateful for the opportunity to pursue her training goals, Ms. S completed her work with Dr. R.

Conclusion

Latinx people represent immigrants and descendants of immigrants from more than 20 countries and 14 territories spanning two continents from Mexico down to Argentina and Easter Island to the Caribbean. Beyond national diversity, the diversity of gender expression, sexual orientation, and racial identity and presentation among Latinx people requires an approach to psychotherapy grounded in critical and culturally humble perspectives. Although this chapter was written from a psychoanalytic perspective, the principles elucidated here are applicable across therapeutic orientations. In stressing that *there is no such thing as Latinx*, I challenge the association between Latin American identities and a "Hispanic" heritage that centers whiteness and erases Blackness and Indigeneity across lines of language, gender, and sexuality. Hence, I have stressed the importance of history, social context, and power in illustrating the complex and even contradictory experiences at the heart of the Latinx Diaspora.

Readers may experience some frustration that in this chapter I raise more questions than provide answers, presenting a picture of Latinx people in psychotherapy as a "moving target." One never quite knows what Latinx even is or means—and it should remain that way. Seeing Latinx identity as a moving target requires us to keep our minds in motion, reflecting on the various meanings, experiences, and challenges of fully understanding what Latinx is or means. That way, our patients can remain free to explore, challenge, and resist in a world that pushes and pulls them across the axes of language and race. Similarly, we should offer that same openness to our Latinx trainees. Rather than boxing them into some image of what Latinx should be like, sound like, and look like, offer Latinx trainees the relational, structural, and cultural resources to be that most elusive of things—themselves. In that vein, I offer a final set of practice recommendations for continued learning to guide clinicians in their work with Latinx patients and to guide supervisors and institutions in their task of training future Latinx psychotherapists.

- Learn about the local Latinx community or communities represented in your clinical setting, city, and state.
- Research the history of immigration and acculturation of your Latinx patient's community.
- Find ways to learn more about your patient's community, culture, and practices (especially if different from your own).
- If you are a white clinician, consider how to position yourself with regard to questions of race, immigration, and identity.
- If you are a non-Latinx clinician of color, consider how your experience of race, immigration, and identity is similar to and distinct from that of your Latinx patient.
- If you are a Latinx clinician, consider how your experience of language, race, immigration, and identity is similar to and distinct from that of your Latinx patient.

Key Points

- Cultural competence is not an endpoint in which one achieves "mastery" but rather an ongoing process of learning, humility, and self-exploration.
- Culturally humble and critical approaches to psychotherapy express curiosity toward the identities that are most salient and important to the patient and invite reflection on how these identities are structured around power.
- The term Latinx is a recent phenomenon in Latin American diasporic identity that is not endorsed by the majority of Latin American people in the United States. Nevertheless, the term evolved within social media and activist academic circles to challenge cisheteronormative and white supremacist assumptions and to make space for LGBTQ+, Indigenous, and Afro-descendant Latin Americans.
- Latin America developed notions of racial *mestizaje*, which acknowledges European, Indigenous, and African heritage so long as the "mixture" produces whiteness.
- The avoidance of Blackness and privileging of whiteness in Latin American cultures has led to a skin color paradox, in which skin color is related to material and psychosocial outcomes but not racial self-identification.
- Latin American countries hold different forms of racial hierarchy organized around white, honorary white, or collective Black caste systems, and these positions may be redefined through immigration and assimilation into U.S. racial hierarchies.
- Indigenous, Afro-descendant, and white or racially ambiguous Latinx people may develop distinct and complex relationships to language, skin color, and national identity, all of which inform the presenting problem.
- Developing clinical and theoretical tools for thinking about race, immigration, and mental health is an ongoing process of learning that should include thinking contextually about the local needs of Latinx communities and how one's own positionality informs this work.
- Given their underrepresentation in psychotherapy training programs, Latinx trainees may feel they do not belong and are not valued, which may affect their academic achievement and well-being.
- Institutional racism within training programs may be exacerbated by national and international crises related to racism, global pandemics (e.g., COVID-19), and anti-immigrant xenophobia.
- Training programs can enhance the well-being of Latinx and other trainees of color by 1) recruiting and retaining Latinx and other faculty of color; 2) developing culture- and language-based affinity groups; and 3) developing sources of funding, mentorship, and professional development.
- Supervision with Latinx trainees should balance relational, cultural, and intellectual humility within a critical decolonial lens that problematizes power relations and constructions of identity and privilege.

- Latinx trainees might operate under additional supervisory threat because of the challenges of becoming a budding clinician, the role of learner in relation to patients, and the disproportionate power relation of the supervisory relationship.
- A critical decolonial lens in supervision necessitates a complex understanding of how the inherent power relation in both patient-therapist and supervisee-supervisor dyads is dynamically nuanced by the specific intersecting identities of each member of the dyad in order to facilitate dialogue exploring and renegotiating power across difference.
- Being a Latinx trainee does not automatically mean that one 1) knows Spanish or another Latin American language or 2) is linguistically competent in delivering psychotherapy in that language. Hence, opportunities for training linguistic competence are necessary in supervision and the curriculum.
- Institutional policies, curriculum, and supervision can enhance the training and well-being of Latinx trainees through 1) supervision that enhances psychological flexibility and 2) structural and communal changes that increase the sense of belongingness and reduce incidences of racial/ethnic microaggressions.

References

Abe J: Beyond cultural competence, toward social transformation: liberation psychologies and the practice of cultural humility. J Soc Work Educ 56(4):696–707, 2020

Adames HY, Chavez-Dueñas NY, Organista KC: Skin color matters in Latino/a communities: identifying, understanding, and addressing mestizaje racial ideologies in clinical practice. Prof Psychol Res Pr 47(1):46–55, 2016

Adames HY, Chavez-Dueñas NY, Sharma S, et al: Intersectionality in psychotherapy: the experiences of an AfroLatinx queer immigrant. Psychotherapy (Chic) 55(1):73–79, 2018 29565624

Airhart-Larraga S, Lloyd-Hazlett J, Purgason LL: Resilience narratives of Hispanic counselors in the Texas Rio Grande Valley. Journal of Professional Counseling: Practice, Theory, and Research 48(1):15–30, 2021

Aranda E, Menjívar C, Donato KM: The spillover consequences of an enforcement-first US immigration regime. Am Behav Sci 58:1687–1695, 2014

Ayala MI, Ramirez C: Coloniality and Latinx college students' experiences. Equity Excell Educ 52(1):129–144, 2019

Bonilla-Silva E: From bi-racial to tri-racial: towards a new system of racial stratification in the USA. Ethn Racial Stud 27(6):931–950, 2004

Bozo J, Revels-Macalinao M, Huynh V: Examining skin color and discrimination among ethnic minority adolescents. Race Soc Probl 10(4):320–331, 2018

Branco SF, Davis M: The Minority Fellowship Program: promoting representation within counselor education and supervision. The Professional Counselor 10(4):603–614, 2020

Brown LS: Cultural competence, in Treating Complex Traumatic Stress Disorders: An Evidence-Based Guide. Edited by Courtois CA, Ford JD. New York, Guilford, 2009, pp 166–182

Capielo Rosario C, Adames HY, Chavez-Dueñas NY, et al: Acculturation profiles of central Florida Puerto Ricans: examining the influence of skin color, perceived ethnic-racial discrimination, and neighborhood ethnic-racial composition. J Cross Cult Psychol 50(4):556–576, 2019

Cardemil EV, Millán F, Aranda E: A new, more inclusive name: The Journal of Latinx Psychology. J Lat Psychol 7(1):1–5, 2019

Chirikov I, Soria KM, Horgos B, et al: Undergraduate and graduate students' mental health during the COVID-19 pandemic. Berkeley, CA, UC Berkeley SERU Consortium Reports, August 17, 2020. Available at: https://escholarship.org/content/qt80k5d5hw/qt80k5d5hw.pdf. Accessed May 31, 2021.
Crenshaw K: Mapping the margins: intersectionality, identity politics, and violence against women of color. Stanford Law Rev 43(6):1241–1299, 1990
Dalal F: Race, Colour and the Processes of Racialization: New Perspectives From Group Analysis, Psychoanalysis and Sociology. New York, Routledge, 2013
Davis DE, DeBlaere C, Owen J, et al: The multicultural orientation framework: a narrative review. Psychotherapy (Chic) 55(1):89–100, 2018 29565626
Delgado-Romero EA, De Los Santos J, Raman VS, et al: Caught in the middle: Spanish-speaking bilingual mental health counselors as language brokers. J Ment Health Couns 40(4):341–352, 2018
Denis N: War Against All Puerto Ricans: Revolution and Terror in America's Colony. New York, Nation Books, 2015
Durston A, Mannheim B (eds): Indigenous Languages, Politics, and Authority in Latin America: Historical and Ethnographic Perspectives. Notre Dame, IN, University of Notre Dame Press, 2018
Faught J, Hunter M: Latinos and the skin color paradox: skin color, national origin, and political attitudes. Sociol Q 53(4):676–701, 2012
Fisher-Borne M, Cain JM, Martin SL: From mastery to accountability: cultural humility as an alternative to cultural competence. Soc Work Educ 34(2):165–181, 2015
Flood D, Rohloff P: Indigenous languages and global health. Lancet Glob Health 6(2):e134–e135, 2018 29389530
Frandsen C, Smith TB, Griner D, et al: Beyond English only: addressing language interpretation in professional psychology training. Train Educ Prof Psychol 13(1):64–71, 2019
Garcia IM: White But Not Equal: Mexican Americans, Jury Discrimination, and the Supreme Court. Tucson, University of Arizona Press, 2009
Garcia JA, Sanchez GR, Sanchez-Youngman S, et al: Race as lived experience: the impact of multi-dimensional measures of race/ethnicity on the self-reported health status of Latinos. Du Bois Rev 12(2):349–373, 2015 26681972
Gaztambide DJ: Reconsidering culture, attachment, and inequality in the treatment of a Puerto Rican migrant: toward structural competence in psychotherapy. J Clin Psychol 75(11):2022–2033, 2019a 31506935
Gaztambide DJ: A People's History of Psychoanalysis: From Freud to Liberation Psychology. New York, Lexington Books, 2019b
Godreau IP: Scripts of Blackness: Race, Cultural Nationalism, and U.S. Colonialism in Puerto Rico. Champaign, University of Illinois Press, 2015
Hordge-Freeman E, Loblack A: "Cops only see the brown skin, they could care less where it originated": Afro-Latinx perceptions of the #BlackLivesMatter movement. Sociol Perspect 64(4):518–535, 2020
Horne G: The Dawning of the Apocalypse: The Roots of Slavery, White Supremacy, Settler Colonialism, and Capitalism in the Long Sixteenth Century. New York, Monthly Review Press, 2020
Jones HA, Perrin PB, Heller MB, et al: Black psychology graduate students' lives matter: using informal mentoring to create an inclusive climate amidst national race-related events. Prof Psychol Res Pr 49(1):75–82, 2018
Limas I: Latinx graduate students' experiences. Long Beach, California State University, 2019
Lloréns H: Identity practices: racial passing, gender, and racial purity in Puerto Rico. Afro-Hispanic Review 37(1):29–47, 2018
Lucana S, Elfers J: Sacred medicine: indigenous healing and mental health. Qual Rep 25(12):4482–4495, 2020
Martín-Baró I: Writings for a Liberation Psychology. Edited by Aron A, Corne S. Cambridge, MA, Harvard University Press, 1994
Miller AN, Orsillo SM: Values, acceptance, and belongingess in graduate school: perspectives from underrepresented minority students. J Contextual Behav Sci 15:197–206, 2020

Miller MG: Rise and Fall of the Cosmic Race: The Cult of Mestizaje in Latin America. Austin, University of Texas Press, 2009

Moncayo R: Cultural diversity and the cultural and epistemological structure of psychoanalysis: implications for psychotherapy with Latinos and other minorities. Psychoanal Psychol 15(2):262–286, 1998

Montero-Hernandez V, Drouin S: The journey into a new me: narratives of self-development and community revitalization among first-generation, Latinx, adult graduate students. Journal of Adult and Continuing Education, May 2020. Available at: https://firstgen.naspa.org/scholarly-article/the-journey-into-a-new-me-narratives-of-self-development-and-community-revitalization-among-first-generation-latinx-adult-graduate-students. Accessed May 31, 2021.

Moon SH, Sandage SJ: Cultural humility for people of color: critique of current theory and practice. J Psychol Theol 47(2):76–86, 2019

Morales E: LatinX: The New Force in American Politics and Culture. New York, Verso, 2019

Mosher DK, Hook JN, Captari LE, et al: Cultural humility: a therapeutic framework for engaging diverse clients. Pract Innov (Wash D C) 2(4):221–233, 2017

Moya J: América Latina y los flujos transatlánticos: una categoría histórica desde una perspectiva global, in Vaivenes del Destino: Inmigrantes Europeos y Latinoamericanos en los Espacios Atlánticos. Edited by Azcue CN, Prado y Arrigo Amadori GH. Madrid, Spain, Ediciones Polifemo, 2014, pp 21–30

Moya J: Migration and the historical formation of Latin America in a global perspective. Sociologias 20(49):24–68, 2018

Muro JA, Martinez LM: Is love color-blind? Racial blind spots and Latinas' romantic relationships. Sociol Race Ethn (Thousand Oaks) 4(4):527–540, 2018

Nadathur S: Therapeutic and cultural factors that enhance therapy outcomes with Latino clients: an exploration of the perceptions of Hispanic clinicians (Order No 13427273). Pro-Quest Dissertations and Theses Global (2281784718), 2019

National Science Foundation: 2017 doctorate recipients from U.S. universities. Alexandria, VA, National Science Foundation, 2017. Available at: https://ncses.nsf.gov/pubs/nsf19301/report. Accessed May 31, 2021.

Noe-Bustamante L, Mora L, Lopez MH: About one-in-four U.S. Hispanics have heard of Latinx, but just 3% use it. Washington, DC, Pew Research Center, 2020

Pedersen D: Reframing political violence and mental health outcomes: outlining a research and action agenda for Latin America and the Caribbean region. Cien Saude Colet 11(2):293–302, 2006

Perez RJ, Robbins CK, Harris L Jr, Montgomery C: Exploring graduate students' socialization to equity, diversity, and inclusion. J Divers High Educ 13(2):133–145, 2020

Perreira KM, Telles EE: The color of health: skin color, ethnoracial classification, and discrimination in the health of Latin Americans. Soc Sci Med 116:241–250, 2014 24957692

Ramírez Stege AM, Chin MY, Graham SR: A critical postcolonial and resilience-based framework of supervision in action. Train Educ Prof Psychol 14(4):316–323, 2020

Rodríguez-Silva I: Silencing Race: Disentangling Blackness, Colonialism, and National Identities in Puerto Rico. New York, Springer, 2012

Salinas C Jr: The complexity of the "x" in Latinx: how Latinx/a/o students relate to, identify with, and understand the term Latinx. J Hispanic High Educ 19(2):149–168, 2020

Salinas C Jr, Lozano A: Mapping and recontextualizing the evolution of the term Latinx: an environmental scanning in higher education. Journal of Latinos and Education 18(4):302–315, 2019

Silva GM, Saldivar E: Comparing ideologies of racial mixing in Latin America: Brazil and Mexico. Sociologia and Antropologia 8(2):427–456, 2018

Soto Vega K, Chávez KR: Latinx rhetoric and intersectionality in racial rhetorical criticism. Communication and Critical/Cultural Studies 15(4):319–325, 2018

Sue DW: Multidimensional facets of cultural competence. Couns Psychol 29(6):790–821, 2001

Sue S: Cultural competency: from philosophy to research and practice. J Community Psychol 34(2):237–245, 2006

Tascon S, Gatwiri K: Towards cultural humility: theorising cultural competence as institutionalised whiteness. Social Work and Policy Studies: Social Justice, Practice, and Theory 3(1):1–16, 2020

Trujillo-Pagán N: Crossed out by LatinX: gender neutrality and genderblind sexism. Lat Stud 16(3):396–406, 2018

Twemlow SW, Fonagy P, Sacco FC: A developmental approach to mentalizing communities I: a model for social change. Bull Menninger Clin 69(4):265–281, 2005 16370789

Valencia-Garcia D, Montoya H: Lost in translation: training issues for bilingual students in health service psychology. Train Educ Prof Psychol 12(3):142–148, 2018

Vargas N: Ideological whitening: does skintone shape colour-blind ideology adherence for Latina/os? Ethn Racial Stud 41(14):2407–2425, 2018

Viego A: Dead Subjects: Toward a Politics of Loss in Latino Studies. Durham, NC, Duke University Press, 2007

Wade P: Degrees of Mixture, Degrees of Freedom: Genomics, Multiculturalism, and Race in Latin America. Durham, NC, Duke University Press, 2017

Watkins CE, Mosher DK: Psychotherapy trainee humility and its impact: conceptual and practical considerations. J Contemp Psychother 50(3):187–195, 2020

Wilderson FB III: Red, White, and Black: Cinema and the Structure of U.S. Antagonisms. Durham, NC, Duke University Press, 2010

Winnicott DW: The Maturational Processes and the Facilitating Environment: Studies in the Theory of Emotional Development (1965). New York, Routledge, 2018

CHAPTER 26

How Our Mind Becomes Racialized

Implications for the Therapeutic Encounter

Beverly J. Stoute, M.D.

No one is born hating another person because of the color of his skin or his background or his religion.

—Nelson Mandela

Race, no matter how hard we consciously fight the reality, is a bedrock descriptor and hierarchical organizer of difference in American society. A dual racial reality in the United States creates dual subjectivities—for Black and for white—and this is foundational. Although race is a biological fiction, it endures as a social construct that defines identity and helps create the social, political, and cultural worlds within which we live. Specific to our discussion here, health care practice and delivery are affected on all levels by racial discrimination. Racism has an effect on people as adults, but the influence begins even before birth. Accumulated interpersonal experience with racism causes chronic stress in Black women, with low birth weights and increased infant mortality for their children (Collins et al. 2004). The damaging health consequences of discrimination and related restrictions on diagnosis and treatment are the subject of current research, but that research has rarely been integrated into the education of mental health clinicians. Signs of change can be found, but how unconscious scripts of the personal, the developmental, the emotional, the cultural, and the historical are integrated will direct how this change plays out on the health care stage.

Elucidating how derivatives of racism and oppression are deeply buried in the collective cultural unconscious of the American psyche would require an exhaustive review of history that is beyond the scope of this chapter. Joel Kovel (1974), in *White Racism: A Psychohistory*, was one of the first American psychoanalysts to discuss racism from a psychohistorical perspective and to formulate that fantasies about race and derogatory images of Blackness are deeply embedded in American collective cultural unconscious. Acknowledging that unconscious racism influences the process of racial-ethnic socialization in American society is vital. How is the concept of self and Other shaped in a child's mind, Black or white, under the influence of a racist society? Are there differentiating nodal points in development for racial-ethnic socialization crucial to developing an ability to engage patients in conversations about race, class, privilege, and racism?

As race awareness evolves from childhood through adolescence into adulthood, the defining impact of the culturally imposed trauma of racism on development for the patient and therapist alike has far-reaching latent and manifest intrapsychic implications. Our individual and group subjectivities become racialized, bringing to bear a sociocultural surround that exerts a powerful impact on the intrapsychic world of the individual. That race is given such defining valence in American society and operates on a structural level precludes our awareness of the ways in which we are socialized additively and perhaps discontinuously along other dimensions such that race, ethnicity, gender, culture, religion, and socioeconomic positioning interrelate. These correlates of identity overlap at the level of *lived experience*, which William Cross postulates according to what he terms a racial-ethnic-cultural identity model that speaks to self-concept as including an individual domain (personal identity) and a reference group orientation (group identity) (Cross 1991; Cross and Cross 2008). How this plays out in the dyadic arena can present rich entry points for psychotherapeutic exploration.

A fundamental understanding of *racial-ethnic socialization* and racial learning, with attention to racial identity formation and the vicissitudes of racial trauma across the developmental spectrum, is necessary, especially when treating children and adults of color. This involves understanding the subtle ways that racism is systemically anchored in our day-to-day experience in American society. Whether one is a person of color or a member of the dominant white culture, race defines the psychosocial position from which we navigate these sociocultural experiences. Large-scale ethnographic studies in the past two decades highlight that the transmission of cultural values to children is a complex interactive process. Rather than promoting the false notion that we can "know" others by labeling their cultural background or that we can be "competent" in other cultures by taking a course, the more relevant question is how do we create a working model of thinking about and being curious about the multidimensional variables involved in constructing racial-ethnic-cultural identities of our individual self and for people we consider to be Other?

Elucidating unconscious racialized attitudes in the therapeutic process presents complex challenges. A developmental perspective is illuminating. Many questions arise. Are there universal ways children come to recognize racial difference, and what developmental experiences have an impact on how racial attitudes evolved in the course of development? For patient and therapist alike, in what ways do unconsciously held racialized attitudes unfold in the psychotherapeutic process on the basis of developmental history? Is racial identity germane to the development of the self, and how does racial trauma affect development? How can the white-identified or dominant culture therapist develop an awareness of the ways race and racism emerge in the therapeutic encounter? Are there transgenerational aspects of the transmission of trauma in families of color and societal attitudes toward children of color of relevant psychotherapeutic import? Although the clinical task is one of interrogating individual subjectivity, understanding racial-ethnic socialization in a multicultural society requires an orientation to the social, cultural, and historical surround. The generalizations made in this chapter with respect to development do not preclude the individual variations that can exist. Although in this chapter I focus on the experience of African Americans, the influence of race, including fantasies about race, is intertwined in psychotherapy for all, including white-identified patients and patients of multicultural backgrounds, as the case vignettes attest.

How Race Awareness and Racialized Attitudes Emerge Across Development

Integrating psychoanalytic theory on the dynamics of unconscious functioning with a developmental understanding of the processes of racial socialization as racial learning emerges in childhood sheds light on how we construct the internal working model that guides us as we evolve from childhood through adolescence into adulthood. Racial-ethnic socialization and racial learning for all children occur in tandem with the unfolding of cognitive capacities to recognize and categorize sameness and difference.

As previously outlined and discussed, to understand how we think about racial difference necessitates understanding the development of race awareness (Stoute 2019). This chapter is an expansion of "Racial Socialization and Thwarted Mentalization: Psychoanalytic Reflections From the Lived Experience of James Baldwin's America," copyright ©2019 Johns Hopkins University Press, which will be quoted extensively with permission. This article first appeared in *American Imago*, Volume 76, Issue 3, Fall 2019, pages 335–337. Drawing on and expanding this previously published work, I incorporate data that demonstrate that awareness of and curiosity about racial difference begin early and occur spontaneously. At age 3 months, infants show a gaze preference for same-race faces, and by age 6 months they recognize racial difference (Katz 1976, 1981). Quintana (2008) asserts from his research that "[r]acial status is one of the first social categories young children learn, probably preceded only by learning to differentiate by sex" (p. 16). The child's developmental perspective on race emerges without the benefit of direct socialization during early childhood.

Children recognize racial difference and are curious about it. As I have demonstrated in prior work (Stoute 2019) through an illuminating series of clinical examples, for children, racial difference arouses curiosity. Kenneth and Mamie Clark's landmark work (Clark 1953; Clark and Clark 1947), which laid the foundation of the data reviewed in 1954 by the U.S. Supreme Court in *Brown v. Board of Education of Topeka* (347 U.S. 483), confirmed these early findings. When given a choice of dolls and asked, "Which is most like you?" 37% of children responded accurately in terms of race at age 3, and 87% of children responded accurately by age 7. As Kenneth Clark put it, "Learning about race and racial differences, learning one's own racial identity, learning which race is preferred and which is rejected—all these are assimilated by the child as part of the total pattern of ideas he acquires about himself" (Clark 1953, p. 23). Clark confirmed that children perceive and internalize the racialized symbols of our society—in his era, segregated schools—and these social symbols demonstrably shape children's view of themselves in relation to others, be they Black or white (Clark 1963). By age 3 years, children develop a sense of "outsiders": people who are different from them (Fishbein 1992, 2002). Mary Ellen Goodman's (1952) classic research on *Race Awareness in Children* demonstrated that preschool-age children ages 3 and 4 years were clearly aware of race—making the connection to appearance and color but not yet to the concept of race as a social construct (Stoute 2019). Both Goodman and Clark demonstrated that children as young as age 4 showed a preference for white skin as superior to Black. In fact, 25% of children sampled in Goodman's study expressed strong entrenched race-related values by age 4.

More recently, Van Ausdale and Feagin (2001), focusing on children's perception of race and ethnicity, reported examples of how children as young as age 3 have an awareness of themselves and others in racial terms and can internalize racist attitudes from parents and the surrounding culture. A notable example was that of a 3-year-old who insisted during naptime in preschool, "I can't sleep next to a n-----" and explained that "n------ are stinky," while her onlooking teacher made no intervention (Van Ausdale and Feagin 2001). (Please note that this derogatory and offensive word is reprinted to be true to the original quotation to demonstrate the extent to which children internalize and imitate adult role models.) Hirschfeld's (2008) research findings dispelled the myth of childhood innocence regarding racial bias, showing that "Three-year-olds generally attribute positive properties to members of the majority race, whereas five-year-olds not only attribute positive properties to majority race, but, by then, also negative properties to minority race" (p. 39).

Stereotypical information about racial groups is also internalized at a surprisingly early age, whether the child becomes the perpetrator or victim of racial prejudice. White children as early as age 3–4 years, for example, express clear preferences for their own racial group (Aboud 2008; Williams and Steele 2019), a finding not observed with Black children (Newheiser and Olson 2012). In his pioneering work *Race Attitudes in Children*, Bruno Lasker revealed that the acquisition of prejudiced attitudes begins in the preschool years and, recent studies confirm, increases with advancing age (Lasker 1929; Skinner and Meltzoff 2019). By age 5 years, children internalize the prejudiced attitudes of parents and teachers (Lasker 1929). Observational studies (e.g., Jernigan and Daniel 2011) have demonstrated that characteristics such as darker skin color and large size can lead to social isolation. In another study, it was notable that "although no child of color used racial epithets to control White children, the same could not be said for White children" (Van Ausdale and Feagin 2001, p. 3).

Because racialized attitudes are clearly evident in preschool- and elementary school–age white children, children of color are exposed to devaluing and toxic messages early. Black children at this developmental juncture often cannot make sense of discriminatory experiences. Children may know, for example, that the teacher treats them in a negative way but may not understand why. Black children internalize these negative racialized experiences, assuming something is wrong with them, not with the teacher. For white children, curiosity about racial difference is thwarted, and being in a society in which the background culture delivers damaging and devaluing messages about Blackness leads to inhibition and distortion, perhaps to negative ideas about "those" people and to a thwarting of interactive curiosity about difference, especially if the child lives in a racially homogeneous environment where experience with people of different cultural backgrounds is limited.

As preschool children evolve from what Piaget termed preoperational thinking (ages 2–7 years) to the stage of concrete operations (ages 7–11 years), the cognitive task of recognizing categories clearly lays the foundation for the capacity to identify the defining attributes of group membership—and later consolidating one's own racial identity in relation to others (Derman-Sparks et al. 1980; Ginsburg and Opper 1979). "As their cognitive development advances, children rely less on appearance and more on the ability to categorize" (Stoute 2019, p. 337). Children internalize the negative social valuation of racial groups from parental cues. By age 7, children can define group preferences and group affiliation and come to appreciate that they are part of a group and that ethnic affiliation is constant (Derman-Sparks et al. 1980; Lieberman et al. 2017). Therefore, how we become aware of sameness and difference, create categories of sameness and difference, and integrate those experiences contributes to our evolving view of self and of others. This affects later functioning in interpersonal relationships.

From early childhood, children are socialized to beliefs, values, and images that reinforce the dominance of the majority white cultural superiority and to the stereotypes and distortions of Black and white. Environmental cues about color are clearly communicated to children, who use them to internalize how Blackness is viewed and thereby internalize the racism of the surrounding culture (Clark 1963; Stoute 2019). Amenable adults can educate young children and dispel distorted and racist attitudes that arise from discriminatory remarks according to the child's cognitive stage by opening up conversations with children even in the school-age years. White teachers and white parents reinforce negative racial attitudes when they minimize and dismiss the meaning of racialized interactions and insist that (white) children are too young to understand the negative meaning of their statements or behavior. When these valuable opportunities are missed, the negative behaviors often go unchecked.

Cross's (1983) work is of particular importance. He showed how Black mothers rear their children from early on to be *biculturally competent* (i.e., aware and comfortable with people of different cultures and practices), whereas white mothers, although not overtly racist, do not. White children, who had limited awareness of and contact with people from different cultural backgrounds, relied more on TV as their primary source of images about people of color and develop what Cross termed a monoracial group orientation. White children, and later white adults, develop social networks with a "white-oriented monoracial reference group orientation," whereas Black children, and later Black adults, develop social networks with a "biracial reference group orientation" or bicultural competence. This gives the latter an advantage when functioning in racially heterogeneous environments.

An adaptive capacity to function across racial social groups has been theorized to require an additional functional component termed *code switching*, which "enhances the ease with which the child of color navigates mainstream academic and social environments" (for a definition of code switching, see Cross and Cross 2008, pp. 156–157).

An intriguing study (Strauss and Cross 2005) described five *identity competencies* that interact in interrelated ways to bolster the adaptive social and academic functioning for children of marginalized identities:

> (1) *buffering*—the transaction of encounters with racism and discrimination; (2) *code switching*—the ability to move in and out of mainstream situations, or stated in another way, move back and forth from one's primary racial-ethnic culture; (3) *bridging*—the desire and competencies related to establishing and sustaining close friendships across racial and cultural divides; (4) *bonding*—attachment to the group; and (5) *individuality*—the transaction of both PI [personal identity] and related interests the person cherished beyond the purview of race and minority culture. (Strauss and Cross 2005, p. 154)

Rather than focusing only on the traumatic aspects, many clinicians and researchers now point to the adaptive tools that make children and adolescents successful in navigating multicultural environments.

Middle childhood represents a developmental fork in the road. Family still plays an important role, but peer relationships grow in importance. In Black families, socialization on the importance of racial bias and discrimination continues. In her riveting study *White Kids: Growing Up With Privilege in a Racially Divided America*, Hagerman (2018) pointed to middle childhood as a pivotal time for education around issues of race and racial socialization for white upper-middle-class children and studied in depth the way that parental attitudes and cultural images shape white children as they acquire prejudiced attitudes about people of color and are inducted into the meaning of the power and privilege of whiteness. The literature on the racial socialization of white children in this area is meager. Hagerman astutely observed that "studies of racial socialization assumed that people of color will encounter racism but did not fully examine the socialization processes among Whites that lead them to discriminate," and "the private world of white families should be studied critically as racialized places where ideas about race get reproduced and reworked by children with racial privilege" (Hagerman 2018, p. 16). As children look more to peer relationships, white families who, at this juncture, choose private schools that are racially and socioeconomically homogeneous are implicitly sentencing their children to environments that limit cross-cultural exposure and foster a white-centered view of Others.

Learned silence on race for white dominant culture children also begins early and is promoted by the culture. This culturally sanctioned learned silence becomes internalized as an unconscious roadblock that for some white therapists later constricts the ability to detect how racism can infiltrate the therapeutic encounter. Research findings (Apfelbaum et al. 2010; Gelman 2003) suggest that non-Black children are more likely to identify and recognize racial discrimination if they have been exposed to "[d]iversity valuing messaging [as opposed to color-blind messages, especially if the messages are] combined with conversations that serve to challenge children's stereotypes and essential thinking will help to decrease implicit racial biases" (Williams and Steele 2019, p. 15). Active intervention is necessary in the form of direct attention to interpretation and discussion of social messaging to interrupt these culturally promoted defensive attitudes that become internalized obstacles later in adulthood.

By adolescence, social factors, including peer influences, shape and consolidate prejudiced thinking as group affiliations are used as a source of identification (the "we") or as an object of projection (the "them"), and individual ethnic identity and the sense of shared ethnic group identity are consolidated (Stoute 2019). Racial identity and in-group and out-group attitudes coalesce in late adolescence, but the process of synthesis and consolidation is dynamic and interactive as the adolescent develops cognitively and emotionally encounters new experiences with peers and forges new relationships independent of parents (Stoute 2019). For adolescents, as the capacity for abstract reasoning matures, they grasp that racial-ethnic designations can affect life choices and social experiences. Further, as their personal identity merges with a group identity, they begin to recognize that group identifications have implications for the future. Umaña-Taylor et al. (2014) refer to this time as a period of *exploration or search* in racial-ethnic identity consolidation. Eventually, this sense of shared ethnic group identity evolves from adolescence into adulthood and becomes invested and transformed into a sense of ethnic and national identity, which creates an individual's *inner working model* or reference point (Volkan 2013).

In covert ways, therefore, from early on, children internalize a socially constructed devaluation of Blackness that has differential consequences depending on one's racial-ethnic-social positioning and identification. Whether one is Black or white, one's subjectivity is profoundly affected by the attitudes and experiences that racialize our thinking in the course of development. Regardless of social class, it is a pervasive aspect of Black subjectivity from which many African Americans operate that they feel that race stratifies how they are viewed and treated and whether they feel under threat and that they must contend with the daily assault of living in a racist society. For whites, especially if they grow up in a homogeneous environment, race does not restrict experience or even seem salient to day-to-day experience; race is not named or discussed. Here, *salience* specifically refers to the extent to which one's ethnicity or race is relevant to one's self-concept in a particular situation; importantly, salience is determined by the interface of the context of the situation and the individual's tendency to define oneself in terms of ethnicity and/or race (Sellers et al. 1998).

As we grow up, a racialized subjectivity subtly develops for Blacks and whites. It collides in school, on the playground, in the workplace, on TV, and in our social circles. As clinicians, we are not exempt. Sometimes we "know" how our experiences growing up have influenced the reference point that is our internal working model for measuring and evaluating sameness and difference. Sometimes we find out only when confronted with difference—often in our consultation rooms.

Outlining the developmental trajectory of how race awareness emerges and racial learning occurs is relevant for the clinician in working with children, adolescents, and adults because racialized attitudes, although unnamed, actively operate in psychic life from early on. If recognized and understood, racial themes can be fertile entry points in psychotherapy regardless of the racial-ethnic composition of the dyad. Unfortunately, many clinicians find themselves drawn into racial scripts in interracial and intercultural dyads without the tools with which to navigate. A colliding of dual racial subjectivities plays out in the therapeutic encounter, complicated by a culturally sanctioned disavowal of racial narratives, supported by culturally accepted, often racist, attitudes that are perpetuated in families of the dominant white culture that make mentalization of the experiences of people of color and attention to the repetitions in the transference so difficult to name.

Parental Socialization on Bias and Discrimination Is Paramount for African American Children

Apartheid-like housing discrimination practices have almost ensured that many American neighborhoods and schools are still largely segregated. As a consequence, zip code and race are interacting and mutually enforcing variables of discrimination. Parental attitudes and socializing environments such as schools are the dominant influences for children: where children live and attend school can be determinative. The impact on racial-ethnic socialization is powerful. Although the differential effects vary, all children are impacted. Greater understanding of this process provides an opportunity for us as clinicians, educators, parents, and racially conscious citizens to clarify how to change racial attitudes in our world.

As children get older, parents' sensitivity to their children's developmental abilities to understand racism can be invaluable. Black parents more often prioritize racial learning, whereas white parents more often do not. Black children come to recognize and understand the dangers of racially imposed stereotyping to which they are subject and must learn how to cope with toxic racialized experiences to which they are often exposed in school environments and through media images. Absorbing the traumatic assault of discriminatory experiences affects health and, later, self-image.

African American parents, especially mothers, who themselves have a strong sense of ethnic pride and who teach their children to understand and to cope with discrimination, can mitigate the impact of racial trauma. In studies of biracial children, the mother was more likely to discuss issues of racial identity and racism if she were Black (Rollins and Hunter 2013). Interestingly enough, Bowman and Howard (1985) reported that African American adolescents "who received messages about racial barriers and who were cautioned about interracial contact had higher grades" (p. 139). Further, positive minority socialization, along with racial identity, promoted resiliency (Miller 1999). For African American parents, the preparation for confronting bias and discrimination is an anxiety-filled lifelong process that often accelerates during these adolescent years. The often-normative adolescent risk taking is met often with significant parental anxiety for Black parents who know the societal consequences for Black children of being seen as older than their actual age.

Developmental theorizing in the past had been woefully inadequate in its attention to the traumatic impact of racism, or as Adams (2021, p. 60) names it, "how the developmentally normal enactments of Black youth are mediated by an often-hostile culture." Adams (2021) points out further that

> [f]or Black youth, age-typical aggression, sexuality and regressive enactments can be very limiting to self-development or be life threatening.... What is often projected into them [by the larger society] are disavowed feelings of carnality and unbounded violence with them being viewed as either children who must be constrained, or adults who must be confronted and subdued." (p. 60)

Ava DuVernay's miniseries commentary *When They See Us*, documenting the racial injustice of the Central Park 5, including Donald Trump's full-page ad calling for the death penalty, documents a poignant contemporary example of the extreme degree to which this racial fantasy of perceived threat dictates a dangerous reality for African American youth. The additional trauma of enduring discriminatory remarks and gestures, especially in school environments, affects the physical and mental health for children and adults of color; latency-age children are especially vulnerable because the degree of traumatic assault can be correlated with depressive and somatic symptoms (Li et al. 2017). One telling longitudinal study found that the 92% of 714 African American children ages 10 or younger followed over 5 years who evidenced conduct and depressive symptoms had experienced repeated episodes of racial discrimination in elementary school (Brody et al. 2006). Studies confirm these findings across ethnic groups for Latinx, Asian American, Caribbean American, and immigrant children (Gee et al. 2009; Liu and Lau 2013; Pachter et al. 2010; Stevens et al. 2020; Sue et al. 2009). Although preparation for racial bias proves helpful in the long term, in the short term, increased awareness of racism is correlated with anxiety and depressive symptoms (Iwamoto and Liu 2010; Seaton 2009), suggesting that this awareness might be overwhelming or challenging for the child or adolescent to metabolize.

Crucial to their development, Black adolescents, especially males, must incorporate the additional burden of legal socialization at an earlier age, and media attention to the murder of African American men, most notably George Floyd in May 2020 during the COVID-19 (coronavirus SARS-CoV-2 disease) pandemic, has elevated "the talk" Black parents have with their children into mainstream discourse. *Legal socialization* is defined as "the process by which individuals come to understand and appreciate the law, the institutions that create those laws, and the people who enforce those laws" (Henning 2017, p. 63). It occurs at a younger age for Black males, especially those who live in urban environments, where there is a significant police presence (Goff et al. 2014; Henning 2017)—a factor of significance impacting parental socialization strategy because of concerns about safety (Stoute 2019; Vaughans 2016; Vaughans and Harris 2016; Vaughans and Spielberg 2014). This complicates the normal adolescent risk taking for children of color, who navigate an often-hostile culture where the consequences can be fatal. For example, was Trayvon Martin, an African American adolescent walking home from the store carrying a bag of Skittles and a soda, a normal teenage boy anticipating the NBA All-Star game while talking to his girlfriend on his cell phone or a dangerous threat that necessitated lethal force, as George Zimmerman contended?

Legal socialization occurs at an earlier age for African American children because understanding the related cautions and prohibitions on behavior is essential to survival. Studies show that police officers view Black children as older—up to 5 years older than white children—and less innocent, and this unconscious racial profiling guides overt behavior, with dire consequences (Goff et al. 2014). Singletary (2020), in his penetrating discussion "Trauma and Black Male Adolescents: A Critical Link," pointed out that adolescence must be negotiated in a safe environment if the usual experimental risk-taking is to occur without adverse result, but the profound effect of negotiating in a racially hostile culture is rarely talked about. As he stated, "No other racial group in America endures more hardships than Black male adolescents." They "experience unique external stressors, including but not limited to police brutality, racism, neglect, abuse, violence, poverty, and academic failure" (Singletary 2020, p. 19) magnified if compounded by lower socioeconomic status or insufficient family emotional support. Singletary made the shattering statement that "Black males in urban areas experience levels of violence and death that are similar to those in active war zones" and underscored the neurobiological insult to the developing brain for children and adolescents exposed to trauma, including racial trauma, during childhood (Bell and Jenkins 1993; Smith and Patton 2016).

Although it is essential for clinicians to understand the developmental impact of racial trauma if they are to understand Black patients' racial identity formation and interpersonal functioning, the topic of racial trauma is rarely discussed in courses on development or in clinical training programs. The day-to-day school environment is a minefield of racialized experiences, whether or not the school is diverse. Overwhelming data reveal that educators often perpetuate negative stereotypes of Black children (Shim and Vinson 2021; Vaughans and Spielberg 2014), affecting academic performance and creating structural inequities that track more Black children into special education than toward enriching college preparatory curricula.

Positive Racial Identifications as a Mitigating Fact in Racial Trauma

Fundamental to racial-ethnic socialization is the reality that one understand that school environments, important places of socialization and learning, often perpetuate racially derogatory stereotypes about children of color. Black youth who have solid positive racial and ethnic identifications fare better when they encounter bias and racism in the world, especially if they have had family support, education, and preparation. Children and adolescents who take pride in their race and ethnicity have higher self-esteem, perform better academically (Hughes et al. 2009), and take greater pride in their academic ability (Murry et al. 2009). This applies cross-culturally, with studies demonstrating the findings not only for African American groups but also with Latinx groups (Altschul et al. 2006) and Asian American groups (Iwamoto and Liu 2010). One study of first and second graders reported that the degree of self-esteem in one's racial identity was a "strong and significant predictor of reading and listening comprehension" (Smith et al. 2009, p. 153). For urban Black children whose families have fewer resources or whose parents may be less able to provide support, the consequences of low self-esteem are more severe. Caught up in a culture and system responding to negative stereotypes of Black children and youth, they often get less support and encouragement from educators, become less engaged, and fall further behind academically and socially.

Racial Trauma as Foundational

Roberts and Rollins (2020) catalogued the innovative biosocial measures of racism that have made it possible to study the health effects of stigma and discrimination. Enduring racism and modulating its intrapsychic load exact a biological toll. African Americans living in states with high levels of structural racism, for example, have a higher incidence of myocardial infarction than those living in states with low levels of structural racism (Lukachko et al. 2014). Perceived discrimination against African American youth (ages 10–15) and adults affects health status from a young age and is correlated with elevated blood pressure (Boen 2019; Goosby et al. 2015; Lewis et al. 2010) and mood and anxiety symptoms across the developmental cycle.

On presentation for treatment, adult patients who have endured racially traumatic experiences endorse an array of symptoms, including depression, suicidality, anxiety, paranoia, phobic reactions, and somatic problems (Hart 2019, in press). These patterns and symptoms, uncovered when adults come into treatment, are not just acute reactions but the posttraumatic result of long-standing and repeated exposure to discriminatory experiences throughout development. For children and adolescents, the psychic consequences manifest similarly in somatic symptoms, depressive symptoms, anxiety, behavioral problems, and posttraumatic symptoms and reactions (Brody et al. 2006). The way in which race, ethnicity, culture, and oppression can be fused in the formation of identity must be analyzed with greater sophistication and nuance if we are to understand the development of racialized attitudes and racial identity over the life cycle.

How children of color manage racial trauma has now received growing attention in the literature. Helms's (1984) and Carter et al.'s (2013) race-based trauma models facilitated a research methodology designed to study the trauma caused by racism in children of color. Carter (2007) applied Carlson's (1997) earlier model of traumatic stress to the study of racial encounters and, integrating the PTSD literature, argued that the stress of memorable race encounters creates emotional pain and trauma, resulting in a cluster of emotional symptoms. Carter et al. (2013) then created an assessment and research tool to characterize this traumatic impact. The tool proved revolutionary to researchers studying discrimination.

During the past two decades, researchers have been developing the methodologies and theory needed to study the racial trauma and racial-ethnic socialization of African American youth. Despite clear data on the damaging effects of racial trauma, the DSM-5 diagnostic criteria for posttraumatic stress disorder define psychological trauma by responses to physical injury, naming "actual or threatened death, serious injury, or sexual violence" (American Psychiatric Association 2013, p. 271) as allowable traumatic causes but excluding the trauma of racism and discrimination. Many researchers interpret this exclusion as a resistance of privilege, an unwillingness to accept the clear correlation documented between racial trauma and posttraumatic reactions (Bryant-Davis and Ocampo 2006).

In their masterful literature review, Jernigan and Daniel (2011) provided a history of our conceptualization of racial trauma. In a now widely accepted conclusion, they stated that racism is a "reality based repetitive trauma" (Daniel 2000; Jernigan et al. 2011, p. 126). Black children are both "observers and victims" and, unfortunately, commonly experience discrimination on individual and systemic levels in their communities and schools. A recent study documented that Black teenagers experience on average five discriminatory encounters per day (English et al. 2020). In a powerful work, Hardy (2013) examined how inner-city Black youth manage racism without having yet achieved the ego resources and developmental strategies to cope with the assault. Pathological symptomatic sequelae include, but are not limited to, mood disorders; acting-out behaviors; suicidal thinking; substance use; and, into adulthood, posttraumatic symptoms and fractured interpersonal functioning (Hardy 2013, 2019; Hart 2019). As Hardy (2013) put it, "Racial oppression is a traumatic form of interpersonal violence which can lacerate the spirit, scar the soul, and puncture the psyche" (p. 24).

The traumatic legacy that African Americans endure permeates the process of therapeutic engagement and necessitates an artful negotiation of the cultural paranoia or cultural mistrust that is an impediment to trust. Shreve (in press) defines cultural mistrust as "a mitigated version of 'healthy cultural paranoia,'" which Grier and Cobbs (1968) define as the conviction shared among many African Americans that "every white [person] is a potential enemy unless proved otherwise and every social system is set against [them] unless [they] personally find out differently" (p. 149). As Harriet Washington (2006) documented in her scholarly work *Medical Apartheid: The Dark History of Medical Experimentation on Black Americans From Colonial Times to the Present*, this normative cultural paranoia has its roots in a long-standing history of discrimination and abuse toward Black, Indigenous, and People of Color (BIPOC) communities.

Understanding the impact of cultural mistrust on the therapeutic process can allow the therapist to recognize the traumatic residue of racism expressed in the form of a racialized transference. Studies looking at the detrimental health impact of discrimination and related stressors across cultures have revealed similar findings. For example, Latinx (Sibrava et al. 2019), Native American (Skewes and Blume 2019), and Asian American (Gee et al. 2009; Iwamoto and Liu 2010) populations studied all showed evidence of posttraumatic stress symptoms that affected health status to a significant degree. These findings point to the need for clinician attention to the impact of discriminatory experiences endured for all patients of color whether the marker of difference is framed in terms of race, ethnicity, culture, language, or immigration status.

In their comprehensive must-read review of this topic, "Racial Trauma in the Lives of Black Children and Adolescents: Challenges and Clinical Implications," Jernigan and Daniel (2011) make crucial points. "Black children and adolescents," they emphasize, "are particularly vulnerable to racial trauma because they may not have yet developed a sophisticated cognitive understanding or the affective language with which to express ongoing effects of racism" (p. 126). Early in development, therefore, the child of color internalizes racist aggressions into a negative self-concept. Later, if parents are available and able to help, children and adolescents can understand and metabolize discriminatory experiences. Keep in mind that a parent's ability to engage in this process of racial socialization on discrimination is affected by the parent's own history of racial trauma, which can be reawakened unconsciously at developmental nodal points. In these cases, parents may need help with or support on the best ways to intervene. A recent community-based prevention program study (Brody et al. 2021) that offered therapeutic support to African American parents in Georgia whose children had endured racial discrimination demonstrated that the negative impact on health can be buffered. Adolescents whose parents underwent a five-session psychoeducational program on limit setting and adaptive racial socialization showed less anxiety, fewer depressive symptoms, and less frequent conduct problems.

Appropriate assessment of racial trauma is crucial to clinicians' ability to identify, conceptualize, and treat intrapsychic and systemic racial dynamics. The Black child will be both victim of and witness to racially traumatic events. Both situations are distressing, especially when they occur in environments where adults cannot intervene or when adults collude, consciously or unconsciously. Early psychic damage from racial trauma is internalized and magnified and is seldom fully understood until disturbances in adult interpersonal functioning are explored in psychotherapy or psychoanalysis. Black subjectivity is constructed under this traumatic influence of discrimination and racism. No reprieve is granted by class, status, or education. Clinicians have a responsibility to learn how to work with issues of race that arise in the consultation room. If race does not come up, the clinician can inquire about it in a supportive and open way but must also ask if they have missed the signals in the clinical material.

A white-centered view can manifest as resistance to recognizing the salience of race and racial trauma for African American patients. In the Black patient–white therapist dyad, the white therapist may miss the salience of race in the patient's developmental experience and the impact of racial trauma on the patient's life, as well as the impact of such oversight on trust. The white patient working with a Black therapist may deny that race has meaning: "It doesn't matter. I don't see color." Not only are there higher dropout rates in interracial therapy dyads (Sue et al. 1991); the quality of care is adversely affected if the BIPOC patient is matched with providers who do not acknowledge the realities of racism in the patient's experience (Jones 2003). Clinician education; cultural sensitivity; and an understanding of racial or ethnic identity, cultural values, and the historical background of cultural mistrust can all moderate the potentially limiting impact of racial differences (Chang and Berk 2009). In the white therapist–white patient dyad, therapist and patient often do not mention race, missing the existence of derivative power dynamics and racialized attitudes. The productive question to ask in all therapeutic dyads is not "Does race matter?" but "How does it matter?"

When taking developmental histories, clinicians should inquire about individual and family cultural background, exposure to people from diverse cultural backgrounds, exposure to racially traumatic events as part of the process of socialization, family immigration history, and any experiences related to diversity and difference across development, including the neighborhoods in which people live, the schools they attend, and transgenerational histories of trauma.

Construction of White Subjectivity

Understanding the traumatic racialized experiences for people of color is imperative, but whiteness must also be interrogated. The bedrock idea that whiteness, functioning as an identity, is constructed, consciously and unconsciously, as the established norm against which all forms of difference are measured and devalued must be named, questioned, and examined because it is subtly internalized in the process of racial-ethnic socialization in American society.

Integrating critical race theory into our working framework allows us to formulate how psychological processes incorporate cultural attitudes about race and then project them back out into society (Rollock and Gillborn 2011). These derogatory ideas are perpetuated intrapsychically and, on the group level, live silently in the collective cultural unconscious (Stoute 2021). In her riveting study "Slavery in the White Psyche," Parker (2019) discusses the defensive purpose that whiteness as a social and identity construct confers: "Not knowing that whiteness, or white privilege, exists means that for the majority of white people, how it functions collectively and individually, externally and internally, is largely unconscious" (p. 1). After recounting the story her father told her of how as an adolescent he had learned of a lynching that occurred in his hometown, Parker poses the penetrating question "What does it do to the minds of white children to realize that they belong to the group that commits these heinous acts of terror and violence?" Further, Parker concludes that "white children learn to disconnect—to stop thinking, to stop noticing, to stop linking reality and history, and to turn off their empathic curiosity and care...when they noticed the racial violence and segregation around them" as they are silenced by their parents on racial issues (p. 8). In Parker's study of white Americans, few could at first even "remember" how or whether they learned about slavery in school, and most never talked about it in their families. Silence, as Parker notes, quoting Leary's (2000) seminal paper, is the most common racial enactment.

In her moving work *Learning to Be White: Money, Race, and God in America*, Thandeka, a theologian and counselor, tells of collecting hundreds of stories over many years from "Euro-American adults" of their earliest memories of the "seemingly inconsequential" events in their childhood reflective of how parental attitudes affected the formation of their white racial identity (Thandeka 1999). Thandeka retells memory after memory: Sarah, who brought home a cherished friend from school only to be told by her parents not to bring home a "colored" child again; Mike, who at age 5 tried to make sense of his father's derogatory remarks about an interracial couple they passed on the street; Dan, a minister who remembered that when he was a child his father explained to him in a matter-of-fact way that "Black people are inferior"; Dorothy, who remembered that when she was 5, her family lived in Mexico and her parents forbade her playing with the Mexican housekeeper's daughter or any Mexican children; and Sally, whose civil rights–supporting parents forbade her to date the Black boy who asked her to the school dance because "What would the neighbors think?" Given the frequency of these mundane day-to-day experiences, is it any wonder that making conscious the effect of these ambivalently held experiences is difficult? As Thandeka puts it, the people she interviewed were forced to think of themselves as white to remain in the good graces of a loved parent: "The Euro-American child, I now believed, is a racial victim of its own white community of parents, caretakers, and peers who attack it because it does not yet have a white racial identity. Rather than continue to suffer such attacks the Euro-American child defends itself by creating a white racial identity for itself" (p. 13). I would add that along with the interviewees thinking of themselves as white, it was also clear that the handmaiden to their sense of white superiority was the inferiority projected onto the racial Other.

Harris (2007), in her insightful formulation stressing the linchpin issue of white subjectivity, calls on us to "approach the project of studying racialized subjectivities through a deconstruction of whiteness," which she powerfully argues involves confronting "that the intergenerational transmissions of guilt and disavowal together leave a blank psychic space [for whites] that makes an authentic expression of racial consciousness and genuine reparation currently difficult and certainly, even if well intentioned, partially compromised" (p. 892). This disavowal, Harris says, creates a resistance to the awareness of how the identification with and entrenchment in racist ways of thinking play out in white psychic life as a collusion and impediment for white clinicians. The disavowal is transgenerationally transmitted in the latent and manifest processes of white racial socialization that are not named or consciously acknowledged. How does this culturally supported, often unconscious, disavowal affect the process of racial learning? How does it later play out in the therapeutic encounter?

While focusing on the impact of racism on youth of color, we must keep in mind that ignoring racism has developmental implications for white youth as well. For example, a 1970 study in Utah of children who lived in homogeneously white communities with no contact with Blacks demonstrated that negative media images played a significant role in organizing children's racial awareness and structuring negative attitudes about race (Withrich 1970). These attitudes persist into adulthood. Critical analysis of related studies reveals that many white Americans who have grown up in homogeneous neighborhoods with limited personal contact with African Americans are significantly influenced by negative media images that portray stereotypes of African Americans as, for example, lazy, less intelligent, and less economically successful and are therefore more likely to endorse the belief that individual failure is more decisive than systemic discrimination as a barrier to social and economic advancement (Stoddard 2015, p. 51). Diversity training programs for college students and adults fail to change these intractable internalized prejudices (Paluck and Green 2009; Dobbin and Kalev 2016a, 2016b).

White families in general talk less about race and ethnicity. A 2007 study conducted by researchers at Vanderbilt University surveyed the parents of 17,372 white, Black, Hispanic, Asian, Native Hawaiian/Pacific Islander, American Indian, and multiracial school-age children (Brown et al. 2007). In the study 57% of the participants were white. Approximately 60% of white parents surveyed reported that they did not discuss race with their children—a number two to five times lower than that of nonwhite parents depending on the reference ethnic group specified, with African American parents the most likely group to discuss race (Brown et al. 2007). Because children and adolescents do internalize implicit social messages and model their parents' behavior, not discussing race conveys that silence on issues of race is an acceptable norm. One can begin to theorize how empathy toward the racial Other is or is not conveyed when such discussions are not prioritized in white families' homes compared with homes of families of color. For Black children and other children of color, understanding and coping with discrimination is necessary, whereas for white children of the dominant culture such aspects of racial socialization, namely, thinking critically about discrimination, are often treated as optional learning. The subtle psychic derivatives of racism and oppression that play out in day-to-day experience go unnoticed and are not critically interrogated by white parents, for whom socialization on racism and discrimination is not generally a priority.

In a small study, Bartoli et al. (2016) presented compelling results in line with other research work on the obstacles for white youth by interviewing white parent-teenager dyads to corroborate parental views about racism and assess the resultant impact of socialization practices on their teenagers. White parents in the study readily admitted that they were not familiar with whiteness as a concept; that they rarely thought about race and focused instead on "good values" of "hard work" and "we are all equal" and "character" matters; and that they tended to think of racism as an individual and overt phenomenon and not as systematic, pervasive, or historical—all findings supported by other researchers on the topic. For the white families studied, lack of attention to social inequity and color blindness was not a default philosophical position but an active tenet of parental socialization; many parents actively taught their children to think of everyone as equal and privilege as earned, stressing meritocracy and egalitarianism. The researchers aptly pointed out that "not seeing race" in a racialized society leaves white children and teenagers unprepared to think about or talk about racism, and white youth are thus often left "unable to detect, understand or intervene with racism" in a society that is structured along racial and class lines (Bartoli et al. 2016, p. 133). Those parents who had Black friends or friends of different cultural backgrounds fared better in recognizing the need to be aware of racism, but most still lacked the skills to engage in conversation with their children on the issues at hand.

Omitting race, denying that race is an important social variable, viewing race in stereotypical ways, and failing to provide an active engagement with understanding racism leaves many white children unprepared. Bartoli et al. (2016) concluded that rather than decreasing the impact of racism, the so called color-blind parental approach "makes race matter more as it leaves common racial stereotypes to persist uninterrogated and makes it impossible for you to talk about their race-related experiences in nuanced and accurate ways" (p. 133).

Diverse academic environments for preadolescents—if white parents do choose them, especially if there is a multicultural curriculum (Banks 2006; Hagerman 2018)—expand children's comfort with difference. A positive feedback loop is created when children attend racially diverse schools because parents also learn from and gain new perspectives from their children (Hughes and Johnson 2001). The idea that one's internal working model may incorporate an awareness of and comfort level with people of different backgrounds has an impact on the comfort with which one negotiates multicultural environments, so it is obvious how important early developmental experiences can be. But the ability to talk about race requires more than exposure in a diverse environment. It involves active engagement and critical thinking about race. Even in diverse school environments, adolescents often do not talk about race across racial lines. One of the earliest studies examining the implicit racial attitudes in interethnic group interactions concluded that

> If interaction is to bring about change, it must be accompanied by emotional insight assimilated at levels deeper than the intellectual. For the irrational and unconscious aspects of mental processes cast doubt on the assumption that mere interaction among adults of dissimilar cultural backgrounds will, in itself, effect positive changes toward out-group persons. (Stoute 1950, p. 145)

In this study of interethnic group interaction with college students, Stoute concluded that modifying subjective beliefs about other ethnic groups in the face of new experiences that challenge subjective beliefs necessitates psychic work in addition to proximity and exposure.

The research endeavor of studying the correlation of white racial identity with racist attitudes was made possible by the development of the White Racial Identity Attitude Scale (WRIAS; Helms and Carter 1990), which assesses five postulated schemas (or attitudes) associated with white racial identity (Helms 1984), and the New Racism Scale (NRS; Jacobson 1985), which measures white attitudes toward Blacks in indirect areas of race relations. A 2004 study of college students' racial attitudes using these two measures demonstrated that white young adults who had no formulation of their racial identity (postulated to be evidence of limited racial socialization) or who had higher attitudinal ambivalence toward Blacks had higher measured racist attitudes (Carter et al. 2004). The converse was also true, namely, that those participants who committed to a specific racial identity (conveying a sense of being able to think about their own racial and ethnic origins) tended to have lower racism scores. These findings indirectly suggest that racial socialization and more differentiated racial identity for whites are correlated with lower scores on scales that measure racist attitudes—a finding of profound significance.

Hagerman's (2018) more recent study, a must read, reveals from interviews how white parents, while believing themselves to be, and teaching their children to be, egalitarian, are surprisingly unaware of how they perpetuate prejudiced ideas that support structural racism and racial inequity in school environments. "Systems (e.g., schools) ascribe racial privilege and power to White youths by reinforcing societal notions of racial oppression through administrative practices and policies and have a negative impact on the racial identity development of White children and adolescents as well" (Hagerman 2018, p. 16). Because most white children are socialized not to think of race as salient or to challenge racist attitudes, they do not develop critical thinking about racial stereotypes. Choosing private schools that are more socioeconomically and racially homogeneous (under the guise of looking for a good school in a nice neighborhood) serves indirectly to reinforce racial stereotypes given that such schools provide limited diversity in thinking and population.

White adults often react with nonverbal expressions of discomfort and silence when children acknowledge racism. The adults' sense of shame and discomfort and the silence that are manifested in this defensive response are communicated and stifle curiosity, even when children and adolescents open up the issue (Clark 2014). White parents, in conversations with children and adolescents, rarely address deconstructing implicit prejudices because the parents may also share those prejudices. It has been well demonstrated that even white adults who experience themselves as egalitarian still harbor prejudiced ideas about people of color. As a result, white children who have very little education on racism and discrimination often have no positive role models on how to think or talk about racist attitudes, so they internalize the racialized thinking and racial attitudes of the surrounding culture that reinforces and supports a defensive disavowal and silence. Unless attitudes about race are interrogated in helpful and supportive ways, discriminatory and racialized derogatory attitudes persist.

This defensive impasse can also play out in the therapeutic arena when white children and adolescents present openings for conversations about racism that adults do not seize as opportunities. Clinicians, especially white clinicians, do not recognize that these are entry points for psychotherapeutic exploration. Such entry points include when the child or adolescent mentions that they witnessed a racist incident or remark in school; when they mention studying civil rights and racism in school; or when they voice stereotypes of people of color or even make racist remarks (Clark 2014). Even if clinicians recognize that these situations could be entry points, they may feel anxious or lacking in the skill needed to navigate these topics. As mental health clinicians, we must challenge ourselves to learn to recognize and to work with the unconscious derivatives of racism that lurk in the therapeutic encounter. This work, if done effectively, can be transformative for individual patients and for the clinicians themselves and advances us all toward the social goal of deconstructing racism in our society.

Implications for Clinical Work

The following case vignettes demonstrate how issues of race, racism, and racial and ethnic identity can be intertwined with other conflicts at different developmental points. Whether you are the therapist or the patient, your internal working model in adulthood harkens back to a foundation constructed across development from childhood to adulthood. The skilled therapist can use racial entry points along the way to negotiate the intrapsychic conflict-laden developmental line and improve the patient's ability to think about difference and identity. However, for a solid self to be constructed, it is crucial that aspects of racial trauma be conceptualized and named. The course of racial identity development must be revisited, understood, and repaired in treatment. In the first two cases that follow, the patients had been treated by white clinicians before treatment with an African American female psychoanalyst.

Cultural Mistrust

Case Vignette 1: "Find Me a Black Child Psychiatrist and I Will Believe You"

The brilliant, successful professional African American parents of 11-year-old Allan were told by the school psychologist that a teacher thought he needed a psychiatric evaluation to rule out an attention-deficit disorder. They were shocked, especially because the psychologist did not mentioned at all how exceptionally bright Allan was. Allan's father told the school psychologist that if she found an African American child psychiatrist who was a graduate of the same Ivy League medical school he had attended, then he would accept the evaluation because he could not be sure if the white teacher in the wealthy white school was stereotyping his son.

The school psychologist called me, and after an extended evaluation, I determined that Allan did have ADHD, inattentive subtype, and that he was an exceptionally bright boy, already reading books at an adult reading level. As Allan talked in the extended evaluation about his anxiety being the only Black boy in the accelerated class and feeling that the teacher was not connected to him, it became clear that an intervention to create greater trust between parents and teachers was indicated. Allan felt ignored, not recognized, and, I postulated, maybe even unmentalized, and he was made more anxious when the teacher did not call on him in class. During my conversations with the teacher and the school psychologist in the course of evaluation and treatment, the psychologist discussed ways she could be helpful to Allan, which allowed me to suggest to her that the academic material was not at all challenging to him. She did not realize that, as a result of this boredom, he was reading books during the lessons to keep himself occupied. As the teacher came to understand Allan better as a result of the intervention, she accepted that Allan was also restless because he was bored. She began to offer more challenging additional material and seemed to behave more empathically, and, as a result, Allan felt more connected to her.

Inadequate Legal Socialization

Case Vignette 2: "Will I Get Killed?"

Jonathan is a 19-year-old African American college student who moved away from home to a Southern college town. He was raised by adoptive college-educated, liberal white parents in a wealthy neighborhood as the second and only adopted child in a highly educated loving family, and he was doted on as the youngest child. He was educated in exclusive private schools. His close friends were all wealthy and all white, as was his family. He had no close African American friends during his development. He had always been anxious as a child and was shielded often in response to the academic pressures in school.

After the murder of George Floyd during the 2020 COVID-19 pandemic and the subsequent Black Lives Matter demonstrations, Jonathan became increasingly more aware of the dangers of what it meant to be a Black man in America. The issue had not been much of a concern for him earlier in development because he was shielded in an upper-middle-class upbringing. His parents were aware of the challenges of discrimination, but the important dangers and risks for him being a Black male had not been emphasized in his early years, and he had not received the education in legal socialization that African American parents often provide beginning early in childhood. Jonathan presented for treatment with panic attacks, obsessive and intrusive thoughts, insomnia with recurring dreams, and worries that he would be pulled over by the police or be the victim of racial profiling, all of which were interfering with his day-to-day functioning to the extent that he was almost agoraphobic.

Dangerous Impact of Race Fantasies

Case Vignette 3: "Why Did His Father Think I Was Dangerous?"

Jordan is a handsome 10-year-old African American boy. At 5′4″, he is tall for his age. His parents, successful African American professionals, are both of Caribbean heritage. They had chosen their son's school, a small, nurturing parochial school with small class size, mindful of the lack of racial, ethnic, and socioeconomic diversity. Overall, Jordan's experience at the school had been good, although he would come home recounting the occasional discriminatory remark, which took the form of a comment from a schoolmate or teacher. His parents considered this manageable and discussed with him what discrimination meant in an age-appropriate way. His parents both knew that Jordan's height made people treat him as if he were older. Jordan's father, a 6′6″ man himself, began early on teaching his son in subtle ways to control his angry reactions to try not to appear angry because "tall Black men who are angry are viewed as threatening"—a prejudice he knew too well.

Of course, when the school started a basketball team, Jordan, a talented athlete, was first pick. One day, the team was playing hard, and a scuffle occurred when three of the boys all went for the ball at once and another boy, a shorter white child, ended up on the floor. Having decided that Jordan had pushed his son, Mr. M, the boy's father, who had not seen the play, ran over to Jordan. Mr. M, who was only an inch taller than Jordan, screamed and threatened Jordan with physical harm, thinking that he had attacked his son. Jordan's father ran to the court and shielded Jordan. After all had settled down, another (white) parent came over and explained that Mr. M's son actually had been the aggressor and had attacked Jordan, and Jordan had just pushed the boy off him, trying to get up off the floor—not as an offensive aggressive move.

The next day, Jordan's mother, an attorney, drafted a letter to the principal naming the event as a racist attack and requested a meeting with him and the father who had threatened her son. In the meeting, Mr. M explained that he was a police officer in a large city and that "I deal with Black boys on the streets all the time." Jordan's mother interrupted and pointed out, "This is not the streets, nor is our son a Black boy on the streets." In the conversation, it became clear that Mr. M's prejudice and perception of Black boys as dangerous and aggressive had provoked his response during the game. His distorted perception that he had to protect his son from aggressive Black boys had led him to overreact to a normal scuffle for the ball. By the end of the meeting, the principal requested that Mr. M apologize to Jordan's parents. At their insistence, Jordan was invited into the room and, with Jordan's parents present, Mr. M apologized to him. Mr. M was put on probation, with the understanding that any further outbursts at sporting events or threats would result in his being barred from all athletic events.

Although the situation came to a positive end, within 2 weeks, Jordan began having recurring nightmares of being attacked. He developed posttraumatic symptoms of anxiety, recurring dreams, a reluctance to play on the team with Mr. M's son, and worry that Mr. M would still come after him. Jordan's parents sought psychotherapeutic intervention. Although Jordan's parents had the wherewithal, clear resources, and education to handle the incident and shield their son to minimize the trauma from the assault, Jordan still was powerfully impacted.

Racialized Perception of Dangerousness

Case Vignette 4: "The Dangerous Black Boy"

Preston, a seriously disturbed 13-year-old tenth-grade African American boy who had experienced many traumas in his life, was hospitalized with depressed mood and disruptive behavior at school after a suicide attempt (case discussed in full in Stoute 2019). Preston's parents met in college, and his mother got pregnant by accident. His mother had a history of serious psychiatric illness and substance use; his father had been inconsistent as a parent throughout his life. When Preston was a young boy, his mother got involved with a new man and dropped Preston off one day with his paternal grandparents. His grandparents had been his consistent caretakers since, but even their consistency could not heal his sense of abandonment and loss.

In the early weeks of his hospital stay, Preston was difficult to manage. His daily aggressive outbursts and suicidal threats and attempts necessitated placement in seclusion and use of restraints. He made a noose out of his bed sheets, tried to break open the window to jump, and flew into a rage at the least provocation. After several incidents requiring four-point restraints to control his aggression, he began to voice how he liked the restraints. This connected to his underlying conflict because the use of restraints drew maximal attention and physical contact, which he craved but could not directly acknowledge. The Black male staff mental health workers were not afraid of Preston and endured his aggression in his many outbursts; the white staff members seemed quietly more cautious.

I met with Preston for sessions daily, Monday through Friday—five sessions a week. We worked on elaborate behavioral contracts and made medication adjustments. Achieving better control and connecting to me in the therapy was the preamble to his organizing, articulating, and voicing his rage. From the outset, the image of him as being dangerous interfered with the staff's ability to see him as a depressed and traumatized boy and to empathize with his trauma. In my mind, he was an angry, insatiably hungry boy who needed to process the painful abandonments by his parents and to understand how he scared away peers and adults in his life with his anger, and this allowed me to mentalize him in a much different way. The challenge was to engage the staff in reflecting on their very different racialized views of him.

Meetings and discussions with the staff focused on helping them to process their frustration with how difficult Preston was to manage and their fear of Preston's "dangerousness." I engaged the staff to reflect on their racialized attitudes by helping them talk about their racialized perceptions, asking them, "How dangerous is he really?" I explained to them how Preston's pain and trauma were undercurrents of his aggressive and self-destructive behavior and how his enactment in the repeated cycles of provoking rejection was a repetition in service of mastering the trauma, abuse, and broken attachments that he had endured. Preston's grandparents, in parallel, were mistrustful of the staff and would follow recommendations about treatment only if I, as the African

American psychiatrist, made the recommendation myself. Over time, after work with Preston's grandparents and the staff, this distrust changed.

Further discussion of this treatment case, including details of how race became an integral part of Preston's identification with me as the therapist and allowed an entry point to his conflicts in the maternal transference, is available in prior work (Stoute 2019). A key component of this treatment, I believe, was how I was able to mentalize Preston despite his many attempts to ward off connection. His so-called dangerousness did not deter me from attempting to develop a treatment relationship, nor did it forestall my using a psychoanalytic framework to make sense of his painful inner world and his hunger for attachment. In the shared reflective mentalization with an important adult, an adolescent like Preston can identify with and internalize aspects of ego functioning and a reflected self-image and go on to develop an ego ideal through identification with that important adult who mentalizes him. This allows the adolescent to connect to and identify with other adults in his life and take in the mentalized image the adult(s) may have of him. Preston's case raises the following question: How can clinicians' anxiety in talking about racialized thinking, and their own racist ideas, impair their availability to engage children and adolescents of color in treatment?

Considerations of Race in the Twenty-First Century

Case Vignette 5: "I Never Knew It Existed"

Miss Z, a 45-year-old Italian American married financial executive, was in treatment for generalized anxiety and obsessive-compulsive disorder. She had been intrigued by the Black Lives Matter demonstrations in the summer of 2020 (after the murder of George Floyd) and had gingerly let me know that she wanted to understand the movement better. When she pointedly asked how she could become more informed, I did interpret, asking if she had previously thought about the racial difference between us, and I also gave her the link to the antiracism education and resources at a local university website.

Miss Z began the next session by saying, "I read those antiracism resources on the university website and watched a documentary. It put it in perspective—I had not understood how wrong things have been for so many years, how hard is it to see people persecuted for so many years. Looking at my family, we are financially privileged because my family owned their own home. Even as an immigrant, my father was able to buy his own property. I realized for the first time that he would not have had that opportunity if he was a different race. I had not thought of this as privilege. I guess this country was really built for white people. For me, America has always been the melting pot and where anyone who was persecuted and wanted freedom could come, but it is not. I guess it is not true. Not everyone is treated equal. I was struggling with it; am I racist?"

In reply, I asked, "You had not known about this?"

She answered, "I knew but never really thought about it. I have never been the type of person to care about history or political things. When I looked at that videotape [of Rodney King being assaulted but the police], I was shocked at how wrong the police were for no clear reason, and it was almost enjoyable to them. It was a side of America I knew it existed, but I did not know the details."

"During the pandemic," she continued, "I have been trying to escape from all of it and distract myself, but it has just been on TV constantly. I have been reflecting on the reality of what is going on." I interpreted to her that it was interesting that she had been so unaware because it was also my understanding that she seemed not to factor in the fact that many Italians who emigrated the same time as her grandparents experienced discrimination; after all, there are Italians with olive complexion—darker skin. She thought about it and "remembered" a distant uncle who had darker skin; no one talked about him. Somehow, she said, things had not gone so well for him. Was it related to his skin color? She had not given it much thought before. "How is that I have been so unaware of racism?" she asked.

Collusion in Thinking About Race

Case Vignette 6: "People Do Not See Me as White"

Sally, a biracial Asian American college student, had been referred as a freshman in college for treatment for depression, social anxiety, and ADHD. She had been receiving solid psychiatric treatment in once-a-week psychotherapy by the referring psychiatrist, who had shepherded her successfully through a severe depression in early adolescence and helped her make the adolescent transition to relocate out of state to attend an elite college that was conveniently located near my office. Sally presented as bright, charming, and likable, but it was clear that profound social anxiety and difficulty with interpersonal interaction lurked beneath the sophisticated intellectual veneer.

Sally began treatment with a long history of depressive symptoms, social anxiety, and family conflict. Her obsessive thinking about social interactions inhibited her daily life, and slightly fragile thinking at first made it unclear how much an insight-oriented approach might be feasible. In college, her social anxiety controlled her. In session one day she expressed surprise that a friend had implied she was a minority, saying, "I am white; why don't other people see me that way?" She clearly looked Asian. This conflict around ethnic and racial aspects of identity and the issue of racial melancholia as it related to seeing herself as white had not been elucidated or explored in her prior treatment (racial melancholia as conceptualized by Eng and Han 2000). I wondered whether she and her therapist had colluded in not naming whiteness an identity construct that invited exploration.

Sally's father was white, her mother Asian. Having attended a diverse school that one had to test into, she was clearly bright, but she felt that she was not "one of those prototypic smart Asians" like her two brothers, who had attended even more prestigious colleges. In the course of our coming to understand her experience of whether or not she fit into groups, it emerged that Sally forged friendships with collegemates and that those friends were of varying ethnic and cultural backgrounds. In true adolescent fashion, these relationships sometimes were a displacement from the transference and developmental working through of her own conflicts of identity, which provided ample material to discuss her struggles with sameness and difference, closeness, and intimacy that took narrative form in racial terms. In the background, she was also able to talk more openly about her attachment to her distant and somewhat schizoid father, a conversation that upstaged deeper oedipal conflicts. As Sally came to a better understanding of her conflicts in her relationship with her mother after her parents divorced, she came to see that her anger was also a displacement from an idealization of her father. When her parents' divorce came to the fore in conversation during the treatment, she saw her mother in more real terms as a woman struggling with a marriage that fell apart rather than the divorce as being completely of her own making. Sally was able to rework and internalize her identification with her Asian mother, a woman of color who also did not talk about race, by using her current therapist, an analyst of color, as the pivot point for reworking the identification.

At one point midway through the treatment, Sally came into session recounting a story with friends and remarked, "That white girl was really annoying" and went on to make a statement regarding "we people of color...." What had happened in the therapeutic process? Was she joining her identification with me as a person of color? Was she using me as a developmental object as a pivot to rework how she saw herself? Being free to discuss racial and ethnic backgrounds of her friendships and romantic partners,

> weaving in and out of the transference as she weaved in and out of her familial identifications, helped Sally rework her own ethnic, racial, and cultural identity. When we terminated after a long treatment, we discussed in our final session how Sally had come to see herself. Her obsessive thinking had lessened as the psychotherapeutic process unfolded. Her social anxiety had abated significantly, and she felt much more comfortable in social relationships. She dated an African American classmate, and although they broke up, they stayed friends. She went on to start and develop a solid relationship with an Asian boyfriend and graduated at the top of her class.

Sally's case provides several questions to consider. The unique issues of racial melancholia for Asian Americans as formulated by Eng and Han (2000) are of import here. Because Sally's prior therapist was not trained to be conversant in how unresolved conflicts around racial identity play out in psychotherapy, this left Sally's foundational conflicts around race untouched. Did the white therapist collude with whiteness as the working identification model that went unnamed and, therefore, uninterrogated? Essentially, Sally identified herself as white, so race—whiteness—went unnamed and identity conflicts were not explored. Did the therapist of color facilitate an exploration of the meanings of race, ethnicity, and identity by recognizing the opportunity to use race as an entry point to the patient's conflicts around identity and even her oedipal rivalry?

The term *race*, to be clear, refers to a social, political, and cultural identification that, although phenotypically correlated with skin color, has no clear biological correlate. Who is defined as Black or a person of color is a social determination carrying significant valence in American society dating back to slavery. Not only is Blackness a defining racial identity in the United States designating the descendants of African slaves; it also came to represent the category of symbolic Other imposed for nonwhite identities. Successive waves of immigrants, deemed as "nonwhite," were inducted into a racialized identity of devalued marginalization in American society. Designation as a person of color carves out a position of Other, and cultural factors influence how that position is experienced and expressed.

Racial Trauma, Immigration Trauma, and Collusion

The following case vignette of Ms. P is particularly illuminating and integrates many of the concepts around a nodal traumatic locus in development. The impact of discrimination on immigrant children also brings to bear the importance of ethnic identity as a stabilizing contribution to a sense of self. All too often, children of immigrant parents, as in the case of Ms. P, are unable to give voice to the traumatic experiences they endure (Stevens et al. 2020). The immigrant child carries the legacy of the family sacrifice and hope in a concrete way because parents often emigrate in service of a better life and opportunity for the family. For the child carrying this legacy (including, but not limited to, Southeast Asian, Chinese American, and Caribbean American children), the challenge of navigating the barriers of language, culture, and societal norms is exponentially difficult given that the immigrant parent may be unfamiliar with or a silent victim to the cultural norm of discrimination in American culture. These parents frequently adopt an ethos of "keep your head down" and do not complain and work even harder in attempting to "prove" themselves as legitimate citizens. Immigrant parents may be unable to negotiate the racial landscape or provide the requisite racial-ethnic socialization safety net or preparation about discrimination and bias that Black American parents are all too familiar with. An understanding of the patient's cultural origins, family structure and supports, immigration experience, and possible immigration trauma is necessary in providing therapeutic space to help children, adolescents, and even adults give voice to these experiences.

Case Vignette 7: "People Thought I Was Different—A Big Black Thing"

Ms. P is a 40-year-old Hindu woman who has achieved professional success but has not married. She had been in psychotherapy, but that treatment had focused on managing work stress and medication as she grieved the loss of her idealized father. She had grown up in the U.S. Deep South, where her parents had immigrated because of a job opportunity for her father without any understanding of the brutality of the racism they would encounter. Ms. P had been born after her parents' arrival in the United States, and in her early years the family traveled regularly to India, the parents' country of origin. The immigration journey had been traumatic; Ms. P's parents were young and lost the needed contact with extended family.

The immigrant journey had been traumatic. Miss P's parents were young and lost the needed contact with extended family. In addition, they met unforeseen challenges after immigrating to the Deep South and were not able to help her, as a child, make sense of the racially toxic environment. Her parents were not able to empathize with the different challenges of their first-generation offspring, who did not internalize the nearby Indian social community as shielding.

In the early stages of the psychotherapy, Ms. P raised the issue of her conflict between two men she was dating: one was a Hindu man of outstanding distinguished pedigree, and the other was an engaging white man to whom she was drawn although he was less financially successful. I interpreted that although this choice involved many issues, Ms. P seemed to be struggling with sameness and difference. She responded by talking about her sadness of how difficult it had been being the only family of color in a Southern rural town. This opened the door to an avalanche of associations, and she recounted experience after experience of exclusion and discrimination. A close white school friend distanced himself from her when they reached middle school and other kids teased him for playing with the "colored girl." In high school, no one asked her to date. Describing how she understood these experiences, she explained that "I felt different, unattractive…inferior." When I referred to her core sense of self that was damaged, she replied, "It goes back to when I was a child." She wanted to try out for the leading role in the school play, but "the other kids said no; they called me a big Black thing." An attractive blonde school friend got the role. "Yeah, they call that a microaggression," I said, "but when you are a child, the aggression is not so micro." She responded, "My early conception of myself was that I was this ugly damaged thing." The coincidence of these racialized experiences with puberty and her physical development merged these issues into a sexual inhibition that she related to her sense of herself as damaged and undesirable. These traumas coincided with key developmental nodal points.

Ms. P's parents' traumatic immigration experiences, and their defensively not knowing how to negotiate being labeled as Black because they had not previously experienced discrimination in this way, left Ms. P without parental guidance or validation to help her negotiate the crushing racism of the Deep South that assaulted her in adolescence. Her parents did not think of themselves as people of color, but she did. However, I clarified for her that Blackness was not a monolithic category and that for her parents, being an immigrant also involved a striving to be part of the newly accepted culture. Therefore, on the basis of her cultural and ethnic background, her experience as a person of color might mean something different from mine.

We were able to explore and unpack Ms. P's conflicts around racial and ethnic identity, and she was able to give voice to her experience as she talked about her sadness that she had not learned to speak her parents' native language fluently and had not internalized the cultural customs of their family heritage despite the trips to India to maintain family connections during her childhood. These intertwined issues were difficult to navigate because her conflict around her racial and ethnic identity had merged with oedipal conflict, and choosing a romantic partner involved teasing this apart. Navigating the multilayered dimensions of the trauma around confronting her difference allowed a revisitation and consolidation of her feeling more solid about who she was on personal and professional levels. It allowed her to unpack her fantasy of me, as an African American woman of color, who, she imagined, could help her negotiate and repair her fractured sense of self and learn to stand up for herself in ways her parents were not able to teach her.

Ms. P's prior psychotherapy with a white therapist was helpful in managing her professional struggles with coworkers and family relationships, but the therapist had not raised these issues of racial trauma or conflict around racial and ethnic identity. There was a collusion in not naming race. The pivotal racial trauma was not discussed as active in Ms. P's psychic experience. Naming the racial trauma that occurred in adolescence as a developmental nodal point facilitated her processing the traumatic experiences that contributed to the deep sense of feeling defective and damaged that played out in her current social and professional arenas. Accessing race as an entry point to these conflicts allowed us to accomplish this transformative therapeutic work.

Conclusion

The U.S. Census Bureau predicts that by 2035, children of color will constitute more than 50% of the American population (Hughes et al. 2006). In light of this reality, we as educators and clinicians must rework our understanding of the complex interplay in development of individual, familial, cultural, and societal factors that enhance children's ability to negotiate multicultural environments with high degrees of racial, ethnic, and cultural diversity. As such, developmental models, having originated from individualistic conflict-based conceptions of intrapsychic development based on acculturation to whiteness as the cultural norm, now require a conceptual reworking to address the dynamic interplay of the multifactorial variables in racial-ethnic socialization in a multiracial society.

Understanding how racism, on an individual and structural basis, impacts us developmentally is crucial to deconstructing the insidious way that racism remains embedded in our thinking on an individual level and in the collective cultural unconscious on the societal level. How we think and talk about race and racism is influenced by early, often traumatic, developmental experiences affected by parental attitudes, cultural socialization, and transgenerationally transmitted attitudes and trauma. Attention to racial identity and trauma is important in development, but it is only through a secure base of having our own solid sense of identity and self, facilitated by internalizing positive role models and critical thinking about structural racism, that we can approach those who are different from us with less conflict and with openness and flexibility. That the resistance to thinking critically about racism is culturally syntonic and culturally sanctioned significantly influences how white subjectivity evolves. This stands in stark contrast to the dominating influence that racism and racialized social realities have on the construction of Black subjectivity. Attention to how this plays out in the therapeutic encounter is crucial. Mental health clinicians can play a critical role in making racialized attitudes and racism a subject of psychotherapeutic inquiry, educational discourse, and active intervention in our work, our professional organizations, our communities, and our world.

Key Points

- A fundamental understanding of racial-ethnic socialization and racial learning, with attention to racial identity formation and the vicissitudes of racial trauma across the developmental spectrum, is necessary, especially when treating children and adults of color.
- All children are socialized from early childhood to beliefs, values, and images that reinforce the dominance of the majority white cultural superiority and to the stereotypes and distortions of Black and white. Environmental cues about color are clearly communicated to children, who use them to internalize how Blackness is viewed.
- White children receive very little education on racism and discrimination and often have no positive role models on how to think or talk about racist attitudes, so they internalize the racialized thinking and racial attitudes of the surrounding culture that reinforces and supports a defensive disavowal and silence. Unless attitudes about race are interrogated in helpful and supportive ways, discriminatory and racialized derogatory attitudes persist.
- Learned silence on race for white dominant culture children begins early and is promoted by the culture. This culturally sanctioned learned silence becomes internalized as an unconscious roadblock that later for some white therapists constricts the ability to detect how racism can infiltrate the therapeutic encounter.
- Racism is a reality-based repetitive trauma. Absorbing the traumatic assault of discriminatory experiences affects health and, later, self-image. Adult patients who have endured racially traumatic experiences endorse an array of symptoms on presentation for treatment, including, but not limited to, mood disorders, physical symptoms, acting-out behaviors, suicidal thinking, substance use, and, into adulthood, posttraumatic symptoms and fractured interpersonal functioning. Children and adolescent patients manifest mood symptoms, anxiety symptoms, and behavior problems. These patterns and symptoms, often uncovered when adults come into treatment, are not just acute reactions, however, but the posttraumatic result of long-standing and repeated exposure throughout development to discriminatory experiences.
- Appropriate assessment of racial trauma is crucial to clinicians' ability to identify, conceptualize, and treat intrapsychic and systemic racial dynamics. Early psychic damage from racial trauma is internalized and magnified and is seldom fully understood until disturbances in adult interpersonal functioning are explored in psychotherapy or psychoanalysis.
- The influence of race, including fantasies about race, and racial themes can be fertile entry points in psychotherapy regardless of the racial-ethnic composition of the dyad. As mental health clinicians, we must challenge ourselves to learn to recognize and to work with the unconscious derivatives of racism that lurk in the therapeutic encounter.

References

Aboud FE: A social-cognitive developmental therapy of prejudice, in Handbook of Race, Racism, and the Developing Child. Edited by Quintana SM, McKown C. Mahwah, NJ, Wiley, 2008, pp 55–71

Adams CJ: Black youth: self-making, creativity and the assertion of hybrid Black identities. Psychoanal Study Child 74(1):59–76, 2021

Altschul I, Oyserman D, Bybee D: Racial-ethnic identity in mid-adolescence: content and change as predictors of academic achievement. Child Dev 77(5):1155–1169, 2006 16999790

American Psychiatric Association: Diagnostic and Statistical Manual of Mental Disorders, 5th Edition. Arlington, VA, American Psychiatric Association, 2013

Apfelbaum EP, Pauker K, Sommers SR, et al: In blind pursuit of racial equality? Psychol Sci 21(11):1587–1592, 2010 20876878

Bartoli E, Michael A, Bentley-Edwards KL, et al: Training for colour-blindness: white racial socialization. Whiteness and Education 1(2):125–136, 2016

Bell CC, Jenkins EJ: Community violence and children on Chicago's southside. Psychiatry 56(1):46–54, 1993 8488212

Boen C: Death by a thousand cuts: stress exposure and Black-white disparities in physiological functioning in late life. J Gerontol B Psychol Sci Soc Sci 75(9):1937–1950, 2019 31127845

Bowman PJ, Howard C: Race-related socialization, motivation, and academic achievement: a study of black youths in three-generation families. J Am Acad Child Psychiatry 24(2):134–141, 1985 3989153

Brody GH, Chen YF, Murry VM, et al: Perceived discrimination and the adjustment of African American youths: a five-year longitudinal analysis with contextual moderation effects. Child Dev 77(5):1170–1189, 2006 16999791

Brody GH, Tianyi Y, Chen E, et al: Family-centered prevention effect on the association between racial discrimination and mental health in Black adolescents. JAMA Netw Open 4(3):e211964, 2021 33760092

Brown TN, Tanner-Smith EE, Lesane-Brown CL, et al: Parent and situational correlates of familial ethnic/race socialization. J Marriage Fam 69(1):14–25, 2007

Bryant-Davis T, Ocampo C: A therapeutic approach to the treatment of racist-incident-based trauma. Journal of Emotional Abuse 6(4):1–22, 2006

Carlson EB: Trauma Assessments: Clinician's Guide. New York, Guilford, 1997

Carter R: Racism and psychological and emotional injury: recognizing and assessing race-based traumatic stress. Couns Psychol 35(1):13–105, 2007

Carter RT, Helms JE, Juby H: The relationship between racism and racial identity profiles. Journal of Multicultural Counseling and Development 30:19–29, 2004

Carter RT, Mazzula S, Victoria R, et al: Initial development of the Race-Based Traumatic Stress Symptom Scale: assessing the emotional impact of racism. Psychological Trauma: Theory, Policy, Research, and Practice 5(1):1–9, 2013

Chang DF, Berk A: Making cross-racial therapy work: a phenomenological study of clients' experiences of cross-racial therapy. J Couns Psychol 56(4):521–536, 2009 20414342

Clark A: Exploring Ways White Children Are Taught About Race and Racism. Master's thesis, Smith College for Social Work, Northamptom, MA, 2014. Available at: https://scholarworks.smith.edu/theses/732. Accessed May 22, 2022.

Clark K: Desegregation: an appraisal of the evidence. J Soc Issues 9(4):1–75, 1953

Clark K: Prejudice and Your Child. Boston, MA, Beacon Press, 1963

Clark KB, Clark MK: Racial identification and preference in Negro children, in Readings in Social Psychology. Edited by Newcomb T, Hartley E. New York, Henry Holt, 1947, pp 602–611

Collins JW Jr, David RJ, Handler A, et al: Very low birthweight in African American infants: the role of maternal exposure to interpersonal racial discrimination. Am J Public Health 94(12):2132–2138, 2004 15569965

Cross W Jr: The ecology of human development for Black and white children: implications for predicting racial preference patterns. Critical Perspectives of Third World America 1(1):177–189, 1983
Cross W Jr: Shades of Black: Diversity in African American Identity. Philadelphia, PA, Temple University Press, 1991
Cross W Jr, Cross TB: Theory, research, and models, in Handbook of Race, Racism, and the Developing Child. Edited by Quintana SM, McKown C. Mahwah, NJ, Wiley, 2008, pp 154–181
Daniel JH: The courage to hear: African American women's memories of racial trauma, in Psychotherapy With African American Women: Innovations in Psychodynamic Perspective and Practice. Edited by Jackson LH, Greene B. New York, Guilford, 2000, pp 126–144
Derman-Sparks L, Higa C, Sparks B: Children, Race, and Racism: How Race Awareness Develops. Washington, DC, Teaching for Change, 1980. Available at: www.teachingforchange.org/wpcontent/uploads/2012/08/ec_childrenraceracism_english.pdf. Accessed May 22, 2022.
Dobbin F, Kalev A: Why diversity programs fail. Harvard Business Review, July–August 2016a, pp 52–60
Dobbin F, Kalev A: Why doesn't diversity training work? The challenge for industry and academia. Anthropology Now 10(2):48–55, 2016b
Eng D, Han S: A dialogue on racial melancholia. Psychoanal Dialogues 10(4):667–700, 2000
English D, Lambert SF, Tynes BM, et al: Daily multidimensional racial discrimination among Black U.S. American adolescents. J Appl Dev Psychol 66:101068, 2020 33994610
Fishbein HD: Factors important in the formation of preschoolers' friendship. J Genet Psychol 146:37–44, 1992
Fishbein HD: Peer Prejudice and Discrimination. Mahwah, NJ, Lawrence Erlbum, 2002
Gee GC, Ro A, Shariff-Marco S, et al: Racial discrimination and health among Asian Americans: evidence, assessment, and directions for future research. Epidemiol Rev 31:130–151, 2009 19805401
Gelman SA: The Essential Child: Origins of Essentialism in Everyday Thought. New York, Oxford University Press, 2003
Ginsburg H, Opper S: Piaget's Theory of Intellectual Development. Englewood Cliffs, NJ, Prentice-Hall, 1979
Goff PA, Jackson MC, Di Leone BA, et al: The essence of innocence: consequences of dehumanizing Black children. J Pers Soc Psychol 106(4):526–545, 2014 24564373
Goodman ME: Race Awareness in Children. Boston, MA, Addison-Wesley Press, 1952
Goosby BJ, Malone S, Richardson EA, et al: Perceived discrimination and markers of cardiovascular risk among low-income African American youth. Am J Hum Biol 27(4):546–552, 2015 25753652
Grier W, Cobbs P: Black Rage. New York, Basic Books, 1968
Hagerman MA: White Kids: Growing Up With Privilege in a Racially Divided America. New York University Press, 2018
Hardy K: Healing the hidden wounds of trauma. Reclaiming Children and Youth 21(4):24–28, 2013
Hardy K: Toward a psychology of the oppressed: understanding the invisible wounds of trauma, in Re-visioning Family Therapy: Addressing Diversity in Clinical Practice, 3rd Edition. Edited by McGoldrick M, Hardy KV. New York, Guilford, 2019, pp 133–150
Harris A: Discussion of "Unraveling Whiteness": commentary of paper by Melanie Suchet. Psychoanal Dialogues 17(6):887–894, 2007
Hart A: The discriminatory gesture: a psychoanalytic consideration of posttraumatic reactions to incidents of racial discrimination. Psychoanalytic Social Work 26(1):5–24, 2019
Hart S: Thinking clinically about post-traumatic reactions to racial trauma, in The Trauma of Racism: Lessons From the Therapeutic Encounter. Edited by Stoute BJ, Slevin M. London, Routledge (in press).
Helms JE: Toward a theoretical explanation of the effects of race on counseling: a Black and white model. Couns Psychol 12(4):153–165, 1984
Helms JE, Carter RT: Development of the White Racial Identity Attitude Inventory, in Black and White Racial Identity: Theory, Research, and Practice. Edited by Helms JE. Westport, CT, Greenwood Press, 1990, pp 67–80

Henning K: Boys to men: the role of policing in the socialization of black boys, in Policing the Black Man: Arrest, Prosecution, and Imprisonment. Edited by Davis AJ. New York, Pantheon Books, 2017, pp 57–94

Hirschfeld LA: Children's developing conceptions of race, in Handbook of Race, Racism, and the Developing Child. Edited by Quintana SM, McKown C. Hoboken, NJ, Wiley, 2008, pp 37–54

Hughes D, Johnson, D: Correlates in children's experiences of parents' racial socialization behaviors. J Marriage Fam 63(4):981–995, 2001

Hughes D, Smith EP, Stevenson HC, et al: Parents' ethnic-racial socialization practices: a review of research and directions for future study. Dev Psychol 42(5):747–770, 2006 16953684

Hughes D, Witherspoon D, Rivas-Drake D, West-Bey N: Received ethnic-racial socialization messages and youths' academic and behavioral outcomes: examining the mediating role of ethnic identity and self-esteem. Cultur Divers Ethnic Minor Psychol 15(2):112–124, 2009 19364198

Iwamoto DK, Liu WM: The impact of racial identity, ethnic identity, Asian values and race-related stress on Asian Americans and Asian international college students' psychological well-being. J Couns Psychol 57(1):79–91, 2010 20396592

Jacobson CK: Resistance to affirmative action: self-interest or racism? J Conflict Resolut 29(2):306–329, 1985

Jernigan MM, Daniel JH: Racial trauma in the lives of Black children and adolescents: challenges and clinical implications. J Child Adolesc Trauma 4:123–141, 2011

Jones J: Constructing race and deconstructing racism, in Handbook of Racial and Ethnic Minority Psychology. Edited by Bernal G, Trimble JE, Burlew AK, Leong FTL. Thousand Oaks, CA, Sage, 2003, pp 276–306

Katz P: The acquisition of racial attitudes in children, in Toward the Elimination of Racism. Edited by Katz P. New York, Pergamon, 1976, pp 125–150

Katz P: Development of children's racial awareness and intergroup attitudes, in Current Topics in Early Childhood Education, Vol 4. Edited by Katz LG. Norwood, NH, Ablex, 1981. Available at: https://files.eric.ed.gov/fulltext/ED207675.pdf. Accessed October 1, 2021.

Kovel J: White Racism: A Psychohistory. New York, Columbia University Press, 1974

Lasker B: Race Attitudes in Children. New York, Henry Holt and Company, 1929

Leary K: Racial enactments in dynamic treatment. Psychoanal Dialogues 10(4):639–653, 2000

Lewis TT, Aiello AE, Leurgans S, et al: Self-reported experiences of everyday discrimination are associated with elevated C-reactive protein levels in older African-American adults. Brain Behav Immun 24(3):438–443, 2010 19944144

Li MJ, Thing JP, Galvan FH, et al: Contextualising family microaggressions and strategies of resilience among young gay and bisexual men of Latino heritage. Cult Health Sex 19(1):107–120, 2017 27426889

Lieberman Z, Woodward AL, Kinzler KD: The origins of social categorization. Trends Cogn Sci 21 (7):556–568, 2017

Liu LL, Lau AS: Teaching about race/ethnicity and racism matters: an examination of how perceived ethnic racial socialization processes are associated with depression symptoms. Cultur Divers Ethnic Minor Psychol 19(4):383–394, 2013 24188535

Lukachko A, Hatzenbuehler ML, Keyes KM: Structural racism and myocardial infarction in the United States. Soc Sci Med 103:42–50, 2014 24507909

Miller DB: Racial socialization and racial identity: can they promote resiliency for African American Adolescents. Adolescence 34(135):493–501, 1999 10658857

Murry VM, Berkel C, Brody GH, et al: Linking parental socialization to interpersonal protective processes, academic self-presentation, and expectations among rural African American youth. Cultur Divers Ethnic Minor Psychol 15(1):1–10, 2009 19209975

Newheiser AK, Olson KR: White and Black American children's implicit intergroup bias. J Exp Soc Psychol 48(1):264–270, 2012 22184478

Pachter LM, Bernstein BA, Szalacha LA, et: Perceived racism and discrimination in children and youths: an exploratory study. Health Soc Work 35(1):61–69, 2010 20218454

Paluck E, Green D: Prejudice reduction: what works? A review and assessment of research and practice. Annu Rev Psychol 60:339–367, 2009 18851685

Parker R: Slavery in the white psyche. Psychoanalytic Social Work 26(1):84–103, 2019
Quintana SM: Racial perspective taking ability: developmental, theoretical and empirical trends, in Handbook of Race, Racism and the Developing Child. Edited by Quintana SM, McKown C. Hoboken, NJ, Wiley, 2008, pp 16–36
Roberts D, Rollins O: Why sociology matters to race and biosocial science. Annu Rev Sociol 46:195–214, 2020
Rollins A, Hunter AG: Racial socialization of biracial youth: maternal messages and approaches to address discrimination. Fam Relat 62(1):140–153, 2013
Rollock N, Gillborn D: Critical race theory (CRT). British Educational Research Association, January 1, 2011. Available at: www.bera.ac.uk/publication/critical-race-theory-crt. Accessed May 25, 2022.
Seaton EK: Perceived racial discrimination and racial identity profiles among African American adolescents. Cultur Divers Ethnic Minor Psychol 15(2):137–144, 2009 19364200
Sellers RM, Smith MA, Shelton JN, et al: Multidimensional model of racial identity: a reconceptualization of African American racial identity. Pers Soc Psychol Rev 2(1):18–39, 1998 15647149
Shim RS, Vinson SY: Social (In)justice and Mental Health. Washington, DC, American Psychiatric Association Publishing, 2021
Shreve G: Get out of my head: experiencing cultural paranoia in Jordan Peele's Get Out, in The Trauma of Racism: Lessons From the Therapeutic Encounter. Edited by Stoute BJ, Slevin M. London, Routledge (in press)
Sibrava NJ, Bjornsson AS, Benitez ACIP, et al: Posttraumatic stress disorder in African American and Latinx adults: clinical course and the role of racial and ethnic discrimination. Am Psychol 74(1):101–116, 2019 30652903
Singletary G: Trauma and Black male adolescents: a critical link. Adolesc Psychiatry 10(1):17–28, 2020
Skewes MC, Blume AW: Understanding the link between racial trauma and substance use among American Indians. Am Psychol 74(1):88–100, 2019 30652902
Skinner AL, Meltzoff AN: Childhood experiences and intergroup biases among children. Soc Issues Policy Rev 13(1):211–410, 2019
Smith CMO, Smith EP, Levine DW, et al: A developmental perspective of the relationship of racial-ethnic identity to self-construct, achievement, and behavior in African American children. Cultur Divers Ethnic Minor Psychol 15(2)145–157, 2009 19364201
Smith JR, Patton DU: Posttraumatic stress symptoms in context: examining trauma responses to violent exposures and homicide death among Black males in urban neighborhoods. Am J Orthopsychiatry 86(2):212–223, 2016 26963344
Stevens GWJM, Boer M, Titzmann PF, et al: Immigration status and bullying victimization: associations across national and school context. J Appl Dev Psychol 66(2020):101075, 2020
Stoddard CN: Cultivating Color-Blindness?: The Impact of TV-Viewing, Racial Policy Reasoning, and Colorblind Racism on Opposition Toward Affirmative Action Policy. MA thesis, University of Massachusetts, Amherst, 2015. Available at: https://scholarworks.umass.edu/masters_theses_2/300. Accessed May 26, 2022.
Stoute A: Implementation of group interpersonal relationships through psychotherapy. J Psychol 30(1):145–156, 1950
Stoute BJ: Racial socialization and thwarted mentalization: psychoanalytic reflections from the lived experience of James Baldwin's America. American Imago 76(3):335–357, 2019
Stoute BJ: Black rage: an adaptation to the trauma of oppression. J Am Psychoanal Assoc 69(2):259–290, 2021 34039068
Strauss LC, Cross WE Jr: Transacting black identity: a two-week daily diary study, in Navigating the Future: Social Identity, Coping, and Life Tasks. Edited by Downey G, Eccles JS, Chatman CM. New York, Russell Sage Foundation, 2005, pp 67–95
Sue S, Fujino DC, Hu LT, et al: Community mental health services of ethnic minority groups: a test of the cultural responsiveness. J Consult Clin Psychol 59(4):533–540, 1991 1918557
Sue DW, Lin AI, Torino GC, et al: Racial microaggressions and difficult dialogues on race in the classroom. Cultur Divers Ethnic Minor Psychol 15(2):183–190, 2009 19364205
Thandeka: Learning to Be White: Money, Race, and God in America. New York: Continuum, 1999

Umaña-Taylor AJ, Quintana SM, Lee RM, et al: Ethnic and racial identity during adolescence and into young adulthood: an integrated conceptualization. Child Dev 85(1):21–39, 2014 24490890

Van Ausdale D, Feagin JR: The First R: How Children Learn Race and Racism. New York, Rowman & Littlefield, 2001

Vaughans K: African-American boys and adolescents under the shadow of slavery's legacy. The American Psychoanalyst 50(3), 2016

Vaughans K, Harris L: The police, Black and Hispanic boys: a dangerous inability to mentalize. J Infant Child Adolesc Psychother 15(3):171–178, 2016

Vaughans K, Spielberg W (eds): The Psychology of Black Boys and Adolescents. Santa Barbara, CA, Praeger, 2014

Volkan V: Large-group-psychology in its own right: large-group identity and peace-making. Internation Journal of Applied Psychoanalytic Studies 10(3):210–246, 2013

Washington H: Medical Apartheid: The Dark History of Medical Experimentation on Black Americans From Colonial Times to the Present. New York, Doubleday, 2006

Williams A, Steele JR: Examining children's implicit racial attitudes using exemplar and category-based measures. Child Dev 90(3):e322–e338, 2019 29115675

Withrich JS: Racial Awareness of Children in a Predominately White Area Compared to an Interracial Area. MS thesis, Logan, Utah State University, 1970. Available at: https://digitalcommons.usu.edu/etd/2447. Accessed May 22, 2022.

PART VIII

Gender and Sexualities in Psychotherapy

Section Editor: Jack Drescher, M.D.

In 2011, the Institute of Medicine (IOM) of the National Academies issued a groundbreaking report on the health (including mental health) of lesbian, gay, bisexual, and transgender (LGBT) people (Institute of Medicine 2011). The IOM organized the findings using a three-part life course framework: childhood/adolescence, early/middle adulthood, and later adulthood. Of concern to mental health practitioners are the following:

Childhood/Adolescence

- LGB youth are at increased risk for suicidal ideation and suicide attempts as well as depression. Small studies suggest that the same may be true for transgender youth.
- Rates of smoking, alcohol consumption, and substance use may be higher among LGB than heterosexual youth. Almost no research has examined substance use among transgender youth.
- The homeless youth population is composed of a disproportionate number of LGB youth. Some research suggests that young transgender women are also at significant risk for homelessness.
- LGBT youth report experiencing elevated levels of violence, victimization, and harassment compared with heterosexual and non-gender-variant youth.

Early/Middle Adulthood

- As a group, LGB adults appear to experience more mood and anxiety disorders, more depression, and an elevated risk for suicidal ideation and attempts com-

pared with heterosexual adults. Research based on smaller convenience samples suggests that elevated rates of suicidal ideation and attempts as well as depression exist among transgender adults; however, little research has examined the prevalence of mood and anxiety disorders in this population.
- LGBT people are frequently the targets of stigma, discrimination, and violence because of their sexual and gender minority status.
- LGB adults may have higher rates of smoking, alcohol use, and substance use than do heterosexual adults. Most research in this area has been conducted among women, with much less being known about gay and bisexual men. Limited research among transgender adults indicates that substance use is a concern for this population.

Later Adulthood

- There is some evidence that LGBT elders exhibit crisis competence (a concept reflecting resilience and perceived hardiness within older LGBT populations).
- LGBT elders experience stigma, discrimination, and violence across the life course.

The IOM report underscored a lack of research needed to address the health and mental health needs of LGBT people. As I write this introduction, now a decade after the report's release, it would be fair to say that the state of research on the needs of this heterogeneous patient population has increased somewhat but is still inadequate. Similarly, training of mental health professions about LGBTQ+ (Q standing for queer/questioning) mental health issues is given minimal attention, if any, in many training programs. Inadequate or perfunctory training about sexual minority populations is consistent with the overall approach to training about human sexuality in general.

On the positive side, increasing efforts are being made to be inclusive of sexual and gender minorities. The chapters in Part VIII (and a few others) in the second edition of this textbook exemplify the growing recognition that issues that come up in treatment of ethnic, racial, sexual, and gender minorities should be part of mainstream textbooks like this one.

Part VIII begins with Chapter 27, "Issues Arising in Psychotherapy With LGBTQ+ Patients," in which Matthew Fadus and I discuss the concept of minority stress and its relationship with mental health conditions. We then review specific issues that may arise with this heterogeneous patient population, including being in the closet, coming out of the closet, the psychotherapeutic search for "causes" of sexual orientation and gender identity, and therapist self-disclosure.

In Chapter 28, "Psychotherapy with Lesbians," Diana Moga and Romy Reading offer an overarching perspective that views patients as having multiple intersecting identities. They emphasize the need to understand how identities can be subject to ongoing development, fluidity, and interaction, depending on external social forces and internal psychodynamics. Their affirmative psychotherapy approach emphasizes a patient's self-acceptance, authenticity, and validation of sexual identity rather than trying to change her sexual desires, attractions, or preferences.

In Chapter 29, "Psychotherapy with Gay Men," Benjamin McCommon emphasizes how gay men come to treatment to work on issues similar to those of other patients. However, their presenting problems often may be influenced by important factors related to being gay: identity; self-esteem; and interpersonal functioning at work, in relationships with family, friends, and intimate partners, and in social and leisure time activities. A goal of psychotherapy is to help patients create an integrated identity. Doing so requires a thorough diagnostic evaluation that includes cultural sensitivity for social and cultural factors, including sexual orientation, behavior, and identity.

In Chapter 30, "Psychotherapy with Bisexual Patients," Barbara Marcus emphasizes the problems inherent in the invisibility of bisexual people. Bisexual individuals are far less often discussed or written about in the psychotherapy literature. In addition, they are often unrecognized, misunderstood, marginalized, or denigrated by others in the LGBTQ+ community. Dr. Marcus reviews a range of theoretical perspectives, both historical and contemporary, regarding bisexuality, including theories that challenge the very existence of bisexuality as an identity. She goes on to review the factors that lead to mental health disparities in this population and presents two detailed clinical vignettes of therapists working with cisgender (having a gender matching their sex assigned at birth) bisexual patients.

In the final chapter in this part, Chapter 31, "Psychotherapy with Trans and Gender Diverse People," Christopher McIntosh and Nicola Brown note that in addition to minority stress, transgender people face unique administrative and policy issues that impede critical aspects of daily living. These include costly and time-consuming barriers to obtaining gender-concordant identity documents, which can affect the ability to travel, seek employment, access education and health care, vote, secure stable housing, and collect social benefits. The authors underscore how transgender patients challenge therapist beliefs not just about gender, the body, and embodiment but about the nature of psychotherapeutic work and its power dynamics, its possibilities, and its limitations.

Reference

Institute of Medicine: The Health of Lesbian, Gay, Bisexual and Transgender People: Building a Foundation for Better Understanding. Washington, DC, National Academies Press, 2011

CHAPTER 27

Issues Arising in Psychotherapy With LGBTQ+ Patients

Jack Drescher, M.D.
Matthew Fadus, M.D.

In a multitude of ways, the practice of psychotherapy with lesbian, gay, bisexual, transgender, and queer/questioning (LGBTQ+) patients does not differ from treatments with heterosexual and cisgender (having a gender matching their sex assigned at birth) patients. LGBTQ+ patients, like everybody else, most commonly enter treatment needing to discuss and receive help in better understanding interpersonal relationships, as well as learning how to navigate stressors related to work, family, and social circumstances.

Although a patient's identity as a sexual or gender minority will undoubtedly come up during treatment, it is unlikely to be the only thing discussed. It bears underscoring that one aspect of a person's identity should never be conflated with the entire individual. A lesbian, gay, bisexual, or transgender identity is inevitably linked to multiple identities: child, parent, spouse, sibling, professional, employer, employee, congregant, patient, and/or citizen.

This chapter was published originally as Drescher J, Fadus M: "Issues Arising in Psychotherapy With Lesbian, Gay, Bisexual, and Transgender Patients." *FOCUS* 18(3):262–267, 2020. The chapter has been edited for consistency with the current publication, and we have taken out the continuing education questions that appeared at the end of the article.

Although an LGBTQ+ identity may not necessarily be the primary focus in many cases, its impact on the course of treatment should not be underestimated or overlooked. Some therapists may believe treating LGBTQ+ patients requires no specialized knowledge. "I treat my LGBTQ+ patients like everyone else" is a laudable attitude. However, it may overlook the fact that growing up lesbian, gay, bisexual, or transgender is a different cultural experience from growing up heterosexual and cisgender.

Specific issues invariably arise when a patient has lived their life as a sexual or gender minority. For example, LGBTQ+ patients often enter treatment following a long period of trying to make sense of feelings they have that are considered unacceptable to themselves and those around them. LGBTQ+ patients' adaptations may range across a spectrum that includes living openly within an LGBTQ+-friendly environment and belonging to communities where people must hide their identities from friends, family, and even themselves.

Consequently, when treating LGBTQ+ patients, it is worth outlining some specific issues that do not typically arise in the treatment of most heterosexual, cisgender patients. Additionally, concepts and considerations that arise in psychotherapy with LGBTQ+ patients can parallel issues that arise in psychotherapy with patients who belong to other stigmatized minority groups. After introducing the concept of minority stress, we go on to review specific issues that often arise with this heterogeneous patient population, which include being in the closet, coming out of the closet, the psychotherapeutic search for "causes" of sexual orientation and gender identity, and therapist self-disclosure.

Minority Stress

The LGBTQ+ community is not a homogeneous group. Members of the community represent a diversity of ethnicity, race, culture, and socioeconomic backgrounds. However, all of the members of the LGBTQ+ community are unified in that they belong to a stigmatized minority group. The *minority stress model* has shown that individuals in a minority group may be at a higher risk for mental health disorders as a result of being subjected to stigmatizing attitudes, discriminatory policies, and other social stressors that are imposed from a majority group. As a result, LGBTQ+ individuals, like other stigmatized minorities, may be subject to significant stress, prejudice, hostility, and expectations of rejection, which can all contribute to a considerable and disparate mental health burden (Meyer 2003).

Studies have shown that cumulative, chronic stress among LGBTQ+ individuals can lead to an increased risk of substance use disorders, depression, anxiety, suicide, self-harm, and many other mental health disorders (Gower et al. 2018; Hafeez et al. 2017; Morton et al. 2018). For example, compared with heterosexual and cisgender individuals, members of the LGBTQ+ community have more than a twofold increase in suicide attempts, and the risk for depression and anxiety disorders is almost double that of individuals who do not identify as LGBTQ+ (Institute of Medicine 2011; King et al. 2008). Substance use is also significantly higher in the LGBTQ+ community, with rates of illicit substance use (particularly cannabis, cocaine, methamphetamine, cigarettes, and opioids) twice as high among LGBTQ+ individuals (Medley et al. 2016).

Despite the significant mental health burden that many members of their community may experience, LGBTQ+ people often delay or forgo seeking treatment as a result of concerns of discrimination or previous mistreatment in a medical setting (Jaffee et al. 2016; Sabin et al. 2015; Samuels et al. 2018). They may specifically avoid mental health treatment as a result of the not-so-distant history of psychiatric pathologizing of LGBTQ+ identities and behaviors (Drescher 2010, 2015). Knowledge of the history of their profession's theorizing about LGBTQ+ individuals (see Drescher 2010) can help psychiatrists better understand the resentment and avoidance that LGBTQ+ patients may have toward mental health practitioners.

The Closet

> *"Closetedness" [is] a performance initiated as such by the speech act of a silence—not a particular silence, but a silence that accrues particularity by fits and starts, in relation to the discourse that surrounds and differentially constitutes it.*
>
> —Eve Kosofsky Sedgwick (1990)

It is not unusual in the developmental histories of LGBTQ+ patients to have experienced some period of difficulty acknowledging to others either their sexual orientation or their gender identity. Colloquially, this state of mind is referred to as "being in the closet," and those who hide their identities are referred to as "closeted."

Having to hide an aspect of one's identity in such a way is not a typical experience for those with heterosexual orientations or cisgender identities. The experience can be analogous to members of other stigmatized groups whose differences from the majority's public expressions are not immediately apparent. For example, persecuted religious minorities may be forced to practice their faith in secret, or individuals of mixed race or ethnicity may need to hide their family origins to "pass" as a member of a religious, racial, or ethnic majority.

However, there is an important difference between the latter minority groups and LGBTQ+ individuals. Members of most minority groups usually learn coping mechanisms to deal with the majority's prejudices from their families and communities. However, only relatively recently have the children who grow up to be LGBTQ+ received family support to deal with antihomosexual prejudices. All too often, their families of origin share the same prejudices as the heterosexual or cisgender majority. As one gay patient put it, "We are the only minority group born into the enemy camp" (Drescher 2001). Lending support to that observation is the fact that 30% of LGBTQ+ individuals are homeless, which is most often the result of being forced out of their home or feeling a need to run away from their home as a result of their sexual orientation and/or gender identity or expression (Choi et al. 2015).

Given the consequences of widespread negative attitudes toward LGBTQ+ individuals, it is not surprising that they may be unable to acknowledge to themselves, or reveal to others, any homoerotic feelings, attractions, or fantasies. Transgender individuals may experience a similar need to hide their gender dysphoria or any gender-nonconforming feelings or behaviors. An individual who finds such thoughts and feelings unacceptable not only may hide them from others, they may keep them out of conscious awareness to themselves in a dissociative manner (Bromberg 1994). Clinical presentations of being in the closet can vary in severity, from the less intense case of a young adult man considering the "possibility" that he might be gay to more severe manifestations in which any hint of same-sex feelings resides totally out of conscious awareness. By dissociating anxiety-provoking knowledge about the self, some individuals may live a whole double life without fully knowing it (Drescher 2001; Drescher and Byne 2017).

From a clinical perspective, it should be noted that keeping aspects of the self hidden or separated is often difficult and harmful. Hiding creates difficulties with, for example, accurately assessing other people's perceptions of oneself or recognizing one's own strengths. The impact of having to dissociate aspects of the self inevitably affects self-esteem, often making it difficult to recognize one's actual accomplishments as reflections of one's own abilities. Nevertheless, some individuals are able to maintain states of closetedness for long periods of time. Sometimes this is done for religious reasons; at other times it is due to an individual's personal choices, as in efforts to maintain a stable heterosexual, cisgender marriage.

Coming Out of the Closet

> *Gay people in the pre-war years, then, did not speak of coming out of what we call the "gay closet" but rather of coming out into what they called "homosexual society" or the "gay world," a world neither so small, nor so isolated, nor, often, so hidden as "closet" implies.*
>
> —George Chauncey (1994)

In contemporary usage, *coming out of the closet* means telling another person that one is lesbian, gay, or bisexual or transgender. A less commonly used term, but one with clinical significance is *coming out to oneself.* Patients often describe this as the first subjective experience of inner recognition. Coming out to oneself as lesbian, gay, or bisexual may precede any sexual contact or may occur in a sexual moment. Some describe the moment as a switch being turned on, "coming home,'" or "discovering who I really am." The experience can be charged with excitement, but at other times it is filled with trepidation. It is a realization that previously unacceptable feelings or desires are part of one's self. It is, in part, a verbal process of putting into words what were previously inarticulate feelings and ideas. Coming out of the closet may also be conceptualized as a recapturing of disavowed experiences. From a psychological perspective, it means a reduction in dissociation and the possibility of integrating previously unacceptable aspects of the self (Drescher 2001, 2012).

Coming out to oneself may be followed by coming out to others. Herdt and Boxer (1993) described coming out as a ritual process of passage requiring a lesbian, gay, or bisexual person to 1) unlearn principles of essentialist heterosexuality, 2) unlearn stereotypes of homosexuality, and 3) learn the ways of LGBTQ+ culture. In coming out, LGBTQ+ individuals must decide, perhaps daily, whether to reveal and to whom they will reveal. Consequently, coming out is a process that never ends. Further, such revelations are not always greeted in a welcoming manner. Fear of rejection often plays a significant role in an LGBTQ+ individual's decision about whom to tell or whether to come out. Further, a need to conceal their identity may be based on reasonable concerns, as in the case of LGBTQ+ individuals living and working in socially and politically conservative religious environments. Clinicians would be unwise to advise a patient to come out to anyone without knowing something about the attitudes and opinions of the intended recipient of a patient's revelation. Even with such knowledge, the therapist cannot always predict accurately the consequences on the relationship of those two people of making such a revelation.

Given the social stigma and the ubiquity of anti-LGBTQ+ attitudes, why come out at all? In most cases, coming out offers LGBTQ+ individuals the possibility of integrating a wider range of previously split-off affects, not just those having to do with sexuality and gender. Coming out can lead to a greater ease in knowing oneself and expressing oneself to others, which in turn can lead to an enormous enrichment of work and relationships. Such activities constitute a reasonable definition of mental health.

Outing

> *What came to be called outing—declaring closeted public figures to be gay—was…a by-product of a revolution [in which] everyone agreed that the closet was an ugly institution that had to be broken down.*
>
> —Michael Signorile (1993)

Outing refers to the involuntary revelation of an individual's LGBTQ+ identity by another party. There are some activists who believe that deliberately exposing a closeted LGBTQ+ person to potential personal or public humiliation is justifiable, particularly if the closeted person is a public figure who espouses anti-LGBTQ+ beliefs and supports anti-LGBTQ+ public policies. This has accounted for revelations of the LGBTQ+ identities of, among others, a conservative U.S. Congressman (Zernike and Goodnough 2006) and an influential megachurch pastor (Banerjee 2007). Sometimes outing is done as an act of revenge by vindictive acquaintances or spurned lovers. Blackmailers may threaten to out an individual for financial or political remuneration. Historically, some politicians have tried to discredit an opponent by exposing them as LGBTQ+ (Progress Queens 2014).

A severe dissociative split between any LGBTQ+ identity and internalized anti-LGBTQ+ attitudes may account for the mental gymnastics of politically and religiously conservative individuals, allowing them to live with such stark contradictions. However, such dissociation often serves as a defense against profound anxiety and shame. In the subjective experience of the outed individual, outing is experienced as a form of psychological violence.

The Search for Causes

Christ, how sick analysts must get of hearing how mommy and daddy made their darlin' into a fairy.

—Mart Crowley (1968)

It is not unusual for LGBTQ+ patients, when first beginning psychotherapy, to have a fantasy of "discovering" the causes of their sexual orientation or gender identity during the process. These fantasized beliefs are often enabled, sometimes even encouraged, by clinicians who believe that two people talking in a room have the necessary tools to discover the origins of either homosexual or transgender identities.

In reality, at present, the "causes" remain unknown (Bailey et al. 2016). This, however, does not stop and will probably never stop continued theorizing by either patients or therapists. However, it should be noted that a therapist's own theories about gender and sexuality can distract from therapeutic goals. Further, a patient's etiological theories, when offered, offer insights into both positive and negative attitudes they may assign, consciously or unconsciously, to their own sexual or gender identity.

It should be noted, in contrast, that heterosexual patients do not come seeking psychotherapeutic treatments to find out why they are "straight." Nor do nontransgender patients expect to learn from a therapist why they are cisgender. Nor are most therapists likely to even raise the question "Do you ever wonder why you are heterosexual?" or "Do you ever wonder why you are cisgender?" with patients. The presumptions are that heterosexuality and cisgender identities are nature's default setting.

Historically, however, it was not altogether unusual for heterosexual, cisgender therapists to bring up questions of etiology to their LGBTQ+ patients. Yet, if a therapist took the unusual step of doing so with heterosexual, cisgender patients, it is unlikely that those patients would be interested in pursuing such a line of inquiry—or paying a therapist for their "insights." Sigmund Freud (1905/1953) once remarked on the need to question the origins of heterosexuality, stating, "Thus from the point of view of psycho-analysis the exclusive sexual interest felt by men for women is also a problem that needs elucidating and is not a self-evident fact based upon an attraction that is ultimately of a chemical nature" (pp. 145–146). Yet, with a few exceptions (e.g., Chodorow 1992; Lewes 1988), psychoanalysts have not concerned themselves with the question nor have they typically offered treatment to find out why their patients are heterosexual or cisgender.

Why would some LGBTQ+ patients put up with such inquiries about the origins of their sexual identity or gender identity? One consequence of belonging to a stigmatized minority is the desire to find a narrative to explain one's "difference" from the majority. In the case of gay people, these etiological narratives take three forms: theories of normal variation, theories of pathology, and theories of immaturity (Drescher 2001, 2002). Transgender narratives define themselves either as normal variation or as pathology.

Theories of pathology first gained prominence in the nineteenth century, most prominently in Krafft-Ebing's (1886/1965) *Psychopathia Sexualis.* These theories define a homosexual or bisexual orientation or a transgender identity as psychopathological, a disease, or an abnormal condition that deviates from biologically predetermined heterosexual, cisgender development. These etiological theories are based on the following assumptions: 1) adult heterosexuality and being cisgender is the normal, nondiseased state; 2) deviations from conventional gender role expectations are symptoms of the disease; and 3) some external pathogenic agent has traumatized an individual, preventing them from becoming heterosexual or cisgender. The external event can occur prenatally or postnatally and may include intrauterine hormonal exposure, excessive mothering, insufficient fathering, seduction, or a decadent lifestyle.

Theories of normal variation regard homosexuality and transgender presentations as phenomena that occur naturally and that are not signs of illness or psychopathology. Left-handedness is often used as an analogy in these narratives. Today, being in the left-handed minority is not defined as illness, although it may have disadvantages. In the past, being left-handed did lead to social opprobrium; the word *sinister* is derived from a Latin root connoting the left side. And historically, left-handed children were often treated as if they were abnormal and were cured of their nonconforming behavior by forcing them to write right-handed. The research of Alfred Kinsey (Kinsey et al. 1948, 1953) played a significant role in the eventual dissemination of theories of normal variation of homosexuality among both professionals and the general public. Today, the belief that one is "born gay" or "born trans" is the most common theory of normal variation.

Theories of immaturity regarding homosexuality are found in psychoanalysis. Freud (1905/1953), for example, saw homosexuality as a developmental arrest or a psychosexual fixation. Immaturity theories are frequently confused with theories of pathology. However, an inability to mature is not necessarily the same thing as being ill. Whereas pathologizing theories treat homosexuality as deviant and abnormal, immaturity theories regard homosexuality as a normal step, ideally a passing phase, to be outgrown on the road to adult (hetero)sexuality. Harry Stack Sullivan (1953) hypothesized that children who ultimately became "homosexuals" as adults were members of the "out-group, if only with respect to so-called mutual masturbation and other presumably homosexual activity which went on in this group of boys as preadolescent pals" (p. 256). In maintaining that homosexuality could be a normal part of the heterosexual's own experience, theories of immaturity were more inclusive and compassionate than theories of pathology. They allowed for the possibility of an LGB person becoming sufficiently mature to become heterosexual, if motivated enough and with adequate adult (meaning heterosexual) guidance. However, etiological theories are not formulated in an objective vacuum. All of them contain underlying value judgments about the impact of being LGBTQ+ on the social order, an individual's worth within that order, or the relationship between being LGBTQ+ and the intent of a higher force (Drescher 2001, 2002). A higher force may include God, other deities, spiritual beings, nature, and even an anthropomorphized conceptualization of evolution. Among the key terms in the *morality tales* underlying etiological theories are social benefit and social harm, good and evil, health and illness, adaptive and maladaptive, holy and sinful, and mature and childish.

For patients, their own etiological theory is likely to have a personal meaning and an affective charge. A therapist who authoritatively claims knowledge of the definitive etiology of being lesbian, gay, bisexual, or transgender would have difficulty appreciating how etiological narratives serve as vehicles for other issues. For example, a gay man asking, "What is the cause of homosexuality?" may simply be asking, "Why do I feel different from everybody else?" It is only by recognizing the often irrational underpinnings of the psychotherapeutic search for origins that clinicians can shift the focus of treatment from trying to figure out *why* patients are LGBTQ+ to helping patients learn *how* to be LGBTQ+.

Therapist Self-Disclosure

> *The doctor should be opaque to his patients and, like a mirror, should show them nothing but what is shown to him.*
>
> —Sigmund Freud (1912/1958)

Today it is not unusual for LGBTQ+ patients to seek out LGBTQ+ therapists, nor is it unusual for LGBTQ+ therapists to come out to patients about their own sexual or gender identity. Richard Isay (1991) reported that the gay male patients he treated often sought him out as an openly gay psychoanalyst because they had concerns that heterosexual therapists might not treat them with appropriate empathy, respect, and neutrality.

One should not assume that because a therapist identifies as LGBTQ+ themself that they will inherently have greater insight into the issues that bring LGBTQ+ patients into treatment. For example, being LGBTQ+ is not a substitute for being trained to do psychotherapy or for undergoing a personal analysis. Further, the therapist's sexual or gender identity may not be the most meaningful way to gauge a therapy's efficacy. One does not need to be LGBTQ+ to treat LGBTQ+ patients any more than one needs a heterosexual and cisgender identity to treat heterosexual and cisgender patients. Psychotherapy's effectiveness is not necessarily determined by any presumed similarities between a patient and therapist. A better way to evaluate effectiveness is by how the similarities and differences between two people are handled in the therapeutic relationship.

Nevertheless, most heterosexual, cisgender therapists are not in the habit of declaring their sexual or gender identities. In a world that naturalizes their sexual and gender identities, many people are unaccustomed to the need for directly making such revelations. Most live in a world where everyone is considered heterosexual and cisgender until declared or labeled otherwise.

Historically, the question of whether therapists should disclose their own sexual or gender identities was rarely discussed for several reasons. These include the traditional psychoanalytic position that all therapists had to be heterosexual (Drescher 2008). If not, they had to pretend they were and hide their true sexual identities or risk professional ostracism and disgrace (Drescher and Merlino 2007; Isay 1996). This began to change toward the end of the twentieth century, which saw a growing literature by openly gay and lesbian therapists (Domenici and Lesser 1995; Isay 1996; Magee and Miller 1997; O'Connor and Ryan 1993; Schwartz 1998). The new century saw the emergence of openly transgender therapists (Hansbury 2005; Pula 2015).

There are practical reasons for therapists to eschew self-disclosure and keep the primary focus of a therapeutic encounter on a patient's inner world. For example, some patients may feel burdened by knowledge of their therapist's sexual or gender identity or other aspects of their personal life. Further, psychodynamic psychotherapy training programs, in teaching fledgling therapists how to set boundaries with patients, advise them to decline to offer any information about themselves while eliciting as much information as they can from their patients.

Coming out to patients is a form of self-disclosure. Whether one should do so is only a small part of the larger issue of therapist self-disclosure, a controversy dating back to technical disagreements between Freud and his close follower, Sándor Ferenczi (1949). For almost a century, the issue of self-disclosure has remained controversial primarily because of unexamined beliefs, ideologies, and allegiances to particular schools of thought. For example, little, if any, empirical evidence supports nondisclosure as a superior therapeutic technique when compared with self-disclosure. No studies showing head-to-head comparisons of the two approaches exist. Further, although withholding of information evokes therapeutic narratives from patients, so does disclosure. Transferences will develop whether or not a patient knows a therapist is LGBTQ+—or whether the patient knows anything else about the therapist, for that matter (Drescher 2013).

In considering self-disclosure with patients, one should consider whether the activity is of therapeutic value to the patient. On the other hand, one should also consider the possible harm of not disclosing. Any therapist, regardless of their own sexual identity or gender, should evaluate a patient's need for them to come out on an individual basis and be prepared to do so when necessary.

Key Points

- The practice of psychotherapy with LGBTQ+ patients does not necessarily differ from clinical work with heterosexual and cisgender patients. Nevertheless, specific issues may arise among sexual and gender minorities.
- Although the LGBTQ+ community is a heterogenous group, its members share the experience of being a stigmatized minority. According to the minority stress model, minority group members are at a higher risk for mental health disorders as a result of being subjected to stigmatizing attitudes, discriminatory policies, and other social stressors that are imposed from a majority group.
- LGBTQ+ patients often experience some period of difficulty acknowledging to others their sexual orientation or gender identity, a state of mind referred to as "being in the closet." Clinical presentations of being in the closet, a dissociative phenomenon, may vary in severity. The impact of having to hide can affect self-esteem.
- In coming out of the closet, LGBTQ+ individuals must decide on a daily basis whether to reveal and to whom they will reveal—it is a process that never ends.

- The "causes" of a person's sexual orientation or gender identity remain unknown. Two people having a conversation in a therapist's offices are discovering not "causes" but rather the meanings of a patient's sexual orientation or gender identity to the two of them.
- Theories of pathology define a homosexual or bisexual orientation or a transgender identity as psychopathological, a disease, or an abnormal condition that deviates from biologically predetermined heterosexual, cisgender development.
- Theories of normal variation regard homosexuality and transgender presentations as phenomena that occur naturally and that are not signs of illness or psychopathology. Left-handedness is often used as an analogy in these narratives.
- Theories of immaturity are found in psychoanalysis and regard homosexuality as a normal step, ideally a passing phase, to be outgrown on the road to adult (hetero)sexuality.
- Coming out to patients is a form of self-disclosure. Whether one should self-disclose to patients is a controversy dating back more than a century, primarily due to unexamined beliefs, ideology, and allegiances to particular schools of thought.

References

Bailey JM, Vasey PL, Diamond LM, et al: Sexual orientation, controversy and science. Psychol Sci Public Interest 17(2):45–101, 2016 27113562

Banerjee N: Ousted pastor "completely heterosexual." The New York Times, February 7, 2007. Available at: www.nytimes.com/2007/02/07/us/07haggard.html. Accessed November 3, 2019.

Bromberg P: "Speak! that I may see you": some reflections on dissociation, reality, and psychoanalytic listening. Psychoanal Dialogues 4(4):517–547, 1994

Chauncey G: Gay New York: Gender, Urban Culture and the Making of the Gay Male World, 1890–1940. New York, Basic Books, 1994

Chodorow NJ: Heterosexuality as a compromise formation: reflections on the psychoanalytic theory of sexual development. Psychoanalysis and Contemporary Thought 15(4):267–304, 1992

Choi SK, Wilson BDM, Shelton J, et al: Serving Our Youth 2015: The Needs and Experiences of Lesbian, Gay, Bisexual, Transgender, and Questioning Youth Experiencing Homelessness. Los Angeles, CA, Williams Institute With True Colors Fund, 2015

Crowley M: The Boys in the Band. New York, Samuel French, 1968

Domenici T, Lesser RC (eds): Disorienting Sexuality: Psychoanalytic Reappraisals of Sexual Identities. New York, Routledge, 1995

Drescher J: Psychoanalytic Therapy and the Gay Man. New York, Routledge, 2001

Drescher J: Causes and becauses: on etiological theories of homosexuality, in The Annual of Psychoanalysis, Vol 30: Rethinking Psychoanalysis and the Homosexualities. Edited by Winer JA, Anderson JW. New York, Routledge, 2002, pp 57–68

Drescher J: A history of homosexuality and organized psychoanalysis. J Am Acad Psychoanal Dyn Psychiatry 36(3):443–460, 2008 18834283

Drescher J: Queer diagnoses: parallels and contrasts in the history of homosexuality, gender variance, and the diagnostic and statistical manual. Arch Sex Behav 39(2):427–460, 2010 19838785

Drescher J: What's in your closet? in The LGBT Casebook. Edited by Levounis P, Drescher J, Barber ME. Washington, DC, American Psychiatric Press, 2012, pp 3–16
Drescher J: Ghosts in the consulting room: a discussion of Anson's "Ghosts in the Dressing Room." J Gay Lesbian Ment Health 17(1):112–120, 2013
Drescher J: Out of DSM: depathologizing homosexuality. Behav Sci (Basel) 5(4):565–575, 2015 26690228
Drescher J, Byne W: Homosexuality, gay and lesbian identities, and homosexual behavior, in Kaplan and Sadock's Comprehensive Textbook of Psychiatry, 10th Edition. Edited by Sadock BJ, Sadock VA, Ruiz P. Philadelphia, PA, Wolters Kluwer, 2017, pp 1982–2013
Drescher J, Merlino JP (eds): American Psychiatry and Homosexuality: An Oral History. New York, Routledge, 2007
Ferenczi S: Confusion of tongues between the adult and the child. Int J Psychoanal 30:225–230, 1949
Freud S: Three essays on the theory of sexuality, I: the sexual aberrations (1905), in Standard Edition of the Complete Psychological Works of Sigmund Freud, Vol 7. Translated and edited by Strachey J. London, Hogarth Press, 1953, pp 135–172
Freud S: Recommendations to physicians practising psycho-analysis (1912), in Standard Edition of the Complete Psychological Works of Sigmund Freud, Vol 12. Translated and edited by Strachey J. London, Hogarth Press, 1958, pp 109–120
Gower AL, Rider GN, McMorris BJ, et al: Bullying victimization among LGBTQ youth: current and future directions. Curr Sex Health Rep 10(4):246–254, 2018 31057341
Hafeez H, Zeshan M, Tahir MA, et al: Health care disparities among lesbian, gay, bisexual, and transgender youth: a literature review. Cureus 9(4):e1184, 2017 28638747
Hansbury G: Mourning the loss of the idealized self: a transsexual passage. Psychoanalytic Social Work 12(1):19–35, 2005
Herdt G, Boxer A: Children of Horizons: How Gay and Lesbian Teens are Leading a New Way Out of the Closet. Boston, MA, Beacon Press, 1993
Institute of Medicine: The Health of Lesbian, Gay, Bisexual and Transgender People: Building a Foundation for Better Understanding. Washington, DC, National Academies Press, 2011
Isay RA: The homosexual analyst: clinical considerations. Psychoanal Study Child 46:199–216, 1991 1788375
Isay RA: Becoming Gay: The Journey to Self-Acceptance. New York, Pantheon, 1996
Jaffee KD, Shires DA, Stroumsa D: Discrimination and delayed health care among transgender women and men. Med Care 54(11):1010–1016, 2016 27314263
King M, Semlyen J, Tai SS, et al: A systematic review of mental disorder, suicide, and deliberate self harm in lesbian, gay and bisexual people. BMC Psychiatry 8:70, 2008 18706118
Kinsey AC, Pomeroy WB, Martin CE: Sexual Behavior in the Human Male. Philadelphia, PA, WB Saunders, 1948
Kinsey A, Pomeroy W, Martin C, et al: Sexual Behavior in the Human Female. Philadelphia, PA, WB Saunders, 1953
Krafft-Ebing R: Psychopathia Sexualis (1886). Translated by Wedeck H. New York, Putnam, 1965
Lewes K: The Psychoanalytic Theory of Male Homosexuality. New York, Simon & Schuster, 1988
Magee M, Miller D: Lesbian Lives: Psychoanalytic Narratives Old and New. New York, Routledge, 1997
Medley G, Lipari R, Bose J, et al: Sexual orientation and estimates of adult substance use and mental health: results from the 2015 National Survey on Drug Use and Health. NSDUH Data Review, October 2016. Available at: www.samhsa.gov/data/sites/default/files/NSDUH-SexualOrientation-2015/NSDUH-SexualOrientation-2015/NSDUH-Sexual Orientation-2015.htm. Accessed November 3, 2019.
Meyer IH: Prejudice, social stress, and mental health in lesbian, gay, and bisexual populations: conceptual issues and research evidence. Psychol Bull 129(5):674–697, 2003 12956539
Morton MH, Dworsky A, Matjasko JL, et al: Prevalence and correlates of youth homelessness in the United States. J Adolesc Health 62(1):14–21, 2018 29153445

O'Connor N, Ryan J: Wild Desires and Mistaken Identities: Lesbianism and Psychoanalysis. New York, Columbia University, 1993
Progress Queens: Three decades later, "Vote For Cuomo, Not The Homo" mailer resurfaces. Progress Queens Transparency Reports, November 14, 2014. Available at: www.progressqueens.com/editorial/2014/11/15/three-decades-later-vote-for-cuomo-not-the-homo-mailer-resurfaces?rq=vote%20for%20cuomo%20not%20the%20homo. Accessed November 3, 2019.
Pula J: Understanding gender through the lens of transgender experience. Psychoanal Inq 35(8):809–822, 2015
Sabin JA, Riskind RG, Nosek BA: Health care providers' implicit and explicit attitudes toward lesbian women and gay men. Am J Public Health 105(9):1831–1841, 2015 26180976
Samuels EA, Tape C, Garber N, et al: "Sometimes you feel like the freak show": a qualitative assessment of emergency care experiences among transgender and gender-nonconforming patients. Ann Emerg Med 71(2):170–182.e1, 2018 28712604
Schwartz AE: Sexual Subjects: Lesbians, Gender, and Psychoanalysis. New York, Routledge, 1998
Sedgwick EK: Epistemology of the Closet. Los Angeles, University of California Press, 1990
Signorile M: Queer in America: Sex, the Media and the Closets of Power. New York, Random House, 1993
Sullivan HS: The Interpersonal Theory of Psychiatry. New York, Norton, 1953
Zernike K, Goodnough A: Lawmaker quits over messages sent to teenage pages. The New York Times, September 30, 2006. Available at: www.nytimes.com/2006/09/30/us/30foley.html. Accessed November 3, 2019.

CHAPTER 28

Psychotherapy With Lesbians

Diana E. Moga, M.D., Ph.D.
Romy A. Reading, Ph.D.

Like other sexual minority groups, the lesbian community is heterogeneous and represents a diversity of race, ethnicity, class, able-bodiedness, neurotypicality, and religious backgrounds. In addition, lesbians have varied gender identities, and not all are cisgender (having a gender matching their sex assigned at birth). In this chapter, we offer an overarching perspective, grounded in this premise of heterogeneity, that encourages clinicians to understand patients as having multiple intersecting identities. This view emphasizes understanding how identities are subject to ongoing development, fluidity, and interaction depending on external social forces and internal psychodynamics.

In this chapter we also offer an affirmative psychotherapy approach emphasizing patient self-acceptance, authenticity, and validation of sexual identity rather than attempting to change the patient's sexual desires, attractions, or preferences. Clinicians from a wide range of theoretical orientations, including behavioral, cognitive-behavioral, counseling, pastoral counseling, and psychodynamic approaches, have contributed to the development of affirmative psychotherapy for LGBTQ+ persons (Brown 2008; DeBord et al. 2017; Johnson 2012; Moradi and Budge 2018). Emphasis is given to strengthening an individual's internal resources and abilities to engage in sustaining interpersonal relationships, allowing them to develop resilience in the face of discrimination and stigma.

In this chapter we discuss applications of psychodynamic psychotherapy with recommendations to assist clinicians in developing effective therapeutic relationships with lesbian patients. These clinical recommendations and guidelines are broadly applicable to work with various sexual minority groups, but specific issues arising in treatment with lesbians—fertility, motherhood, and trauma—are highlighted. Additionally, psychodynamic perspectives on development and "coming out," guidelines regarding countertransference issues likely to arise with lesbian patients, and an affirming intersectional perspective that underscores the pathologizing effects of discrimination and stigma are emphasized. The central importance of a strong therapeutic alliance is highlighted because the clinical recommendations to be discussed can be helpful in fostering an affirming and positive therapeutic relationship.

Use of Terms

The use of appropriate terms in lesbian, gay, bisexual, transgender, queer, questioning, intersex, asexual, pansexual, and ally communities is ever-changing and fraught with political and emotional complexity (DeBord et al. 2017). No term is all-inclusive or wholly representative. Furthermore, today's terms likely will evolve with future generations. The changeability of terms related to sexual identity, sexuality, and gender identity can cause confusion and anxiety for clinicians. However, fluidity of language in this context is representative of and parallels the fluidity of sexuality.

Among sexual minority women (SMW), many view sexual identity as *fluid*, on a continuum, and oppose using specific labels (Wignall and Driscoll 2020). They view sexuality as subject to change, depending on time, context, and situation. For some, internalized stigma and reluctance to group-affiliate inhibit using self-identifying labels such as lesbian, gay, or queer. Others hold these terms with great conviction because they reinforce feelings of positive self-regard and self-expression.

Some commonly used terms include lesbian, gay, queer, mostly lesbian, and homoflexible. *Lesbian* is used to describe the female-identified person's sexual identity and experience of having a same-gender attraction. *Gay* is used interchangeably with lesbian by some individuals and may be the preferred term. One reason for this preference is the belief that it helps overcome the gender divide within sexual minority communities. *Queer* can be viewed as an umbrella term for sexual minorities and/or anyone who is not cisgender. It was initially used by the heterosexual majority as a pejorative, but political activists reclaimed this term after the 1969 explosion of the gay civil rights movement in the United States. It now carries political connotations and evokes nonnormative sexuality, gender, and/or politics. Although it is more commonly used by younger people, older generations may also self-refer with the term queer.

Mostly lesbian and *homoflexible* are increasingly popular terms used to describe an individual's experience of nonexclusive same-gender attraction. In one study examining the attitudes of individuals using these identifiers, investigators found that many feel these terms more accurately describe their experience and thus diminish feelings of inauthenticity (Wignall and Driscoll 2020). Useful sources for the latest information on identity terms are the websites of GLAAD and the Williams Institute.

Prevalence of Mental Health Issues in the Lesbian Population

Meyer's (2003) *minority stress model* posits an elevated risk for mental health issues due to stressors related to holding a minority identity. The concept of *insidious trauma*

(Root 1992) describes the trauma of ongoing daily encounters with stigma, oppression, objectification, prejudice, and othering that cause cumulative stress that result in negative effects on mental health. It is well documented that LGBTQ+ individuals exhibit an increased frequency of substance use disorders, depression, anxiety disorders, PTSD, suicidality, and self-harm (DeBord et al. 2017; Gower et al. 2018; Morton et al. 2018). In spite of an increase in civil and legal rights in the past decade, LGBTQ+ individuals still experience higher rates of interpersonal trauma, harassment, and stress related to stigma (DeBord et al. 2017).

Historically, most mental health prevalence studies grouped all sexual minorities into one population. Few studies exist exploring specific differences between lesbians and other populations. Nonetheless, a growing body of literature examining differences reports some consistent findings. For example, there is widespread consensus that gay women are at increased risk for alcohol abuse or dependence when compared with heterosexual women and bisexual women (Hughes et al. 2010; Lewis et al. 2019; Roberts et al. 2004). This is likely due to increased rates of depression, anxiety, and PTSD; greater exposure to discrimination; increased frequency of sexual abuse; and the higher frequency of socializing in bar settings. Additionally, consistent with findings concerning LGBTQ+ individuals more broadly, studies demonstrate that lesbians, when compared with heterosexual women, exhibit higher rates of PTSD, depression, anxiety, suicidality, and self-harm (Everett et al. 2019; Straub et al. 2018).

Multiple Marginalized Identities and Intersectionality

A dearth of research exists on mental health disparities among individuals with multiple marginalized identities. It is reasonable to hypothesize that effects of minority stress and insidious traumatization would be compounded in complex ways when individuals hold multiple marginalized identities with regard to gender, sexual identity, race, ethnicity, and able-bodiedness. In recent decades, *intersectional* methodologies and studies have increased exponentially (Dess et al. 2018; Shangani et al. 2020). A study by Shangani and colleagues (2020) demonstrated a complex intersection with regard to minority stress when examining race and socioeconomic status in SMW. Unsurprisingly, Black and Latinx SMW experienced greater stigma than did their white counterparts. Additionally, for Black and Latinx SMW, higher socioeconomic status was associated with higher stigma, whereas among white SMW it was associated with lower stigma.

In another study examining the intersection of race and gender nonconformity in SMW, Everett and colleagues (2019) demonstrated that gender nonconformity worked in opposite directions for white and Black or Latinx SMW in that greater gender nonconformity, specifically greater presentations of masculinity among white SMW, increased victimization and discrimination, whereas it decreased them for Black and Latinx SMW. These studies illustrate how an intersectional perspective can illuminate the complexity of ways in which differing combinations of discrimination and oppression interact and create effects that are not merely additive but result in distinct outcomes in which the whole is greater than the sum of its parts.

Intersectionality, rooted in the work of Black and Latinx feminist social activism, later migrated to academia. Law professor Kimberle Crenshaw (1989) first popularized the term, highlighting how the unique combination of racism and sexism is obscured when these two forms of discrimination are treated separately by the law. It is a framework for examining the matrix of *both* oppression and privilege that interact and mutually affect individuals and populations. An intersectional framework also takes into account the ways in which privilege and power present in a person's experience. The aforementioned studies by Dess et al. (2018), Everett et al. (2019), and Shangani et al. (2020) demonstrate that certain forms of privilege, such as high socioeconomic status, have differing effects depending on the intersection with race and ethnicity. The holistic and multivariate aspects of an intersectional framework of understanding align well with psychodynamic approaches that emphasize understanding of the individual as shaped and continuously influenced by internal dimensions of mind, as well as by interactions with the external world of people *and* systems.

Theoretical Overview of Developmental Considerations

Developmental theories of homosexuality have traditionally been pathologizing and reflected the values of their authors rather than scientific neutrality (Drescher 2002). Unfortunately, psychodynamic psychotherapists' thinking about adult sexuality remains heavily influenced, implicitly or not, by heteronormative (Warner 1991), phallocentric developmental models dating back to Freud. These models assume first that healthy, mature sexuality is heterosexual and second that there are only two genders, male and female, that "naturally" complement each other. When patients seek treatment to understand their sexuality, their choice of partners, or conflicts in their relationships and sex life, psychotherapeutic efforts to make connections to childhood can be tinged with such biases.

Having a wider range of developmental models can help clinicians imagine childhood experiences different from their own and increase empathy for patients' experiences. Updated models can also help clinicians and patients understand otherwise overwhelming or shame-filled experiences. Finally, they can clarify the role of childhood experience in current conflicts without the assumption that such conflicts led to a same-sex partner choice. Instead, all partner choices result from compromises among conflicting feelings and self-other representations stemming from experiences and identifications with early caregivers (Benjamin 1991; Chodorow 1992; Fast 1990).

In writing about the Oedipus complex, Freud (1905/1962) theorized that mature sexuality involves the genitals and the other sex; its goal is procreation. He described female sexual development as the little girl perceiving the little boy's penis and wondering why she does not have one, feeling herself to be lacking or "castrated" (Freud 1924/1962). The psychoanalytic canon maintained this view of female sexual development, conceptualizing female sexuality as based on absence rather than presence and as being inherently passive and submissive. Women who did not accept this state of affairs were said to suffer from "penis envy," turning disappointment into an identification with their fathers and a wish to possess a penis themselves. Lesbian women were thought to suffer from penis envy, to have masculine identifications with their fathers, and to be fixated at the oedipal stage of development—if not earlier.

Female psychoanalysts' writing and the entrance of feminist and queer theory into analytic discourse drastically changed psychodynamic understanding of female sexuality and eventually lesbian sexuality. Some theorists elaborated on the little girl's experiences of her own genitals—their interiority, their multiple areas of sensory pleasure—and specific developmental anxieties and conflicting feelings about her female body (Bernstein 1993; Elise 1997). Adult female sexuality shifted from being seen as passive and receptive to a highly diversified sexuality located all over the female body and allowing for multiple orgasms (Irigaray 1985). Women's sexuality could be a source of pride and showing off (Balsam 2008), a source of tomboyishness and physical prowess (Harris 2005), or a source of power and generativity (Balsam 2019), and it could be manifested in a wide array of erotic signatures: individual scripts that elicit erotic desire (Person 1980).

Developmental theories of sexuality have also undergone a sea change while retaining Freud's insight that the parent-child relationship is the template for future intimate love relationships. They describe a multitude of identificatory and complementary love bonds that children navigate with both parents, as well as with siblings, important caregivers, and the culture at large. These identifications and complementary roles form the templates of future partner choices and erotic signatures (Benjamin 1991; Fast 1990). For instance, Elise (2002) described the little girl's primary desire for her mother. Benjamin (1991) described how identification with a second parent, often the father, during rapprochement, is important for both boys and girls in their struggle to separate from their primary caregiver and locate their own agency and desire.

Writings by lesbian psychoanalysts illustrate what it may be like for lesbians to grow up, come out, fall in love, and raise children in a heteronormative world. These narratives include the young girl's intense emotional investment in her female friends and the shame about the intensity of her longing and rejection sensitivity; the adolescent girl's need to navigate confusion about her attractions in the face of internalized homophobia; and the lesbian woman's anxieties and conflicts about outing her relationship in daily life or when becoming a parent, given the assumption that she is straight (Magee and Miller 1997; O'Connor and Ryan 1993; Schwartz 1998, 2004; Vaughan 2007).

From this perspective, the goal of thinking about the role of development in patients' current conflicts is not to understand why they are gay. Rather, it is to help them understand how old childhood templates and internalized homophobia may be interfering with their current ability to love and to embrace their sexuality.

Coming Out

"Coming out" experiences for lesbians also vary. No typical scenario or single prescription exists for how, when, and why an individual might or should come out. Nonetheless, some important issues arise for gay women with regard to this process.

First, many SMW view sexual orientation and identity as fluid (Diamond 2008; Wignall and Driscoll 2020). Holding such a view can affect coming-out decisions because many SMW do not want to declare themselves to be gay or lesbian, feeling that the label is too fixed and confining. Consequently, some women prefer to self-identify as mostly lesbian or heteroflexible. Others may choose to define themselves as a person who experiments. In fact, women are more likely than men to accept experimentation as a normative part of sexual experience (Denes et al. 2020).

Although SMW may hold positive views regarding experimentation and fluidity, the role of internalized stigma and homophobia should not be disregarded. For many, there are reasonable concerns about coming out depending on how conservative the individual's immediate family and/or community environment is. Therefore, when advising a patient about coming out, clinicians should aim to fully understand the individual's perspective on fluidity and experimentation, as well as gather detailed information about the views on homosexuality of their communities and family. The latter is especially true when treating adolescents. If family and community are either overtly or covertly homophobic, coming out may increase the risk of experiencing discrimination, harassment, and violence in home and school environments (D'Augelli et al. 1998; Robohm et al. 2003). Careful assessment can help therapists make a determination about the degree to which internalized stigma and the individual's views on sexuality are affecting the process of coming out. Only then can a clinician wisely guide a patient toward a decision that will support positive mental health. Additionally, an intersectional framework can be extremely useful in this context because it aids in understanding the multiple dimensions of stigma and bias a person may be experiencing as well as illuminates an individual's potential sources of resilience and privilege.

Another important issue is what a patient imagines about the clinician's actual or perceived views on lesbian identity and sexuality. A patient may have reasonable concerns about critical judgments from the clinician given the extremely pathologizing history of mental health professions. In addition, a female-identified patient may feel uncertain about disclosing her sexual identity and/or sexual history to a male clinician, given the prevalence of men's sexual objectification of lesbians (Fredrickson and Roberts 1997; Szymanski et al. 2011). Careful exploration of patient attitudes and beliefs about the clinician's views can be helpful in overcoming possible anxieties and concerns, as long as the clinician is able to honestly self-reflect, identify, and modify any potentially detrimental biases.

General Psychodynamic Issues

Countertransference

The concept of countertransference has been extensively discussed and its definition widely debated in psychoanalytic literature. Here, countertransference is defined as the sum total of a therapist's thoughts, emotions, fantasies, and beliefs that emerge in reaction to the patient, the therapeutic relationship, and the overall treatment. This broad general definition of countertransference has clinical utility. In drawing on contemporary conceptualizations, it includes therapists' beliefs, biases, and understanding of sexual identity and other identity experiences, as well as their understanding of social systems of discrimination and power that affect patients' lives. It is important to highlight that countertransference reactions to a patient's sexual identity are not solely indicative of a specific patient's presentation but also reflect the therapist's own views, cultural background, and implicit and explicit biases.

One important bias that all individuals, regardless of sexual identity, can and do internalize is heteronormativity. Heteronormative assumptions can include, but are not limited to, a belief in monogamy as the standard for healthy relationships; how, when, and where one should find a sexual and/or relationship partner; how one engages in sex and with whom; and norms regarding how a "healthy" person should end a relationship. Both patients and therapists grapple with external and internal heteronormative biases. For patients, the conflict between these assumptions and the realities of how they love can generate a chronic and distinct form of stress (Meyer 2003). Clinicians can aid patients in unpacking these assumptions to reduce such stress. In order to do so, clinicians must identify their own biases to better understand if they are impeding a capacity for empathy and understanding. A clinical vignette illustrates some potential pitfalls of heteronormative bias.

Case Vignette 1

Ms. K, a 48-year-old cisgender Indian American female, self-identified as a lesbian, sought treatment in the context of ending a long-term relationship. She described the relationship as warm and supportive, yet she and her partner had not engaged in sexual activity for more than 5 years. Ms. K reported no longer experiencing feelings of attraction toward her partner. She began dating and having sex with other women in order to satisfy her unmet sexual and romantic needs. Ms. K also continued to share a home with her long-term partner and expected to do so for several months until they could "sort out the housing situation." Understandably, she was tormented by feelings of shame and guilt and would at times wonder, "Am I some kind of sociopath?" Of note, Ms. K described having supportive parents who accepted her sexual identity. She described her parents, who had immigrated to the United States from India in their 20s, as "quite modern."

In this vignette, numerous questions and assumptions immediately form about Ms. K's life. However, heteronormative judgments may interfere with gaining a deeper understanding of the particulars of her situation. For example, many psychodynamic theories about enmeshment are based on Western heteronormative values of individualism and self-sufficiency. In this case, the therapist was aware of holding a possible bias against interdependence or communality that could lead to viewing Ms. K's decision to continue living with her girlfriend as toxic enmeshment. Additionally, the therapist sensed that internalized heteronormative views were likely at play for Ms. K with regard to her shame and guilt. The therapist examined both her own and Ms. K's views in this regard in order to avoid aligning with the patient's self-loathing. Using an intersectional lens, the therapist was able to explore Ms. K's views about community and interdependence. Given that *both* Indian culture and certain subgroups of lesbian culture prize these values, it is quite normative to remain in a relationship with a partner after ending the romantic or sexual aspects of the relationship.

This vignette illustrates the importance of thoughtful self-examination when encountering what may on the surface seem like maladaptive behavioral patterns. Such self-examination can provoke anxiety. However, if it is approached with openness and understanding that mistakes can be made and then repaired, much can be gained from unpacking one's own heteronormative assumptions. This vignette also demonstrates another countertransference issue: at times, a clinician's desire to be culturally competent can cloud their ability to fully acknowledge and attend to patients' issues and pathology. In this clinical situation, the therapist was aware of the possibility of an overly strong desire to identify with the lesbian and Indian norms of interdependence. However, doing so would have thwarted the discovery of self-beliefs that the patient eventually expressed.

Over the course of several sessions, a detailed inquiry about Ms. K's self-critical question, "Am I some kind of a sociopath?" revealed a complex layer or beliefs. Ms. K gradually expressed that she did not believe she was capable of taking care of herself because she had never had "any independent women in my life as role models." Also, Ms. K expressed deeply embedded insecurity about her capacity to self-soothe when alone for extended periods of time.

Ms. K's self-beliefs might have remained unarticulated if the therapist had thought that the self-criticism had resulted only from internalized heteronormativity and social norms of individualism. When a patient's self-beliefs are examined from a both/and approach, it becomes evident that they emerge from a complex intersection of social, familial, and internal pressures and dynamics.

Fluidity

The Urban Dictionary (www.urbandictionary.com) defines *hasbian* as "1) a woman who used to be a lesbian but is now dating a man. Ellen Degeneres' former girlfriend." Anne Heche famously dated Ellen DeGeneres and then reportedly said she "closed that door" and dated only men. Kelly McGillis, the blonde bombshell in the film *Top Gun*, came out as a lesbian at age 52 after two long-term marriages to men. Multiple studies, most notably Diamond's (2008) longitudinal study, show that women's sexuality is more fluid than that of men.

Diamond (2008) followed 100 young women self-identified as heterosexual, bisexual, lesbian, or "unlabeled" with detailed interviews regarding their sexuality every 2 years over the span of 10 years. Between each 2-year span, one-fourth to one-third of the women changed identity labels. By the end of the 10-year period, two-thirds of women had changed identity labels at least once after the first interview. Furthermore, the women's arousal patterns did not necessarily align with their subjective self-identification. Heterosexual and lesbian women were equally likely to become genitally aroused (as measured by increased blood flow to the vaginal wall) by watching videos of two men having sex, two women having sex, or a man and a woman having sex (Chivers et al. 2004). Thus, most women have a physiological capacity for arousal to either gender but may have subjective desires toward one gender or the other or toward both. In Diamond's study, all women, including lesbians, reported physical attraction to men at some point in time. In Rust's (2000) survey of more than 300 adult lesbians, more than 40% had other-sex relationships at some point since identifying as lesbian.

In considering what is currently known about genetic, hormonal, psychological, and cultural influences on female sexuality, Diamond (2008) concluded that female sexuality can best be understood as a variability around a "malleable core" (quoting Rust's [2006] paper). Aware of this fluidity, many young people today refuse to label themselves altogether, perceiving their sexuality as an ongoing exploration. Thus, siloed categories may no longer adequately capture people's experiences, nor do they reflect current scientific knowledge.

Motherhood and Fertility

Advancements in reproductive technology and legal rights and the growing acceptance of gay relationships have contributed to a widening range of parenting options available to lesbian couples. Today, gay women can adopt as a couple, use anonymous or known sperm donors with intrauterine insemination, or use in vitro fertilization to implant either of the women's embryos in either womb. The latter allows both women to contribute biologically to their offspring, even if not strictly genetically. With the multitude of options available, the process of creating a family involves greater planning. With each potential decision (Anonymous sperm donor versus known friend or relative? Whose egg? Whose womb?) there is potential for creativity and increased intimacy but also for conflict.

Although data about children growing up with gay parents are consistently reassuring (American Psychiatric Association 2002; Biblarz and Stacey 2010; Gartrell et al. 2011; Perrin et al. 2004), lesbian couples still present with conscious and unconscious anxieties and conflicts around fertility and motherhood, often resulting from internalized homophobia. In her comprehensive paper on the topic, Vaughan (2007) outlined a number of concerns lesbian individuals and couples bring to treatment:

1. Fear of not being a fit parent by virtue of one's identity: Lesbians who may have been tomboys growing up or who are driven to prioritize their careers may worry they are not feminine enough to mother. Undergoing fertility treatments can also exacerbate anxieties about one's fertility that were already driven by internalized bias about one's gender as it relates to one's sexuality (i.e., "If I love women, am I too masculine to be fertile?").
2. Fear that a child's gender expression or sexual orientation may be adversely affected by having lesbian mothers: Some lesbians may worry that they are not feminine enough to model womanhood for a girl, may be concerned about not having a male role model to model manliness for a boy, or may fear creating gay children.
3. Concerns about picking a sperm donor: If picking a known sperm donor, what will be the psychological and legal ramifications of involving him in the child's life? What will this mean to the couple? If picking an anonymous sperm donor, should he be picked on the basis of heritage or desirable traits? What should the child be told about the donor? For a more detailed discussion, see Mamo (2004).
4. Issues of competition, envy, and/or exclusion within the couple: Questions may arise about who is the "real mother." The nonbiological mother may worry that she will not bond with the baby because of a lack of genetic inheritance. She may also worry she will be excluded and lose her partner's love. These worries are common with egg donation and surrogacy in general and are not exclusive to lesbian mothers. However, the added burden of internalized homophobia can contribute to excessive shame around the issue.

One goal of treatment is to facilitate awareness of heteronormative values and internalized homophobia leading to idealization of heterosexual couples as ideal parents.

Treatment may also involve mourning the inability to combine genetic material with the loved partner. Once internalized homophobia and heterosexism have been worked through, lesbian couples can recognize that difference does not have to be problematic. Once they can free themselves from the confines of cultural stereotypes about gender, they can embrace a wider range of complementary and identificatory relationships with their children and creatively respond to the gendered needs of the child.

Trauma

Recent studies show higher rates of childhood and adult sexual and physical abuse in lesbian women compared with heterosexual counterparts (Austin et al. 2008; Balsam et al. 2005; Corliss et al. 2002; Stoddard et al. 2009; Tjaden et al. 1999). The perpetrator of childhood sexual abuse is most often, as with heterosexual women, a male relative (Stoddard et al. 2009). Research suggests that the reasons for this disparity are complex and multifactorial. Studies of LGBTQ+ youth suggest that sexual minority youth who are out are more likely to be targeted for violence by parents, other adults, and peers (D'Augelli et al. 1998; Pilkington and D'Augelli 1995). Furthermore, lesbian women are more likely than heterosexual women to express gender atypicality in childhood, which has been linked to higher rates of abuse (Bailey and Zucker 1995; D'Augelli et al. 2006). Finally, sexual minority adolescents may be more likely to experience social isolation and internalized homophobia and thus may be more prone to engage in risky behaviors (Garofalo et al. 1998; Russell et al. 2002).

A history of childhood sexual abuse can also complicate women's feelings about their sexual identity and about how and when to come out and can affect their sexual behavior. Robohm et al. (2003) found a strong association between childhood sexual abuse and sexual risk taking in lesbian and bisexual young women. Nearly half the women reported that this history affected their feelings about their sexuality and coming out in diverse ways. Some women felt that it delayed their coming out because they felt disempowered, that they did not want to fit into the stereotype of an abused girl becoming a lesbian, or because they avoided sexual feelings altogether. Others reported that their history made them aware of sexuality at a younger age, which ultimately helped them to consolidate their sexual identity.

Clinicians need to be mindful of any possible history of abuse in lesbian patients, especially when symptoms of PTSD and/or substance abuse are present. However, such history may not be disclosed right away, and a good deal of trust and alliance usually is required before it is revealed. SMW may be especially wary of disclosing such a history, given the long-standing pathologizing of homosexuality in the mental health field and given the fear that clinicians may perceive childhood sexual abuse as the "cause" of their sexual orientation (Morris and Balsam 2003).

As with any traumatized patient, emphasis should be placed first on establishing alliance and trust; bolstering the patient's resilience; and addressing any symptoms of anxiety, depression, or substance abuse. Only then should the clinician deepen the work around trauma (unless the patient wants to discuss it earlier). Even then it is crucial to ensure that the patient is not retraumatized by telling her story. This can be accomplished by frequently checking in with the patient's present emotional state and attending to any anxiety and/or dissociation. It is especially important to check in well before the end of the session so that the patient is not left in a dysregulated state. Helping the patient ground herself by offering to do some mindfulness exercises together (e.g., progressive muscle relaxation, deep breathing) can be beneficial. Often just the act of checking in and the patient naming her emotions can bring her back to the present. Many women will volunteer their trauma stories once they develop sufficient trust in the therapist and feel emotionally ready to do so. In some cases, the traumatic incident(s) may be revealed at the very beginning of treatment in a dissociated or disavowed way. Only later, when the patient is ready to reexperience the trauma in her own shoes, will the full extent of the experience and its aftermath be revealed.

Case Vignette 2

Alice is a 23-year-old lesbian woman who presented for symptoms of depression since moving back home after graduating college. During the evaluation phase, when asked about traumatic events, she mentioned an incident with a woman who tried to "take advantage" of her online. The therapist was puzzled by the nature of the trauma but sensed that Alice was uncomfortable discussing these episodes any further. Treatment initially focused on her depression and individuation from her family's expectations. The therapist encouraged her to seek out social venues where she felt accepted, which improved her self-esteem.

After a year of treatment, Alice revealed that while feeling like a "social pariah" in elementary and middle school, she received significant attention from boys after puberty. She started dressing "girly" and drinking heavily in order to feel she fit in and to alleviate anxiety. At times, while she was drinking and having foreplay with male peers, they would push her to perform sexual acts that made her uncomfortable, leaving her feeling humiliated. However, the incident she considered traumatic occurred online with an older girl when Alice was 11. At the time, she had difficulty making female friends, feeling hypersensitive to their feedback. "I felt this desperate need to be with them, to have them like me." When an online friendship with an 18-year-old girl budded around a mutual interest in manga, Alice was thrilled. During a video chat, the other girl asked Alice to model a bathing suit and then gradually encouraged her to undress and masturbate.

It was important for the therapist to allow Alice to gradually unravel what that experience was like *for her*. Alice felt deeply humiliated: "Here I thought she actually liked me, found me interesting, but all she wanted was to use me." This episode was deeply shameful because it involved someone she idealized and whose affirmation and friendship she craved. This incident and the rejection by girlfriends she experienced as a child led to significant inhibition in her current romantic life. Discussing what her experience had been helped her realize that she was now an adult and no longer had to hide her desire, which in turn made her more confident and attractive to other women.

Conclusion

Good psychodynamic psychotherapy requires sensitivity, tact, and a willingness to look honestly at one's own countertransference, assumptions, and biases. These skills are crucial when treating any minority population, but especially so when treating lesbian women, who at a minimum are doubly discriminated against because of both their gender and sexual orientation and perhaps face further discrimination based on other identities as well. The result of effective psychodynamic psychotherapy is increased flexibility and freedom to create oneself as a unique individual along with the acceptance and mourning of realities that cannot be changed. However, "reality" is much more problematic when treating SMW, whose views of reality are often unconsciously constrained by internalized misogyny, racism, and homophobia.

To further complicate matters, clinicians' understanding of reality often includes blind spots as to what their patients may be dealing with based on unconscious assumptions and biases. Thus, to effectively work with SMW, clinicians need to be aware of, or at least be curious about, the intersection of discriminatory societal forces faced by their patients as well as the internalized biases that may be constraining the possibility of growth and change.

Efforts to understand the way societal forces interact with psychodynamic ones to affect sexuality may leave clinicians feeling perplexed. A limitation of *cultural competence* is its assumption that a static body of knowledge can be acquired and then used in treatment with patients. A more helpful concept is that of *cultural immersion*. Immersion involves learning as much as possible about patients' identities and backgrounds and then immersing oneself in the therapeutic experience with them while keeping in mind one's own background and biases. We must keep in mind that we are all subject to societal and unconscious forces and that we are all swimming in slightly different waters, and swimming against the tide requires resilience.

Key Points

- The lesbian community is heterogeneous and represents a diversity of race, ethnicity, gender identity, class, able-bodiedness, neurotypicality, and religious backgrounds. Lesbians may face added discrimination as a result of the intersection of gender and other minority statuses.
- Psychodynamic psychotherapy with a lesbian patient should be grounded in an affirmative approach. Its goal is to strengthen her internal resources and ability to engage in sustaining interpersonal relationships in order to bolster her resilience in the face of discrimination.
- Discrimination and stigma as well as gender atypicality increase lesbian youth's susceptibility to abuse. Clinicians should be mindful of the possibility of a trauma history or PTSD. It is strongly advised that the clinician first gain a patient's trust *and* support her decision-making about when and how to explore her traumatic history.
- The goal of conceptualizing a patient's developmental history is not to find out why she is gay but rather to understand how childhood templates and internalized homophobia may be interfering with her current ability to love and to embrace her sexuality.
- Sexual identity in women is not a choice, but it can be subject to a certain amount of fluidity around a malleable core throughout the life span.
- Coming out may increase the risk of experiencing discrimination, harassment, and violence in home and school environments for LGBTQ+ adoles-

cents; clinicians should take into account not only the patient's views but also those of her community, family, and primary supports.

- In treating lesbians, clinicians need to be aware of their heteronormative biases regarding what constitutes healthy sexuality and how, when, and where one finds a sexual and/or relationship partner.
- The goal of discussing fertility with lesbian patients or couples is to facilitate awareness of gender stereotypes and internalized homophobia, which can lead to idealizing heterosexual parents.

References

American Psychiatric Association: Adoption and co-parenting of children by same-sex couples: position statement. November 2002. Available at: www.clearinghouse.net/chDocs/public/PB-MI-0004-0016.pdf. Accessed October 3, 2020.

Austin SB, Jun HJ, Jackson B, et al: Disparities in child abuse victimization in lesbian, bisexual, and heterosexual women in the Nurses' Health Study II. J Womens Health (Larchmt) 17(4):597–606, 2008 18447763

Bailey JM, Zucker JJ: Childhood sex-typed behavior and sexual orientation: a conceptual analysis and quantitative review. Dev Psychol 31(1):43–55, 1995

Balsam KF, Rothblum ED, Beauchaine TP: Victimization over the life span: a comparison of lesbian, gay, bisexual, and heterosexual siblings. J Consult Clin Psychol 73(3):477–487, 2005 15982145

Balsam RH: Women showing off: notes on female exhibitionism. J Am Psychoanal Assoc 56(1):99–121, 2008 18430704

Balsam RH: On the natal body and its confusing place in mental life. J Am Psychoanal Assoc 67(1):15–36, 2019 30880415

Benjamin J: Father and daughter: identification with difference: a contribution to gender heterodoxy. Psychoanal Dialogues 1(3):277–299, 1991

Bernstein D: Female Identity Conflicts in Clinical Practice. Northvale, NJ, Jason Aronson, 1993

Biblarz TJ, Stacey J: How does the gender of parents matter? J Marriage Fam 72(1):3–22, 2010

Brown L: Cultural Competence in Trauma Therapy: Beyond the Flashback. Washington, DC, American Psychological Association, 2008

Chivers ML, Rieger G, Latty E, et al: A sex difference in the specificity of sexual arousal. Psychol Sci 15(11):736–744, 2004 15482445

Chodorow N: Heterosexuality as a compromise formation: reflections on the psychoanalytic theory of sexual development. Psychoanalysis and Contemporary Thought 15(3):267–304, 1992

Corliss HL, Cochran SD, Mays VM: Reports of parental maltreatment during childhood in a United States population-based survey of homosexual, bisexual, and heterosexual adults. Child Abuse Negl 26(11):1165–1178, 2002 12398854

Crenshaw K: Demarginalizing the intersection of race and sex: a Black feminist critique of antidiscrimination doctrine, feminist theory and antiracist politics. University of Chicago Legal Forum 1989(1):139–168, 1989

D'Augelli AR, Hershberger SL, Pilkington NW: Lesbian, gay, and bisexual youth and their families: disclosure of sexual orientation and its consequences. Am J Orthopsychiatry 68(3):361–371, discussion 372–375, 1998 9686289

D'Augelli AR, Grossman AH, Starks MT: Childhood gender atypicality, victimization, and PTSD among lesbian, gay, and bisexual youth. J Interpers Violence 21(11):1462–1482, 2006 17057162

DeBord KA, Bieschke KJ, Perez RM: Introduction: the pace of change and the challenge to keep up, in Handbook of Sexual Orientation and Gender Diversity in Psychotherapy and Coun-

seling, 3rd Edition. Edited by DeBord KA, Fischer AR, Bieschke KJ, et al. Washington, DC, American Psychological Association, 2017, pp 3–16
Denes A, Dillow MR, Lannutti PJ, et al: Acceptable experimentation? Investigating reasons for same-sex infidelity and women's anticipated responses to a male partner's hypothetical same-sex infidelity. Pers Individ Dif 160:109929, 2020
Dess NK, Marecek J, Bell LC: Gender, Sex, and Sexualities: Psychological Perspectives. New York, Oxford University Press, 2018
Diamond LM: Sexual Fluidity: Understanding Women's Love and Desire. Cambridge, MA, Harvard University Press, 2008
Drescher J: Causes and becauses: on etiological theories of homosexuality, in The Annual of Psychoanalysis, Vol 30: Rethinking Psychoanalysis and the Homosexualities. Edited by Winer JA, Anderson JW. New York, Routledge, 2002, pp 57–68
Elise D: Primary femininity, bisexuality, and the female ego ideal: a re-examination of female developmental theory. Psychoanal Q 66(3):489–517, 1997 9259037
Elise D: The primary maternal oedipal situation and female homoerotic desire. Psychoanal Inq 22(2):209–228, 2002
Everett BG, Steele SM, Matthews AK, et al: Gender, race, and minority stress among sexual minority women: an intersectional approach. Arch Sex Behav 48(5):1505–1517, 2019 31144216
Fast I: Aspects of early gender development: toward a reformulation. Psychoanal Psychol 7(suppl):105–117, 1990
Fredrickson BL, Roberts TA: Objectification theory: toward understanding women's lived experiences and mental health risks. Psychol Women Q 21(2):173–206, 1997
Freud S: Three essays on the theory of sexuality (1905) in Standard Edition of the Complete Psychological Works of Sigmund Freud, Vol 7. Translated and edited by Strachey J. London, Hogarth Press, 1962, pp 123–246
Freud S: The dissolution of the Oedipus complex (1924) in The Standard Edition of the Complete Psychological Works of Sigmund Freud, Vol 19. Translated and edited by Strachey J. London, Hogarth Press, 1962, pp 173–179
Garofalo R, Wolf RC, Kessel S, et al: The association between health risk behaviors and sexual orientation among a school-based sample of adolescents. Pediatrics 101(5):895–902, 1998 9565422
Gartrell NK, Bos HM, Goldberg NG: Adolescents of the U.S. National Longitudinal Lesbian Family Study: sexual orientation, sexual behavior, and sexual risk exposure. Arch Sex Behav 40(6):1199–1209, 2011 21057866
Gower AL, Forster M, Gloppen K, et al: School practices to foster LGBT-supportive climate: associations with adolescent bullying involvement. Prev Sci 19(6):813–821, 2018 29032496
Harris A: Gender as Soft Assembly. Hillsdale, NJ, Analytic Press, 2005, pp 131–154
Hughes T, Szalacha LA, McNair R: Substance abuse and mental health disparities: comparisons across sexual identity groups in a national sample of young Australian women. Soc Sci Med 71(4):824–831, 2010 20579794
Irigaray L: This sex which is not one, in This Sex Which Is Not One. Translated by Porter C, Burke C. Ithaca, NY, Cornell University Press, 1985, pp 23–33
Johnson SD: Gay affirmative psychotherapy with lesbian, gay, and bisexual individuals: implications for contemporary psychotherapy research. Am J Orthopsychiatry 82(4):516–522, 2012 23039349
Lewis RJ, Ehlke SJ, Shappie AT, et al: Health disparities among exclusively lesbian, mostly lesbian, and bisexual young women. LGBT Health 6(8):400–408, 2019 31738644
Magee M, Miller DC: Lesbian Lives: Psychoanalytic Narratives Old and New. Hillsdale, NJ, Analytic Press, 1997
Mamo L: The lesbian "Great American Sperm Hunt:" a sociological analysis of selecting donors and constructing relatedness, in Uncoupling Convention: Psychoanalytic Approaches to Same-Sex Couples and Families. Edited by D'Ercole A, Drescher J. New York, Routledge, 2004, pp 115–140
Meyer IH: Prejudice, social stress, and mental health in lesbian, gay, and bisexual populations: conceptual issues and research evidence. Psychol Bull 129(5):674–697, 2003 12956539

Moradi B, Budge SL: Engaging in LGBQ+ affirmative psychotherapies with all clients: defining themes and practices. J Clin Psychol 74(11):2028–2042, 2018 30238455
Morris JF, Balsam KF: Lesbian and bisexual women's experiences of victimization: mental health, revictimization, and sexual identity development. J Lesbian Stud 7(4):67–85, 2003 24831385
Morton MH, Dworsky A, Matjasko JL, et al: Prevalence and correlates of youth homelessness in the United States. J Adolesc Health 62(1):14–21, 2018 29153445
O'Connor N, Ryan J: Wild Desires and Mistaken Identities: Lesbianism and Psychoanalysis. New York, Columbia University, 1993
Perrin EC, Cohen KM, Gold M, et al: Gay and lesbian issues in pediatric health care. Curr Probl Pediatr Adolesc Health Care 34(10):355–398, 2004 15570222
Person ES: Sexuality as the mainstay of identity: psychoanalytic perspectives. Journal of Women in Culture and Society 5(4):605–630, 1980
Pilkington NW, D'Augelli AR: Victimization of lesbian, gay, and bisexual youth in community settings. J Community Psychol 23(1):34–56, 1995
Roberts SJ, Grindel CG, Patsdaughter CA, et al: Lesbian use and abuse of alcohol: results of the Boston Lesbian Health Project II. Subst Abus 25(4):1–9, 2004 16172087
Robohm JS, Litzenberger BW, Pearlman LA: Sexual abuse in lesbian and bisexual young women: associations with emotional/behavioral difficulties, feelings about sexuality, and the "coming out" process. J Lesbian Stud 7(4):31–47, 2003 24831383
Root MP: Reconstructing the impact of trauma on personality, in Personality and Psychopathology: Feminist Reappraisals. Edited by Brown LS, Ballou M. New York, Guilford, 1992, pp 229–265
Russell ST, Driscoll AK, Truong N: Adolescent same-sex romantic attractions and relationships: implications for substance use and abuse. Am J Public Health 92(2):198–202, 2002 11818291
Rust PC: Bisexuality: a contemporary paradox for women. J Soc Issues 56(2):205–221, 2000
Rust PC: Reparative science and social responsibility: the concept of a malleable core as theoretical challenge and psychological and psychological comfort, in Ex-Gay Research: Analyzing the Spitzer Study and Its Relation to Science, Religion, Politics, and Culture. Edited by Drescher J, Zucker KJ. Binghamton, NY, Haworth Press, 2006, pp 171–177
Schwartz AE: Sexual Subjects: Lesbians, Gender, and Psychoanalysis. New York, Routledge, 1998
Schwartz AE: Ozzie and Harriet are dead: new family narratives in a postmodern world, in Uncoupling Convention: Psychoanalytic Approaches to Same-Sex Couples and Families. Edited by D'Ercole A, Drescher J. New York, Routledge, 2004, pp 13–29
Shangani S, Gamarel KE, Ogunbajo A, et al: Intersectional minority stress disparities among sexual minority adults in the USA: the role of race/ethnicity and socioeconomic status. Cult Health Sex 22(4):398–412, 2020 31144598
Stoddard JP, Dibble SL, Fineman N: Sexual and physical abuse: a comparison between lesbians and their heterosexual sisters. J Homosex 56(4):407–420, 2009 19418332
Straub KT, McConnell AA, Messman-Moore TL: Internalized heterosexism and posttraumatic stress disorder symptoms: the mediating role of shame proneness among trauma-exposed sexual minority women. Psychol Sex Orientat Gend Divers 5(1):99–108, 2018
Szymanski DM, Moffitt LB, Carr ER: Sexual objectification of women: advances to theory and research. Couns Psychol 39:6–38, 2011
Tjaden P, Thoennes N, Allison CJ: Comparing violence over the life span in samples of same-sex and opposite-sex cohabitants. Violence Vict 14(4):413–425, 1999 10751048
Vaughan SC: Scrambled eggs: psychological meanings of new reproductive choices for lesbians. J Infant Child Adolesc Psychother 6(2):141–155, 2007
Warner M: Introduction: fear of a queer planet. Social Text 29:3–17, 1991
Wignall L, Driscoll H: Women's rationales and perspectives on "mostly" as a nonexclusive sexual identity label. Psychol Sex Orientat Gend Divers 7(3):366–374, 2020

CHAPTER 29

Psychotherapy With Gay Men

Benjamin McCommon, M.D.

Effective psychotherapy for LGBTQ+ patients, including gay men, begins with general psychotherapy practices applicable to all patients. Knowledge about gay men and specific adaptations of psychotherapy for them serve as a complement to, not a substitute for, education about general psychotherapeutic techniques. Gay men come to treatment wishing to work on issues similar to those of other patients, but their problems often are influenced by important factors related to being gay: identity; self-esteem; and interpersonal functioning at work, in relationships with family, friends, and intimate partners, and in social and leisure time activities. Forming or reinforcing an integrated identity that incorporates gay sexual orientation and identity with other aspects of life is likely to be an important goal of psychotherapy (Drescher 2001).

Gay men, like other LGBTQ+ people, are a diverse group made up of different races, ethnicities, religions, and socioeconomic classes. Nonetheless, the lifetime experiences of gay men are colored by the impact of *minority stress:* ingrained negative attitudes (or relative lack of positive attitudes) toward gay men from society at large leading to stigma and discrimination (Meyer 2003). The resulting prejudice and expectations of hostility and rejection contribute to negative self-assessments and negative attitudes toward oneself in relation to others. The pervasiveness of minority stress in gay men provides a reasonable explanation for increased risk of negative health outcomes, including certain psychiatric disorders.

Gay men, compared with the general population, have been found to have higher rates of mood and anxiety disorders, suicidal behaviors and self-harm, and substance use disorders (Bostwick et al. 2010; Lee et al. 2017; McCabe et al. 2009; Wang et al. 2014). Higher rates of some personality disorders have been found in a few studies, although results are inconsistent (Sandfort et al. 2014; Wang et al. 2014). The most common causes of depression in gay men are experiences of prejudice contributing to fear in public spaces; expectations of rejection and discrimination; concealment of identity (being closeted), including not sharing intimate relationships with family, friends, or work colleagues; and internalized antigay attitudes (also called internalized homophobia) (Lee et al. 2017; Meyer 2003). Standard approaches to these disorders, including psychotherapeutic treatments, may be insufficiently effective or ineffective for gay men if core aspects of identity and self-esteem are not also addressed.

Cultural Sensitivity in Evaluation and Treatment

All psychiatric treatment, including psychotherapy, begins with a thorough diagnostic evaluation that includes cultural sensitivity for social and cultural factors, which include sexual orientation, sexual behavior, and sexual identity (Silverman et al. 2015). Sexual orientation for gay men is a pattern of sexual, romantic, and emotional attraction toward men that usually, but not always, leads to sexual behaviors with other men. Sexual identity, calling oneself "gay," is the subjective acceptance of being gay and the sharing of this identity with others. Sexual orientation and sexual identity should be distinguished from gender identity and gender expression. For a gay man, his gender identity as a man is compatible with a range of possible masculine and feminine gender expressions. In particular, aspects of feminine gender expression are compatible with a gay man's gender identity as being male.

All patients, but especially LGBTQ+ patients, benefit from early establishment of an atmosphere during evaluation that is empathic, open, and nonjudgmental. This makes it more likely that patients will share potentially sensitive clinical information, including sexual feelings, behavior, orientation, and identity. This will help clinicians make accurate diagnoses, elicit patient goals, and consider effective treatment approaches. In addition, tactful inquiry, combined with assurances of confidentiality, which are especially important to many gay men, can begin to help establish a treatment alliance.

For instance, in obtaining initial personal information, rather than asking, "Are you married?" a clinician communicates more openness by asking, "Are you single or married, or do you have a partner?" Similarly, the psychotherapist can ask, "Do you live alone or with other people?" and then inquire about the patient's relationship with anyone else living with him. This approach may help with gay men worried about the possibility of antigay attitudes in their evaluating clinician; patients may be familiar with the extensive history in psychiatry and psychoanalysis of such attitudes.

Of course, cultural sensitivity to gay men requires a psychotherapist who, in accord with scientific evidence and an increasingly dominant legal and social consensus, does not view gay sexual orientation or identity as pathological or worthy of rejection. Clinicians who hold a different position or feel that they lack the necessary tact and knowledge to evaluate and treat gay men are advised to seek consultation or consider referral of gay male patients to appropriate clinicians.

Common Presenting Problems

Being gay can be an important factor in evaluation of problems that gay men might want to work on in psychotherapy. Examples include the following:

- Mood and anxiety symptoms emerging from rejection sensitivity
- Suicidal feelings in the context of coming out to oneself or others
- Problems with substances commonly available in the gay community, related to reliance on bars and clubs as places for socializing possibly contributing to higher rates of alcohol and substance use disorders
- Impulsive sexual behaviors possibly contributing to risk for HIV and other sexually transmitted diseases
- Self-esteem problems from internalized antigay attitudes or overt experiences of prejudice leading to difficulties in work and relationships
- Cultural factors such as a focus on appearance that may contribute to eating disorders or misuse of anabolic steroids

Patients may need education and help adhering to safer sex practices and accessing appropriate medical care, including HIV testing and consideration of preexposure prophylactic treatment (PrEP) to prevent HIV seroconversion. Gaps in safer sex practices are more likely with mood disorders and problems with alcohol and substance use, self-esteem, internalized antigay attitudes, and social support (Batchelder et al. 2017). Particular substances associated with lack of safer sex and HIV seroconversion in gay men are stimulants, methamphetamines (including crystal meth), cocaine (including "crack"), and volatile inhalants (including amyl nitrate or "poppers"); use of three or more substances is also associated with higher risk (Skeer et al. 2012). Issues related to HIV may include fear of being HIV positive, fear of having exposed others informing them, and shame about having engaged in risky sexual behaviors.

Psychosocial Functioning and Social Supports

A thorough evaluation is best achieved with information obtained from collateral sources, especially if safety issues are present. Patients may be more likely to share these sources with clinicians who have established trust and confidentiality. These additional sources might include other medical professionals, such as primary care physicians, same-sex partners or spouses, and family members who may or may not be aware of the patient's sexual orientation. Necessary collateral information, which might be needed to establish patient safety, can be obtained without necessarily disclosing a patient's sexual orientation or identity.

When collateral information is not immediately needed for safety reasons, clinicians should identify sources of support for their patients. Some patients may be estranged from their families of origin, may be in the closet at work, or may belong to unwelcoming religious or community organizations. They may depend more on alternative sources of support such as friends (sometimes referred to as *families of choice*), or they might lack support, in which case pursuing sources of support may be an important psychotherapy goal. This requires either a clinician already knowledgeable about sources of support for a gay male patient or a clinician willing to help a patient investigate and learn about such resources.

Evaluation of psychosocial functioning includes a history of past relationships and any children. For some gay men, this may include a history of past or current heterosexual marriages. Sexual orientation may be relevant to other psychosocial factors, such as work, education, housing, health care, financial status, and legal issues, including partner or spousal abuse or antigay violence.

Talking About Sex

Clinicians must strive to be comfortable asking and talking about sex. As with all aspects of psychotherapeutic technique, this requires practice. A good beginning for clinicians to use with all patients is "Please tell me about your sexual interests and behavior." If the patient responds, "What would you like to know?" that is a good start and provides an opening for the clinician to say, "I'm interested in your sexual desires and fantasies, who you're attracted to—men, women, or both—and your sexual behaviors, both now and in the past, including when you were growing up."

For a patient who is reticent or unwilling, a gentle push is appropriate: "A lot of people have difficulty talking about this. However, it is important information for me to get to know you and be able to help you with your problems. There are no wrong or bad answers here." Specific questions such as "How do you identify your sexual orientation and identity?" are likely to be helpful in communicating openness and eliciting full answers. Of course, the clinician should be prepared to explain what is meant by sexual orientation and sexual identity further, if asked.

Clinicians should be familiar with the range of common sexual practices of gay men, including penetrative and receptive anal sex ("topping" and "bottoming"), oral sex, and mutual masturbation. This is important not only for obtaining a sexual history but also to assess and provide education about safer sex, especially condom use during anal sex. Therapists may experience countertransference anxiety in asking about sexual practices that differ from their own. However, keeping to a goal of nonjudgmental inquiry without making assumptions about the sexual practices of any patient will likely reduce the chance of a patient experiencing shame in talking about sexual desires or behavior.

Gay Men and Choosing a Psychotherapist

Some gay patients may seek a gay male psychotherapist. They may have hope of being better understood by someone like themselves, or they might fear being shamed or pathologized by nongay clinicians. If a gay male therapist decides to self-disclose his sexual orientation to a patient, the therapist should include guidance that there are likely to be similarities and differences related to being gay and that the therapist will be interested in any ideas and feelings that the patient has about the therapist's sexual orientation. Gay male therapists may need to be especially vigilant to avoid imposing on their patients their own ideas of what it means to be gay. The patient's values and beliefs should be explored, and psychoeducation can be considered if these values and beliefs are overly harsh or distorted.

For therapists who are not gay themselves, sharing this difference nondefensively may be helpful to some gay patients. This can include sharing, if possible, the therapist's knowledge and experience in treating gay men with an expectation of being helpful. In general, whether the therapist has the same or a different sexual orientation as a patient, the therapist should communicate comfort and interest in difference and how this affects the patient's experience of treatment.

In any event, a psychotherapy's effectiveness is not necessarily determined by any presumed similarities between patient and therapist. A better way to evaluate its effectiveness is by how similarities and differences between two people are handled in the therapeutic relationship (Drescher 2001). Ultimately, each patient gets to decide whether he feels comfortable working with a particular therapist, and a therapist's openness, skill, and empathy are likely to be more important factors contributing to a successful treatment than the therapist's sexual orientation or identity.

Psychoeducation About Sexual Orientation

For patients with overt negative attitudes about being gay, which may include an idea that something wrong in their development "made them gay," psychoeducation about the origins of sexual orientation may be useful. In general, conveying an attitude of humility about the limits of scientific knowledge about all sexual orientations is appropriate. The main point to impart is that the origins of sexual orientation, for LGBTQ+ people and heterosexual and cisgender people alike, are unknown. The best scientific evidence suggests that both genetic and environmental factors play roles in the development of sexual orientation, but no evidence supports theories about the influence of parenting or social pressure on subsequent sexual orientation (Bailey et al. 2016).

Kinsey et al. (1948) conceptualized sexual orientation as existing on a continuum from heterosexual to homosexual. From that perspective, no sexual orientation is abnormal. Nor does a homosexual orientation represent an immature or arrested stage of development in which a person fails to achieve heterosexuality (Drescher 2002). Sexual orientation is most likely the culmination of a developmental process rather than the result of a "choice" made by an individual. A person with a same-sex sexual orientation can choose only whether or not to affirm these feelings as part of their sexual identity and sexual behavior.

The Closet and Coming Out

Gay men show a range of openness, from living fully openly as gay to living completely in the closet with difficulty acknowledging being gay even to themselves. Through dissociation, patients who feel identifying as gay is unacceptable may temporarily ward off full awareness of their sexual orientation. Some will be aware of their sexual orientation but take steps to keep it hidden from others, an understandable response to fears of social stigma and discrimination.

Minority stress may be acute for gay men because they may not have the support of their families in being openly gay, either during childhood and adolescence or in adulthood. Coming out to oneself, often the precursor to exploration and coming out to others, is usually harder without family or social support. Coming out to others may lead to problems with family, workplaces, housing, and finances. This, in turn, may lead to adjustment disorders, mood and anxiety disorders, and suicidal thoughts and behaviors. Risking rejection from others by coming out of the closet is likely to be made more tolerable to a patient if he can be helped beforehand to achieve a nonrejecting attitude toward himself. For each patient, respectful exploration of his particular situation and possible risks and benefits of coming out is appropriate.

This respectful approach extends to those patients with a same-sex sexual orientation who nonetheless decide not to pursue same-sex sexual activity or relationships. This may be for religious reasons or to preserve a heterosexual marriage. Informed consent for these men would include psychoeducation that purported treatments to change sexual orientation are ineffective and may be harmful, in addition to being illegal in many localities (Drescher et al. 2016); sexual orientation is unlikely to change with or without treatment, and possible harms of not acknowledging and living a life congruent with one's sexual orientation include certain psychiatric disorders and suicidality. In this case, one goal of psychotherapy might be to accept and mourn the loss involved in living a life that is incongruent with one's sexual orientation. This might help reduce symptomatology otherwise resulting from dissociation from one's sexual orientation and loss.

Developing a Gay Identity

Retrospective accounts confirm that there is no single pathway to developing a gay male identity. Many gay men have early memories of sexual attraction to other boys or men and feelings of difference. Many recall gender-atypical play, including a lack of interest in rough-and-tumble play with other boys and a preference for playing with girls and girl-identified toys. They may have been bullied for effeminate behaviors by family, peers, and even teachers. In the absence of any explanation having been offered by families or society at large for these differences, some questioned their male gender because of social expectations of "normal" feelings and behavior assigned to boys. Some find it hard to trust authority figures, including psychotherapists.

Even with today's progress in openness to LGBTQ+ sexual orientation and sexual identity, gay men often did not have opportunities to date as adolescents, missing early chances to learn about intimate relationships in the socially sanctioned way available to heterosexual adolescents. Instead, they may have been exposed to confusing and shaming sexual overstimulation (e.g., in the school locker room). Awareness of same-sex attraction and sexual orientation may have long preceded acceptance of a gay identity. Exploration and coming out may have been postponed to young adulthood or later, after the patient had achieved a greater degree of autonomy, therefore limiting the distress of disapproval of family and earlier social milieus.

For some older gay men, establishing a gay identity will have taken place during the early emergence of the AIDS epidemic in the 1980s and 1990s. Many will have lost partners, friends, and acquaintances, and some might never have fully reestablished support networks in subsequent years, resulting in isolation and aspects of complicated bereavement and PTSD.

Internalized Antigay Attitudes

Some patients accept intellectually that being gay is a normal variant of human sexuality but nonetheless describe an experience of being different in a negative way that leads to feelings of badness, shame, and inferiority. This can be conceptualized as a tendency toward self-rejection that is manifested less in thinking and more in feelings. This attitude may interfere, in overt and subtle ways, with a patient's being able to use knowledge about himself, including his desires and his values, to know what constitutes a full life for himself and take steps to pursue it.

As with all patients, gay male patients should be asked about their longer-term goals for relationships, parenthood, and work. Does a single gay man want to find a long-term intimate partner or spouse? Is he interested in children and parenting, including through adoption or surrogacy? What are his career goals? These questions can elicit below-the-surface negative attitudes about being gay that might lead a patient to feel that opportunities are unavailable to him. These attitudes are often informed by negative stereotypes that include the likely instability of gay relationships, the inherent unsuitability of gay men as parents, and the possibility that certain vocational opportunities should not be open to gay men. This creates a valuable opportunity for psychoeducation, and addressing such stereotyped concerns and beliefs could be an important psychotherapy goal.

Some gay men may present for psychotherapy treatment with little sense that being gay has any impact on their problems. They may see themselves as completely accepting of themselves, without any negative internalized attitudes, surrounded by communities of accepting families and friends. Some of these patients even may feel ashamed if they have any antigay feelings, as if they are letting down their community, and strive to put them out of mind. Psychotherapists would be wise to keep an open mind about the possibility of less overt manifestations of internalized antigay attitudes. Such attitudes might include devaluation of feminine-identified sexual or interpersonal characteristics, which may be seen as weak, submissive, or inferior. These attitudes may coexist with self-defeating attitudes toward dating and forming an intimate relationship or toward work and career advancement.

Double Minorities

Gay men who are members of another minority (e.g., those who are Black, Hispanic, Asian American, or Indigenous), are known as *double minorities* and are likely to have experienced even more minority stress than white gay men. Men who are double minorities require a clinician's cultural sensitivity to race and ethnicity and the effect of these factors on sexual orientation and identity. Experiences of antigay prejudice may be exacerbated by ethnic and racial prejudice, and minority stress has been shown to be correlated with depressive and anxiety symptoms in lesbian, gay, and bisexual people of color (Ramirez and Paz Galupo 2019).

Problems associated with being a double minority include lack of acceptance or overt antigay discrimination from families and racially or ethnically based supports, without help for bias related to race and ethnicity. Gay men who are double minorities also may experience lack of acceptance or overt racist discrimination from the dominant gay community of white men. Some may feel forced to choose one aspect of their identity over another in order to keep ties to a community for support, and psychotherapy may help with developing a positive, integrated identity of being both gay and a member of a racial or ethnic minority.

Adapting Psychotherapy Treatments for Use With Gay Men

Currently, few randomized studies of specific psychotherapy treatments targeting problems in gay men are available. Some evidence, including one randomized trial, exists for the use of lesbian, gay, and bisexual affirmative therapy in gay men (O'Shaughnessy and Speir 2018; Pachankis 2018; Pachankis et al. 2015). This treatment adapts cognitive-behavioral psychotherapy to target mood and anxiety symptoms, substance use, sexual compulsivity, and condomless anal sex (*barebacking*) in gay men. These symptoms and problematic behaviors are considered to be caused by rejection sensitivity, internalized antigay attitudes, and concealment, which are manifestations of minority stress. Adapted treatment principles include awareness and normalization of the adverse impact of minority stress, restructuring of minority stress cognitions, validation of the unique strengths of LGBTQ+ people and communities, and affirmation of healthy expressions of sexuality.

In the absence of a strong evidence base guiding psychotherapy practice specific to gay men, it is also reasonable to consider using principles developed originally for disorders that overlap with common problems encountered in psychotherapy with gay men. In particular, diagnostic criteria for borderline personality disorder (BPD) include several problems, at varying degrees of severity, relevant to many gay male patients. These include 1) identity problems and self-esteem difficulties; 2) mood reactivity related to interpersonal stressors, including perceived or actual rejection; 3) suicidal behavior and self-injury; 4) impulsive sexual behaviors and use of substances; and 5) dissociation.

I should emphasize clearly that use of these principles does not mean that gay men should be viewed as having BPD or any personality disorder. Nor does it mean that being gay itself represents a personality disorder, as espoused in the past by psychiatric and psychoanalytic authorities (Drescher 2001). Rather, the model of minority stress can be used to understand the development of certain overly rigid aspects of self and personality, influenced by experiences of social stigma and discrimination forming a patient's perceptions of himself and perceptions of others as well as interactions with others. Indeed, all patients, and all people, are likely to have aspects of personality rigidity, which becomes a focus of treatment only if it contributes to distressing symptoms or problems in functioning. The goal of psychotherapy treatment, if this is the case, is to introduce greater flexibility into conceptions of the self and others and interactions between the two, leading to reductions in symptoms and better interpersonal functioning. This provides a relevant model for approaching psychotherapy treatment in gay men.

Good psychiatric management (GPM) for BPD, for example, is an evidence-supported treatment that may be especially useful in adapting approaches to psychotherapy for gay men. Designed for generalist practitioners without extensive specialist training, GPM is built around a model of interpersonal hypersensitivity to rejection that guides a combination of psychodynamically informed supportive psychotherapy, case management, and limited medication management. Although GPM was originally targeted to psychiatrists, nonpsychiatrist clinicians can provide the psychotherapy and case management viewed as the core aspects of treatment in collaboration with a physician providing medication management if needed (Gunderson and Links 2014; McMain et al. 2009).

In the model of interpersonal hypersensitivity, patients are conceptualized as cycling among four self-states: 1) *connectedness* to others, which can develop into 2) *feeling threatened* with actual or perceived rejection; if reassurance or support are not forthcoming, this can lead to remaining self-states of 3) *aloneness* and 4) *despair*. When therapeutic support is given and experiences of rejection are ameliorated, connectedness can be quickly reestablished. However, because of persistent rejection sensitivity, a patient may cycle back to feeling threatened, feeling aloneness, and feeling despair. Treatment is targeted at helping patients interrupt this cycle by developing alternative ways of thinking about their self-states and engaging in behaviors more likely to elicit support from others. Setting goals for treatment is collaborative and emphasizes improvements in functioning, and symptom relief is expected to follow functional improvement. In patients with BPD, collaboration also is encouraged in addressing possible risky behaviors and suicidality ahead of time.

The model of interpersonal hypersensitivity to rejection may be particularly valuable to adapt for use in LGBTQ+ populations, where expectations of rejection from others are a common result of minority stress. GPM also has been adapted to address *intra*personal hypersensitivity to rejection, which can occur in patients with self-esteem and narcissistic problems who attack and reject themselves when they do not meet excessively high or distorted internal standards (Bernanke and McCommon 2018; McCommon 2018). I have found this approach useful for higher-functioning gay patients who do not have BPD but who hold antigay attitudes and are excessively self-rejecting about their sexual orientation. Patients can be helped to develop alternative ways of thinking about minority stress and their internalized antigay attitudes and to identify and pursue sources of support available to gay men. Use of case management principles, in which clinicians actively help patients with specific problems, may be useful for gay men with work, financial, medical, or legal issues related to the impact of minority stress.

Case Vignette

Mr. D, a gay man in his early 30s, works as a salesman in a large company. He sought evaluation from a psychiatrist because he wanted to "feel better" and "not be so stuck." He described intermittent depressive and anxiety symptoms and chronic bouts of low self-esteem. On a few occasions in the prior several years, Mr. D had had receptive anal intercourse without a condom after going home with someone from a bar. Usually, this occurred after having "three or four" drinks during the night.

Mr. D did not come out as gay until after college because he "did not feel comfortable being gay back then," although he had been aware of being "different" as a small boy and began noticing attraction to other boys before puberty. He remembers his parents making antigay remarks despite having some gay friends. He felt they disliked the way he spoke and his taste in clothes and music, which they associated with gayness, although nothing was ever explicitly said directly to him. Since coming out to his parents a few years earlier, Mr. D never talked about being gay or anyone he was dating when he visited them.

A year prior to his initial consultation, Mr. D tried an antidepressant prescribed by his primary care physician, but he stopped it after developing sexual side effects and was not interested in trying medication again. He and his psychiatrist agreed to weekly psychotherapy with goals of addressing his depressive and anxiety symptoms and his low self-esteem while working on his problems with dating and intimate relationships. Mr. D agreed to limit his alcohol intake to one or two drinks in an evening, which both he and his psychiatrist thought might help him adhere to safer sex practices. He also agreed to make an appointment with his primary care physician to discuss starting PrEP medication treatment.

During the first month of treatment, sessions were focused on an upcoming visit to his parents and whether Mr. D might bring up being gay with them. He now avoided alcohol entirely, which he was pleased about, but he felt that going out with friends was less fun and talked about disappointments with them. He had not pursued any dating opportunities, which he attributed to heavy work demands. He also had not scheduled an appointment with his primary care physician to discuss PrEP because of being "too busy."

Then Mr. D missed a session because of conflict with a work event. At the next session, appearing downcast and ashamed, he told the psychiatrist that two weekends earlier he had met a man at a bar. Although he had had only one drink that night, Mr. D had bottomed bareback. He was alarmed and scheduled an urgent appointment with his primary care physician. He was HIV-negative but tested positive for syphilis and received penicillin. He also started PrEP. Sounding somewhat discouraged, Mr. D said, "I really messed up."

The psychiatrist responded without judgment, and the following exchange occurred.

Psychiatrist: I'm not sure I look at it quite that way. Yes, you did have a real problem, and you did something about it. There is a genuine way in which you strive to act positively toward yourself, including by seeking out medical care and starting PrEP, and also by talking about this problem here with me.

(*Mr. D brightens somewhat.*)

Psychiatrist: Yet it does seem there is another way you can act, as if there is something in you that has an unprotective, destructive attitude toward yourself.

Mr. D: I know (*almost bewildered*). Why do I do that?

Psychiatrist: Do you have any ideas?

Mr. D: No, it doesn't make any sense. Why would I want to do that?

Psychiatrist: Well, I'm wondering whether you might have some negative attitudes toward pursuing other men or being gay. That's when risky behaviors seem to happen.

Mr. D (*answering quickly*): My family has never liked my being gay. I wish I weren't; it's so much harder.

Psychiatrist: Yes, those seem like ways to start having a negative attitude about being gay. But I wonder if something in you might be holding a negative view about yourself more strongly than you need to. If that's the case, that would be good for us to try to help you with.

Mr. D: How do we do that?

Psychiatrist: Well, what comes to your mind when you think about the possibility of strongly holding on to a negative view of yourself?

Mr. D (*after prolonged thought*): I don't know if this answers your question, and I'm embarrassed to talk about this. But I had a flash to how bad I feel when I'm prepping to bottom. It just seems so gross. I really enjoy being the bottom, but I feel bad too.

Psychiatrist: Yes, you look like you feel bad just telling me about it. Perhaps that could be something we consider working on together, trying to understand better your negative feelings about bottoming. Maybe that would not only help you enjoy sex more but also stay safe doing it.

> **Mr. D:** It feels weird to talk about feeling better about bottoming. I'm thinking, good luck with that, that's a hard one.
>
> **Psychiatrist:** It seems worth the effort.
>
> **Mr. D** (*with a bit of a skeptical smile*): OK, I guess we'll see.

This vignette illustrates principles of effective psychotherapy adapted for use with gay men. In the evaluation, the clinician elicits important information about sexual orientation, sexual identity, and sexual behavior. Mr. D's low self-esteem, in the context of lack of family support for his being gay, is plausibly related to his risky sexual behavior. Treatment goals extend beyond symptoms to target functioning in life, including dating. Safety planning is addressed with appropriate limits on alcohol and an agreement for the patient to investigate PrEP and could include case management strategies if needed. This initial safety plan supports Mr. D in taking appropriate action when he engages in risky behavior again during treatment. Having a reasonable approach to safety allows the focus in the session to include exploration of Mr. D's shame and low self-esteem.

The clinician first acknowledges positive behaviors that Mr. D is overlooking. This supports Mr. D's ability to *think* about his problematic behavior rather than simply use it to excoriate himself. In encouragement of exploration, the clinician offers as a hypothesis his idea of Mr. D's having antigay attitudes, which would not be forced if it did not resonate with Mr. D. The psychiatrist's comfort in talking about sex is demonstrated, fostering an atmosphere in which Mr. D also can talk about sex despite his discomfort. The clinician offers to help address Mr. D's low self-esteem and antigay attitudes and links them to improved sexual functioning and reduced risky behaviors, and Mr. D responds in a way that suggests a sufficient early treatment alliance.

Key Points

- Effective psychotherapy for gay men builds on psychotherapeutic practices applicable to all patients.
- Growing up gay has an impact on identity, self-esteem, and interpersonal functioning that is relevant to problems gay men work on in psychotherapy.
- Higher rates of some psychiatric disorders in gay men are likely a result of *minority stress* caused by negative attitudes in society leading to stigma and discrimination.
- Standard psychotherapeutic approaches may be insufficiently effective for gay men if core aspects of identity and self-esteem are not addressed.
- Cultural sensitivity to sexual orientation, sexual behavior, and sexual identity is necessary for effective diagnostic evaluation and establishment of a treatment alliance.
- Clinicians should be familiar with common sexual practices of gay men and be able to talk comfortably about sex.
- There are many pathways to developing a gay identity, and patients have different experiences of the closet and coming out.

- Internalized antigay attitudes are common in gay men, in both overt and subtle manifestations, and may lead to low self-esteem and difficulty in pursuing life opportunities.
- Psychoeducation can address patients' inaccurate ideas that being gay represents an abnormality of development and that psychotherapy can change sexual orientation.
- Gay men who are members of a racial or ethnic minority may experience additional prejudice and discrimination because they may face lack of acceptance in the white gay male community as well as their racial or ethnic community of origin.
- Evidence-supported psychotherapy treatments developed for general populations can be adapted for use with gay men, incorporating techniques that address rejection sensitivity and internalized antigay attitudes.

References

Bailey JM, Vasey PL, Diamond LM, et al: Sexual orientation, controversy and science. Psychol Sci Public Interest 17(2):45–101, 2016 27113562

Batchelder AW, Safren S, Mitchell AD, et al: Mental health in 2020 for men who have sex with men in the United States. Sex Health 14(1):59–71, 2017 28055823

Bernanke J, McCommon B: Training in good psychiatric management for borderline personality disorder in residency: an aide to learning supportive psychotherapy for challenging-to-treat patients. Psychodyn Psychiatry 46(2):181–200, 2018 29809114

Bostwick WB, Boyd CJ, Hughes TL, et al: Dimensions of sexual orientation and the prevalence of mood and anxiety disorders in the United States. Am J Public Health 100(3):468–475, 2010 19696380

Drescher J: Psychoanalytic Therapy and the Gay Man. New York, Routledge, 2001

Drescher J: Causes and becauses: on etiological theories of homosexuality, in The Annual of Psychoanalysis, Vol 30: Rethinking Psychoanalysis and the Homosexualities. Edited by Winer JA, Anderson JW. New York, Routledge, 2002, pp 57–68

Drescher J, Schwartz A, Casoy F, et al: The growing regulation of conversion therapy. J Med Regul 102(2):7–12, 2016 27754500

Gunderson JG, Links PS: Handbook of Good Psychiatric Management for Borderline Personality Disorder. Washington, DC, American Psychiatric Publishing, 2014

Kinsey AC, Pomeroy WB, Martin CE: Sexual Behavior in the Human Male. Philadelphia, PA, WB Saunders, 1948

Lee C, Oliffe JL, Kelly MT, et al: Depression and suicidality in gay men: implications for health care providers. Am J Men Health 11(4):910–919, 2017 28103765

McCabe SE, Hughes TL, Bostwick WB, et al: Sexual orientation, substance use behaviors and substance dependence in the United States. Addiction 104(8):1333–1345, 2009 19438839

McCommon B: Borderline personality disorder with narcissistic features, in Borderline Personality Disorder: A Case-Based Approach. Edited by Palmer B, Unruh B. Cham, Switzerland, Springer International, 2018, pp 151–162

McMain SF, Links PS, Gnam WH, et al: A randomized trial of dialectical behavior therapy versus general psychiatric management for borderline personality disorder. Am J Psychiatry 166(12):1365–1374, 2009 19755574

Meyer IH: Prejudice, social stress, and mental health in lesbian, gay, and bisexual populations: conceptual issues and research evidence. Psychol Bull 129(5):674–697, 2003 12956539

O'Shaughnessy T, Speir Z: The state of LGBQ affirmative therapy clinical research: a mixed-methods systematic synthesis. Psychol Sex Orientat Gend Divers 2018(5):82–98, 2018

Pachankis JE: The scientific pursuit of sexual and gender minority mental health treatments: toward evidence-based affirmative practice. Am Psychol 73(9):1207–1219, 2018 30525805
Pachankis JE, Hatzenbuehler ML, Rendina HJ, et al: LGB-affirmative cognitive-behavioral therapy for young adult gay and bisexual men: a randomized controlled trial of a transdiagnostic minority stress approach. J Consult Clin Psychol 83(5):875–889, 2015 26147563
Ramirez JL, Paz Galupo M: Multiple minority stress: the role of proximal and distal stress on mental health outcomes among lesbian, gay, and bisexual people of color. J Gay Lesbian Ment Health 23(2):145–167, 2019
Sandfort TGM, de Graaf R, Ten Have M, et al: Same-sex sexuality and psychiatric disorders in the second Netherlands Mental Health Survey and Incidence Study (NEMESIS-2). LGBT Health 1(4):292–301, 2014 26609539
Silverman JJ, Galanter M, Jackson-Triche M, et al: The American Psychiatric Association practice guidelines for the psychiatric evaluation of adults. Am J Psychiatry 172(8):798–802, 2015 26234607
Skeer MR, Mimiaga MJ, Mayer KH, et al: Patterns of substance use among a large urban cohort of HIV-infected men who have sex with men in primary care. AIDS Behav 16(3):676–689, 2012 21234666
Wang J, Dey M, Soldati L, et al: Psychiatric disorders, suicidality, and personality among young men by sexual orientation. Eur Psychiatry 29(8):514–522, 2014 24972914

CHAPTER 30

Psychotherapy With Bisexual Patients

Barbara F. Marcus, Ph.D.

Bisexuality remains the nearly silent B in the now well-known acronym LGBT. More recent additions, such as Q (queer), Q (questioning), I (intersex), and A (asexual), have only further obscured bisexuality's communality with other sexual and gender identities. Within scholarly sociopolitical, philosophy, religious, and literary discourse; across the biomedical and social sciences and their empirical research; and among psychological professional organizations, until very recently and largely still, bisexuality has stood in the shadows compared with its more visible and outspoken L, G, T, and Q siblings (Layton 2000; Young-Bruehl 2001).

Further, not only are bisexual individuals far less often discussed or written about, often they are unrecognized, misunderstood, marginalized, or overtly denigrated by those within the LGBTQ+ community (Ross et al. 2018). As Hemmings (2002) chronicles, the very legitimacy of bisexuality as an identity and practice has been challenged in scholarly theoretical discussions, as well as social and political discourse, for embracing a traditional binary view of gender seen by some as reactionary. Doubly stigmatized, bisexuals experience higher levels of minority stress than gay and lesbian individuals (Brewster and Moradi 2010; Feinstein et al. 2019).

According to Feinstein and Dyar (2017), *bisexuality* is "[t]he capacity for emotional, romantic, and/or physical attraction to more than one sex or gender," and "that capacity for attraction may or may not manifest itself in terms of sexual interaction" (quoted in American Psychiatric Association 2020, p. 1). Yoshino (2000) differentiates bisexual identity, bisexual attraction, and/or bisexual behavior, each of which can be considered independently. In this chapter, a bisexual person is defined as an individual, regardless of gender identity, whose erotic interests include both men and women.

Helpful Definitions

Terms used in this chapter can be defined as follows:

- *Sex* includes the biological attributes of being male or female.
- *Gender* includes the psychological and social qualities attributed to the sexes.
- *Sexual orientation* refers to a person's erotic response tendency or sexual attractions, be they directed toward individuals of the same sex (homosexual), the other sex (heterosexual), both sexes (bisexual), or neither (asexual). *Sexual identities*, or *sexual orientation identities*, constitute the subjective experiences and meanings of one's sexual desires or attractions (Drescher et al. 2019). In this chapter, *bisexuality* can refer to both a sexual identity and a sexual orientation.
- *Bigender* is defined as having a gender identity that is psychologically both male and female. Androgyny is an older synonym.
- *Biphobia* is dislike of or prejudice against bisexual people.

Theoretical Models

Early Psychoanalysis

Bisexuality was an essential element of Freud's (1937/1964) theory of mind, identity formation, neurosis, and relatedness. He believed in a universal psychic or constitutional bisexuality, in which every individual has a certain component of masculine (active) as well as feminine (passive) tendencies and the capacity for interpersonal connections with either or both sexes. Although he believed bisexual tendencies were universal, Freud also believed some people were constitutionally endowed with more of one tendency than the other. Later British and American theorists proposed revisions of his theory. However, Rado (1940), an important influence in the mid-twentieth century, refuted the existence of normal bisexuality. Whether or not mainstream analysts of that time accepted bisexuality conceptually, they believed that psychological maturity and mental health required the acquisition of a stable, fixed, heterosexual identity.

Contemporary Psychoanalysis

Contemporary psychoanalytic writers acknowledge the absence of a model for a normative or successful bisexual trajectory and recognize the possibility of healthy bisexual adaptations, and their work underscores the paucity of discussions about bisexuals in clinical literature. Elise (1998) argued that bisexuality "should illuminate the wish to *be* both sexes (self-representation) and to *have* both sexes" (p. 354) and that "the gendered psyche can lead to a split, and therefore constricted, experience of sexuality for the two sexes—one that can creatively expand, or not, depending on access to psychic bisexuality in the gendered mind of the self and of the partner" (p. 355). Her case material of a bisexual woman illustrates creative sexual variations that emerge when one has access to fluid gender identifications for both oneself and one's partners.

Layton (2000) noted that many contemporary psychoanalytic feminist contributions and scholarly cultural discourse both within and outside psychoanalysis have "no use for actual bisexuals; many of them, in fact, keep bisexuality firmly rooted in fantasy, not reality" (p. 43). While noting rare exceptions, regarding approaches to bisexuality within recent psychoanalytic writing, she concluded, "In general, however, the psychoanalytic literature neither discusses bisexuality as an identity nor legitimates, except in fantasy and transference, fluid object choice. And so contemporary psychoanalysis is one of the discourses that renders the practice of bisexual sexuality invisible" (p. 44). She faults most models of bisexuality for failing to consider the subjective experience of bisexual desires and its actual practice. When bisexual desires or object choices are considered, they are often viewed pejoratively, as the "narcissistic wish to have everything" (p. 50) or as unresolved conflicts (Roughton 2001).

Young-Bruehl (2001) was among the first to identify the persistent problematic conflation of bisexuality as gender identity with bisexual choices of partner. "In my view, understanding of the bisexualities would be deepened considerably by recognizing that the most underestimated and thus understudied of the three Freudian bisexuality domains—sex, gender, kind of object choice—[i]s the last where the emphasis has always fallen on the choice not the object" (pp. 201–202). Her case vignettes of two female patients and one male patient exemplify the difficulties that individuals with bisexual inclinations face in developing a positive bisexual identity.

Roughton (2001) traced the evolution of his own understanding of homosexuality and bisexuality by illustrating earlier "unrecognized heterosexist assumptions" imposed on his therapeutic efforts with four male patients. His case histories provide a window into different expressions of bisexuality and their unique life courses. Drescher (2007) argued for a shift away from questions of causation and toward helping patients understand what their same-sex feelings mean. His critiques of etiological theories of homosexuality (Drescher 2002) are equally applicable to assumptions implicit in models of bisexuality. Blechner (2016) noted that countertransference obstacles were common in treating patients with unusual presentations of gender and sexuality, to avoid detailed inquiry, and an overreliance on early history as explanatory of their gender or sexual variance. Gulati and Pauley (2019) commented on the stubbornness of culturally embedded heteronormative prescriptions: "A more embracing vision of bisexuality would seek to 'hold' rather than enact, the grief and anxiety associated with the development of myriad diverse personal patterns" (p. 97).

Modern Empirical Research: The Twentieth Century to the Present

Sexology Research

The work of Kinsey and colleagues (Kinsey et al. 1948, 1953) placed bisexuality along a normal continuum of sexuality. Their typology of sexuality, although based almost entirely on overt sexual behavior, regarded a bisexual orientation and its various forms of expression as normal variations within a broader spectrum of sexual behavior. Their model viewed sexuality as existing along a seven-point continuum from exclusively heterosexual (Kinsey 0) to exclusively homosexual (Kinsey 6), with "equally heterosexual and homosexual" (Kinsey 3), that is, bisexual, occupying the midpoint. In their extensive cross-cultural study, Ford and Beach (1951) found that bisexual behavior was common across the 191 cultures studied.

Klein (1978) critiqued Kinsey's scale for not taking into account the ways in which sexual orientation, or its variety of expressions, might change over the course of a lifetime. He proposed four ways of categorizing bisexuality:

1. Historical—past bisexual activity in someone currently monosexual (meaning only heterosexual or only homosexual)
2. Transitional—having been bisexual for a time-limited phase of life during which one was transitioning from heterosexuality to homosexuality or vice versa
3. Concurrent—having both homosexual and heterosexual partnerships at the same time (i.e., triadic bisexuality)
4. Sequential—having several phases of exclusive monosexuality in which one's partner is sometimes male and sometimes female.

Prevalence

Methodological limitations make the actual prevalence of bisexuality difficult to gauge and likely to be underestimated (Ross et al. 2018; Swan and Habibi 2018). First, bisexuality is defined differently across studies. Further, studies typically either do not differentiate exclusively homosexual from bisexual persons or group LGBTQ+ individuals under the broad heading of sexual minorities.

Copen et al. (2016) reported that bisexual and other plurisexual (i.e., attracted to people of more than one sex or gender) individuals make up the largest proportion of sexual minority individuals in the United States. They also reported that 3.9% of the adult population in the United States self-identify as bisexual (5.5% of females, 2% of males). Kann et al.'s (2011) report on bisexuality cited about double these percentages for U.S. high school students. When using a measure of bisexual attraction in a large representative sample of Australian adults, Richters et al. (2014) estimated a greater prevalence of 10% (14.2% of females, 5.8% of males). Although data show that more women than men identify as bisexual, it is unclear whether the reports reflect actual differences rather than other factors such as inherent biases in research methods, participants' differing internalized biases, or patterns of concealment of women and men.

Disparities in Mental Health

Research devoted to the study of bisexuals' mental health has been disproportionately small (Ross et al. 2018; Swan and Habibi 2018). More recently, however, bisexuality has received more attention. Literature reviews, meta-analyses, and research studies have revealed that bisexuals are at increased risk for poor mental health and substance abuse compared with heterosexuals (Conron et al. 2010; Feinstein and Dyar 2017; Pompili et al. 2014). In their systematic literature review, Pompili et al. (2014) concluded that despite wide variations in samples and methods, people with a bisexual orientation were at higher risk of psychological distress and poor mental health when compared with either homosexuals or heterosexuals and were at greater risk than heterosexuals of both substance abuse and suicidality.

When compared with monosexuals (gay men, lesbian women, and heterosexuals), bisexuals showed elevated risks for both overall mental health problems and suicidality (Bauer et al. 2016; Conron et al. 2010; Pakula et al. 2016). Ross et al. (2010) found consistently higher rates of anxiety and depression among bisexuals as compared with heterosexuals and higher or equivalent rates as compared with lesbian and gay individuals.

Although research that differentiates groups by both gender and sexual orientation are relatively few in contrast with those that group LGB data, studies that have been conducted found differences between subgroups. Bisexual women were found to have substantially greater risk of mood and anxiety disorders and poorer mental health than their lesbian or female heterosexual counterparts (Bostwick et al. 2010; Feinstein and Dyar 2017; Kerr et al. 2013). Conron et al.'s (2010) analysis of aggregated survey data found that bisexual women were 21 times more likely than heterosexual women to have considered suicide in the prior year. Behaviorally, bisexual females have shown higher rates of substance use and dependence than monosexual women (Feinstein and Dyar 2017). Women bisexuals are also twice as likely than lesbian women to report eating disorders (Koh and Ross 2006).

In research examining males grouped by their sexual orientation, men with bisexual behavior or attractions had poorer mental health than did monosexual men (Bostwick et al. 2010). Bisexual-identified men, like gay-identified men, have a greater likelihood of mood and anxiety disorders (Brennan et al. 2010; Feinstein and Dyar 2017) and higher rates of alcohol or drug dependence than do heterosexual men (Feinstein and Dyar 2017). In reporting on research that differentiated the dimensions of identity, attraction, and behavior of sexual orientation, Feinstein and Dyar's (2017) review found higher rates of substance dependence for behaviorally bisexual men than for behaviorally gay men but similar rates for men self-identified as bisexual or gay. Results of a study by Brennan et al. (2010) showed a higher prevalence of both lifetime suicidality and of ever having seriously considered suicide among bisexual men as compared with monosexual men. In comparison with heterosexual men, both bisexual and gay men have shown an especially high lifetime risk of suicide attempts (King et al. 2008).

Taylor et al.'s (2020) study, a large online survey of Australian adults, systematically examined distinctions according to Yoshino's (2000) three dimensions of bisexuality: bisexual identity, bisexual attraction, and bisexual behavior. Individuals with a bisexual identity were found to be more likely to experience psychological distress than those who reported bisexual attractions or bisexual behavior.

Causes of Mental Health Disparities

Invisibility

One aspect of bisexuality's invisibility is disbelief in its very existence, often reflected in the frequent assumption that bisexual people are "really gay" (Yost and Thomas 2012). Questioning the legitimacy of a bisexual orientation in women has typically taken the form of either doubts about its stability or a belief that bisexuality in women reflects a greater capacity for and/or acceptance of sexual fluidity in women as compared with men. Diamond (2008), for example, argued that the distinction between lesbianism and bisexuality is a matter of degree rather than kind.

Contributing to the invisibility of bisexuality, bisexual individuals, both male and female, are less likely to disclose their sexual orientation than are gay men or lesbian women (Balsam and Mohr 2007; Dyar et al. 2015; Lewis et al. 2009; Mohr et al. 2017; Pachankis et al. 2020). Negativity among lesbian and gay individuals, although lesser than among heterosexuals, contributes to greater challenges to coming out as bisexual as compared with coming out as gay or lesbian (Friedman et al. 2014).

Stigma and Victimization

Some researchers believe that the existence of greater mental health issues among bisexuals is primarily due to societal stigma and its internalization by bisexuals (Feinstein et al. 2019; Meyer 2003)—that bisexuality is a stigmatized identity leading first to fear of discrimination and rejection and then to more concealment or more selective self-disclosure (Jones and King 2014; Kase and Mohr 2020). In several studies, bisexual individuals reported significantly more discrimination from the heterosexual community in comparison with the gay or lesbian community (Friedman et al. 2014; Roberts et al. 2015) and reported that they encounter negative stereotypes from potential and actual partners (Armstrong and Reissing 2014; Bostwick and Hequembourg 2014; Hequembourg and Brallier 2009; Ross et al. 2010). In their comprehensive survey of intimate partner violence and sexual orientation, Walters et al. (2013) concluded that bisexual women had a significantly higher prevalence of nearly all forms of intimate partner violence when compared with monosexual women. Among males, bisexual men encountered more frequent intimate partner violence (other than rape) than did heterosexual men.

Bisexuals are more often subjected to microaggressions (Flanders 2015; Ross et al. 2010) and victimization (Katz-Wise and Hyde 2012; Sweet and Welles 2012; Walters et al. 2013). Bisexuals have more often experienced childhood sexual abuse than both homosexuals and heterosexuals (Sweet and Welles 2012). Katz-Wise and Hyde (2012) found that whereas lesbian, gay, and bisexual individuals were victimized more often than heterosexuals, bisexuals were somewhat more frequently the victims of certain types of aggression, particularly violent threats, physical assault, and weapons assault than either lesbian or gay subjects. Friedman et al. (2011) found that male bisexuals were more likely than heterosexual males to experience physical abuse or nonconsensual sex in childhood and to have a much higher incidence of both threat or injury with a weapon. They were also more likely than homosexual males to be subjected to bullying. Bisexual men and women were more likely than gay men or lesbians to report a history of sexual assault or coercion. Both male and female bisexuals were more likely than either gay men or lesbians to report a history of rape (Balsam et al. 2005). In a study comparing women according to their sexual orientation, bisexual females were at greater risk of rape or sexual violence compared with both heterosexual and lesbian women (Walters et al. 2013).

Minority Stress

Minority stress (Meyer 2003) describes the range of interpersonal, social, and systemic stressors to which LGBTQ+ individuals are subjected. Relative to other sexual orientations, bisexual individuals encounter greater prejudice and discrimination from both heterosexuals and gay or lesbian individuals (Brewster and Moradi 2010). Compared with their gay and lesbian peers, bisexual individuals encounter greater barriers to health care (Conron et al. 2010), may seek mental health services less often, and are more likely to find the services received less useful. Research shows that bisexuals often feel marginalized or excluded, even within the gay and lesbian community, resulting in lessened feelings of belonging, and that they have greater difficulty finding bisexual communities (Dyar et al. 2015; Feinstein and Dyar 2017; Hayfield et al. 2014; Hequembourg and Brallier 2009). Some studies find that bisexuals' sexual identities are less central to their overall identities than are gay men and lesbian women's sexual identities (Dyar et al. 2015), especially among racial and ethnic minorities, who may be additionally stigmatized (Akerlund and Cheung 2000).

Case Examples

Case Example 1

Initial Assessment

Ms. E was a middle-aged attorney, self-described bisexual, and divorced mother of adult fraternal twins when she entered treatment with Dr. A to help with an increase in her lifelong struggles with anxiety and depression. Although her marriage had been a happy one for the first decade, the recent divorce from her husband of more than 20 years felt like it was "a long time in coming." After some "postdivorce manic-type flings" with both men and women, she felt dispirited about her relational future and had taken a pause from seeking another life partner. She explained, "I don't know what I am looking for and whether the gender of my partner matters—or should matter. I guess I'm still stuck in the binary. Unlike my younger years, I worry about what other people will think."

As a child, Ms. E was a tomboy who imagined herself an FBI agent, presenting incognito as male. She loved engaging in all forms of athletic play with boys and was ushered into their circle by her older brother. "I played football games, had rock-skimming contests, and built model cars." However, she also loved playing with her baby doll, dressing up in her mother's high heels and feather boas, and doing handcrafts with female friends. She recognized she was different from her peers in crossing stereotypical gender lines, and she thought of this proudly, as a measure of her broader range and superior talents.

Her brother had been the "golden boy," much admired, who in his teenage years began showing signs of what later emerged as psychotic illness. In later years, after Ms. E garnered her parents' pride and her brother's resentment about her successes, they grew apart.

Beginning in early adolescence, Ms. E was aware of attractions to both boys and girls. Her masturbatory fantasies involved both, often together in some sort of scrum or wrestling match that led to clothes being torn asunder and a mélange of bodies being caressed or entered in ways without knowing where one body ended and another began.

Ms. E's conscious awareness of romantic interest in women began with "a serious crush" on a middle school teacher, a vivacious, ostensibly heterosexual single woman who took a special interest in helping Amy develop her nascent musical talent. Amy became aware of a "stirring, down there" that became actualized in sexual explorations with her female best friend. At the same time, she was also "head over heels" in love with Bruce Springsteen, a crush that evolved into her earliest heterosexual romance with a slightly older boy. In early high school she dated mostly boys and one girl, but then settled into a "steady relationship" with a girl that spanned the remainder of high school.

In college, early on Ms. E dated mostly women, occasionally a man, but then had a 2-year relationship with a young man. She met her husband-to-be, James, an attorney a few years her senior, at a summer clerkship during law school. They began dating once she graduated and then married after she established herself professionally.

Dr. A asked Ms. E if the tragic course of her relationship with her brother paralleled the trajectory of her marriage—a thrilling relationship with an admired older man, her success in the wake of his disappointing career, then his withdrawal from her. She burst into tears, suddenly aware of the unconscious role her sadness and guilt over her brother's deterioration had played in her retreat from her depressed husband.

James had accepted her bisexual past, expressing appreciation of her openness to playful sexual experimentation. Their erotic connection was thrilling to her, a fluid, sensual, and adventurous exploration of the many possibilities for pleasure that allowed her to express a wide range of wishes for initiative, surrender, penetrating and being penetrated, and trying on various personae. She mused, "Kind of like being undercover, like the secret agent I fantasized about becoming when I was a kid."

Ms. E had fraternal twins, and motherhood had been and continued to be enormously fulfilling. She felt fortunate for the opportunity to parent both a son and a daughter whose commonalities and differences she enjoyed. She relished bringing to child-rearing what she called "her androgynous sensibilities."

However, creative marital sex play became gradually more restricted and routinized. When Ms. E's efforts to renew her sexual bond with her husband failed, she lamented what ultimately was "a seemingly mutual waning in both sexual and emotional intimacy." With the children grown and on their own, she became increasingly aware of wanting more out of the second half of her life. After a year of couple therapy, she and James divorced amicably and maintained a distant but cordial relationship.

Course of Treatment

The mourning of Ms. E's marriage and its impact on her children was the primary focus for the first year of a 4-year therapy. Ms. E struggled to come to terms with feelings of failure and loneliness and fears of aging alone. She was hesitant at first, but a new way of life began to emerge, and her professional and social life was reinvigorated. She resumed dating both men and women and found that affectionate connections were easier with women, whereas sexual excitement was easier with men. Dr. A wondered aloud whether Ms. E's relationships with men were colored by her failed marriage or reflected her fears of stigmatization. Ms. E considered both dating alternatives with curiosity, suggesting a more analytic approach: "Let's keep both hypotheses open and interrogate them together."

After a year of uninspiring dating experiences, Ms. E and Dr. A had the following conversation:

Ms. E: I still find closeness easier with a woman. Women's boundaries are less strenuously defended, more porous. Men seem to have to assert themselves to defend their masculine prerogatives. But sex with men is more, I don't know, edgy. Maybe it's their physical strength or size. Or is this just some sexist holdover? Is an emotional bond more important in later adulthood, or is that just succumbing to old age, like maybe you have to just give up on having a sex life?

Dr. A: Essentially, your relationship with James was a bisexual one; it transcended your genders. Now you fear having to sacrifice your bisexual self as penance for having wanted *too* much, as though you failed because you wanted it all—the prerogatives of men as well as women and to be with a partner who could also inhabit both.

Ms. E (*sobbing*): Yes, someone who embodies both and can play creatively with any or all of the possibilities for giving and receiving pleasure whether gendered or not. Maybe I won't give up on that quite yet.

In the third year of treatment, Ms. E began an exciting romantic relationship with an older widower, Paul, an educated and cosmopolitan man. Sexually, he was more aggressive than she had been accustomed to, but he could be tender as well. She felt freer to be more expressive of her own desires than previously. Their relationship continued to deepen until hitting a "speed bump" when Paul became aware of not having fully mourned his wife and shared his sense of disloyalty in falling in love with another woman. He announced wanting to take a hiatus from their relationship. Ms. E was heartbroken.

In therapy, Ms. E revisited her divorce, wondering again whether she was to blame for the marriage's demise—unable to re-enliven her deadened husband. Several months were spent exploring ways she had withdrawn from him and become more invested in her career and their children—a posture that at the time she felt had been reactive to his growing distance from her. In retrospect, she considered that perhaps she had taken his emotional flatness too personally and had not recognized his withdrawal as a sign of depression.

Ms. E also realized that she had always been more motivated to please James sexually and was less attuned to her own pleasure. "I enjoyed our sensual connection, but often I didn't come when we made love. I told myself that reaching an orgasm wasn't that important to me. Paul was more patient. He wanted very much for me to be satisfied."

While keeping in touch with Paul, Ms. E began dating Marie. She felt happy and safe with "my sista-from-another-motha," and the sex was "great." But when Paul expressed a wish to resume their relationship, Ms. E struggled. Was he really able to love another woman? Could she invest in a relationship with a man again? Could she tolerate hurting Marie?

Dr. A remained neutral about whom Ms. E should choose while questioning her conflicts that centered on concerns about her own self-assertion and guilt about its consequences. They reflected again on Ms. E's now-conscious belief that she had caused her brother's psychological collapse. She felt that she and Paul had the potential for a fuller, richer relationship. After working through their separation, his need to mourn his wife, and her need to accept her role in the demise of her marriage, she felt confident they could weather future relationship storms.

As Ms. E's treatment approached termination, although her concerns about the social consequences of her bisexuality had largely receded, that subject once again returned to the conversation. She reflected back on her journey:

> **Ms. E:** I guess I'd describe myself as a bisexual who is homosocial and heteroerotic. But who cares about labels? At the end of the day, it's not about choosing the preferred genitals of a partner—all of them are quite wonderful. To me, it boils down to the individual and the relationship between two very unique and particular people. I just hope that Paul and I can explore new things and share an erotic, enduring attachment. I don't think that's too much to ask.

Case Commentary

Dr. A never questioned Ms. E's long-standing self-definition as bisexual. She was respectful of her patient's early history of androgynous interests as enhancing her stable and confident sense of self, understood as important sources of strength, pride, and pleasure. Nor did Dr. A seek to explain Ms. E's history of relationships with men and women as a developmental arrest, instead recognizing her concerns that stigma might be greater later in life.

Ms. E's marital difficulties were not attributed to her bisexuality. Instead, her dual sexual desires were explored as part of a complex picture. Dr. A conveyed a nonjudgmental attitude toward Ms. E's interest in a wide variety of sexual activities. Her struggles were understood as organized around survivor guilt for having become favored over her brother and succeeding beyond her once-heralded older brother, who declined into severe mental illness. Another therapeutic focus was appreciation for midlife challenges that Ms. E's divorce posed as she sought to reconstitute her life and to overcome discouragement about pursuing new relationships.

Ms. E was allowed to work through and mourn the end of her marriage and to accept her own role in the problems and their roots in her personal history. In revisiting her bisexual desires, she was able to reaffirm her bisexual identity, address ways that issues of aging interfaced with her feelings about sexual self-image, and make relational choices that felt true to both lifelong dearly held values and enduring aspirations as well as the new challenges and opportunities of later life.

Case Example 2

Initial Assessment

Mr. R, a single man in his 30s, had begun wondering about his sexual orientation in college. For much of his adolescence and adult life, he had been sexually involved only with women. Although these heterosexual relationships were gratifying, he had become aware of attractions to men when watching heterosexual pornography. During the assessment, Mr. R said that a former girlfriend had anally penetrated him with a sex toy, giving rise to the idea he was "probably gay." However, he had not acted on his attractions to men until recently.

In the 2 years prior to initiating therapy, Mr. R developed a few platonic friendships with gay men and engaged in occasional "hook-ups" with men, usually after going to a gay bar or meeting men online. He was disappointed that these were only one-night stands, although he was aware that the thought of pursuing a fuller gay relationship made him apprehensive. In order to overcome his anxiety and feelings of disgust and self-recrimination, he engaged in sex with men only when inebriated. Mr. R saw his aversions to his homosexual attractions and practices as hurdles he hoped to overcome while continuing to enjoy sexual relations with women. He presented with an unremitting self-criticism over his indecision about his sexual identity.

Course of Treatment

Dr. B, noting Mr. R's extreme anxiety and the obsessional quality of his thoughts about sexual identity, elicited a history of compulsive handwashing. Mr. R's "germophobia" also played a role in his fear of same-sex activity and the possibility of getting HIV or another sexually transmitted disease. Dr. B suggested a diagnosis of obsessive-compulsive disorder (OCD), wondering aloud whether it might have contributed to Mr. R's painfully long inability to establish his sexual identity. Dr. B recommended a selective serotonin reuptake inhibitor to help allay obsessionality and compulsive behavior, but Mr. R declined initially. However, months later he agreed to the medication trial, which succeeded in reducing his anxiety-related symptoms.

Given Mr. R's greater ease with women and uneasiness with homosexual attractions, Dr. B asked why he did not simply identify as heterosexual and work on relationships with women. Mr. R protested. By not integrating his same-sex feelings into his life and identity, he said, he might be "living a lie" that would be "inexcusably homophobic."

Mr. R's reply prompted Dr. B to explore an aspect of his own countertransference regarding Mr. R's evident bisexuality—a belief that no one who could function heterosexually would ever choose a homosexual identity. Now aware of both his own and Mr. R's binegativity, Dr. B suggested that some people, like Mr. R, are attracted to, are sexually excited by, and have sex with both men and women. "Why not identify as bisexual?"

Mr. R was initially taken aback by the idea. He did not believe "true bisexuals" existed. Only one set of feelings could be authentic, so he must make a definitive choice. Dr. B remarked on the rigidity of Mr. R's thinking, suggesting that it ran counter to the facts. Over time, such interventions helped Mr. R relax his self-critical attitude. He showed more openness to embracing his bisexuality. He placed a personal profile on a mixed-orientation dating site, indicating in his profile that he was a bisexual man looking for a woman. This led to several encounters that challenged his belief that no woman would want him if she knew he was also attracted to men. Despite what he was experiencing, he remained skeptical of being "truly bisexual" or of being accepted as such.

Dr. B continued to question Mr. R's ability to distinguish his genuine sexual desires from his presumptions about others' judgments or from his own internalized biphobia. Mr. R reiterated his earlier conviction that his authentic feelings were gay. He questioned whether Dr. B's agenda was intended to discourage him from what he viewed as his emergent gay identity. Dr. B clarified that he was accepting of whatever identity and sexual interests best suited Mr. R. Explaining that it is entirely possible to have multiple, contradictory feelings, Dr. B said that the therapeutic goal was to discourage Mr. R from disavowing feelings he felt were unacceptable—anger, revulsion, disapproval—that were knotted up with his desires. Tolerating a fuller spectrum of feelings might help untangle these feelings and help free Mr. R from his inhibitions.

This more complicated view of himself confused Mr. R. He preferred to think of his feelings as obstacles preventing him from moving forward toward a singular authentic feeling that would define him. However, he acknowledged that he experienced attraction and discomfort about both gay sex and sex with women.

Over time, Mr. R developed an ability to experience a fuller range of feelings that included his various attractions and apprehensions. Although, at times, Mr. R found it was distressing to see himself in more complex ways, Dr. B's challenges to his constricted thinking were always in the context of an explicitly therapeutic posture that was accepting of whatever identity he chose. Dr. B pointed out that disavowal of any of Mr. R's feelings might ultimately derail a fuller acceptance of himself.

Mr. R gradually gained a growing awareness of his conflicting desires, each having its own authenticity. Dr. B offered Mr. R a different way to think—not either/or and good/bad but rather both/and. He suggested that Mr. R might develop a more benevolent mediating third voice to help him deal with the duality of internal contradictions.

After 3 years of treatment, Mr. R was dating both men and woman. He could own his ambivalence. This fuller acceptance of himself held the hope that whatever his partners' gender, he could pursue a relationship less encumbered by doubt, anxiety, and self-recrimination.

Case Commentary

In his therapeutic posture, Dr. B showed awareness and acceptance that bisexual identities normally evolve over the course of development and may change in relation to life circumstances or in the context of particular relationships. His nonjudgmental attitude allowed his patient to share his sexual history and current experiences openly.

Dr. B also demonstrated a capacity to consider his own countertransference. His willingness to consider his own biases about bisexuality created a psychological space for complexity and ambiguity, despite Mr. R's pressuring to foreclose the subject prematurely.

Dr. B was able to actively address Mr. R's internalized biphobia and binegativity. He accepted Mr. R's uncertainty about his sexual identity respectfully, keeping its resolution as an open question and expressing openness to any identity Mr. R might embrace.

Although questioning of his sexual identity was primary in Mr. R's mind, it was not necessarily the only important clinical focus. Together, Mr. R and Dr. B were able to sustain an inquiry into issues that underlay Mr. R's sexual anxieties, homophobia, "authentic repulsions" that interfaced with OCD symptoms, sexual inhibitions, and chronic ambivalence. Mr. R's anxiety, OCD, and alcohol use were problematic both with respect to his general well-being and, more specifically, with respect to his difficulty resolving questions about his sexual identity and unease in acting on his desires.

Key Points

- Research about sexual orientation often has conflated gender identity and sexual orientation or rarely focused on bisexuality until recently.

- Bisexual individuals are more likely to experience poorer mental health than heterosexuals or individuals of other nonconforming sexual identities or orientations.
- Issues of invisibility, stigma and victimization, minority stress, and intersectionality are salient factors in the increased risk for mental health problems among bisexual individuals.
- Bisexual individuals encounter unique family, intimate partnership, and societal issues that isolate them, complicate the process of coming out, and limit the availability of support and social opportunities.
- Bisexual individuals encounter greater challenges than do monosexual individuals in the treatment setting, including less access, assessment biases and barriers, prejudice, professionals' lack of education and training, and a lack of needed family and social interventions.

References

Akerlund M, Cheung M: Teaching beyond the deficit model. J Soc Work Educ 36(2):279–292, 2000

American Psychiatric Association: Mental Health Facts on Bisexual Populations. Washington, DC, American Psychiatric Association, 2020

Armstrong HL, Reissing ED: Attitudes toward casual sex, dating, and committed relationships with bisexual partners. J Bisex 14(2):236–264, 2014

Balsam KF, Rothblum ED, Beauchaine TP: Victimization over the life span: a comparison of lesbian, gay, bisexual, and heterosexual siblings. J Consult Clin Psychol 73(3):477–487, 2005 15982145

Balsam KF, Mohr JJ: Adaptation to sexual orientation stigma: a comparison of bisexual and lesbian/gay adults. J Couns Psychol 54(3):306–319, 2007

Bauer GR, Flanders C, MacLeod MA, Ross LE: Occurrence of multiple mental health or substance use outcomes among bisexuals: a respondent-driven sampling study. BMC Public Health 16(1):1–11 2016 27287188

Blechner MJ: Psychoanalysis and sexual issues. Contemp Psychoanal 52(4):502–546, 2016

Bostwick W, Hequembourg A: "Just a little hint": bisexual-specific microaggressions and their connection to epistemic injustices. Cult Health Sex 16(5):488–503, 2014 24666221

Bostwick WB, McCabe SE, Horn S, et al: Drinking patterns, problems, and motivations among collegiate bisexual women. J Am Coll Health 56(3):285–292, 2007 18089511

Bostwick WB, Boyd CJ, Hughes TL, et al: Dimensions of sexual orientation and the prevalence of mood and anxiety disorders in the United States. Am J Public Health 100(3):468–475, 2010 19696380

Brennan DJ, Ross LE, Dobinson C, et al: Men's sexual orientation and health in Canada. Can J Public Health 101(3):255–258, 2010 20737821

Brewster ME, Moradi B: Perceived experiences of anti-bisexual prejudice: instrument development and evaluation. J Couns Psychol 57(4):451–468, 2010

Conron KJ, Mimiaga MJ, Landers SJ: A population-based study of sexual orientation identity and gender differences in adult health. Am J Public Health 100(10):1953–1960, 2010 20516373

Copen CE, Chandra A, Febo-Vazquez I: Sexual behavior, sexual attraction, and sexual orientation among adults aged 18–44 in the United States: data from the 2011–2013 National Survey of Family Growth. Natl Health Stat Rep (88):1–14, 2016 26766410

Diamond LM: Female bisexuality from adolescence to adulthood: results from a 10-year longitudinal study. Dev Psychol 44(1):5–14, 2008 18194000

Drescher J: Causes and becauses: on etiological theories of homosexuality, in The Annual of Psychoanalysis, Vol 30: Rethinking Psychoanalysis and the Homosexualities. Edited by Winer JA, Anderson JW. New York, Routledge, 2002, pp 57–68

Drescher J: From bisexuality to intersexuality: rethinking gender categories. Contemp Psychoanal 43(2):204–228, 2007

Drescher J, Roberts LW, Termuehlen G: Lesbian, gay, bisexual, and transgender patients, in The American Psychiatric Publishing Textbook of Psychiatry, 7th Edition. Edited by Roberts LW. Washington, DC, American Psychiatric Association, 2019, pp 1185–1212

Dyar C, Feinstein BA, London B: Mediators of differences between lesbians and bisexual women in sexual identity and minority stress. Psychol Sex Orientat Gend Divers 2(1):43–51, 2015

Elise D: Gender repertoire: body, mind, and bisexuality. Psychoanal Dialogues 8(3):353–371, 1998

Feinstein BA, Dyar C: Bisexuality, minority stress, and health. Curr Sex Health Rep 9(1):42–49, 2017 28943815

Feinstein BA, Dyar C, Pachankis JE: A multilevel approach for reducing mental health and substance use disparities affecting bisexual individuals. Cognit Behav Pract 26(2):243–253, 2019 31160876

Flanders CE: Bisexual health: a daily diary analysis of stress and anxiety. Basic Appl Soc Psych 37(6):319–335, 2015

Ford CS, Beach FA: Patterns of Sexual Behavior. New York, Harper, 1951

Freud S: Analysis terminable and interminable (1937), in Standard Edition of the Complete Psychological Works of Sigmund Freud, Vol 23. Translated and edited by Strachey J. London, Hogarth Press, 1964, pp 209–253

Friedman MR, Dodge B, Schick V, et al: From bias to bisexual health disparities: attitudes toward bisexual men and women in the United States. LGBT Health 1(4):309–318, 2014 25568885

Friedman MS, Marshal MP, Guadamuz TE, et al: A meta-analysis of disparities in childhood sexual abuse, parental physical abuse, and peer victimization among sexual minority and sexual nonminority individuals. Am J Public Health 101(8):1481–1494, 2011 21680921

Gulati R, Pauley D: The half embrace of psychic bisexuality. J Am Psychoanal Assoc 67(1):97–121, 2019 30880410

Hayfield N, Clarke V, Halliwell E: Bisexual women's understandings of social marginalization: "The heterosexuals don't understand us but nor do the lesbians." Fem Psychol 24(3):352–372, 2014

Hemmings C: Bisexual Spaces: A Geography of Sexuality and Gender. New York, Routledge, 2002

Hequembourg AL, Brallier SA: An exploration of sexual minority stress across the lines of gender and sexual identity. J Homosex 56(3):273–298, 2009 19319738

Jones KP, King EB: Managing concealable stigmas at work: a review and multilevel model. J Manage 40(5):1466–1494, 2014

Kann L, Olsen EO, McManus T, et al: Sexual identity, sex of sexual contacts, and health-risk behaviors among students in grades 9–12—youth risk behavior surveillance, selected sites, United States, 2001–2009. MMWR Surveill Summ 60(7):1–133, 2011 21659985

Kase CA, Mohr JJ: Within-person predictors and outcomes of daily sexual orientation self-presentation among plurisexual women. J Counseling Psych 68(2):156–167, 2020 21659985

Katz-Wise SL, Hyde JS: Victimization experiences of lesbian, gay, and bisexual individuals: a meta-analysis. J Sex Res 49(2–3):142–167, 2012 22380586

Kerr DL, Santurri L, Peters P: A comparison of lesbian, bisexual, and heterosexual college undergraduate women on selected mental health issues. J Am Coll Health 61(4):185–194, 2013 23663122

King M, Semlyen J, Tai SS, et al: A systematic review of mental disorder, suicide, and deliberate self harm in lesbian, gay and bisexual people. BMC Psychiatry 8:70, 2008 18706118

Kinsey A, Pomeroy WB, Martin CE: The Sexual Behavior in the Human Male. Philadelphia, PA, WB Saunders, 1948

Kinsey A, Pomeroy W, Martin CE, et al: Sexual Behavior in the Human Female. Philadelphia, PA, WB Saunders, 1953

Klein F: The Bisexual Option. New York, Arbor House, 1978
Koh AS, Ross LK: Mental health issues: a comparison of lesbian, bisexual and heterosexual women. J Homosex 51(1):33–57, 2006 16893825
Layton LB: The psychopolitics of bisexuality. Stud Gend Sex 1(1):41–60, 2000
Lewis RJ, Derlega VJ, Brown D, et al: Sexual minority stress, depressive symptoms, and sexual orientation conflict: focus on the experiences of bisexuals. J Soc Clin Psychol 28:971–992, 2009
Marshal MP, Friedman MS, Stall R, et al: Sexual orientation and adolescent substance use: a meta-analysis and methodological review. Addiction 103(4):546–556, 2008 18339100
Meyer IH: Prejudice, social stress, and mental health in lesbian, gay, and bisexual populations: conceptual issues and research evidence. Psychol Bull 129(5):674–697, 2003 12956539
Mohr JJ, Jackson SD, Sheets RL: Sexual orientation self-presentation among bisexual-identified women and men: patterns and predictors. Arch Sex Behav 46(5):1465–1479, 2017 27502348
Pachankis JE, Mahon CP, Jackson SD, et al: Sexual orientation concealment and mental health: a conceptual and meta-analytic review. Psychol Bull 146(10):831–871, 2020 32700941
Page EH: Mental health services experiences of bisexual women and bisexual men. J Homosex 4(1–2):137–160, 2004
Pakula B, Shoveller J, Ratner PA, Carpiano R: Prevalence and co-occurrence of heavy drinking and anxiety and mood disorders among gay, lesbian, bisexual, and heterosexual Canadians. Am J Public Health 106(6):1042–1048, 2016 26985615
Paul R, Smith NG, Mohr JJ, et al: Measuring dimensions of bisexual identity: initial development of the Bisexual Identity Inventory. Psychol Sex Orientat Gend Divers 1(4):452–460, 2014
Pompili M, Lester D, Forte A, et al: Bisexuality and suicide: a systemic review of the current literature. J Sex Med 11(8):1903–1913, 2014 24839908
Rado S: A critical examination of the concept of bisexuality. Psychosom Med 2:459–467, 1940
Richters J, Altman D, Badcock PB, et al: Sexual identity, sexual attraction and sexual experience: the Second Australian Study of Health and Relationships. Sex Health 11(5):451–460, 2014 25376998
Roberts TS, Horne SG, Hoyt WT: Between a gay and a straight place: bisexual individuals' experiences with monosexism. J Bisex 15:554–569, 2015
Ross LE, Dobinson C, Eady A: Perceived determinants of mental health for bisexual people: a qualitative examination. Am J Public Health 100(3):496–502, 2010 20075326
Ross LE, Salway T, Tarasoff LA, et al: Prevalence of depression and anxiety among bisexual people compared to gay, lesbian, and heterosexual individuals: a systematic review and metaanalysis, J Sex Res 55(4-5):435–456, 2018 29099625
Roughton RE: Four men in treatment: an evolving perspective on homosexuality and bisexuality, 1965 to 2000. J Am Psychoanal Assoc 49(4):1187–1217, 2001 11809020
Swan DJ, Habibi S: Bisexuality: Theories, Research, and Recommendations for the Invisible Sexuality. Cham, Switzerland, Springer, 2018
Sweet T, Welles SL: Associations of sexual identity or same-sex behaviors with history of childhood sexual abuse and HIV/STI risk in the United States. J Acquir Immune Defic Syndr 59(4):400–408, 2012 22083072
Taylor J, Power J, Smith E: Experiences of bisexual identity, attraction, and behavior and their relationship with mental health findings from the Who I Am Study. J Psychosoc Nurs Ment Health Serv 58(3):28–37, 2020 31846045
Walters ML, Chen J, Breiding MJ: The National Intimate Partner and Sexual Violence Survey (NISVS): 2010 findings on victimization by sexual orientation. Atlanta, GA, National Center for Injury Prevention and Control, Centers for Disease Control and Prevention, 2013. Available at: www.cdc.gov/violenceprevention/pdf/nisvs_sofindings.pdf. Accessed November 14, 2020.
Yoshino K: The epistemic contract of bisexual erasure. Stanford Law Rev 52(2):353–461, 2000
Yost MR, Thomas GD: Gender and binegativity: men's and women's attitudes toward male and female bisexuals. Arch Sex Behav 41(3):691–702, 2012 21597943
Young-Bruehl E: Are human beings "by nature" bisexual? Stud Gend Sex 2(3):179–213, 2001

CHAPTER 31

Psychotherapy With Trans and Gender Diverse People

Christopher McIntosh, M.D., FRCPC
Nicola Brown, Ph.D., C.Psych.

The past decade has been a decade of new transgender visibility. A systematic review of recent studies assessing population demographics suggested that, narrowly defined, transgender adults may comprise 0.3%–0.5% of the population; when using the more inclusive definition of *gender diverse*, they may comprise perhaps 0.5%–4.5% of the population (Zhang et al. 2020). As recently as 2007, estimates of prevalence were more than 35 times lower than these recent figures (De Cuypere et al. 2007). The improvement of social conditions is undoubtedly one of the reasons more people are coming out as transgender (Nolan et al. 2019). This parallels in some ways a similar phenomenon that occurred in the 1990s for lesbians and gay men.

Similarly, the diversity of the trans community has also become more apparent. In the past, the most visible members of the trans community were people seeking gender-affirming hormones and surgery. Today, the term *transgender* includes people who simply wish to express their gender in a different manner than the binary designations of *man* or *woman*. In this chapter we provide a guide to helping transgender people presenting for psychotherapeutic care.

The authors wish to thank Dr. Jack Pula for his review and feedback on this chapter.

Situating the T in LGBTQ

Historically, mental health professions stigmatized trans people as psychologically immature or perverse, similar to past approaches to lesbian, gay, and bisexual (LGB) identities (Drescher 2010; Drescher and Byne 2017). In the 5th edition of the *Diagnostic and Statistical Manual of Mental Disorders* (DSM-5; American Psychiatric Association 2013), the diagnostic category was revised from gender identity disorder to gender dysphoria, with less focus on the notion of *disorder* of transgender identity and instead focusing on distress caused by incongruence between one's gender and one's body. In 2019, the World Health Organization went a step further. The diagnoses of transsexualism and gender identity disorder of childhood were reconceptualized as gender incongruence of adolescence and adulthood and gender incongruence of childhood. ICD-11 moved these diagnoses out of the mental disorders section and into a new chapter called "Conditions related to sexual health" (Drescher et al. 2012, 2016; Reed et al. 2016). Today, even in countries where human rights protections for gender identity exist and universal health care is provided, research shows that when compared with cisgender populations, trans people are medically underserved and have significantly more unmet health needs, and research about their health and mental health care needs is sorely lacking (Brown and Jones 2016; Giblon and Bauer 2017; Institute of Medicine 2011).

In recent years, the minority stress model (Meyer 2003) has spurred research demonstrating associations between social stress endured by LGB people and higher rates of mental health issues. Trans communities, however, differ significantly from LGB populations with respect to minority stress—both structurally and by a matter of degree. On a structural level, trans people have fewer legal protections than do cisgender LGB people. For example, LGB people can now marry, but trans people are currently fighting legal battles to be able to use a public bathroom (New York Times 2017).

Trans people also face unique administrative and policy issues that impede critical aspects of daily living. Costly and time-consuming barriers to obtaining gender-concordant identity documents affect the ability to travel, seek employment, access education and health care, vote, secure stable housing, and collect social benefits (Malta et al. 2020, p. e178). A large U.S.-based research study linking this access with mental health found that compared with respondents who lacked gender-concordant identification, respondents whose documents were fully gender-concordant had a significantly lower prevalence of serious psychological distress and suicidal ideation (Scheim et al. 2020).

Further, given that one's identity is multidimensional, additional aspects of identity, such as gender, race, ethnicity, class, and (dis)ability, can mean trans people navigate multiple sources of marginalization. This can intensify their level of social exclusion and their vulnerability to mental health problems.

These are important contextual factors, both in conceptualizing a patient's mental health and in considering how one's work with a trans patient may differ substantially from the usual practice of psychotherapeutic work with cisgender patients. For example, it may be necessary for the therapist to write letters supporting change of identity documents or to become involved in preassessment for trans-related surgery.

Language and Defining Terms

Work with transgender people involves learning new terms and paying closer attention to unarticulated, dissociated, and possibly unconscious assumptions about gender embedded within everyday language. The most common example of this is the use of pronouns, which in English are gender neutral in the first, second, and plural third person. Pronouns are conventionally gendered in the singular third person (e.g., he/she, him/her, his/her). One should always use and respect a patient's chosen pronouns, including the use of the increasingly popular singular they/them/their. Other terms requiring explanation include the following:

- *Gender identity*—the intrapsychic experience of one's gender; can be masculine, feminine, both, neither, or on a spectrum between a male/female binary
- *Gender expression*—how one demonstrates one's gender externally (appearance) to oneself and to others
- *Trans/transgender*—adjective describing a person whose gender identity is not concordant with the gender assigned at birth
- *Gender diverse*—a broad term encompassing people who have nonconventional gender identities, gender expressions, and life courses
- *Trans woman/transfeminine*—a trans person assigned male at birth whose felt sense of gender is feminine/feminine spectrum; historically male to female
- *Trans man/transmasculine*—a trans person assigned female at birth whose felt sense of gender is masculine/masculine spectrum; historically female to male
- *Nonbinary/genderqueer*—adjective referring to a trans or gender diverse person (assigned male or female at birth) who identifies their gender as neither exclusively male nor exclusively female. Such a person may choose the singular "they" for their pronouns
- *Cis or cisgender*—adjective describing the majority of the population whose gender identity is concordant with the gender assigned at birth. The term was originally coined from the cis/trans isomer distinction in organic chemistry.
- *Gender dysphoria*—distress about incongruence between one's experienced or expressed gender and one's gender assigned at birth. Gender dysphoria is also a DSM-5 diagnosis; the equivalent ICD-11 diagnosis is gender incongruence, reflecting the clinical reality that some trans people do not experience the distress associated with the term dysphoria.
- *Gender-affirming surgery*—surgical interventions to reduce gender dysphoria and gender incongruence; historically referred to as sex reassignment surgery

Presenting for Psychotherapeutic Care

The role and importance of gender-related issues in the presentation of trans people for psychotherapeutic treatment should be neither underemphasized nor overemphasized. Frequently, trans and gender diverse people wish to engage in psychotherapy for a host of reasons having nothing to do with their gender identity or expression

(Mizock and Lundquist 2016). Nevertheless, gender-related issues typically have some saliency, even if in the background, insofar as patients will have coped with or are still coping with high levels of social exclusion and the greater mental health burdens and risks of minority stress (Hendricks and Testa 2012; Meyer 2003) (see also Chapter 27, "Issues Arising in Psychotherapy with LGBTQ+ Patients").

Prior to 1998, psychotherapy was a required part of the evaluative process for gender-affirming medical and/or surgical procedures (Fraser 2009b; Levine et al. 1999). Even subsequently, the requirement of an evaluating mental health professional in some parts of this process can be a barrier to establishing a trusting therapeutic relationship. Tensions related to the role of "gatekeeping" for gender-affirming medicosurgical care may emerge as one of the early issues in treating trans people in psychotherapy.

Sometimes, the goal of a trans patient seeking psychotherapeutic consultation is obtaining a letter of support for surgical intervention. In some cases, one of the letters must come from a physician. At other times, the letter may require a formal diagnosis, which may be a restricted scope of practice in one's jurisdiction. It is best at the outset for patient and clinician to collaborate on understanding the goals of treatment. Where does the patient want to go? What are the barriers to getting there? How can the psychotherapist help?

For those trans patients seeking therapy for issues more directly connected to their gender, a phased approach, outlined in the following subsections, can be useful. These phases are gender questioning, coming out, and transitioning. Patients may come to treatment during any of these phases, and the phases are not necessarily linear, nor are they presented as a developmental schema. Each involves legitimate choices, dilemmas, nuances, and endpoints. According to trans-identified psychiatrist and psychoanalyst Jack Pula (2017), "Coming out is a liberating and frightening process for most trans people...transition is a source of relief and stress...[and hormones and surgery] can be a mix of life-promotion, enhancement and disappointment."

Gender Questioning

One of the most important therapeutic tasks during the gender questioning phase is creating an open space for patients to focus, allowing patients to reach a place of greater clarity. A curious stance is helpful in asking questions and exploring gendered feelings or experiences that patients may find confusing or be ambivalent about. How do they feel about their bodies? What has been their relationship to their body over time—and at particular times, such as puberty or pregnancy, or for particularly gender-charged experiences such as sexual activity? What exploration have they done thus far and how do they feel about it? As in any psychotherapy, gender questioning exploration is fundamentally about a process rather than a particular outcome.

Coming Out

If and when a patient decides they are trans or gender nonconforming, *coming out* may be an entirely private experience. *Coming out to oneself* is about self-acknowledgment. Subsequently, coming out to others may be partially or fully public. It may or may not involve a transition.

For some people, being out improves mental health. However, this may not be true for everyone. For some patients, it is not about "wanting" or "deciding" to come out but rather is a feeling that they must come out. For others, it is a volitional decision whether or not to come out. In such cases, some people's reasons may be uniquely personal, whereas for others it may involve cultural or religious considerations. Ideally, everyone gets to decide how, when, and whether they come out. Patients should be encouraged to find their own way, although learning about how others have come out may be helpful (Rohrer and Keig 2010; Testa et al. 2014).

Disclosure to others can be frightening. Words, once spoken, cannot be taken back. The truth may indelibly change relationships. Coming out may have a smoother path if the individual starts by telling people they think are most likely to be supportive. An incremental approach can help build a base of support to fall back on if needed. Psychotherapeutic aspects of this phase can include perspective taking, anticipating reactions, and managing distress.

Pacing is also a significant consideration. Coming out can be an emotionally exhausting process. Other people may have a lot of questions and feelings about the patient coming out as trans, and the patient will be dually managing their own and others' reactions.

Coming out should also involve considerations of safety, particularly the possible risk of losing relational supports, housing, or employment. Some patients, acutely aware of these risks, may feel paralyzed. The perception of risk can be realistic, underestimated, or exaggerated. Psychotherapeutic work often involves figuring out the difference.

In this stage, patients feel vulnerable and are highly attuned to signs of withdrawal or rejection. They may find it difficult to be patient and generous with recently enlightened loved ones just beginning to process new information that affects their lives as well. If a patient comes out in a public manner, their loved ones will have a coming out of their own in their social and family circles, as in the following vignette.

Case Vignette 1

Jala desperately wished to come out and had the support of her immediate family. However, she recognized it would likely mean they would all be shunned by the extended family. In therapy, she wrestled with the complex ethics of coming out publicly. Ultimately, she realized her own integrity required that she have her immediate family's support and assent before proceeding.

However, support from family in the coming-out process often is not possible. Patients may instead seek community and professional support, so it is important that therapists become familiar with local trans support services and groups.

Deciding to Transition

Not all patients seek transition. Transition-related decisions depend on a patient's age, stage of life, personality, financial resources, and partnership status as well as where they live and the risks or protections of their immediate environment. Ideally, good planning precedes a social and medical transition and includes establishing a timeline; organizing medical care; and saving for significant financial costs of necessary aspects of transition, some of which may not be covered by medical insurance.

There are many uncertainties involved in a transition, including one's final appearance and the level of acceptance afterward. Inevitably, many patients wonder whether the relief they might find in reducing gender dysphoria is worth the potential losses that may accompany transition. These concerns parallel the dilemmas of coming out, although patients may experience the stakes as being significantly higher. When patients can imagine what this life might look like, it can provide reassurance and hope. This might entail finding first-person narratives of life after transition or before-and-after media of others' transition processes.

Transition

Navigating Early Stages of Transition

When a transgender person seriously considers changing their public gender expression, issues of gender identity cease to be solely internal and intrapsychic and become external and relational. Some patients adopt an "I don't give a damn what others think" attitude during the phase of gender expression and early transition. At the other end of the spectrum are individuals who are "people pleasing" in their relationships. They may be unwilling to take necessary steps toward self-expression that require assertiveness and courage in their relational world. There is also a range of possibilities between the two poles. Consequently, a psychotherapist can play a vital role helping patients navigate these challenges.

Many patients begin by making subtle changes to their public presentation, exhibiting greater androgyny where possible. However, in working environments requiring gendered uniforms or regulation haircuts (e.g, police and military settings), a gradual transition is difficult. During these periods, patients may practice at home and in select settings where they feel safe. After patients begin living continuously in their experienced gender, there are a host of practical considerations they may wish psychotherapeutic help in navigating.

Patients often wish to prepare for family gatherings. The importance of these events may relate to such an event being the first time they present to family as themselves or may relate to particular features of gatherings such as holidays, weddings, and deaths that typically involve gendered formal dress, seating arrangements, or activities. If they are dating or starting to date, they are often contemplating if and when to tell a potential partner. Patients often struggle with when to start using different washrooms or changing rooms. They are also coping with changes in how they are perceived by others, including gains and losses in social privilege. For example, trans men describe being bestowed greater authority, respect, and rewards at work, even in the same jobs they had prior to transition (Schilt 2006), advantages found to be mediated by race and to be greater for white men than Black men. Other research and the media have highlighted that for Black trans men, presenting as male magnifies the dangers of anti-Black racism, including being targeted by police (Alter 2016; Dozier 2005). Likewise, some trans women go through a challenging time as they face loss of social privilege. Supportive community, friends, and family are crucial for helping individuals navigate these changes, as is the therapist's ability to empathically understand these struggles.

Hormone Therapy

An important and often first medical intervention in transition is starting hormone therapy (HT). Coming to this decision means different things for different patients.

Some, particularly transfeminine patients, may use hormones to resolve any remaining ambivalence while still in a gender questioning phase. Some begin HT feeling certain about the decision but before making a social transition in order to "pave the way." Still others begin HT in conjunction with a social transition. Some nonbinary or genderqueer patients take low-dose hormone therapy only for a discrete amount of time to bring about certain changes.

Because hormones alter fertility, decisions regarding fertility preservation ideally should be made before beginning HT. The decision to start HT can be experienced as incredibly meaningful and satisfying, while also surprising and challenging. Hormone effects on internal mental life and external appearance are different for the masculinizing hormone testosterone and for the feminizing hormone estrogen.

From the perspective of external appearance, trans men appear to have a more robust response to hormone therapy than do trans women. Testosterone therapy produces several characteristics relatively quickly (and with more permanence) that most people construe as unequivocally masculine, such as facial hair and a voice pitch drop into a tenor or bass register. Testosterone increases upper body strength and facilitates a gain of lean muscle mass, and bodybuilding activities can quicken further masculinization. Also possible are less desired effects such as androgenic alopecia and abdominal adiposity.

Trans women taking estrogen experience skin changes leading to smoother skin and a softening of facial features as well as finer body hair. They also experience breast growth, although the amount of growth is often less than expected, which can be disappointing. Because estrogen does not alter bone structure or voice pitch, this often leaves aspects of appearance that are more visibly mixed in terms of gender signals, particularly for women starting treatment in adulthood. Because of this differential visibility, as a group, trans women are more vulnerable to experiencing stigmatizing social exchanges, discrimination, and threats to their safety. Some patients may need help building coping skills and resiliency in the face of these risks.

The subjective experience of taking hormones can vary. Some patients report a positive change in their mood or reduction of gender dysphoria after just one dose. Such a euphoric response is seen not as physiological but as the result of having achieved a long-wished-for step in transition. More commonly, the positive psychological effects coincide with the development of physical changes that allow a patient to increasingly recognize themselves in their experienced gender. Relief from gender incongruence they have had for much of their lives can be profound.

A psychotherapy patient starting HT will have much to explore about the multiply determined meaning(s) of these changes. As they feel more themselves, they may also experience a shift in their relationship with their parents and their internal representations.

Case Vignette 2

Jayden grew up resenting his mother's expectations that he would be more like her rather than like his brothers and father, whom he idolized. This led to much conflict in his teenage years. After testosterone treatment allowed him to feel more settled in his own gender identity, he was able in psychotherapy to examine these feelings with greater perspective and realize the ways in which he did resemble his mother. This shift enabled him to become closer to her in his adult years.

Complex identifications can also be influenced by emotional changes brought on by hormone therapy. For example, some transmasculine individuals report increased aggressive feelings from testosterone, whereas others report feeling calmer and more settled (Rubin 2003). The former may be anxiety-provoking for those who have experienced overly aggressive or abusive men in their family. In addition to work on processing the impact of these changes, reassurance about the usually time-limited nature of this response to HT can be helpful, as can building skills in moderating emotional reactivity (Devor 2010).

Research on the effects of hormone therapy has reliably shown significant reductions in anxiety and social distress, as well as improvements in measures of self-esteem and subjective well-being (Costa and Colizzi 2016; White Hughto and Reisner 2016). Clinically, some trans women report increased emotional lability. Some trans men taking testosterone experience the opposite, feeling unable to access feelings in the same way. Depending on the individual, these developments may be either welcomed or experienced as a loss. Processing these experiences with patients will present an opportunity to explore their varied meanings.

Surgery

Having a surgical intervention is a personal decision. Surgery does not necessarily follow HT. Some trans people who identify as nonbinary or genderqueer may want top surgery and never take hormones. For some, certain surgeries are more important than others. Some patients will not be interested in surgery at all. Others may want surgery, but the associated costs are prohibitive or surgery may be too medically risky because of co-occurring health problems. For many trans people, surgery brings a significant sense of peace and "rightness." Research shows that a very small minority of patients (<2%) regret surgery (Ruppin and Pfäfflin 2015). Often, these regrets relate to a poor surgical result or unfulfilled expectations. Far fewer have regrets about transition in general (Danker et al. 2018).

A psychotherapist supporting a patient's planned surgery, despite having no assessor role, should know enough about the surgery to have a sense of a patient's understanding of the risks and benefits. It is also helpful for therapists to know what kind of support the patient will need in the recovery process.

If the psychotherapist is trained and qualified to write a letter of recommendation, knowledge about surgeries will better enable them to address relevant diagnostic, eligibility, and readiness criteria as set out by the World Professional Association for Transgender Health (WPATH), which publishes broadly recognized standards of care (Coleman et al. 2012). The psychotherapist would offer an opinion about whether any mental health issues, if present, are *relatively well controlled*, the usual criterion for top surgeries, or *well controlled*, the usual criterion for gonadal or genital surgeries.

This distinction reflects the fact that top surgeries involve less risk and a less demanding recovery period than do bottom surgeries. Well controlled means improvement and stability of mental health symptoms and establishment of alternative means of handling stress other than the use of substances, if not complete sobriety. If a patient has been engaged in psychotherapeutic or medical treatment for mental health symptoms and is actively working on any problematic substance use disorders, that is sufficient for being described as relatively well controlled. Longer periods of abstinence from substances are needed for genital surgeries.

On Mourning and Celebration

Transition can involve aspects of grief and mourning (Fraser 2009a; Gozlan 2018; Lemma 2013; Saketopoulou 2014). Patients may have missed out on a childhood in which they felt fundamentally recognized and embodied. They may have also missed out on dating and sexual experiences in their experienced gender and the body in which they wanted to have these experiences. Some, aware of feeling different and fearful of discovery, withdrew from social life and missed out on having close friends. They may now be trying to catch up but may feel developmentally behind. Some mourn the distancing or ending of relationships following a transition not everyone understands or supports. Many regret not having transitioned earlier in life. There may be a feeling of grief in never having had the body they wished to have been born with and understanding that the body they have through hormones and surgery may fall short of all that they wished for (e.g., giving birth to a child, having full-sized and spontaneous erections).

Accompanying grief and mourning may be a deep sense of joy and liberation. Patients describe a profound sense of "rightness" and greater embodiment as transition progressed. Mock (2014) described transition as "an evolution from me to closer-to-me-ness" and a "reconciliation with myself" (p. 227). Benaway (2018) described surgery as allowing her body to be "reimagined," to be a body that "feels like home," a place of possibility, pleasure, and joy through which she could feel both more present and also ordinary. Increasingly, such personal reflections have become more intersectional and nuanced (Shraya 2018; Thom 2019).

The Patient and the Psychotherapist

Co-occurring Issues

People's preexisting personality traits may become exaggerated in the transition process. During this process, clinicians can provide a psychotherapeutic perspective on how one may, at times, be getting in one's own way.

Case Vignette 3

Quentin, a trans man with significant narcissistic traits, aims to move quickly through the milestones of transition and is unable to listen to the expressed concerns of their lesbian partner or allow her more time to adjust.

Case Vignette 4

Kris has long-standing tendencies of catastrophizing when anxious and struggles with mental images of transition leading to abandonment and homelessness. They focus overly on the question of what could go terribly wrong and can barely contemplate what could go right.

If co-occurring mental health issues are related to gender dysphoria, significant changes may be seen after beginning hormone therapy (Keo-Meier et al. 2015). Sometimes improvement can be seen in areas generally thought to be intractable, such as eating disorders. Disorders involving both overeating and undereating reflective of gender dysphoria often begin when patients try to control their body shape. In some cases, HT can give them a more desirable body shape, and eating issues improve. For others, disordered eating persists and may even worsen, requiring more specialized or intensive treatment. Even if there is no or little improvement of co-occurring issues, with the lessened dysphoria, the patient will have greater emotional capacity for subsequent work.

Countertransference Issues

It is important to be aware of ways in which clinician attitudes and knowledge of gender identity affect the nature and quality of care provided (American Psychological Association 2015). A number of possible countertransferential responses in working with trans and gender diverse patients exist. Novice cis clinicians working with trans people may experience a novelty countertransference in which enthusiasm for learning becomes voyeuristic. Clinicians should consider whether the questions they ask patients are clinically meaningful ones intended to better understand the patient or are being asked to satisfy the clinician's own curiosity. On the other hand, clinicians invested in being seen as an ally may take on a deferential or cheerleading role, accepting what the patient says at face value without exploring or examining contradictions. This can result in perfunctory care, lacking the due diligence patients deserve (Mizock and Lundquist 2016).

Relational clinicians have provided candid reflections on their countertransferential responses to patient disclosures and transitions in long-term therapies. These accounts suggest that case conceptualization, a therapist's own identification with the patient, or a therapist's own bodily changes may make therapists more vulnerable to countertransference.

Suchet (2011) and Silverman (2015) adopted analytic stances that intrapsychic conflict was to be "worked through" and conceptualized patient dysphoria as largely psychic. Suchet's formulation was that a patient's history of sexual abuse and intrusion had unduly linked femaleness with vulnerability, and transition was the patient's attempt to disidentify with this vulnerability. Silverman's formulation was one of intergenerational transmission of trauma, whereby a patient stored the mother's disavowed experiences of gender and sexuality. These accounts suggest a warning regarding case conceptualization: if the therapist believes, consciously or unconsciously, that a patient's transition means psychotherapy has fallen short, this can lead to gender policing (Drescher 2015). One example of such policing is a power struggle between the therapist and the patient about how and when transition proceeds (Pula 2017). At times, a therapist may experience a patient's differing subjective experience as a personal affront. This is seen in Suchet's wish that her patient, like her, could "feel, psychologically, both boy and girl" (Suchet 2011, p. 175). Offman (2014) expressed dismay with her patient's increasing masculinization, which she saw as a devaluation of her own femininity, engendering in the therapist a sense of betrayal because the patient was "switch[ing] gender 'teams'" (p. 80).

Therapists' countertransferential reactions may be particularly heightened in times of the therapist's own bodily or gendered vulnerability. For example, in a case presented by Marcus and McNamara (2013), Marcus felt conflicted about her own bodily changes as she provided therapy during her first pregnancy. Marcus would slip and forget to use the patient's new name and pronouns. She attributed this to the patient's descriptions of intense body dysphoria and violent wishes to be rid of his breasts, which she experienced as an assault on her own "engorged" body (p. 60). In the case discussed by Offman (2014), Offman's irritation intensified as the patient enthusiastically contemplated his chest surgery while she herself awaited genetic testing results that might dictate an unwanted, prophylactic double mastectomy. Offman noted that her patient had made his medical decisions without informing her until after the fact. She wondered what space she had made (or not made) for the patient to talk about the decision. As she shared some aspects of her personal struggle with the patient, both patient and clinician experienced greater recognition of each other's subjectivities and an increased ability to explore shared similarities and tolerate felt differences.

Trans-Trans Therapy Dyads

Trans therapists illuminate other therapeutic possibilities. For example, Hansbury (2011) noted that trans patients sought him out for identificatory needs, "looking for an experience of twinship and mirroring" they lacked growing up (p. 212). Some of his patients developed more idealized transferences, and some differences with, or empathic failures by, the therapist were felt more keenly. Working with a trans man patient dealing with ambivalence about his masculinity, Hansbury strove to be simultaneously both and neither parent in the transference so that the patient could figure out "where it might be safe enough to land" in terms of their own gender identity (p. 213).

Conclusion and Resources

Working with trans and gender diverse people in psychotherapy can be both rewarding and unsettling. Accompanying a person on a gender transitioning journey can be as profound an experience for the psychotherapist as it is for the patient. At the same time, trans patients challenge beliefs not just about gender, the body, and embodiment but also about the nature of psychotherapeutic work, its power dynamics, its possibilities, and its limitations. Clinicians at all levels of experience can find their assumptions challenged, sometimes even about their own personal relationship to sex, gender, and gender roles.

Clinicians working with trans and gender diverse patients can refer to the WPATH Standards of Care (Coleman et al. 2012) and the practice guidelines of their professional associations (e.g., American Psychological Association 2015). In addition, clinicians are encouraged to pursue basic specialized training, either through WPATH, the American Psychiatric Association's course on transgender mental health, or opportunities offered locally. Another valuable resource is *Trans Bodies, Trans Selves: A Resource by and for Transgender Communities*, 2nd Edition (Erickson-Schroth 2022), written collectively by queer and trans community members and covering many areas of trans lives.

Key Points

- Trans communities differ significantly from LGB ones with respect to the nature and degree of social stress they endure.
- Trans people are a heterogeneous group and vary widely in their experiences, needs, and therapeutic goals; these variations often relate to multiple intersecting identities.
- Therapists should have no stake in any particular outcome, while attending empathically to how transition may both relieve and generate stress.
- Transition sometimes brings about shifts in a patient's object relations, an important avenue of exploration in psychotherapy.
- People's preexisting personalities inevitably display themselves in the transition process. A therapist can help a patient see where they may be getting in their own way.
- Hormones and surgery can be effective treatments for gender dysphoria, and psychotherapists should be mindful of conscious or unconscious beliefs that such treatments represent a "failure" of psychotherapy.
- Countertransferential responses can include clinical voyeurism, a wish for patient approval, identification with the patient, and a therapist's feelings about their own bodily changes.
- Profession-based guidelines, international standards of care, training, and supervision can help support psychotherapists in work with transgender patients.

References

Alter C: Seeing sexism from both sides: what trans men experience. Time, June 16, 2016. Available at: https://time.com/transgender-men-sexism. Accessed September 13, 2020.

American Psychiatric Association: Diagnostic and Statistical Manual of Mental Disorders, 5th Edition. Arlington, VA, American Psychiatric Association, 2013

American Psychological Association: Guidelines for psychological practice with transgender and gender nonconforming people. Am Psychol 70(9):832–864, 2015 26653312

Benaway G: A body like a home. Hazlitt Magazine, May 30, 2018. Available at: https://hazlitt.net/longreads/body-home. Accessed August 22, 2020.

Brown GR, Jones KT: Mental health and medical health disparities in 5135 transgender veterans receiving healthcare in the Veterans Health Administration: a case-control study. LGBT Health 3(2):122–131, 2016 26674598

Coleman E, Bockting W, Botzer M, et al: Standards of Care for the Health of Trans, Transgender, and Gender Nonconforming People. East Dundee, IL, World Professional Association for Transgender Health, 2012. Available at: www.wpath.org/publications/soc. Accessed March 1, 2020.

Costa R, Colizzi M: The effect of cross-sex hormonal treatment on gender dysphoria individuals' mental health: a systematic review. Neuropsychiatr Dis Treat 12:1953–1966, 2016 27536118

Danker S, Narayan SK, Bluebond-Langner R, et al: Abstract: a survey study of surgeons' experience with regret and/or reversal or gender-confirmation surgeries. Plast Reconstr Surg Glob Open 6(9 Suppl):189, 2018

De Cuypere G, Van Hemelrijck M, Michel A, et al: Prevalence and demography of transsexualism in Belgium. Eur Psychiatry 22(3):137–141, 2007 17188846

Devor AH: Learned along the way, in Letters for My Brothers: Transitional Wisdom in Retrospect, 4th Edition. Edited by Rohrer MM, Keig Z. San Francisco, CA, Wilgefortis, 2010, pp 48–62

Dozier R: Beards, breasts, and bodies: doing sex in a gendered world. Gend Soc 19:297–316, 2005

Drescher J: Queer diagnoses: parallels and contrasts in the history of homosexuality, gender variance and the Diagnostic and Statistical Manual. Arch Sex Behav 39(2):427–460, 2010 19838785

Drescher J: Gender policing in the clinical setting: discussion of Sandra Silverman's "The Colonized Mind: Gender, Trauma, and Mentalization." Psychoanal Dialogues 25(1):67–76, 2015

Drescher J, Byne W: Gender identity, gender variance and gender dysphoria, in Kaplan and Sadock's Comprehensive Textbook of Psychiatry, 10th Edition. Edited by Sadock BJ, Sadock VA, Ruiz P. Philadelphia, PA, Wolters Kluwer, 2017, pp 2023–2039

Drescher J, Cohen-Kettenis P, Winter S: Minding the body: situating gender identity diagnoses in the ICD-11. Int Rev Psychiatry 24(6):568–577, 2012 23244612

Drescher J, Cohen-Kettenis PT, Reed GM: Gender incongruence of childhood in the ICD-11: controversies, proposal, and rationale. Lancet Psychiatry 3(3):297–304, 2016 26946394

Erickson-Schroth L (ed): Trans Bodies, Trans Selves: A Resource by and for Transgender Communities, 2nd Edition. New York, Oxford University Press, 2022

Fraser L: Depth psychotherapy with transgender people. Sex Relationship Ther 24:126–142, 2009a

Fraser L: Psychotherapy in the World Professional Association for Transgender Health's Standards of Care: background and recommendations. Int J Transgenderism 11:110–126, 2009b

Giblon R, Bauer GR: Health care availability, quality, and unmet need: a comparison of transgender and cisgender residents of Ontario, Canada. BMC Health Serv Res 17(1):283, 2017 28420361

Gozlan O: From continuity to contiguity: a response to the fraught temporality of gender. Psychoanal Rev 105(1):1–29, 2018 29364080

Hansbury G: King Kong and Goldilocks: imagining transmaculinities through the trans-trans dyad. Psychoanal Dialogues 21(2):210–220, 2011

Hendricks M, Testa R: A conceptual framework for clinical work with transgender and gender nonconforming clients: an adaptation of the minority stress model. Prof Psychol Res Pr 43(5):460–467, 2012

Institute of Medicine: The Health of Lesbian, Gay, Bisexual, and Transgender People: Building a Foundation for Better Understanding. Washington, DC, National Academies Press, 2011

Keo-Meier CL, Herman LI, Reisner SL, et al: Testosterone treatment and MMPI-2 improvement in transgender men: a prospective controlled study. J Consult Clin Psychol 83(1):143–156, 2015 25111431

Lemma A: The body one has and the body one is: understanding the transsexual's need to be seen. Int J Psychoanal 94(2):277–292, 2013 23560903

Levine SB, Brown GR, Coleman E, et al: The standards of care for gender identity disorders. J Psychol Human Sex 11(2):1–34, 1999

Malta M, LeGrand S, Turban J, et al: Gender-congruent government identification is crucial for gender affirmation. Lancet Public Health 5(4):e178–e179, 2020 32192576

Marcus BF, McNamara S: "Strange and otherwise unaccountable actions": category, conundrum, and trans identities. J Am Psychoanal Assoc 61(1):45–66, 2013 23197166

Meyer IH: Prejudice, social stress, and mental health in lesbian, gay, and bisexual populations: conceptual issues and research evidence. Psychol Bull 129(5):674–697, 2003 12956539

Mizock L, Lundquist C: Missteps in psychotherapy with transgender clients: promoting gender sensitivity in counseling and psychological practice. Psychol Sex Orientat Gend Divers 3(2):148–155, 2016

Mock J: Redefining Realness: My Path to Womanhood, Identity, Love and So Much More. New York, Atria, 2014

New York Times: Understanding transgender access laws. New York Times, February 24, 2017. Available at: www.nytimes.com/2017/02/24/us/transgender-bathroom-law.html. Accessed August 1, 2020.

Nolan IT, Kuhner CJ, Dy GW: Demographic and temporal trends in transgender identities and gender confirming surgery. Transl Androl Urol 8(3):184–190, 2019 31380225
Offman H: The princess and the penis: a postmodern queer-y tale. Psychoanal Dialogues 24(1):72–87, 2014
Pula J: Increasing clinical and cultural competency in psychotherapeutic work with transgender patients. Invited speaker, 46th Scientific Session of the Toronto Psychoanalytic Society and Institute, Toronto, ON, Canada, March 4, 2017
Reed GM, Drescher J, Krueger RB, et al: Disorders related to sexuality and gender identity in the ICD-11: revising the ICD-10 classification based on current scientific evidence, best clinical practices, and human rights considerations. World Psychiatry 15(3):205–221, 2016 27717275
Rohrer MM, Keig Z (eds): Letters for My Brothers: Transitional Wisdom in Retrospect, 4th Edition. San Francisco, CA, Wilgefortis, 2010
Rubin H: Self-Made Men: Identity and Embodiment Among Transsexual Men. Nashville, TN, Vanderbilt University Press, 2003
Ruppin U, Pfäfflin F: Long-term follow-up of adults with gender identity disorder. Arch Sex Behav 44(5):1321–1329, 2015 25690443
Saketopoulou A: Mourning the body as bedrock: developmental considerations in treating transsexual patients analytically. J Am Psychoanal Assoc 62(5):773–806, 2014 25277869
Scheim AI, Perez-Brumer AG, Bauer GR: Gender-concordant identity documents and mental health among transgender adults in the USA: a cross-sectional study. Lancet Public Health 5(4):e196–e203, 2020 32192577
Schilt K: Just one of the guys?: How trans men make gender visible at work. Gend Soc 20:465–490, 2006
Shraya V: I'm Afraid of Men. New York, Penguin Random House, 2018
Silverman S: The colonized mind: gender, trauma, and mentalization. Psychoanal Dialogues 25(1):51–66, 2015
Suchet M: Crossing over. Psychoanal Dialogues 21(2):51–66, 2011
Testa RJ, Jimenez CL, Rankin S: Risk and resilience during transgender identity development: the effects of awareness and engagement with other transgender people on affect. J Gay Lesbian Ment Health 18(1):31–46, 2014
Thom KC: I Hope We Choose Love: A Trans Girl's Notes From the End of the World. Vancouver, BC, Canada, Arsenal Pulp Press, 2019
White Hughto JM, Reisner SL: A systematic review of the effects of hormone therapy on psychological functioning and quality of life in transgender individuals. Transgend Health 1(1):21–31, 2016 27595141
Zhang Q, Goodman M, Adams N, et al: Epidemiological considerations in transgender health: a systematic review with focus on higher quality data. Int J Transgend Health 21(2):125–137, 2020 33015664

PART IX

Special Issues in Psychotherapy

Section Editors: Holly Crisp, M.D., and Glen O. Gabbard, M.D.

In the final part of this textbook, we want to emphasize a variety of topics that are pertinent across different types of psychotherapy. As we have seen in this volume, psychotherapy is practiced using varied schools of thought and clinical approaches. Across all approaches, however, fundamental concepts can be applied to all psychotherapies. In this part, we include chapters on fundamental concepts such as boundaries and ethics as well as supervision and consultation. In addition, we include a chapter on the interface between neuroscience and psychotherapy. In an era in which virtual communication has become commonplace, psychotherapy in cyberspace has greatly broadened the context of our scientific understanding of how therapy works while also offering us a host of modifications of the therapeutic frame, so one chapter is devoted to this topic. The remaining chapter in this part is on combining medications and psychotherapy in the various forms of combined treatment.

In Chapter 32, "Professional Boundaries and Ethics in Psychotherapy," we include a succinct overview of key principles involving professional boundaries and ethical concepts that apply broadly to therapeutic practice.

In Chapter 33, "Neuroscience of Psychotherapy," Susan Vaughan and Mohsin Ahmed outline the contemporary understanding of how psychotherapy affects the brain and the neuroscience underlying the changes psychotherapy brings about.

In Chapter 34, Peter Yellowlees and Jay Shore author a new chapter for this volume, "Psychotherapy and Cyberspace." Before the coronavirus SARS-CoV-2 disease (COVID-19) era, psychotherapists were already employing modalities that took advantage of the internet, and these authors address some of the basic concepts and approaches to working virtually. With the abrupt shift to online practice for many therapists during the pandemic, a significant increase in awareness of virtual therapies and technologies for the delivery of health care remotely occurred. In addition, a massive rethinking in how we adjust what we do in our day-to-day experience to the frame of teletherapy took place. Yellowlees and Shore provide an overview and explanation of the issues that may arise in working with patients virtually, as well as possible frameworks for virtual therapies in the future.

In Chapter 35, "Combining Medications and Psychotherapy," David Mintz provides an approach to thinking about the use of medications in conjunction with psychotherapy for the benefit of the patient. In addition, he outlines both common technical issues and practical issues that may unfold in combined treatment with psychotherapy and medications.

Finally, we include the chapter "Supervision and Consultation in Psychotherapy" to serve as an overview of the functions and roles of supervisors and consultants in psychotherapy. Psychotherapy is both a skill and an art, and the importance of supervision during training and lifelong consultation after training cannot be emphasized enough in our field.

CHAPTER 32

Professional Boundaries and Ethics in Psychotherapy

Glen O. Gabbard, M.D
Holly Crisp, M.D.

Psychotherapy, regardless of orientation, must take place in an ethical context that is safe and conducive to therapeutic possibilities. Psychotherapy is a professional relationship that, above all, is focused on helping patients with problems that they identify. Psychotherapeutic treatments occur within an envelope that is often referred to as the *therapeutic frame*. However, the metaphor of a frame implies a rigidity that may not be in the best interest of the process.

At the heart of the psychotherapeutic experience is a dyad of two different people with different personal experiences and different backgrounds. Hence, one must keep in mind that ethnicity, culture, religion, gender, and sexuality are critical aspects to be understood in the context of a therapeutic process. These crucially important factors have been underemphasized in psychotherapy and psychotherapy education. In this volume, outstanding parts spearheaded by Dionne Powell (Part 7, "Racial and Ethnic Diversities in Psychotherapy") and Jack Drescher (Part 8, "Gender and Sexualities in Psychotherapy") are specifically devoted to human diversities and how to approach patients with these important factors in mind. Hence, we touch on these subjects briefly in this chapter but defer to the authors in those parts for a more thoroughgoing treatment of these topics. Similarly, not all ethical issues that arise in psychotherapy grow out of a dyad. For therapists engaging in couple therapy, family therapy, or group therapy, the ethics issues extend beyond the dyad and involve complex systemic issues. These dynamics are addressed in greater depth in Part 6, "Family, Couple, and Group Psychotherapy," edited by Alison Heru.

Professional Boundaries in Psychotherapy

The concept of *professional boundaries*, with some degree of inherent flexibility, may be more suited than the concept of therapeutic frame to most discussions of sound psychotherapeutic practice. A simple definition of professional boundaries is that they are the parameters defining the limits of a fiduciary relationship in which one person (a patient) entrusts their welfare to another (a psychotherapist), who is paid for the provision of a service (Gabbard and Nadelson 1995). Boundaries suggest a professional distance and respect that are characteristic of ethical professional behavior, but they also allow for some degree of bending in the service of individualizing treatment.

The concept of professional boundaries grew out of concern about sexual misconduct, which led to malpractice suits, serious harm to patients, and severe damage to the reputation of the mental health professions (Gutheil and Gabbard 1993). Studies of cases of sexual misconduct, however, led to a growing awareness that instances in which psychotherapists engage in sexual relations with patients are typically preceded by a slippery slope involving a progressive series of nonsexual boundary violations (Gabbard 2017; Gutheil and Gabbard 1993; Strasburger et al. 1992). As a result, increasing attention has been focused on such matters as the location of sessions, confidentiality, excessive self-disclosure, the professional role of the therapist, length and time of sessions, fees, the exchange of gifts and services, appropriate clothing and language, and nonsexual physical contact (Table 32–1).

Boundary Crossings Versus Boundary Violations

Nonsexual boundary violations are less absolute than sexual boundary violations. All practitioners can think of instances in which the transgression of a boundary led to productive therapeutic work and caused no harm. Therefore, the definitions involved in professional boundaries must take into account that both boundary crossings and boundary violations exist in the practice of psychotherapy.

Boundary crossings are generally benign phenomena that do not occur repetitively, are discussable between the therapist and the patient, and are not exploitative (Gabbard 2016; Gutheil and Gabbard 1993, 1998). Inherent in the notion of a boundary crossing is the idea that rigidity is generally antitherapeutic. A good psychotherapist adjusts the treatment to the patient rather than expecting the patient to adjust to the treatment. Beginning psychotherapists sometimes practice with such great concern about maintaining proper boundaries that they become remote and overly formal in their way of relating to the patient. Some patients will feel that they are talking to an automaton and will not return for the next visit. Rigidity about boundaries can lead to a failure to engage the patient.

In most therapeutic dyads, a period of adjustment occurs in which a sensitive psychotherapist implicitly negotiates with the patient a comfortable level of closeness or distance so that an optimal context for the therapy is jointly constructed. Some patients are much more comfortable with a more talkative therapist, whereas others need a good listener. Some patients appreciate the use of humor, whereas others feel they are being laughed at when the therapist jokes. Good psychotherapists often com-

TABLE 32–1. **Dimensions of professional boundaries**
Maintenance of professional role
Avoidance of dual relationships
Appropriate location, time, and length of sessions
Appropriate professional attire and language
Professional fees
Ethical handling of gifts and services
Importance of confidentiality
Avoidance of excessive self-disclosure
Limited physical contact
Absence of sexual contact
Avoidance of business transactions

ment that they are different with each patient during the course of a workday. They vary their therapeutic style depending on the particular patient's needs. Obviously, these variations are within the general parameters of ethical behavior and do not involve outrageous conduct.

Another aspect of boundary crossings is the recognition that extraordinary events occur that require humane responses. If the patient experiences a tragic loss and reaches out to the therapist for an embrace, most therapists will return the embrace, knowing that pushing the patient away might permanently destroy the therapeutic alliance. Moreover, no therapist is perfect, and at times even the best of therapists unconsciously enact something with the patient that may be outside the usual technique. These enactments often reflect significant internal object relationships that have been mobilized within the therapeutic dyad.

One psychotherapist who had seen a depressed man in therapy for several weeks noted to herself that she was becoming increasingly bored with the sessions. The patient frequently fell silent, tended to make repeated self-recriminations, and referred to his situation as "hopeless." Even though he had improved with antidepressants, the patient seemed to be characterologically entrenched in his depression, and the therapist found him frustrating and irritating. She often dreaded the sessions and felt bored with the content. On one occasion, she announced that the session was over and said to the patient, "I'll see you next week." The patient hesitated and then left the room with a strange expression on his face. The therapist suddenly realized that she had ended the session 15 minutes early, thinking that 45 minutes had elapsed. She felt mortified, and she began reflecting on her own motives for such a countertransference enactment. She was able to acknowledge to herself that she really did not want to hear him drone on and on, and she was acting out of her own needs rather than on the basis of what the patient needed. When the patient returned the following week, she apologized for the mistake and offered to make up for the time. The patient forgave her, but he then said it reminded him of how his wife frequently interrupted him during a conversation and said she had to do something else. When the therapist and the patient explored the two separate phenomena, the patient began to see a pattern of how his negativity might lead others to feel alienated or irritated with him. Hence, a boundary crossing based on unconscious factors in the therapist as well as certain characteristics of the patient led to a productive discussion in the therapy about an issue that had not been directly addressed.

Boundary violations, however, represent egregious phenomena that are usually repetitive, harmful to the patient, and exploitative of the patient's dependent position. Engaging in a sexual relationship with a patient is the most extreme example, but taking financial advantage of the patient by soliciting money for an investment scheme may be just as exploitative. Another feature of boundary violations is that the therapist often refuses to discuss them with the patient. Therapists may claim that the unorthodox behavior is part of the "real relationship" and therefore no discussion is required.

The psychotherapeutic relationship is, by definition, a relationship with a power imbalance. The psychotherapist is being paid to deliver a service based on a special set of skills and a knowledge base acquired by specialized training. The patient entrusts the therapist to function with the patient's best interest in mind. Hence, the patient may assume that whatever the therapist says or does is designed to help the patient. As a result, even an intelligent, nonpsychotic patient may agree to egregious boundary violations under the influence of that power differential and vulnerability. Moreover, transferences to the therapist may resemble past relationships with parents and other authority figures and can set up a situation in which the patient feels that saying no is not an option. Some nefarious therapists have suggested that sexual relations might be helpful to the patient in the service of overcoming sexual inhibitions, and patients have complied under the assumption that they are receiving a therapeutic intervention.

Some therapists start to feel that the rules do not apply to them. This may be an example of moral hypocrisy, defined as an individual's ability to hold a belief while acting in discord with it. Most individuals evaluate their own transgressions as being less egregious than the same transgressions enacted by others. Some people who are generally moral find it fairly easy to justify immoral behavior under certain circumstances (Gabbard 2016).

At times, *boundary transgression* is used as an umbrella term that encompasses both boundary crossings and boundary violations. Another term in the literature is *boundary blurring*, which is used to describe instances in which the boundaries are confused but not necessarily enacted in the form of a boundary crossing or boundary violation.

Specific Dimensions of Professional Boundaries

Location

In any consideration of the professional boundaries that define psychotherapy, one dimension that must be taken into account is where the therapy takes place. Therapy usually takes place in an office, a clinic, or a hospital setting that is sufficiently private that the patient feels comfortable disclosing embarrassing and shameful wishes, fears, and fantasies. However, the location of psychotherapy may vary within a setting. In a psychiatric hospital environment, for example, disturbed patients may feel confined and uncomfortable in a closed room and may find it much easier to talk while taking a walk on the hospital grounds. A medically ill patient in a general hospital may require therapy at the bedside.

The location of the psychotherapy also varies with the type of therapy that is indicated by the nature of the patient's pathology. A patient with an elevator phobia, for example, may require a behavioral approach that includes in vivo exposure. Hence, the therapist may drive the patient to a skyscraper and spend time riding up and down the elevator during the therapy hour. This form of treatment is entirely within the community standards of behavioral approaches and has been shown to be efficacious.

In general, when one is contemplating a departure from community standards in terms of the setting, one must consider one's rationale for the departure. Therapists may usefully ask themselves, "Is this part of a thoughtfully considered treatment plan?" Therapists may also wish to engage a consultant before making such a departure to make sure that they are not acting on unconscious countertransference needs of their own.

Many psychotherapists are embracing online and phone therapies as modalities of connecting with patients in the virtual space. In Chapter 34, "Psychotherapy and Cyberspace," Peter Yellowlees and Jay Shore present the current thinking about teletherapies and how these established modes of therapeutic practice have evolved rapidly since the beginning of the coronavirus SARS-CoV-2 disease (COVID-19) pandemic. The widespread use of both in-person and virtual therapies is now well established in psychiatric and psychotherapeutic practice.

Confidentiality

The fundamental principle that what is heard in psychotherapy is not repeated elsewhere makes the therapeutic process possible. Patients who come to psychotherapy, for whatever reasons, are often struggling with shame, guilt, remorse, self-loathing, fears of disapproval, and a host of other anxieties. The reassurance that what they say will be kept private between the two people in the consulting room allows them to open up in a manner that would not be possible otherwise. Hence, *confidentiality* is one of the most sacred professional boundaries.

The principle of confidentiality extends beyond simply not repeating what the patient says. Therapists are ethically bound not to act on information they receive in a therapeutic session. For example, a therapist should not act on a stock market tip from a patient. Similarly, if a therapist hears from a patient that a colleague of the therapist is going through a divorce and her only source of information is that patient, the therapist must not acknowledge that she knows about the divorce in any other context. Numerous cases exist in which a third party realized that the only source of specific information could have been from the patient, leading to justifiable feelings of violation or breach of privacy. Confidentiality is protected by state statutes and ethics codes as well. A breach of confidentiality can make one vulnerable to litigation or to sanctions from professional boards or organizations.

Taking confidentiality seriously entails deception at times. Ironically, in the interest of maintaining privacy, therapists may have to deceive those they encounter outside the consulting room. If, for example, the therapist noted above knows about a colleague's divorce only through her patient and she then encounters the colleague, she must pretend that she does not know, and if she is asked if she has heard the news, she must deny it. Otherwise, the patient's confidentiality is violated. Over time, psychotherapists develop the capacity to compartmentalize certain information to keep it sequestered in a private sector of the psyche belonging to information heard in psychotherapy (Gabbard 2016).

Confidentiality is not an absolute boundary. In all states, one is required to break confidentiality to report child abuse. In some venues, a threat of imminent violence to an individual requires a *duty to warn* exception to confidentiality. Similarly, when a patient appears acutely suicidal and likely to act on the wish to die, many therapists choose to disclose suicidality to family members in the interest of saving the patient's life by enlisting a support system to monitor the patient's potentially lethal behavior. In a small number of states, therapists who hear of sexual misconduct by a fellow professional from a confidential source are required to report this matter to a licensing board. However, these regulations vary from state to state, and psychotherapists are well advised to consult their own state statutes when in doubt and to consult an attorney or knowledgeable colleague about the implications of a breach of confidentiality. Clinicians who decide to report without checking their regulatory statutes may think they are doing the right thing, only to end up with a lawsuit based on violation of confidentiality.

Gossiping psychotherapists are ubiquitous, and the delight in treating a well-known patient often leads certain psychotherapists to confide in colleagues about their secret pleasure of treating an illustrious person. However, the notion of confidentiality should be construed as meaning that one cannot even reveal whether a specific patient is in treatment or not. A formal consultation with a colleague is a different matter, of course, and requires the same level of confidentiality as treatment. The same is true of supervision. In most cases, the supervisee or consultee does not need to reveal the patient's name; in certain circumstances, however, doing so may be necessary for the supervisor or colleague to fully appreciate the difficulties the therapist is experiencing. There is nothing unethical about that type of revelation in the context of supervision or consultation.

However, when one presents a psychotherapy case for educational purposes or chooses to use clinical material in a publication, one must be careful to disguise identifying features of the patient. There are pros and cons of obtaining consent from the patient to present or publish, and those considerations have been thoroughly discussed elsewhere (Gabbard 2000b). Some people will argue that patients cannot provide truly informed consent because of the power differential and the difficulty of refusing the therapist who requests that permission. Moreover, even if consent is offered, identifying features must still be disguised so that an audience or reader does not recognize the patient. Some professional organizations have specific criteria that must be followed in publications or presentations, and members of each professional discipline must consult those guidelines before making a decision on how to proceed. Similarly, professional journals may have specific guidelines that must be followed.

Excessive Self-Disclosure

The classical principle of psychoanalytic psychotherapy known as *anonymity* has undergone a significant rethinking in recent years. Therapists cannot be anonymous to the patient, no matter how hard they may try. The way they dress, the way they decorate their offices, their facial expressions in response to what the patient says, and the issues they choose to address when they speak all reveal a great deal about the therapists' subjectivity. Hence, the idea of the therapist as a blank screen is a myth that is no longer endorsed by mainstream therapists of any persuasion. The issue for the contemporary psychotherapist is not whether to self-disclose. The technical and boundary concern is how much, what, and when to self-disclose.

Feelings that the therapist may experience in the here and now with the patient may be revealed at times in a way that advances the therapy and provides useful feedback for the patient. For example, when a provocative patient is insulting or devalues the therapist over and over again, the patient may pick up on the fact that the therapist is becoming angry. If, in such situations, the patient asks the therapist, "Are you angry at me?" the therapist may be far better off answering honestly than concealing true feelings in an effort to avoid self-disclosure (Gabbard and Wilkinson 1994). A therapist in that situation might choose to say something like "Yes, I think you're picking up on something. Let's look at the interaction and try to figure out what is going on between us that provoked feelings of irritation in me." In this way, the therapist transforms the countertransference anger into a topic that can be productively explored between the two parties in the therapeutic dyad. It would be far better to be honest in that situation than to be deliberately deceptive. Therapists often communicate feelings nonverbally, so the patient may know what the therapist feels before the patient asks.

Not all feelings that the therapist has toward a patient are helpful to self-disclose. For example, even if a therapist feels genuine feelings of hate toward the patient, the act of saying "I hate you" to the patient is unlikely to help the therapy or lead to further self-understanding on the part of the patient. Similarly, saying to a patient "I have sexual feelings for you" is also unlikely to be useful and might even be experienced as traumatizing or violating to some patients. In society, when one person says to another, "I have sexual feelings for you," an action is usually implied to follow, namely, sexual engagement. On the other hand, it is not true that physical involvement follows an expression of irritation. Therefore, one must be wary of the implications of any type of self-disclosure.

One way of implementing a boundary on self-disclosure is to deliberately avoid sharing with the patient any details about one's personal life or family. Superficial elements of one's personal life may be helpful at times. For example, a therapist working with an adolescent boy may find that forming a therapeutic alliance requires some chitchat about sports that are of mutual interest, so the therapist might tell a patient about a football game he went to the previous weekend, to strike up a relationship with the patient.

Self-disclosures about personal problems must be rigorously monitored, however, because they are frequently the first step on the slippery slope (Gabbard 1996; Gabbard 2016). Some disclosures may be initially received with open arms by the patient and therefore mislead the therapist into thinking that such information is productive and should be continued.

Case Vignette

Dr. F, a male therapist in his 40s, came to a session with Ms. J, a female patient in her 30s. He seemed excessively tired and inattentive. Ms. J eventually said to him, "Are you okay? You look distracted today." Dr. F responded, "No, I don't think I could conceal anything from you. You read me like a book. My wife left me, and I'm struggling to stay at work in the midst of a huge personal crisis in my life." Ms. J paused for a moment and then said, "I am so honored that you would tell me about what is happening in your life so I can help you. You're always the one helping me, and it feels great for me to be able to offer you support for a change. I feel it's easier to open up to you when you open up to me." At the end of the session, Ms. J gave Dr. F a hug and told him, "You'll get through this. Hang in there." After she left, Dr. F thought to himself, "That went much better than I thought it would. She was so understanding about it." Having entered into this self-deception about the value of burdening the patient with his personal problems, Dr. F continued to disclose the details of the divorce to Ms. J at each session of the therapy, until they were sitting on the couch together embracing, meeting outside for coffee, and, ultimately, entering into a sexual relationship. During the course of an evaluation ordered by a licensing board, Ms. J told the evaluator that she realized she was paying a fee to Dr. F to hear about his personal problems. She said it didn't seem right to her in retrospect, even though she wanted to help him.

This vignette illustrates how a single self-disclosure can escalate into major boundary violations because of the therapist's neediness and the capacity for self-deception about who is helping whom. As always, consultation with a colleague may be essential in a life crisis to prevent this type of transgression from occurring.

Professional Role

The concept of *professional role* is fundamental to boundaries. Because of the fiduciary relationship, the therapist functions as one who tries to help the patient address symptoms or problems that have been brought to treatment. That is the therapist's sole purpose. The therapist is not a mother, a father, a priest or rabbi, a lover, a friend, or a sibling. In the initial therapist-patient meeting, some discussion of the professional role is usually necessary to clarify what therapy is and what therapy is not.

The therapist's professional role does not require that the therapist be excessively formal or inordinately depriving. Although it is entirely appropriate to begin a first meeting by referring to the patient as "Mr. Smith" or "Ms. Jones," if the patient prefers to be called by their first name, the therapist may accommodate the patient's wish to help the patient feel comfortable in the therapeutic setting. Similarly, the therapist should not hesitate to be warm and emotionally available to help the patient grow and to provide empathic resonance that may have been missing in the patient's development.

Length and Time of Sessions

Another limit imposed on the therapist-patient relationship involves the length and time of sessions. Winnicott (1954/1958) once noted that both love and aggression are communicated in the treatment relationship. The therapist communicates the loving component by listening empathically and providing an opportunity for the patient to grow and change in the context of an accepting relationship. On the other hand, the therapist communicates the aggressive part of the equation by ending the hour on time and charging a fee for the services.

The time of the session is often 45–50 minutes but can be as brief as 15 minutes or as long as 90 minutes. In any case, the time parameters must be clear to the patient, and it is useful for the patient to understand from the beginning of the therapy that time constraints will always apply. Patients generally understand if the therapist explains that the session cannot be extended because there are other patients waiting to be seen. One cannot be totally rigid, however, and occasionally may need to go over a few minutes to accommodate an intense emotional reaction by a patient or other unusual circumstances.

Another important factor related to time is the hour of the day when the patient is seen. A number of cases of boundary violations have been preceded by scheduling a patient during the last hour of the day, when the office personnel in the clinic may have gone home and no other people are around. This setting may communicate to the patient that there is a potential for something other than a professional relationship (Gutheil and Gabbard 1993). Therefore, one should be mindful about scheduling patients at such times.

Fees

That therapists are paid for their services underscores the fact that the therapist is working. Therapy is hard work, and the therapist deserves to be paid. In many settings, the patient does not hand the therapist a check or is not even charged a fee. However, therapists are, nevertheless, paid a salary by the clinic or organization for which they work, and the patient is aware that the therapist makes a living through seeing patients.

The fact of being paid further differentiates the therapist from parent, lover, friend, and so on. When patients pay a fee, they are reminded that they have "rented" the therapist's time and should use it productively. One of the most common steps in the descent down the slippery slope is for the therapist to stop charging a fee or to allow the bill to accumulate. Another variation is to allow the patient a double session but expect payment for only one. In any case, therapists should carefully monitor their attitude about the patient's payment and the fee they are charging as a way of examining countertransference wishes to give the patient something for nothing. Billing problems often relate to feelings that the therapy is not worth anything or that the clinician is doing a poor job. Beginning therapists are typically conflicted about deserving a fee, and in training settings, supervisors should include collecting the fee as part of the training of future therapists.

Exchange of Gifts and Services

Grateful patients often wish to express their appreciation by bringing surprise gifts to their therapists. Some wealthy patients may wish to make a donation to the institution where a therapist works or to a project with which a therapist is involved. Accepting large gifts from patients opens the door to a variety of complications. Patients may consciously or unconsciously feel that they are entitled to special dispensation because they have given money or other material gifts to a therapist. Gifts may also mask aggression and negative feelings that the patient prefers to conceal. Sometimes the gift is an "unconscious bribe" to influence the therapist in one way or another (Gutheil and Gabbard 1993). Patients may think, "Maybe the therapist will not bring up shameful or unpleasant topics," "Maybe the therapist won't expect me to change things that I really don't want to change," or "Maybe a check written out to the therapist's research project will stop the therapist from pushing me in directions I do not want to go."

Because of concerns about the potential of gifts to corrupt the therapeutic process, the historical tendency has been to refuse all gifts. However, in recent years, the view on accepting small gifts has shifted to a much more reasonable perspective, with the recognition that some patients will be devastated when a small gift is refused. When a patient brings something handmade, a recommended book, or a small memento, many therapists simply thank the patient for the gift and talk about the particular meaning or symbolism of the gift. At the end of therapy, a patient may want to express appreciation with a small gift, and if the therapist refuses it, there may be no opportunity to discuss the impact of that refusal on the patient. Sometimes, the therapist may have doubts about whether it is right to accept the gift and may share the dilemma with the patient. In some instances, the therapist may explain that they would like to have the opportunity to think about it or talk about the gift with a consultant before making a decision.

Despite the complexity of the problem of gifts, therapists can follow several rules of thumb:

- Do not accept donations to your projects or the institution's projects during treatment.
- Do not accept cash gifts.
- Avoid accepting expensive gifts, and when the expense is in doubt, consider delaying the decision and possibly consulting with a colleague.
- Always explore the meaning of any gift to see whether the act of offering the present to the therapist can open up new areas for exploration in the therapy.

A corollary to gift giving is the offering of services. Patients who may not be able to afford a gift or who feel that gifts are inappropriate will sometimes offer to provide services for the therapist. These may include such activities as painting a house, babysitting, enhancing features on the therapist's computer, or redecorating the therapist's office. These types of services are fraught with difficulties because the therapist is stuck if the service is done badly. What therapist would feel free to complain or critique the service or refuse to pay? In general, services from patients blend into the area of business transactions and dual relationships, which are almost always problematic in psychotherapy.

Clothing and Language

Both clothing and language are aspects of the psychotherapist role that are often underemphasized as part of professional boundaries. Dressing in a professional manner conveys that the therapist does not consider the meeting to be recreation. Patients sometimes quit after an initial meeting with a mental health professional because they feel that the clinician does not appear to be professional. Besides casual dress, seductive clothing can also create a problem in conveying professionalism to the patient. Some clinicians dress in a way that appears seductive to others without knowing it themselves. It is sometimes useful for therapists to speak to one another when they perceive a problem with the way a colleague dresses.

Informal or crude language can also work against professionalism. The use of slang to refer to genitals or sexuality may be problematic for some patients, and therapists must attempt to mentalize a patient's probable response before choosing to speak in such terms. Generally, one is on much firmer ground when using more technical terms for sex acts and anatomical parts. Language can also be experienced as abusive by some patients, particularly those who have experienced verbal abuse in the past. Hence, thoughtful attention to language is part of effective technique in psychotherapy.

Physical Contact

In general, psychotherapy proceeds without physical contact. Sometimes a handshake takes place when a therapist and patient first meet. However, in most cases, the handshakes do not continue throughout the treatment. There are exceptions, of course, often based on cultural practices, so that some patients will initiate a handshake at the beginning and end of each session. Psychotherapists can return the handshake without concerns about boundaries in most cases. The only exception is if there is erotization in the transference and the patient is using the handshake as a way of having sexualized physical contact with the therapist. Hence, these judgments must be made on a case-by-case basis.

As noted in the section "Boundary Crossings Versus Boundary Violations," one cannot make an absolutist statement that hugs are never acceptable in psychotherapy. In unusual situations, such as a significant loss, therapists may return a hug initiated by a patient. However, hugs on a regular basis are not part of psychotherapy and may cause the patient to misinterpret the therapist's intentions. Some therapists argue that a hug is sometimes needed by a patient, but people's capacity for self-deception is extraordinary. What a therapist may think is best for the patient may actually be a way of fulfilling the therapist's own needs.

It is important to remember that psychotherapists have chosen their profession for a myriad of unconscious reasons that may be incompletely understood (Gabbard 1996). A therapist may have a conscious intention of demonstrating caring to a patient. However, a hug, for example, that is intended by a male therapist to provide nurturance may be perceived by the female patient as a sexual overture, particularly if there is a history of sexual violation in that patient's past. The concept of a nonsexual hug is usually in the mind of the therapist but not necessarily in the mind of the patient.

This consideration of hugs leads to a basic tenet of psychotherapy that must be part of the training of every psychotherapist: The therapist's intent when engaging in a particular behavior may not be the same as the impact that behavior has on the patient. A corollary to this tenet is that therapists cannot always know the unconscious intent. The road to hell is paved with good intentions, and many serious boundary violations have begun with what the therapist thought was a benign hug or a pat on the shoulder.

The following are useful guidelines regarding physical contact:

- Do not initiate hugs.
- Respond to hugs initiated by a patient only under extraordinary circumstances.

- If the patient is clearly expressing an erotic transference, physical contact should be avoided.
- Explore the meaning of any physical contact with the patient as part of the therapeutic process.

Posttermination Professional Boundaries

Although broad consensus exists that sexual contact between the psychotherapist and a patient is always unethical, the idea of posttermination sexual relationships has historically been more controversial. The major mental health organizations have agreed that sexual contact between a clinician and a current or former patient is unethical (American Psychiatric Association 2013). Social workers have also declared that engaging in sexual activities with a client or former client is unethical (National Association of Social Workers 2021). The American Psychological Association has similar ethical standards regarding current and former patients for at least 2 years. However, they allow for exceptions in unusual cases after 2 years (American Psychological Association 2017). As discussed in the following subsections, several sound arguments are useful in supporting the idea of an absolute prohibition against sexual relationships between a therapist and former patient (Gabbard 2002; Gabbard et al. 2015).

Persistence of Transference

Transference involves the reexperiencing of the therapist as a powerful and authoritative figure from the past. Cognitive neuroscience suggests that representations of parents are laid down in neural networks that represent self and other from early in childhood and then are activated again and again by specific characteristics of current figures in one's life (Westen and Gabbard 2002). One implication of this understanding of transference is that transference is never completely resolved. Follow-up research has confirmed that transference persists long after the therapist-patient relationship is terminated. A series of studies (Buckley et al. 1981; Norman et al. 1976; Pfeffer 1963, 1993) demonstrated that transference is instantly reestablished when patients are followed up after the ending of treatment, and an active effort to process and work through persistent transference issues still occurs. In other words, the patient's dependency and vulnerability to exploitation do not disappear at termination of therapy. Even in psychotherapies that eschew transference work, the phenomenon of transference is activated.

Power Differential

Patients place their mental health in the hands of a therapist and offer a fee for the therapist's expertise. In a psychotherapeutic relationship, regardless of the age, gender, or professional credentials, there is always, consciously or unconsciously, a power differential between the two participants in the therapeutic dyad. The psychiatrist or therapist inevitably holds the power within the therapeutic dyad, while the patient remains in a vulnerable position. Even when patients feel they are on equal ground with the therapist, the power differential remains present, even if unconscious, and must be respected and held in mind by the therapist. That power differential, once established, will continue after the therapeutic relationship has ended (Gabbard 2016).

Destruction of the Therapeutic Relationship

Above all, psychotherapists wish to avoid harm to the patient. An ethics code is constructed to identify situations of potential harm and prevent them from entering into a therapeutic relationship. Hence, another argument in favor of an absolute prohibition is that the knowledge of that prohibition may prevent a corruption of the therapeutic process.

If posttermination sexual relationships were acceptable, one could imagine a scenario with a single therapist and a single patient that would involve a growing attraction to one another that confounded the therapeutic purpose (Gabbard 2002). The therapist might begin to think that the patient is someone ideally suited as a romantic partner and try to foster idealization. The therapist might, for example, avoid confrontation of any undesirable features to gain the patient's love and respect. The patient, if also attracted, might decide to conceal certain shameful episodes from the past so as not to disgust or turn off the therapist. The patient might even curry favor by expressing to the therapist great admiration of the therapist's skill. The result might be a mutual admiration society in which important therapeutic issues are kept out of the dialogue.

If one or both members of the therapeutic dyad are aware that a romantic relationship is forever off-limits, this knowledge frees the therapeutic dialogue from interference from that hoped-for future relationship. Indeed, the essence of the therapeutic relationship is that it will never be anything but psychotherapy, so patients are free to say whatever they like without repercussions in another context in which they will see the therapist.

Possible Return of the Patient

As all experienced clinicians know, patients who terminate psychotherapy frequently return for further therapeutic work in the midst of a life crisis or a struggle with a new developmental phase that must be mastered. Kantrowitz (2015) conducted a systematic study that followed up 82 patients who were former analysands. She found that 51 out of 82 of the subjects sought out further help from their analyst after termination. Hence, another argument for an absolute prohibition against romantic involvement following termination is that the therapist may be needed again in the professional role of psychotherapist rather than as a friend, business partner, or lover.

When the professional boundaries do not involve considerations of sexual contact, posttermination relationships are much less clearly defined. Psychotherapists may see former patients in various social situations and certainly should feel free to be warm and friendly with them. Areas of common interest may bring them together periodically as well. For example, patients and mental health professionals may serve on committees together or may be involved in organizing a conference. Nevertheless, therapists are well advised to maintain some boundary involving personal problems such that they remain available as a potential therapist in the future.

Prevention of Boundary Violations

Education about professional boundaries is essential in the training of psychotherapists, but one must face the fact that serious boundary violations will never be eliminated entirely from the practice of psychotherapy. By its very nature, psychotherapy involves a radical form of privacy. Two people are meeting each other regularly behind closed doors, and one of them is confessing their darkest and most shameful secrets to the other. The atmosphere of emotional confession and acceptance fosters a rare kind of intimacy not often available outside therapy. Some therapists will rationalize to themselves that a romantic relationship is possible and acceptable because there is no exploitation of the patient.

Nevertheless, education about professional boundaries may be useful in preventing some instances of boundary transgressions by providing therapists with a framework for thinking about the nature of a professional relationship versus a personal one. Boundaries cannot be taught simply as a list of rules. They need to be taught as part of clinical wisdom, integrating boundary notions into discussions of technique and the choices a therapist must make.

Ongoing consultation throughout their career is probably the best preventive measure that psychotherapists can build into their professional lives. There is something quasi-incestuous about sexual relations between therapist and patient. Like incest, the sexual behavior occurs in a dyad outside the view of any third party. By introducing a consultant into that dyad, the dynamics of the relationship change in such a way that the therapist has a colleague or partner to discuss the case with, and the radical privacy shifts. In training, therapists are accustomed to a triad rather than a dyad: patient-therapist-supervisor. This triad builds in a quality control factor: the therapist knows that they are being "observed" by the supervisor and can talk to someone when anything unusual is happening in the therapy.

Isolation is a risk factor for professional boundary violations (Gabbard 2016), and the use of consultation, either individually or in a group format, also serves to relieve that isolation. The therapist must be sure to choose a consultant who is not simply a friend who will confirm the value of whatever the therapist is doing. Consultants must have two key qualities: the capacity to make the therapist feel comfortable and the capacity to confront the therapist when things are heading in problematic directions (Gabbard 2000a). One must always keep in mind that this preventive measure is not foolproof because consultation can be misused. The therapist can conceal information from the consultant. The therapist can select a consultant who will confirm the course of the therapy. The therapist can even use consultation informally in a way that is not effective—the so-called curbside consultation.

In any case, prevention depends to a large extent on what the therapist does in private moments. A useful monitoring tool is for therapists to ask themselves, "Is what I'm doing something I can tell my consultant?" If the answer is no, the therapist knows that this behavior is the very thing that *should* be brought up to the consultant. In the final analysis, therapists must be their own watchdogs to avoid professional boundary violations.

Ethics in Psychotherapy

Following on the heels of this discussion of boundaries and boundary violations in psychotherapy, we now turn to some broader ethical issues in the therapeutic encounter. Drozek (2019) roots his views on the psychotherapeutic and psychoanalytic understanding of ethics in moral philosophy. He outlines a system in which the "ethical development of both therapist and patient serves as the fulcrum of psychic change" (p. 7). He emphasizes the following basic principles as being fundamental to the human experience: the assumption of freedom, the importance of behavior and consequences, the notion of dignity, the possibility of altruism, and the connection between ethical living and psychological well-being (Drozek 2019). In psychotherapy, he challenges clinicians to bring these practical ethical commitments into their daily psychotherapeutic work with patients.

In addition to boundaries, ethical conceptualizations of psychotherapy include attention to issues of informed consent, nonmaleficence, confidentiality (or the informed consent to disclose), and the values of the patient and psychotherapist (Adshead 2005). Clinicians have an ethical responsibility to be guided by research and practice guidelines and to stay up-to-date on the literature. Various types of therapy may focus on ethical issues specific to that particular line of therapy, for example, psychoanalytic psychotherapy (Brenner and Cather 2015) and cognitive-behavioral therapy (Sookman 2015).

Therapists (and their patients) benefit from supervision and/or consultation with an experienced therapist to maintain the therapeutic focus, navigate rough waters in the therapy, and prevent boundary violations. It can be helpful for the therapist to raise ethical issues with which they may be grappling with a consultant of their choosing (Gabbard 2000a). Such issues for consultation may include when one should contact the patient's family, when one needs to disclose to preserve the patient's safety, and what could be considered an emergency. Therapists must navigate the conflict between the patient's right to privacy and autonomy and the patient's safety. Although the answer to this dilemma may be clear in a case of true, immediate emergency, many of the clinical situations therapists face are more chronic, challenging gray areas in which it is useful to have another mind with whom to collaborate.

For couple, family, and group therapies, the ethical issues at stake must be at once individualized to each participant and broad enough to encompass the entire system. A couple therapist has two patients, not one, and similarly, the family or group therapist must attend to the needs of the individual along with the needs of others in the group and the group as whole.

In family or couple therapy, the therapist must manage each family member's conflicting goals for therapy and differing perspectives or narratives about the family story, as well as attend to each member of the family or group so that each person feels heard and seen (Margolin et al. 2015). Furthermore, it can be challenging to decide to hold and/or share information that has been obtained privately from one member of the couple or group. Often, the guidelines about what types of information may be held privately by the therapist with only one member versus shared together with the couple, family, or group are clearly established at the beginning of a therapeutic process as the frame of therapy is set. In some cases, a consultant can be helpful in making the decision if it is complicated. Family or group members may be at risk of feeling their confidentiality has been betrayed. Therapists should use sensitivity and a forthright manner to communicate these possible conflicts at the outset of the therapy, both verbally and in writing in the therapist's policies and practices in terms of managing the confidentiality and disclosure of all participants. It is essential to avoid any real or perceived collusions with one participant in the family at the expense of another (Margolin et al. 2015). The assessment of safety and risk for each family member must be in the family therapist's mind because of the risk of undisclosed or developing physical aggression and violence within the family. Family members should understand the limits of confidentiality from the beginning of the therapy. Examples are legal proceedings with divorce, child custody, or forensic documents (Gottlieb et al. 2008; Margolin et al. 2015).

Similarly, group therapists must navigate the needs of the individual versus the needs of the group as a whole, including the thoughtful management of any private information that group therapists may know from meetings outside the group setting. A group agreement can be helpful in assisting members of the group to learn the expectations around ethics and boundaries that are part of participating in the group. As in couple or family therapy, policies and procedures regarding the roles of the group members and the role of the therapist must be presented in a clear and forthright manner.

Ethics and Diversities

As therapists, we have entered into a vocation in which every day we value our curiosity and wonder how others' experiences may be similar to or different from our own. We marvel at the workings of the minds of others; we want to learn their narratives and hear their stories. It is an ethical duty to practice with a respect for the experience and autonomy of each person, attending to the nuances of their personal identity and cultural context, trying to understand how the world looks through their eyes.

In the narrowness of one person's experience, harm can be done by not understanding or making space for experiences different from our own. We must tune into and embrace a curiosity about the self and the other. As Dionne Powell reminds us eloquently in the introduction to Part 7, "Racial and Ethnic Diversities in Psychotherapy," in order to be competent therapists, we are ethically required to have "cultural humility, informed inquiry, and open curiosity" about our own views of self and other, in addition to curiosity about how those views shape the therapeutic alliance, transference, and countertransference (p. 460).

It is incumbent on therapists to educate themselves and become aware of the conscious and unconscious aspects of their awareness of their own ethnicity, culture, gender, and sexuality, as well as those dynamics in their patients. Power and privilege have long been part of psychotherapeutic training institutions, psychiatry and psychology departments, and clinical settings, and these dynamics must be understood, reflected on, and changed in both individuals and systems. Systemic racism and prejudice have clearly caused harm historically in medicine and in psychotherapy. Furthermore, the pathologizing of gay, lesbian, bisexual, and transgender people by psychiatrists and therapists has been a shameful part of our history as a profession, as Jack Drescher and colleagues outline in Part 8, "Gender and Sexualities in Psychotherapy." We have an ethical duty to be actively curious about the identity and experience of each person with whom we engage in a therapeutic process and to understand how power and privilege play out in the psychotherapeutic encounter as well as in the day-to-day experiences of our patients.

Ethics and Virtual Therapies

During the past two decades the amount of psychotherapy that is practiced in virtual formats has grown. Therapists who had begun the foray into teletherapies and have been on the forefront of these ideas have been outlining ethical modes of interacting with patients as well as attending to the boundaries that shift in an electronic format (Perez-Garcia 2015; Russell 2015; Yellowlees and Shore 2018). The onset of the COVID-19 pandemic in 2020 brought an immediate and wide-scale shift to the virtual delivery of all types of therapy across the world. This sea change inevitably and importantly brought into focus for all therapists the ethical issues at stake for teletherapies. The necessity of providing confidentiality and privacy in a new, distanced location across time and space and in the home or workplace of the patient necessitated that therapists consider new ethical issues related to privacy, confidentiality, the development of the therapeutic alliance, access to care, and issues of safety. For a more detailed look at the issues regarding teletherapy, see Chapter 34, "Psychotherapy and Cyberspace," by Yellowlees and Shore.

Conclusion

In this overview of ethics and professional boundaries in psychotherapy, we have provided a set of helpful guidelines that should be used flexibly by psychotherapists. Different forms of psychotherapy require different emphases on the way that professional boundaries are implemented. Within different techniques, the therapist adjusts the boundaries to make the patient more accessible and more capable of collaborating with the therapist.

One of the most difficult aspects of psychotherapeutic practice is our incapacity to know the ultimate impact of departing from boundaries. We can rationalize rather dramatic exceptions to boundaries in certain situations, and although we may think we are being humane, the patient may feel they are no longer safe. Hence, frank discussion of the boundaries between therapist and patient must be part of the therapeutic dialogue on a regular basis.

Along with boundaries in psychotherapy, it is wise to consider ethical dilemmas that may arise around issues of confidentiality, privacy, autonomy, access to care, and varying goals for therapy. All of us, patients and therapists, are alike in our fundamental humanity, and we must approach our patients with an ethical attitude of respect, humility, and compassion.

Key Points

- Professional boundaries are the parameters defining the limits of a fiduciary relationship in which one person (a patient) entrusts their welfare to another (a psychotherapist), who is paid for the provision of a service.
- Boundary crossings are generally benign phenomena that do not recur repetitively, are discussable between the therapist and the patient, are not exploitative, and may even help the therapeutic process.
- Boundary violations are egregious phenomena that are usually repetitive, harmful to the patient, and exploitative of the patient's vulnerable position. They are also generally not discussable with the therapist.
- Specific dimensions of professional boundaries include location, confidentiality, excessive self-disclosure, professional role, time of sessions, payment, gifts and services, clothing, language, and nonsexual physical contact.
- Posttermination sexual contact is generally considered unethical because of the persistence of transference, the power differential, the potential to destroy the therapeutic nature of the relationship, and the possible return of the patient.
- Education about professional boundaries is essential in the training of all psychotherapists, even though it will not entirely eliminate the problem.
- Ongoing consultation throughout one's career is probably the best preventive measure that psychotherapists can use to avoid serious boundary violations.
- In addition to boundaries, ethical issues for therapists include privacy and confidentiality, disclosure, autonomy, and addressing the values of the patient.
- Therapists who do couple, family, or group therapies have a broader set of ethical obligations and tensions to attend to than those focused only on individuals.
- Attention to experiential diversities of ethnicity, culture, gender, and sexualities is an important ethical issue for therapists and in psychotherapy education.
- Ongoing attention to ethics as psychotherapy continues to expand into teletherapies is an important current and future consideration.

Recommended Readings

Epstein R: Keeping Boundaries: Maintaining Safety and Integrity in the Psychotherapeutic Process. Washington, DC, American Psychiatric Press, 1994

Gabbard GO, Lester E: Boundaries and Boundary Violations in Psychoanalysis, 2nd Edition. Washington, DC, American Psychiatric Publishing, 2016

References

Adshead G: Ethics and psychotherapy, in Oxford Textbook of Psychotherapy. Edited by Gabbard GO, Beck JS, Holmes J. Oxford, UK, Oxford University Press, 2005, pp 477–485

American Psychiatric Association: The Principles of Medical Ethics: With Annotations Especially Applicable to Psychiatry, 3rd Edition. Arlington, VA, American Psychiatric Association, 20131

American Psychological Association: Ethical Principles of Psychologists and Code of Conduct. Washington, DC, American Psychological Association, 2017. Available at: www.apa.org/ethics/code. Accessed May 19, 2022

Brenner A, Cather JC: Using a "virtues" approach to ethical challenges in psychoanalytic psychotherapy, in The Oxford Handbook of Psychiatric Ethics. Edited by Sadler JA, Van Staden CW, Fulford KWM. New York, Oxford University Press, 2015, pp 1264–1275

Buckley P, Karasu TB, Charles E: Psychotherapists view their personal therapy. Psychotherapy (Chic) 18(2):299–305, 1981

Drozek RP: Psychoanalysis as an Ethical Process. New York, Routledge, 2019.

Gabbard GO: Lessons to be learned from the study of sexual boundary violations. Am J Psychother 50(3):311–322, 1996 8886231

Gabbard GO: Consultation from the consultant's perspective. Psychoanal Dialogues 10(2):209–218, 2000a

Gabbard GO: Disguise or consent: problems and recommendations concerning the publication and presentation of clinical material. Int J Psychoanal 81 (Part 6):1071–1086, 2000b 11144850

Gabbard GO: Post-termination sexual boundary violations. Psychiatr Clin North Am 25(3):593–603, 2002 12232973

Gabbard GO: Boundaries and Boundary Violations in Psychoanalysis, 2nd Edition. Arlington, VA, American Psychiatric Association Publishing, 2016

Gabbard GO: Sexual boundary violations in psychoanalysis: a 30-year retrospective. Psychoanal Psychol 34(2):151–156, 2017

Gabbard GO, Nadelson C: Professional boundaries in the physician-patient relationship. JAMA 273(18):1445–1449, 1995 7723159

Gabbard GO, Wilkinson SM: Management of Countertransference With Borderline Patients. Washington, DC, American Psychiatric Press, 1994

Gabbard GO, Crisp-Han H, Hobday G: Professional Boundaries in Psychiatric Practice, in The Oxford Handbook of Psychiatric Ethics. Edited by Sadler JA, Van Staden CW, Fulford KWM. New York, Oxford University Press, 2015, pp 1160–1174

Gottlieb MC, Lasser J, Simpson GL: Legal and ethical issues in couple therapy, in A Clinical Handbook of Couple Therapy, 4th Edition. Edited by Gurman AS. New York, Guilford, 2008

Gutheil TG, Gabbard GO: The concept of boundaries in clinical practice: theoretical and risk-management dimensions. Am J Psychiatry 150(2):188–196, 1993 8422069

Gutheil TG, Gabbard GO: Misuses and misunderstandings of boundary theory in clinical and regulatory settings. Am J Psychiatry 155(3):409–414, 1998 9501754

Kantrowitz JL: Myths of Termination: What Patients Can Teach Psychoanalysts About Endings. New York, Routledge, 2015

Margolin G, Shapiro LS, Miller KF: Ethics in couple and family psychotherapy, in The Oxford Handbook of Psychiatric Ethics. Edited by Sadler JA, Van Staden CW, Fulford KWM. New York, Oxford University Press, 2015, pp 1306–1314

National Association of Social Workers: Code of Ethics 2021. Washington, DC, National Association of Social Workers, 2021. Available at: www.socialworkers.org/about/ethics/code-of-ethics/code-of-ethics-english. Accessed May 19, 2022

Norman HF, Blacker KH, Oremland JD, et al: The fate of the transference neurosis after termination of a satisfactory analysis. J Am Psychoanal Assoc 24(3):471–498, 1976 965699

Perez-Garcia GJ: Ethics of telepsychiatry, in The Oxford Handbook of Psychiatric Ethics. Edited by Sadler JA, Van Staden CW, Fulford KWM. New York, Oxford University Press, 2015, pp 1346–1359

Pfeffer AZ: The meaning of the analyst after analysis: a contribution to the theory of therapeutic results. J Am Psychoanal Assoc 11:229–244, 1963 13943055

Pfeffer AZ: After the analysis: analyst as both old and new object. J Am Psychoanal Assoc 41(2):323–337, 1993 8478512

Russell GI: Screen Relations: The Limits of Computer-Mediated Psychoanalysis and Psychotherapy. New York, Karnac, 2015

Sookman D: Ethical practice of cognitive behavioral therapy, in The Oxford Handbook of Psychiatric Ethics. Edited by Sadler JA, Van Staden CW, Fulford KWM. New York, Oxford University Press, 2015, pp 1293–1301

Strasburger LH, Jorgenson L, Sutherland P: The prevention of psychotherapist sexual misconduct: avoiding the slippery slope. Am J Psychother 46(4):544–555, 1992 1443284

Westen D, Gabbard GO: Developments in cognitive neuroscience II: implications for theories of transference. J Am Psychoanal Assoc 50(1):99–134, 2002 12018876

Winnicott DW: Metapsychological and clinical aspects of regression within the psycho-analytic set-up (1954), in Collected Papers: Through Paediatrics to Psycho-analysis. New York, Basic Books, 1958, pp 278–294

Yellowlees P, Shore JH: Telepsychiatry and Health Technologies: A Guide for Mental Health Professionals. Arlington, VA, American Psychiatric Association Publishing, 2018

CHAPTER 33

Neuroscience of Psychotherapy

Susan Vaughan, M.D.
Mohsin Ahmed, M.D., Ph.D.

The deficiencies in our description would probably vanish if we were already in a position to replace the psychological terms with physiological or chemical ones.

—Sigmund Freud (1920/1955)

I would argue that it is only insofar as our words produce changes in each other's brains that psychotherapeutic intervention produces changes in patients' minds. From this perspective the biologic and psychologic approaches are joined.

—Eric Kandel (2001)

Although we cannot yet explain the workings of the mind in the language of the brain or the process of psychotherapy in the language of the neuron, we are closer than ever before to being able to do so. The challenge for any chapter on neuroscience as it relates to psychotherapy is to demonstrate the tantalizing connections between the two without shifting into neuroscience as metaphor, on the one hand, and without forcing premature closure between the fields, on the other. In this chapter we examine a number of known neuroscience mechanisms and explore their relevance to various forms of psychotherapy.

Molecular Mechanisms of Memory

Neurobiological Mechanisms

Although pioneering physicians and neuropsychologists such as Brenda Milner had begun to disentangle the differences in various types of memory as early as the 1950s (Scoville and Milner 1957), little was known about how memory is acquired, modified, or disrupted. Eric Kandel and his associates uncovered the molecular basis of memory at the level of the individual neuron using the sea slug *Aplysia* as their animal model (Kandel et al. 2014). *Aplysia* has the advantage of having large neurons visible under a dissecting microscope, which allows scientists to record the strength of synapses during simple reflex behaviors. Kandel demonstrated that short-term changes to memory, lasting from a few minutes to an hour, resulted from changes in the strength of certain critical synapses via the modulation of synaptic transmission. When a slug's sensory-motor neuronal path was stimulated repeatedly with a harmless stimulus (shrimp juice), fewer and fewer vesicles of neurotransmitter were released gradually, and the synapse became less likely to drive the postsynaptic cell to fire. This phenomenon is habituation. In contrast, when the stimulus was harmful (electric shock to the tail), release of a neurotransmitter in the synapse between sensory and motor neurons was increased, with more vesicles released. This response is sensitization (Castellucci and Kandel 1976; Glanzman et al. 1989). For the first time, psychological concepts inferred from behavioral studies about classical and operant conditioning, nonassociative and associative learning, could be explained in molecular and cellular terms, demonstrating that synaptic plasticity is the basis for learning.

Relevance to Psychotherapy

Laying down traces of short-term memory is how we begin to learn, regardless of what we are learning. The same is true in psychotherapy, which is a form of learning involving pattern recognition. All forms of psychotherapy consist of repeated exploration of patterns, and multiple trials are required to convert short-term memory to long-term memory. However, at heart, all psychotherapy is the "psychotherapy of the single synapse" (Kandel 2001, p. 1036) and begins with a short-term memory trace that can be converted into a long-term memory.

Consolidation of Short-Term Memory Into Long-Term Memory

Neurobiological Mechanisms

Kandel and colleagues turned next to how these short-term changes are encoded and stored as long-term memories, demonstrating that as trials of learning continue over weeks, increased release of neurotransmitter, operating via the cyclic adenosine monophosphate (cAMP) second messenger system in neurons, leads to activation of gene expression via cAMP response element binding protein 1 (CREB1) (Abrams et al. 1991; Guan et al. 2002). CREB1 in turn triggers gene transcription to messenger RNA (mRNA) and to new protein synthesis that can serve as the scaffolding for new neuronal connections to form (Barco et al. 2002). Another type of cAMP response element binding protein, CREB2, acts as a memory suppressor gene. If CREB2 is removed, then a single exposure to serotonin, which would normally create an increase in synaptic strength lasting only minutes, will increase synaptic strength for days and induce the robust growth of new synaptic connections (Bartsch et al. 1995).

In essence, Kandel and colleagues' work demonstrated that both short- and long-term memories arise from synaptic modulation by Ca^{2+}/calmodulin and ras pathways that activate the brain-derived neurotrophic factor (BDNF), followed by the sprouting and growth, via CREB1 and other proteins, of new synaptic connections (Kandel et al. 2014). A single neuron can have up to a thousand synapses, which are the units of information storage. Communications between the synapse and cell nucleus result in production of neurotrophins that permit the growth of new neuronal connections via the transcription of genes and the translation of new proteins. This work conclusively demonstrated that synaptic connections are a primary basis of all long-term learning in *Aplysia*. In mammals, the combination of changes in synaptic strength and growth of new connections and synapses contributes to learning and memory.

Implications for Psychotherapy

Change in psychotherapy arises from the storage of new information about thoughts, feelings, and behaviors in memory, which requires multiple trials, protein synthesis, and neuronal growth. Thus, continued pattern recognition of whatever patterns a particular psychotherapy examines is essential. Learning takes multiple repetitions across time. Insight, although important, is only one piece of what creates change in psychotherapy. Interestingly, because selective serotonin reuptake inhibitors (SSRIs) can boost the production of BDNF, which leads to CREB1 production and dendritic sprouting, it may be possible to use medications to put the patient's brain in "high gear" for change (Duman and Aghajanian 2012).

Memory Reconsolidation

Neurobiological Mechanisms

Nader et al. (2000) and Sara (2000) demonstrated that reactivation of the long-term memory trace on its retrieval can result in transient destabilization of the memory that may lead to its change. This phenomenon is called reconsolidation. In fact, in *Aplysia* it has been shown that the same sensory-motor synapses that store long-term memories are destabilized by protein degradation on reactivation and restabilized by protein synthesis afterward. In other words, long-term memories, once formed, remain potentially dynamic even in simple reflexes in *Aplysia* (Kandel et al. 2014).

In humans, determining cues that are associated with neuronal changes and finding the neuron that changes within a large neuronal network are daunting. In addition, mammalian plasticity can be modulated by other transmitter and hormonal systems as well as by the past activation history of the individual synapse itself, which is known as metaplasticity (Abraham and Tate 1997). To make matters more complex still, reconsolidation does not seem to occur after each memory reactivation (Tronson and Taylor 2007). It is more likely to occur when the memory is strong, when the duration between memory formation and reactivation is shorter, and when the memory retrieval task includes the presence of new information (Kandel et al. 2014).

Relevance to Psychotherapy

Although memory is central in psychoanalytic theory, the focus on memory has shifted several times. First, in the topographic model, Freud's goal was to make the disavowed sexual memories (or, later, fantasies) of early life conscious, thereby alleviating symptoms. In the structural model, the focus was on defenses, especially repression, that operate to keep painful, conflicted content and dangerous affective states out of awareness via defense mechanisms. Analysis of the resistance to this material was the focus, although bringing the underlying unconscious mental content and its associated affects into awareness was also important. More recently, focus has shifted to the patient's life narrative and how life narratives may be permeated with unconscious distortions and fears. The reworking of these life narratives and bringing self-deceptions into awareness allow for a differently reconsolidated narrative of the patient's life (Gorman and Roose 2011).

Neurobiological work on memory reconsolidation has some important implications for psychotherapy. First, all memory is susceptible to change via memory reconsolidation. Second, memories formed in earliest life appear to be the most difficult to change with reconsolidation. Finally, certain conditions such as providing new information in the context of the activation of a memory (in the form of an interpretation or other intervention) should be part of all therapeutic techniques, harnessing what we know about memory reconsolidation to make the affective associations of memories more amenable to change. What is reawakened in memory and reconsolidated may differ in different forms of psychotherapy, but many types of psychotherapy create long-term change by reconsolidating memory and its associated affects in a different form. As we learn more, it may also be possible to increase neural plasticity using plasticity-enhancing agents such as D-cycloserine, a partial agonist of the *N*-methyl-D-aspartate receptor, to synergistically speed learning-related synaptic changes using medications alongside psychotherapy (Gabriele and Packard 2007).

Fear Circuitry and Memory Reconsolidation

Neurobiological Mechanisms

Perhaps the most important determinant of whether an activated memory can be reconsolidated, however, is the presence or absence of a strong emotional response, such as fear. Studies of fear conditioning in rodents by LeDoux (1995, 2003) have used classical conditioning paradigms that pair neutral stimuli, such as tones (the conditioned stimulus), with aversive or fear-inducing stimuli, such as mild electric shocks (the unconditioned stimulus). After pairings, the animal learns that the conditioned stimulus predicts the unconditioned stimulus and will display an innate fear response (such as freezing) to the conditioned stimulus alone. This conditioned response can be extinguished by repeated presentation of the tone without an accompanying shock. This is the paradigm of treatment for many phobias. However, this extinction learning does not erase the learned association driving the conditioned response. Indeed, the conditioned response may be immediately and strongly reawakened by even one exposure to the tone-shock pair itself, even after years. Unlike extinction, however, the fear-laden memory of the tone-shock experience *can* be completely eliminated by chemically blocking memory reconsolidation via various chemical pathways (Phelps and Hofmann 2019).

In addition, a fascinating study by Schiller et al. (2010) demonstrated that reconsolidation of a fear memory also can be inhibited in humans using purely *psychological* intervention. By pairing colored squares (conditioned stimulus) with mild electric wrist shock (unconditioned stimulus) and examining the skin conductance response (SCR), researchers found that subjects responded with increased SCR in response to the colored squares alone, as expected with classical conditioning.

One day later, the subjects underwent extinction by presentation of colored squares without wrist shocks. However, some subjects underwent a presentation of a reminder of the paired shock and colored square in the 10 minutes before their fear was extinguished, a period known as the reconsolidation window. A day later, subjects were again presented with the colored squares paired with wrist shocks. The group with no reminder before extinction showed a strong SCR response with a single presentation of the colored squares (consistent with spontaneous recovery of extinguished response, as expected). However, those who had the reminder manifested no change in SCR. These results remained the same 1 year later when some subjects returned to the laboratory for follow-up testing. The molecular biology, neural circuitry, and brain areas involved in these processes are quite well understood and have been reviewed elsewhere (Gorman and Roose 2011).

In terms of trauma, memory reconsolidation is also relevant to treatment of the resultant increased startle, hypervigilance, increased heart rate and respiration, dry mouth, emotional reactivity, defensive behaviors, and flashbacks to the original trauma. At a circuit level, the influence of the hypothalamic-pituitary-adrenal (HPA) axis and the sympathetic nervous system in PTSD suggests that the stress response system is hyperreactive to triggers, both in the magnitude of the response and in the time it takes this response to return to baseline. During stress, activation of the limbic system inhibits prefrontal cortical response, so the prefrontal cortex is unable to inhibit the amygdala and reduce the stress response (Ross et al. 2017). Amygdala hyperreactivity can be reduced by SSRIs (Shin et al. 2006).

Relevance to Psychotherapy

If, as the neurobiology seems to show, the presence of strong emotion is the most important determinant of whether an activated memory can be reconsolidated, therapists should adjust their technique to wait to intervene until the patient has a strong affective response in combination with a memory. Psychoanalysts have always included this idea in their technique, but now a neural basis exists for asserting that interpretations will have more impact if they are made in the presence of associated reawakened affective states.

Because many patients in therapy suffer from relational trauma caused by problematic interactions with caregivers in early life and their associated fantasies and emotions, the use of SSRIs may be indicated to help allow the prefrontal cortex to more effectively inhibit hyperreactive fear circuitry enough to facilitate effective engagement in psychotherapy, whether by exposure or by other cognitive-behavioral techniques. In psychodynamic therapy and psychoanalysis, the analyst may, perhaps, serve a function in regulating the amygdala through therapeutic reliance and the analytic witnessing of childhood trauma.

It seems clear that the mechanism of memory reconsolidation may reinforce traumatic memories through repeated recall of traumatic memories and their negative effects. In contrast, memory recall accompanied by fear that results in a different outcome (e.g., a triggering stimulus without a bad outcome in PTSD or the fact that the therapist responds differently to patients in psychotherapy than parental figures did) may be therapeutic.

Implicit and Explicit Memory Systems

Neurobiological Mechanisms

The case of H.M., whose traumatic brain injury occurred in 1954, provided fascinating clues about memory that started a new era of psychological (Scoville and Milner 1957) and, later, neurobiological inquiries (Kandel et al. 2014) into these two different memory systems. H.M., whose real name was Henry Molaison, had intractable epileptic seizures that made it impossible for him to function and underwent a bilateral resection of his medial temporal lobes (containing his hippocampi) at age 27 after his seizures were localized to those areas. Following the procedure, his seizures ceased, but he was no longer able to form specific and long-lasting memories of events that occurred after the surgery. He was, however, able to improve over time on a difficult motor task of drawing of a star using a mirror as his guide, even though each day he did not remember having done the task the day before. Investigation of his capacities led to a new taxonomy of long-term memory systems into explicit (also called semantic or declarative) memory and implicit (also known as procedural) memory.

Explicit memory is memory for facts and events, which is localized to the medial temporal lobe and diencephalon and depends on having an intact hippocampus, which H.M. lacked. Explicit memories can be formed in one trial; we can potentially be told someone's name once and remember it years later. Implicit memory, in contrast, is memory for procedures, skills, and habits and is dependent on the striatum (which contains the nucleus accumbens, caudate nucleus, and putamen) and not on the hippocampus. Implicit memory is the memory used when we learn a new skill, such as riding a bike. As you may know if you have ever tried to change your golf swing, changing a procedural memory can take a long time because it usually involves translating what is wrong with your swing into words, then repeatedly doing it differently until your new swing becomes "natural," meaning it has been returned to long-term procedural memory storage in a different form that no longer requires conscious thought to make the now internalized adjustment. As with memory reconsolidation more generally, the longer you have been practicing doing something sub-

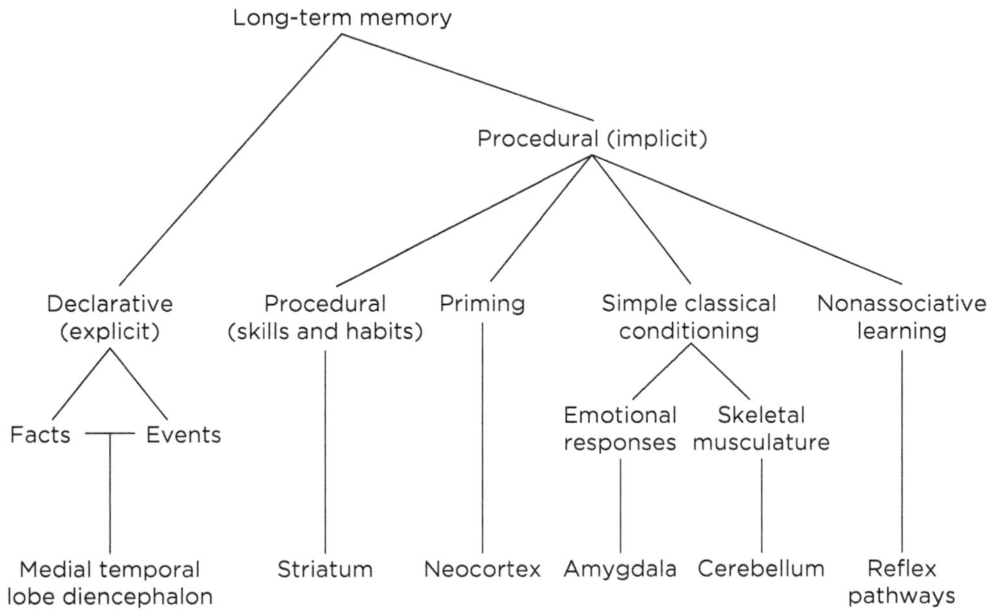

FIGURE 33–1. Taxonomy of memory systems.
Source. Adapted from Kandel ER: Biology and the future of psychoanalysis: a new intellectual framework for psychiatry revisited. *Am J Psychiatry* 156(4):505–524, 1999.

optimally, the longer it will take to change and reconsolidate in a different and better form. Figure 33–1 describes the taxonomy of memory systems that has been established to date. Despite this division between explicit and implicit memories, rat pups exposed to a single threat prior to hippocampal development demonstrate that latent memories of the event can be reinstated later in life if the correct reminders are provided (Alberini 2005; Alberini and Travaglia 2017; Bessières et al. 2020).

Relevance to Psychotherapy

Psychoanalysts have long thought that understanding more about how memory works is key to theoretical shifts, technical interventions, and the process of psychotherapeutic change. Moreover, understanding that the hippocampus is not fully formed and functional in the first 18 months or so of life means that implicit memory may have important implications for how we encode the procedure of how to have a relationship with early caregivers based on how they relate to us and our reactions to them. For example, Hans Loewald, in his paper "On the Therapeutic Action of Psychoanalysis" (Loewald 1960), explored transference as a form of enactive memory. The task of psychoanalysis, he argued, was the translation of enactive (i.e., implicit) memory, which is unconscious and nonverbal, into representational (i.e., explicit) memory, which is conscious and verbal. He suggested that the transference is, at its essence, an enactive form of memory that gradually comes to light between patient and analyst. Exploration of the transference is key in dynamic psychotherapies because assumptions about the self and others in relation to one another can be made explicit.

Gorman and Roose (2011) concurred with Loewald's ideas, proposing that the transference "involves in part the reactivation of sets of unconscious fantasies that influence conscious experience and behavior. Once brought into awareness through the process of free association and interpretation of the transference it is possible to uncouple a patient's emotions, cognitions and behaviors from the existing narrative…then co-construct a revised narrative that sheds pathogenic elements and incorporates reconsolidated memory" (Gorman and Roose 2011, p. 1210) a process that analysts call *working through*. Psychoanalytic therapy, therefore, is a process that "at its core involves learning about the self, by facilitating reconsolidation of previously harmful psychological material after it has been reworked into a less toxic state by treatment" (Gorman and Roose 2011, p. 1212).

Social Buffering

Neurobiological Mechanisms

Moving from a molecular, synaptic, and circuit approach to examining the systems of social buffering means looking at relationships between organisms rather than within an individual. Social buffering is a phenomenon in which a social partner can attenuate the release of stress hormones in response to a threatening or challenging situation.

In rodent models, prolonged separation of the infant rat pup from its mother causes the pup to increase its stress response, whereas reunion with the mother rat or even stimuli (such as smells, warmth, fur, or an anesthetized mother) reminiscent of the real mother can decrease the stress response. Additionally, maternal presence causes social buffering in the face of traumatic events, diminishing cortisol release in the pup. The pup still responds behaviorally to the pain or trauma producing the stress, but the effect is not further amplified through the stress response (Sullivan and Perry 2015). Even the most attentive mother rats commonly cause brief pain as they handle the pups roughly or step on them entering and leaving the nest (Roth and Sullivan 2005). In earliest life, rat pups approach rather than avoid painful stimuli, presumably to help foster attachment to the mother. Then during a period of early life, the presence of the mother and interactions with the mother mediate cortisol responses in the pup. As the pup nears independence from the mother around weaning, fear learning occurs by the same amygdala-dependent pathways that are important in adulthood.

Interestingly, although the mother rat is a good social buffer from birth until weaning, after weaning, peers become a potent source of social buffering (Hennessy et al. 2009). Social buffering also highlights the dependence of mammals on their caregivers and the necessity of attachment, even to mothers that are abusive or neglectful caretakers. Simply put, the quality of parental care determines the effectiveness of social buffering. However, adverse rearing conditions limit a caregiver's ability to socially buffer their young and have ubiquitous and deleterious effects on neural development as a result of increased cortisol levels, which in turn make the amygdala more reactive and, subsequently, the pup harder to buffer. Precocious emergence of the prefrontal cortex related to early life adversity increases the ability of the offspring to detect threat, but this mechanism is maladaptive when no threat is present, such as later in life when a person may be in a comparatively safe situation. Much of the neural control of the HPA axis occurs via neurons in the paraventricular nucleus of the hypothalamus, which regulates both the corticotropin-releasing factor and vasopressin, which in turn signal the release of adrenocorticotropic hormone, which activates cortisol secretion from the cortex of the adrenal gland. Biological mediators of social buffering involve both hormones and neurotransmitters, including oxytocin, dopamine, serotonin, and opioids (Hostinar et al. 2014).

Relevance to Psychotherapy

The importance of social buffering in mammals in early life is clear, with the mother figure being a key regulator of early fear and anxiety experiences in an infant. Child studies in human infants have long shown that the mother functions as a kind of emotional pacemaker for the infant; examining the mother's face for fear and anxiety allows the infant, in part, to judge how large the threat creating the anxiety or fear really is. In addition, studies by Beebe and Lachmann (1994, 2002, 2014) demonstrated that all maternal-child interactions are co-constructed, albeit not necessarily in symmetrical, equal ways. They demonstrated that this co-construction or coregulation is simultaneous, is complementary, and has an optimal dynamic balance, and they proposed three principles of salience—ongoing regulation, disruption and repair, and heightened affective moments—that refine the understanding of the nature of self- and interactive regulation. They also demonstrated that these principles extend to the coregulation between analyst and patient by examining vocal rhythm coordination, facial mirroring, and distress regulation in pairs of patients and analysts in dynamic psychotherapy. In infants they demonstrated that these same factors, examined in the early months of life, can predict attachment style at 1 year and organize the nonverbal implicit dimension of relatedness. They also proposed that these implicit relational patterns constitute an important dimension of transference (Beebe and Lachmann 2014).

The implications of the neurobiological mechanisms previously described and these developmental findings that have been related to the therapeutic relationship suggest that co-construction of self and other in the context of a relationship with a therapist is built from microscopic moments of relatedness in which both partners react to and interact with the other. They suggest that part of the exploration of transference must involve attention, insofar as is possible, to this coregulatory function by which the analyst may represent and be incorporated as a different model of relatedness. Over time, this process can be generalized and can affect relationships beyond the psychotherapeutic one. These findings may also suggest an important role of the analyst's calming presence as patient and analyst explore deeply traumatic and often emotionally frightening material within sessions, where the analyst's ability to regulate aspects of the patient's HPA axis and arousal of the amygdala may allow reworking of traumatic experience.

Finally, these findings all suggest a crucial role for early intervention, such as that of parent-infant psychotherapy. Here maternal modes of relatedness are explored and linked to the mother's own traumatic experiences in early life, with emphasis on microanalysis of maternal-infant interactions via video proving crucial to the work. One example is showing a mother whose infant is at risk of disorganized attachment how she is unable to tolerate the child looking away from her, a form of self-regulation in infants that gives their nascent and easily overexcited nervous systems an opportunity to return to baseline. By repeatedly not allowing the infant to disengage because she cannot tolerate the separation herself, the mother can create an attachment situation in which the baby is constantly avoiding eye contact and the associated intensity of the mother's gaze. The infant here may learn that relationships with others are intrusive and dysregulating. A few months of work on these patterns with mothers and with the mother-infant dyad can greatly change the trajectory of the relationship and hence the relationship model the child internalizes in their implicit memory, avoiding years of psychotherapeutic work in adulthood.

Looking Toward the Future

The final three examples of connections between neuroscience and psychotherapy are the most speculative of all but are well worth watching in the future. They consist of 1) epigenetics and the intergenerational transmission of trauma, 2) mirror neurons and the neurobiological basis of empathy, and 3) the role of the default mode network in the creation of a cohesive sense of self.

Epigenetics

Neurobiological Mechanisms

The role of life experience on the human genome has been debated since Darwin and Lamarck differed in their ideas about evolutionary biology in the 1850s. Although Darwin believed that changes in the overall gene pool that promoted survival of the fittest shifted over time to favor positive adaptations, Lamarck believed that physical changes in organisms during their lifetime, such as greater development of an organ or a part through increased use, could be transmitted to their offspring. For years it looked like Darwin was right until epigenetics brought Lamarck's ideas back into focus.

Epigenetics is the study of chemical marking and modification of DNA by mechanisms such as methylation and acetylation of the DNA itself, changes that affect the ease with which certain portions of the genes that code for various proteins are expressed. When DNA is transcribed, the histones on which the genetic sequence is wrapped may spool it tightly or loosely according to how heavily marked it is; the more methylation, the more the gene is transcribed to mRNA and the greater the synthesis of the protein for which the gene codes becomes—the more the tags, the looser the DNA (Levenson and Sweatt 2005). Thus, for example, adding methyl groups may turn a gene on, whereas demethylating it may turn it off; if it is methylated, the gene portion produces more mRNA and more protein synthesis.

Research on maternal behavior in rodents has helped to elucidate the connection between the effects of maternal behavior on adult anxiety as well as on epigenetic DNA markings passed to the offspring. Although some mother rats spend a lot of time licking, grooming, and nursing their pups, other mother rats seem to largely ignore their pups. The highly groomed and licked rats tend to grow into calm adults, whereas those who do not receive adequate nurturing tend to be anxious. The nurturing behavior of a mother rat during week 1 of life shapes the pups' epigenetics in a way that tends to persist into adulthood. If the environment surrounding the rat pups is safe and comfortable, calmness is a benefit as they age.

In contrast, rats with low grooming tend toward exhibiting stress-related behaviors. If the environment has food scarcity and more danger, the low-nurture rat may do better, however. Thus, in this circumstance the low-nurture rats are best prepared for a harsh environment. But the high-nurture rats are more likely to have higher social standing as well as fewer stress-related behaviors in adulthood. However, one can transform low-nurture rats into rats that act as if they were highly nurtured via the injection of a drug that removes methyl groups. With demethylation of DNA, the glucocorticoid receptor gene *GR* is turned on, cells make more GR protein, and the rat exhibits more relaxed behaviors. Conversely, injecting relaxed, high-nurture rats with methionine (a source of methyl groups) makes them act more anxious, similar to the behavior of low-nurture rats. Through her licking behavior, a mother rat can thus write information onto her pups' DNA in a way that completely bypasses eggs and sperm, and thus, the epigenetic code gives the genome a level of flexibility that enables it to be sensitive to changing environmental conditions such as the availability of food, threat from predators, or nurturing versus neglect.

These effects are not limited to the injection of drugs and can also derive from life experiences that similarly mark and tag DNA. For example, exposure of adolescent female mice to an enriched environment consisting of novel objects, exercise, and increased capacity for social interaction is known to have a beneficial effect on synaptic long-term plasticity induction and learning ability in their offspring. Further, this is true even when the female has had a low-nurture upbringing that has resulted in stress-induced decreases in learning ability (Arai et al. 2009).

There is also fascinating work in epigenetics about the way that chronic exposure to the experience of social defeat can be transmitted transgenerationally. Specifically, adult male mice that were exposed to chronic social defeat stress and control mice were bred with female mice that had never experienced any type of stress. Offspring were then assessed for anxiety- and depressive-like behaviors. Not only did chronic exposure to social defeat produce social avoidance behavior in fathers, but also both their male and female offspring showed greater amounts of social avoidance behavior. Offspring of defeated fathers also showed reduced preference for sucrose and decreased latencies in immobility in the forced swim test, suggestive of depressive-like behavior. Remarkably, some of the transgenerational effects could even be replicated with in vitro fertilization experiments using the father's sperm (Dietz et al. 2011).

Disruptions in social hierarchy in adolescent mice (modeled through repeatedly changing a rodent's cage mates) have also been shown to increase anxiety-like behaviors in both mothers and first-generation females. Fathers from this paradigm also appear able to transmit the anxiety and defective social interaction phenotypes to subsequent generations, such as their F2 and F3 daughters (Saavedra-Rodríguez and Feig 2013). Finally, environmental information experienced later in life can also be inherited; remarkably, subjecting mice to fear conditioning with a novel odor before conception can alter behavioral sensitivity to that same odor (but not other odors) in F1 and F2 generation offspring (Dias and Ressler 2014).

Relevance to Psychotherapy

Psychodynamic theory dating back to Freud has long proposed that the impact of early childhood experiences can affect adult behavior. These beliefs have been strengthened by studies of attachment and maltreatment of children (Schwartz et al. 1994). Epigenetics suggests a molecular underpinning for this belief and also raises the idea that the new and different relationship with the therapist or important others later in life can effect changes in the patient's DNA marking that can then be conveyed to the patient's offspring, raising the tantalizing concept of breaking the cycle of intergenerational transmission of trauma (Yehuda and Lehrner 2018).

Mirror Neurons and the Basis of Empathy

Rizzolatti et al. (1996) described that in the monkey premotor cortex, there are neurons that discharge both when the monkey performs an action and when it observes a similar action made by another monkey or by the experimenter. They claimed that mirror neuron activity "represents" the observed action. This motor representation is at the core "of the understanding of motor events" (p. 137). Some scientists quickly moved to claim that in humans, the observation of motor actions activates the posterior part of inferior frontal gyrus and this primitive system of communication based on recognition of hand and face gestures is the basis of empathy in humans. They further asserted that this motor system finding and the capacity for imitation found in early life together constituted biological building blocks of empathy, using the concept of *embodied simulation*, in which internal representations of the body states associated with actions, emotions, and sensations are evoked in the observer as if the observer were experiencing a similar emotion or sensation (Ammaniti 2009; Iacoboni 2005, 2009).

This hypothesis has also led to some fascinating research in which 16 mothers were instructed to actively imitate or to feel empathy for pictures of their own or of an unknown child. Pictures were divided in distinct groups according to infants' facial expressions (joy, distress, ambiguous, and neutral). The functional MRI data showed that when mothers felt empathy with infants' emotional expressions, this significantly activated a large cluster of mirror neuron areas that were especially more active when mothers felt empathy with their own child. In these studies, mirror neurons were proposed to represent the neurobiological substrate of maternal responsivity, playing a significant role during the baby's first year and facilitating the dyadic exchange in a developmental stage when language has not developed yet (Lenzi et al. 2009).

The mirror neuron system is certainly fascinating and possibly related to the capacity for empathy, providing an intriguing potential mechanism for how we intuit how others feel by putting ourselves in their neurological "shoes," but it is premature to conclude on the basis of current evidence that this is definitively the case. Such generalization from a motor neuron mechanism to the human capacity for empathy highlights the warning in the beginning of this chapter that neuroscience findings not be used as metaphor. We can imagine the exciting potential of mirror neurons for explaining aspects of empathy and even transference and countertransference in psychotherapy, but concluding that this work is relevant to psychotherapy is currently too big a leap.

Default Mode Network

Most functional MRI research began with tasks, examining what areas of the brain were active when performing a particular task. Researchers therefore sought to subtract the activation of the resting brain, in the process learning that the resting brain, which has come to be called the default mode network (DMN): "a large-scale brain circuit that is activated during quiet wakefulness and deactivated during goal-directed tasks which evoke cognitive load" (Hanson 2021, p. 4). Because the DMN accounts for 20% of the brain's energy consumption, researchers began to study its function. Some researchers noted that the DMN may have a fundamental role to play in our sense of a continuous self, providing the building blocks for consciousness, introspection, self-reflection, and empathy for others (Hanson 2021). Such high energy usage caused researchers to become curious about this resting DMN in the brain and began to study it, and an interesting story has begun to emerge about the function of the DMN in the process.

One intriguing possibility is that the DMN accounts for our sense of self, constantly reminding us over and over that we are a continuous self and rendering our experience of self a seamless one. More recently, the DMN has also been implicated in psychiatric disorders such as depression and social anxiety disorder (Aguilar and McNally 2022; Dixon et al. 2022), with one researcher describing it as the place where "the idiosyncratic self meets the shared social world" (Yeshurun et al. 2021, p. 181). It is not yet clear whether the DMN is relevant in psychotherapy or how it might relate, but it is a tantalizing neuroscience window into the mind during self-reflection or introspection.

Conclusion

Neuroscience findings are already relevant for understanding the neural underpinning of how psychotherapy acts on the brain to create change. Recent work in learning and memory, especially memory reconsolidation, represents a series of exciting new confluences of understanding the brain and mind as connections between the two fields emerge. Through careful review and without jumping to premature conclusions or using neuroscience as a metaphor for psychotherapeutic processes, these connections are likely to be further strengthened and clarified in the years ahead. We look forward to these developments in understanding the mind and brain together, a pursuit that has always excited and invigorated psychotherapeutic quests.

Key Points

- Psychotherapy is a process of learning that depends on pattern recognition and repetition to change the brain.
- Memories and their associated emotions are best changed when they are reconsolidated differently, which is more likely to happen in states of heightened emotion.
- Memories that have been laid down for longer (i.e., memories from earlier in life) will take longer to alter in psychotherapy.
- Memories are more likely to be reconsolidated differently in the presence of new information.

- The procedure for how to relate to others is laid down during the first year of life, which is largely preverbal; it is likely stored in procedural or enactive memory and can be reawakened in intensive psychotherapeutic treatment in the relationship with the therapist.
- The therapist likely provides social buffering of the patient's HPA axis, which plays a role in stress and glucocorticoid production during the process of exploring painful memories in psychotherapy.

References

Abraham WC, Tate WP: Metaplasticity: a new vista across the field of synaptic plasticity. Prog Neurobiol 52(4):303–323, 1997 9247968

Abrams TW, Karl KA, Kandel ER: Biochemical studies of stimulus convergence during classical conditioning in Aplysia: dual regulation of adenylate cyclase by Ca2+/calmodulin and transmitter. J Neurosci 11(9):2655–2665, 1991 1679120

Aguilar DD, McNally JM: Subcortical control of the default mode network: role of the basal forebrain and implications for neuropsychiatric disorders. Brain Res Bull 185:129–139, 2022 35562013

Alberini CM: Mechanisms of memory stabilization: are consolidation and reconsolidation similar or distinct processes? Trends Neurosci 28(1):51–56, 2005 15626497

Alberini CM, Travaglia A: Infantile amnesia: a critical period of learning to learn and remember. J Neurosci 37(24):5783–5795, 2017 28615475

Ammaniti MT: How new knowledge about parenting reveals the neurobiological implications of intersubjectivity: a conceptual synthesis of recent research. Psychoanal Dialogues 19(5):537–555, 2009

Arai JA, Li S, Hartley DM, et al: Transgenerational rescue of a genetic defect in long-term potentiation and memory formation by juvenile enrichment. J Neurosci 29(5):1496–1502, 2009 19193896

Barco A, Alarcon JM, Kandel ER: Expression of constitutively active CREB protein facilitates the late phase of long-term potentiation by enhancing synaptic capture. Cell 108(5):689–703, 2002 11893339

Bartsch D, Ghirardi M, Skehel PA, et al: Aplysia CREB2 represses long-term facilitation: relief of repression converts transient facilitation into long-term functional and structural change. Cell 83(6):979–992, 1995 8521521

Beebe B, Lachmann FM: Representation and internalization in infancy: three principles of salience. Psychoanal Psychol 11(2):127–165, 1994

Beebe B, Lachmann F: Organizing principles of interaction from infant research and the lifespan prediction of attachment: application to adult treatment. J Infant Child Adolesc Psychother 2(4):61–89, 2002

Beebe B, Lachmann FM: The Origins of Attachment: Infant Research and Adult Treatment. New York, Routledge, 2014, pp xxiii, 231

Bessières B, Travaglia A, Mowery TM, et al: Early life experiences selectively mature learning and memory abilities. Nat Commun 11(1):628, 2020 32005863

Castellucci V, Kandel ER: Presynaptic facilitation as a mechanism for behavioral sensitization in Aplysia. Science 194(4270):1176–1178, 1976 11560

Dias BG, Ressler KJ: Parental olfactory experience influences behavior and neural structure in subsequent generations. Nat Neurosci 17(1):89–96, 2014 24292232

Dietz DM, Laplant Q, Watts EL, et al: Paternal transmission of stress-induced pathologies. Biol Psychiatry 70(5):408–414, 2011 21679926

Dixon ML, Moodie CA, Goldin PR, et al: Frontoparietal and default mode network contributions to self-referential processing in social anxiety disorder. Cogn Affect Behav Neurosci 22(1):187–198, 2022 34341966

Duman RS, Aghajanian GK: Synaptic dysfunction in depression: potential therapeutic targets. Science 338(6103):68–72, 2012 23042884

Freud S: Beyond the pleasure principle (1920), in Standard Edition of the Complete Psychological Works of Sigmund Freud, Vol 18. Translated and edited by Strachey J. London, Hogarth Press, 1955, pp 1–64

Gabriele A, Packard MG: D-Cycloserine enhances memory consolidation of hippocampus-dependent latent extinction. Learn Mem 14(7):468–471, 2007 17600116

Glanzman DL, Mackey SL, Hawkins RD, et al: Depletion of serotonin in the nervous system of aplysia reduces the behavioral enhancement of gill withdrawal as well as the heterosynaptic facilitation produced by tail shock. J Neurosci 9(12):4200–4213, 1989 2592997

Gorman JM, Roose SP: The neurobiology of fear memory reconsolidation and psychoanalytic theory. J Am Psychoanal Assoc 59(6):1201–1220, 2011 22080504

Guan Z, Giustetto M, Lomvardas S, et al: Integration of long-term-memory-related synaptic plasticity involves bidirectional regulation of gene expression and chromatin structure. Cell 111(4):483–493, 2002 12437922

Hanson A: Spontaneous electrical low-frequency oscillations: a possible role in Hydra and all living systems. Philos Trans R Soc Lond B Biol Sci 376(1820):20190763 2021 33487108

Hennessy MB, Kaiser S, Sachser N: Social buffering of the stress response: diversity, mechanisms, and functions. Front Neuroendocrinol 30(4):470–482, 2009 19545584

Hostinar CE, Sullivan RM, Gunnar MR: Psychobiological mechanisms underlying the social buffering of the hypothalamic-pituitary-adrenocortical axis: a review of animal models and human studies across development. Psychol Bull 140(1):256–282, 2014 23607429

Iacoboni M: Neural mechanisms of imitation. Curr Opin Neurobiol 15(6):632–637, 2005 16271461

Iacoboni M: Imitation, empathy, and mirror neurons. Annu Rev Psychol 60:653–670, 2009 18793090

Kandel ER: Psychotherapy and the single synapse: the impact of psychiatric thought on neurobiological research. J Neuropsychiatry Clin Neurosci 13(2):290–300, discussion 289, 2001 11449037

Kandel ER, Dudai Y, Mayford MR: The molecular and systems biology of memory. Cell 157(1):163–186, 2014 24679534

LeDoux JE: Emotion: clues from the brain. Annu Rev Psychol 46:209–235, 1995 7872730

LeDoux J: The emotional brain, fear, and the amygdala. Cell Mol Neurobiol 23(4–5):727–738, 2003 14514027

Lenzi D, Trentini C, Pantano P, et al: Neural basis of maternal communication and emotional expression processing during infant preverbal stage. Cereb Cortex 19(5):1124–1133, 2009 18787229

Levenson JM, Sweatt JD: Epigenetic mechanisms in memory formation. Nat Rev Neurosci 6(2):108–118, 2005 15654323

Loewald HW: On the therapeutic action of psycho-analysis. Int J Psychoanal 41:16–33, 1960 14417912

Nader K, Schafe GE, Le Doux JE: Fear memories require protein synthesis in the amygdala for reconsolidation after retrieval. Nature 406(6797):722–726, 2000 10963596

Phelps EA, Hofmann SG: Memory editing from science fiction to clinical practice. Nature 572(7767):43–50, 2019 31367027

Rizzolatti G, Fadiga L, Gallese V, et al: Premotor cortex and the recognition of motor actions. Brain Res Cogn Brain Res 3(2):131–141, 1996 8713554

Ross DA, Arbuckle MR, Travis MJ, et al: An integrated neuroscience perspective on formulation and treatment planning for posttraumatic stress disorder: an educational review. JAMA Psychiatry 74(4):407–415, 2017 28273291

Roth TL, Sullivan RM: Memory of early maltreatment: neonatal behavioral and neural correlates of maternal maltreatment within the context of classical conditioning. Biol Psychiatry 57(8):823–831, 2005 15820702

Saavedra-Rodríguez L, Feig LA: Chronic social instability induces anxiety and defective social interactions across generations. Biol Psychiatry 73(1):44–53, 2013 22906514

Sara SJ: Retrieval and reconsolidation: toward a neurobiology of remembering. Learn Mem 7(2):73–84, 2000 10753974

Schiller D, Monfils M-H, Raio CM, et al: Preventing the return of fear in humans using reconsolidation update mechanisms. Nature 463(7277):49–53, 2010 20010606
Schwartz S, Dohrenwend BP, Levav I: Nongenetic familial transmission of psychiatric disorders? Evidence from children of Holocaust survivors. J Health Soc Behav 35(4):385–402, 1994 7844332
Scoville WB, Milner B: Loss of recent memory after bilateral hippocampal lesions. J Neurol Neurosurg Psychiatry 20(1):11–21, 1957 13406589
Shin LM, Rauch SL, Pitman RK: Amygdala, medial prefrontal cortex, and hippocampal function in PTSD. Ann NY Acad Sci 1071:67–79, 2006 16891563
Sullivan RM, Perry RE: Mechanisms and functional implications of social buffering in infants: lessons from animal models. Soc Neurosci 10(5):500–511, 2015 26324338
Tronson NC, Taylor JR: Molecular mechanisms of memory reconsolidation. Nat Rev Neurosci 8(4):262–275, 2007 17342174
Yehuda R, Lehrner A: Intergenerational transmission of trauma effects: putative role of epigenetic mechanisms. World Psychiatry 17(3):243–257, 2018 30192087
Yeshurun Y, Nguyen M, Hasson U: The default mode network: where the idiosyncratic self meets the shared social world. Nat Rev Neurosci 22(3):181–192, 2021 33483717

CHAPTER 34

Psychotherapy and Cyberspace

Peter Yellowlees, M.D., M.B.B.S.
Jay Shore, M.D., M.P.H.

The practice of telepsychiatry is usually defined as the use of videoconferencing to perform psychiatric consultations. In this chapter we are more inclusive and include any clinical interactions that are mediated or enabled by technology in which the doctor or therapist and the patient are not physically together. So although the practice of using videoconferencing for psychiatric assessment and treatment is more than 60 years old and telephony has been used for more than a century, email, secure texting, and home monitoring using multiple smartphone-based mobile devices are much more recent.

In the past decade the technical and economic barriers that have slowed the adoption of telepsychiatry have almost disappeared with the advent of web- and cloud-based systems, mobile computing, the impact of commercial telemedicine service companies, and a growing body of evidence and telehealth research. Now we can see patients securely and in high definition on a laptop, tablet, or smartphone at minimal cost using video systems that function well in parallel with most electronic medical records and, in many cases, are already integrated into them. As of 2020 mobile devices dominate the global market for internet access and will soon become the primary way that digital technologies are used to deliver mental health care.

At the same time, with the rise in younger, more technologically savvy providers and patients from the millennial and Generation Z populations, expectations about how psychotherapy and other medical and mental health treatments can be provided are changing. These younger generations are beginning to influence how health care is delivered (Nakagawa and Yellowlees 2020) as patients and providers expect care to be available anytime, anywhere, just like most other services in their lives. Using technology to deliver mental health care, including psychotherapy, aligns with the integration of technology in their day-to-day life.

Finally, the advent of coronavirus SARS-CoV-2 disease (COVID-19), a tragic global pandemic that is still raging at the time of writing, has been a major driver of the use of telepsychiatry and other mental health technologies. In the United States, most psychiatrists and therapists have taken to using technologies, especially video and telephony, to connect with their patients and to continue therapy with those who are sheltering in place. This has allowed both therapists and patients to remain separated and safe from infection while enabling continuing mental health care to be provided.

The opportunity for mental health professionals to engage in psychotherapy with their patients is here, and many thousands of patients have already benefited. The future will likely bring many mental health professionals working increasingly in a hybrid model, both in person and online, using the strengths of both approaches to improve patient care. Technologies are gradually changing the therapist-patient relationship, softening its boundaries, and making it more of an anytime, anywhere collaborative partnership, something that will be especially helpful when practicing the range of psychotherapies described throughout this book.

A significant amount of research has demonstrated the advantages of telepsychiatry beyond increasing access to care, and since 2015, the scientific literature has dramatically expanded, so that discussion of the use of technologies in mental health care has now become mainstream in almost all academic and clinical settings. Post COVID-19 this will continue.

The use of videoconferencing leads to high patient and provider satisfaction ratings and achieves health outcomes equivalent to in-person care (Bashshur et al. 2016; Hilty et al. 2013). Trials of multiple types of brief therapy, particularly dynamic and cognitive-behavioral approaches, have demonstrated outcomes equivalent to those of in-person care, and some studies with veterans using evidence-based prolonged exposure therapy for PTSD have led to better outcomes than in-person therapy (Fortney et al. 2015a). Younger patients often prefer telepsychiatry over in-person encounters, and it has been noted that telepsychiatry encourages intimate conversations (Yellowlees et al. 2015) and unique clinical observational opportunities such as the patient's home environment. Indeed, telepsychiatry may be preferable to traditional clinic consultations for patients who have paranoia, anxiety, or PTSD (Chan et al. 2015). A number of dynamic issues in psychoanalytically oriented therapy have been examined and discussed (Kocsis and Yellowlees 2018), especially some advantages of seeing patients on video through the use of virtual space.

An increasing number of textbooks have been written describing the use of telepsychiatry (Yellowlees and Shore 2018), and other texts on mental health topics now frequently include chapters summarizing the major technological issues of importance and relevance (Saeed et al., in press; Waugh et al. 2018; Yellowlees 2018; Yellowlees and Liu 2020; Yellowlees and Shore 2019). Finally, several mental health journals have published collections of papers focused on telepsychiatry, telepsychology, and other mental health technologies (Shore 2019; Shore et al. 2020a), and the two major telemedicine journals, the *Journal of Telemedicine and eHealth* and the *Journal of Telemedicine and Telecare*, routinely publish papers about telemental health.

Telepsychiatry is already used in a wide variety of settings beyond the home, and during the COVID-19 pandemic many patients have been receiving care in their parked vehicles using mobile phones, often outside their clinics, so much so that some have said that the car is the new therapy room. In outpatient clinics, many of which have become virtual hubs, with providers and patients all based in their homes, telepsychiatry is used for diagnosis and treatment, which can include medication management, individual psychotherapy, and group psychotherapy from a range of mental health professionals (Yellowlees et al. 2020). At the beginning of the pandemic, when hospitals were being overwhelmed by patients, group sessions for health care workers, using the principles of psychological first aid, were commonly offered by videoconferencing. One of us (P.Y.) cofacilitated a number of these "Zoom debriefing" sessions with groups of surgeons who were very committed to providing excellent care in situations that were potentially dangerous for themselves and their families. For these physicians the risk of spreading infections to their own families was substantial and frightening, and they were relieved to be able to ventilate and discuss their emotional responses to their situation via video.

Telemental health can also be used for consultations in primary care; with the emergency department; and with specialist clinics, including pain, obesity, and surgery clinics. Apps are increasingly being integrated into standard inpatient and outpatient treatment programs for both monitoring and therapy. Elsewhere, telepsychiatry is being used in colleges, universities, medical and nursing schools, and mental health facilities for consultation and education, as well as in correctional, substance use, and rehabilitation settings, and by pharmaceutical companies in drug trials. The technologies and processes have been implemented and used for all ages (children, adults, elderly people) and have been especially useful for language and sign interpretation to cross cultures and aid deaf people. Automated language interpretation systems are being developed that transcribe and interpret languages in near–real time from recorded asynchronous telepsychiatry conversations, and avatar therapists, trained to react to patients' movement and language, are no longer a fantasy of the future but are being developed to deliver treatment for PTSD to veterans.

What Drivers Are Causing the Doctor-Patient Relationship to Change and Encourage the Use of All Types of Online and Hybrid Psychotherapy?

There are three main drivers of change: 1) technological improvements and the move to mobile devices, 2) changing demographics as younger populations dominate the health care market, and 3) the COVID-19 global pandemic, which is requiring social distancing and care in the home to ensure the safety of providers and patients.

Technological Changes

Advances in technology are rapidly changing the practice of mental health professionals. These advances include the development of the internet, increasingly ubiquitous broadband access, and the miniaturization of computers and integration of computing power in smartphones and smartwatches. Altered patient expectations and a shift toward consumer-driven health care, as well as the decreasing cost of technology and increasing need for better access to psychiatrists, who are in increasingly short supply, are other change drivers. Much of what is true of videoconferencing on fixed and mobile devices also applies to telephony and email, both of which are equally important in their impacts on the therapist-patient relationship.

Since 2015, the typical smartphone has been equipped with forward-facing and rear-facing high-resolution video cameras, a high-resolution display, internet connectivity, audio inputs and outputs—via a microphone, speaker, headset port, and Bluetooth connections—and advanced processing power. All of these features make smartphones ideal for a new class of applications providing on-the-go mobile telemental health (Chan et al. 2014).

One of us (P.Y.) has taken advantage of the dramatic improvements in mobile devices and no longer owns a desktop computer or a fixed telephone line at home. Instead, he use three wireless mobile devices—laptop, iPad, and iPhone—with a large computer screen that any of these devices can be plugged into if preferred for all his professional and personal activities. During the COVID-19 pandemic, P.Y. has seen all of his patients at home.

P.Y. uses three types of videoconferencing with patients (Extended Care via Epic, Zoom, and Webex) and three versions of the Epic electronic medical record (Epic, Haiku, and Canto), available on his three mobile devices, all connected via apps or a virtual private network to UC Davis Health servers. He is able to see patients and supervise residents, often situated in three different home environments at once, while using apps for education and monitoring.

Why does he do all of this? In reality all that P.Y. is doing is following international trends on the use of mobile devices, as described by Deyan G (2020). Although most mental health professionals likely still use fixed computers, younger generations of physicians and mental health clinicians are rapidly switching to fully mobile devices. The global figures, as described by Deyan G (2020), are astonishing and explain why such devices are the future of mental health in cyberspace.

Worldwide in 2020 there were 3.5 billion smartphone users, with 1.5 billion new smartphone sales and 7.9 billion mobile broadband subscriptions (104% of the world's population), with almost 10 billion smartphones in use. Globally, 67% of all users access the internet by smartphone; 81% of Americans own smartphones, and 47% of them say they could not live without them. In China (the leader in smartphone traffic) 99.3% of internet users go online using mobile devices, and globally, 56% of all website traffic in 2019 was generated by smartphones (Deyan G 2020).

The value of mobile apps and advertising is astonishing. In America, of the internet time spent on smartphones, 90% is via an app, with only 10% being via the general internet. In 2019 there were 204 billion app downloads globally, and revenue from advertising in those apps was worth $201 billion (Deyan G 2020). App store revenue itself was worth more than $100 billion in 2020, with 76% from games and 24% from app sales, with apps projected to generate $190 billion in direct revenue in 2020.

Seventy percent of YouTube traffic is mobile, and 70% of time spent watching or listening to media is spent on smartphones or mobile devices. Not surprisingly, 68% of Twitter users are on smartphones. The consequence of this is that the average user checks their phone 58 times per day, and 66% report being addicted to their phones. Globally, 14 million jobs are directly related to the mobile industry currently, and by 2025, it is projected that 80% of global connections will be by smartphones (Deyan G 2020).

It is hardly surprising that we conclude that most mental health care in the future, when it is online, will be delivered in mobile environments, especially when we look at how smartphones are used today (Deyan G 2020). Currently, 49% of emails are already read on smartphones, and 90% of internet searches use Google. Female college students average 10 hours per day on their cell phones. For consumers in the United States, YouTube is their favorite app (81%), followed by Facebook (76%). Forty percent of all products in the United States are purchased via smartphone; 80% of shoppers use phones inside stores for reviews and to check prices, and 85% of travelers use mobile devices to book travel (Deyan G 2020).

What other advantages do mobile devices bring? They not only provide an audiovisual medium for mobile telepsychiatry but also serve as intelligent information-gathering devices for objective data. The typical smartphone is equipped with accelerometers to detect the position of the smartphone and estimate the activity of the user and Wi-Fi and GPS to locate the user, as well as software that can capture the user's interactions. These devices already provide even more, and more accurate, patient-reported data than do standard paper assessments, and wearable devices extend the functionality of smartphones with additional Bluetooth-enabled sensors that can be worn as jewelry or embedded in smartwatches or in clothing. These sensors can provide quantified data that can detect gait and movement disorders.

Novel forms of interventions are more accessible. A vast body of literature discusses computerized and internet therapeutic interventions, including improving cognition with video games, the use of virtual reality equipment for the treatment of anxiety disorders and PTSD, and internet-based cognitive therapies (Chan et al. 2017). Smartphone apps have made these interventions more portable, more accessible, and more affordable for typical users. Psychoeducation materials and bibliotherapy are more interactive on mobile platforms, and traditional worksheets and therapy homework, such as those found in cognitive-behavioral therapy (CBT), can be made interactive to increase patient engagement and retention. Wearable apps for heads-up displays have been developed to analyze facial emotions and track vital signs, and apps can even intervene in a patient with a substance use disorder at risk of relapse, alerting its user when they approach a liquor store and coaching them through difficult social situations where alcohol is readily available, such as weddings.

The common theme with these applications is the digitization and automation of much of the range of traditional therapies, making them available to patients between sessions with the therapist or perhaps supplementing traditional therapy with an "avatar therapist" between sessions. Good examples built by the U.S. Department of Veterans Affairs that act like a "therapist in the pocket" are CBT-i Coach and PTSD Coach. The potential also exists for the human therapist to be replaced entirely with a technology-based avatar that is trained to respond therapeutically to movements and language (Yellowlees et al. 2012).

Unfortunately, a downside to all these applications is that they are only occasionally backed by the latest research. The amount of financial capital flowing into the development of such devices has increased faster than the amount of research, meaning that clinical validation is not yet ready for most, and new unvetted technologies should be approached with caution despite a number of methodologies being developed to enable users to objectively evaluate them (Torous et al. 2018). In summary, the combination of massive increases in the number of mobile devices and the widespread development of multiple apps and sensors will increasingly affect the mental health professional–patient relationship, potentially making it a 24-7 cross-cultural anytime, anywhere hybrid process (Chan et al. 2015).

Intergenerational Changes

The health care industry has been relatively slow in adapting to the social and technological changes of the past 50 years, especially at the doctor-patient interface, but that is changing with the advent of the millennial and Generation Z groups of clinicians and patients. Most of the impact of information technology in health care until the last decade has been through administrative, population-based, and electronic record systems. Hence, despite the emergence of many telemedicine and mobile technologies—and the development of more patient-centric policies and movements—the conventional in-person doctor-patient interaction is still the core of most clinical practice. Prior to the COVID-19 pandemic, most physicians and mental health professionals still practiced by preference in a broadly conservative provider-centric manner, in which communication with patients was generally in person and the use of information and communication technologies for clinical care directly with patients was still less than many patients would like (Yellowlees and Shore 2018).

The advent of advanced information and communication technologies has led to dramatic changes in all aspects of human life, so much so that young people born after the advent of the internet in 1989 are often referred to as *digital natives*. This generation was raised in an environment in which living in both real and virtual worlds simultaneously is commonplace and accepted. Many see the traditional approach to health care—in which the patient always has to physically travel to consult with a doctor—as outmoded and inconvenient, costly, and excessively time-consuming. They want to be able to receive their health care in a more accessible and immediate manner, like most other services in their lives. Nakagawa and Yellowlees (2020) documented the differences between the various generations involved in health care and the impact that these differences are having on the use of technology for patient care, across medicine, and especially for mental health purposes. They summarized their conclusions as follows:

> Younger physicians will drive technological advancement and integration faster than previous generations, allowing technology to adapt more quickly to serve the needs of clinicians and patients. These changes will improve efficiency, allow more flexible working arrangements, and increase convenience for patients and physicians. The next generation of physicians will use technology to support their work and lifestyle preferences, making them more resilient to burnout than previous generations. (Nakagawa and Yellowlees 2020)

Nakagawa and Yellowlees (2020) noted that baby boomers and Gen Z are quite different in their cognitive styles, communication preferences, and information consumption; older generations such as traditionalists and baby boomers lived in a world with less digital technology and more limited sources of information to focus on. Younger generations have more digital distractions with the internet, social media, and many potential sources of information to manage. However, they are also better suited to cognitively multitask, and because the current health care system requires physicians to process and manage so much digital information, they are naturally more adept and efficient at managing the digital aspects of their work.

Unfortunately, most technology-related decisions in health care are still made by baby boomers, leaders who shepherded the use of faxes, pagers, and electronic medical records and who had to learn and understand the technologies as they were being developed rather than being enveloped by them since birth. When digital natives are finally in the position to craft policies and champion technologies in health care, their approach will likely be very different from that of prior generations. As such, the millennials and Gen Z, the first groups of practicing mental health professionals who are digital natives, will likely manage technology, and technological change, very differently and will greatly enhance the use of cyberspace for mental health practice and psychotherapy.

COVID-19-Related Changes

COVID-19 triggered an unprecedented easing of inhibitory regulations in relation to reimbursement for video and telephony, licensing, technical security, and geography. This dramatically accelerated telemedicine adoption, ensuring that patients and mental health professionals were able to keep physically safe in the new era of social distancing, as described in the Telepsychiatry Toolkit on the American Psychiatric Association website (www.psychiatry.org/psychiatrists/practice/telepsychiatry/toolkit). At the University of California, Davis, for example, the psychiatry outpatient service converted from mostly in-person office visits to fully virtual in 3 days, and the rest of the health system converted to a largely virtual operation in 1 week (Yellowlees et al. 2020). As the pandemic continued, 8 months later in November the UC Davis psychiatric outpatients remained 100% virtual, with not only no loss of patients but also half the prior number of no-show appointments, whereas only 15%–20% of all patients attending medical and surgical outpatient appointments continued to be seen on video. In the psychiatric clinic, all long-term therapy patients had converted to video, and psychiatry and psychology residents were being fully trained to deliver both dynamic and cognitive-behavioral psychotherapy via video by their usual faculty supervisors, all working from home. A series of previously in person trauma groups was successfully transitioned to video group meetings.

Similar accounts have been published about the transition to telemedicine for other psychiatric services, including advice on the use of video visits for psychotherapy (Cowan et al. 2020). At the Centre for Addiction and Mental Health, the largest psychiatric hospital in Canada, virtual care visits increased from approximately 350 per month to almost 3,000, an increase of more than 850%, from March to April 2020. Kaiser Permanente, the largest managed care organization in the United States, with 12 million plan members, moved rapidly to deliver 90% of its psychiatric care virtually, and an unpublished survey of 20 American psychiatrists by Peter Yellowlees found that all of them changed to fully virtual practices because of the COVID-19 pandemic, although most had not used telepsychiatry previously. Others have noted how apps and other forms of online care rapidly grew more popular, with Talkspace, an app offering text messages and therapy sessions, reporting a 65% increase in clients since the pandemic started (Perrone 2020).

In the United States, just 5% of Medicare psychiatrists provided at least one telemedicine visit in 2018. With COVID-19, the workload of many physicians changed dramatically, as did the way that they performed their work, and on the whole, physicians took to using video very well. The number of video visits paid for by insurers increased nationally by more than 4,000% in March 2020 in comparison with previous years and then by 8,800% to more than 14% of total reimbursed visits in April (FAIR Health 2020), with about half of these visits being for mental health needs.

This is progress, and these advances should not be temporary. Although COVID-19 was the trigger, the underlying benefits of increased telemedicine and remote care should be made permanent, and many patients and mental health clinicians, having now experienced the ease of virtual visits without artificial regulatory barriers, want to retain the positive consequences of this rapid technological adoption and a more consumer-driven care model. All types of therapy as described throughout this book can be delivered online, and following the start of the COVID-19 emergency, it is likely that all of them have already been so delivered.

Technologies such as telemedicine were also used to enable altered clinical workflows in response to COVID-19. These included hybrid rounding, which became popular with inpatient medical and psychiatric teams divided in space but connected by video in order to minimize exposure and use of personal protective equipment. Hybrid rounding has been in practice for quite some time in intensive care units, but COVID-19 expanded the potential of this practice across many inpatient services and also enabled services to be conferenced to and from community sites, such as dialysis or hospice care units, where a number of psychiatrists and other mental health professionals work.

COVID-19-related school closures also created an unexpected strain on working parents. The use of telemedicine allowed many clinicians, including some residents and fellows, to work at least part-time from home, alleviating some childcare burdens—a move that would have been unimaginable before COVID-19. Residents continued their training programs, with virtual didactics and mentoring; meetings and social gatherings over video; and regular check-ins and buddy systems via email, phone, and text, all rapidly put in place. These changes, driven by COVID-19 speeding up the adoption of teleworking for all clinicians during conventional office hours, at night, and on weekends, are also a reflection of generational shifts as more millennials become practicing clinicians and demand such choices, as described in the subsection "Intergenerational Changes." COVID-19 offered an opportunity to test more time and geographically flexible working arrangements that will likely lead to long-term workplace solutions that offer increased flexibility and further support the well-being of clinicians and their families, allowing clinicians to offer online psychotherapies literally anytime, anywhere.

The COVID-19 increase in videoconferencing has highlighted several issues associated with telemental health. Many patients still face challenges using and accessing videoconferencing due to both comfort and capacity as well as the *digital divide*, namely, bandwidth limitations constricting patients' access to technology. This concept also includes the wider impacts of social determinants of health that restrict access, including social and community context, education, economics, and health care systems issues (Ramsetty and Adams 2020). The consequence is that COVID-19 has also led to a significant increase in the use of the telephone to manage patients, with a recent survey of American Psychiatric Association members indicating that up to 25% were using only the telephone for telehealth encounters because of either access or other patient barriers (American Psychiatric Association 2020b). The literature on psychiatric treatments via telephone has been limited to structured evidence-based therapies (Everitt et al. 2019) and interactive voice response treatments (Rose et al. 2017). This literature is sparse or absent with regard to the ability of therapists to complete full psychiatric assessments, conduct treatments, and administer the full range of psychotherapy via the telephone compared with in-person or video interactions outside the aforementioned areas. Current clinical activity in this area appears to be occurring on a case-by-case basis depending on provider comfort, patient characteristics, technology access, and social circumstances. It remains in the domain of the individual provider to weigh the benefits of phone-based treatment (access and availability) compared with the risks (sparse guides on pairing appropriate treatments with patients) and to exercise their judgment on providing the best treatment possible during COVID-19.

Another major COVID-19-related issue is a concept getting wide attention: *videoconferencing fatigue* or *Zoom fatigue*, named by the press after a popular videoconferencing platform. The media and public have associated this concept specifically with videoconferencing, and because it is new to the vernacular, the current data for this are largely anecdotal. Given the need to make large aspects of work and personal life virtual, some fatigue with technologies is not surprising, but arguably, the causation is more complex and multifactorial. Possible contributors to this fatigue include having to rapidly adapt to a new set of clinical and administrative skills (e.g., videoconferencing) without a full implementation process or training. One also cannot discount the impact that living in quarantine during an international pandemic has on overall stress and energy. Although no single solution for this fatigue exists, using best practices for videoconferencing, including the following, may help to alleviate some of these issues:

- Assure adequate training, knowledge, and skills in the use of videoconferencing.
- Develop comfortable work spaces with attention to lighting, air flow, and ergonomics (e.g., chairs, monitors).
- Take breaks and schedule a diversity of work (e.g., administrative, calls) throughout the day between videoconferences and vary the types of videoconferencing.
- Use team-based approaches to virtual work, making sure to connect as a team with additional time for team bonding and informal discussions.
- Work to reach out and connect with team members at a human level; according to Mark Twain, "Against the assault of laughter, nothing can stand."

Organizations should make sure they offer training in best practices for virtual group meetings and facilitations (e.g., have an agenda, draw out quiet individuals, attempt to have equal participation).

How Can Patients Be Matched With Virtual Therapies?

A growing and robust literature demonstrates the effectiveness of all therapy in general delivered over videoconferencing (Bashshur et al. 2014; Chherawala and Gill 2020; Hubley et al. 2016) as well as therapy tailored to specific diagnoses (Shore et al. 2020a) and specific therapies or modalities (Wright and Mishkind 2020). A crucial task for the therapist is to appropriately pair the patient's problem with the planned therapy and determine the best technology to deliver the treatment. This should be accomplished in an organized and stepwise fashion by first assessing the patient and then matching the treatment and selecting the delivery method.

An initial session, which can be conducted over video, should include assessments of the patient's history and diagnosis and the problem to be addressed as well as their technology access (bandwidth, equipment, privacy), setting (office, home, other), therapy and technology preferences, and prior experience and comfort with technology. The therapist should recognize that prior experience with technology and the type of technology used may affect the therapeutic alliance, rapport, and engagement (Hubley et al. 2016; Lopez et al. 2019). This information can then be synthesized with the clinician's training, experience, and knowledge to recommend specific treatment.

Evidence is variable across different types of therapies regarding their use in videoconferencing, with some having a more robust literature base and documentation, such as the literature around CBT for depression, and others having scant or no description in the telepsychiatry literature, such as dynamic psychotherapy. The COVID-19 pandemic and subsequent public health response have caused widespread virtualization of health care to address social distancing requirements. Under the COVID-19 emergency almost all therapies have been virtualized to some extent, even those lacking a more detailed formal literature and evidence base (Chherawala and Gill 2020; Shore et al. 2020a). It is anticipated that the literature will continue to catch up with current practice in the coming years as the experience of therapy during the COVID-19 pandemic is described and documented. Because we know that psychotherapy can be delivered over video, it is reasonable to argue that an individual literature exploration consisting of randomized controlled trials for each individual type of therapy is not required at this point. Indeed, even before COVID-19, research in this area had moved beyond effectiveness trials comparing in-person to virtual treatments to new treatments in which technology is an integral part of the intervention.

Delivery through videoconferencing has been investigated for a number of structured evidence-based psychotherapies. Medication management, with its associated psychoeducation and supportive therapies, was one of the first applications of telepsychiatry (Hubley et al. 2016). Many of these have modifications and adaptations for remote delivery, including cognitive-behavioral therapy, family-focused therapy, and prolonged exposure therapy (Dausch et al. 2009; Hubley et al. 2016; Olden et al. 2017). Often, these therapies have specified and manualized adaptations for their administration through videoconferencing or other technologies that can guide the clinician. Other types of individual psychotherapies, including dynamic, psychoanalytic, and supportive therapies, have been successfully completed via videoconferencing, although the literature is less complete outside descriptive papers and proffered best practices. A small but longer-standing body of literature discusses group modalities for telepsychiatry, including structured or limited group treatments, supportive groups, and marital and family treatments (Dausch et al. 2009; Lopez et al. 2019; Van Voorhees et al. 2019). Team-based approaches to treatment that blend in-person and virtual visits with behavioral health team members to deliver an array of interventions, including group and individual therapy, have been well documented and include virtual integrated care services and substance use interventions (Shore 2019).

When selecting the recommended psychotherapy, clinicians should also strongly consider the technology used for the treatment. Although the majority of the literature has focused on synchronous videoconferencing, experience with web-based therapies, apps, text, and email in both real time (synchronous) and asynchronous time is emerging and expanding (Chan et al. 2017). These interventions can be standalone, such as a randomized controlled trial that demonstrated the effectiveness of a text message–based maintenance intervention for major depressive disorder after inpatient CBT (Schlicker et al. 2018). Alternatively, technologies or modalities can be combined together or used in conjunction with in-person treatment. For example, a CBT web-based treatment model that covers a range of cognitive-behavioral skills (Shi et al. 2019) was shown to be effective for outpatient substance use treatment as an add-on and as a stand-alone treatment. Other web-based treatments have been developed to support in-person treatment (computer-assisted therapy) such as in the case of psychotherapy for depression (Thase et al. 2018). Mobile apps offer promise in terms of variety, portability, and conveyance but remain in the early stage of development, with limited information on their effectiveness (Wright et al. 2019).

What Are the Practical and Psychotherapeutic Advantages of Telehealth for Patients and Therapists?

Convenience, Safety, and Satisfaction

In this era of an increasingly patient-focused approach to care, the scientific literature on telemedicine for many years has shown the remarkable trend that patients express continuously high satisfaction rates once they have experienced telemedicine in many different clinical specialties, from psychiatry to surgery (Hilty et al. 2013). Although many factors contribute to patient satisfaction, one that is repeatedly mentioned in the literature is the convenient empathic connection that patients feel that they can make with their telemedicine providers. This may be because of the greater and more direct amount of eye contact that tends to occur in telemedicine consultations compared with the typical in-person consultation. Other reasons for the high satisfaction rates include reduced patient anxiety resulting from patients being seen in or close to their homes in personally comfortable and nonintimidating surroundings, with added benefits from savings in reduced travel time and cost as their therapists are "beamed in" from afar. Psychiatrists and other mental health professionals have certainly found delivering online therapies to be more convenient and physically safe during COVID-19, although some have expressed doubts about efficacy. The U.S. Department of Health and Human Services (2020) was unequivocal in its advice:

> We encourage health care providers to adopt and use telehealth as a way to safely provide care to your patients in appropriate situations, including: routine health care, like wellness visits; medication consultation; dermatology (skin care); eye exams; nutrition counseling; mental health counseling.

Power

A subtler issue concerns the power relationship between doctor and patient; in the in-person relationship, the doctor typically has more authority and the psychological advantage of being in their own clinic or environment. Patients tend to feel more in control during video consultations and can, if they wish, literally switch off the doctor on their end and leave the consultation without any physical embarrassment or loss of face. Much has been written about the power issues between doctors and patients (Yellowlees and Shore 2018), but it seems clear that the online relationship, in most situations, tends to be more egalitarian than the one that occurs in person. This is something that today's patients, with their need for more patient-focused care approaches, greatly value. The environment of the patient's home or workplace, by virtue of its familiarity, likely has a containing effect for the patient, which may help the patient to feel more at ease both in initiating therapy and in being honest and forthcoming with the therapist. Similarly, the therapist has the option to see the patient from a setting that is more containing for them, such as the comfort of the therapist's own desk space at their office—which is not typically a portion of the office shared with the patient—or even from the therapist's home. This geographical relocation may help both parties to feel more relaxed or settled and could foster the development of psychotherapeutic intimacy.

Kocsis and Yellowlees (2018) noted that the patient frequently experiences a greater sense of physical and psychological control over the session in online psychotherapy; simultaneously, the therapist is less likely to be successful with a paternalistic approach. This combination means that in general, treatment styles are more likely to be patient centered. Traditional in-person psychotherapy gives the therapist the advantage of conducting sessions from the familiarity of their office or clinic, which is an unfamiliar space for the patient. Coupled with the increased eye contact and the use of the virtual space, as described in the subsection "Virtual Space," all of these factors combine to drive the relationship into a more egalitarian space (Yellowlees 2018).

Hybrid Care

The use of a hybrid model combining in-person therapy and telepsychotherapy was described in detail by Yellowlees and Shore (2018, p. 254), who defined a hybrid psychiatrist as a clinician who

> interacts with patients both in person and online so that their doctor-patient relationship crosses both environments. The addition of interactions via videoconferencing, e-mail, text messaging and telephony leads to improved access and interactions at times and places not possible with care restricted to the in-person venue. This hybrid practice is becoming a preferred model of care for many physicians as secure messaging is incorporated into electronic medical record (EMR) systems. It is especially relevant to telepsychiatry as a range of video technologies, text-based systems, and apps can readily complement in-person care depending on the psychiatrist's and patient's preferences.... The incorporation of online models of care into practice can strengthen the doctor-patient relationship by increasing empathy and forming a trusting therapeutic bond.

The American Psychiatric Association (2020a) has published a guidance document for members about opening their practice during COVID-19 with the following advice:

> The safest way to continue providing treatment is through telehealth when feasible, particularly if this has been a viable option to date. Many patients may want to continue working in a hybrid way, with a mix of in-person and telehealth visits.

It is likely that in the post-COVID-19 world, many, if not most, mental health professionals will continue to practice in this hybrid manner, seeing patients both online and in person, depending on mutual convenience and preference. This may well lead to the development of a number of novel future psychotherapies that take the best aspects of both in-person and online models of care and therapy and combine them. This is already happening, with Fortney et al. (2015a) describing the use of online video sessions with veterans who have PTSD as an engagement strategy to eventually lead to them attending in-person group sessions.

Teamwork

Another significant advantage of video consultations over traditional in-person clinical care is that they give us the ability to work more effectively in teams; across disciplines; and with patients, their families, and local providers (Fortney et al. 2015a; Hilty et al. 2013; Yellowlees and Shore 2018) in a collaborative care model, especially in primary care. This involves working within the concept of the primary care medical home, for which Myers et al. (2015) showed how short-term therapies can be integrated into a collaborative team-based model of care for children with ADHD. Fortney et al. (2015b) demonstrated that online video cognitive-behavioral psychotherapy sessions can actually lead to enhanced in-person care if they are added to usual care. Their research showed that video-based psychotherapy was actually more effective than in-person psychotherapy with patients with PTSD and that the evidence-based psychotherapy given online had better fidelity than that given in person. In some of his studies Fortney also showed that in this group of typically avoidant veterans with PTSD, the use of this hybrid model of online and in-person care actually led to enhanced patient engagement, as well as improved clinical outcomes. This work has led to the Study to Promote Innovation in Rural Integrated Telepsychiatry (SPIRIT) trial, for which Fortney and his team have been funded to compare the outcomes of team-based telepsychiatry collaborative care with traditional telepsychiatry individual referrals and treatments (Fortney et al. 2020). It will be fascinating to see whether the telepsychiatry team-based care in this pragmatic comparative effectiveness trial for patients with bipolar disorder or PTSD has better outcomes than the traditional telemental health treatment process.

Clearly, many of the therapies described in this book involve the use of groups or teams of therapists or patients, and the ability to bring everyone together in a single online video room makes group sessions very much more convenient and easy to attend. A number of studies have examined group therapy delivered by video, ranging from that of Xie et al. (2013), who demonstrated the effectiveness of video for teaching parent training skills to parents of children with ADHD, to numerous papers examining the effectiveness of video group therapy in veterans with PTSD (Morland et al. 2015).

A final recent example is the group therapy meetings delivered over video by Alcoholics Anonymous and related organizations that were introduced as a result of COVID-19. These have been taken up enthusiastically by many patients with alcohol and substance use disorders, with some meetings involving more than 500 attendees from many states or countries. Anecdotal stories given to us by some attendees indicate that these meetings have been very positive.

Virtual Space

Online consultation addresses the two major weaknesses of in-person consultation, *physical access* and the *power differential*, as already described in the subsections "Convenience, Safety, and Satisfaction" and "Power," and adds a third component that is clinically useful: the existence and use of a *virtual space* between the patient and therapist. There are two components of the virtual space that affect both provider and patient: physical and psychological, as described in detail by Yellowlees and Shore (2018) and Yellowlees et al. (2015).

At the most basic level, the *physical space* and separation for providers enhance a feeling of safety, particularly when seeing patients who are physically dangerous or who inhabit potentially dangerous environments, such as correctional institutions. Interestingly, this feeling of safety also allows providers to give much more direct feedback to patients about their diagnosis and treatment plan than they might give in consultations where the patient is physically present in the room. This is especially true if this feedback involves comments on substance-related, behavioral, or personality-focused issues that the patient may not wish to hear about or may disagree with. From the patient's perspective, it is also common for patients living in small communities, which are increasingly being serviced by telemedicine, to prefer to see a physician who does not live in their community to decrease the probability of a loss of confidentiality.

The *psychological space* and distancing are much more important and have differing impacts on providers and patients. It is possible to have intense, intimate, and empathic relationships over videoconferencing. Many long-distance relationships are started and maintained on easily available videoconferencing software platforms all around the world and in all cultures. These systems allow users to clearly show and detect emotions, connect with each other, and interact empathically on today's high-quality video systems with which they can see and hear each other over video and audio that have the quality of high-definition television. The psychological extra distance that both partners in the consultation frequently initially notice tends to reduce markedly after a few minutes.

The psychological space is especially important for patients and frequently allows them to have more intimate conversations with their providers than they would have in a physical consultation. Religions around the world have understood the importance of this virtual space for centuries, with parishioners in a confessional box telling intimate stories about themselves to a priest who is close by and who they know is listening but who is distant and not physically seen. Similarly, when the topic of conversation is possibly embarrassing, stigmatizing, or awkward, people find it easier to discuss it on video or online and respond more honestly when there is a small amount of virtual distance or virtual space, compared with an in-person interview (Yellowlees and Shore 2018). For instance, a woman who has just been raped may feel uncomfortable talking to a male therapist in the same room. The extra distance of a video consultation makes even someone who is well known and trusted appear just a bit more distant and therefore the discussion is less threatening or potentially embarrassing.

For providers, the psychological space allows them to be simultaneously part of the consultation but also more of an objective observer of the consultation. This occurs most commonly when seeing children with behavioral disorders; often, mental health professionals engage the child's parents initially to take a history from them, but at the same time they can observe through the video the child's behavior, the interactions between the child and the parents, and the parents' parenting and disciplinary skills. Such objective observation is more difficult in the in-person consultation because the family in this situation tends to be much more aware of the physician's physical presence (Pakyurek et al. 2010).

Return of the Home Visit

Since the introduction of smartphones and mobile devices such as tablets in about 2007, it has suddenly become possible to easily connect with patients directly in their homes, their workplaces, social environments, and their vehicles rather than having to see them in primary care clinics, which has been the case with traditional telepsychiatry. This has revolutionized the practice of telemental health, especially following the adaptation of American Telemedicine Association guidelines for delivering video mental health care at home or in community settings (Shore et al. 2018). These guidelines importantly included standard operating procedures to ensure patient safety.

Most telepsychiatrists now deliver care direct to patients in nonclinical community settings routinely. It should be noted that patient privacy still warrants careful attention even in home settings because many patients live in space shared with others, and ensuring the availability of a quiet, secluded space in the patient's home is essential. The home offers many more opportunities to get to know patients and to further deepen understanding and the level of the doctor-patient relationship. It is possible to take a tour of the home and garden and thereby discover a patient's interests such as art, from pictures on the walls, or sports, from memorabilia on counters. Equally, it is possible to see how a patient lives more easily than when meeting them only in a clinic. Is their home neat and tidy or chaotic? Do they have personal space? Do they have pets, and how do they look after them? What about others in the family? Can you speak to parents, partners, and children and perhaps get a better idea of the patient's relationships and the views of people important in their lives about how the patient is coping? Does the patient have food in the house? Is there a surprising number of bottles of alcohol in evidence? Is there a suggestion of disorganization, with unwashed plates in the kitchen and dirty clothes on the floor? Does the patient have a sense of pride and commitment to their home, and are they interested in gardening and prepared to show you around not just the house but also the garden and immediate locality to give you more of an idea of how and where they live?

Answers to these sorts of questions used to be obtained only by literally making physical home visits, but now that making such visits virtually is possible, this extra knowledge can often be easily obtained and used to help the patient. We mentioned at the beginning of this chapter how the new therapy room is the equivalent of the car and how the ability to connect to people's homes during the COVID-19 pandemic has allowed many thousands of patients to continue receiving psychotherapy in many different forms, and it will continue to do so in future.

Why Do Some Patients Prefer Telepsychiatry to In-Person Care for Therapy?

Increasing numbers of patients prefer to be seen through telemedicine rather than in person for a range of reasons, including personal preference, convenience, cost, and stigma minimization. These individuals include not only patients who are anxious, avoidant, shy, or paranoid but also those who are reticent to see physicians at the best of times, such as young males, as well as many from younger generations who see video interactions as being not only normal but preferred. Some new telemedicine services specifically target people with stigmatized disorders, such as erectile dysfunction, baldness, and HIV, offering a combination of highly private medical assessments, prescribing, and counseling. Many patients are still afraid of seeing psychiatrists, but some feel calmer about the process if they can have the consultation at a distance on video, either from their primary care clinic or, increasingly, from home. Obviously, with the recent drivers of telepsychiatry, namely, COVID-19, mobile devices, and the younger age demographics of both patients and therapists, these patients have been joined by many others for whom telepsychiatry initially became essential to continue their care but who now have become accustomed to this modality.

A number of video consultation services to the home that are offered as part of concierge practices or through privately owned telepsychiatry companies have emerged and are marketed as a more convenient time-saving service that improves access to physicians and therapists. These services tend to attract as patients individuals who are VIPs or celebrities, as well as doctors, lawyers, and businesspeople who have psychiatric or substance-related disorders or who just prefer more privacy for all of their health care, perhaps because they have a stigmatized disorder. These people prefer to have their consultations in extreme privacy for many reasons and often wish to be seen from their homes, which has been possible via mobile devices in recent years, as well as pay cash for services. This ensures that their psychiatric history is not potentially available to insurance company databases and ends the possibility of the VIP being photographed and "outed" outside a therapist's office.

Finally, increasing numbers of patients are seeking video opinions from physicians who are known to be national or international experts in a particular area but who are otherwise inaccessible. This is especially important for patients with rare diseases, those who wish to receive unusual or highly specialized treatments from acknowledged national experts, or those who wish to have an unusual therapy for which no locally licensed or trained practitioners are available.

After years of practice by many psychiatrists and psychotherapists, the consensus of the field is clear that any type of patient may be seen using videoconferencing (Bashshur et al. 2016). The only absolute contraindications to a psychiatric interview are if the patient refuses to attend, as some do, or if they are actively acting out and demonstrating dangerous behavior to themselves or others at the time of the interview. However, a number of groups of patients have other specific psychotherapeutic issues that are of importance and should be considered, as described by Kocsis and Yellowlees (2018).

Patients With Psychotic Disorders

Some patients with psychotic disorders may do better receiving therapy by video than in person because they often feel unsafe by virtue of their illness and may feel more at ease when the provider is not in the room and they are distanced by video. Sharp et al. (2011) found that psychiatric care through videoconferencing was well tolerated by patients with psychotic disorders and that the increased physical and psychological distance afforded by the modality may reduce anxiety in this population. For especially paranoid patients, offering to temporarily point the camera away from them (so that the provider has only audio information but the patient can still both see and hear the provider) may provide enough distance that the patient feels safer. Additionally, the therapist may feel safer with the removal of the threat of physical harm by patients with psychotic disorders who are potentially assaultive. This enables the therapist to be both more relaxed and more direct when communicating with such patients. Many county mental health systems now routinely hold telepsychiatry clinics for patients with chronic psychoses where supportive psychotherapy and medication management are provided by a psychiatrist from afar, often in tandem with a local caseworker sitting in with their patient.

Highly Anxious Patients

Psychotherapy over video may be particularly helpful for anxious patients who have difficulty with leaving the home, especially if their difficulty is related to agoraphobia or other phobias (Morland et al. 2015), which has been the case with many patients during the COVID-19 pandemic. With a video-based modality, patients who might otherwise delay or forego treatment can access a therapeutic relationship in a way that feels safe for them. If a cognitive-behavioral therapeutic model is used for treatment, having the patient eventually come to the therapist's office could be set as a goal for therapy or could specifically serve as one of the steps in a set of gradually escalating exposures (Kocsis and Yellowlees 2018).

Autistic Patients

Autistic patients struggle with tolerating novel environments, and many have difficulty with the social norms and sensory experience of visiting the office of a doctor or therapist. Many higher-functioning autistic persons enjoy using computers and find a sense of community online, such that they may feel more comfortable with this modality for receiving psychiatric and psychotherapeutic care, and a number of such programs have transitioned to an online modality during the COVID-19 pandemic.

Children and Teens

Younger children may be less nervous at home than in a therapist's office, and thus the therapist may get a more accurate picture of the child's everyday behavior from the less intrusive vantage of telepsychotherapy (Pakyurek et al. 2010). Additionally, many teens today spend a considerable amount of time online, and they may be more comfortable using online modalities to obtain mental health services.

Traumatized Patients

Patients with significant childhood abuse histories may have an especially difficult time feeling safe around the authority figure of the doctor or therapist. For victims of sexual abuse or rape, the intimate setting of the therapist's office and the potential gender difference between patient and provider may cause considerable anxiety. An online approach may help to build important initial rapport and safety. Morland and colleagues (2015) conducted several studies examining the use of teleconferencing for delivery of psychotherapeutic treatments in both veteran and nonveteran populations with PTSD. This work has shown that cognitive processing therapy (both individual and group) and CBT over videoconference are not inferior to in-person delivery of these modalities. The advantages of telepsychotherapy, as well as the potential for increased privacy, may make this modality preferable for treatment of some patients with PTSD.

Patients With Personality Disorders

Telepsychiatry for patients with personality disorders has been discussed in detail by Kocsis and Yellowlees (2018), who concluded that more research is needed to assess the particular aspects of caring for this group of patients online. They suggested that a hybrid approach or exclusively in-person sessions may be necessary for some patients at the beginning of treatment because many patients with personality disorder may struggle without the literal, concrete presence of the therapist in the room. They noted that when caring for these patients, the therapist will have to be attentive to setting boundaries and maintaining a consistent frame just as in person. Morland et al. (2015) noted that a specific discussion of boundaries is important for the effective delivery of psychotherapy over video because Morland observed some of her patients engaging in multitasking activities such as cooking during therapy sessions taking place at home. An area of particular importance for this group of patients is the maintenance of boundaries around times of access to the therapist to ensure that the therapist does not become burned out responding to every patient contact any time of the day or night.

What Clinical and Organizational Skills Do Therapists Require to Work Successfully Online With Their Patients?

For any therapist wanting to work in this area, the first thing to review is the website for the American Telemedicine Association (www.americantelemed.org). The most important document to download is the mental health guidelines from 2018, which cover in detail all the technical, clinical, administrative, and legal issues anyone will need to be aware of to successfully practice online mental health and to provide short-term online psychotherapy. Equally important is a detailed downloadable list of state and licensing regulations and rules for all 50 states available from the American Telemedicine Association (www.americantelemed.org). The other key website is the American Psychiatric Association's (2021) Telepsychiatry Toolkit, which includes multiple written resources and more than 30 video clips describing differing aspects of telepsychiatry practice. A textbook covering most aspects of telepsychiatry, from planning to implementation, describes the following practical issues (Yellowlees and Shore 2018):

- Planning the overall implementation of video services and teleconsultations to provide the therapy that you wish to undertake
- Type of technology to be used and a needs analysis
- Technical and media training, clinical policies required, knowledge and implementation of administrative and safety guidelines, possible staffing, and role changes in the clinic
- Business aspects (e.g., understanding legal, licensing, and local regulations; credentialing; and billing and payment issues)

The key clinical policies that most practices will need to address are as follows:

- Release of information and informed consent as required by your state
- Intake procedures, appointment scheduling, synchronizing schedules at all sites, and staff roles and responsibilities
- Ensuring privacy and confidentiality; use of electronic medical records; and the transmission of prescriptions, laboratory orders, and progress notes as necessary

How Will We Practice in the Future?

Telepsychiatry allows practitioners to practice routinely in a hybrid manner, with patients seeing individuals both in person and online, depending on the practitioner's and patient's mutual convenience and wishes. In the future telepsychiatry will increasingly be considered a best practice that improves, augments, and replaces some of our current in-person practices with primarily mobile technologically driven and supported interventions, as described in this chapter.

The future psychiatrist-patient relationship will be a hybrid form, both in person and online. This relationship will include the core strengths of the traditional in-person medical consultation, which has long been the gold standard for practice, in which there is immediacy and trust in the personal interaction and use of the relationship, through transference and countertransference, can lead to healing and support. This will be supplemented and improved by online interactions through multiple modalities: video, text, apps, virtual reality, and artificial intelligence. These provide patients better convenience and improved access to their providers, potentially anytime, anywhere, and make the whole relationship more egalitarian, whatever the type of psychotherapy being used. For providers the online component of the relationship may also be more convenient, allowing them to work from home at preferred times and freeing them from the typical business week practice while also enhancing their safety with certain patient groups.

The practice of psychiatry, and mental health more generally, is changing and promises to be very different in future decades. Even more nascent, but potentially more intriguing, is the future use of automated computerized programs such as chatbots to provide psychotherapy by using ever-expanding artificial intelligence (AI) technologies. These chatbots are AI programs that attempt to simulate human conversation and interactions (Moore and Caudill 2019), and although AI is still in a conceptual and experimental stage, the potential for AI collaboration and support of traditional therapists both brings with it an exciting potential but also raises a host of ethical, quality-of-care, and workforce issues that will need to be appropriately addressed and navigated.

Some therapists will, of course, always prefer to practice completely or almost entirely in person, and many patients will prefer this modality. Ensuring that such choices continue to be available is important, whatever revolutionary changes in mental health practice in cyberspace become available over time. Ensuring that AI is used to enhance and support the human connection between therapist and patient and not to diminish it will be important.

Key Points

- Telepsychiatry outcomes and patient satisfaction rates are similar to in-person care, with some patients and providers preferring online care, especially when delivered to and from their homes.
- The hybrid doctor-patient relationship, both in-person and online, in the post-pandemic world is likely to become increasingly common.
- Online psychotherapy has become common in recent years, driven by technological improvements and the move to mobile devices, changing demographics with younger patients and providers, and the need for safety and social distancing during the pandemic.
- Online psychotherapy has a number of advantages over in-person therapy, especially the use of the "virtual space" in the consultation, and differing technologies can be matched to the needs of individual patients.

References

American Psychiatric Association: Guidance document on reopening practices. Washington, DC, American Psychiatric Association, 2020a. Available at: www.psychiatry.org/psychiatrists/covid-19-coronavirus. Accessed August 24, 2020.

American Psychiatric Association: Psychiatrists use of telepsychiatry during COVID-19 public health emergency: survey results. Washington, DC, American Psychiatric Association, June 2020b. Available at: www.psychiatry.org/File%20Library/Psychiatrists/Practice/Telepsychiatry/APA-Telehealth-Survey-2020.pdf. Accessed August 28, 2020.

American Psychiatric Association: Telepsychiatry Toolkit. Washington, DC, American Psychiatric Association, 2021. Available at: www.psychiatry.org/psychiatrists/practice/telepsychiatry/toolkit. Accessed October 11, 2021.

Bashshur RL, Shannon GW, Smith BR, et al: The empirical foundations of telemedicine interventions for chronic disease management. Telemed J E Health 20(9):769–800, 2014 24968105

Bashshur RL, Shannon GW, Bashshur N, et al: The empirical evidence for telemedicine interventions in mental disorders. Telemed J E Health 22(2):87–113, 2016 26624248

Chan SR, Torous J, Hinton L, et al: Mobile tele-mental health: increasing applications and a move to hybrid models of care. Healthcare (Basel) 2(2):220–233, 2014 27429272

Chan S, Parish M, Yellowlees P: Telepsychiatry today. Curr Psychiatry Rep 17(11):89, 2015 26384338

Chan S, Godwin H, Gonzalez A, et al: Review of use and integration of mobile apps into psychiatric treatments. Curr Psychiatry Rep 19(12):96, 2017 29082425

Chherawala N, Gill S: Up-to-date review of psychotherapy via videoconference: implications and recommendations for the RANZCP Psychotherapy Written Case during the COVID-19 pandemic. Australas Psychiatry 28(5):517–520, 2020 32689815

Cowan A, Johnson R, Close H: Telepsychiatry in psychotherapy practice. Innov Clin Neurosci 17(4–6):23–26, 2020 32802589

Dausch BM, Miklowitz DJ, Nagamoto HT, et al: Family focused therapy via videoconferencing. J Telemed Telecare 15(4):211–214, 2009 19471035

Deyan G: 67+ revealing smartphone statistics for 2020. Techjury, July 31, 2020. Available at: https://techjury.net/blog/smartphone-usage-statistics/#gref. Accessed October 8, 2021.

Everitt HA, Landau S, O'Reilly G, et al: Assessing telephone-delivered cognitive-behavioural therapy (CBT) and web-delivered CBT versus treatment as usual in irritable bowel syndrome (ACTIB): a multicentre randomised trial. Gut 68(9):1613–1623, 2019 30971419

FAIR Health: Monthly telehealth regional tracker. New York, FAIR Health, 2020. Available at: www.fairhealth.org/states-by-the-numbers/telehealth. Accessed February 14, 2022.

Fortney JC, Pyne JM, Kimbrell TA, et al: Telemedicine-based collaborative care for posttraumatic stress disorder: a randomized clinical trial. JAMA Psychiatry 72(1):58–67, 2015a 25409287

Fortney JC, Pyne JM, Turner EE, et al: Telepsychiatry integration of mental health services into rural primary care settings. Int Rev Psychiatry 27(6):525–539, 2015b 26634618

Fortney JC, Heagerty PJ, Bauer AM, et al: Study to Promote Innovation in Rural Integrated Telepsychiatry (SPIRIT): rationale and design of a randomized comparative effectiveness trial of managing complex psychiatric disorders in rural primary care clinics. Contemp Clin Trials 90:105873, 2020 31678410

Hilty DM, Ferrer DC, Parish MB, et al: The effectiveness of telemental health: a 2013 review. Telemed J E Health 19(6):444–454, 2013 23697504

Hubley S, Lynch SB, Schneck C, et al: Review of key telepsychiatry outcomes. World J Psychiatry 6(2):269–282, 2016 27354970

Kocsis BJ, Yellowlees P: Telepsychotherapy and the therapeutic relationship: principles, advantages, and case examples. Telemed J E Health 24(5):329–334, 2018 28836902

Lopez A, Schwenk S, Schneck CD, et al: Technology-based mental health treatment and the impact on the therapeutic alliance. Curr Psychiatry Rep 21(8):76, 2019 31286280

Moore JR, Caudill R: The bot will see you now: a history and review of interactive computerized mental health programs. Psychiatr Clin North Am 42(4):627–634, 2019 31672212

Morland LA, Poizner JM, Williams KE, et al: Home-based clinical video teleconferencing care: clinical considerations and future directions. Int Rev Psychiatry 27(6):504–512, 2015 26619273

Myers K, Vander Stoep A, Zhou C, et al: Effectiveness of a telehealth service delivery model for treating attention-deficit/hyperactivity disorder: a community-based randomized controlled trial. J Am Acad Child Adolesc Psychiatry 54(4):263–274, 2015 25791143

Nakagawa K, Yellowlees P: Inter-generational effects of technology: why millennial physicians may be less at risk for burnout than baby boomers. Curr Psychiatry Rep 22(9):45, 2020 32661817

Olden M, Shingleton R, Finkelstein-Fox L, et al: Telemedicine exposure therapy and assessment for PTSD: a systematic clinical practice narrative review. J Technol Behav Sci 1(1–4):22–31, 2017

Pakyurek M, Yellowlees P, Hilty D: The child and adolescent telepsychiatry consultation: can it be a more effective clinical process for certain patients than conventional practice? Telemed J E Health 16(3):289–292, 2010 20406115

Perrone M: Virus drives new demand for Talkspace's online therapy. May 10, 2020. Available at: https://abcnews.go.com/US/wireStory/virus-drives-demand-talkspaces-online-therapy-70603681. Accessed October 8, 2021.

Ramsetty A, Adams C: Impact of the digital divide in the age of COVID-19. J Am Med Inform Assoc 27(7):1147–1148, 2020 32343813
Rose GL, Badger GJ, Skelly JM, et al: A randomized controlled trial of brief intervention by interactive voice response. Alcohol Alcohol 52(3):335–343, 2017 28069598
Saeed SA, Shore JH, Yellowlees P: Using technology for providing care, in Textbook of Psychiatric Administration and Leadership, 3rd Edition. Edited by Saeed S, Lauriello J, Roberts LW. Washington, DC, American Psychiatric Association Publishing, in press
Schlicker S, Ebert DD, Middendorf T, et al: Evaluation of a text-message-based maintenance intervention for major depressive disorder after inpatient cognitive behavioral therapy. J Affect Disord 227:305–312, 2018 29132073
Sharp IR, Kobak KA, Osman DA: The use of videoconferencing with patients with psychosis: a review of the literature. Ann Gen Psychiatry 10(1):14, 2011 21501496
Shi JM, Henry SP, Dwy SL, et al: Randomized pilot trial of web-based cognitive-behavioral therapy adapted for use in office-based buprenorphine maintenance. Subst Abus 40(2):132–135, 2019 30714880
Shore JH: Best practices in tele-teaming: managing virtual teams in the delivery of care in telepsychiatry. Curr Psychiatry Rep 21(8):77, 2019 31286277
Shore JH, Yellowlees P, Caudill R, et al: Best practices in videoconferencing-based telemental health April 2018. Telemed J E Health 24(11):827–832, 2018 30358514
Shore JH, Schneck CD, Mishkind M, et al: Advancing treatment of depression and other mood disorders through innovative models of telepsychiatry. Focus Am Psychiatr Publ 18(2):169–174, 2020a 33162854
Shore JH, Schneck CD, Mishkind MC: Telepsychiatry and the coronavirus disease 2019 pandemic: current and future outcomes of the rapid virtualization of psychiatric care. JAMA Psychiatry 77(12):1211–1212, 2020b 32391861
Thase ME, Wright JH, Eells TD, et al: Improving the efficiency of psychotherapy for depression: computer-assisted versus standard CBT. Am J Psychiatry 175(3):242–250, 2018 28969439
Torous J, Firth J, Huckvale K, et al: The emerging imperative for a consensus approach toward the rating and clinical recommendation of mental health apps. J Nerv Ment Dis 206(8):662–666, 2018 30020203
U.S. Department of Health and Human Services: Telehealth: delivering care safely during COVID-19. Washington, DC, U.S. Department of Health and Human Services, July 15, 2020. Available at: www.hhs.gov/coronavirus/telehealth/index.html. Accessed October 11, 2021.
Van Voorhees EE, Dillon KH, Wilson SM, et al: A comparison of group anger management treatments for combat veterans with PTSD: results from a quasi-experimental trial. J Interpers Violence 36(19–20):NP10276–NP10300, 2019 34523367
Waugh M, Yellowlees PM, Dixon R, et al: Telepsychiatry, in Understanding Telehealth. Edited by Rheuban KS, Krupinski EA. New York, McGraw Hill, 2018, pp 125–132
Wright JH, Mishkind M: Computer-assisted CBT and mobile apps for depression: assessment and integration into clinical care. Focus Am Psychiatr Publ 18(2):162–168, 2020 33162853
Wright JH, Mishkind M, Eells TD, et al: Computer-assisted cognitive-behavior therapy and mobile apps for depression and anxiety. Curr Psychiatry Rep 21(7):62, 2019 31250242
Xie Y, Dixon JF, Yee OM, et al: A study on the effectiveness of videoconferencing on teaching parent training skills to parents of children with ADHD. Telemed J E Health 19(3):192–199, 2013 23405952
Yellowlees P: Telepsychiatry, in The Art and Science of Brief Psychotherapies: A Practitioner's Guide, 3rd Edition. Edited by Dewan M, Steenbarger B, Greenberg R. Washington, DC, American Psychiatric Association Publishing, 2018, pp 303–314
Yellowlees PM, Liu B: Suicide prevention programs, in The American Psychiatric Association Publishing Textbook of Suicide Risk Assessment and Management, 3rd Edition. Edited by Gold L, Frierson RL. Washington, DC, American Psychiatric Association Publishing, 2020, pp 391–402
Yellowlees PM, Shore J: Telepsychiatry and Health Technologies: A Guide for Mental Health Professionals. Washington, DC, American Psychiatric Association Publishing, 2018

Yellowlees PM, Shore JH: Hybrid practitioners and digital treatments, in The American Psychiatric Assocation Publishing Textbook of Psychiatry. Edited by Roberts LW. Washington, DC, American Psychiatric Association Publishing, 2019, pp 1041–1056

Yellowlees PM, Holloway KM, Parish MB: Therapy in virtual environments—clinical and ethical issues. Telemed J E Health 18(7):558–564, 2012 22823138

Yellowlees P, Chan SR, Parish MB: The hybrid doctor-patient relationship in the age of technology—telepsychiatry consultations and the use of virtual space. Int Rev Psychiatry 27(6):476–489, 2015 26493089

Yellowlees P, Nakagawa K, Pakyurek M, et al: Rapid conversion of an outpatient psychiatric clinic to a 100% virtual telepsychiatry clinic in response to COVID-19. Psychiatr Serv 71(7):749–752, 2020 32460683

CHAPTER 35

Combining Medications and Psychotherapy

David Mintz, M.D.

The human and societal toll of mental illness remains significant, despite advances in understanding and treatment. For all the optimism promised by the "Decade of the Brain" (Gabbard 1992), little evidence suggests that pharmacotherapy outcomes have improved substantially in the past four decades. As former National Institute of Mental Health director Thomas Insel noted at the conclusion of his tenure, "The unfortunate reality is that current medications help too few people to get better and very few people to get well" (Insel 2009, p. 704). Neither are psychological treatments a panacea, and too many patients are left with a burden of suffering, despite receiving skilled psychotherapy.

The combination of medications and psychotherapy is one strategy for optimizing outcomes for patients with psychiatric distress. Evidence suggests that the combination of medications and psychotherapy is a powerful tool in our treatment armamentarium. Patients also often prefer combining medications and psychotherapy over unimodal treatments (Seligman 1995).

The practicalities of limited resources mean that uniform provision of combined medications and psychotherapy may be cost prohibitive, and such a strategy risks overwhelming an already burdened system. There are some conditions for which the evidence and treatment guidelines suggest that combined treatment should be considered as a first-line approach (Table 35–1). For other highly prevalent conditions, such as depression, that show modest benefit from either medications or psychotherapy, consideration of limited resources suggests a more tailored approach to the unique characteristics of the patient and their illness.

In this chapter we survey the indications for combined treatment and the possible mechanisms by which medications and pharmacotherapy interact, generally, but not always, to the patient's benefit. In addition, we explore common technical and practical issues involved in combined treatment.

When to Offer Combined Treatment

Conditions for Which Combined Treatment Should Be Considered as a First-Line Approach

With some psychiatric conditions, the evidence clearly suggests that combined treatment with some form of psychotherapy is preferential to monotherapy with either psychotherapy or medications. American Psychiatric Association (APA) practice guidelines include both substance use disorders and schizophrenia on this list (American Psychiatric Association 2007a, 2021). These conditions have both high rates of treatment discontinuation and high rates of relapse. Combined treatment not only improves functioning but also reduces nonadherence and preserves a connection to treatment if the patient becomes nonadherent with one treatment modality. For patients with eating disorders, combined treatment is also recommended (American Psychiatric Association 2007b).

Although pharmacotherapy is the recommended first-line approach for patients in an acute manic episode, APA practice guidelines recommend combined approaches in the maintenance phase (American Psychiatric Association 2010). Combined treatment with psychotherapy can address interpersonal issues that are exacerbated by bipolar symptoms or are triggers for increased symptoms. Psychotherapy can also foster the patient's agency in illness management by supporting the patient in developing a healthier and more stable lifestyle, addressing psychological factors affecting medication adherence, and increasing awareness of bipolar triggers and prodromal symptoms.

Conditions for Which Combined Treatment Is Not Recommended as an Initial Approach

Treatment guidelines recommend first-line monotherapy for other psychiatric conditions (Table 35–2). In the case of PTSD, APA practice guidelines (Ursano et al. 2004) recommend evidence-based psychotherapeutic approaches as a first line of response, to be followed with pharmacotherapy in the context of treatment nonresponse. Psychotherapeutic approaches also represent the core approach to significant personality disorders such as borderline personality disorder, although adjunctive, symptom-targeted pharmacotherapy may prove helpful (American Psychiatric Association 2001).

Conditions for Which a More Tailored Approach to Combining Treatments Is Appropriate

Many of the most common psychiatric conditions, such as anxiety disorders, obsessive-compulsive disorder, and depression, are known to respond both to psychotherapy and to pharmacotherapy, although it is also not unusual for the response to be limited or partial. As noted at the beginning of this chapter, the high prevalence of these conditions means that routine provision of combined treatment would risk taxing system resources while not always clearly offering added benefit. Treatment guidelines (American Psychiatric Association 1998, 2009; Koran et al. 2007) suggest

Table 35–1. Common conditions for which combined treatment is the recommended first-line approach

Schizophrenia
Substance use disorders
Bipolar disorder, maintenance phase

Table 35–2. Common conditions for which monotherapy is recommended as a first-line approach

PTSD
Personality disorders

Table 35–3. Common conditions for which monotherapy progressing to combined treatment is recommended

Obsessive-compulsive disorder
Panic disorder
Major depression

starting with one treatment or the other for treatment-naive patients and progressing to combined treatment in the context of inadequate response to monotherapy (Table 35–3). Guidelines leave much to clinical judgment in the selection of an initial treatment. Evidence shows a significant role for patient preference in promoting positive outcomes (Kocsis et al. 2009), suggesting that this should be an important factor in selecting initial treatments.

Major Depression

In the case of major depression, which is among the most common and most researched psychiatric condition with regard to combined treatment, evidence points to a modest short-term benefit over unimodal treatment. The breadth of research illustratively reveals the true complexity of issues involved in combining treatments because illness severity, phase of illness, different psychotherapies, comorbidities, and other factors affecting depression outcome are considered.

Some meta-analyses do not show superiority for combined treatment over psychotherapy alone but do show improved outcomes compared with antidepressant monotherapy (Blom et al. 2007; Karyotaki et al. 2016). However, most meta-analyses demonstrate improved remission rates with combined treatment over monotherapy of any sort (Cuijpers et al. 2009, 2012, 2014, 2015; Oestergaard and Møldrup 2011). This finding applies to heterogeneous samples of depressed patients and to patients with more severe depressive symptoms.

Although much early research into combined treatment for depression focused on cognitive-behavioral therapy (CBT) and its derivatives or interpersonal psychotherapy (IPT) (Cuijpers et al. 2011; Thase et al. 1997), more recent research into combined treatments with psychodynamic psychotherapies (de Jonghe et al. 2001; Molenaar et al. 2007) demonstrated similar benefits. In a large trial in which short-term dynamic supportive psychotherapy with medications was compared with antidepressant monotherapy (de Jonghe et al. 2001), 37% of patients remitted with combined treatment, compared with 16% receiving monotherapy.

More impressive benefits of combined treatment of depression appear when considering long-term outcomes (Blackburn et al. 1986; Oestergaard and Møldrup 2011) and when looking at subpopulations with a poorer prognosis. In addition to higher rates of remission, numerous studies suggest that combined treatment yields lower risk of relapse and higher rates of long-term recovery, particularly when compared with medications alone.

CBT added to antidepressant pharmacotherapy reduces relapse rates (Evans et al. 1992; Simon et al. 1986). A meta-analysis of 13 studies examining the addition of CBT to treatment of medication responders found that added psychotherapy led to an absolute reduction of relapse recurrence of 22%, whether patients were maintained on medications (19% risk reduction) or tapered off of medications (33% risk reduction) (Guidi et al. 2016).

Similarly, IPT added to medications substantially reduces relapse rates. In one study, in the 3 months after hospital discharge, only 3% of patients receiving IPT relapsed, compared with 25% who had received only antidepressants and treatment as usual (Schramm et al. 2007). In another trial, even after 5 years of naturalistic follow-up, hospitalized patients receiving combined treatment with IPT for depression demonstrated significant ongoing benefits, with 28% remaining free of recurrence with combined treatment versus 11% experiencing sustained remission with pharmacotherapy alone (Zobel et al. 2011).

Brief dynamic therapies also contribute to better long-term outcomes compared with medications alone. In a study of brief dynamic therapy administered concurrently with medications for depression, patients receiving dynamic therapy in the acute phase of treatment did not show statistically significant benefit during acute phase treatment. However, measured at 1 year, 75% of patients receiving combined treatment had remitted, compared with only 12.5% of patients with antidepressant monotherapy (Maina et al. 2007). These patients then halved their relapse rate over a 4-year period following treatment discontinuation (46.9% vs. 27.5%) (Maina et al. 2009). Taken together, the research suggests that evidence-based psychotherapy administered in conjunction with pharmacotherapy in the acute phase of treatment is one helpful approach to reducing later risk of depressive relapse.

Although combined treatment appears to improve remission rates, combined treatment is not recommended as a first-line approach for all patients with depression. Both pharmacotherapy and mainstream psychotherapies are modestly effective for depression as monotherapy, and the benefits of combined treatment are modest themselves. Given the high prevalence rates of depression, providing combined treatment for all cases of depression would burden the current health care system. Consequently, monotherapy is recommended for treatment-naive depressed patients and patients with milder forms of depression. Given the potent role of patient preference in shaping treatment outcomes (Kocsis et al. 2009), patient preference should be a major factor in treatment selection. The prognostic importance of patient expectations also suggests that a strong preference for combined treatment would be sufficient reason to provide combined treatment.

TABLE 35–4. Specific populations for whom combined treatment of depression is recommended

Patients with severe depression
Patients with chronic depression
Patients at high risk of depressive relapse
Patients with a history of trauma
Patients with comorbid personality disorders
Patients with dysfunctional attitudes about treatment or illness

Current guidelines (American Psychiatric Association 2009) suggest that combined approaches to the treatment of depression are most efficiently applied to specific populations (Table 35–4). Patients at high risk of relapse—including patients with a history of relapse, patients with residual depressive symptoms after antidepressant treatment, and patients with other complicating and confounding factors—are prime candidates for combined treatment.

More severe depression is optimally treated with a combination of pharmacotherapy and psychotherapy. In a large study of IPT added to medications (Thase et al. 1997), remission rates were improved by about 15% with combined treatment, with more pronounced benefit for patients with more severe depression. Combined approaches may also lead to faster remission when coadministering IPT for severe depression (Zobel et al. 2011) or the cognitive-behavioral analysis system of psychotherapy (CBASP) for double depression (Manber et al. 2008). As with less severe depression, combined approaches may also produce higher rates of sustained remission, with one prospective, naturalistic study showing a 28% sustained remission rate at 5 years, compared with 11% sustained remission for patients receiving antidepressant monotherapy (Zobel et al. 2011).

Early adversity indicates poor prognosis with pharmacotherapy alone. Although one important study demonstrated a substantial benefit for combined treatment with IPT over antidepressants alone (Zobel et al. 2011), that study did not have a psychotherapy-only arm, so it was not possible to draw conclusions about whether combined treatment was superior to psychotherapy alone for this population. An earlier study (Nemeroff et al. 2003) similarly found that combined treatment with CBASP was superior to pharmacotherapy alone but not superior to CBASP alone. As in previous examples, however, there is evidence that even if combined treatment does not yield superior results in the acute phase of depression treatment, lasting benefits may occur; for example, one study showed that a combination of pharmacotherapy and mindfulness-based cognitive therapy appeared to protect against recurrence of depression in patients with a history of childhood trauma (Williams et al. 2014).

Multiple lines of evidence suggest poorer antidepressant outcomes in patients with comorbid personality disorders (Grilo et al. 2010; Gunderson et al. 2004; Skodol et al. 2011). CBT, IPT, and psychodynamic treatments have all been shown to improve outcomes in this population when used in conjunction with pharmacotherapy. When short-term dynamic supportive therapy was added to antidepressants in patients with underlying personality disorder, remission rates increased 2.5-fold, from 19% to 47% (Kool et al. 2003). IPT added to medications produced superior results after 32 weeks

(Bozzatello and Bellino 2016). Patients responding to combined treatment with CBT had much lower relapse rates than patients receiving only medications (Fournier et al. 2008).

Beyond Symptom Reduction

Combined treatment compared with antidepressant monotherapy offers benefits beyond symptom reduction. Meta-analyses suggest that the addition of psychotherapy to pharmacotherapy appears to improve quality of life, even in the absence of measurable reduction in depressive symptoms (von Wolff et al. 2012). If psychiatric prescribers are to think of themselves as mental health providers and not just mental illness providers (Mintz and Flynn 2012), a patient-centered approach requires consideration of not only symptoms but also the patient's general level of functioning and overall developmental aims. Certainly, this is also important to patients, who appear to prioritize quality of life and functional outcomes over symptom reduction (IsHak et al. 2011; McKnight and Kashdan 2009; Zimmerman et al. 2006).

Combined treatment of depression with short psychodynamic supportive psychotherapy, in addition to reducing symptoms more than antidepressant treatment alone, produced significant functional improvements (Molenaar et al. 2007). CBT added to medications for patients with residual depression led to improved relationships with self (e.g., less guilt and hopelessness, better self-esteem) and with others (less friction and dependency, improved interpersonal behavior) (Scott et al. 2000). Similarly, IPT may be combined with medications for depression. As a whole, the evidence supports the proposition that both medications and psychotherapy improve quality of life for depressed patients, but the combination of the two produces more substantial benefits, as was demonstrated in a meta-analysis of 153 outcome studies involving a total of 29,879 patients (Kamenov et al. 2017).

Not surprisingly, these results seem to be more robust in patients with personality disorders, for whom functional impairments are often more pronounced than specific symptoms. IPT in combination with medications in patients with depression and personality disorder produced enduring benefits for impulsivity and relationships (Bellino et al. 2006; Bozzatello and Bellino 2016).

Although functional outcomes with combined treatment of depression have been a particular focus of research, long-term functional outcomes are improved in other conditions when psychotherapy is added to medications. Even in conditions for which cognitive-behavioral approaches are recommended for symptom reduction, such as obsessive-compulsive disorder, when dynamic therapy was added to clomipramine, patients demonstrated better occupational adjustment, improved global functioning, and reduced rates of hospitalization (Burnand et al. 2002).

New Directions in the Combination of Psychotherapy and Pharmacotherapy

After nearly 50 years during which most research with psychedelic medications was prohibited, a resurgence in interest in and research on these medications has occurred in the past decade. In particular, 3,4-methylenedioxymethamphetamine (MDMA), psilocybin, and lysergic acid diethylamide (LSD) have been investigated for their therapeutic properties, and MDMA and psilocybin have been designated by the FDA as *breakthrough therapies* for PTSD and treatment-resistant depression, respectively, easing the way for further research. Benefits for classical psychedelics have also been found for some conditions, including substance use disorders and anxiety related to terminal illness (Johnson et al. 2019). According to Google Scholar (https://scholar.google.com, accessed October 10, 2020), in the 5-year period from 2016 to 2020, more than 3,000 articles were published that were identified under the search terms *psychedelic* and *psychotherapy*.

Research suggests that the combination of psychotherapy and psychedelic treatment is important for achieving optimal therapeutic benefit from psychedelic medications, with a higher incidence of adverse outcomes experienced when these medications are used in nonclinical settings and in the absence of psychotherapy (Reiff et al. 2020). Psychedelic-assisted psychotherapy appears to offer potentially lasting benefits with a relatively small number of treatments (two to three sessions of psychedelic-assisted psychotherapy as well as several preparatory and integrative sessions without psychedelics).

Although it is not yet clear how, precisely, psychedelics amplify gains in psychotherapy, it is known that these substances produce lasting personality changes, such as openness to new experiences (Erritzoe et al. 2018), that may promote learning in psychotherapy. Psychedelic experiences appear to enhance access to autobiographical memory (Carhart-Harris et al. 2012). Mystical experiences also appear to be associated with more significant gains in psychedelic-assisted psychotherapy (Roseman et al. 2018). It is intriguing to speculate that psychedelic-assisted psychotherapy may be one avenue by which psychotherapy becomes reestablished more squarely within the clinical practice of psychiatry.

Combined Treatment: Modes of Interaction

Pharmacotherapy and psychotherapy can have either antagonistic or synergistic interactions, either interfering with or enhancing each other's efficacy.

Antagonistic Effects

Old psychoanalytic concerns that pharmacotherapy undercuts motivation and learning, lessening lasting benefits of deeper and more meaningful treatment, have generally not borne out. One important exception appears to be the antagonistic effects that benzodiazepines show in relation to exposure therapies. Although some initial benefits of combined treatment may occur with regard to symptom reduction, the long-term course suggests that patients treated concurrently with benzodiazepines have worse outcomes than patients treated with CBT alone (Başoğlu et al. 1994; Marks et al. 1993).

Antagonism may also emerge from the level of meaning. Such may be the case when the patient uses one treatment to devalue the other (e.g., holding that one treatment is real and the other is unimportant). Similarly, the meaning of treatment may be wielded defensively, which might occur when patients equate biological treatment with a biogenic theory of illness and conclude that they cannot be held responsible for their own recovery in therapy. Generally, when such resistances to optimal treatment emerge from the level of meaning, they are best addressed at the level of meaning (Mintz 2022; Mintz and Belnap 2006, 2011; Mintz and Flynn 2012).

Additive Effects

The combination of pharmacotherapy and psychotherapy may derive potency from combining distinct biological and psychological effects, addressing different aspects of symptomology. For example, in depression, pharmacotherapy may target more neurovegetative aspects of illness, whereas psychotherapy targets depressogenic thoughts and interpersonal issues that perpetuate depression. Neuroimaging in part supports this hypothesis. Antidepressants seem to work in a bottom-up fashion, with effects spreading upward from the lower brain, whereas meaning-induced changes in brain function move in a top-down manner, spreading from cortical areas into deeper brain structures (Mayberg et al. 2002).

Synergies

Pharmacotherapy and psychotherapy may also work synergistically, with one modality supporting or amplifying the effectiveness of the other. These synergies may move in either direction, from medications to psychotherapy or vice versa.

Medications may directly prime the brain for new learning in psychotherapy by enhancing neural plasticity. Antidepressants, for example, increase hippocampal brain-derived neurotrophic factor (BDNF) (Chen et al. 2001) and neurogenesis (Castrén 2004; Castrén and Rantamäki 2010), potentially facilitating new learning in psychotherapy. Recently, Hutten et al. (2020) proposed that an increase in BDNF and increased neural plasticity are one mechanism by which psychedelic-assisted psychotherapy exerts such long-term effects.

Psychological effects of medications may also support a patient's ability to engage effectively in psychotherapy. Pharmacotherapy may improve impaired cognition, for example, when effectively used in the treatment of depression or anxiety (Wright 2004) or psychotic illnesses. Antidepressants appear to enhance emotional processing of positive information, such as what might be experienced in psychotherapy (Wells et al. 2014). Medications that decrease autonomic reactivity may increase fear extinction in response to exposure to anxiogenic internal or external stimuli. Similarly, medications may decrease arousal states, allowing patients (particularly patients with affective dysregulation) to more effectively mentalize and make better use of psychotherapy (Gabbard 2005).

Likewise, psychotherapy may enhance a patient's capacity to make healthy use of medications in a number of ways. Combined treatment appears to contribute to increased adherence to medications (Gabbard and Kay 2001) and therefore may be recommended as a first-line approach in patients for whom problems with medication adherence are anticipated. Patients participating in research trials of psychiatric medications drop out at much lower rates when they receive concurrent psychotherapy (Manber et al. 2008; Pampallona et al. 2004). When medications are a nonpreferred treatment, combined treatments may support adherence by ensuring that patients receive their preferred intervention (at the cost of receiving the nonpreferred intervention) (Swift et al. 2017).

Psychotherapy can also support pharmacotherapy when used to address dysfunctional attitudes toward medications (Shankman et al. 2013) or negative transferences that adversely affect healthy use of medications (Mintz 2022; Mintz and Belnap 2006; Mintz and Flynn 2012). Concurrent psychotherapy, through the effort to find meaning in illness, may also counter a semiotic pull toward reductionistic biogenic explanations of illness, such as what may be implied with unimodal treatment with pharmacotherapy. Biogenic theories of illness, although enhancing acceptance of pharmacotherapy (Pescosolido et al. 2010) and sometimes reducing self-blame (Deacon and Baird 2009; Kvaale et al. 2013), also appear to risk worsening outcomes with pharmacotherapy (Sullivan et al. 2003). In one study, depressed college students were randomly assigned to a situation in which, after a mock genetic test, they were informed that their depression was either biological or nonbiological in nature (Kemp et al. 2014). Patients experiencing their depression as biological exhibited higher levels of prognostic pessimism and negative mood regulation expectancies. Concurrent psychotherapy can counter such negative effects on agency and self-efficacy by highlighting the role of patients' agency (and blocks to experiencing it) in their own recovery.

Treatment Integration

Treatments may be integrated at many different levels. Note that combining treatments does not necessarily make them integrated. Combination and integration are independent dimensions (Figure 35–1).

Unintegrated Care

A split treatment may be unintegrated when the prescriber and psychotherapist each has their own treatment plans and targets, with little or no coordination. In a worst-case scenario, such approaches may even be in opposition (Busch and Gould 1993; Gould and Busch 1998), such as when the therapist is working to allow the patient to mobilize and release affect while the prescriber is aiming to help the patient suppress affect. When goals of treatment are in conflict, the prospects for successful treatment are dimmed.

Psychotherapy and psychopharmacology by a single provider may also be poorly integrated if the provider has dual approaches that are largely divorced. The therapy may address developmental goals while the pharmacotherapy remains disease focused or symptom focused, with little reference to the larger psychotherapeutic goals.

It is not unusual for a mind-body split to be manifested in the structure of the treatment frame, such as when the treatment hour is divided starkly into a psychotherapy portion and a pharmacotherapy portion, both reflecting and facilitating a split in the work. Recent innovations in psychiatric coding that account for the minutes devoted to each task may further contribute to the impulse to divide the appointment into distinct parts. Optimally, statements about medications made in the context of a combined treatment will be heard by the therapist-prescriber as carrying important, but

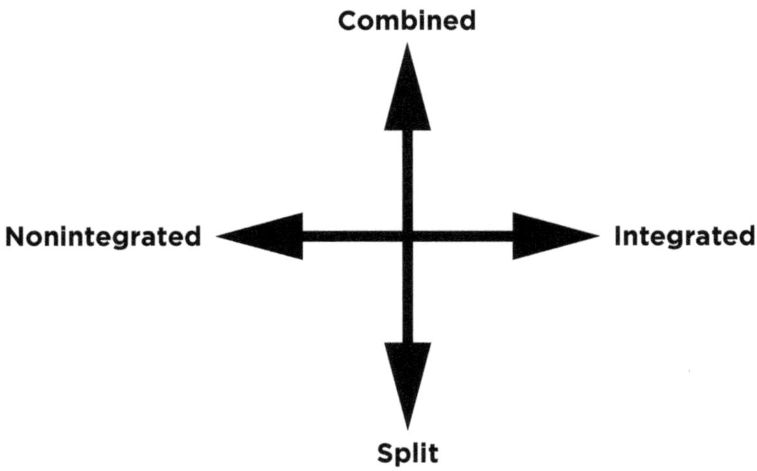

FIGURE 35–1. Combined, split, and integrated treatment.

possibly obscure, meanings, addressing deeper concerns about the self and the transference to the therapist-prescriber.

Truly Integrating Pharmacotherapy and Psychotherapy

An integrated treatment frame optimally includes awareness of the role played by the other treatment and a concordance of goals. In highly integrated approaches, intentional synergies are incorporated into the treatment frame (Mintz 2022; Mintz and Belnap 2006; Mintz and Flynn 2012), with a focus on the triadic alliance (Kahn 1991). For example, the prescriber explicitly states as a goal that pharmacotherapy should optimize a patient's ability to engage in and use psychotherapy. In turn, if the patient does not adhere to the prescribed regimen, the therapist is in a position to experience medication nonadherence as a therapy-interfering behavior and to engage the patient from that position. Thus, just as the pharmacotherapist supports the therapist's work, the psychotherapist directly support the pharmacotherapist's work. This highly integrated approach works best in the context of established treatment teams.

Technical Issues in Combining Treatments When There Are Two or More Clinicians

Apart from broader issues of when to combine treatments and what treatments to combine, issues of how to combine treatments also exist.

Task, Role, and Boundaries

When two or more clinicians are providing mental health care, having a shared understanding of both the distinct and shared responsibilities of the two roles is useful. Clearly delineated distinctions between roles can prevent conflict and confusion at the boundaries between roles. However, sharp and exclusive role distinctions often do not reflect the clinical complexity at the border between meaning and medication. Complicated issues risk falling into the gap between the two roles (Mintz 2019, 2022). Particularly when medications have developed pathogenic meanings to the patient (e.g., I am defective or helpless) or are used in countertherapeutic and defensive ways (Mintz and Belnap 2006), avoidance of boundary tensions in split treatments may leave important issues unaddressed, contributing to chronicity (Mintz 2022).

In one case, for example, a young woman with borderline tendencies has been prescribed a sedating antipsychotic, which she uses regularly to manage episodes of emotional dysregulation. The psychotherapist occasionally wonders whether this is interfering with her development of other coping skills but is reluctant to suggest that the patient might benefit from using less medication for fear of impinging on the psychiatrist's role. In consequence, the patient becomes progressively emotionally deskilled. In another case, the psychiatrist feels that the patient may be using a defensively biologized understanding of illness (i.e., "I am not responsible for my interpersonally destructive behavior because I have a mental illness"). At times the psychiatrist wants to interpret the patient's defensive interpretation of psychiatric treatment but refrains because of concerns that this would encroach on the psychotherapist's role. The therapist avoids the topic out of a similar concern, and the patient's defensive use of treatment goes unaddressed.

In cases in which one treater feels that it is clinically important to make an intervention that potentially encroaches on the role of the other clinician, the meaning of this impulse should be considered before acting (Busch and Sandberg 2014). Are there underlying motives besides good clinical care, such as competitiveness or mistrust? Has the patient induced such feelings? Are there ways that the clinicians have been induced to enact some conflictual aspect of the patient's history or internal world? Such impulses also suggest opportunities for treatment integration that can improve clinical care.

Communication in Combined Treatment

A central issue to the competent provision of combined treatment is communication between treaters. Communication serves to promote a triadic alliance, ensures that the approaches are concordant (or, if they are not, provides opportunities to work through the meaning of discordances), provides an avenue for addressing treatment-interfering dynamics in the patients and providers, and mitigates risk when there are concerns about a patient. Nonetheless, in practice, communication between treaters is often suboptimal (Gitlin and Miklowitz 2016; Hansen-Grant and Riba 1995). Time pressures are a major impediment to communication in split treatments. For the sake of efficiency, communication need not be frequent, but having an idea of when communication is necessary is important.

In beginning a new treatment, working toward a shared understanding of the trouble and goals of treatment is useful, although therapist and prescriber may address different aspects of the patient's trouble. If the psychotherapist and pharmacotherapist do not have an established working relationship, negotiating treatment boundaries (e.g., Who holds primary responsibility in a crisis? Is it acceptable for the prescriber to make psychotherapeutic interventions relevant to the patient's use of medication?) is also useful. Whenever possible, consent allowing treaters to communicate should be obtained at the outset of combined treatment. A crisis in the treatment (because of either symptomatic decompensation or splitting) is not the time to be trying to negotiate such consent.

In ongoing treatment, certain situations call for communication between treaters (Table 35–5). When important clinical concerns emerge or notable changes in the patient's clinical presentation are present, communication between treaters can provide context, ensure concordance and collaboration, and decrease risk, both clinically and medicolegally. Similarly, when one treater makes a major revision in the understanding of the patient's difficulties (changes in diagnosis or important changes in the formulation), communication between treaters helps maintain concordance in treatment approaches. When there appear to be important disagreements between treaters, communication between psychotherapist and pharmacotherapist is crucial. When treaters are working at cross-purposes, patients are unlikely to benefit substantially from combined treatment.

Addressing Splitting in Split Treatments

Discordance may be real or illusory, seen through the filter of the patient who offers distorted reports of the work of one clinician to the other. Patients who rely on splitting as a primary defense mechanism will experience treaters in distorted ways that conform to stark impressions of clinicians as either good/helpful/understanding or bad/dangerous/authoritarian. Then, when they characterize the work of one treater to the other, this will often be done in a way that casts suspicion on the work of one treater, who may be seen as dangerous, domineering, neglectful, blinded, or overly protective and infantilizing. When the patient complains directly about the work of one treater to another or more indirectly raises suspicions about the other treater's work, addressing this with the other treater is especially important to avoid getting caught up in a splitting dynamic. Unless other evidence casts doubt on the work of the other treater, it is best to remain curious about whether the conflict experienced with the other treater is real or is a product of the patient's defensively distorted perceptions.

Such patients may respond to treaters as either helpful or persecutory in ways that induce corresponding behaviors and attitudes, leading to actual splitting in the treatment team. Although it may serve the patient's defensive needs to have treaters pitted against each other, the patient is unlikely to get better in this context. Treaters may gain some perspective by understanding how they may be enacting roles projected onto them from the patient's inner world and/or reflecting an aspect of the patient's history (Kayatekin and Plakun 2011). Sometimes it is helpful for the psychotherapist and pharmacotherapist to meet together with the patient when splitting is recognized but remains disruptive. At times, treaters in conflict may seek to detoxify their relationship by blaming the patient, in essence putting all of the badness back into and onto the patient. This, however, often misses the fact that the patient's splitting was unconscious rather than intentional. An understanding of the underlying dynamics may help preserve a modicum of empathy for the patient's plight (Treloar 2009). When treaters are unable to integrate a pronounced split, frequently, a consultation by a third party is needed to help establish distance and heal the split (Muller 2011) to avoid fostering treatment resistance.

TABLE 35–5. Situations requiring communication between treaters

Major clinical concerns
Major revision in the understanding of the patient's difficulties
Significant changes in the treatment plan that have the potential to affect the other clinician's work
Disagreement between treaters
Patient complaints about one clinician to the other

Conclusion

With the severe burden of illness imposed by common psychiatric conditions and frequently incomplete results with either pharmacotherapy or psychotherapy, combined treatment with medications and pharmacotherapy remains an important tool in our armamentarium. For many of the most common and burdensome psychiatric conditions, combined treatment with psychotherapy and pharmacotherapy has effect sizes greater than treatment with either modality alone. Benefits of combined treatment are often particularly pronounced in the context of more severe illness, psychiatric chronicity, and complex comorbidities. Inadequate response to a single modality is another possible indication for combined treatment, as is treatment nonresponse related to medication nonadherence, given that combined treatment is correlated with improved medication adherence.

In addition to benefits for the treatment of acute psychiatric episodes, combined treatment may support longer-term recovery in the maintenance phase, with lower long-term rates of symptomatic relapse. Further benefits of combined treatment include additive effects; for example, medications address neurovegetative symptoms of depression, whereas psychotherapy promotes improved affective coping, better interpersonal functioning, and an enhanced sense of personal agency, with improved quality of life protecting against subsequent relapse.

Although combining treatment modalities (and different treaters) generally promotes effectiveness, doing so introduces a potential for covert conflict between modalities, requiring greater attention to integration of care. Integrative efforts may be particularly important when patients rely on primitive defenses, unconsciously driving splits in the treatment team or using one modality as a defense against the other. When medications (or their meanings) serve defensive ends, there is a risk that this may go unexplored and unaddressed if the prescriber and psychotherapist both avoid exploring the meaning of medication out of a concern that to do so would encroach on the domain of the other treater. Periodic communication between treaters in such situations is essential.

Key Points

- Combined pharmacotherapy-psychotherapy is often more effective than either modality alone.
- Potential benefits of combined treatment include improved acute treatment response and decreased risk of relapse.
- Addition of psychotherapy to pharmacotherapy may confer additional benefits, such as improved relationship to self and other, better interpersonal functioning, and overall improved quality of life.
- Effects of combined psychotherapy and pharmacotherapy are particularly pronounced in severe illness, chronic and treatment-refractory psychiatric conditions, complex comorbidities, and conditions for which medication adherence is crucial.
- In some situations, pharmacotherapy or psychotherapy may lessen the effect of the other treatment, including when benzodiazepines are used in the context of exposure therapies or when patients use one treatment to devalue the other treatment.
- Providers should be attentive to those situations where treatments are potentially in conflict and should maintain communication in such situations to enhance treatment integration.

References

American Psychiatric Association: Practice guideline for the treatment of patients with panic disorder. Work Group on Panic Disorder. American Psychiatric Association. Am J Psychiatry 155(5 suppl):1–34, 1998 9585731

American Psychiatric Association: Practice guideline for the treatment of patients with borderline personality disorder. American Psychiatric Association. Am J Psychiatry 158(10 suppl):1–52, 2001 11665545

American Psychiatric Association: Practice Guideline for the Treatment of Patients With Substance Use Disorders, 2nd Edition. Washington, DC, American Psychiatric Association, 2007a

American Psychiatric Association: Practice Guideline for the Treatment of Patients With Eating Disorders, 3rd Edition. Washington, DC, American Psychiatric Association, 2007b

American Psychiatric Association: Practice Guideline for the Treatment of Patients With Major Depressive Disorder, 3rd Edition. Washington, DC, American Psychiatric Association, 2009

American Psychiatric Association: Practice Guideline for the Treatment of Patients With Bipolar Disorder, 2nd Edition. Washington, DC, American Psychiatric Association, 2010

American Psychiatric Association: The American Psychiatric Association Practice Guideline for the Treatment of Patients With Schizophrenia, 3rd Edition. Washington, DC, American Psychiatric Association, 2021

Başoğlu M, Marks IM, Kiliç C, et al: Alprazolam and exposure for panic disorder with agoraphobia: attribution of improvement to medication predicts subsequent relapse. Br J Psychiatry 164(5):652–659, 1994 7921716

Bellino S, Zizza M, Rinaldi C, Bogetto F: Combined treatment of major depression in patients with borderline personality disorder: a comparison with pharmacotherapy. Can J Psychiatry 51(7):453–460, 2006 16838827

Blackburn IM, Eunson KM, Bishop S: A two-year naturalistic follow-up of depressed patients treated with cognitive therapy, pharmacotherapy and a combination of both. J Affect Disord 10(1):67–75, 1986 2939125
Blom MB, Jonker K, Dusseldorp E, et al: Combination treatment for acute depression is superior only when psychotherapy is added to medication. Psychother Psychosom 76(5):289–297, 2007 17700049
Bozzatello P, Bellino S: Combined therapy with interpersonal psychotherapy adapted for borderline personality disorder: a two-years follow-up. Psychiatry Res 240:151–156, 2016 27107668
Burnand Y, Andreoli A, Kolatte E, et al: Psychodynamic psychotherapy and clomipramine in the treatment of major depression. Psychiatr Serv 53(5):585–590, 2002 11986508
Busch FN, Gould E: Treatment by a psychotherapist and a psychopharmacologist: transference and countertransference issues. Hosp Community Psychiatry 44(8):772–774, 1993 8375839
Busch FN, Sandberg LS: Psychotherapy and Medication: The Challenge of Integration. New York, Routledge, 2014
Carhart-Harris RL, Leech R, Williams TM, et al: Implications for psychedelic-assisted psychotherapy: functional magnetic resonance imaging study with psilocybin. Br J Psychiatry 200(3):238–244, 2012 22282432
Castrén E: Neurotrophic effects of antidepressant drugs. Curr Opin Pharmacol 4(1):58–64, 2004 15018840
Castrén E, Rantamäki T: The role of BDNF and its receptors in depression and antidepressant drug action: reactivation of developmental plasticity. Dev Neurobiol 70(5):289–297, 2010 20186711
Chen B, Dowlatshahi D, MacQueen GM, et al: Increased hippocampal BDNF immunoreactivity in subjects treated with antidepressant medication. Biol Psychiatry 50(4):260–265, 2001 11522260
Cuijpers P, Dekker J, Hollon SD, et al: Adding psychotherapy to pharmacotherapy in the treatment of depressive disorders in adults: a meta-analysis. J Clin Psychiatry 70(9):1219–1229, 2009 19818243
Cuijpers P, Geraedts AS, van Oppen P, et al: Interpersonal psychotherapy for depression: a meta-analysis. Am J Psychiatry 168(6):581–592, 2011 21362740
Cuijpers P, Reynolds CF III, Donker T, et al: Personalized treatment of adult depression: medication, psychotherapy, or both? A systematic review. Depress Anxiety 29(10):855–864, 2012 22815247
Cuijpers P, Sijbrandij M, Koole SL, et al: Adding psychotherapy to antidepressant medication in depression and anxiety disorders: a meta-analysis. World Psychiatry 13(1):56–67, 2014 24497254
Cuijpers P, De Wit L, Weitz E, et al: The combination of psychotherapy and pharmacotherapy in the treatment of adult depression: a comprehensive meta-analysis. J Evid Based Psychother 15:147–168, 2015
Deacon BJ, Baird GL: The chemical imbalance explanation of depression: reducing blame at what cost? J Soc Clin Psychol 28(4):415–435, 2009
de Jonghe F, Kool S, van Aalst G, et al: Combining psychotherapy and antidepressants in the treatment of depression. J Affect Disord 64(2–3):217–229, 2001 11313088
Erritzoe D, Roseman L, Nour MM, et al: Effects of psilocybin therapy on personality structure. Acta Psychiatr Scand 138(5):368–378, 2018 29923178
Evans MD, Hollon SD, DeRubeis RJ, et al: Differential relapse following cognitive therapy and pharmacotherapy for depression. Arch Gen Psychiatry 49(10):802–808, 1992 1417433
Fournier JC, DeRubeis RJ, Shelton RC, et al: Antidepressant medications v. cognitive therapy in people with depression with or without personality disorder. Br J Psychiatry 192(2):124–129, 2008 18245030
Gabbard GO: Psychodynamic psychiatry in the "Decade of the Brain." Am J Psychiatry 149(8):991–998, 1992 1353321
Gabbard GO: Mind, brain, and personality disorders. Am J Psychiatry 162(4):648–655, 2005 15800133

Gabbard GO, Kay J: The fate of integrated treatment: whatever happened to the biopsychosocial psychiatrist? Am J Psychiatry 158(12):1956–1963, 2001 11729008

Gitlin MJ, Miklowitz DJ: Split treatment: recommendations for optimal use in the care of psychiatric patients. Ann Clin Psychiatry 28(2):132–137, 2016 27285393

Gould E, Busch FN: Therapeutic triangles: some complex clinical issues. Psychoanal Inq 18(5):730–745, 1998

Grilo CM, Stout RL, Markowitz JC, et al: Personality disorders predict relapse after remission from an episode of major depressive disorder: a 6-year prospective study. J Clin Psychiatry 71(12):1629–1635, 2010 20584514

Guidi J, Tomba E, Fava GA: The sequential integration of pharmacotherapy and psychotherapy in the treatment of major depressive disorder: a meta-analysis of the sequential model and a critical review of the literature. Am J Psychiatry 173(2):128–137, 2016 26481173

Gunderson JG, Morey LC, Stout RL, et al: Major depressive disorder and borderline personality disorder revisited: longitudinal interactions. J Clin Psychiatry 65(8):1049–1056, 2004 15323588

Hansen-Grant S, Riba MB: Contact between psychotherapists and psychiatric residents who provide medication backup. Psychiatr Serv 46(8):774–777, 1995 7583476

Hutten NRPW, Mason NL, Dolder PC, et al: Low doses of LSD acutely increase BDNF blood plasma levels in healthy volunteers. ACS Pharmacol Transl Sci 4(2):461–466, 2020 33860175

Insel TR: Disruptive insights in psychiatry: transforming a clinical discipline. J Clin Invest 119(4):700–705, 2009 19339761

IsHak WW, Greenberg JM, Balayan K, et al: Quality of life: the ultimate outcome measure of interventions in major depressive disorder. Harv Rev Psychiatry 19(5):229–239, 2011 21916825

Johnson MW, Hendricks PS, Barrett FS, et al: Classic psychedelics: an integrative review of epidemiology, therapeutics, mystical experience, and brain network function. Pharmacol Ther 197:83–102, 2019 30521880

Kahn DA: Medication consultation and split treatment during psychotherapy. J Am Acad Psychoanal 19(1):84–98, 1991 1676395

Kamenov K, Twomey C, Cabello M, et al: The efficacy of psychotherapy, pharmacotherapy and their combination on functioning and quality of life in depression: a meta-analysis. Psychol Med 47(3):414–425, 2017 27780478

Karyotaki E, Smit Y, Holdt Henningsen K, et al: Combining pharmacotherapy and psychotherapy or monotherapy for major depression? A meta-analysis on the long-term effects. J Affect Disord 194:144–152, 2016 26826534

Kayatekin S, Plakun EM: From acting out to enactment in treatment-resistant disorders, in Treatment Resistance and Patient Authority: The Austen Riggs Reader. Edited by Plakun EM. New York, WW Norton, 2011, pp 24–41

Kemp JJ, Lickel JJ, Deacon BJ: Effects of a chemical imbalance causal explanation on individuals' perceptions of their depressive symptoms. Behav Res Ther 56:47–52, 2014 24657311

Kocsis JH, Leon AC, Markowitz JC, et al: Patient preference as a moderator of outcome for chronic forms of major depressive disorder treated with nefazodone, cognitive behavioral analysis system of psychotherapy, or their combination. J Clin Psychiatry 70(3):354–361, 2009 19192474

Kool S, Dekker J, Duijsens IJ, et al: Efficacy of combined therapy and pharmacotherapy for depressed patients with or without personality disorders. Harv Rev Psychiatry 11(3):133–141, 2003 12893503

Koran LM, Hanna GL, Hollander E, et al: Practice guideline for the treatment of patients with obsessive-compulsive disorder. Am J Psychiatry 164(7 suppl):5–53, 2007 17849776

Kvaale EP, Haslam N, Gottdiener WH: The "side effects" of medicalization: a meta-analytic review of how biogenetic explanations affect stigma. Clin Psychol Rev 33(6):782–794, 2013 23831861

Maina G, Rosso G, Crespi C, et al: Combined brief dynamic therapy and pharmacotherapy in the treatment of major depressive disorder: a pilot study. Psychother Psychosom 76(5):298–305, 2007 17700050

Maina G, Rosso G, Bogetto F: Brief dynamic therapy combined with pharmacotherapy in the treatment of major depressive disorder: long-term results. J Affect Disord 114(1–3):200–207, 2009 18728001
Manber R, Kraemer HC, Arnow BA, et al: Faster remission of chronic depression with combined psychotherapy and medication than with each therapy alone. J Consult Clin Psychol 76(3):459–467, 2008 18540739
Marks IM, Swinson RP, Başoğlu M, et al: Alprazolam and exposure alone and combined in panic disorder with agoraphobia: a controlled study in London and Toronto. Br J Psychiatry 162:776–787, 1993 8101126
Mayberg HS, Silva JA, Brannan SK, et al: The functional neuroanatomy of the placebo effect. Am J Psychiatry 159(5):728–737, 2002 11986125
McKnight PE, Kashdan TB: The importance of functional impairment to mental health outcomes: a case for reassessing our goals in depression treatment research. Clin Psychol Rev 29(3):243–259, 2009 19269076
Mintz D: Recovery from childhood psychiatric treatment: addressing the meaning of medications. Psychodyn Psychiatry 47(3):235–256, 2019 31448987
Mintz D: Psychodynamic Psychopharmacology: Caring for the Treatment-Resistant Patient. Washington DC, American Psychiatric Association Publishing, 2022
Mintz D, Belnap B: A view from Riggs: treatment resistance and patient authority: III. What is psychodynamic psychopharmacology? An approach to pharmacologic treatment resistance. J Am Acad Psychoanal Dyn Psychiatry 34(4):581–601, 2006 17274730
Mintz D, Belnap BA: What is psychodynamic psychopharmacology? An approach to pharmacological treatment resistance, in Treatment Resistance and Patient Authority: The Austen Riggs Reader. Edited by Plakun EM. New York, WW Norton, 2011, pp 42–65
Mintz DL, Flynn DF: How (not what) to prescribe: nonpharmacologic aspects of psychopharmacology. Psychiatr Clin North Am 35(1):143–163, 2012 22370496
Molenaar PJ, Dekker J, Van R, et al: Does adding psychotherapy to pharmacotherapy improve social functioning in the treatment of outpatient depression? Depress Anxiety 24(8):553–562, 2007 17131302
Muller J: Why the pair needs the third, in Treatment Resistance and Patient Authority: The Austen Riggs Reader. Edited by Plakun EM. New York, WW Norton, 2011, pp 97–120
Nemeroff CB, Heim CM, Thase ME, et al: Differential responses to psychotherapy versus pharmacotherapy in patients with chronic forms of major depression and childhood trauma. Proc Natl Acad Sci USA 100(24):14293–14296, 2003 14615578
Oestergaard S, Møldrup C: Improving outcomes for patients with depression by enhancing antidepressant therapy with non-pharmacological interventions: a systematic review of reviews. Public Health 125(6):357–367, 2011 21600619
Pampallona S, Bollini P, Tibaldi G, et al: Combined pharmacotherapy and psychological treatment for depression: a systematic review. Arch Gen Psychiatry 61(7):714–719, 2004 15237083
Pescosolido BA, Martin JK, Long JS, et al: "A disease like any other"? A decade of change in public reactions to schizophrenia, depression, and alcohol dependence. Am J Psychiatry 167(11):1321–1330, 2010 20843872
Reiff CM, Richman EE, Nemeroff CB, et al: Psychedelics and psychedelic-assisted psychotherapy. Am J Psychiatry 177(5):391–410, 2020 32098487
Roseman L, Nutt DJ, Carhart-Harris RL: Quality of acute psychedelic experience predicts therapeutic efficacy of psilocybin for treatment-resistant depression. Front Pharmacol 8:974, 2018 29387009
Schramm E, van Calker D, Dykierek P, et al: An intensive treatment program of interpersonal psychotherapy plus pharmacotherapy for depressed inpatients: acute and long-term results. Am J Psychiatry 164(5):768–777, 2007 17475736
Scott J, Teasdale JD, Paykel ES, et al: Effects of cognitive therapy on psychological symptoms and social functioning in residual depression. Br J Psychiatry 177:440–446, 2000 11059998
Seligman ME: The effectiveness of psychotherapy: the Consumer Reports study. Am Psychol 50(12):965–974, 1995 8561380

Shankman SA, Campbell ML, Klein DN, et al: Dysfunctional attitudes as a moderator of pharmacotherapy and psychotherapy for chronic depression. J Psychiatr Res 47(1):113–121, 2013 23102821

Simons AD, Murphy GE, Levine JL, Wetzel RD: Cognitive therapy and pharmacotherapy for depression: sustained improvement over one year. Arc Gen Psychiatry 43(1):43–48, 1986 3942473

Skodol AE, Grilo CM, Keyes KM, et al: Relationship of personality disorders to the course of major depressive disorder in a nationally representative sample. Am J Psychiatry 168(3):257–264, 2011 21245088

Sullivan MD, Katon WJ, Russo JE, et al: Patient beliefs predict response to paroxetine among primary care patients with dysthymia and minor depression. J Am Board Fam Pract 16(1):22–31, 2003 12583647

Swift JK, Greenberg RP, Tompkins KA, et al: Treatment refusal and premature termination in psychotherapy, pharmacotherapy, and their combination: a meta-analysis of head-to-head comparisons. Psychotherapy (Chic) 54(1):47–57, 2017 28263651

Thase ME, Greenhouse JB, Frank E, et al: Treatment of major depression with psychotherapy or psychotherapy-pharmacotherapy combinations. Arch Gen Psychiatry 54(11):1009–1015, 1997 9366657

Treloar AJC: Effectiveness of education programs in changing clinicians' attitudes toward treating borderline personality disorder. Psychiatr Serv 60(8):1128–1131, 2009 19648203

Ursano RJ, Bell C, Eth S, et al: Practice guideline for the treatment of patients with acute stress disorder and posttraumatic stress disorder. Am J Psychiatry 161(11 suppl):3–31, 2004 15617511

von Wolff A, Hölzel LP, Westphal A, et al: Combination of pharmacotherapy and psychotherapy in the treatment of chronic depression: a systematic review and meta-analysis. BMC Psychiatry 12:61, 2012 22694751

Wells TT, Clerkin EM, Ellis AJ, et al: Effect of antidepressant medication use on emotional information processing in major depression. Am J Psychiatry 171(2):195–200, 2014 24030200

Williams JMG, Crane C, Barnhofer T, et al: Mindfulness-based cognitive therapy for preventing relapse in recurrent depression: a randomized dismantling trial. J Consult Clin Psychol 82(2):275–286, 2014 24294837

Wright JH: Integrating cognitive-behavioral therapy and pharmacotherapy, in Contemporary Cognitive Therapy: Theory, Research, and Practice. Edited by Leahy RL. New York, Guilford, 2004, pp 341–366

Zimmerman M, McGlinchey JB, Posternak MA, et al: How should remission from depression be defined? The depressed patient's perspective. Am J Psychiatry 163(1):148–150, 2006 16390903

Zobel I, Kech S, van Calker D, et al: Long-term effect of combined interpersonal psychotherapy and pharmacotherapy in a randomized trial of depressed patients. Acta Psychiatr Scand 123(4):276–282, 2011 21231926

CHAPTER 36

Supervision and Consultation in Psychotherapy

Holly Crisp, M.D.
Glen O. Gabbard, M.D.

In mental health education, supervision has long been a primary way of conveying information to the next generation of therapists. Psychotherapy is both a skill and an art, and therapists in training must learn both practical tools and nuances of tone, affect, voice, timing, and insight. Psychotherapy supervision is a core practice that is integral to training and development as a psychotherapist. The work of therapy for therapists in training is inherently both dyadic and triadic—the dyad of patient and therapist in training is in the foreground, and the psychotherapy supervisor is generally in the background (Kantrowitz 2002).

The role of the supervisor is complex and multifaceted. The supervisor is responsible for teaching the fundamentals of psychotherapy to the supervisee and for helping the neophyte therapist manage challenges that arise. The supervisor provides a framework and education for the supervisee and also may serve as a mentor and professional role model. At the same time, supervisors are tasked with oversight of the trainee therapist's treatment of the patient and must be aware of their own role as the more experienced clinician involved in the patient's care. Moreover, in many educational programs, supervisors are responsible for the evaluation of the supervisee. It is imperative that supervisors know the context and environment in which they are serving as a supervisor, including expectations regarding the trainee's level of experience and the supervisor's evaluative function (De Golia 2019a). These multiple responsibilities require a complex, straightforward, and open attitude on the part of the supervisor.

An undeniable power differential exists between the supervisee and the supervisor. As a result, supervisors must balance their various roles, be cognizant of the trainee's transferences to those who are observing their work, and be aware of their responsibility with regard to the patient while avoiding dual relationships and maintaining clear boundaries (De Golia 2019a; Gabbard 2017). Effective supervisors are generally more democratic than autocratic in terms of their engagement with the supervisee (Gabbard 2017; Greben and Ruskin 1994). Supervisors must create a sense of safety for those being supervised so that supervisees can openly disclose their work in therapy and the two professionals can collaborate on the challenging task of becoming a skilled therapist.

Supervision may shift over time depending on the ability and training level of the supervisee. Beginning therapists may require more overt guidance from the supervisor on developing a professional relationship with the patient, setting up the frame of psychotherapy, and formulating the case in a complex manner that transcends a simple DSM diagnosis. As trainees progress in their psychotherapeutic education with didactic instruction, the psychotherapy supervision increases in depth, with discussions of ongoing cases and playing with different therapeutic interventions (Lomax et al. 2005). Over time the supervisor may become internalized as a background figure in the therapist's mind on whom the supervisee relies as a guide. Many supervisees find themselves "trying on" the words of *their* supervisors in sessions with their patients, to greater or lesser success. They may feel fraudulent or as if they are "playing supervisor" (Gabbard 2017). Over time and with practice, supervisees transform the internalized phrases or interventions modeled by the supervisor to fit their own style. All therapists learn the practice of psychotherapy by listening to and modeling the internalized therapists who have been their supervisors and teachers.

Tasks of Supervision

The tasks of supervision vary with different modalities of individual therapy, including, for example, psychodynamic psychotherapy (Binder and Strupp 1997; Cabaniss 2019; Gabbard 2017), supportive therapy (Welton and Rueve 2019), cognitive-behavioral therapy (Liese and Beck 1997; Sudak 2019; Sudak et al. 2015), and time-limited therapy (Levenson 2019). In the supervision of group therapy the supervisor provides education regarding group dynamics and how to intervene in the group setting, including establishing group norms, dealing with group conflict and scapegoating, and managing situations involving friction in which the group challenges the supervisee or a cotherapist (Malat 2019). In couple and family therapies, the supervisor is also tasked with guiding supervisees as they recognize family roles and developmental and cultural influences, understand systemic patterns, and apply a systemic model of change. These clinicians may help the supervisees navigate when they feel overidentified with one family member or too focused on being an individual therapist, rather than taking a systems view (Rait 2019a).

Supervisory Dyad

The supervisory alliance (Lomax et al. 2005) has much in common with the therapeutic alliance, and it must be developed and attended to as the supervisor and supervisee work together. As one would expect, there is a vulnerability inherent in the supervisory dyad similar to the vulnerability in the therapist-patient dyad (Gabbard 2017). Supervision is not mentorship or psychotherapy, although it may embody aspects of both while also having an evaluative component (De Golia 2019a). Supervisees are asked to disclose their clinical work and how they assess and intervene in the treatment of their patient. They are also asked to reveal in supervision their anxieties, fears, obstacles, self-doubts, and mistakes. Many of those disclosures place the supervisee in a vulnerable position vis-à-vis the supervisor, who is often responsible for writing an evaluation of the supervisee. It is often challenging for supervisees to bring these insecurities into this new educational setting, when for much of their lives as students they have tried to present themselves in the best possible light. This challenge is even greater if the supervisor behaves in a way that is critical, condescending, or dismissive. Hence, the challenge for the supervisor is to create safety and invite openness while also finding ways to make recommendations and to further the supervisee's insight without wounding the learner. The expectation for the supervisees, on the other hand, is to bring questions, problems, self-doubts, and successes to the supervision while also trying to avoid concealment of the very things that the supervisor could help them understand.

Boundaries in Supervision

Supervision is a fiduciary relationship, much like the therapeutic relationship. Education about boundaries, how to manage them, and how to avoid boundary violations is an important function of supervision. Two basic axioms can guide supervisees as they are navigating the boundaries with their patients and figuring out what to bring to their supervisors (Gabbard 1996, 2016, 2017):

1. If anything you are doing with a patient cannot be shared with a supervisor or consultant, you may be starting a dangerous descent down the slippery slope of boundary violations.
2. The thing that you most wish to avoid sharing in supervision is probably the most important issue to discuss with your supervisor.

In Chapter 32, "Professional Boundaries and Ethics in Psychotherapy," we provide an extensive discussion of boundaries in psychotherapy, so we will not repeat the same precepts here. Rather, we are simply underscoring the absolute necessity of bringing boundary concerns with a patient to one's supervisor. Boundary crossings can be addressed in supervision and with the patient before they become boundary violations. The supervisor can assist the supervisee in looking at the supervisee's countertransference responses to the patient that could be leading to boundary permeability. A supervisor can also be helpful in discussing some of the common challenges that beginning therapists have in maintaining the frame, such as starting and ending the sessions on time, making sure to stay with the agenda of the therapy, and learning how to navigate between appropriate and excessive self-disclosure. Furthermore, the supervisor must maintain appropriate professional boundaries between the supervisor and supervisee, both for the safety of the supervisee-supervisor relationship and for the purpose of modeling healthy boundaries for the developing therapist (Gabbard 2017; Waldinger 1994).

Data for Supervision

A wide variety of tools are used to transmit data from the patient-supervisee session back to the supervisor. Transcripts (De Golia et al. 2019); process notes (Wideman 2019); role-playing (Bullock 2019); modeling, rehearsing, and feedback (Jarecki et al. 2019); and audio or video recordings (Abbass 2004; Alpert 1996; De Golia 2019a; Funkenstein et al. 2014) are all used by various training programs to provide a window for the supervisor into what is happening in the therapy. Some supervisors may address issues of countertransference in an effort to understand the unconscious communications in psychotherapy (Gabbard 2017; Greaves 2019; Issacharoff 1984). All the data communicated about the session guide the supervisor to understand how the trainee is progressing as a therapist and what aspects of the trainee's work need attention. Live supervision may occur in some settings, either with the supervisor behind a one-way mirror (Rait 2019b) or in the form of cotherapy with supervisor and supervisee together (Lee et al. 2019). No form of data recording in the process of learning the skills of psychotherapy is perfect. Each of these different methods has advantages and disadvantages.

Specific schools of psychotherapy may use different methods for collecting data. Psychodynamic therapy may be particularly suited to the presentation of process notes because some of the data gathered in psychodynamic therapy reflect the countertransference of the therapist. In addition, process notes may also clarify the therapist's considerations of possible interventions, that is, why the therapist said or did not say certain things at particular junctures in the session (Gabbard 2017). Trainees can be encouraged to write about their thinking, not just what they said, in process notes. For example, supervisory review of process notes (or recordings) may include a comment by the supervisee such as "I was thinking about the patient's tendency to see failure around every corner, but I didn't say that. Instead, I encouraged her to tell me more about her experiences." The supervisor and supervisee can then address the timing of such a comment and investigate why the supervisee hesitated in pointing out the patient's expectations of failure. Was the supervisee accurately tuning in to a moment in which the patient would not have been receptive to such feedback? Was the supervisee hesitating out of fear that the interpretation was mistaken? How can the supervisor and supervisee work together to address issues of timing and tact with this specific patient?

These same themes, of course, can be assessed in a conversation between the supervisor and supervisee while they watch a video or listen to an audio recording of a session. Realizing that the therapist was using a condescending tone or that the therapist's voice contained an encouraging inflection may also provide insight for the supervisor and supervisee about how the therapist is coming across in the here and now of the session. How the session became derailed from the agenda in cognitive-behavioral therapy can be recognized in a recording. However, video and audio recordings both present the challenge of consent. For example, patients may feel pressured to consent because they want to please the therapist or because they assume that their therapy is possible only if they participate. In addition, session recordings can also take up a great deal of time in a supervision, and both supervisor and supervisee can become focused on the minute details of the interactions at the expense of understanding broader themes in the therapy. It is a challenge for the supervisor and supervisee to see *both* the forest and the trees, to make time to look at the small details of interactions and absorb the larger picture of the patient's trajectory as a whole (Gabbard 2017).

One of the challenges for therapists in training is to find the right balance of recording the information from the session. If process notes are kept, many beginning therapists will keep their eyes glued to the paper or computer and will be frantically writing or typing, diligently trying to capture every word. This strategy may be harmful if it cuts off the therapist from the in-the-moment interactions with the patient. Other therapists may write nothing, then struggle to reconstruct the session in their notes afterward. Finding the balance of recording a few notes or points to help them remember the flow of the interchanges afterward—that is, writing down important shifts, interventions, and reactions—may help supervisees avoid losing themselves in the computer or notebook. We recommend that therapists attempt to reconstruct the session immediately afterward by writing notes that can then be taken to supervision. If audio or video recordings are used, some therapists will become nervous or robotic in their efforts to do a good job and may feel that they are more inhibited and less free than usual in the recorded session. Moreover, if the patient also feels anxious or constrained by the video or audio recording, both members of the dyad may feel that the whole experience was performative and not reflective of their usual way of interacting (Gabbard 2017).

Role-playing can be an excellent learning experience. The supervisor and supervisee can alternate playing the roles of the patient and the therapist, trying on different approaches and interventions. If supervisees feel stuck, enacting how the patient behaves while the supervisor tries on some different approaches may be useful for them. They can then switch roles once the supervisor has a sense of how the patient might respond, and the supervisee can practice interventions as well (Bullock 2019; Gabbard 2017). Modeling, rehearsing, and deliberate practice are other forms of developing skills-based goals, seeking feedback, practicing skills, and trying on interventions (Jarecki et al. 2019; Rousmaniere 2019).

Cotherapy may also occur with a therapist in training. In this approach, both the supervisor and beginning therapist function as therapists. This approach can take place in individual therapy but most often occurs in group therapies, with both supervisor and supervisee serving as group leaders. This form of cotherapy has the advantage of providing real-time interaction between the supervisor and supervisee with the group members, and the supervisor can see in vivo how the supervisee works. However, a disadvantage is that the group members may experience and be shaped by the considerable differences in experience and authority between the two different group leaders. Unfortunately, supervisees can feel stilted or anxious in the face of the power differential in this context. Sometimes patients can also feel hesitant with two therapists. They may decide to talk to only one of the cotherapists, an issue that can be addressed directly with the patient in therapy (Lee et al. 2019).

Appreciating Diversities

The supervisor and supervisee can be of the same or different genders, sexualities, ethnic/cultural backgrounds, religions, or ages. These overlapping or differing aspects of identity can play a role in how the supervisee experiences supervision. They can also affect how the patient's clinical material is examined, considered, and understood by the two parties. In an optimal setting, supervisors try to foster a "safe and productive learning climate for supervisees to discuss uncomfortable topics related to race, ethnicity, class, gender, sexual orientation, nationality, age, identity or other categories of cultural belonging" (Shah et al. 2019, p. 338). Supervisees of one gender identity may see or experience a clinical issue differently than a supervisor of a different gender identity when evaluating a patient, yet they may be inhibited about bringing up the differences in supervision. The same dilemma can be played out in terms of ethnicity, culture, religion, nationality, class, or age. One of the most important attitudes to cultivate in supervision is curiosity, not only about the patient but also about the unique perspectives on the patient from both the supervisor and the supervisee (Bandstra et al. 2019).

For too long intersectionalities and cultural diversities have been overlooked or ignored in psychotherapy education. As a result, this notable absence has been problematic in both psychotherapy and supervision. If the supervisors are not educated and adept in their own approach to issues of diversity, how can they possibly expect to help their supervisees navigate these complex and deeply important waters (Bandstra et al. 2019; Roberts et al. 2014)? Supervisors should explore their own cultural biases and be willing to discuss explicit and implicit bias with supervisees (Shah et al. 2019). It is imperative that training program leaders and supervisors learn about the intersectional experiences of diversities so they can also bring these important concepts into supervision.

Maximizing the Educational Value of Supervision

Supervisors and supervisees can achieve a satisfying educational experience by setting goals for the supervision. At the beginning of the supervision, it is useful for the supervisor to explain the frame of supervision, the expectations, and some of the challenges they will face together. Supervisees can also conceptualize their goals and what they hope to learn from the collaboration. Supervisors will want to get to know the basics about who their supervisees are, including some details of their educational background, their career goals, and who they are as a person. Similarly, the supervisee will want to know the same from the supervisor. From the outset, supervisors must set a frame that avoids delving too deeply into the supervisee's intrapsychic struggles. Good supervisors balance supportive listening with insights about what might be going on with the therapist's countertransference, an ongoing tension in supervision (De Golia 2019a). The boundary between supervision and therapy must be clear to both parties (Gabbard 2016, 2017). This careful dance to avoid a clinical role with the supervisee takes diligence on the part of the supervisor, especially because the supervisor's daily work with patients may pull them toward a more therapeutic role. Supervisees may also attend to this boundary by sharing more of their here-and-now reactions to the patient rather than too much of their childhood or developmental backgrounds. Nevertheless, moments when the countertransference reactions of the supervisee to the patient have palpable roots in the developmental experiences of the supervisee may arise. When this occurs, both supervisor and supervisee must remember that supervision is not a therapeutic relationship, and the supervisor can both encourage the supervisee to use their countertransference to generate understanding about the patient and gently redirect supervisees to their own therapists. Supervisors may clarify the boundaries of the supervision if necessary.

A broad view of transference and countertransference is that both are ubiquitous in all human relationships and are largely unconscious. Although psychodynamic psychotherapy addresses transference and countertransference explicitly, these concepts arise in all treatment relationships. Hence, we expect that some form of transference and countertransference will arise in supervisory relationships between supervisor and supervisee. The countertransference reactions of the supervisee to the patient may be powerful at times, and the supervisor can come to share and contain these reactions. The concept of parallel process (Gabbard 2016, 2017; Gediman and Wolkenfeld 1980; Gross Doehrman 1976) arises when the supervisee and supervisor begin to interact with the same dynamics as the patient and supervisee. In the parallel process paradigm, supervisees unconsciously enact with their supervisors their experiences in the therapy rather than putting them into words. The supervisor then expands the experience by replicating a countertransference that is similar to the patient's countertransference to the supervisee. When supervisors are able to see what is occurring, they can put it into words so that the supervisee can grasp what is going on. The supervisor's self-disclosure can provide a framework for the supervisee to understand what is happening in the therapy (Gabbard 2017; Sarnat 2014).

Another possible path toward a positive experience in supervision lies in the therapeutic experience of rupture and repair. First outlined in Kohut's (1971, 1977) work on self psychology, the concept of rupture and repair is now used by object relations therapists and relational therapists and in mentalization-based therapies. Rupture and repair are regarded as a major mode of action in most psychotherapies (Gabbard and Crisp 2018). Supervision, like psychotherapy, features moments of rupture, disappointment, and frustration that can arise in the dyad (Watkins 2019). Supervisees may feel that the supervisor is not valuing their perspective. Supervisors can find themselves overly critical or didactic if they are getting uncomfortable with their supervisee's management of the patient. From both perspectives, tensions and disappointments can lead to ruptures. The process of apologizing, being actively curious about the other person's perspective, and seeking common ground in supervision is akin to the process of rupture and repair that can be healing in psychotherapy. The ability to talk through problems in supervision creates a pathway for the supervisee to learn that rupture and repair can be an important tool in therapy as well.

Problems That Can Arise in Supervision

The Chatty Supervisor

In a good supervision, the supervisee and supervisor are engaged in a mutual project to understand the patient, educate the supervisee, and share in an interactive dialogue about the supervisee's questions and interventions. One problem arises when the supervisor takes over too much of the conversation with chitchat about issues separate from the supervisee's learning. Supervisors are clinicians who spend much of their days listening to their patients and can be starved for conversation with other therapists or professionals. Furthermore, supervisors may be curious about the inner workings of the training program or other colleagues. Although it is understandable to chitchat for a couple of moments of greeting, it is not a good use of the supervisee's time, nor does it meet their needs for education if the conversation is sidetracked by such things. It is the duty of the supervisor to keep the conversation on track, but if the supervisor veers away, the supervisee can bring it back with a question about the patient or with a direct request for help regarding a particular issue. Many supervisees are reluctant to confront supervisors because of the vast differences in experience and knowledge, not to mention their inherent power in evaluating the supervisee. However, most supervisors will quickly recognize that they have gotten off track and remember their obligation for the education of the supervisee. Of course, if the problem persists, the supervisee can bring up the issue with the training director (Gabbard 2017).

The Didactic or Authoritarian Supervisor

Some supervisors behave as if they know exactly how to manage every clinical situation. This seemingly omniscient supervisor can be appealing to a supervisee who is seeking certainty about how to work as a therapist in a formulaic manner that removes all guesswork. However, authoritarian supervisors can also impede supervisees from learning how to do therapy in their own way—to make mistakes, to try different tactics, and to learn from their errors. Some supervisors have a specific theoretical position of "truth" from which they teach. Others tend to launch into long didactic speeches rather than engaging in a back-and-forth dialogue with the supervisee. Although it can be beneficial for supervisees to learn particular theoretical models, it is also imperative that supervisees feel that they can ask questions about why particular theories apply or how to use them with their patients. Supervisees sometimes feel they are being pressured to apply the supervisor's preferred theoretical model to their patients even when the supervisee does not agree with the supervisor. They may feel too intimidated to question the supervisor. Some supervisees may end up presenting an edited version of their work or their thinking in order to try to please the supervisor. Recognizing the transference dynamics of authority between supervisee and supervisor is important. In an optimal supervision, the supervisor should open up a dialogue with the supervisee that invites questions and different theoretical approaches (Gabbard 2017).

The Sleepy Supervisor

Clinicians are notorious for not taking care of themselves. Some supervisors may have overloaded clinical schedules and, unfortunately, may find themselves sleepy or distracted during their working hours. They may feel a sense of decreased pressure with supervisees, as opposed to sitting with their own patients, and, unfortunately, may let their attention lapse or may drift off into sleepiness. Sitting in an office with a sleeping supervisor is understandably disconcerting and uncomfortable to the supervisee, who is likely to imagine that the supervisor is bored. Just as patients have no obligation to entertain their therapists, supervisees have no obligation to entertain their supervisors. It is the supervisor's responsibility to maintain alertness, engagement, and curiosity. If the supervisee notices a sleepy supervisor, the supervisee might ask the supervisor if there is a better way to discuss the material that would be livelier. However, we must be clear that it is *not* the job of the supervisee to keep the supervisor awake. If the supervisor notices somnolence in themselves, they can try to engage supervisees in more interactive techniques such as role-play. Similarly, supervisors may become disengaged if there is something in their countertransference to the supervisee (or the supervisee's patient) that is distancing to the supervisor. The supervisor must internally examine this disengaged countertransference so it is not enacted in the supervision. Supervisors may also be disengaged in the face of their own personal stressors or if they are preoccupied by a troubling patient of their own. If a supervisor's somnolence or disengagement develops into a continuous problem, the supervisee should discuss the problem with leaders in the training program.

The Boundaryless Supervisor

Professional boundaries are at the heart of what we do as therapists and should be carried with us into our work with supervisees. As therapists, we are curious about our patients and may ask probing personal questions. As supervisors, we must deliberately shift gears to avoid asking deeply personal questions about our supervisee, such as whether the supervisee is single or married and questions about sexual orientation or historical personal and familial experiences. The focus of the supervision must be on the work of the supervisee in therapy.

It is also important for the supervisor to set clear physical professional boundaries in the supervision. One trainee arrived at her supervisor's office, and the supervisor asked her to sit next to him on the couch. She simply stated that she preferred the chair. This interaction shows a way to handle inappropriate interactions with a boundaryless supervisor, but many supervisees may not have the presence of mind to respond with clarity in the face of intrusive or uncomfortable interactions. Furthermore, given the power differential in supervision, they may fear negative evaluations if they do not comply with the wishes of the supervisor. Like in psychotherapy with patients, we encourage supervisors not to initiate hugs with their supervisees. The role of the supervisor is to set appropriate boundaries in the supervision—not only appropriate physical boundaries but also appropriate boundaries regarding self-disclosure or too much talk of the supervisor's own patients (Wallace and Alonso 1994). One supervisee reported hearing more about her supervisor's patients than spending time discussing the patients she was treating. Although an occasional clinical example from the supervisor's practice may be helpful, the overall balance should weigh much more on the side of discussing the trainee's cases. Serious concerns about a supervisor's boundaries should be discussed with the training director (Gabbard 2017).

Differences Between Supervisee and Supervisor

Supervisor and supervisee are sometimes separated by age, gender, sexuality, religion, culture, or ethnicity in ways that can feel distancing to each member of the supervisory dyad. An older supervisor may feel generationally far away from a young supervisee, whose experiences in training and in the world may be quite different. We have all heard some form of "back in my day…" when in training, usually expressed by a senior supervisor or mentor in a manner that conveys how much easier things are for trainees today or how an idealized experience has shifted over time. This does not usually go over well with the supervisee. Conversely, there can be a real pleasure and appreciation that some things have changed for the better for both trainees and patients.

Differences in gender, sexuality, ethnicity, and cultural background between supervisor and supervisee provide significant underpinnings to the supervisory relationship. It is incumbent on the supervisor to be open to discussing differences in perspective regarding the supervisee's patient. Variances in cultural identity may also be usefully discussed between supervisor and supervisee (Bandstra et al. 2019). Supervisees may feel uncomfortable bringing up with their supervisors sensitive topics in their clinical work around issues of sexuality, gender, culture, ethnicity, or class, but to leave out these important topics is to perpetuate the perception of them as being off-limits within psychotherapy and detrimental to psychotherapeutic education.

The Disengaged or Absent Supervisee

One of the more frustrating experiences for a supervisor is to have a supervisee who appears to be uninterested or does not come consistently to supervision. Supervisors are often donating their time to supervisees and may be quite passionate about the work they do. Working with a supervisee who is uninterested in learning therapy or does not arrive to supervision sessions can be a vexing problem. Supervisors can work to engage the supervisee by developing a supervisory alliance, asking directly what supervisees want to learn, what kinds of patients puzzle them, and perhaps what might be keeping them from engaging more deeply in their work with patients. The more the supervisor is able to cultivate insight and curiosity in thinking about the patients in supervision, the more curiosity the supervisee carries into the consulting room. If the supervisee is not attending supervision, asking whether the supervisor can do anything to make the supervisory experience more useful to the supervisee or whether the supervisee has concerns about the supervision that are getting in the way can also be helpful. Although the supervisor may wonder whether something in the supervisee's personal life is preventing regular attendance at supervision, it is best not to probe too much into the supervisee's personal life. The supervisor can reach out to the training leadership to let them know if there is a problem with attendance or engagement and gain some ideas about how best to handle it with the individual supervisee.

The Advice-Giving Supervisee

Supervisors may struggle when trying to work with a supervisee who is bent on giving advice to their patients. These supervisees may pepper their psychotherapy sessions with advice that they would give a friend, beginning with "You should" or "If I were in your shoes." This is not to say that one should never give advice in therapy, but one of the important tasks of beginning supervisees is to learn to engage with patients differently than they would engage with friends or loved ones. Supervisors can find themselves engaged in a parallel process with such supervisees, finding themselves giving advice to the supervisee in much the same way the supervisee gives advice to the patient. When the supervisor recognizes this dynamic, it is a valuable moment to shift gears and encourage the supervisee to explore their own solutions rather than feed them a diet of perpetual advice. Both supervisor (to supervisee) and therapist (to patient) must step out of solely advice-giving roles.

One supervisor observed to her supervisee that he was giving quite a bit of advice to the patient, and she asked why he thought he might be taking that approach. The supervisee expressed that he felt a powerful need to be "doing something." The patient had come to therapy to get better, and he felt he needed to make recommendations in order for that to happen. The supervisor and supervisee looked at the dynamics with the patient, in which the patient was devaluing the therapist for being in training and was sure he would not be able to help her. Hence, the therapist was trying to give lots of advice so that the patient felt he had something useful to contribute and she would stop criticizing him for being inexperienced. The supervisor and supervisee were able to look together at the patient's devaluing transference and how it was getting in the way of the therapist's attempt to help the patient find agency in her own life rather than pull for wise advice and guidance. The supervisor normalized the supervisee's countertransference anxiety about being in training, and they were able to think together about how to move away from so much advice giving in the therapy.

The Boundaryless Supervisee

Like supervisors, supervisees can also struggle with boundaries. Indeed, professional boundaries are limits to be learned in a training program as part of one's educational process. Boundaries are taught in didactic education and modeled in supervision. Supervisees may have insight about their challenges with boundaries, such as self-disclosure or keeping the time of the session. Other supervisees may lack insight into their slippery boundaries, and supervisors may need to be directive in teaching appropriate boundaries. Discussing with supervisees the reasons for maintenance of boundaries and exploring issues of countertransference that arise in the particular therapy that may lead to blurred boundaries can be helpful. Supervisees who struggle with boundaries may benefit from reading material about professional boundaries (Gabbard 2017).

Impression Management by the Supervisee

Supervisees sometimes lie in supervision (Hantoot 2000). Many beginning supervisees massage or edit the clinical data in order to produce a better fit. By making their observations more palatable to the supervisor, they hope to impress the supervisor and avoid the embarrassment of reporting what actually happened in the session. Some supervisees fear the judgment of the supervisor and attempt to contrive the material into the preferred theoretical model of the supervisor. In this context, the idea of impression management is apt to describe a repackaging of what was said and done with the patient. The problem with these edits or deceptions is that they do not serve the supervisee or the patient. The moments that the supervisee most wants to conceal are the most important moments to discuss in supervision. The mistakes or failures are *exactly* the clinical moments that should lead the supervisee to ask for help from the supervisor. Once a supervisee can be open, the supervisor and supervisee can strategize together. In addition, supervisors should do their best to convey a nonjudgmental attitude to supervisees and to explain that the things the supervisee may want to hide the most are the things that should be shared and discussed together. Of course, any pervasive pattern of deception about clinical work should be discussed with the training director.

Mutual Influence in the Supervisory Dyad

It is worth noting that many of the problems described in previous subsections in either the supervisor or the supervisee may be created in the dyad. In other words, an authoritarian attitude in a supervisor may contribute to the creation of a disengaged or deceptive supervisee, and then in response, the supervisor can become even more authoritarian in an effort to try to compel the supervisee to comply. Similarly, a disengaged or disinterested supervisee may contribute to a supervisor becoming sleepy or disengaged as well, leaving the supervisee to feel alone and perhaps even less motivated or interested. In this way, both parties are influenced and shaped by each other's disinterest. On a positive note, if both supervisor and supervisee engage the patient's clinical material with curiosity and enthusiasm, this engagement can create the type of rich, educational, and lively dynamic we aim for in the supervisory process.

One other issue that must be addressed is what to do if there is a serious concern from the perspective of either supervisor or supervisee. Because the therapist in training always has an educational administrator or program director overseeing educational experiences, it makes sense to reach out to that person if there are serious concerns from either party. If supervisors have concerns about the performance, engagement, professionalism, or competence of the supervisee, they should seek out further clarification and support from the program. Similarly, if supervisees are having difficulties with their supervisor and have serious concerns that they have not been able to address directly, bringing the problem to the training leaders for further guidance is important.

Evaluation

The evaluative function of supervision is a common aspect of education in training programs. The role of the supervisor as evaluator may come into conflict with the aspect of the supervisor whose goal is to support beginning clinicians in their struggles and clinical doubts. "Tell me your worst mistakes even though I am grading you" does not always bode well for supervisory honesty. Indeed, some studies show that supervisees lie in supervision (Hantoot 2000). One of the challenges of the evaluative function is ambivalence on the part of supervisors, who may not want to be in an evaluative role. Supervisees may want a good evaluation and so may hold back on disclosures of mistakes in order to protect the evaluation because of the narcissistic vulnerability of the supervisee. We all want to be seen in a positive light. Paradoxically, the looming evaluation may also disincentivize the supervisee from presenting their problems or questions for fear of being judged harshly in the evaluation. Supervisors can help solve this conundrum by being forthright from the beginning of the supervision about how they see their role in terms of teaching versus evaluation, what the expectations of the training program are in terms of evaluation, and what their primary goals are in terms of helping the therapist in training with their questions and mistakes. It can be helpful to say "I know it's a challenge to ask you to be completely honest and to tell me the things you are most insecure about when I am evaluating you." The supervisor can then be clear that mistakes are inevitable and that evaluations are based on the supervisee's efforts to learn and to be open and self-reflective, *not* on their missteps.

Consultation

Long after training, therapists continue to need the input, support, and perspectives of wise mentors and clear-eyed peers. Although the task of supervision is one rooted in psychotherapy training, one cannot overestimate the value of ongoing consultation after training is complete. All therapists benefit from a consultant to help them think through difficult therapies, challenging patients, or clinical impasses. Consultation may be done one-on-one or in a peer or group consultation setting. Often, long relationships with consultants that are both grounding and enriching to the therapist's professional identity and working relationships can develop. Although in most cases the consultant is paid, if finances are an issue, peer consultation relationships or groups can provide a similar support and accountability in a confidential setting (Gabbard 2000, 2017).

The ideal consultant is one who creates an atmosphere of acceptance but is also willing to confront the therapist about problematic comments or behaviors in the therapy (Gabbard 2017). Boundary violations are an ever-present risk to all therapists. Clinicians work behind closed doors in private relationships in which the most painful and intimate details of people's lives are considered. The risk of sliding down the slippery slope of boundary violations can be guarded against by encouraging all therapists to seek consultation, remain open about what they are doing, and be honest about mistakes and challenges. Telling a consultant one's fantasies about wanting to rescue a patient or sleep with a patient or even slap a patient can transform private countertransference feelings into words as part of a conversation between the therapist and the consultant. When these fantasies are out in the open, they can be discussed, reflected on, and understood, rather than put into action in an unethical manner with a patient. Boundaries can be discussed and agreed on between the consultant and the therapist. Subsequently, the therapist takes back to the therapy the internalized representation of the consultant as a third member of the treatment setting, helping to manage the fantasies that were leading down the slippery slope or veering on the edge of inappropriateness.

Some therapists may experience the seeking out of consultation as a narcissistic injury. They have a feeling that they should know how to function independently, or they do not want to risk having their judgment being questioned by a colleague. Others may feel that they cannot seek out consultation because they are too senior or are seeing patients who are public figures. These rationalizations prevent therapists from getting the support that would greatly benefit them and the patient. If the patient is known in a particular community, the therapist can seek out consultation from a colleague in another area or consult while keeping the patient's name and identifying information disguised. Furthermore, consultants have the same ethical obligation regarding confidentiality that therapists have for therapy. Hence, they cannot disclose the contents of consultation to others (Gabbard 2017).

Finally, whether in supervision or consultation, the consultant is able to work with only what the supervisee or therapist provides. Therapists can know only what the patient brings into the room, consciously for the most part, but sometimes unconsciously. Patients can limit what they tell therapists and present a distorted or minimized version of their struggles. Similarly, supervisees and therapists can present a narrow or edited version of what is happening in the room with the patient in a manner that serves to limit the consultant's usefulness. Some therapists who know they are engaging in problematic behavior with a patient will choose a consultant who they believe will agree with them or will share only partial information (Gabbard 2017). The best consultations, like the best therapies, are conducted when both therapist and consultant attempt to be open, honest, and self-reflective.

Finally, for the consultant, a potential dilemma arises if there is grave concern regarding ethics and/or boundaries that would require a mandatory report to a licensing board. The consultant may need to seek information about reporting to authorities such as an ethics board, licensing board, colleague assistance program, or physician health program if there are concerns at this level. It is wise to know the legal obligations in the state or country of practice as well as within the particular discipline, and it is important to seek out that information and assistance should it become necessary.

Conclusion

In summary, supervision and consultation are similar constructs, but each of them has its own set of challenges. Although supervision is vital for the beginning of a psychotherapist's education, consultation is a lifelong process. Although in this chapter we have listed a number of the common challenges encountered by supervisors, supervisees, and consultants, one has to be aware that idiosyncratic situations will arise that do not necessarily fit neatly into any category. The essence of supervision and consultation is that all of us have vulnerabilities and weaknesses, and we must be able to rely on teachers, mentors, and colleagues to help us with our struggles.

Key Points

- The role of the psychotherapy supervisor is complex, encompassing teaching the fundamentals of psychotherapy, supporting the trainee's skill development, overseeing the trainee's care of the patient, and evaluating the supervisee.
- The supervisory alliance must be developed and attended to because there is vulnerability for the supervisee in the dyad, much as there is vulnerability in the relationship between therapist and patient.
- Boundaries in supervision must be both taught and modeled.
- Data for supervision may be gathered through process notes; role-play; modeling, rehearsal, and feedback; video or audio recordings; cotherapy; or live observation of therapy.

- Diversities between supervisor and supervisee must be appreciated and attended to in order to create an optimal learning environment for the supervisee and foster understanding of the dyad between supervisee and patient.
- Clear goals for the supervision are important, as are frame setting and attention to the development of skills, transference, countertransference, parallel process, and rupture and repair.
- Problems that arise in supervision should be reflected on by the supervisor and supervisee, and if the need arises, involvement of a training director or educational leaders may be helpful.
- Consultation is an ongoing process following training that is beneficial to therapists at all stages of development.

References

Abbass A: Small-group videotape training for psychotherapy skills development. Acad Psychiatry 28(2):151–155, 2004 15298869

Alpert MC: Videotaping psychotherapy. J Psychother Pract Res 5(2):93–105, 1996 22700270

Bandstra BS, Shah R, Tan M: Cultural issues within the supervisory relationship, in Supervision in Clinical Practice: Practical Approaches Across Venues and Providers. Edited by De Golia SG, Corcoran KM. Washington, DC, American Psychiatric Association Publishing, 2019, pp 293–297

Binder JL, Strupp HH: Supervision of psychodynamic psychotherapies, in Handbook of Psychotherapy Supervision. Edited by Watkins CE. New York, Wiley, 1997, pp 44–62

Bullock KD: Role-play, in Supervision in Clinical Practice: Practical Approaches Across Venues and Providers. Edited by De Golia SG, Corcoran KM. Washington, DC, American Psychiatric Association Publishing, 2019, pp 69–77

Cabaniss DL: Psychodynamic supervision, in Supervision in Clinical Practice: Practical Approaches Across Venues and Providers. Edited by De Golia SG, Corcoran KM. Washington, DC, American Psychiatric Association Publishing, 2019, pp 179–186

De Golia SG: Elements of supervision, in Supervision in Clinical Practice: Practical Approaches Across Venues and Providers. Edited by De Golia SG, Corcoran KM. Washington, DC, American Psychiatric Association Publishing, 2019a, pp 3–24

De Golia SG: Video recordings: learning through facilitated observation and feedback, in Supervision in Clinical Practice: Practical Approaches Across Venues and Providers. Edited by De Golia SG, Corcoran KM. Washington, DC, American Psychiatric Association Publishing, 2019b, pp 85–95

De Golia SG, Williams KE, Safer DL: Working with transcripts, in Supervision in Clinical Practice: Practical Approaches Across Venues and Providers. Edited by De Golia SG, Corcoran KM. Washington, DC, American Psychiatric Association Publishing, 2019, pp 57–62

Funkenstein AB, Kessler KA, Schen CR: Learning through the lens: ethical considerations in videotaping psychotherapy. Harv Rev Psychiatry 22(5):316–322, 2014 25188735

Gabbard GO: Lessons to be learned from the study of sexual boundary violations. Am J Psychother 50(3):311–322, 1996 8886231

Gabbard GO: Consultation from the consultant's perspective. Psychoanal Dialogues 10(2):209–218, 2000

Gabbard GO: Boundaries and Boundary Violations in Psychoanalysis, 2nd Edition. Arlington, VA, American Psychiatric Association Publishing, 2016

Gabbard GO: Long-Term Psychodynamic Psychotherapy: A Basic Text, 3rd Edition. Arlington, VA, American Psychiatric Association Publishing, 2017, pp 201–215

Gabbard GO, Crisp H: Narcissism and Its Discontents: Diagnostic Dilemmas and Treatment Strategies With Narcissistic Patients. Washington DC, American Psychiatric Association Publishing, 2018

Gediman HK, Wolkenfeld F: The parallelism phenomenon in psychoanalysis and supervision: its reconsideration as a triadic system. Psychoanal Q 49(2):234–255, 1980 7375592

Greaves CC: The supervision of countertransference, in Supervision in Clinical Practice: Practical Approaches Across Venues and Providers. Edited by De Golia SG, Corcoran KM. Washington, DC, American Psychiatric Association Publishing, 2019, pp 305–310

Greben SE, Ruskin R: Introduction: significant aspects of the supervisor-supervisee relationship and interaction, in Clinical Perspectives on Psychotherapy Supervision. Edited by Greben SE, Ruskin R. Washington, DC, American Psychiatric Press, 1994, pp 1–10

Gross Doehrman MJ: Parallel processes in supervision and psychotherapy. Bull Menninger Clin 40(1):1–104, 1976 1252650

Hantoot MS: Lying in psychotherapy supervision. Acad Psychiatry 24:179–187, 2000

Issacharoff A: Countertransference in supervision: therapeutic consequences for the supervisee, in Clinical Perspectives on the Supervision of Psychoanalysis and Psychotherapy. Edited by Caligor L, Bromberg PM, Meltzer JD. New York, Plenum, 1984, pp 89–105

Jarecki J, McNair F, Ruzhynsky J, et al: Modeling, rehearsal, and feedback: a simple approach to teaching complex skills, in Supervision in Clinical Practice: Practical Approaches Across Venues and Providers. Edited by De Golia SG, Corcoran KM. Washington, DC, American Psychiatric Association Publishing, 2019, pp 79–84

Kantrowitz JL: The triadic match: the interactive effect of supervisor, candidate, and patient. J Am Psychoanal Assoc 50(3):939–968, 2002 12434877

Kohut H: The Analysis of the Self: A Systematic Approach to the Psychoanalytic Treatment of Narcissistic Personality Disorders. New York, International Universities Press, 1971

Kohut H: The Restoration of the Self. New York, International Universities Press, 1977

Lee A, Isaac S, Stubbe D, et al: Cotherapy: Observing and modeling in real time, in Supervision in Clinical Practice: Practical Approaches Across Venues and Providers. Edited by De Golia SG, Corcoran KM. Washington, DC, American Psychiatric Association Publishing, 2019, pp 113–118

Levenson H: Time-limited psychotherapy supervision, in Supervision in Clinical Practice: Practical Approaches Across Venues and Providers. Edited by De Golia SG, Corcoran KM. Washington, DC, American Psychiatric Association Publishing, 2019, pp 187–193

Liese BS, Beck JS: Cognitive therapy supervision, in Handbook of Psychotherapy Supervision. Edited by Watkins CE. New York, Wiley, 1997, pp 114–133

Lomax J, Andrews LB, Burruss JW, et al: Psychotherapy supervision, in Oxford Textbook of Psychotherapy. Edited by Gabbard GO, Beck JS, Holmes J. New York, Oxford University Press, 2005, pp 495–506

Malat J: Group psychotherapy supervision: working at multiple levels, in Supervision in Clinical Practice: Practical Approaches Across Venues and Providers. Edited by De Golia SG, Corcoran KM. Washington, DC, American Psychiatric Association Publishing, 2019, pp 195–202

Rait D: Couples and family therapy supervision: learning to work systematically, in Supervision in Clinical Practice: Practical Approaches Across Venues and Providers. Edited by De Golia SG, Corcoran KM. Washington, DC, American Psychiatric Association Publishing, 2019a, pp 203–209

Rait D: Live supervision: behind the one-way mirror, in Supervision in Clinical Practice: Practical Approaches Across Venues and Providers. Edited by De Golia SG, Corcoran KM. Washington, DC, American Psychiatric Association Publishing, 2019b, pp 105–111

Roberts LW, Maldonado Y, Coverdale JH, et al: The critical need to diversity the clinical and academic workforce. Acad Psychiatry 38(4):395–397, 2014

Rousmaniere T: Deliberate practice for clinical supervision and training, in Supervision in Clinical Practice: Practical Approaches Across Venues and Providers. Edited by De Golia SG, Corcoran KM. Washington, DC, American Psychiatric Association Publishing, 2019, pp 97–103

Sarnat J: Disruption and working through in the supervisory process: a vignette from supervision of a psychoanalytic candidate. Psychoanal Dialogues 24(5):532–539, 2014

Shah R, Tan M, Bandstra BS: Supervising cross-cultural topics in a clinical setting, in Supervision in Clinical Practice: Practical Approaches Across Venues and Providers. Edited by De Golia SG, Corcoran KM. Washington, DC, American Psychiatric Association Publishing, 2019, pp 337–343

Sudak DM: Cognitive-behavioral therapy supervision: enhancing learning and promoting expertise, in Supervision in Clinical Practice: Practical Approaches Across Venues and Providers. Edited by De Golia SG, Corcoran KM. Washington, DC, American Psychiatric Association Publishing, 2019, pp 171–177

Sudak DM, Codd RT, Ludgate JW, et al: Teaching and Supervising Cognitive Behavioral Therapy. New York, Wiley, 2015

Waldinger RJ: Boundary crossings and boundary violations: thoughts on navigating a slippery slope. Harv Rev Psychiatry 2(4):225–227, 1994 9384906

Wallace E, Alonso A: Privacy vs. disclosure in psychotherapy supervision, in Clinical Perspectives on Psychotherapy Supervision. Edited by Greben SE, Ruskin R. Washington, DC, American Psychiatric Press, 1994, pp 211–230

Watkins CE: Ruptures in the supervisory alliance, in Supervision in Clinical Practice: Practical Approaches Across Venues and Providers. Edited by De Golia SG, Corcoran KM. Washington, DC, American Psychiatric Association Publishing, 2019, pp 299–304

Welton RS, Rueve ME: Supportive psychotherapy supervision, in Supervision in Clinical Practice: Practical Approaches Across Venues and Providers. Edited by De Golia SG, Corcoran KM. Washington, DC, American Psychiatric Association Publishing, 2019, pp 163–170

Wideman D: Working with process notes, in Supervision in Clinical Practice: Practical Approaches Across Venues and Providers. Edited by De Golia SG, Corcoran KM. Washington, DC, American Psychiatric Association Publishing, 2019, pp 63–68

Index

Page numbers printed in **boldface** type refer to figures and tables.

www.ingramcontent.com/pod-product-compliance
Ingram Content Group UK Ltd.
Pitfield, Milton Keynes, MK11 3LW, UK
UKHW050418080526
5582IPUK00012B/7

9 781615 37326(